D0811326

LIBRARY
Tel: 329241 Ext. 2

must be returned

000

0

Management of Diabetes Mellitus

Perspectives of Care Across the Life Span

Management of Diabetes Mellitus
Perspectives of Care Across the Life Span

DEBRA HAIRE-JOSHU, RN, MSEd, MSN, PhD
Research Associate Professor of Medicine
Center for Health Behavior Research
Washington University School of Medicine
St. Louis, Missouri

SECOND EDITION
With 75 illustrations

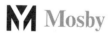 Mosby

St. Louis Baltimore Boston Carlsbad Chicago Naples New York Philadelphia Portland
London Madrid Mexico City Singapore Sydney Tokyo Toronto Wiesbaden

030026I

Mosby

Dedicated to Publishing Excellence

A Times Mirror
Company

Vice President and Publisher: Nancy L. Coon
Editor: Barry Bowlus
Senior Developmental Editor: Nancy C. Baker
Project Manager: Patricia Tannian
Senior Production Editor: Betty Hazelwood
Book Design Manager: Gail Morey Hudson
Manufacturing Manager: David Graybill
Cover Design: Teresa Breckwoldt

SECOND EDITION

Copyright © 1996 by Mosby–Year Book, Inc.

Previous edition copyrighted 1992

All rights reserved. No part of this publication may be reproduced,
stored in a retrieval system, or transmitted, in any form or by any
means, electronic, mechanical, photocopying, recording, or otherwise,
without prior written permission from the publisher.

Permission to photocopy or reproduce solely for internal or personal
use is permitted for libraries or other users registered with the Copyright
Clearance Center, provided that the base fee of $4.00 per chapter plus $.10
per page is paid directly to the Copyright Clearance Center, 27 Congress
Street, Salem, MA 01970. This consent does not extend to other kinds
of copying, such as copying for general distribution, for advertising or
promotional purposes, for creating new collected works, or for resale.

Printed in the United States of America
Composition by Graphic World, Inc.
Printing/binding by Maple-Vail Book Mfg Group

Mosby–Year Book, Inc.
11830 Westline Industrial Drive
St. Louis, Missouri 63146

Library of Congress Cataloging in Publication Data

Management of diabetes mellitus : perspectives of care across the life
  span / [edited by] Debra Haire-Joshu.—2nd ed.
    p.   cm.
   Includes bibliographical references and index.
   ISBN 0-8151-4223-4
   1. Diabetes.   I. Haire-Joshu, Debra.
   [DNLM: 1. Diabetes Mellitus.   WK 810 M266 1996]
  RC660.M333 1996
  616.4'62—dc20
  DNLM/DLC
  for Library of Congress   95-26440
                                                  CIP

96 97 98 99 00 / 9 8 7 6 5 4 3 2 1

1 1 APR 1997

Contributors

WENDY AUSLANDER, PhD

Associate Professor of Social Work
George Warren Brown School of Social Work
Washington University
St. Louis, Missouri

CHRISTINE A. BEEBE, MS, RD, CDE

Director, Diabetes Center
St. James Hospital and Health Centers
Chicago Heights, Illinois

R. KEITH CAMPBELL, RPh, BPharm, MBA, FASHP

Associate Dean, Professor of Pharmacy Practice
College of Pharmacy
Washington State University
Pullman, Washington

WILLIAM C. COLEMAN, DPM

Podiatrist, Department of Endocrinology
Ochsner Clinic
New Orleans, Louisiana

DANIELE CORN, MSW

Study Coordinator
George Warren Brown School of Social Work
Washington University
St. Louis, Missouri

DENIS DANEMAN, MB, BCh, FRCP(C)

Professor of Pediatrics
Chief, Division of Endocrinology
Department of Pediatrics
University of Toronto
The Hospital for Sick Children
Toronto, Ontario, Canada

GAIL D'ERAMO-MELKUS, RN, EdD, CDE

Associate Professor
Chair, Primary Care Division
Yale University School of Nursing
New Haven, Connecticut

JAMES A. FAIN, RN, PhD

Associate Professor
Director, Collaborative PhD Program in Nursing
Graduate School of Nursing
University of Massachusetts Medical Center
Worcester, Massachusetts

MARCIA FRANK, RN, MHSc, CDE

Clinical Nurse Specialist
Diabetes Service
The Hospital for Sick Children
Toronto, Ontario, Canada

MARION J. FRANZ, MS, RD, CDE

Director, Nutrition and Publications
International Diabetes Center
Minneapolis, Minnesota

MARTHA MITCHELL FUNNELL, RN, MS, CDE

Associate Director for Administration
Michigan Diabetes Research and Training Center
University of Michigan
Ann Arbor, Michigan

JEFFREY A. GAVARD, PhD

Research Fellow in Medicine
Department of Internal Medicine
Washington University School of Medicine
St. Louis, Missouri

DOUGLAS A. GREENE, MD

Professor of Internal Medicine
Chief, Division of Endocrinology and
Metabolism
Director of Michigan Diabetes Research and
Training Center
University of Michigan Medical Center
Ann Arbor, Michigan

DEBRA HAIRE-JOSHU, RN, MsEd, MSN, PhD

Research Associate Professor of Medicine
Center for Health Behavior Research
Washington University School of Medicine
St. Louis, Missouri

JOAN M. HEINS, MA, RD, CDE

Research Nutritionist
Center for Health Behavior Research
Washington University School of Medicine
St. Louis, Missouri

DOUGLAS N. HENRY, MD, CDE

Assistant Professor
Physiology, Pediatrics and Human Development
College of Human Medicine
Michigan State University
East Lansing, Michigan

WILLIAM H. HERMAN, MD, MPH

Associate Professor of Internal Medicine
Associate Professor of Epidemiology
University of Michigan
Ann Arbor, Michigan

IRL B. HIRSCH, MD

Associate Professor of Medicine
Division of Metabolism, Endocrinology, and
Nutrition
University of Washington
Seattle, Washington

PRISCILLA HOLLANDER, MD

Diabetologist, International Diabetes Center
Park Nicollet Clinic
St Louis Park, Minnesota

CHERYL A. HOUSTON, MS, RD

Research Instructor of Medicine
Center for Health Behavior Research
Washington University School of Medicine
St. Louis, Missouri

JENNIFER HAYDEN MERRITT, RN, MSN

Gerontological Clinical Nurse Specialist
Geriatrics Ambulatory Care (Turner Clinic)
University of Michigan Medical Center
Ann Arbor, Michigan

JILL M. NORRIS, MPH, PhD

Assistant Professor
Department of Preventive Medicine and
Biometrics
University of Colorado Health Sciences Center
Denver, Colorado

SHARON L. PONTIOUS, RN, PhD

President, Dean, and Professor
Jewish Hospital College of Nursing and Allied
Health
St. Louis, Missouri

ROBERT E. RATNER, MD, CDE

Director, Clinical Research Center
Medlantic Research Institute;
Associate Professor of Medicine
George Washington University Medical School
Washington, DC

LINDA K. SUSSMAN, PhD

Medical Anthropologist
Diabetes Research and Training Center
Center for Health Behavior Research
Washington University School of Medicine
St. Louis, Missouri

FRANK VINICOR, MD, MPH

Director, Division of Diabetes Translation
NCCDPHP
Centers for Disease Control and Prevention
Atlanta, Georgia

JOHN R. WHITE, Jr., PharmD

Associate Professor
Director, Drug Studies Unit
Sacred Heart Medical Center
Washington State University
Spokane, Washington

NEIL H. WHITE, MD, CDE

Associate Professor of Pediatrics
St. Louis Children's Hospital
Washington University School of Medicine
St. Louis, Missouri

Consultants

JEAN BETSCHART, RN, MN, CDE

Coordinator, Diabetes Program
Department of Endocrinology
Children's Hospital of Pittsburgh
Pittsburgh, Pennsylvania

DARLENE E. BIGGS, RN, MS, CDE

Program Manager, Endocrine Division
Baystate Medical Center
Springfield, Massachusetts

PEGGY BOURGEOIS, RN, MN, CDE

Team Leader, Diabetes Services
Diabetes Center
Baton Rouge General Medical Center
Baton Rouge, Louisiana

JOHN M. BURKE, PharmD, BCPS

Associate Professor of Pharmacy Practice
St. Louis College of Pharmacy
St. Louis, Missouri

PATRICIA M. BUTLER, RN, PhD, CDE

Educational Specialist
University of Michigan Medical Center;
Adjunct Assistant Professor
University of Michigan School of Nursing
Ann Arbor, Michigan

GREGORY A. CASALENUOVO, RN, CS, MSN

Clinical Specialist, Department of Diabetes
Methodist Medical Center
Oak Ridge, Tennessee

SUSAN M. CHAPPELL, RN, MSN, CDE

Specialist, School of Nursing
University of Texas at Arlington
Arlington, Texas

CATHERINE COWIE, PhD, MPH

Senior Epidemiologist
Social & Scientific Systems, Inc.
Bethesda, Maryland

DEE DEAKINS, RN, MS, CDE

Diabetes Specialist, Department of Nursing
Department of Veterans Affairs Medical Center
Lexington, Kentucky

MARIANNE GERGELY, RN, MS, CDE

Program Director, Indiana Diabetes Center
Indiana University Medical Center
Indianapolis, Indiana

MARILYN GRAFF, RN, BSN, CDE

Diabetes Program Coordinator
Diabetes Care Team
Longmont Clinic
Longmont, Colorado

JOHN P. GRAHAM, PharmD

Assistant Professor of Pharmacy Practice
St. Louis College of Pharmacy
St. Louis, Missouri

LINDA B. HAAS, RN, PhC, CDE

Endocrinology Clinical Nurse Specialist
Department of Nursing
Seattle Department of Veterans Affairs Medical
Center, Seattle, Washington

SUSAN HENDERSHOTT, RN, MSN, CDE

Diabetes Educator, Division of Nursing
Hoag Memorial Hospital
Newport Beach, California

DEBORAH HINNEN HENTZEN, RN, MN, ARNP, CDE

Program Coordinator
Diabetes Treatment and Research Center
St. Joseph Medical Center
Wichita, Kansas;
Assistant Clinical Professor
Department of Pediatrics
University of Kansas, School of Medicine
Wichita, Kansas

ELIZABETH (LIBBY) HUGHES, RN, MSN, CDE

Manager, Diabetes Services
Department of General Medicine
Barnes Hospital
St. Louis, Missouri

CHERYL HUNT, MSEd, CDE

Certified Diabetes Educator
Health Education and Resources
Alexandria, Virginia

PATRICIA S. MOORE, RN, MSN, CDE

Research Associate
Diabetes Clinical Nurse Specialist
Department of Medicine
Indiana University
Indianapolis, Indiana

CHARLOTTE NATH, RN, EdD, CDE

Professor, Department of Family Medicine
Robert C. Byrd Health Sciences Center
West Virginia University
Morgantown, West Virginia

DARLENE J. PADUANO, RN, MSN, CS, CDE, CETN

Director, Diabetes Nursing Practice
Department of Nursing
University Medical Center
Stonybrook, New York

DEBORAH L. PATNODE, RD, CDE

Diabetes Specialist, Diabetes Center
Michael Reese Hospital and Medical Center
Chicago, Illinois

CYNTHIA W. SANBORN, RN, MN, CDE

Diabetes Nurse Specialist
Department of Internal Medicine
School of Medicine
University of Virginia
Charlottesville, Virginia

LOIS SCHMIDT, RD, MPH, CDE

Senior Scientist/Study Coordinator
Diabetes Prevention Trial—Type 1
Department of Medicine
University of Minnesota
Minneapolis, Minnesota

STEPHANIE SCHWARTZ, RN, MPH, CDE

Diabetes Nurse Specialist
Children's Diabetes Center
The Children's Mercy Hospital
Kansas City, Missouri

SUSAN SHERMAN SINGER, RN, MSN

Professor, Department of Nursing
Bucks County Community College
Newtown, Pennsylvania

DONNA J. GRYCTZ THOMAS, RN, MSN

Nurse Educator, School of Nursing
Ohio Valley Hospital
Steubenville, Ohio

JUDITH WYLIE-ROSETTE, EdD, RD

Professor of Epidemiology and Social Medicine
Associate Director of Diabetes and Training Center
Albert Einstein College of Medicine
Bronx, New York

TIM WYSOCKI, PhD

Chief Psychologist
Division of Behavioral Pediatrics and Psychology
Nemours Children's Clinic
Jacksonville, Florida

TO
COJO and JOELY

TO
ERIC

Preface

The second edition of *Management of Diabetes Mellitus: Perspectives of Care Across the Life Span* expands on the primary themes of the first edition. These themes are that self-management by the person with diabetes is the optimal goal of care, that achievement of this goal requires diabetes care designed to meet the physical and psychosocial needs of the individual, and that such care reflects the collaborative input of multidisciplinary health care providers.

This book is designed for health care professionals who are dedicated to the delivery of comprehensive diabetes care. Information will be of benefit to clinicians working with individuals with diabetes and their families. The content will enhance education of the professional interested in lifelong learning. This book will also assist faculty responsible for the development of future diabetes experts.

NEW TO THIS EDITION

Three general areas are addressed in the 21 chapters of this book. Several chapters have been added to ensure a comprehensive approach to diabetes care. Part One provides an overview of diabetes from diagnostic, physical, and management perspectives. Two chapters have been added that provide detailed content related to the epidemiology of IDDM and NIDDM. This section also now includes a chapter addressing surgical management of diabetes. Part Two focuses on contexts of diabetes care and education. A chapter addressing sociocultural aspects of care expands on the content in this section. Content related to family and community environments has been expanded. Part Three addresses issues of diabetes management across the life span. These chapters focus on the individualization of care across the stages of growth and development.

The content and references in each chapter have been revised and updated. Many chapters have been extensively revised to reflect the rapid changes in diabetes care and research that occurred since the publication of the first edition. Several chapters now include case studies to reflect application of content. Preventive and educational aspects of care are also stressed throughout the chapters and appendixes.

CONTRIBUTORS

The strength of this book lies in the broad spectrum and expertise of the contributors. The contributors are nationally known experts who set the standards for quality diabetes care. Each chapter reflects content, issues, and practice implications that are critical to achieving the optimal goal of diabetes self-care and management. The diverse professional backgrounds result in the presentation of information that mirrors the interdependent nature of diabetes self-care.

ACKNOWLEDGMENTS

As always, this book would not have been possible without the assistance and hard work of numerous colleagues and contributors. Many of my colleagues offered their time, ideas, and patience to this project, and for that I am grateful.

I cannot express enough thanks to the reviewers of this book. These professionals donated their time and expertise, which proved to be invaluable in enhancing the content. Their assistance to the contributors and me in revising this text cannot be overestimated.

I would also like to thank many of the staff at Mosby–Year Book, Inc. who worked so closely with me on this revision. A special thanks to Nancy Baker and Brian Morovitz at Mosby for their invaluable coordinating assistance and patience. My gratitude is also extended to Tylisa Jones for her assistance in keeping everything in my immediate environment organized throughout this process.

Finally, this book is a reflection of the extensive research, education, practice, and dedication of the diabetes community to the ongoing care of those with diabetes. *Management of Diabetes Mellitus: Perspectives of Care Across the Life Span* is intended to serve as acknowledgment of that work.

Debra Haire-Joshu

Contents

PART THREE
INDIVIDUALIZING DIABETES CARE ACROSS THE LIFE SPAN

21   Diabetes Mellitus and the Older Adult, 755

Martha Mitchell Funnell and Jennifer Hayden Merritt

APPENDIX

PART ONE

Overview of Diabetes Care

1 Review of Diabetes Mellitus

Robert E. Ratner

INTRODUCTION

Diabetes has long been a clinical model for general medicine. The primary defect in fuel metabolism results in widespread, multiorgan complications that ultimately encompass virtually every system of the body and every specialty of medicine. It has been said that to know diabetes is to know medicine and health care. Although from a clinical standpoint this may be true, our increasing knowledge of the pathophysiology of the syndrome, together with the mechanisms of long-term complications, has placed diabetes research at the frontier of immunology and molecular biology. In addition, implementation of clinical care for the individual with diabetes is now serving as the paradigm for a chronic disease model of health care delivery. In no other health care setting is an individual with a disorder incorporated more into his or her own clinical care plan. Involving the individual in his or her health care is the first step toward implementing preventive medicine and is revolutionizing the concept of health care delivery. In essence, the individual with diabetes is becoming his or her own primary health care provider. Thus the evolution of diabetes care and research places diabetes at the forefront of both scientific and social advances in the health care sciences.

EPIDEMIOLOGY AND DEMOGRAPHICS

Diabetes mellitus is a clinical syndrome characterized by inappropriate hyperglycemia caused by a relative or absolute deficiency of insulin or by a resistance to the action of insulin at the cellular level. It is the most common endocrine disorder, affecting approximately 16 million individuals in the United States and perhaps as many as 200 million worldwide. Perhaps more importantly, individuals with diabetes are disproportionate users of the health care system. In 1992 health care expenditures per individual with diabetes were more than three times greater than per capita expenditure for those without diabetes.[107] As a result, 4.5% of the general population (those with diabetes) accounted for 14.6%, or $105 billion, of total health care

---

CHAPTER OBJECTIVES

- Know the groups at risk for the development of diabetes.
- Understand the impact of diabetes care on health care delivery and financing.
- Know the diagnostic criteria for diabetes mellitus.
- Know the differences among the various forms of diabetes mellitus.
- Understand the stages of development of insulin-dependent diabetes mellitus and the implications for early intervention and prevention.
- Understand the mechanisms by which non-insulin-dependent diabetes mellitus occurs, the risk factors for its development, and mechanisms for its potential prevention.
- Understand the findings and implications of the Diabetes Control and Complications Trial as they relate to standards of diabetes care and the importance of the team approach.
- Be aware of the available technologies for assessing long-term glycemic control and their limitations and clinical usefulness.
- Be aware of the available systems for self-monitoring of blood glucose levels and the importance of appropriate instruction, proper operation, and use of the data that the systems provide.
- Understand the interrelationships among the various health care providers involved in the team approach to diabetes care.
- Know the legal restrictions and liability concerns involved in diabetes education.
- Understand the health care financing ramifications of diabetes education and the implications for the chronic care model.

---

expenditures in the United States. This excess cost is seen across the spectrum of health care delivery. Physician visits for individuals with diabetes totaled more than 15.8 million, or 2.2 visits per average individual with diabetes per year.[105] Almost 500,000 home health care visits are made to individuals with diabetes, and more than 600,000 emergency room visits are required annually. In addition to this high rate of outpatient care, individuals with diabetes are hospitalized twice as often as age-matched control subjects. Once hospitalized, individuals with diabetes also have disproportionately long hospital stays—almost 3 days longer than for patients without diabetes but with similar disorders.[105] As a result, financial expenditures for hospitalization of individuals with diabetes accounts for 66% of total health care costs for this population.[107] This suggests that a potentially enormous health care cost savings can be accrued by moving toward outpatient health care delivery and institution of preventive care to minimize long-term complications of diabetes.

These disproportionate costs attributed to diabetes must be borne by society in general. However, those within our society who are least capable of paying are those most often affected. Non-insulin-dependent diabetes mellitus (NIDDM or type II diabetes), which is discussed in detail in a later section, accounts for approximately 90% of diabetes cases in the United States and increases significantly with age. According to the Second National Health and Nutritional Examination Survey (NHANES II), 18% of Americans ages 65 to 74 have diabetes.[80] Perhaps most alarming is that half this population was undiagnosed before this broad-based screening study. Subsequent studies have substantiated this high prevalence of diabetes in older adults, with a symptomatic increase in prevalence at each decade after the sixth.[137] Even assuming no increase in the prevalence of diabetes, the number of individuals affected yearly by diabetes is expected to grow at an annual rate of 2.8%, or about 69,000 additional individuals, for the next 25 years.[52] Thus more than 3.7 million additional individuals will be requiring care for diabetes and diabetes-related complications by the year 2020.

Although some argue that carbohydrate intolerance is a natural consequence of aging, it still requires intervention because of the short-term disabilities and acute complications, as well as the potential for exacerbation of macrovascular disease.[98] Underlying defects in carbohydrate handling with aging include delays in glucose-induced insulin secretion, impaired insulin-mediated glucose uptake, and ineffective intracellular glucose transport.[54] As discussed in the following section, these mimic the defects noted in type II diabetes. The high prevalence of diabetes in the older adult population also raises questions about specific educational needs. Cognitive abilities, physical constraints, and social and financial status must be considered in the context of modifying lifelong health beliefs and practices.[34]

In addition, minority populations have significantly higher relative rates of NIDDM when compared with an age-matched white population. Specifically, diabetes is two times more common in African Americans, two and one-half times more common in Hispanics, and five times more common in Native Americans.[51,138] African Americans have undergone a progressive increase in the prevalence, morbidity, and mortality associated with diabetes since the turn of the twentieth century.[93] Although obesity certainly contributes to these increased risks, African Americans are more likely to have diabetes even when adiposity and socioeconomic status are controlled.[87] Some authors suggest that specific forms of diabetes selectively affecting blacks may mimic either maturity-onset diabetes of young persons or atypical type I diabetes.[12,138] Educational techniques must be adapted to the specific social, financial, and educational context of these minority populations.[63]

DIAGNOSIS AND CLASSIFICATION

Any efforts, whether social or medical, to improve the care and prognosis of individuals with diabetes require precise definitions and classifications of that disease. Although not ideal, the National Diabetes Data Group (NDDG) classification has provided a framework for both diagnosis and classification.[81] Appendix C gives three independent criteria for diagnosing diabetes mellitus. Any *one* of these criteria is sufficient to establish a firm diagnosis, pending further classification in type. For patients with classic signs and symptoms of diabetes, including polydipsia, polyuria, and unexplained weight loss, random serum glucose determinations in excess of 200 mg/dl (11 mmol/L) are sufficient to make the diagnosis. In asymptomatic individuals, fasting glucose determinations must be performed; levels in excess of 140 mg/dl (7.7 mmol/L) on two occasions are necessary to meet diagnostic criteria. In those unusual circumstances in which the fasting glucose level is normal but there is a high index of suspicion that diabetes exists (i.e., family history or other risk factors or clinical signs suggestive of long-term diabetic complications), then and only then is a glucose tolerance test (GTT) necessary. In the nonpregnant adult, this test is a standardized 75 g liquid glucose challenge extending for 2 hours. This test should be limited to individuals who are ambulatory and have no intercurrent illness, and it should be performed only after a 3-day diet consisting of at least 150 g of carbohydrate and only in the morning after an overnight fast. Criteria to establish the diagnosis of diabetes include a 2-hour post–glucose load, serum glucose value in excess of 200 mg/dl (11 mmol/L), with one intervening value also greater than 200 mg/dl. In general the GTT is rarely necessary to identify individuals with diabetes and is most valuable in proving that an individual at risk *does not* have the disorder.

Diagnostic criteria for diabetes in the pregnant woman remain controversial. The NDDG-accepted diagnostic criteria were originally established by O'Sullivan and Mahan in 1964,[88] and these modified criteria continue to be used for diagnosis. Current recommendations include screening all pregnant, nondiabetic women for gestational diabetes. This involves a 50 g glucose challenge test (GCT), typically performed between 24 and 28 weeks of gestation, as an initial screening test for identification of patients at risk. Definitive diagnosis of gestational diabetes involves a 100 g liquid GTT followed over 3 hours. Diagnostic criteria require that two values, including baseline, 1-hour, 2-hour, and 3-hour values, exceed the modified O'Sullivan and Mahan limits of fasting, 105 mg%; 1 hour, 190 mg%; 2 hours, 165 mg%; and 3 hours, 145 mg%.

Gestational diabetes is defined as the diabetic condition that initially manifests during pregnancy.[3] Some authors have suggested that a substantial percentage of diabetes is only the identification of preexisting carbohydrate intolerance because of increased surveillance.[46] Although this may be true in a large percentage of individuals, the subsequent normalization of carbohydrate tolerance postpartum would suggest that impaired glucose handling or metabolism is an acquired defect inherent in the pregnant state. Despite its temporary diabetogenic state, pregnancy itself is not associated with an increased risk of subsequent NIDDM.[71] The occurrence of gestational diabetes, however, is a strong indicator of future progression to NIDDM. As many as 50% of women will develop NIDDM after a pregnancy complicated by gestational diabetes, with obesity and the fasting glucose value being the strongest predictors.[23,76]

Once the diagnosis of diabetes is established by NDDG criteria, it is imperative to subsequently classify this syndrome into specific disorders. Although rather primitive, the NDDG classification does serve as a model for differentiation. The historic classification of "juvenile-onset" versus "adult-onset" diabetes eroded with the realization that both forms of diabetes may occur in any age-group. The newer classification is an attempt to define the specific diseases according to an etiologic mechanism. The disorder previously described as juvenile-onset diabetes is now more appropriately described as *insulin-dependent diabetes mellitus* (IDDM), or *type I diabetes*. Adult-onset diabetes mellitus is now more appropriately described as *non-insulin-dependent diabetes mellitus* (NIDDM), or *type II diabetes*.

Two major problems emerge from this diagnostic classification system. First, the terms *IDDM* and *NIDDM* tend to suggest that the disease classification depends on whether insulin is used in the treatment. This is not the case. Approximately 50% of all individuals with diabetes currently being treated with insulin have NIDDM, or type II diabetes.[73] This remains a major stumbling block in the effective education of health professionals and patients as to appropriate classification and prognosis of the disorder. Second, the descriptions of type I and type II diabetes in no way suggest the etiologic mechanism underlying the disorder. It is a firm belief and hope that future efforts to standardize diagnosis and classification will establish designations relevant to the pathophysiology of any given disorder rather than to descriptive terms of therapy. From a social standpoint, the societal limitations and activities of an individual with diabetes are now predominantly decided on the basis of whether the individual is using insulin in his or her therapeutic management. This is most inappropriate because individuals with type I diabetes have an extremely different response to insulin therapy and a unique prognosis compared with insulin-treated, non-insulin-dependent individuals.

The NDDG classification also calls for the identification of other forms of diabetes, particularly secondary forms of the disease. These may include diabetes occurring as a complication of the following:

- Pancreatic disease or surgery
- Complications of endocrine disorders, such as acromegaly, pheochromocytoma, or Cushing syndrome
- Complications of pharmacologic therapy, such as glucocorticoids, streptozotocin, or pentamidine

These are potentially reversible forms of diabetes, with no genetic linkage. The historic description of borderline or chemical diabetes has now been eliminated. To remove the stigma of a diagnosis, including the term *diabetes,* this status is now defined as *impaired glucose tolerance.* These individuals may be diagnosed only by glucose tolerance testing and, according to NDDG criteria, are classified by the findings of a 2-hour post–glucose load, serum glucose value less than 200 mg/dl (11 mmol/L), but with one intervening value in excess of 200 mg/dl. Approximately one third of these individuals will subsequently develop carbohydrate intolerance, meeting criteria for diabetes mellitus. In addition, these individuals remain at risk for the development of severe macrovascular complications. As a result, the National Institutes of Health (NIH) has embarked on a long-term diabetes prevention program to target individuals with impaired glucose tolerance and to intervene with both life-style modification and pharmacologic intervention in an effort to prevent the future progression to NIDDM.

PATHOGENESIS AND PATHOPHYSIOLOGY: IDDM

Our current understanding of the pathogenesis of the different forms of diabetes should serve as a framework for the development of nomenclature more descriptive of the etiology. For example, it is known that type I or IDDM is a result of an autoimmune attack on the beta cell.[121] Thus the ultimate designation of IDDM as autoimmune diabetes would be much more descriptive and better understood than either insulin-dependent or type I diabetes mellitus.

Putting aside these problems with nomenclature, however, IDDM is characterized by the abrupt onset of clinical signs and symptoms associated with marked hyperglycemia and the strong propensity for the development of ketoacidosis. Classic studies performed at the Joslin Clinic demonstrated pathologic and biochemical changes as long as 9 years before the clinical onset of disease.[111] Type I diabetes may now be broken down into five stages of development (Box 1-1).

It has long been known that a genetic propensity exists for the occurrence of IDDM. The risk of IDDM in the general population ranges from 1 in 400 to 1 in 1000. That risk is substantially increased in the offspring of individuals with diabetes, to approximately 1 in 20 to 1 in 50.[100] Subsequent studies examining the genetics of IDDM have focused on the histocompatibility locus, or HLA system, on the sixth chromosome. Early studies of class I antigens within the HLA system revealed a greatly elevated relative risk of developing IDDM in those individuals found to be positive for B-8 and Bw-15.[84] Analyses of this sort do not identify the specific locus resulting in the disease but rather identify a linkage disequilibrium at that area. Subsequent analyses of class II antigens found the B-8 and Bw-15 association to be in linkage disequilibrium with DR-3 and DR-4. Positivity at DR-3 and DR-4 loci confers a higher degree of relative risk than does positivity at B-8 or B-15, suggesting that DR-3 and DR-4 are more important for the genetic predisposition to the disorder.

As more and more HLA genes are identified, molecular geneticists have moved from a serologic definition (e.g., HLA DR-3 or DR-4) to a genomic typing of HLA loci according to the specific genes encoded. Therefore the DQ serologic locus may consist of multiple specific genes, all with differential transmission of diabetes (Table 1-1). Thus HLA DR-4 is associated with both DQ A-1 0301 and DQ B-1 0302. Using this genomic terminology allows a more precise definition of the potential gene(s) leading to the development of IDDM. HLA DR-3 and/or DR-4 appear to be present in greater than 90% of Caucasians with IDDM. However, 95% of these are found to have the genomic definition DQ A-1 0301, DQ B-1 0302. This HLA genotype is strongly associated with the occurrence of IDDM among African-American, Caucasian, and Japanese populations.[122] Additional DQ associations with the occurrence of IDDM include the observation that 96% of IDDM patients are homozygous for the absence of the amino acid aspartate at position 57 of the DQ beta chain, compared with 19% in the general population.[124] In addition to the presence of the aspartate acid codon 57

BOX 1-1

PATHOPHYSIOLOGIC STAGES IN THE DEVELOPMENT OF IDDM

Stage 1: genetic predisposition
Stage 2: environmental trigger
Stage 3: active autoimmunity
Stage 4: progressive beta-cell dysfunction
Stage 5: overt diabetes mellitus

Table 1-1   Genetic Risk for Development of IDDM

DQ A-1, DQ B-1	DQ serology	Associated DR	Relative risk
0102, 0602	DQ-6	DR-2, DR-11	0.02
0103, 0603	DQ-6	DR-6	0.02
0501, 0301	DQ-7	DR-5	0.02 to 0.04
0501, 0201	DQ-2	DR-3	3 to 5
0301, 0302	DQ-8	DR-4	8 to 12
0301, 0402			5 to 15
0301, 0201			5 to 20
0501, 0302			8 to 35

Modified from Thorsby E, Ronningen KS: *Diabetologia* 36:371-377, 1993.

of the DQ beta chain, dominant protection also appears to be conferred by the presence of the antigen DQ B-1 0602 or DQ W-1.2.[11] The genetic predisposition to develop IDDM is the result of the combination of HLA DQ–coded genes for disease susceptibility offset by these genes related to disease resistance. Available data would further suggest that genes conferring resistance are frequently dominant over those conferring disease susceptibility.[122] Thus our understanding of the genetics of IDDM is leading to the identification of markers of susceptibility and resistance for the disorder.

However, not all individuals at genetic risk for IDDM ultimately develop it. Epidemiologic surveys reveal that 40% of Caucasian individuals express the DR-3 or DR-4 haplotype, but despite this high prevalence, fewer than 1% ultimately develop diabetes.[121] Further convincing evidence that genetics is not sufficient for the development of the disease is the finding of a 50% discordance rate of IDDM between identical twins.[117] This would suggest that specific alleles within the class II antigens of the histocompatibility complex on chromosome 6 are *necessary but not sufficient conditions* for the development of IDDM. In particular, some trigger is necessary for the expression of this genetic propensity.

Environmental triggers for the development of IDDM have long been suspected. Epidemiologic studies have suggested that the incidence of IDDM is increased in both spring and fall and is coincidental with epidemics of various viral disorders.[35] Past studies relating apparent epidemic outbreaks of IDDM in populations previously affected by outbreaks of mumps provide strong circumstantial evidence. The finding of activated T cells and active autoimmunity in as many as one third of individuals with congenital rubella syndrome further supports a viral etiology.[99] The finding of a beta-cell cytotropic coxsackie virus B in a young child dying of ketoacidosis when presenting with IDDM was the first apparent demonstration of direct viral attack on the beta cells.[139] Although this direct viral hypothesis remains controversial, it is evident that several viruses have the potential either to destroy islet cells directly or to induce changes leading to a slow autoimmune destruction of the beta cell.[116] The dilemma in identifying specific triggers involves the apparent long latency period between the triggering of active autoimmunity and the subsequent clinical development of diabetes mellitus. Thus it is extremely difficult to identify which insult over the past 7 to 10 years may have been the actual trigger of the disease process. More likely is the possibility that a variety of viral or environmental agents may trigger expression of the genetic predisposition to the disease.

One such environmental antigen receiving much attention is bovine serum albumin (BSA). An early report of the finding of BSA-specific antibodies in most children with newly diagnosed diabetes triggered the interest in molecular mimicry as a modulator for active autoimmunity.[58] A comprehensive review of this issue suggests that early exposure to cow's milk is an important determinant of subsequent IDDM, increasing disease risk as much as 1.5 times.[37] This window of risk is thought to be during the first 3 to 4 months of life, during which diabetes risk declines with the duration of exclusive breastfeeding.[129] The potential role of BSA as an environmental trigger of IDDM became more provocative with the identification of the molecular similarity between BSA and a cell surface antigen found on the islet cell, which has subsequently been named ICA-69.[91] The cross-reactivity with circulating anti-BSA antibodies to ICA-69 would provide the linkage between the environmental trigger and the subsequent development of autoimmunity causing IDDM. Additional environmental factors suggested as triggers for IDDM include sex steroids, as seen in puberty and during pregnancy; environmental toxins, including *N*-nitroso derivatives and vacor; or possibly insulin itself.[67]

Regardless of the trigger, early IDDM is first identified by the appearance of active autoimmunity directed against the beta cells of the pancreas and their products. Various immunologic markers occur in individuals before the development of carbohydrate intolerance in diabetes. International standardization of islet cell antibody (ICA) assays has finally been achieved to promote comparisons among laboratories. Standardization of the ICA assay with expression of values in JDF units has defined ICA-"positive" individuals as having greater than 40 JDF units. Life table analyses reveal that 50% of relatives with high-titer ICAs become diabetic within 5 years of follow-up. Approximately 10% of ICA-positive relatives develop diabetes per year, with the interval as long as 8 years between detection of ICAs and onset of diabetes.[140] In the largest prospective study, 4800 Dutch schoolchildren were followed for 10 years. ICA positivity was found in 0.24%, with 50% of these individuals ultimately developing IDDM. ICA negativity conferred a 99.9% probability of freedom from the development of IDDM.[17]

ICAs are composed of a variety of specific islet cell antigens with which diabetic serum is capable of interacting. Of particular interest among this family of autoantigens is a 64,000 M_r protein called *glutamic acid decarboxylase* (GAD).[9] This particular autoantigen has been found to precede the development of IDDM by many years.[10] It appears to be the best immunologic predictor for the future development of IDDM.[8] At least in an animal model, autoimmunity to GAD triggers T cell responses to other beta-cell antigens with subsequent beta-cell destruction. This process can be prevented with the induction of tolerance to GAD and the prevention of this step in autoimmunity.[59] In addition to basic immunologic dysfunction and direct immunologic attack on the beta cell, there appears to be an immunologic attack on insulin, the product of the beta cell.[89] Table 1-2 shows additional islet cell autoantigens that may be playing a permissive or pathologic role in the causation of IDDM. Although each antibody confers an increased relative risk for the development of IDDM, the combination of positive antibody titers provides both increased sensitivity and increased specificity for disease progression. Seventy-eight percent of future cases of IDDM

Table 1-2 Islet Cell Antibodies (ICAs) Observed in IDDM

Autoantigen	T cell reactivity	Description
GM2-1	?	Nonspecific; in all islet cells
Glutamic acid decarboxylase (GAD)	Positive	Present as GAD-65, GAD-67, and 64,000 M_r antibodies
Insulin	Positive	Insulin autoantibodies (IAAs)
ICA-69 (PM-1)	?	Homologous to bovine serum albumin (BSA)
38,000 M_r	Positive	Secretory granule related
52,000 M_r	?	Rubella associated
Carboxypeptidase H	?	Secretory granule related
GLUT	?	Inhibition of glucose-stimulated insulin secretion

Modified from Atkinson MA and others: *Lancet* 35:1357-1360, 1990.
M_r, Relative molecular mass; molecular weight.

found in ICA-positive individuals arose from the subset with multiple autoantibodies composing only 27% of the population.[14]

The combination of autoimmune attack on the beta cell and on insulin by insulin autoantibodies (IAAs) progressively diminishes the effective circulating insulin level. Before the clinical onset of diabetes mellitus, intravenous (IV) GTT demonstrates a progressive decrease in first-phase insulin secretion in those individuals with positive immunologic markers.[112] More than 50% of individuals with positive islet cell antibodies but normal GTTs have first-phase insulin secretion falling within the tenth percentile of the normal population.[70] In a prospective study of 53 subjects, a regression equation has been developed to predict the time to onset of diabetes in individuals with high-titer ICA, IAA, and impaired first-phase insulin secretion:

$$\text{Years to diabetes} = -0.86 - 1.23 \, [\log(\text{IAA} + 40)] + 2.41[\log(1 \text{ minute} + 3 \text{ minutes IV GTT insulin})]$$

This formula correctly predicted the onset of hyperglycemia in 18 individuals.[110]

As is clear from this regression model, it is not until greater than 90% of the secretory capacity of the beta-cell mass has been destroyed that the patient will ultimately manifest hyperglycemia and symptoms consistent with the diagnosis of diabetes mellitus. Thus the clinical onset may be abrupt, but the pathophysiologic insult is a slow, progressive phenomenon. At any time during this progressive fall in beta-cell function, overt diabetes may be precipitated either by acute illness or by stress, increasing the insulin demand beyond the reserve of the damaged islet cell mass. Hyperglycemia will ensue until the acute illness or stress is resolved; then the patient may revert to a compensated state for a variable time, during which the beta-cell mass is sufficient to maintain normal glycemia. This has been referred to as the "honeymoon period" and is a variable period of non–insulin dependency following acute decompensation. It is now apparent that continued beta-cell destruction occurs and that these patients ultimately require insulin within 3 to 12 months and then have diabetes permanently.

The identification of these multiple stages of development of IDDM has provided a provocative framework for potential interventions for its prevention and cure. The identification of HLA markers may allow recognition of populations at risk at birth. Further delineation of environmental triggers may allow the development of specific vaccines for prevention or the simple avoidance of environmental toxins such as BSA. If prevention of the trigger is ineffective, the identification of active autoimmunity by the measurement of islet cell antibodies may serve as a marker for those individuals destined ultimately to develop diabetes. First, one must have both sensitive and specific markers of disease risk to identify individuals at high risk for disease progression.[13] Then, one must be able to apply this technology in a cost-effective manner to identify individuals for testing, based on their relative risk of developing IDDM. Finally, safe and effective interventions must be developed for application to this population who, although not currently affected, is at extremely high risk for the ultimate development of IDDM.[30] At present the NIH has embarked on the Diabetes Prevention Trial—Type I (DPT-1) to include the screening of first-degree relatives of IDDM probands with measurement of ICAs, including anti-GAD, and the ultimate performance of IV GTTs with measurement of first-phase insulin release. Individuals are stratified according to risks and to interventions with either oral insulin or subcutaneous insulin in an effort to prevent the ultimate development of IDDM.

Finally, our understanding of the basic autoimmune pathogenesis of IDDM sheds great light on the potential use of transplantation as a modality of ultimate therapy for individuals with IDDM. The simple transplantation of islet cells apparently is insufficient for curing individuals with IDDM. The subsequent anamnestic immunologic response seen after pancreas transplantation between HLA identical twins reveals the underlying nature of the disorder and the likelihood of the immunologic attack simply destroying subsequent islet cell transplants.[115] Future considerations may include the use of HLA nonidentical islet cell tissue, transplantation of islet cells into immunologically privileged sites, microencapsulation of islets to prevent immune attack, or preparation of transplanted islets with masking of cell surface antigens to prevent immunologic attack. Finally, the identification of a prediabetic state, together with specific immunosuppressive therapy, may provide the best opportunity for preventing the disease.

PATHOGENESIS AND PATHOPHYSIOLOGY: NIDDM

Type II diabetes, or NIDDM, is a very distinctive disorder from IDDM. NIDDM classically develops in an older patient population and may or may not require the use of therapeutic insulin. As previously mentioned, approximately 90% of diabetes in the United States is of the type II variety, with disproportionate representation among older adults and ethnic minority communities. Ascertainment of type II diabetes remains extremely poor, with almost 50% of those affected being undiagnosed.[47] This apparent failure to identify individuals with NIDDM results in progressive morbidity and mortality. Extrapolation based on the prevalence of retinopathy at the time of clinical diagnosis of NIDDM suggests that the disease has been present for 6.5 years before its clinical identification and treatment.[50] The prevalence of coronary artery disease appears to be twice that of the nondiabetic population, and cardiovascular and total mortality are twofold to threefold greater.[32,55]

Identification of these currently undiagnosed individuals with NIDDM is a critical public health problem. Use of simple fasting plasma glucose determinations greater than 100 mg% yields a sensitivity of 83% with a specificity of 76% for identifying these individuals.[47] A 2-hour plasma glucose determination after a 75 g glucose load in excess of 200 mg% provides a sensitivity of 97% with a 100% specificity and definitive criteria for the diagnosis. The yield on identifying individuals at risk has improved by examining individuals who are obese and/or have a family history of diabetes. Therefore testing of individuals with an ideal body weight in excess of 120% would detect 67% of all cases of undiagnosed NIDDM. The prevalence of undiagnosed NIDDM in this population, however, would only be 9%. By altering screening criteria to examination of those with greater than 140% of ideal body weight with a family history of diabetes, fully 25% of those screened would be found to have NIDDM.[47]

NIDDM is a heterogeneous disorder characterized by variable plasma insulin levels associated with hyperglycemia and peripheral insulin resistance. Heredity plays a major role in its transmission. Although there is no recognized HLA linkage, the offspring of a patient with type II diabetes has a 15% chance of developing NIDDM and a 30% risk of developing impaired glucose tolerance.[100] In addition, a greater than 90% concordance rate exists between monozygotic twins if one has type II diabetes, suggesting the primacy of the genetic defect in this form of disease.[117] The heterogeneity of NIDDM further complicates the identification of the genetic linkage for this syndrome, but the GENNID study sponsored by the American Diabetes Association (ADA) may shed light on the genetics of a large series of families with NIDDM.

Unusual cohorts with an exceptionally high prevalence of NIDDM have provided some insight into potential genetic linkages for NIDDM. For example, the Pima Indians of North America have a 50% prevalence of NIDDM, with insulin resistance and hyperinsulinemia inherited as an autosomal trait.[15] In a familial form of NIDDM, known as *maturity-onset diabetes in the young* (MODY), diabetes was closely associated with alterations of chromosome 7 in proximity to the glucokinase gene.[33] Unfortunately, screening of larger populations with NIDDM failed to reveal any association with glucokinase gene variants.[18] Recent reports of genetic linkages to obesity may provide insight into both the pathogenesis of NIDDM and innovative approaches to its treatment. Specific studies of defects in genes coding for the OB protein leptin in the genetically obese mouse, with the resultant weight loss after treatment with leptin, provide provocative evidence of the genetic link among food intake, obesity, and diabetes.[45] Mutations in the beta$_3$-adrenergic receptor correlate with decreased energy expenditure, obesity, and diabetes.[130]

Research into the etiology of NIDDM is currently proceeding along two complementary tracks. Population genetics, with formal screening of candidate genes, in small inbred communities potentially identifies gene products involved in carbohydrate intolerance. Similarly, physiologic approaches in the examination of beta-cell activity in insulin action ultimately lead to the identification of the molecular mechanisms underlying these defects and the subsequent genetic factors controlling them.[56] Recent reviews describing the current state of the art in the genetics of NIDDM emphasize the paucity of generalizable genetic information, while also emphasizing the important potential for understanding NIDDM.[31,74,125]

Multiple theories exist to explain the defects observed in NIDDM.[56,95,119] It is one opinion that NIDDM will ultimately be broken down into several specific defects, which may include (1) primary beta-cell dysfunction, (2) rare insulin receptor abnormalities, and (3) specific postreceptor defects, including altered glucose transporter function and specific enzymatic defects modulating intracellular insulin activity. At present, however, clinical observations would suggest several phenomena at work in NIDDM. Limitation in beta-cell response to hyperglycemia appears to be the cornerstone of the pathophysiology of NIDDM. Regardless of the degree of peripheral insulin resistance, if the islets have an unlimited capacity to secrete insulin, sufficient insulin should be available to overcome any degree of resistance. However, the beta cell apparently is unable to respond appropriately to a hyperglycemic challenge.[97] Morphologic studies have revealed an approximate 50% reduction in beta-cell mass in individuals with NIDDM compared with control subjects, particularly when the degree of obesity is also taken into account.[62] No evidence of autoimmune insulitis is found within these beta cells, but the expected degree of hypertrophy and hyperfunction caused by chronic hyperglycemia is distinctly absent.

Alterations in the gene coding for insulin are a rare but well-defined cause of NIDDM.[113] Beta-cell recognition of glucose and its subsequent linkage to insulin synthesis and secretion have also been identified as specific mechanisms by which the beta cell plays a critical role in NIDDM.[101] Furthermore, intrinsic abnormalities in patterns of insulin secretion are noted in most individuals with NIDDM.[96,97] Ultimately, the packaging and secretion of insulin appear to be progressive abnormalities as one moves from normal to impaired glucose tolerance and subsequently to NIDDM. Abnormal secretion of the insulin precursor proinsulin has been noted in multiple populations. Thus the secretion of proinsulin (with only 10% to 15% of the biologic activity of insulin) would result in apparent decreased insulin action.[44,57,104,120]

Finally, acquired defects in beta-cell activity have been noted in response to hyperglycemia and are referred to as *glucose toxicity*. In essence, it has been found that beta cells chronically exposed to hyperglycemia become progressively less efficient in responding to subsequent glucose challenges.[26] This is a reversible phenomenon in which normalization of ambient glucose produces a dramatic improvement in insulin secretory response to a fixed glucose challenge.[66] Thus beta-cell dysfunction may be either primary or acquired in the pathogenesis of NIDDM; however, it remains a necessary component to carbohydrate intolerance.

A second hallmark of NIDDM is the presence of resistance to the biologic activity of insulin noted in both liver and peripheral tissues.[106] Longitudinal studies in populations at high risk for the development of NIDDM have revealed the preexistence of severe insulin resistance years before the onset of hyperglycemia.[132] Longitudinal follow-up revealed those individuals with impaired insulin sensitivity (i.e., insulin resistance) cluster within families and subsequently predict the onset of NIDDM.[72] This is further supported by longitudinal studies in high-risk patient populations such as the Pima Indians and Hispanic Americans.[43,69] Such resistance to the biologic activity of insulin may result in hyperglycemia, with progressively increased requirements for insulin secretion, and promote the expression of either glucose toxicity or some genetic limitation in beta-cell activity. The relative roles of insulin resistance and insulin deficiency remain highly controversial and are frequently presented in the literature.[119]

Nevertheless, the capability of insulin to suppress glucose production at the level of the liver has been well documented in individuals with NIDDM. In the fasting state, circulating blood glucose is maintained by hepatic glucose production via glycogenolysis and gluconeogenesis. Insulin suppresses these processes in a sharp dose-response manner. Those with NIDDM have a substantial shift to the right of these curves, with a decrease in both the sensitivity and the response of the system.[77] Thus regardless of circulating insulin levels, individuals with NIDDM have a persistent hepatic glucose production that increases fasting glucose levels. Ordinarily this would not result in circulating hyperglycemia unless the periphery, specifically muscle and fat, were unable to compensate with increased glucose uptake. Similar studies using a euglycemic hyperinsulinemic clamp show both decreased sensitivity and decreased response in peripheral glucose disposal in individuals with NIDDM compared with nondiabetic control subjects.[27]

The mechanism by which the peripheral insulin resistance occurs is not entirely clear. Early suggestions of impaired insulin receptor function have not been borne out. Although rare individuals have been identified as having altered insulin receptor structure or function, in the vast majority of individuals with NIDDM, insulin binding to its receptor, insulin receptor number, and insulin receptor activity appear to be entirely normal.[118] Elucidation of the specific mechanisms by which insulin resistance occurs requires a better understanding than current knowledge of normal insulin action. The proximal pathway of insulin action via binding to the insulin receptor and the subsequent tyrosine kinase activity have been elegantly described.[56] This results in a phosphorylation cascade through insulin receptor substrate 1 (IRS-1) and a family of enzymes referred to as mitogen-activated protein (MAP) kinase. This cascade process subsequently leads to the biologic effectors of insulin action, including glucose transporter synthesis and translocation; the enzymatic machinery for glycogen, protein, and lipid synthesis; and mitogenic activity. These more distal effector mechanisms appear to play a predominant role in human insulin resistance.[135]

Further delineation of the pathophysiologic pathways underlying NIDDM and subclassification according to the specific defect should allow for a more refined definition of the disease and more directed therapeutic approaches. For example, individuals with predominant beta-cell defects may clearly require intervention with insulin to overcome the absolute deficiency in beta-cell insulin secretion. In contrast, individuals with predominant peripheral insulin resistance may respond more efficiently to interventions that improve insulin response at the target tissue. Direct inhibition of hepatic glucose production tends to lower fasting blood glucose levels and reduce the effects of glucose toxicity on the beta cell, thus allowing for more efficient insulin response to a subsequent meal. Likewise, an increase in non-insulin-mediated glucose disposal in the periphery (e.g., by exercise) lowers circulating glucose levels independent of beta-cell function.

These premises, together with the public health demands of recognizing an insidious disorder that carries substantial morbidity and mortality, have led the NIH to propose a prevention trial for NIDDM. The Diabetes Prevention Program (DPP) intends to screen high-risk populations for the presence of impaired glucose tolerance. It is hoped that subsequent intervention with intensive life-style (diet, exercise, and subsequent weight loss) versus pharmacologic interventions to improve endogenous insulin action will ameliorate the specific defects before decompensation to a hyperglycemic state. Health care professionals anxiously await the outcomes of both DPT-1 and DPP for guidance in the ultimate prevention of diabetes mellitus.

DIABETES CONTROL AND COMPLICATIONS

With the discovery of insulin and the ability to avoid acute complications of diabetes, the relationship between glycemic control and complications has become the seminal issue in the care of the individual with diabetes. The following question arises: are the chronic complications of diabetes mellitus independently inherited, or are they the consequence of the metabolic state found in diabetes mellitus? Independent inheritance is suggested by the finding of thickened basement membranes in nondiabetic family members of probands with type I diabetes. However, the preponderance of evidence would suggest that the chronic complications are indeed the consequence of the altered metabolic milieu inherent in diabetes. Support for this hypothesis is found in secondary forms of diabetes, such as hemochromatosis, hypercortisolism, and acromegaly, and in individuals with diabetes secondary to either surgical or inflammatory destruction of the beta cells of the islet cells. In these noninherited forms of diabetes, both microangiopathy and nephropathy can be demonstrated.

If one accepts that the long-term consequences of diabetes result from the altered metabolic state, the next obvious question is whether current efforts at glycemic control are sufficient in preventing the development of the complications. Proving that hypothesis has been more difficult than originally anticipated. Difficulties involved are questioned as follows:

1. Is control of plasma glucose alone sufficient to prevent the development of the complications?
2. How tightly controlled must the plasma glucose be?
3. At what stage in the development of the complications must glycemic control be initiated?
4. Is there a critical period during which development of the complications is irreversible?

The completion of the Diabetes Control and Complications Trial (DCCT) has provided definitive evidence of not only the relationship between longstanding complications of diabetes and hyperglycemia, but also the potential ability to prevent or slow the progression of those complications by achieving intensive glycemic control.[29] In the DCCT, more than 1400 patients with IDDM were followed for as long as 9 years in a randomized, controlled trial of intensive versus conventional therapy.

Intensive therapy was defined as use of three or four injections of insulin per day or use of an insulin pump and daily self-monitoring of blood glucose (SMBG), with the patient using insulin-adjustment algorithms in an effort to achieve normalization of both fasting and postprandial glucose determinations. At the termination of the study, clinical and statistical differences were seen in mean glucose determinations and hemoglobin (Hb) A_{1c} between the two treatment groups. Although the intensively treated group was able to lower their Hb A_{1c} from 8.9% to 7.2% during the study, they were unable to normalize completely either glucose or Hb A_{1c} determinations. The limiting factor in achieving improved glycemic control appeared to be hypoglycemia. The incidence of severe hypoglycemia was approximately three times higher in the intensive therapy group than in the conventional therapy group, with 62 episodes per 100 patient years compared with 19 episodes per 100 patient years, respectively. Incidence of both hypoglycemic coma and seizure increased threefold in the intensive therapy group. Clustering of these episodes of severe hypoglycemia in a relatively small cohort of individuals was noted early in the DCCT.[28] Risk factors for severe hypoglycemia included a history of hypoglycemic unawareness or coma and, not surprisingly, intensive efforts to achieve normal glycemia with near-normal glycohemoglobin levels. Clearly, any efforts to normalize glycemic control in individuals with IDDM must be tempered by the risk and subsequent occurrence of severe hypoglycemia. Understanding of these mechanisms and modalities for minimizing the occurrence of severe hypoglycemia received recognition with a recent ADA Banting Lecture.[24]

Despite the inability to normalize glucose homeostasis completely, the DCCT demonstrated a reduction in development and progression of end-organ damage. The primary end point in the study was the development of retinopathy, and a 60% to 76% reduction in the risk of both new-onset and progression of diabetic retinopathy was noted in the intensively treated group. Nephropathy was similarly reduced, with the risk of developing microalbuminuria reduced by 35% and the risk of developing fixed proteinuria reduced by 56%. Intensive treatment reduced the risk of experiencing onset of new neuropathy by 70% and the risk of progressive neuropathy by 58%. Surprisingly, even in this cohort of young individuals, the risk of macrovascular disease (predominantly myocardial infarctions) was reduced by 44% with intensive therapy.

It is important to realize that the DCCT was undertaken exclusively in adolescents and young adults with IDDM. Some believe that the applicability of these findings to the much larger population with NIDDM is problematic. In most cases, however, clinical and pathologic manifestations of microvascular disease are identical in the two forms of diabetes.[79] The proposed mechanisms by which these complications occur are also thought to be similar.[16,20] Efforts to study specifically the relationship between glycemic control and complications in NIDDM, however, are further complicated by the heterogeneity in the disease itself, the difficulty in intervening at disease onset, the highly variable treatment approaches found to achieve near-normal glycemia, and the high degree of covariants, such as hypertension, obesity, and dyslipidemia. Nonetheless, three separate studies have attempted to delineate this relationship. The UGDP Study of the late 1960s and early 1970s was sufficiently flawed as to render it uninterpretable. The Veterans Administration (VA) Cooperative Study was designed to complement the DCCT in studying NIDDM. These investigators were able to demonstrate short-term differences in glycemic control, but the study failed to reach any statistical conclusions because of premature termination for lack of funding.[1] The United Kingdom Prospective Diabetes Study (UKPDS) remains an ongoing protocol attempting to answer this question. These investigators have used a "give them everything including the kitchen sink" approach. As a result, differences in glycemia among the group are minimal, and no differences in chronic complications have been discernible to date.[127]

Nonetheless, in the absence of data to the contrary, it is logical to assume that improved glycemia will have a similar effect on microvascular complications in NIDDM as they do in IDDM. The available modalities for intervention to achieve near-normal glycemia, however, are much greater in the NIDDM population. Weight loss and life-style modifications with increased physical activity become the hallmark of therapy, and the options of sulfonylureas, biguanides, glucosidase inhibitors, and insulin are all available. It is reasonable to conclude, therefore, that similar efforts in glycemic control should be applied to patients with NIDDM as to those with IDDM.[78,94] This position has further been codified by both the ADA in its statement, "Many otherwise healthy patients with NIDDM should strive to achieve tight control,"[5] and the American Association of Clinical Endocrinologists (AACE), who agreed and stated, "A system of intensive control of diabetes mellitus would likely decrease the rate of complications, improve patients' quality of life, and decrease the total cost of care associated with both IDDM and NIDDM."[2]

The 70-year debate addressing the relationship between diabetes control and complications is now clearly resolved based on observational studies from the Joslin Clinic[60] and Pirart,[92] meta-analyses,[131] and now the definitive prospective, randomized DCCT study. Perhaps equally as important, however, is how health care providers proceed from here with such data in hand. Several questions arise, such as the following[102]:

1. How does one achieve strict glycemic control in a clinical setting without the expertise and personnel of the research center?
2. How does one improve the adherence to treatment regimens that are expensive and intrusive and require sophisticated self-management techniques?
3. How does one avoid hypoglycemia?
4. In view of complications, cost, and difficulty of intensive insulin therapy, how does one predict which individuals are at greatest risk for developing late complications and thus would benefit from this intervention?

Translating research to practice is particularly problematic when a multispecialty team is necessary to demonstrate efficacy for a disease that is usually managed by a general internist in 90% of patients. Necessary steps include convincing patients of the importance of glycemic control, convincing physicians of the importance of control and instructing them in the tools necessary to achieve it, and facilitating patient acceptance and adherence, including reduction in the costs of intensive therapy or third-party reimbursement for them.[128] Efforts to include such measures in health care reform proposals of the mid-1990s have not always been received favorably.[65] Short-term fiscal constraints together with a highly volatile health care financing system have effectively paralyzed implementation of DCCT standards within the medical community.

With these data in hand, implementation of intensive management remains considerably more problematic. Translation efforts are underway, but patient acceptability, availability of experienced health care providers, and adequate reimbursement for these services are all lacking.[108] The first step in patient acceptance requires extensive patient education, motivation, and provision of the tools necessary for accomplishing intensive therapy goals. Psychosocial support is imperative at those times when less than optimal glycemia is achieved.[75] Only a small minority of patients are aware of the value of glycated hemoglobin or practice SMBG.[49]

Motivating physicians is even more problematic. With more than 90% of patients in the United States receiving care from primary care providers, it is distressing to find that only half are aware or believe in the importance of glycemic control.[126] Review of almost 100,000 Medicare patients with diabetes seen in office-based physician practices revealed only 16% receiving optimal care.[134] Finally, the impact of health care reform on implementation of intensive therapy remains the ultimate financial stumbling block. Current economic policy mandates reduction in medical expenditures, even when those initial expenditures may result in long-term health care gains and cost savings. It is hoped, however, that incorporation of intensive therapy goals into practice guidelines and standards of care will allow for better accountability in the era of managed care.[114] Grading of health care plans according to their routine assessment of glycated hemoglobin, referral to ophthalmologists and podiatrists, and avoidance of hospitalization for acute and chronic complications may allow consumers to control the provision of diabetes care. Consumer-directed health care management may play directly into the hands of those advancing the cause of intensive diabetes management.[65]

CLINICAL CHEMISTRY ASSESSMENT

Diabetes management historically has been a hospital-based system, necessitating frequent visits for venipuncture to measure serum glucose and electrolytes and to determine appropriate pharmacologic intervention. Two laboratory components have become standards of care by providing both immediate and longer-term information regarding glucose control.[40] These innovations made the DCCT possible by allowing immediate information feedback for adjustment of glucose by use of insulin algorithms and the ability to measure glycemic control over time.

Self-monitoring of blood glucose (SMBG) technology allows more realistic management of glycemia on an outpatient basis and facilitates implementing intensive insulin regimens. The growth and use of this technology have been consumer driven. Physicians were initially skeptical of the utility and acceptability of whole blood testing of glucose on a daily basis. They presumed that pain, inconvenience, and expense would all be impediments to widespread clinical use. It quickly became apparent that individuals with diabetes sought precise information concerning ambient glucose levels and accepted the minor discomfort, annoyance, and cost in exchange for an improved sense of well-being and control. In community-based intervention programs the use of SMBG over the last decade has increased threefold in the IDDM population, fourteenfold in an insulin-using NIDDM population, and fifteenfold in the non-insulin-using NIDDM populations.[6] Despite this impressive growth in use, only 33% of all patients with diabetes perform SMBG. Of those IDDM patients who performed monitoring, only half monitor on a daily basis. The use of SMBG within NIDDM is even lower, with 26% of insulin-treated patients monitoring daily and only 5% of those treated with diet or oral agents.[48] This dismal utilization of a remarkable diagnostic technique is related to both physician bias and financial restraints. Box 1-2 lists potential indications for the use of SMBG, as outlined by the ADA consensus statement.

BOX 1-2

INDICATIONS FOR SELF-MONITORING OF BLOOD GLUCOSE (SMBG)

Achieve and maintain specific levels of glycemic control.
Prevent and detect hypoglycemia.
Avoid severe hyperglycemia.
Adjust management in response to changes in life-style.
Determine the need for insulin therapy in gestational diabetes.

———

From American Diabetes Association: *Diabetes Care* 17:81-86, 1994.

Various technologies rapidly became available, using dry reagents in either a colorimetric or ion exchange methodology.[40] It is almost impossible to provide a comprehensive listing of available systems, since new meters are entering the marketplace at an astounding rate. Nonetheless, Table 1-3 provides an abridged listing. The certified diabetes educator is best prepared to evaluate the accuracy, precision, and applicability of any given monitoring system for a particular patient. Matching monitors to the individual's needs and technical capabilities is imperative to ensure proper use of SMBG technology.

Numerous manuscripts can be cited to validate the precision and accuracy of various systems. User variability remains the major stumbling block in the proper operation and use of SMBG technology.[42,83,85] These findings underscore the critical importance of diabetes education in the use of particular monitors and the interpretation and application of the data provided. Despite the potential pitfalls of the clinical implementation of SMBG technology, the methodology exists for assessing the clinical accuracy and importance of the information provided which makes SMBG indispensable to patient care.[6,21]

Glycated hemoglobin determinations are an additional clinical laboratory assessment that have become invaluable in both research and clinical care. This measurement is predicated on the nonenzymatic, irreversible binding of glucose to the amino terminus of the beta chain of hemoglobin. This reaction depends solely on the ambient glucose concentration during the life of the red cell, reflecting past glucose control and modeling the cellular effects of hyperglycemia.[36] The implications of advanced glycosylated end products is beyond the scope of this chapter, but excellent reviews are available in the recent literature.[16] The more relevant application of glycated hemoglobin is the assessment of long-term glycemic control. At a clinical level, it allows the health care provider to validate the results of SMBG and reinforce the means of achieving glycemic control. From a research perspective, it is an indispensable parameter in relating glycemic control and long-term diabetic complications.[39] In addition, recent studies suggest that glycated hemoglobin results can be used as a very effective educational and motivational tool to improve overall diabetes control.[64]

Table 1-3   Systems for Self-Monitoring of Blood Glucose (SMBG)

Product	Manufacturer
Visual	
Chemstrips bG	Boehringer-Mannheim
Monitors with internal memory	
Accu-Chek Advantage	Boehringer-Mannheim
Accu-Chek III	
Accu-Chek Easy	
Tracer II	
Ultra	HDI
One-Touch II	Lifescan
One-Touch Profile	
Glucometer M+	Miles
Glucometer Encore	
Monitors down-loading to computer-based managers	
Merlin	Boehringer-Mannheim
Accu-Chek III	
Accu-Chek Advantage	
Accu-Chek Easy	
One-Touch II	
Glucofacts: Glucometer M+	Miles
Humabase	Lilly
One-Touch II	
One-Touch Profile	
Monitors using no-wipe technology	
Accu-Chek Easy	Boehringer-Mannheim
Accu-Chek Advantage	
One-Touch II	Lifescan
One-Touch Basic	
One-Touch Profile	
Companion II Pen	Medisense
Companion II Card	
Ultra	HDI
Glucometer Elite	Miles
Glucometer Encore	
Supreme bG	Chronomed

Modified from Buyer's guide update, *Diabetes Forecast,* January 1995.

Multiple methodologies, with varying normative values, exist for measuring glycated hemoglobin. As a result, comparisons among laboratories are hazardous at best and probably inaccurate. Characteristics of the assay critical to interpretation are as follows[61]:

1. Whether the assay measures HbA_{1c} or total HbA_1
2. The ability to separate the labile from the stable fraction of glycated hemoglobin

Table 1-4   Characteristics of Glycated Hemoglobin (Hb) Assays

Method	Measures	CV (%)	Interferences
Ion exchange (HPLC)	Hb A$_{1c}$	3%	Hb C and F
Ion exchange (Minicolumn)	Hb A$_{1c}$ or Hb A$_1$*	2%-16%	Hb C, S, and F
Affinity column	Total glycated Hb†	1%-3%	None
Affinity binding	Total glycated Hb†		None
Immunoassay	Hb A$_{1c}$		None
Electrophoresis	Hb A$_{1c}$ or Hb A$_1$*	4%-10%	Hb F

Modified from Goldstein DE and others: *Diabetes Care* 18:896-909, 1995.
CV, Coefficient of variation; *HPLC,* high-performance liquid chromatography.
*Varies depending on system.
†Reports total glycated Hb or is internally calibrated to report an Hb A$_{1c}$ standardized value.

3. The temperature dependance of the system
4. The degree of interference by Hb F

No standardization of the assay exists at present, although the NDDG has been addressing the issue for a decade. Recently, standardization has been attempted using calibrators determined by high-performance liquid chromatography (HPLC) on standard samples to correct for varying methodologies. As a result, some comparison among laboratories and among varying techniques can be achieved with the coefficient of variation (CV) in the range of 5%.[136] Nevertheless, knowledge of the specific assay being used for measurement of glycosylated hemoglobin, its normative values, and comparison of longitudinal data obtained by the same laboratory using the same technique remain imperative. Table 1-4 provides a compilation of assay characteristics.

ROLE OF THE HEALTH CARE TEAM IN DIABETES MANAGEMENT

Despite rapid advances in medical research exploring the outer limits of molecular biology and immunology, pharmacologic intervention in individuals with diabetes has remained virtually unchanged over the last 20 years. Interventions with diet, exercise, sulfonylureas, biguanides, and insulin are different only in degree from those used in the 1960s. The greatest advance in clinical care since the discovery of insulin has been the development and improvement of SMBG techniques. SMBG not only has allowed for improved glycemic control, but also has revolutionized the approach to clinical care. Although Elliot Joslin had advocated diabetes education in the 1920s, it was not until SMBG technology was introduced into clinical care that the individual with diabetes was integrated into the therapeutic decision-making process. It is now apparent that a well-educated individual with diabetes is much more capable of caring for his or her diabetes than the most expert health care delivery systems. To allow for optimal use of this remarkable tool, a health care team encompassing the physician, nurse educator, nutritionist, exercise physiologist, pharmacist, and psychosocial professionals must interact with the patient for beneficial outcomes. This team approach was effectively implemented in the DCCT, with the success of intensive therapy clearly being attributed to the efforts of the diabetes educators. Two specific studies have demonstrated the efficacy of clinical care by diabetes educators in reducing glycated hemoglobin levels and avoiding hospitalization for individuals with diabetes.[90,133] Diabetes is now the prototypic model for integration of individuals into their own health care. This will become the cornerstone for preventive measures in a health care model for chronic disease.

With integration of the individual with diabetes into the health care delivery team, individualized goals of therapy may be determined. Establishing goals depends on the individual's ability to learn in his or her psychosocial environment and on determination of specific outcome variables. Applying education techniques to various populations is described in greater detail in other chapters of this text; however, it is the responsibility of the members of the health care team to work directly with the individual with diabetes to determine both the goals and the approaches to diabetes therapy.

The necessity of the team approach to diabetes care has further been codified in the ADA standards of care for individuals with diabetes mellitus.[7] The need for a team approach to the care of diabetes may appear self-evident to those in the field, but it is frequently *not* implemented in the community. In a review of community diabetes care in Michigan in 1991, Hiss and colleagues[53] found that 20% of insulin-requiring patients received no diet instruction by a dietitian, 23% received no diabetes education, and 33% were not seen by an ophthalmologist in the previous 2 years. In a larger nationwide study,[22] only 35% of individuals with diabetes had attended a class or program about diabetes during the course of their disease. This included 59% of individuals with IDDM, 49% of insulin-treated individuals with NIDDM, and 24% of non-insulin-requiring individuals with NIDDM. Individuals most likely to have participated in a diabetes education program included younger individuals with higher levels of education and those with diabetes complications. Although income was not an independent determinant for having received diabetes education, this is complicated by the unknown factor of third-party reimbursement. In a separate study, degree of third-party reimbursement for services played a critical role in facilitating patient care.[86]

Added patient responsibility demands that education and psychologic support be provided as an integral part of health care delivery. Diabetes education is now firmly entrenched as the cornerstone of diabetes care. As such, members of the health care team function as an integrated unit to meet the specific ongoing needs of the individual with diabetes. These needs may change over time, with emphasis directed sequentially from survival skills to the effects of diet, to psychologic support, to pharmacologic intervention, to foot care, and ultimately to coping with chronic complications. Depending on the specific needs of the patient, various members of the health care team may play the dominant interventional role.

Client needs change through the life span as consideration of issues such as growth and development change to issues of pregnancy or management of chronic complications. The health care team undertakes continuous needs assessment to determine educational goals and the most appropriate techniques with which to achieve them. Concerns of reading level, social support systems, and financial ramifications must all be weighed in the most appropriate educational approach to the individual client at any particular time.

LEGAL RAMIFICATIONS OF DIABETES EDUCATION

The introduction of the health care delivery team and increased patient responsibilities for self-care have introduced a unique medical model and potential legal ramifications. Two practical issues readily become apparent: (1) are the nonphysician members of the treatment team practicing medicine without appropriate licensure? and (2) with whom does the civil liability for such practice reside? The first issue pertains to criminal activity independent of the quality of care. The second is a civil concern that addresses negligence in the performance of a duty. To date there have been no legal challenges to the expanding role of diabetes educators in health care management of individuals with diabetes.[103]

The practice of medicine has traditionally been limited to individuals holding doctorates of medicine or osteopathy. However, the definition of the practice of medicine has remained fluid throughout the years, and with the expansion of responsibilities, it is apparent that more and more activities are falling within the purview of other health professionals. Ultimately, the limits of activities of health professionals are delineated by their state's licensure requirements, and criminal practice is defined as activities specifically requiring a specialized degree. For example, licensure within a state may limit the parenteral administration of pharmacologic agents to either physicians or nurses; therefore, nutritionists and exercise physiologists may not administer an insulin injection to an individual with diabetes. However, it is unclear whether or not the recommendation of insulin adjustments with alterations in eating patterns or exercise would also be precluded by these restrictions. With the growth of diabetes team intervention, those team members not *traditionally* allowed to administer pharmacologic agents most likely may be allowed to make such recommendations according to an established protocol. This view has been supported in the courts to a limited extent.[109]

The second issue, civil liability for negligent performance, is a more difficult problem. Clearly, anyone can be sued for virtually any reason. Typically, those named in malpractice cases are those who are able to pay the most. Rapport and communication with the patient may be the best recommendations for avoiding malpractice litigation, but once a suit is filed, identification of those liable for negligent performance of duty and standards of care are the critical issues.

Precedent teaches that health professionals may be held independently liable for negligent practice, independent of the action of the responsible physician.[25] If a diabetes educator acting within the scope of his or her responsibilities performs in a negligent manner, liability for the negligence should be borne by the educator directly. This is especially important as diabetes educators become independent providers of health care outside of the hospital or physician's office. Because of this, diabetes educators may be held independently liable for negligent acts stemming from improper instruction in insulin administration or adjustment, poor implementation or understanding of the prescribed therapy, or negligent assessment of the patient's comprehension of instruction.

To provide the best service and to avoid litigation, members of a diabetes treatment team first should ensure that both their program and their individual educators are recognized and certified by the ADA and The National Certification Board for Diabetes Educators (NCBDE), respectively. This identifies the expanded responsibilities of the team members and their specialty expertise. The responsibilities of each person should be viewed as legal requirements. Depending on the expertise of the educators, written outlines of procedure and content of instruction should be centrally developed and categorically implemented. These programs should adhere to ADA standards of medical care.[7] In one review of diabetes-related malpractice claims, 85% of claims stemmed directly from failure to provide care consistent with national professional standards.[19]

Educators must ensure sufficient patient comprehension of instructions in self-care techniques to implement therapy both safely and effectively. In addition, they have an ongoing responsibility to reassess the effectiveness of instruction and thoroughly document all information concerning the patient's therapy. Although litigation may be brought against the diabetes care team for any number of reasons, thoughtful attention to the national practice standards may serve as a potent defense against claims of negligent patient care.

IMPACT OF TEAM CARE ON HEALTH CARE DELIVERY AND FINANCING

The emphasis on team management and patient education has made the individual with diabetes an active participant in the health care process. As such, the team may be less likely to use the passive health care delivery inherent in a hospital situation. In general, patients sick enough to require hospitalization are not in a situation conducive to learning anything more than survival skills. On the other hand, outpatient diabetes education may provide sufficient care to preclude the necessity for routine hospitalization of individuals with diabetes for problems such as initiation of insulin management, difficulties with uncontrolled diabetes, and prevention of chronic complications.[4] As a result, the ultimate costs of health care delivery should be reduced substantially. To the extent that expenditures for hospitalization account for approximately two thirds of the direct cost of diabetes, a reliance on outpatient education and management should be expected to reduce substantially the frequency of hospitalization, the duration of hospital stays, and consequently health care costs.[107] In addition, the institution of an inpatient diabetes health care team may reduce hospital stays by as much as 56%.[68] Time spent in the hospital with a primary diagnosis of diabetes in the absence of being seen by a diabetes treatment team is essentially lost time. Length of stay is consistent from the moment of diabetes team consultation until discharge. Thus time spent before that consultation is without hospital benefit.

The reliance on diabetes education as a primary modality of therapy forces health care providers to reevaluate their means of health care reimbursement and financing. By defining diabetes education as diabetes care, direct third-party reimbursement for such services would be logical. However, this may require an entire restructuring of health care financing in the United States to move away from the acute care model, with its emphasis on palliative and sometimes curative procedures, toward a chronic care model of prevention of disease and complications. The systematic collection of clinical outcomes data together with cost-effectiveness and cost-benefit analyses are critical to this effort. Numerous studies are ongoing in an effort to collect such data prospectively.[41] A compendium of available data is available through the National Diabetes Information Clearing House.[82]

Unfortunately, reimbursement is "spotty" nationwide and depends on specific health care plans and the tenacity of both patient and health care provider.[123] Receiving payment for services relative to diabetes education and care requires the providers to familiarize themselves with the archaic language of the insurance industry and government. Appropriate coding may make the difference whether or not one is paid for necessary services provided.[38] Diabetes care providers can no longer avoid entering the forum of health care financing reform. Rather, it is imperative that all providers speak up in support of established standards of care and their appropriate coverage within health care plans for outpatients.

SUMMARY

Exploration of the pathophysiology of type I diabetes (IDDM) has taken health care providers to the frontiers of genetics, immunology, and immunomodulation. Exploration of type II diabetes (NIDDM) is at the forefront of molecular biology and physiology. Diabetes education and a health care team directed toward patient involvement in self-care and prevention of complications constitute a model for a revolution in health care delivery and financing within the United States. At all levels, including research, education, and clinical care, diabetes intervention is progressing rapidly and is at the forefront of its prospective discipline.

REFERENCES

1. Abraira C and others: VA Cooperative Study on Glycemic Control and Complications in Type II Diabetes: results of the feasibility trial, *Diabetes Care* 18:1113-1123, 1995.
2. American Association of Clinical Endocrinologists: *AACE guidelines of the management of diabetes mellitus,* Jacksonville, Fla, 1995, AACE.
3. American Diabetes Association, Freinkel N, editor: Summary and recommendations of the 2nd International Workshop Conference on Gestational Diabetes Mellitus, *Diabetes* 34 (suppl 2):123-126, 1985.
4. American Diabetes Association: Hospital admission guidelines for diabetes mellitus, *Diabetes Care* 18 (suppl 1):35, 1995.
5. American Diabetes Association: Implications of the Diabetes Control and Complications Trial, *Diabetes* 42:1555-1558, 1993.
6. American Diabetes Association: Self-monitoring of blood glucose consensus statement, *Diabetes Care* 17:81-86, 1994.
7. American Diabetes Association: Standards of medical care for patients with diabetes mellitus, *Diabetes Care* 18 (suppl 1):8-15, 1995.
8. Atkinson MA and others: 64k M_r auto antibodies as predictors of insulin-dependent diabetes, *Lancet* 35:1357-1360, 1990.
9. Baekkeskov S and others: Antibodies to a M_r 64,000 human islet cell antigen precede the clinical onset of insulin dependent diabetes, *J Clin Invest* 79:926-934, 1987.
10. Baekkeskov S and others: Identification of the 64-K auto-antigen in insulin-dependent diabetes as the GABA-synthesizing enzyme glutamic acid decarboxylase, *Nature* 347:151-156, 1990.
11. Baisch JM and others: Analysis of HLA DQ genotypes and susceptibility in insulin-dependent diabetes mellitus, *N Engl J Med* 322:1836-1841, 1990.
12. Banerji MA and others: GAD antibody negative NIDDM in adult black subjects with diabetic ketoacidosis and increased frequency of human leukocyte antigen DR3 and DR4: flatbush diabetes, *Diabetes* 43:741-745, 1994.
13. Bingley PJ, Bonifacio E, Gale EAM: Can we really predict IDDM? *Diabetes* 42:213-220, 1993.
14. Bingley PJ and others: Combined analysis of autoantibodies improves prediction of IDDM in islet cell antibody positive relatives, *Diabetes* 43:1304-1310, 1994.
15. Bogardus C and others: Distribution of in vivo insulin action in Pima Indians as a mixture of 3 normal distributions, *Diabetes* 38:1423-1432, 1989.
16. Brownlee M: Glycation and diabetic complications, *Diabetes* 43:836-841, 1994.
17. Bruining GJ and others: Ten year follow up of islet cell antibodies in childhood diabetes mellitus, *Lancet* 1:1100-1102, 1989.
18. Chiu KC, Tanizawa Y, Permutt MA: Glucokinase gene variance in the common form of NIDDM, *Diabetes* 42:579-582, 1993.

19. Clark CM Jr, Kinney ED: The potential role of diabetes guidelines in the reduction of medical injury and malpractice claims involving diabetes, *Diabetes Care* 17:155-159, 1994.

20. Clark CM Jr, Lee DA: Drug therapy: prevention and treatment of the complications of diabetes mellitus, *N Engl J Med* 332:1210-1217, 1995.

21. Clarke WL, Cox D, Gonder-Frederick LA: Evaluating clinical accuracy of systems for self-monitoring for blood glucose, *Diabetes Care* 10:622-628, 1987.

22. Coonrod BA, Betschart J, Harris MI: Frequency and determinants of diabetes patient education among adults in the U.S. population, *Diabetes Care* 17:852-858, 1994.

23. Coustan DR and others: Gestational diabetes: predictors of subsequent disordered glucose metabolism, *Am J Obstet Gynecol* 168:1139-1145, 1993.

24. Cryer PE: Banting Lecture: Hypoglycemia, the limiting factor in management of IDDM, *Diabetes* 43:1378-1389, 1994.

25. *Darling v Charleston Community Memorial Hospital,* 33 Ill 2nd 326, 211, NE 2nd 253, cert denied 383 US 946, 1965.

26. DeFronzo RA, Ferrannini E, Koivisto V: New concepts in the pathogenesis and treatment of non-insulin dependent diabetes mellitus, *Am J Med* 74(suppl 1A):52-81, 1983.

27. DeFronzo RA, Bonadonna RC, Ferrannini E: Pathogenesis of NIDDM: a balanced overview, *Diabetes Care* 15:318-368, 1992.

28. Diabetes Control and Complications Trial Research Group: Epidemiology of severe hypoglycemia in the diabetes control and complications trial, *Am J Med* 90:450-459, 1991.

29. Diabetes Control and Complications Trial Research Group: The effect of intensive treatment of diabetes on the development and progression of long-term complications in insulin-dependent diabetes mellitus, *N Engl J Med* 329:977-986, 1993.

30. Eisenbarth GS and others: The design of trials for prevention of IDDM, *Diabetes* 42:941-947, 1993.

31. Elbein SC and others: The genetics of NIDDM, *Diabetes Care* 17:1523-1533, 1994.

32. Eschwege E and others: Coronary heart disease mortality in relation to diabetes, blood glucose, and plasma insulin levels, the Paris Prospective Study 10 years later, *Horm Metabol Res* 15(suppl):41-46, 1985.

33. Froguel PH and others: Close linkage of glucokinase locus on chromosome 7P to early onset non-insulin dependent diabetes mellitus, *Nature* 356:162-164, 1992.

34. Funnell MM: Role of the diabetes educator for older adults, *Diabetes Care* 13(suppl 2):60-65, 1990.

35. Gamble DR, Taylor KW: Seasonal incidence of diabetes mellitus, *Br J Med* 3:631-633, 1969.

36. Garlick RL and others: Characterization of glycosylated hemoglobin: relevance to diabetic control and analysis of other proteins, *J Clin Invest* 71:1062-1072, 1983.

37. Gerstein HC: Cow's milk exposure in type I diabetes mellitus, *Diabetes Care* 17:13-19, 1994.

38. Gillespie S: Coverage, coding, and reimbursement, *Diabetes Spectrum* 6:228-232, 1993.

39. Goldstein DE and others: Feasibility of centralized measurements of glycated hemoglobin in the diabetes control and complications trial: a multi-center study, *Clin Chem* 33:2267-2271, 1987.

40. Goldstein DE and others: Technical review: tests of glycemia in diabetes, *Diabetes Care* 18:896-909, 1995.

41. Greenfield S and others: The uses of outcomes research for medical effectiveness, quality of care, and reimbursement in type II diabetes, *Diabetes Care* 17 (suppl 1):32-39, 1994.

42. Greyson J: Quality control in patients self-monitoring of blood glucose, *Diabetes Care* 16:1306-1308, 1993.

43. Gulli G and others: Metabolic profile of NIDDM is fully established in glucose tolerant offspring of 2 Mexican American NIDDM parents, *Diabetes* 41:1575-1586, 1992.

44. Haffner SM and others: Proinsulin and specific insulin concentrations in high and low risk populations for NIDDM, *Diabetes* 43:1490-1493, 1994.

45. Halaas JL and others: Weight reducing effects of the plasma protein encoded by the *obese* gene, *Science* 269:543-546, 1995.

46. Harris MI: Gestational diabetes may represent discovery of preexisting glucose intolerance, *Diabetes Care* 11:402-411, 1988.

47. Harris MI: Undiagnosed NIDDM: clinical and public health issues, *Diabetes Care* 16:642-652, 1993.

48. Harris MI, Cowie CC, Howie LJ: Self-monitoring of blood glucose by adults with diabetes in the United States population, *Diabetes Care* 16:1116-1123, 1993.

49. Harris MI, Eastman RC, Siebert C: The DCCT in medical care for diabetes in the U.S., *Diabetes Care* 17:761-764, 1994.

50. Harris MI and others: Onset of NIDDM occurs at least 4 to 7 years before clinical diagnosis, *Diabetes Care* 15:815-819, 1992.

51. Harris MI and others: Prevalence of diabetes and impaired glucose tolerance and plasma glucose

levels in the U.S. population age 20-74 years, *Diabetes* 36:523-534, 1987.

52. Helms RB: Implications of population growth on prevalence of diabetes, *Diabetes Care* 15 (suppl 1):6-9, 1992.

53. Hiss RG and others: Community diabetes care: a ten-year perspective, *Diabetes Care* 17:1124-1134, 1994.

54. Jackson RA: Mechanisms of age-related glucose intolerance, *Diabetes Care* 13 (suppl 2):9-19, 1990.

55. Jarrett RJ, Shipley MJ: Type II diabetes mellitus and cardiovascular disease: putative association via common antecedents: further evidence from the Whitehall Study, *Diabetologia* 31:737-740, 1988.

56. Kahn CR: Insulin action, diabetogenes and the cause of type II diabetes, *Diabetes* 43:1066-1084, 1994.

57. Kahn SE and others: Proinsulin as a marker for the development of NIDDM in Japanese American men, *Diabetes* 44:173-179, 1995.

58. Karjalainen J and others: A bovine albumin peptide is a possible trigger of insulin dependent diabetes mellitus, *N Engl J Med* 327:302-307, 1992.

59. Kaufman DL and others: Spontaneous loss of T-cell tolerance to glutamic acid decarboxylase in murine insulin-dependent diabetes, *Nature* 366:69-72, 1993.

60. Keiding NR, Root HF, Marble A: Importance of control of diabetes and prevention of vascular complications, *JAMA* 150:1964-1969, 1962.

61. King ME: Glycosylated hemoglobin. In Kaplan LA, Pesce AJ, editors: *Clinical chemistry; theory, analysis, and correlation,* ed 2, St Louis, 1989, Mosby.

62. Kloppel G and others: Islet pathology in the pathogenesis of type I and type II diabetes mellitus revisited, *Surv Synth Pathol Res* 4:110-125, 1985.

63. Kuminyika SK, Ewart CK: Theoretical and baseline considerations for diet and weight control of diabetes among blacks, *Diabetes Care* 13 (suppl 4):1154-1162, 1990.

64. Larsen ML, Horder M, Mogensen EF: Effective long-term monitoring of glycosylated hemoglobin levels in insulin dependent diabetes mellitus, *N Engl J Med* 323:1021-1025, 1990.

65. Lasker RD: The Diabetes Control and Complications Trial: putting prevention into practice under health care reform, *Diabetes Rev* 2:350-358, 1994.

66. Leahy JL: Natural history of beta cell dysfunction in NIDDM, *Diabetes Care* 13:992-1010, 1990.

67. Leslie RDG, Elliott RB: Early environmental events as a cause of IDDM, *Diabetes* 43:843-850, 1994.

68. Levetan CS and others: Impact of endocrine and diabetes team consultation on hospital length of stay for patients with diabetes, *Am J Med* 99:22-28, 1995.

69. Lillioja S and others: Insulin resistance and insulin secretory dysfunction as precursors of non-insulin dependent diabetes mellitus: prospective studies in Pima Indians, *N Engl J Med* 329:1988-1992, 1993.

70. MacLaren NK: How, when and why to predict IDDM, *Diabetes* 37:1591-1594, 1988.

71. Manson JE and others: Parity and incidence of non-insulin dependent diabetes mellitus, *Am J Med* 93:13-19, 1992.

72. Martin BC and others: Role of glucose and insulin resistance in development of type II diabetes mellitus: results of a 25 year follow-up study, *Lancet* 340:925-929, 1992.

73. Martin DB, Quint AR: Therapy for diabetes. In National Diabetes Data Group: *Diabetes in America,* NIH Pub No 85-1468, Washington, DC, 1985, US Government Printing Office.

74. McCarthy MI, Froguel P, Hitman GA: The genetics of non-insulin dependent diabetes mellitus: tools and aims, *Diabetologia* 37:959-968, 1994.

75. McCulloch DK and others: A systematic approach to diabetes management in the post DCCT era, *Diabetes Care* 17:765-769, 1994.

76. Metzger BE and others: Pre-pregnancy weight and ante-partum insulin secretion predict glucose tolerance five years after gestational diabetes mellitus, *Diabetes Care* 16:1598-1605, 1993.

77. Mitrakou A and others: Contribution of abnormal muscle and liver glucose metabolism to postprandial hyperglycemia in NIDDM, *Diabetes* 39:1381-1390, 1992.

78. Nathan DM: Do results from the Diabetes Control and Complications Trial apply in NIDDM? *Diabetes Care* 18:251-257, 1995.

79. Nathan DM: Long-term complications of diabetes mellitus, *N Engl J Med* 328:1676-1685, 1992.

80. National Center for Health Statistics: *The Second National Health and Nutrition Examination Survey, 1976-1980,* Vital and Health Statistics Series 10, No 15, DHHS-PHS Pub No 81-1317, Hyattsville, Md 1981, US Government Printing Office.

81. National Diabetes Data Group: Classification and diagnosis of diabetes mellitus and other categories of glucose intolerance, *Diabetes* 28:1039-1057, 1979.

82. National Diabetes Information Clearing House: *Cost effectiveness of diabetes patient education,* Bethesda, Md, 1993, National Institutes of Health, National Institute of Diabetes and Digestive and Kidney Diseases.

83. National Steering Committee for Quality Assurance in Glucose Monitoring: Proposed strategies for reducing user error capillary monitoring, *Diabetes Care* 16:493-498, 1993.

84. Nerup J, Mandrup-Poulsen T, Molvig J: The HLA-IDDM association: implications for etiology and pathogenesis of IDDM, *Diabetes Metab Rev* 3:779-802, 1987.

85. Nettles A: User error in blood glucose monitoring: National Steering Committee for Quality Assurance Report, *Diabetes Care* 16:946-948, 1993.

86. Nordberg BJ and others: Effect of third-party reimbursement on use of services and indexes of management among indigent diabetic patients, *Diabetes Care* 16:1076-1080, 1993.

87. O'Brien TR and others: Are racial differences in the prevalence of diabetes in adults explained by differences in obesity? *JAMA* 262:1485-1488, 1989.

88. O'Sullivan JB, Mahan CM: Criteria for the oral glucose tolerance test in pregnancy, *Diabetes* 13:278-285, 1964.

89. Palmer JB and others: Insulin antibodies in insulin-dependent diabetics before insulin treatment, *Science* 222:1337-1339, 1983.

90. Peters AL, Davidson MB, Ossorio RC: Management of patients with diabetes by nurses with support of subspecialists, *HMO Pract* 9:8-13, 1995.

91. Pietropaolo M and others: Islet cell auto-antigen 69-KD [ICA-69], *J Clin Invest* 92:359-371, 1993.

92. Pirart J: Diabetes mellitus and its degenerative complications: a prospective study of 4,400 patients observed between 1947-1973, *Diabetes Care* 1:168-188, 252-263, 1978.

93. Pi-Sunyer FX: Obesity and diabetes in blacks, *Diabetes Care* 13 (suppl 4):1144-1149, 1990.

94. Pollet RJ, El-Kebbi IM: The applicability and implications of the DCCT to NIDDM, *Diabetes Rev* 2:413-427, 1994.

95. Polonsky KS: The Lilly Lecture: the beta cell in diabetes: from molecular genetics to clinical research, *Diabetes* 44:705-717, 1995.

96. Polonsky KS and others: Abnormal patterns of insulin secretions in non-insulin diabetes mellitus, *N Engl J Med* 318:1231-1239, 1988.

97. Porte DJ Jr: Banting Lecture: beta cells in type II diabetes mellitus, *Diabetes* 40:166-180, 1991.

98. Porte DJ Jr, Kahn SE: What geriatricians should know about diabetes mellitus, *Diabetes Care* 13 (suppl 2):47-54, 1990.

99. Rabinowe SL and others: Congenital rubella: mono-clonal antibody defined T-cell abnormalities in young adults, *Am J Med* 81:779-782, 1986.

100. Raffel LJ, Rotter JI: The genetics of diabetes, *Clin Diabetes* 3:49-54, 1985.

101. Randle PJ: Glucokinase and candidate genes for type II (non-insulin dependent) diabetes mellitus, *Diabetologia* 36:269-275, 1993.

102. Ratner RE: Diabetes control and complications:

where do we go from here? *Online J Curr Clin Trials (Serial Online),* June 5, 1993.

103. Ratner RE, El-Gamassey ER: Legal aspects of the team approach to diabetes treatment, *Diabetes Educ* 16:113-116, 1990.

104. Ratner RE and others: Proinsulin and specific insulin patterns with respect to glucose tolerance in African American and Caucasian populations, *Diabetes* 44(suppl 1):227A, 1995.

105. Ray NF, Wills S, Thamer M: *Direct and in-direct costs of diabetes in the United States in 1992,* Alexandria, Va, 1993, American Diabetes Association.

106. Reaven GM: Role of insulin resistance in human disease, *Diabetes* 37:1595-1607, 1988.

107. Rubin RJ, Altman WM, Mendelson DN: Health-care expenditures for people with diabetes mellitus, *J Clin Endocrinol Metab* 78:809a-809f, 1994.

108. Rubin RR, Peyrot M: Implications of the DCCT, looking beyond tight control, *Diabetes Care* 17:235-236, 1994.

109. *Sermchief v Gonzales,* 660 SW 2nd 683, 684, Mo Banc 2, 1983.

110. Skyler JS, Marks JB: Immune intervention in type I diabetes mellitus, *Diabetes Rev* 1:15-42, 1993.

111. Srikanta S and others: Islet cell antibodies in beta cell function in monozygotic triplets and twins initially discordant for type I diabetes, *N Engl J Med* 308:322-325, 1983.

112. Srikanta S and others: Type I diabetes mellitus in monozygotic twins: chronic progressive beta cell dysfunction, *Ann Intern Med* 99:320-326, 1983.

113. Steiner DF and others: Lessons learned from molecular biology of insulin gene mutation, *Diabetes Care* 13:600-609, 1990.

114. Stolar MW: Clinical management of the NIDDM patient: impact of the American Diabetes Association guidelines, 1985-1993, *Diabetes Care* 18:701-707, 1995.

115. Sutherland DER and others: Twin to twin pancreas transplantation: reversal and reenactment of the pathogenesis of type I diabetes, *Trans Assoc Am Phys* 97:80-87, 1984.

116. Szopa TM and others: Diabetes mellitus due to viruses: some recent developments, *Diabetologia* 36:687-695, 1993.

117. Tattersall RB, Pyke DA: Diabetes in identical twins, *Lancet* 2:1120-1125, 1972.

118. Taylor SI: Lilly Lecture: molecular mechanisms of insulin resistance: lessons from patients with mutations in the insulin-receptor gene, *Diabetes* 41:1473-1490, 1992.

119. Taylor SI, Accili D, Imai Y: Insulin resistance or insulin deficiency, which is the primary cause of NIDDM? *Diabetes* 43:735-740, 1994.

120. Temple RC and others: Insulin deficiency in

non-insulin dependent diabetes, *Lancet* I:293-295, 1989.

121. Thai A-C, Eisenbarth GS: Natural history of IDDM, *Diabetes Rev* 1:1-14, 1993.

122. Thorsby E, Ronningen KS: Particular HLA-DQ molecules play a dominant role in determining susceptibility or resistance to type I diabetes mellitus, *Diabetologia* 36:371-377, 1993.

123. Tobin CT: Third party reimbursement coverage for diabetes outpatient education program, *Diabetes Care* 15 (suppl 1):41-43, 1992.

124. Todd JA, Bell JI, McDevitt HO: HLA DQ B gene contributes to susceptibility and resistance to insulin-dependent diabetes mellitus, *Nature* 329: 599-604, 1987.

125. Turner RC and others: Type II diabetes: clinical aspects of molecular biological studies, *Diabetes* 44:1-10, 1995.

126. Tuttleman M, Lipsett L, Harris MI: Attitudes and behaviors of primary care physicians regarding tight control of glucose in IDDM patients, *Diabetes Care* 16:765-762, 1993.

127. UK Prospective Diabetes Group: UKPDS: study design, progress and performance, *Diabetologia* 34:877-890, 1991.

128. Vinicor F: Barriers to the translation of the Diabetes Control and Complications Trial, *Diabetes Rev* 2:371-383, 1994.

129. Virtanen SM and others: Early introduction of dairy products associated with increased risk for insulin dependent diabetes mellitus in Finnish children, *Diabetes* 42:1786-1790, 1993.

130. Walston J and others: Time of onset of non-insulin-dependent diabetes mellitus and genetic variation in the beta$_3$ adrenergic receptor gene, *N Engl J Med* 333:343-347, 1995.

131. Wang PH: Tight glucose control and diabetic complications, *Lancet* 342:129, 1993.

132. Warram JH and others: Slow glucose removal rate and hyperinsulinemia precede the development of type II diabetes in the offspring of diabetic parents, *Ann Intern Med* 113:909-915, 1990.

133. Weinberger M and others: A nurse-coordinated intervention for primary care patients with non-insulin dependent diabetes mellitus: impact on glycemic control and health-related quality of life, *J Gen Intern Med* 10:59-66, 1995.

134. Weiner JP and others: Variation in office-based quality. A claims-based profile of care provided to Medicare patients with diabetes, *JAMA* 273:1503-1508, 1995.

135. Wells AM and others: Abnormal activation of glycogen synthesis in fibroblasts from NIDDM subjects: evidence for an abnormality specific to glucose metabolism, *Diabetes* 42:583-589, 1993.

136. Weykamp CW and others: Standardization of glycohemoglobin results and reference values in whole blood studied in 103 laboratories using 20 methods, *Clin Chem* 41:82-86, 1995.

137. Wingard DL and others: Community-based study of prevalence of NIDDM in older adults, *Diabetes Care* 13 (suppl 2):3-8, 1990.

138. Winter WE and others: Maturity onset diabetes of youth in Black Americans, *New Engl J Med* 316:285-291, 1987.

139. Yoon JW and others: Isolation of a virus from the pancreas of a child with diabetic ketoacidosis, *N Engl J Med* 300:1173-1179, 1979.

140. Ziegler AG and others: Predicting type I diabetes, *Diabetes Care* 13:762-775, 1990.

2 Epidemiology of Insulin-Dependent Diabetes Mellitus

Jeffrey A. Gavard

INTRODUCTION

The establishment of population-based IDDM registries worldwide in recent years has enabled the incidence of the disease to be monitored through intracountry and intercountry comparisons. The geographic disparity is evident in that a child in Finland has a seventy-fold higher risk of IDDM than a child in Mexico City. Europe generally has the highest incidence rates and Asia the lowest incidence rates. The geographic pattern in incidence rates, the assimilation of ethnic and immigrant groups to the host country's IDDM risk, and increasing and epidemic fluctuations in IDDM incidence over time implicate environmental factors in the causes of the disease. Coxsackie, encephalomyocarditis, mumps, congenital rubella, and Cytomegalovirus infection have been found to be associated with IDDM. Chemicals, stressful events, food additives, and consumption of cow's milk in early infancy have also been implicated as potential causative agents. Breastfeeding may have a protective effect against IDDM development, perhaps because of immunologic factors. A genetic predisposition through HLA antigens, particularly DR3, DR4, and DQB1, has been

---

CHAPTER OBJECTIVES

- Report the incidence of IDDM related to geographic variation.
- Overview the incidence of IDDM related to gender and ethnic differences and temporal patterns.
- Describe the environmental etiology of IDDM.
- Describe the genetic etiology of IDDM.
- Present conclusions about genetic-environmental interactions.
- Summarize the familial risks associated with IDDM.
- Describe the prevalence of psychiatric disorders in adult IDDM populations.

documented through population, family, and twin studies. The genetic susceptibility may code for a propensity of the beta cells of the endocrine pancreas to damage by an environmental agent, a defective ability to regenerate themselves after attack, or vulnerability to an autoimmune defect. Secondary attack rate studies can generate hypotheses for both genetic and environmental etiologies for the disease. Siblings of cases are at greatest risk for the disease and afford a unique opportunity to study genetic-environmental interactions in IDDM development. Persons with IDDM have also been found to be at increased risk for psychiatric disorders, particularly depression. Family studies will again prove useful in examining whether depression is caused by biologic changes of IDDM, a psychologic response to living with IDDM, an antecedent risk factor for IDDM, or the result of a shared etiology with IDDM.

INCIDENCE OF IDDM
Geographic Variation

The past 15 years of diabetes research has seen a proliferation of population-based IDDM registries worldwide* (Table 2-1). These registries were conceptualized by the necessity of having standardized rates for international comparisons of IDDM risk. Cross-cultural examination of IDDM incidence in 15 countries[30,126] and mortality in four countries[31a,158] was completed in the mid-1980s by the Diabetes Epidemiology Research International Group (DERI). The highest incidence rates were noted in Scandinavia, and the lowest incidence rate was in Japan. An apparent increasing gradient in IDDM incidence from south to north was noted in Europe, implicating the possibility of environmental factors dependent on cooler temperatures in the etiology of the disease. The EURODIAB study was begun in 1988 to monitor the prospective surveillance of IDDM within Europe, to examine the north-south gradient of risk, and to collect descriptive epidemiologic data to investigate genetic and environmental causes of IDDM.[55] The World Health Organization Study, the Multinational Project for Childhood Diabetes (DIAMOND), was initiated in 1990.[174] The main purpose of DIAMOND is surveillance of IDDM incidence worldwide through the year 2000. Other aims include the monitoring of temporal patterns of IDDM incidence and mortality, availability of insulin, and costs of diabetes through intracountry and intercountry comparisons. The geographic and racial differences in incidence will form the basis for generating hypotheses to be tested at the population and family level concerning particular environmental exposures and genetic markers as causative agents for the disease. The recurrence risk among siblings of index cases, as well as familial aggregation among parents and offspring, will especially provide insight in terms of how environmental determinants interact with host susceptibility in IDDM.

The highest incidence of IDDM was seen in Finland (42.9/100,000) and the lowest incidence was noted in Mexico City (0.6/100,000), representing over a seventyfold difference in risk (Table 2-1). Very low rates were also found in Shanghai, China (0.7/100,000) and Seoul,

---

*References 11, 14, 17, 24, 37, 39, 42, 55, 56, 58, 63, 71, 74, 77, 78, 88, 96, 98, 107, 126, 139, 142-145, 155, 157, 159, 160, 161, 164, 177.

Text continued on p. 37.

Table 2-1   Worldwide Incidence of IDDM in Persons 0-14 Years of Age (per 100,000 population)

Country and area	Study period	Degree of ascertainment (%)	Mean annual incidence			Male/Female incidence ratio	IDDM cases		
			Males	Females	Total		Males	Females	Total
Asia									
China									
Hong Kong[177]	1986-1990	94	1.5	2.4	2.0	0.6	—	—	22
Shanghai[63]	1980-1991	85	0.6	0.8	0.7	0.8	35	40	75
Israel[126]	1975-1980	—	4.4	4.6	4.5	1.0	142	154	296
Japan									
Hokkaido[126]	1974-1986	100	1.3	2.1	1.7	0.6	112	171	283
Kuwait[144]	1992-1993	92	16.6	14.1	15.4	1.2	47	39	86
South Korea									
Seoul[77]	1985-1988	—	0.6	0.8	0.7	0.8	32	39	71
Russia									
Novosibirsk[145]	1983-1989	96	4.4	4.7	4.6	0.9	101	104	205
Africa									
Mauritius[159]	1986-1990	>95	1.8	2.5	2.1	0.7	14	18	32
Sudan									
Khartoum[37]	1987-1990	95	—	—	8.0	—	—	—	327
Tanzania									
Dar es Salaam[96]	1982-1991	—	0.8	0.9	0.8	0.9	45	41	86
South America									
Argentina									
Avellaneda[142]	1985-1990	89	—	—	6.7	—	—	—	29
Brazil									
Sao Paulo[39]	1987-1991	95	5.7	9.5	7.6	0.6	20	32	52
Chile[14]	1990-1991	100	2.2	2.8	2.5	0.8	35	43	78

Continued.

Table 2-1   Worldwide Incidence of IDDM in Persons 0-14 Years of Age (per 100,000 population)—cont'd

Country and area	Study period	Degree of ascertainment (%)	Mean annual incidence			Male/Female incidence ratio	IDDM cases		
			Males	Females	Total		Males	Females	Total
Oceania									
Australia									
New South Wales[164]	1990-1991	99	14.2	14.8	14.5	1.0	181	180	361
Western Australia[74]	1985-1989	99	—	—	13.2	—	—	—	235
New Zealand[126]	1968-1972	—	8.6	9.1	8.9	0.9	212	216	428
Auckland[126]	1978-1985	—	9.0	10.5	9.8	0.9	109	124	233
Canterbury[126]	1981-1986	100	10.2	12.9	11.6	0.8	18	21	39
North America									
Barbados[71]	1982-1991	94	5.2	4.7	5.0	1.1	31	28	59
Canada									
Montreal[126]	1971-1985	94	9.6	10.0	9.8	1.0	461	458	919
Prince Edward Island[126]	1975-1986	99	27.0	20.8	23.9	1.3	53	39	92
Cuba[126]	1978-1980	—	2.5	2.8	2.7	0.9	128	139	267
Mexico									
Mexico City[126]	1984-1986	—	0.4	0.7	0.6	0.6	38	62	100
Puerto Rico[42]	1985-1989	—	—	—	10.0	—	—	—	—
United States									
Allegheny Co., Penn.[126]	1965-1985	>90	15.1	16.0	15.6	0.9	568	580	1148
Colorado[126]	1978-1983	>95	14.8	15.2	15.0	1.0	304	300	604
Jefferson Co., Ala.[126]	1979-1985	96	9.9	14.9	12.4	0.7	52	76	128
North Dakota[126]	1980-1986	—	21.6	16.2	18.9	1.3	120	84	204
Philadelphia, Penn.[88]	1985-1989	93	11.6	15.2	13.4	0.8	98	117	215
Rochester, Minn.[126]	1965-1979	100	15.8	18.4	17.1	0.9	18	20	38
San Diego, Calif.[126]	1978-1981	—	9.6	9.1	9.4	1.1	25	23	48
Wisconsin (part)[126]	1970-1979	>90	20.2	16.2	18.2	1.2	94	72	166
Virgin Islands[157]	1979-1988	92	—	—	7.2	—	—	—	27

Europe

Austria[55]	1989-1990	94	7.9	7.5	7.7	1.1	107	98	205
Belgium									
Antwerp[55]	1989-1990	100	9.2	10.4	9.8	0.9	15	16	31
Denmark									
3 Counties[55]	1989-1990	99	21.5	21.4	21.5	1.0	34	32	66
Estonia[161]	1983-1988	95	10.7	10.0	10.4	1.1	110	98	208
Finland[160]	1987-1989	100	38.4	32.2	35.3	1.2	563	451	1014
2 Regions[55]	1989-1990	100	47.0	38.8	42.9	1.2	84	67	151
France									
4 Regions[55]	1989-1990	100	7.8	7.8	7.8	1.0	134	127	261
Greece[24]	1992	100	6.2	6.3	6.3	1.0	75	62	137
Athens[55]	1989-1990	99	10.9	7.7	9.3	1.4	72	50	122
5 Northern Regions[55]	1989-1990	100	5.3	3.8	4.6	1.4	9	6	15
Hungary[55]	1989-1990	99	7.7	7.5	7.6	1.0	132	124	256
Iceland[58]	1970-1989	100	9.9	8.8	9.4	1.1	65	55	120
Italy									
Eastern Sicily[55]	1989-1990	100	11.2	9.0	10.1	1.2	29	23	52
Region of Lazio[55]	1989-1990	100	7.2	5.8	6.5	1.2	66	51	117
Region of Lombardy[55]	1989-1990	100	7.6	5.9	6.8	1.3	110	83	193
Region of Marche[17]	1990-1992	100	7.7	8.1	7.9	1.0	25	25	50
Province of Pavia[155]	1988-1992	100	10.2	8.8	9.5	1.2	17	14	31
Sardinia[55]	1989-1990	95	33.5	26.9	30.2	1.2	126	95	221
Province of Turin[11]	1984-1986	99	7.6	8.5	8.1	0.9	21	22	43
Latvia[161]	1983-1988	80-99	6.4	6.9	6.6	0.9	106	109	215
Lithuania[161]	1983-1988	—	6.5	7.0	6.7	0.9	165	171	336
Luxembourg[55]	1989-1990	100	12.1	12.6	12.4	1.0	8	8	16
Macedonia[78]	1985-1991	97	2.4	2.5	2.5	1.0	55	57	112

Continued.

Table 2-1 Worldwide Incidence of IDDM in Persons 0-14 Years of Age (per 100,000 population)—cont'd

Country and area	Study period	Degree of ascertainment (%)	Mean annual incidence			Male/Female incidence ratio	IDDM cases		
			Males	Females	Total		Males	Females	Total
Malta[139]	1980-1987	—	12.7	14.6	13.6	0.9	28	38	66
Netherlands[55]	1989-1990	99	11.2	10.8	11.0	1.0	30	28	58
Norway									
8 Counties[55]	1989-1990	100	22.3	19.3	20.8	1.2	87	71	158
Poland									
3 Cities[55]	1989-1990	100	5.7	6.0	5.8	1.0	51	51	102
9 Western Provinces[55]	1989-1990	100	5.3	5.8	5.5	0.9	80	84	164
Province of Rzeszow[56]	1980-1992	99	5.4	4.8	5.1	1.1	67	55	122
Portugal									
3 Regions[55]	1989-1990	91	10.1	4.9	7.5	2.1	17	8	25
Romania									
Bucharest[55]	1989-1990	100	4.6	5.7	5.1	0.8	22	25	47
Slovenia[55]	1989-1990	100	5.2	7.7	6.5	0.7	23	33	56
Spain									
Catalonia[55]	1989-1990	95	10.5	10.6	10.6	1.0	151	146	297
Madrid[143]	1985-1988	90	11.3	10.5	10.9	1.1	267	234	501
Sweden[107]	1978-1987	99	25.0	23.8	24.4	1.1	2012	1824	3836
United Kingdom[98]	1988	90	13.8	13.3	13.5	1.0	837	763	1600
Ireland[98]	1988	90	—	—	6.8	—	—	—	71
Leicestershire[126]	1965-1981	>90	8.7	8.6	8.7	1.0	140	132	272
Northern Ireland[55]	1989-1990	95	17.8	15.4	16.6	1.2	71	59	130
Oxford[55]	1989-1990	98	17.8	14.9	16.4	1.2	90	71	161
Scotland[126]	1976-1983	100	20.0	19.4	19.7	1.0	966	890	1856
Tayside[126]	1980-1983	100	19.7	22.1	20.0	0.9	36	28	64

South Korea (0.7/100,000). The highest rates were generally found in Europe, followed by North America, Oceania, South America, Africa, and Asia. Although genetic variation is certainly likely to account for a portion of the incidence differences, the influence of viral infections, diet, temperature, cultural practices, and other environmental factors cannot be excluded.[87] The north-south gradient in Europe was generally seen with some notable exceptions. Iceland, despite being the northernmost island in Europe, had an incidence one fourth that of Finland and one half that of Norway, despite sharing ancestral heritage with the latter. Similarly, Estonia, despite geographic proximity and common descendents, also had an incidence roughly one fourth that of Finland. Poland had a relatively low incidence compared with countries at similar latitudes. The most striking exception was found in Sardinia in southern Europe, which had the second highest rate in the continent after Finland. The high risk of IDDM in Malta also did not support the north-south gradient.

The comparability of incidence rates in Table 2-1 is enhanced by the inclusion criteria employed by the registries: (1) a diagnosis of IDDM made by a physician, (2) on insulin therapy at time of registration, and (3) diagnosis of IDDM from birth to 14 years of age where age at onset is taken to be the age at first insulin administration. Residence in the area in question at the time of diagnosis is also a requirement, thus strengthening the validity of the rates by generalizing them to a particular population base. The completeness of case identification was maximized as much as possible by employing various primary and secondary ascertainment sources (e.g., hospitals, clinics, endocrinology centers, physicians, schools, central record offices, insulin records, diabetes camps). Most registries reported case ascertainment greater than 90%. The degree of ascertainment, however, was not reported for 12 registries.* Incidence rates based on small sample sizes also should be interpreted with caution. An additional potential difficulty for some rate comparisons lies in the lack of age-adjustment. Most rates were adjusted to the age composition of the world population. Some registries, however, adjusted their incidence rates to the 1983 census population of Khartoum,[37] the 1980 population of Finland,[160] or the 1992 European population,[24] or they did not age-adjust their rates at all.[142,144,145]

Gender Differences

Males generally tended to have higher incidence rates than females in countries of high IDDM incidence; the reverse was true in countries of low IDDM risk (see Table 2-1). Both could indicate differential distribution of high-risk susceptibility genes or environmental agents within particular countries.

Race and Ethnic Differences

Whites were found to be at highest risk for IDDM of all race groups examined† (as shown in Table 2-2). Although whites generally had incidence rates 1.5 to 2 times greater than blacks,

---

*References 42, 77, 96, 126, 139, 161.
†References 82, 88, 128, 157, 168.

Table 2-2   Race Differences in Incidence of IDDM in Persons 0-14 Years of Age (per 100,000 population)

Country and area	Study period	Degree of ascertainment (%)	Mean annual incidence			Male/Female incidence ratio	IDDM cases		
			Males	Females	Total		Males	Females	Total
Allegheny Co., Penn.[128]									
White	1970-1985	>90	17.0	17.5	17.3	1.0	389	383	772
Black	1970-1985	>90	9.7	13.3	11.5	0.7	33	45	78
Colorado[82]*									
Hispanic	1978-1988	93	7.1	10.5	8.8	0.7	47	70	117
Non-Hispanic†	1978-1988	93	16.4	14.5	15.5	1.1	560	488	1048
Jefferson Co., Ala.[168]									
White	1979-1985	96	15.1	16.2	15.6	0.9	66	68	134
Black	1979-1985	96	3.4	10.6	7.0	0.3	10	31	41
Philadelphia, Penn.[88]									
White	1985-1989	93	12.8	13.7	13.3	0.9	54	55	109
Black	1985-1989	93	8.9	13.0	11.0	0.7	35	51	86
Hispanic	1985-1989	93	10.7	19.6	15.2	0.5	6	11	17
Virgin Islands[157]									
White	1979-1988	92	—	—	28.9	—	—	—	6
Black	1979-1988	92	6.9	4.8	5.9	1.4	10	7	17
Hispanic	1979-1988	92	—	—	7.2	—	—	—	4

*0-17 years of age.
†Includes whites and blacks; blacks represented only 4.7% of this study population.

Hispanics and blacks were relatively similar. The higher rate among Hispanics in Philadelphia can be attributed to the presence of a large Puerto Rican population, a high-risk Hispanic group[88] (see Table 2-1). Whites had a very high rate in the Virgin Islands; the incidence, however, was based on only six cases over the 10-year study period. Blacks and Hispanics who had IDDM in this study were found to have a greater number of white ancestors than their nondiabetic counterparts, thus providing evidence that IDDM in these two races was partly attributed to the greater presence of IDDM susceptibility genes from whites because of racial admixture.[157]

Migration Studies

Migration studies afford the opportunity to investigate the role of environmental factors in the etiology of IDDM through a "natural experiment." Genetically homogeneous groups in different locations or the monitoring of one such immigrant group over time in a single location enables the influence of environmental factors in different host countries to be examined. French children living in Montreal had twice the risk of IDDM than French children living in France (8.2/100,000 versus 3.7/100,000, Table 2-3).[146] The disparity was even greater for Ashkenazi Jews in Montreal (17.2/100,000) than for Ashkenazi Jews in Israel (6.8/100,000). The incidence among first-generation children of Pakistani and Indian immigrants to Bradford, England, increased nearly fourfold until it was virtually equivalent to that of the host country (Table 2-3).[9] Both studies point to the importance of environmental agents as causative factors for IDDM.

Temporal Patterns

There is evidence that the incidence of IDDM is increasing in many parts of the world, particularly in Europe.* In Finland alone the incidence increased 57% from 1965 to 1984.[46,163] A doubling of incidence rates over time was seen in registries in Africa,[37] Oceania,[74] and North America[88] (Table 2-4). The incidence of IDDM in children from birth to 14 years of age in Kuwait quadrupled from 1980 to 1993, but the greatest change was seen in the birth to 4-year age-group, where a ninefold increase occurred over the same period. Scandinavian and northern European countries also showed increases in IDDM incidence over time[70,98,135,162] (see Table 2-4). Genetic explanations for the rising incidence could be either a change in susceptibility or an increased penetrance of the diabetes genes in the populations in question. An increase in the pool of genetically susceptible individuals also may have occurred. Because the rising incidence has been most prolific in Scandinavian countries that have relatively homogeneous populations, the above occurrences are not probable. Environmental factors are likely responsible for some rises in incidence.

Temporal patterns in IDDM risk, however, may also take the form of rapid fluctuations in incidence† (Table 2-5). Six of the nine registries listed indicated an increase in IDDM

---

*References 7, 31, 35, 54, 107, 138, 163.
†References 32, 71, 118, 127, 141, 145.

Table 2-3   Migration Studies in IDDM

Location and ethnic group	Study period	Age (yr)	IDDM cases	Mean annual incidence of IDDM (per 100,000 population)	Location	Study period	Age (yr)	IDDM cases	Mean annual incidence of IDDM (per 100,000 population)
Montreal, Canada[146]									
French	1971-1985	0-14	491	8.2	France	1975	0-14	467	3.7
Ashkenazi Jews*	1971-1985	0-14	48	17.2	Israel	1975-1980	0-20	183	6.8
Bradford, England[9]									
Pakistani and Indian	1978-1981	0-16	3	3.1	Bradford, Eng.	1988-1990	0-16	12	11.7
Non-Asian	1978-1981	0-16	46	11.8	Bradford, Eng.	1988-1990	0-16	31	12.0

*Jews with national origins in middle and eastern Europe. Rate includes the very small minority of non-Ashkenazi Jews living in Montreal.

Table 2-4   Temporal Trends in IDDM: Increasing Incidence

Location	Age (yr)	Group	Study period	Mean annual incidence of IDDM (per 100,000 population)	Study period	Mean annual incidence of IDDM (per 100,000 population)
Asia						
Kuwait[144]	0-14	Males and Females	1980-1981	4.0	1992-1993	15.4
	0-4	Males and Females	1980-1981	1.4	1992-1993	12.0
Africa						
Sudan[37]	0-14	Males and Females	1987	5.9	1990	10.1
Oceania						
Western Australia[74]	0-14	Females	1985	10.2	1989	18.0
North America						
United States						
Philadelphia, Penn.[88]	0-14	Whites	1985-1986	8.3	1987-1988	16.8
Europe						
Finland[162]	0-14	Males and Females	1980-1982	29.6	1986-1988	35.7
Leicestershire, Eng.[98]	0-16	Males and Females	1961-1970	5.3	1971-1980	10.6
Netherlands[135]	0-14	Males and Females	1978-1980	11.1	1988-1990	12.9
Norway[70]	0-14	Males and Females	1973-1977	18.5	1978-1982	22.7
United Kingdom[98]	0-16	Males and Females	1973-1974	7.7	1988	13.5

Table 2-5 Temporal Trends in IDDM: Epidemic Fluctuations in Incidence

Location	Age (yr)	Group	Study period	Mean annual incidence of IDDM (per 100,000 population)	Study period	Mean annual incidence of IDDM (per 100,000 population)
Asia						
Russia						
Novosibirsk (city)[145]	0-14	Males and Females	1983-1989	4.6	1985	8.9
Oceania						
New Zealand[141]	0-19	Males and Females	1982-1990	12.7	1990	21.2
North America						
Barbados[71]	0-14	Males and Females	1982-1991	5.0	1985	9.4
United States						
Allegheny Co., Penn.[32]	0-19	White Males	1965-1989	15.1	1985-1989	20.0
	0-19	Black Males	1965-1989	8.5	1985-1989	16.2
Virgin Islands[157]	0-14	Males and Females	1979-1988	7.2	1984	28.4
Europe						
Estonia[118]	0-14	Native Estonians	1980-1989	11.8	1982	13.0
	0-14	Russian Immigrants	1980-1989	7.6	1982	14.5
Poland (midwestern)[127]	0-16	Males and Females	1970-1981	3.5	1982-1984	6.6

incidence of roughly double the rate for the overall study period. A seventh registry documented a fourfold increase during 1 year.[157] The greatest increase appeared to occur between 1982 and 1985. Inasmuch as the genetic composition of a population cannot undergo rapid change, such fluctuations clearly implicate the involvement of environmental determinants for IDDM.

The geographic disparity in incidence rates, the differential risk of similar racial groups in different locations, the assimilation of immigrants to the host country's risk of IDDM, and the temporal patterns of the disease all point to an environmental etiology for IDDM. Perhaps the strongest evidence for such an etiology is provided through identical twin studies, which display less than 50% concordance.[72,108,122,154] A concordance rate of 100% in identical twins would be expected if the disease were determined entirely by genetic factors. Environmental and genetic factors interact to yield insulin-dependency through decompensation of the beta cells of the endocrine pancreas. Their primacy in etiology is the focus of much debate. The environmental theory states that some environmental agent is ultimately responsible for beta-cell destruction. The genetic theory states that IDDM is essentially determined by a genetic propensity for the disease. Both may involve the triggering of autoimmunity where the beta cells become recognized as foreign to the body and are consequently destroyed by the immune system. Although each addresses a primary focus, the theories are not mutually exclusive and extensive overlap exists between them.

GENETIC-ENVIRONMENTAL INTERACTIONS

Environmental Etiology

Introduction

Environmental factors may initiate beta-cell destruction, which may not result in overt diabetes for years or may quickly precipitate the diabetic condition through rapid beta-cell destruction. Various environmental agents have been proposed as etiologic factors; these include infectious agents, chemicals, stress, food additives, breastfeeding, and cow's milk proteins. Infectious agents and cow's milk proteins have received the most investigative scrutiny of all purported environmental factors.

Infectious agents

A considerable amount of evidence has implicated infectious agents in the etiology of IDDM. General epidemiologic characteristics of most infectious diseases, particularly viral illnesses, are similar to those of IDDM, including seasonality, socioeconomic gradient, and age of onset in mainly younger age-groups. The overall evidence for an infectious etiology in IDDM, however, has been both supportive and contradictory.

Seasonality. Seasonality studies have supported an infectious etiology for IDDM. Most studies that have investigated the seasonality of onset of IDDM have discovered that the disease parallels that of common viral infections with peaks of incidence occurring in late autumn and winter and few cases occurring in the summer months. Studies in the northern hemisphere* and in the southern hemisphere[36,41,141,164] have supported this pattern, indicating that seasonality, rather than calendar time, is the influential factor.

The above seasonal pattern has not been found in all studies.† No significant overall seasonal pattern was found for a population-based group of 901 persons whose age at onset of IDDM was 19 years or younger and who were diagnosed from 1965 to 1976 in Allegheny County, Pennsylvania.[40] A nonsignificant overall trend toward the expected seasonality pattern, however, was present. Significant seasonal patterns were found for the 5- to 9-year age-group and the 10- to 14-year age-group. The 10- to 14- year age-group, however, did not follow a typical pattern for viral infections in that the fewest cases of IDDM occurred in late autumn. No epidemic years were apparent; each year had approximately the same number of newly diagnosed cases. This does not suggest a true viral etiologic pattern of seasonality where high numbers of cases and low numbers of cases would be expected to occur in alternate time periods. The investigators proposed that if a viral etiology for IDDM did exist, it would likely involve multiple viruses or a single virus that had uniform transmission throughout the year.

Socioeconomic status. Information on the influence of socioeconomic status on the incidence of IDDM has been equally inconclusive regarding an infectious etiology for the disease. Certain infectious diseases, such as polio, are known to have specific epidemiologic patterns of occurrence by socioeconomic status.[104] This model purports that the ratio of cases to infections will be larger in high socioeconomic groups than in low socioeconomic groups because of the spread of the virus through low socioeconomic groups at younger ages. Subclinical cases and acquired immunity will occur in the low socioeconomic group, resulting in fewer cases diagnosed within this group at older ages. The low socioeconomic group will thus have a younger mean age at onset of disease than the high socioeconomic group. Such a pattern of age at onset and incidence of new cases would be expected to occur in IDDM if the disease were influenced by a viral etiology similar to polio. This pattern was not found in the Pittsburgh study.[86] Socioeconomic differences were not related to the incidence of IDDM when persons within various socioeconomic levels were age-adjusted and analyzed by race. Nor was age at onset found to vary significantly by socioeconomic status within race-gender groups. Other studies have not found any significant relationship between socioeconomic status and IDDM.[88,155,168] Although such evidence does not support the polio model, it does not negate the possibility of other viral etiologies for IDDM.

Other studies have yielded opposite findings for the relationship of IDDM to socioeconomic status. Low socioeconomic status was associated with greater incidence of IDDM in Copenhagen,[18] whereas high socioeconomic status was associated with greater incidence of the disease in Montreal.[22,173] These studies could have been influenced by underascertainment of cases; age at onset by socioeconomic class also was not measured. Inconsistencies in the definition of socioeconomic status also hinder comparability of studies. Socioeconomic status was defined as property assessment value in the Copenhagen study and as average household income within particular census tracts in the Montreal studies. Such

---

*References 18, 37, 41, 56, 57, 71, 77, 78, 98, 107, 155, 168, 173.
†References 11, 17, 24, 40, 91, 101, 142, 157.

factors prohibit these studies from being fully compared with the polio epidemiologic model to determine if a socioeconomic gradient is associated with IDDM.

Perhaps one explanation for the lack of any consistent relationship between socioeconomic status and IDDM is that by restricting the studies to urban populations, the studies are too homogeneous to show any real differences between various socioeconomic levels and the disease. If overcrowding with resultant greater spread of infection and other factors that are associated with high population density influence IDDM risk, such factors would perhaps mask the role of socioeconomic status. Differences in risk of IDDM by socioeconomic status could become apparent when comparisons are made between areas of differing population densities, such as urban-rural studies. The relationship between population density and IDDM has been examined in numerous investigations.

The incidence of IDDM for children from birth to 14 years of age in Sweden for 1977 to 1980 and for 1980 to 1983 did not differ significantly by counties of varying population densities.[26] There was also no difference in risk of IDDM for persons from birth to 29 years of age in Denmark when the Copenhagen metropolitan area (measured during 1970 to 1974) was compared with the 14 times less densely populated areas of West and South Jutland (measured during 1970 to 1976).[19] Other studies have documented no association between IDDM risk and population density.* An inverse correlation between IDDM and population density was actually noted in Scotland.[115] Other studies, however, have found a positive relationship between IDDM risk and population density.†

Mean annual incidence rates of IDDM in children from birth to 14 years of age in Finland for 1970 to 1979 followed a positive population gradient: 31.6/100,000 in eastern Finland and 24.4/100,000 in northern Finland.[125] A similar pattern was found in Norway from 1973 to 1977 for children from birth to 14 years of age, with the northern and southern areas of the country having mean annual incidence rates of IDDM of 6.8/100,000 and 20.0/100,000, respectively.[69]

Significant differences in risk of IDDM by population density have also been found in Poland. The city of Poznan, Poland, with a population of over 300,000, had significantly higher incidence rates of IDDM than towns and villages in the region with populations less than 100,000 during a low overall incidence period for midwestern Poland from 1970 to 1981.[127] Although IDDM incidence rates during the high incidence period from 1982 to 1984 were not significantly different between the two areas, Poznan had a higher overall rate (9.54/100,000 compared with 6.02/100,000). Similar findings were noted in an urban-rural study of IDDM incidence in Wisconsin from 1970 to 1979.[1] Although nonsignificant, age-specific incidence rates were always higher for urban males than rural males. There was no consistent pattern of IDDM incidence differences between urban and rural females. The most striking finding from this study, however, was the seasonal variation in incidence. Urban cases of IDDM had virtually constant rates throughout the year, whereas rural cases had high rates throughout the summer months and a very high incidence peak in late autumn. This pattern was especially pronounced among rural males ages 10 to 19 years; 52% of IDDM cases

---

*References 56, 57, 155, 160, 164.
†References 1, 24, 69, 125, 127, 145.

within this group were diagnosed during the fourth quarter. The seasonal variation among rural IDDM cases suggests an infectious component. The authors concluded that several initiating and precipitating infectious factors operating concurrently could explain the lack of an apparent seasonal pattern among urban IDDM cases.

The socioeconomic component of IDDM needs much additional investigation. The very lack of a consistent relationship between socioeconomic status and IDDM, however, could indicate the differential population distribution and influence of other environmental factors in similar socioeconomic levels.

Age at onset. The age-at-onset patterns of IDDM also support an infectious etiology for the disease. IDDM occurs infrequently in the first 9 months of life. Most infectious diseases also follow this pattern because of protection afforded by maternal antibodies.[46a] An initial rise in IDDM incidence occurs at age five, which coincides with the spread of infectious diseases at the commencement of school attendance. Viral illnesses such as mumps and Coxsackie B also have peak periods of incidence at 5 years of age.[46a,156] This distribution pattern has been found in Allegheny County, Pennsylvania,[85] in Denmark,[18] in Chile,[36] and in the United Kingdom.[47] Data regarding age at onset of IDDM in ages beyond 30 have been scarce and suspect because true IDDM is often difficult to distinguish from NIDDM, which utilizes insulin as part of the treatment regimen.

The incidence of IDDM continues to rise in both males and females until a peak is reached in both genders around the age of puberty. Although hormonal factors are impaired by this pattern, they cannot explain the rising occurrence of IDDM in ages below puberty. A major weakness of an infectious etiology for IDDM is the difficulty in ascertaining an infectious agent that has peak activity at the age of puberty. Varying incubation periods, slow virus infections, reinfection, and cumulative beta-cell damage from several infections could perhaps reconcile this fallacy. Nevertheless, why all such possibilities should culminate within the narrow age range of puberty in virtually all populations studied remains unknown.

Viruses

Introduction. Most of the seasonality and socioeconomic studies just discussed have investigated the plausibility of viruses as precipitating agents for IDDM through rapid direct destruction of the beta cells. Several isolated cases of IDDM have been causally linked to viruses in this manner. Coxsackie,[15,16,179a] mumps,[61] and infectious mononucleosis[12] have all been documented in newly diagnosed IDDM cases.

The role of viruses, however, may also be that of merely damaging the beta cells, which initiates a slow diabetogenic process, which becomes overt disease only after the action of additional environmental stressors. Although metabolic stress has been purported to be the final step in eliciting clinical IDDM in persons who have had islet cell damage caused by viral infection, few studies have been done to identify what environmental stressors could be operating during the peak seasonality periods for IDDM.[46a] The role of viruses in the etiology of IDDM also may not involve destruction of the beta cells at all; the viral agents themselves may be the metabolic stressors that bring on IDDM in a person who has had previous beta-cell damage.

Other evidence has shown that viruses may also act directly on the DNA of the host to facilitate increased susceptibility to IDDM.[113] A portion of the viral DNA genome becomes inserted into the host DNA sequence; such insertion may be followed by autoimmune destruction of the beta cells. It is unknown if this process would be quickly precipitated after viral infection or would be characterized by a long diabetogenic period.

Viruses that have been commonly implicated in IDDM include Coxsackie, encephalomyocarditis (EMC), mumps, congenital rubella, and Cytomegalovirus (CMV).

Coxsackie. Coxsackie has been perhaps the virus most frequently linked with IDDM. Coxsackie B4 and B5 viruses, when extracted from the pancreas of newly diagnosed IDDM cases, were found to initiate IDDM when injected into mice.[15,179a] Other newly diagnosed cases of IDDM have indicated recent Coxsackie B4 infection.[76,111] Insulitis and beta-cell damage in four of seven neonates who died of Coxsackie B1 or B4 viral infections further depict the destructive tropism of the viruses for the insulin-producing cells.[67] Coxsackie viruses, however, have lacked consistent support as etiologic agents for IDDM.

Some of the strongest evidence linking Coxsackie viruses with IDDM concerns an epidemic of Coxsackie viruses in Sweden in 1983. Twenty-four consecutive newly diagnosed IDDM patients exhibited recent Coxsackie B1-B5 antibodies.[44] Most serologic studies for Coxsackie B viruses, however, have provided unconvincing and even contradictory results. Schmidt and others[137] studied 83 newly diagnosed IDDM cases and found no evidence of Coxsackie B viral infection. Gamble and others[48] found that Coxsackie B4 antibodies occurred more frequently in persons with IDDM who were 10 to 19 years old and more than 20 years old than in age-matched controls; this relationship was actually reversed in the birth to 9-year-old group. Similar results were found in a study of newly diagnosed IDDM cases in Copenhagen.[26a] Persons with onset of IDDM at ages 15 to 29 years had a greater prevalence of Coxsackie B4 antibodies than did age-matched nondiabetic controls; this relationship was again reversed in persons with onset at birth to 14 years of age. In contrast, findings from Finland have implicated intrauterine exposure to Coxsackie B5 and enteroviruses in general with the development of IDDM before 3 years of age.[65]

The incidence of IDDM in Jefferson County, Alabama, increased 57% from 11.7/100,000 in 1979 to 1983 to 18.4/100,000 in 1983 to 1984 after an epidemic of Coxsackie B5 in 1983.[169] This study was an ecologic analysis, however, and it is unknown if newly diagnosed IDDM cases had a greater prevalence of recent Coxsackie B5 infection than nondiabetic controls. The diabetogenic influence of Coxsackie viruses may further depend on genetic factors. Recent Coxsackie B1-B5 infection was found to be significantly associated only in IDDM individuals positive for the HLA DR3 antigen in a controlled study in Wisconsin.[27]

One explanation for the inconsistent nature of the above findings could be indiscriminate Coxsackie B4 antibody testing. Only if IgM antibodies, typifying recent infection, were found in recently diagnosed IDDM cases could Coxsackie B4 be evoked as a likely precipitating etiologic agent. The presence of IgG long-lasting antibodies could indicate that infection occurred many years before onset of IDDM, which would support the possibility that the virus could be part of a slow prediabetogenic process or that it is unrelated to IDDM. Many studies of viral agents do not discriminate between such antibody fractions.[182] The lack of such differentiation renders it impossible to determine if IDDM is associated with early or recent viral infection. It is possible that a heterogeneous viral etiology for IDDM exists, with some viruses acting as precipitating agents and other viruses as slow-acting initiating agents.

Table 2-6   Diabetogenic Activity of Variants of Coxsackie B4

Variant	Glucose index (mean ± SD)	Percent mice developing IDDM*
Coxsackie B4-NP	165 ± 27	0
Coxsackie B4-FP	156 ± 19	0
Coxsackie B4-MK	149 ± 21	0
Coxsackie B4-BP	245 ± 103	60

Modified from Yoon JW, Bachurski CJ, McArthur RG: *Diabetes Res Clin Prac* 2(letter):365-366, 1986.
*The mean glucose index of 110 uninfected SJL/J mice was 145 ± 19 mg/dl. Any mouse with a glucose index above 240 mg/dl (5 SD above the mean) was scored as diabetic.
SD, Standard deviation.

Indiscriminate measurement of the variants of Coxsackie B4 virus may also explain the lack of a consistent relationship between the virus and IDDM. Coxsackie B4 can be implicated as a causal agent in IDDM only if the particular diabetogenic variant of the virus is identified through monoclonal antibody testing. There are 13 variants of Coxsackie B4 virus, only one of which appears to be diabetogenic.[180]

Studies that do not use recently diagnosed IDDM cases further contain the possibility that infection occurred after the diagnosis of diabetes, thus having nothing to do with the onset of the disease. Numerous other serologic studies have suffered from not being undertaken until years after diagnosis of IDDM, when evidence of a possible infectious etiology may no longer be detectable through antibody titers.

The diabetogenicity of particular variants of Coxsackie B4 virus has been examined in animal studies. The pathogenicity of the virus is that of direct beta-cell destruction. Only the Coxsackie B4-BP variant was found to be diabetogenic when injected into SJL/J male mice.[180] Onset occurred in a matter of days after injection. The diabetogenicity of particular variants of Coxsackie B4 is given in Table 2-6.

Although apparently being capable of quickly precipitating IDDM through direct beta-cell destruction and being the most frequently linked viral agent with the disease, Coxsackie viruses are unlikely to account for a sizeable portion of all IDDM cases. Many of the associations just mentioned likely involve indiscriminate Coxsackie antibody testing. If animal findings are extrapolated to humans, only one variant of the virus is capable of eliciting IDDM; the diabetogenicity of Coxsackie B4-BP in humans, however, lacks direct evidence. To be implicated as an etiologic factor in IDDM, monoclonal antibody testing must identify the presence of the Coxsackie B4-BP variant in persons with the disease. Prospective studies involving such testing on recently diagnosed IDDM cases are needed to ascertain the importance of this viral agent in the etiology of IDDM.

Encephalomyocarditis. The encephalomyocarditis virus is a murine picornavirus, which is similar to the Coxsackie viruses found in man. Inasmuch as the activity of the virus is confined to such animals as household mice and rats, this viral agent has been used in animal models as an analog to Coxsackie-mediated IDDM in man. The pathogenicity of the virus is also that of direct beta-cell destruction.

Table 2-7 Diabetogenic Activity of Variants of Encephalomyocarditis Virus

Variant	Glucose index (mean + SD)	Percent mice developing IDDM*
EMC-M	252 ± 136	47
EMC-B	164 ± 12	0
EMC-D	430 ± 51	100

Modified from Yoon JW, Bachurski CJ, McArthur RG: *Diabetes Res Clin Prac* 2(letter):365-366, 1986.
*The mean glucose index of 110 uninfected SJL/J mice was 145 ± 19 mg/dl. Any mouse with a glucose index above 240 mg/dl (5 SD above the mean) was scored as diabetic.
SD, Standard deviation.

The diabetogenicity of variants of encephalomyocarditis (EMC) virus has been illustrated in animal studies. The EMC-M variant was found to produce IDDM in approximately 47% of injected SJL/J male mice.[183] The EMC-M variant was later found to be composed of two distinct variants, EMC-B and EMC-D.[179] The EMC-B variant produced no diabetes when injected into mice, whereas the EMC-D variant produced IDDM in virtually 100% of the infected mice. The onset of IDDM again occurred in a matter of days after injection. When a live-attenuated vaccine of EMC-B was given, followed by injection of EMC-D, none of the immunized mice developed diabetes.[184] Interferon was further found to prevent development of IDDM in mice injected with EMC-D.[181] Apparently a specific diabetogenic variant of EMC is needed to elicit IDDM; if prior infection with a nondiabetogenic variant of the same virus has taken place, the diabetogenic variant is unlikely to have any effect. The diabetogenicity of variants of EMC is given in Table 2-7.

Certain strains of mice that had been susceptible to induced IDDM from Coxsackie B4-BP were also found to be susceptible to induced IDDM from EMC-D; other strains of mice were found to be resistant to induced IDDM from both viruses. A genetic predisposition in addition to initial infection with the particular diabetogenic variant is thus required for viral-induced IDDM to occur.

EMC-D has naturally lacked direct evidence in humans with diabetes. Its usefulness is to probe possible analogous mechanisms for IDDM via Coxsackie viruses.

Mumps. Mumps has been implicated with IDDM but not as strongly as Coxsackie and EMC viruses. Unlike the latter two viral agents, there is no known diabetogenic variant of mumps. New cases of IDDM, however, have occurred rapidly after mumps infection.[61] The United Kingdom study of 1663 cases of childhood diabetes found that the cases had more than five times the number of episodes of mumps in the month before onset than did the general population.[46] Although the latter study strongly implicates the virus as an etiologic agent for IDDM, mumps was estimated to account for only 2% to 3% of all cases.

Much research concerning mumps has focused on the plausibility of the virus as a triggering agent for an autoimmune response. If such a relationship were true, serologic evidence of islet cell antibodies (ICA) and islet cell surface antibodies (ICSA) would be expected to be present in persons with recent mumps infection, as well as in persons with recently diagnosed IDDM. Such evidence has been found in few studies.

Palmer and others[114] found no relationship between ICA and mumps antibody titers in either nondiabetic patients or newly diagnosed IDDM cases. Helmke[61] did detect ICA in a child who developed IDDM 3 weeks after mumps infection. As part of this same study, ICA was found in 14 of 30 nondiabetic children who had recently been infected with mumps. The mumps antibody titers and ICA titers were not correlated, however, and the ICA disappeared in 12 of the 14 patients within 14 months. No abnormal glucose tolerance was apparent at the time of ICA detection.

Islet cell surface antibodies have been found to be common in children after mumps infection. Islet cell surface antibodies are relatively long-lasting; more than 50% of ICSA-positive individuals remain positive for as long as 26 months after mumps infection.[124]

Detectable ICSA titers were found in 42 of 68 nondiabetic children (62%) with recent mumps infection.[60] The prevalence of ICSA in healthy children free of mumps infection has been found to be only approximately 5%.[140] Such findings lend support for a mumps-mediated effect on the immune system that is targeted for the islet cells. It is unknown, however, whether such an effect is widely manifested in IDDM. When Helmke and others[60] followed 127 nondiabetic children who tested ICSA-positive after mumps infection prospectively for a 3- to 5-year period, only one child developed diabetes.

Mumps may be correlated in some fashion with IDDM but apparently accounts for only a small number of cases. If truly implicated as an etiologic factor in the disease, its effect is likely to be that of an initiator of a slow diabetogenic process or as an environmental stressor that elicits IDDM in persons with prior beta-cell damage.

Congenital rubella. Perhaps the strongest viral etiology that has been implicated with increased risk of IDDM is *in utero* exposure to rubella. The maternal acquisition of rubella infection during pregnancy allows for transplacental transfer of the virus from mother to fetus. The association of congenital rubella exposure with later development of IDDM has been established through numerous studies.

Rubella virus has been isolated from the beta cells of IDDM patients.[29,99] An infant with congenital rubella syndrome who died 5 days after the onset of acute diabetes displayed insulitis and complete beta-cell destruction.[116] Menser and others[97] examined 87 patients with congenital rubella syndrome and found 8 to be diabetic (4 being IDDM), while another 10 were found to have abnormal glucose tolerance. The four NIDDM individuals all had onset of their disease in their late twenties, while the four persons with IDDM had onset occurring at 1.5, 12, 12, and 24 years of age. These findings support not only the influence of *in utero* exposure with the future development of diabetes, but also the fact that a long diabetogenic process may precede clinical onset of the disease. Because the great majority of persons with congenital rubella syndrome did not develop diabetes, these findings further suggest a "two-hit" theory in that apparently some additional environmental factor is necessary to elicit IDDM.

Evidence exists that congenital rubella syndrome may exert its effect through a genetic susceptibility for an autoimmune defect. Islet cell surface antibodies were found in 20% of nondiabetic persons with congenital rubella but in less than 4% of the control group.[52] When persons with IDDM and congenital rubella syndrome were examined, 37% were ICSA-positive. A slow, progressive, autoimmune destructive process for IDDM is supported by this study inasmuch as the mean duration of diabetes in ICSA-positive persons was 12 years. Such an etiology cannot be conclusively supported, however, because no information on ICSA status at time of IDDM onset is known for these persons.

Certain HLA antigens also appear to be strongly associated with IDDM development in persons exposed to congenital rubella. Persons having the congenital rubella syndrome who had IDDM had a significantly lower frequency of DR2 and a significantly higher frequency of DR3 than either the control group or congenital rubella patients who were nondiabetic.[134] Such findings suggest that a genetic susceptibility for an autoimmune defect must be inherited for congenital rubella to act as a diabetogenic agent.

While congenital rubella may be associated with IDDM through initiation of a slow autoimmune process, other genetic factors for such a predisposition besides the HLA findings just mentioned remain undiscovered. Congenital rubella, as with most purported viral etiologies, also is not likely to account for a sizeable number of IDDM cases.

Cytomegalovirus. The plausibility of Cytomegalovirus (CMV) as an etiologic agent in IDDM is supported by the fact that beta-cell destruction was found in 20 of 45 children with fatal infections of the virus.[67] Cytomegalovirus infection has also been documented in persons who developed IDDM. Evidence exists that this virus inserts part of its genome directly into the host DNA sequence.[113] Autoimmunity is the suspected mechanism by which such insertion results in decompensation of the beta cells to yield IDDM.

The frequency of CMV infections in newly diagnosed IDDM individuals has been found to be three times higher than in controls.[113] When DNA was extracted from the lymphocytes of both groups, approximately 55% of the IDDM patients who were positive for CMV infection possessed DNA nucleotide sequence homology to the CMV genome. None of the controls possessed homology to the CMV genome. It was further found that approximately 80% of patients with IDDM who were positive for both CMV antibodies and the CMV genome possessed ICSA. Diabetic patients not possessing the CMV genome did not display ICSA. Apparently viral insertion into the host DNA sequence may be associated with initiation of autoimmunity directed against the beta cells. Such an etiology is again likely to be mediated only in a genetically susceptible individual.

Other viruses. Other viral agents including influenza, Epstein-Barr, and hepatitis B have been implicated in case studies of IDDM.[34] Influenza virus infection has been documented in newly diagnosed IDDM cases.[111] No relationship was found, however, between ICA titers and influenza A and B antibody titers in either newly diagnosed IDDM cases or in nondiabetic persons with documented influenza infection.[114] Reovirus type I has also been found to produce IDDM in animal models.[110] In contrast to EMC-D and Coxsackie B4-BP, which directly attack the beta cells, the action of Reovirus type I appears to be that of autoimmunity, resembling congenital rubella in this regard. Mice infected with Reovirus type I exhibited autoantibodies directed against the islets of Langerhans, anterior pituitary, and gastric mucosa. The viral-induced IDDM was found to be prevented through administration of immunosuppressant drugs.[109] No other variants of Reovirus were found to produce IDDM. The above reported doubling of the incidence of IDDM in midwestern Poland from 1982 to 1984 further coincided with enteroviral meningitis epidemics in that country.[127] The meningitis epidemics regularly preceded periods of increased IDDM incidence by 4 to 6 months.

Table 2-8   Purported Pathogeneses for Viral-Induced IDDM

Virus	Pathogenic mechanism	Autoantibodies
EMC-D	Cytolytic destruction	Absent
Coxsackie B4-BP	Cytolytic destruction	Absent
Reovirus Type I	Autoimmune polyendocrine disease	Present

Modified from Yoon JW: *Pediat Adolesc Endocr* 15:64-73, 1986.

Conclusions about viruses. A major problem with the viral studies just mentioned is that many are individual cases that prohibit conclusions from being generalized to the majority of persons with IDDM. Many other studies have simply shown association rather than causality. The exact pathogenesis of the viral-mediated IDDM process also remains unclear.

A key finding with most purported viral etiologies for IDDM is that a diabetogenic variant of a virus may elicit IDDM in a genetically susceptible individual through a mechanism characteristic of that particular virus. The purported mechanisms of viral-induced IDDM based on the animal studies of Yoon and his colleagues at the University of Calgary, Alberta, Canada, are given in Table 2-8. The implied pathogeneses of mumps and congenital rubella, although largely undeveloped through animal studies, have been documented above as likely involving autoimmunity.

Yoon's studies, as well as several of the aforementioned investigations, have pertained to animal studies. If extrapolation of these findings is made to humans, two possible mechanisms for viral-induced IDDM are (1) direct destruction of the beta cells apart from autoimmunity and (2) viral initiation of an autoimmune response resulting in beta-cell decompensation. Genetic factors, evidenced by susceptibility of different strains of mice to the particular diabetogenic variants, undoubtedly influence both mechanisms in animals and likely would affect susceptibility to IDDM in human populations.

A third possible mechanism for viral-induced IDDM is that of insertion of part of the viral genome into the DNA of a genetically susceptible host. This mechanism, as evidenced in human studies with Cytomegalovirus, also likely involves autoimmunity. Much research is needed in all three purported areas of viral-induced IDDM.

Chemicals

Studies of chemical agents have, for ethical reasons, dealt largely with animals. Alloxan[46a] and streptozotocin[46a] have been found to destroy the beta cells of animals, resulting in insulin dependency. Prednisone and other glucocorticoids have also been found to produce insulin resistance in dogs,[13] healthy nondiabetic human volunteers,[112] and nondiabetic human renal transplant recipients.[4] The resulting diabetes, however, was not true IDDM; the diabetes was either transient or resembled non-insulin-dependent diabetes, which included insulin as part of the treatment regimen. A rodenticide, N-3 pyridylmethyl, N-p-nitrophenyl (PNU), has been shown to induce IDDM in humans after accidental ingestion.[121] Chronic arsenic exposure in artesian well drinking water was found to be significantly associated with diabetes in southern Taiwan.[83] Although chemicals can cause IDDM, they do not explain a sizeable number of cases in any given population. It is unlikely that chemicals would affect only certain persons within family units while leaving other members untouched. Nor would chemicals be expected to exert a diabetogenic influence only within young populations.

Stress

Stress has been implicated as an etiologic agent in IDDM. Stein and Charles[151] found that a significantly greater proportion of adolescents with diabetes had suffered parental loss before onset than had nondiabetic chronically ill adolescents. Parental loss was defined as deaths, separations, or divorces. Thirty-four percent of the diabetic adolescents had suffered parental loss before clinical onset of their disease compared with only 11% of the control subjects. Similarly, Robinson and Fuller[130] in the Barts-Windsor-Middlesex Prospective Family Study found that a significantly greater proportion of IDDM subjects had undergone severe life events in the 3 years before onset than had nondiabetic siblings of similar age or age- and sex-matched neighborhood control subjects. Severe life events included highway accidents and breaking off significant relationships with the opposite sex. Seventy-seven percent of the IDDM subjects had undergone one or more severe life events in the 3 years before onset compared with 39% of the siblings and 15% of the neighborhood controls. Such findings indicate that stress may serve as an inciting factor for IDDM in a genetically susceptible individual.

Food additives

Maternal consumption of smoked meats containing N-nitroso compounds during pregnancy has been correlated with increased risk of IDDM in the progeny of Icelandic mothers, raising further speculation on the influence of environmental agents operating in utero.[59] Weekly nitrosamine consumption in food before onset was also significantly associated with risk of IDDM in a controlled study in Sweden.[26a] An ecologic analysis found a significant correlation between nitrate levels in drinking water and IDDM incidence rates in Colorado.[81] No direct measurement of nitrate exposure with IDDM cases and nondiabetic controls was naturally obtained in this study. Nutritional factors are unlikely to account for a sizeable proportion of all IDDM cases and would not explain the age at onset or seasonality patterns seen in the disease.

Breastfeeding

Borch-Johnsen and associates[10] found that a smaller proportion of IDDM children had been breast-fed and for a shorter period than their nondiabetic siblings. Similar findings were obtained for IDDM subjects and unrelated control groups in Colorado.[94] Breast milk may provide some protective effect, perhaps immunologic, against IDDM. The protection against IDDM, however, may not come directly from breast milk but indirectly through delay of introduction of other milk products, particularly cow's milk.

Bovine milk protein consumption

Recent studies in Finland[165-167] and in the United States[79,80] have documented an increased risk of IDDM with the introduction of breast milk substitutes before 3 months of age. The association held when only cow's milk was considered.[25,80] The focus of these studies has been the potential initiation of an autoimmune response directed against the beta cells. The infant gut is in an immature state for approximately 3 months after birth. Bovine serum albumin (BSA) chains may pass directly into the bloodstream where sensitization to the infant immune system may occur. An immunologic reaction against a similar protein homology on the surface of the beta cells may then take place through molecular mimicry.[73] Elevated BSA antibodies in children with recently diagnosed IDDM compared with nondiabetic controls support this theory.[73,136] It was not known, however, if the antibodies were present before IDDM onset. The antibodies may thus indicate (1) a generalized antibody response, (2) a response to excess milk intake before onset, or (3) a long, prediabetic period of autoimmunity culminating in IDDM. A genetic susceptibility for such an autoimmune response appears to be necessary. Children possessing the HLA-DQB1 antigen who were exposed to cow's milk before the age of 3 months had 11 times the risk of developing IDDM compared with children not possessing the antigen who were not exposed to cow's milk at that early age.[79]

Cow's milk proteins, as well as purported viral etiologies for IDDM, apparently depend on a critical time frame of exposure. Although consistent and intriguing, the findings just mentioned should be interpreted with caution. All infant dietary histories were assessed retrospectively as many as 20 years after the fact. Prospective infant dietary collection is needed to accurately relate exposure to IDDM risk.

Conclusions

The geographical differences, temporal trends, and assimilated risk of IDDM of migrants to the host country all support the role of environmental factors in the etiology of the disease. If such factors could be identified and controlled, a sizeable amount of IDDM would likely be prevented. The proportion of IDDM cases on a worldwide basis that are attributed to environmental factors and thus are potentially preventable has been estimated to be at least 60%; the actual proportion could be as high as 95%.[84]

Although the discordance seen in identical twin studies undoubtedly implicates environmental factors in IDDM, many questions remain to be answered. Infectious agents have epidemiologic plausibility of being implicated in the disease. Certain viral agents are known to precipitate insulin dependency through rapid beta-cell destruction in animals. Many studies, however, have involved only individual cases. The degree to which viral, chemical, and other environmental factors account for IDDM on a population basis is virtually unknown. Other studies have not conclusively supported seasonal or socioeconomic patterns of IDDM with those of known infectious diseases such as polio. The lack of consistent seasonality and socioeconomic patterns, however, provides support for the influence of other environmental factors besides infectious agents, as well as infectious agents dissimilar to polio. Several environmental factors may be involved in the etiology of IDDM, either as precipitating or initiating factors.

Variants of a particular virus would be difficult to be implicated as etiologic agents in IDDM because of the possible negating effect of nondiabetogenic variants of the same virus. A child first exposed to a nondiabetogenic variant of a particular virus may be protected from the influence of later exposure to the diabetogenic variant of the same virus. Evidence for such a possible protection is based only on animal studies. If such protection were analogous in man, specific viral associations with IDDM in human beings could be difficult to determine. The influence of a diabetogenic variant may further be prolific in some populations and inconsequential in others because of varying genetic factors.

Many possibilities exist for the study of environmental etiologies in IDDM. Retrospective studies on recently diagnosed IDDM cases and age- and sex-matched neighborhood control subjects could continue to investigate whether stressful events undergone in the years before onset could be associated with IDDM. Stress could be viewed as either multiple "hits" or the final event that precipitates clinical diabetes. Research should continue in the development of animal models to determine which variants of a particular virus are diabetogenic. Once these variants have been identified, future studies on recently diagnosed human cases of IDDM can measure the prevalence of antibody titers to such variants versus their prevalence in nondiabetic controls. Prospective studies may also be employed after outbreaks of an infectious disease, where the risk of development of IDDM is measured in persons affected with the diabetogenic and nondiabetogenic variants. Animal studies should also continue to investigate whether protection against IDDM is afforded by prior infection with particular nondiabetogenic variants of a virus. If such a phenomenon was true with many viruses and if the sequence of infection in recently diagnosed IDDM cases was not known, associations of particular viral variants with diabetes would be difficult to be ascertained.

Two major problems exist in any study involving environmental etiologies of IDDM. One is the ascertainment of an environmental factor that could have propagated a long prediabetogenic period of decompensation of the beta cells through autoimmunity many years before clinical onset of diabetes. Evidence of such a factor, if it were viral, would probably not be detected through antibody titers if titers were measured at the onset of IDDM. The second major problem is that if case-control studies were performed, it would be extremely difficult to identify all environmental factors that could have provided cumulative insults to the beta cells over a person's entire lifetime. Such considerations would make prospective studies the studies of choice to investigate environmental etiologies of IDDM.

The ideal prospective study would involve persons who are at high risk to develop IDDM, such as siblings of cases. Siblings would be HLA typed and monitored periodically for evidence of viral infections, stressful events, chemical exposure, and other environmental factors. Monitoring of glucose tolerance and ICA would also take place. Such a study would afford accurate and proper sequencing of viral infections and would enable the influence of other environmental stressors on glucose tolerance to be ascertained. Siblings who develop IDDM would have environmental exposures contrasted with those of siblings who do not develop IDDM. The major drawback to such a study is that a very large study population would have to be followed for a sufficient number of cases of diabetes to develop. Based on the conversion rates of the Pittsburgh study, 2040 HLA identical siblings to the index cases would be required for 50 secondary cases of IDDM to develop over a 5-year period.[106] This restriction necessitates the use of family data from many research centers.

The evidence for an environmental etiology in IDDM is strong and intriguing; much work, however, remains to be done. The pathologic sequence of beta-cell destruction, the stage at which an infectious agent exerts its influence, under what conditions a viral agent could slowly initiate or rapidly precipitate insulin dependency, and host characteristics that are amenable to such an etiology are all unknown. The environmental component in IDDM appears to be supported; the specifics of the identity, nature, and extent of that involvement await future research.

Genetic Etiology

A genetic component for IDDM has long been well established, with strong associations being found between the disease and certain human leukocyte histocompatibility antigens (HLA) that are coded for by loci on chromosome 6.[20] The genes of primary interest in IDDM are class I genes (HLA, A, B, and C), that code for transplantation antigens that appear on the surface of all nucleated bodily cells, and class II genes (HLA DR and DQ) that code for antigens that appear on the surfaces of B lymphocytes, activated T cells, and several other specialized cells that are involved in the immune response. Associations of HLA with IDDM have been documented in population, family, and twin studies.

Initial associations of HLA B8 and B15 with increased risk of IDDM that were found in population studies[105,147] were later attributed to HLA DR3 and DR4 that were inherited via linkage disequilibrium with the B8 and B15 antigens.[117,152] Wolf and associates[176] in a study of 122 Caucasian IDDM probands and 110 unrelated persons without diabetes, found that 98% of the probands were positive for either HLA DR3 or DR4 and that over 50% of the probands were positive for both antigens. Compared with persons without the respective antigens, persons possessing DR3 were over five times more at risk for IDDM, whereas persons possessing DR4 were almost eight times more at risk for the disease. The combination of both DR3 and DR4 was found to increase the risk of IDDM over 14 times. These findings imply that HLA DR3 and DR4 could increase the risk of IDDM independently by different mechanisms that act synergistically with each other. Rotter and associates[133] have speculated that the HLA DR3 form of IDDM is an autoimmune disorder that destroys the beta cells, whereas the HLA DR4 form of the disease is a defect in insulin release. These mechanistic theories, however, have largely lacked supporting data. The synergistic risk of DR3/DR4 does suggest at least a two-gene system involvement for susceptibility for IDDM.

Plausibility for a genetic etiology for IDDM is also provided through familial occurrence of the disease. Age-specific incidence rates of IDDM among siblings of cases have been found to be 6 to 18 times those in the general population.[2] Studies involving haplotype sharing status among families containing multiple sibling cases of IDDM have indicated that approximately 58% of the cases were haploidentical, 37% shared one parental haplotype, and 5% did not share either parental haplotype.[2,152] Since proportions in the ratio $1:2:1$ would be expected to occur if the HLA haplotype followed a random segregation within families, the observed frequencies indicate a strong relationship between HLA antigens and the occurrence of IDDM.

Haplotype sharing status is also related to the risk of IDDM. Siblings of an IDDM case have a 10% to 20% risk of developing the disease if they share both haplotypes with their diabetic sibling. The risk of development of IDDM in siblings reduces to 5% if only one haplotype is shared with the IDDM sibling and to 1% if neither haplotype is shared.[23,123]

Similar risk of development of IDDM by haplotype sharing status was found by Wagener and others in the Pittsburgh study.[2] The cumulative incidence of IDDM by age 20 was found to be 6/1000 for HLA nonidentical siblings to the proband, 24/1000 for HLA haploidentical siblings, and 76/1000 for HLA identical siblings. These risks were approximately 2, 8, and 25 times the rate of IDDM by age 20 in the general population.

Support for an HLA-linked genetic mechanism is also provided through rates of concordance involving identical twins. Such rates have been found to be approximately 50%.* The concordance rate increases to 70% when twins possess the HLA DR3/DR4 phenotype.[68] Because the above family studies document a concordance rate of IDDM in HLA identical siblings of only 10% to 20%, some other genetic mechanism besides HLA appears to be responsible for susceptibility to IDDM.

The incidence of IDDM varies greatly worldwide, with children living in Finland being 70 times more likely to develop IDDM than children living in Mexico City.[55,126] Studies have supported that this disparity in risk may be attributed to genetic differences at the molecular level, namely, to the differential distribution of a single amino acid residue at position 57 of the HLA DQ beta chain (non-Asp-57 homozygosity).[5,33,100]

There can be little doubt of a genetic etiology for IDDM. The true nature of the association of HLA with the disease, however, remains unclear. The HLA associations could indicate increased susceptibility for IDDM, which is conveyed by the antigens themselves, by immune-response genes linked to the HLA region, or by other genes that are inherited in linkage disequilibrium with those genes coding for the HLA antigens.

Conclusions About Genetic-Environmental Interactions

Environmental agents, genetic susceptibility, dysfunctional immunity, and autoimmunity all appear to be related to the etiology of IDDM. There is no denying that environmental factors can quickly precipitate direct destruction of the beta cells. Environmental agents may also initiate a slow diabetogenic process that manifests itself as clinical diabetes only after many years, serve as an outside stressor to elicit IDDM in an already damaged or compromised beta-cell mass, or realize a genetic susceptibility for an autoimmune defect that results in overt diabetes. If environmental factors do act as slow initiating agents for IDDM, identifying them at the onset of disease may be difficult.

The occurrence of IDDM within families, the increased risk to siblings of IDDM cases, and the association of IDDM with HLA antigens—especially DR3 and DR4—however, all point to a genetic influence. Insulin-dependent diabetes, nevertheless, cannot be considered strictly a genetic disease, since HLA DR3 and DR4 are common in the general population and the great majority of persons positive for these antigens do not develop IDDM. A susceptibility for the disease, rather than the disease itself, must be inherited. Genetic susceptibility to IDDM may again mean a propensity of the beta cells to damage by an environmental agent, a defective ability of the beta cell to regenerate itself after attack, or susceptibility to an autoimmune defect.

---

*References 6, 72, 108, 122, 154.

Numerous plausible pathogeneses exist that could encompass various aspects of genetic-environmental interactions for IDDM. Environmental agents may quickly precipitate or slowly initiate direct beta-cell destruction in a genetically susceptible individual. A genetically inherited dysfunctional immune system may render the beta cells particularly vulnerable to such damage. The environmental factors could initiate autoimmunity directed against the beta cells or serve as stressors that elicit IDDM in an individual with prior beta-cell damage. Insertion of part of a viral homology into the genome of a genetically susceptible host could initiate an autoimmune reaction directed against the beta cells. Molecular mimicry of an antigen such as cow's milk, which is introduced early in life, may initiate a similar autoimmune response. The majority of IDDM cases are likely to have extensive overlap from the components of both environmental and genetic etiologies.

FAMILIAL RISK OF IDDM
Secondary Attack Rate Studies

Several studies have examined the risk of IDDM among siblings of probands* (Table 2-9). The variability in study period, participation rate, insulin requirement, and age at onset should dictate caution when comparing the findings. Despite the inconsistencies in measurement, the secondary attack rates were remarkably similar. The Allegheny County study was the only study that had a high response rate, had insulin and age at onset requirements for both probands and IDDM siblings, validated IDDM sibling cases through corroboration with family members and physicians, and was representative of a particular population base. Family history information was further collected over several decades, enabling the risk of IDDM to be calculated in siblings through older ages. The overall secondary attack rate estimates through 10, 20, and 30 years of age were 1.6%, 4.1%, and 6.3%, respectively.[50] Male and female siblings had equivalent risks of IDDM through 15 years of age (3.0%). Males had a significant increase in risk of 4.0% at 16 to 30 years of age compared with only 2.5% for females. This could indicate an increased exposure to environmental factors at those ages in males or could reflect a protective effect, perhaps hormonal, in females. No significant gender concordance was found between proband and IDDM siblings, thus providing no evidence that environmental etiologic agents in IDDM include those that are likely to be shared by siblings of the same gender.[50]

Nondiabetic siblings are frequently chosen to be partial pancreatic donors for their IDDM brothers and sisters. A triad criteria has been employed to select potential donors: the interval between diagnosis of IDDM in the recipient and hemipancreatectomy in the donor is at least 10 years, the age of the donor must be at least 10 years older than the age at which IDDM developed in the recipient, and the donor must be an adult (≥18 years of age).[75] Such criteria have been used to minimize the chance of selecting siblings at high risk to develop IDDM themselves. The appropriateness of these selection criteria was tested with 156 multiple case families of IDDM in Allegheny County[49] (Table 2-10). The data did not validate the selection

---

*References 28, 45, 50, 53, 173.

Table 2-9   Secondary Attack Rate of IDDM Studies

Study	Study period	Participation rate (%)	Number of IDDM probands (families)	Number of IDDM siblings	Insulin requirement		Age at onset		Secondary attack rate (%)
					Proband	IDDM sibling	Proband	IDDM sibling	
Allegheny Co., Penn.[50]	1950-1981	94	1774	169	yes	yes	<17	≤30	6.3
Montreal, Canada[173]	1971-1977	99	518	44	yes	yes	<17	<30	4.1
United Kingdom[45]	1973-1976	74	4868	184	no	no	<16	<16	5.6
Denmark[28]	1932-1946	97	187	—	no	no	<20	<20	5.1
Joslin Clinic[53]	1928-1939	36	259	—	yes	yes	<20	—	4.5

Table 2-10   Duration Between Intrasibship Case Diagnosis of IDDM in 156 Families

Duration (yr)*	Number	Percent	Duration (yr)*	Number	Percent
<1	4	2.4	13	6	3.6
1	17	10.1	14	3	1.8
2	8	4.7	15	4	2.4
3	13	7.7	16	4	2.4
4	19	11.2	17	6	3.6
5	10	5.9	18	2	1.2
6	9	5.3	19	1	0.6
7	7	4.1	20	1	0.6
8	14	8.3	21	—	—
9	10	5.9	22	3	1.8
10	12	7.1	23	1	0.6
11	7	4.1	24	1	0.6
12	6	3.6	25	1	0.6

From Gavard JA and others: *Lancet* 341:303-304, 1993.
*Rounded to whole years except for <1 category.

criteria in that over a quarter of the IDDM sibling cases were diagnosed more than 10 years after onset of the index case. It is unlikely, however, that the criteria would result in the selection of a sibling who would develop IDDM later in life in the absence of hemipancreatectomy. The secondary attack rate of 6.3% through 30 years of age for siblings of probands would be reduced to 0.7% if only siblings who fit the three criteria were included.[49,50]

Secondary attack rate studies can also furnish clues about environmental factors in IDDM. Male siblings younger than their probands who were born within 1 year, greater than 1 year but within 2 years, and greater than 2 years before their proband diagnosis date had secondary attack rates through 20 years of age of 13.4%, 11.0%, and 5.3%, respectively; the corresponding risks for females were 2.3%, 8.2%, and 5.5% (Gavard and others unpublished data). These findings indicate that siblings born close to their proband diagnosis date have the highest risk of IDDM, with sharing of environmental agents especially likely between proband and young male sibling cases.

Parent-Offspring Studies

An intriguing finding about familial aggregation of IDDM is the differential risk to offspring of diabetic parents. Children of a father with IDDM have a risk of the disease of 6.0% through 20 years of age, whereas children of a mother with IDDM have a risk of 2.0% through 20 years of age.[170,171] Explanations could be a loss of progeny likely to develop IDDM later in life in diabetic mothers, the greater likelihood of delivering an intact multiple gene diabetogenic system during gametogenesis from diabetic fathers, or immune tolerance protection to high-risk HLA antigens *in utero* in diabetic mothers.

PREVALENCE OF PSYCHIATRIC DISORDERS IN ADULT IDDM POPULATIONS

Major Depressive Disorder

Numerous studies investigating the comorbidity of mental illness and IDDM have occurred during the past decade.[51] Depression may have special clinical relevancy in diabetes through its purported association with poor glycemic control and decreased adherence to treatment modalities. Five controlled studies* (Tables 2-11, 2-12) and eight uncontrolled studies† (R.B. Montague, M.I. Harris, unpublished observations; Table 2-13) have been performed to investigate the prevalence of depression in adult IDDM populations. These studies addressed two issues: (1) whether diabetes was associated with an increased prevalence of depression; and (2) whether diabetes could be differentiated from other somatic illnesses in the risk of depression.

The range of the prevalence of current depression obtained from structured diagnostic interviews in IDDM or mixed diabetic samples was 8.5% to 10.7% ($\bar{X} = 9.6\%$) in controlled studies (see Table 2-12) and 11.0% to 16.5% ($\bar{X} = 13.8\%$) in uncontrolled studies (see Table 2-13). These rates are approximately three times the 3% to 4% prevalence of major depressive disorder found in the general adult population of the United States. Studies using depression symptom scales corroborated these findings, as the range of clinically significant depression symptomatology in diabetic samples was 21.8% to 60.0% ($\bar{X} = 40.9\%$) in controlled studies (Table 2-12) and 10.0% to 28.0% ($\bar{X} = 19.8\%$) in uncontrolled studies (see Table 2-13). An increased prevalence of depression in IDDM relative to the general adult population is highly suggested by these studies.[51]

Whether depression is more common in IDDM than in other chronic diseases is far less supported by the literature. The controlled community interview study by Wells and associates[172] found a significantly increased prevalence of lifetime depression for diabetes (14.4%), as well as for arthritis (14.3%), heart disease (18.6%), hypertension (16.4%), and chronic lung disease (17.9%), relative to healthy control subjects (6.9%). This study, however, suffered from numerous biases and methodologic problems (Table 2-14). An increased prevalence of depression in diabetes relative to other somatic illnesses remains unproven until further research is performed.[51]

Spurious depression prevalence estimates could have resulted if diabetic and control samples differed significantly on variables known to be associated with an increased risk of depression.[51] Such factors include 30 to 44 years of age, female, low socioeconomic status, obesity, assortative mating, concomitant medical illness in the diabetic or control sample, and disease severity (see Table 2-14). Methodologic issues, such as a lack of physician verification of self-reported IDDM, variability in the time frame of depression being assessed, small sample sizes, and low participation rates could have also hindered the validity of findings.[51] Although all five controlled studies accounted for some factors

---

*References 43, 103, 119, 131, 172.
†References 89, 90, 93, 95, 102, 148, 175.

Text continued on p. 66.

Table 2-11   Controlled Studies of Depression in Adult IDDM Populations: Methods Employed

| Study | Diabetic sample | | | Control sample | | Method |
	Type	Size	Source	Size	Source	
Structured diagnostic interviews						
Wells and others, 1989[172]	IDDM and NIDDM	154	Los Angeles community, U.S.A.	1353	Medically well	DIS/DSM-II*
Popkin and others, 1988[119]	IDDM	75	Pancreatic transplantation candidates	34	First-degree relatives	DIS/DSM-III*
				9543	General population	
Robinson and others, 1988[131]	IDDM and NIDDM	130	Outpatients	130	Medically well	PSE† ID ≥ 5
Depression symptom scales						
Friis and Nanjundappa, 1986[43]	IDDM and NIDDM	56	Outpatients	56	Medically ill	CES-D Scale‡ ≥16
Murrell and others, 1983[103]	IDDM and NIDDM	179	Community sample, Kentucky, U.S.A.	2338	Community sample	CES-D Scale‡ ≥20

*Diagnostic Interview Schedule for diagnosis of major depressive disorder by lay interviewers, based on criteria specified in the Diagnostic and Statistical Manual of Mental Disorders of the American Psychiatric Association (DSM-III).

†Present State Examination, which assesses the present mental state. An Index of Definition Score ≥5 designates a psychiatric case; a diagnosis of depression is subsequently based on equivalent ICD-9 criteria.

‡Center for Epidemiologic Studies-Depression Scale.

Table 2-12   Controlled Studies of Depression in Adult IDDM Populations: Prevalence Findings*

Study	Overall		Males		Females		Mean depression scale scores
	Current	Lifetime	Current	Lifetime	Current	Lifetime	
Structured diagnostic interviews: prevalence of major depressive disorders							
Wells and others, 1989[172]							
Diabetes†	9.6%	14.4%	—	—	—	—	—
Controls†	4.4%NS	6.9%‡	—	—	—	—	—
Popkin and others, 1988[119]							
Diabetes	10.7%	24.0%	3.7%	25.9%	14.6%	22.9%	—
Relatives	2.9%NS	5.9%‡	0.0%NS	6.7%NS	5.3%NS	5.3%NS	—
Gen. Pop.	3.1%§	5.5%§	1.7%NS	3.1%§	4.0%§	7.1%§	—
Robinson and others, 1988[131]							
Diabetes	8.5%	17.7%	—	—	—	—	—
Controls	8.5%NS	NotMeas.	—	—	—	—	—
Depression symptom scales: prevalence of clinically significant depression symptomatology							
Friis and Nanjundappa, 1986[43]							
Diabetes	60.0%	—	—	—	—	—	20.4
Controls	50.0%NS	—	—	—	—	—	14.2‡
Murrell and others, 1983[103]							
Diabetes	21.8%	—	15.5%	—	25.4%	—	—
Controls	16.0%‡	—	13.4%NS	—	17.6%‡	—	—

*Prevalence findings reflect those of major depressive disorder for structured diagnostic interviews and clinically significant depression symptomatology for depression symptom scales.

†Prevalences reflect those of any affective disorder, which include major depression, dysthymia, and mania. Mania represented only 2.9% of all affective disorders in this study sample.

‡p < 0.05

§p < 0.001

NS, Not significant. Each control group was compared with its respective overall or sex-specific diabetic group in assessing significant differences in the prevalence of depression.

Table 2-13 Uncontrolled Studies of Depression in Adult IDDM Populations

Study	Diabetes type	Sample size	Sample source	Method	Prevalence of depression*	
					Current	Lifetime
Structured diagnostic interviews: prevalence of major depressive disorder						
Mayou and others, 1991[95]	IDDM	109	Clinic outpatients	PSE† ID ≥ 5	11.0%	—
Wilkinson and others, 1988[175]	IDDM	194	Clinic outpatients	GHQ‡ ≥12	16.5%	—
Lustman and others, 1986[93]	IDDM and NIDDM	114	Clinic outpatients	CIS§ DIS/DSM-III‖	14.0%	32.5%
Depression symptom scales: prevalence of clinically significant depression symptomatology						
Lloyd and others, 1992[90]	IDDM	175	Hospital-based registry, duration of diabetes ≥ 25 yr	BDI¶ ≥16	12.7%	—
Littlefield and others, 1990[89]	IDDM	158	Diabetes education and renal dialysis patients	BDI¶ ≥16	10.0%	—
Murawski and others, 1970[102]	IDDM and NIDDM	112	Clinic outpatients, duration of diabetes ≥25 yr	MMPI-D Scale** ≥70	21.0%	—
Slawson and others, 1963[148]	IDDM and NIDDM	25	Inpatients and outpatients	MMPI-D Scale** ≥70	28.0%	—
Montague and others, 1992 (unpublished observations)	IDDM	92	Clinic outpatients	CES-D Scale†† ≥16	27.2%	—

*Prevalence findings reflect those of major depressive disorder for structured diagnostic interviews and clinically significant depression symptomatology for depression symptom scales.
†Present state examination, which assesses the present mental state. An Index of Definition Score ≥5 designates a psychiatric case; a diagnosis of depression is subsequently based on equivalent ICD-9 criteria.
‡General health questionnaire.
§Clinical interview schedule for diagnosis of major depressive disorder by psychiatrists and psychologists.
‖Diagnostic interview schedule for diagnosis of major depressive disorder by lay interviewers, based on criteria specified in the Diagnostic and Statistical Manual of Mental Disorders of the American Psychiatric Association (DSM-III).
¶Beck depression inventory scale.
**Minnesota Multiphasic Personality Inventory-Depression Scale.
††Center for Epidemiologic Studies-Depression Scale.

Table 2-14   Adjustment for Potential Biases and Summary of Methodologic Problems: Controlled Studies

Study	Age	Sex	SES	Obesity	Assortative mating	Concomitant medical illness		Severity*	Verification of diabetes	Time frame of current depression	Participation rate (%)
						in diabetic sample	in control sample				
Structured Diagnostic Interviews											
Wells and others, 1989[172]	+	+	–	–	n/a	–	+	–	–	Last 6 months	68
Popkin and others, 1988[119]	–†	+	–	–	n/a	+	–	+	+	Last 6 months	100 (D,R)
Robinson and others, 1988[131]	–‡	+	–§	–	n/a	–	–	+	+	Last month	85 (D), nr (C)
Depression Symptom Scales											
Friis and Nanjundappa, 1986[43]	+	+	–‖	–	n/a	–	–	–	+	Last 7 days	nr
Murrell and others, 1983[103]	+	+	–	–	–	–	–	–	–	Last 7 days	80

*Diabetes severity was unrelated to depression, which minimizes an ascertainment bias from the use of treatment samples.[119,131]

†The 25-44 year category contained 76% of the IDDM pancreatic recipients, 62% of the family donors, and 39% of the general population (p < 0.001).

‡The mean age was 51 ± 6.6 years in the diabetic sample and 44 ± 10.4 years in the control sample (p < 0.01).

§The proportion of low SES occupations represented in the diabetic and control samples was 63% and 45%, respectively (p < 0.01).

‖The proportion unemployed was 75% in the diabetic sample and 37% in the control sample (p < 0.01).

+ = Potential bias adjusted for in either sample selection or analyses.

– = Potential bias not adjusted for in either sample selection or analyses, or no significant differences found between diabetic and control groups.

n/a, Bias not applicable to study; nr, not reported; D, diabetes; C, controls; R, relatives; SES, socioeconomic status.

through either sample selection or analyses, many potential biases were not addressed (see Table 2-14).

Despite the potential biases and methodologic difficulties, the increased prevalence of depression in IDDM relative to the general adult population likely signifies a true association.[51] The relationship was found for two of three interview studies and both corroborating depression symptom scale studies, despite the variety of diabetic and control samples used and the different depression assessment methods employed. Future studies are needed that will address the potential biases and methodologic issues just outlined to identify the absolute strength of the association. Research is also needed that investigates depression according to gender, emphasizes lifetime depression, and further discriminates between nonspecific effects of chronic illness and depression specifically related to diabetes.[51] Family studies would be extremely useful for studying genetic-environmental interactions of IDDM and depression. Such studies could examine if depression is caused by biologic changes of IDDM, a psychologic response to living with IDDM, an antecedent risk factor for IDDM, or the result of a shared etiology with IDDM.

Eating Disorders

Eating disorders such as anorexia nervosa and bulimia have been poorly studied in persons with diabetes. The former is characterized by extreme aversion to food resulting in radical weight loss. Self-induced vomiting, vigorous exercise, and diuretic abuse may also help to accomplish that end. Bulimia is identified by frequent binge eating with accompanying purging usually by self-induced vomiting. Fasting between binges and laxatives also may be used to maintain weight at normal or below normal levels. Anorexia nervosa and bulimia in diabetes predominantly occur in young women, and the onset of diabetes generally precedes the onset of the eating disorder.[120,153] Both eating disorders are aided through specific utilization of the diabetic condition with accompanying harmful sequelae.[62] Diabetic individuals with anorexia nervosa may fail to eat after taking insulin, resulting in hypoglycemia. Diabetic patients with bulimia may intentionally lower their insulin dosage during binging to avoid weight gain, resulting in acute hyperglycemia, glycosuria, and ketoacidosis. Such binging and purging frequently results in wildly varying blood glucose levels and poor glycemic control. An increased risk of diabetic complications may be the result.[21,150]

The prevalence of anorexia nervosa and bulimia in diabetes is currently unknown. Diabetic women with eating disorders may be reluctant to talk about them, and physicians may not ask about aberrant eating patterns unless severe emaciation is present or glycemic control is poor with no apparent cause. The few prevalence studies that have been performed have varied greatly in their estimates mainly as a result of differences in case definition. Controlled studies that used psychiatric diagnostic interviews with DSM-III-R criteria found no difference in the prevalence of bulimia between diabetic and nondiabetic groups (5.6% versus 3.0%[38] and 1.8% versus 0.0%[129]). These differences were based on very small case numbers of 3 versus 2[38] and 1 versus 0.[129] Another controlled study examined anorexia nervosa and bulimia symptomatology on a single continuum.[132] Diabetic women were found to have a

Table 2-15   Psychiatric Disorders Other Than Depression in Adult IDDM Populations: Prevalence Findings

Study	Disorder		Overall		Males		Females	
			Current	Lifetime	Current	Lifetime	Current	Lifetime
Controlled studies: structured diagnostic interviews								
Wells and others, 1989[172]	Anxiety	Diabetes	15.7%	26.2%	—	—	—	—
		Controls	5.3%†	10.5%†	—	—	—	—
	Substance use	Diabetes	5.7%	21.6%	—	—	—	—
		Controls	6.0%NS	17.3%NS	—	—	—	—
Popkin and others, 1988[119]	Simple phobia	Diabetes	18.7%	21.3%	—	3.7%	—	31.3%
		Relatives	0.0%*	0.0%†	—	0.0%NS	—	0.0%*
		Gen. Pop.	9.0%†	14.9%NS	—	9.5%NS	—	18.4%*
	Antisocial personality	Diabetes	—	6.7%	—	14.8%	—	2.1%
		Relatives	—	11.8%NS	—	26.7%NS	—	0.0%NS
		Gen. Pop.	—	2.3%*	—	4.6%*	—	0.8%NS

*p < 0.05
†p < 0.01
NS, Not Significant. Each control group was compared with its respective overall or sex-specific diabetic group in assessing significant differences in the prevalence of each psychiatric disorder.

greater prevalence of clinically significant anorexic-bulimic symptomatology than nondiabetic women (4.9% versus 0.0%, p < 0.05). This finding was based on case numbers of 2 versus 0 and was not diagnostic for an eating disorder.

Uncontrolled studies using DSM-III diagnostic criteria in self-report questionnaires found much higher prevalences of bulimia in diabetic women. The estimates ranged from 11.9% to 35.0%.[8,64,149] One explanation is that the more stringent DSM-III-R criteria required quantification of binging episodes (at least two a week for at least 3 months), as well as some method of purging (self-induced vomiting, laxatives or diuretics, fasting, or vigorous exercise), whereas DSM-III criteria did not.[8] The prevalence of eating disorders in diabetes may thus vary widely depending on which diagnostic criteria are employed. Greater reporting of bulimia may have also occurred owing to the anonymity of a questionnaire. Response rates, however, were as low as 30%.[64] An increased prevalence of eating disorders in diabetes relative to the general population remains unproven.

Other Psychiatric Disorders

Two controlled diagnostic interview studies have examined the prevalence of psychiatric disorders other than depression in adult IDDM or mixed diabetic populations[119,172] (Table 2-15). Popkin and associates[119] found that diabetic individuals who were candidates for pancreatic transplantation had a significantly greater prevalence of current simple phobia than the general population (18.7% versus 9.0%; p < 0.01). Significant differences were found for females for lifetime simple phobia (31.3% versus 18.4%; p < 0.05). Male transplantation candidates were at higher risk for lifetime antisocial personality than males in the general population (14.8% versus 4.6%; p < 0.05). Wells and others[172] found that diabetic subjects had almost three times the rate of current anxiety (15.7% versus 5.3%; p < 0.05) and lifetime anxiety (26.2% versus 10.5%; p < 0.01) than the general population. Corroboration was provided by an uncontrolled study of Lustman and associates,[92] which found a prevalence of lifetime anxiety disorder of 40.9% in diabetic patients.

REFERENCES

1. Allen C, Palta M, D'Alessio DJ: Incidence and differences in urban-rural seasonal variation of type I (insulin-dependent) diabetes in Wisconsin, *Diabetologia* 29:629-633, 1986.
2. Anderson CE, and others: A search for heterogeneity in insulin dependent diabetes mellitus (IDDM): HLA and autoimmune studies in simplex, multiplex, and multigenerational families, *Metabolism* 32:471-477, 1983.
3. Andersen OO, Christy M, Buschard AK: Viruses and diabetes. In Bajaj JS, editor: Diabetes. Proceedings of the IX Congress of the International Diabetes Federation, Amsterdam-Oxford, 1977, Excerpta Medica.
4. Arner P and others: Some characteristics of steroid diabetes: a study in renal-transplant recipients

receiving high-dose corticosteroid therapy, *Diabetes Care* 6:23-25, 1983.
5. Bao MZ and others: HLA-DQ beta non-Asp-57 allele and incidence of diabetes in China and the U.S.A. *Lancet* 2:497-498, 1989.
6. Barnett AH and others: Diabetes in identical twins: a study of 200 pairs, *Diabetologia* 20:87-93, 1981.
7. Bingley PJ, Gale EAM: Rising incidence of IDDM in Europe, *Diabetes Care* 12:289-295, 1989.
8. Birk R, Spencer ML: The prevalence of anorexia nervosa, bulimia, and induced glycosuria in IDDM females, *Diabetes Educator* 15:336-341, 1989.
9. Bodansky HJ and others: Evidence for an environmental effect in the aetiology of insulin dependent diabetes in a transmigratory population, *Br Med J* 304:1020-1022, 1992.

10. Borch-Johnsen K and others: Relation between breast-feeding and incidence rates of insulin-dependent diabetes mellitus: a hypothesis, *Lancet* 10:1083-1086, 1984.

11. Bruno G and others: Incidence of IDDM during 1984-1986 in population aged <30 yr: residents of Turin, Italy, *Diabetes Care* 13:1051-1056, 1990.

12. Burgess JA, Kirkpatrick KL, Menser MA: Fulminant onset of diabetes mellitus during an attack of infectious mononucleosis, *Med J Austr* 2:706-707, 1974.

13. Campbell KL, Latimer KS: Transient diabetes mellitus associated with prednisone therapy in a dog, *JAVMA* 185:299-302, 1984.

14. Carrasco E and others: Incidence of insulin-dependent diabetes mellitus in 1990-1991, Santiago, Chile, *Rev Soc Argent Diabetes* 26(suppl.): 14-15, 1992.

15. Champsaur HF and others: Virologic, immunologic, and genetic factors in insulin-dependent diabetes mellitus, *J Pediatr* 100:15-20, 1982.

16. Champsaur H and others: Diabetes and Coxsackie virus B5 infection, *Lancet* 1:251, 1980.

17. Cherubini V and others: Incidence of IDDM in the Marche region, Italy, *Diabetes Care* 17:432-435, 1994.

18. Christau B and others: Incidence, seasonal, and geographical patterns of juvenile-onset insulin-dependent diabetes mellitus in Denmark, *Diabetologia* 13:281-284, 1977.

19. Christau B and others: Incidence of insulin-dependent diabetes mellitus (0-29 years at onset) in Denmark, *Acta Med Scand* 624(suppl.):54-60, 1979.

20. Christy M and others: Studies of the HLA system and insulin-dependent diabetes mellitus, *Diabetes Care* 2:209-214, 1979.

21. Colas CL, Mathieu P, Tchobroutsky G: Eating disorders and retinal lesions in type I (insulin-dependent) diabetic women, *Diabetologia* 34:288, 1991.

22. Colle E and others: Incidence of juvenile onset diabetes in Montreal—demonstration of ethnic differences and socio-economic class differences, *J Chron Dis* 34:611-616, 1981.

23. Cudworth A, Wolf E: Genetic susceptibility to Type I (insulin-dependent) diabetes mellitus, *Clinics Endo Metab* 11:389-408, 1982.

24. Dacou-Voutetakis C, Karavanaki K, Tsoka-Gennatas H: National data on the epidemiology of IDDM in Greece, *Diabetes Care* 18:552-554, 1995.

25. Dahlquist G, Savilahti E, Landin-Olsson M: An increased level of antibodies to lactoglobulin is a risk determinant of early-onset type I (insulin-dependent) diabetes mellitus independent of islet cell antibodies and early introduction of cow's milk, *Diabetologia* 35:980-984, 1992.

26. Dahlquist G and others: The epidemiology of diabetes in Swedish children 0-14 years—a six-year prospective study, *Diabetologia* 28:802-808, 1985.

26a. Dahlquist GG and others: Dietary factors and the risk of developing insulin dependent diabetes in childhood, *Br Med J* 300:1302-1305, 1990.

27. D'Alessio DJ: A Case-control study of group B Coxsackievirus immunoglobulin M antibody prevalence and HLA-DR antigens in newly diagnosed cases of insulin-dependent diabetes mellitus, *Am J Epidemiol* 135:1331-1338, 1992.

28. Degnbol B, Green A: Diabetes mellitus among first- and second-degree relatives of early onset diabetes, *Ann Hum Gen* 42:25-47, 1978.

29. DePrins F, Van Assche FA, Desmyter J: Congenital rubella and diabetes mellitus, *Lancet* 1:439-440, 1978.

30. Diabetes Epidemiology Research International Group: Geographic patterns of childhood insulin-dependent diabetes mellitus, *Diabetes* 37:1113-1119, 1988.

31. Diabetes Epidemiology Research International Group: Secular trends in incidence of childhood IDDM in 10 countries, *Diabetes* 39:858-864, 1990.

31a. Diabetes Epidemiology Research International Mortality Study Group: International evaluation of cause-specific mortality and IDDM. *Diabetes Care* 14:55-60, 1991.

32. Dokheel TM: An epidemic of childhood diabetes in the United States: evidence from Allegheny County, Pennsylvania, *Diabetes Care* 16:1606-1611, 1993.

33. Dorman JS and others: Worldwide differences in the incidence of type I diabetes are associated with amino acid variation at position 57 of the HLA-DQ beta chain, *Proc Natl Acad Sci USA* 87:7370-7374, 1990.

34. Drash A and others: Pittsburgh diabetes mellitus study: studies on the etiology of insulin-dependent diabetes mellitus with special reference to viral infections, *Acta Paediatr Jpn* 26:306-321, 1984.

35. Drykoningen CEM and others: The incidence of male childhood type I (insulin-dependent) diabetes mellitus is rising rapidly in the Netherlands, *Diabetologia* 35:139-142, 1992.

36. Durruty P, Ruiz BQ, Garcia de los Rios M: Age at onset and seasonal variation in the onset of insulin dependent diabetes, *Diabetologia* 17:357-360, 1974.

37. Elamin A and others: Epidemiology of childhood type I diabetes in Sudan, 1987-1990, *Diabetes Care* 15:1556-1559, 1992.

38. Fairburn CG and others: Eating disorders in young adults with insulin-dependent diabetes mellitus: a controlled study, *Br Med J* 303:17-20, 1991.

39. Ferreira SRG and others: Population-based incidence of IDDM in the state of Sao Paulo, Brazil, *Diabetes Care* 16:701-704, 1993.

40. Fishbein HA and others: The Pittsburgh insulin-dependent diabetes mellitus registry: seasonal incidence, *Diabetologia* 23:83-85, 1982.

41. Fleegler FM and others: Age, sex, and season of onset of juvenile diabetes in different geographic areas, *Pediatrics* 63:374-379, 1979.

42. Frazer de Llado T and others: Incidence of youth-onset insulin-dependent diabetes mellitus in Southern and Western Puerto Rico (Abstract), *Diabetes* 40(suppl. 1):316A, 1991.

43. Friis R, Nanjundappa G: Diabetes, depression, and employment status, *Soc Sci Med* 23:471-475, 1986.

44. Friman G and others: An incidence peak of juvenile diabetes: relation to Coxsackie B virus immune response, *Acta Paediatr Scand* 320(suppl.):14-19, 1985.

45. Gamble DR: An epidemiological study of childhood diabetes affecting two or more siblings, *Diabetologia* 19:341-344, 1980.

46. Gamble DR: Relation of antecedent illness to development of diabetes in children, *Br Med J* 281:99-101, 1980.

46a. Gamble DR: The epidemiology of insulin-dependent diabetes, with particular reference to the relationship of virus infection to its etiology, *Epidemiol Rev* 2:49-70, 1980.

47. Gamble DR, Taylor KW: Seasonal incidence of diabetes mellitus, *Br Med J* 3:631-633, 1969.

48. Gamble DR, Taylor KW, Cumming H: Coxsackie viruses and diabetes mellitus, *Br Med J* 4:260-262, 1973.

49. Gavard JA and others: Familial insulin-dependent diabetes mellitus and hemipancreatectomy, *Lancet* 341:303-304, 1993.

50. Gavard JA and others: Sex differences in secondary attack rate of IDDM to siblings of probands through older ages: Pittsburgh etiology of IDDM study, *Diabetes Care* 15:559-561, 1992.

51. Gavard JA, Lustman PJ, Clouse RE: Prevalence of depression in adults with diabetes: an epidemiological evaluation, *Diabetes Care* 16:1167-1178, 1993.

52. Ginsberg-Fellner F and others: Congenital rubella syndrome as a model for type I (insulin-dependent) diabetes mellitus: increased prevalence of islet cell surface antibodies, *Diabetologia* 27:87-89, 1984.

53. Gottlieb MS: Diabetes in offspring and siblings of juvenile- and maturity-onset type diabetics, *J Chron Dis* 33:331-339, 1980.

54. Green A and others: Increasing incidence of early onset type I (insulin-dependent) diabetes mellitus: a study of Danish male birth cohorts, *Diabetologia* 35:178-182, 1992.

55. Green A, Gale EAM, Patterson CC: Incidence of childhood-onset insulin-dependent diabetes mellitus: the EURODIAB ACE Study *Lancet* 339:905-909, 1992.

56. Grzywa MA, Sobel AK: Incidence of IDDM in the Province of Rzeszow, Poland, 0 to 29 year old age group, 1980-1992, *Diabetes Care* 18:542-544, 1995.

57. Hamman RF and others: Colorado IDDM registry: incidence and validation of IDDM in children aged 0-17 yr, *Diabetes Care* 13:499-506, 1990.

58. Helgason T, Danielson R, Thorsson AV: Incidence and prevalence of type I (insulin-dependent) diabetes mellitus in Icelandic children 1970-1989, *Diabetologia* 35:880-883, 1992.

59. Helgason T, Jonasson MR: Evidence for a food additive as a cause of ketosis-prone diabetes, *Lancet* 2:716-720, 1981.

60. Helmke K and others: Islet cell antibodies and the development of diabetes mellitus in relation to mumps infection and mumps vaccination, *Diabetologia* 29:30-33, 1986.

61. Helmke K, Otten A, Willems W: Islet cell antibodies in children with mumps infection, *Lancet* 2:211-212, 1980.

62. Hillard JR, Hillard PJA: Bulimia, anorexia nervosa, and diabetes: deadly combinations, *Psychiatr Clinics North Am* 7:367-379, 1984.

63. Hua F and others: Shanghai, China, has the lowest confirmed incidence of childhood diabetes in the world, *Diabetes Care* 17:1206-1208, 1994.

64. Hudson JI and others: Prevalence of anorexia nervosa and bulimia among young diabetic women, *J Clin Psychiatry* 46:88-89, 1985.

65. Hyoty H and others: A prospective study of the role of Coxsackie B and other enterovirus infections in the pathogenesis of IDDM, *Diabetes* 44:652-657, 1995.

66. Deleted in proofs.

67. Jenson AB and others: Pancreatic islet cell damage in children with fatal viral infections, *Lancet* 2:354-358, 1980.

68. Johnston C and others: HLA-DR typing in identical twins with insulin-dependent diabetes: differences between concordant and discordant pairs, *Br Med J* 286:253-255, 1983.

69. Joner G, Sovik O: Incidence, age at onset, and seasonal variation of diabetes mellitus in Norwegian children 1973-1977, *Acta Paediatr Scand* 70:329-335, 1981.

70. Joner G, Sovik O: Increasing incidence of diabetes mellitus in Norwegian children 0-14 years of age 1973-1982, *Diabetologia* 32:79-83, 1989.

71. Jordan OW and others: Incidence of type I diabetes in people under 30 years of age in Barbados, West Indies, 1982-1991, *Diabetes Care* 17:428-431, 1994.

72. Kaprio J and others: Concordance for type I (insulin-dependent) and type 2 (non-insulin-dependent) diabetes mellitus in a population-based cohort of twins in Finland, *Diabetologia* 35:1060-1067, 1993.

73. Karjalainen J and others: A bovine albumin peptide as a possible trigger of insulin-dependent diabetes mellitus, *N Engl J Med* 327:302-307, 1992.

74. Kelly HA, Byrne GC: Incidence of IDDM in Western Australia in children aged 0-14 yr from 1985-1989, *Diabetes Care* 15:515-517, 1992.

75. Kendall DM and others: Effects of hemipancreatectomy on insulin secretion and glucose tolerance in healthy humans, *N Engl J Med* 322:898-903, 1990.

76. King ML and others: Coxsackie-B-virus specific IgM responses in children with insulin-dependent diabetes mellitus, *Lancet* 1:1397-1399, 1983.

77. Ko KW, Yang SW, Cho NH: The incidence of IDDM in Seoul from 1985 to 1988, *Diabetes Care* 17:1473-1475, 1994.

78. Kocova M and others: A cold spot of IDDM incidence in Europe: Macedonia, *Diabetes Care* 16:1236-1240, 1993.

79. Kostraba JN and others: Early exposure to cow's milk and solid foods in infancy, genetic predisposition, and risk of IDDM, *Diabetes* 42:288-295, 1993.

80. Kostraba JN and others: Early infant diet and risk of IDDM in blacks and whites, *Diabetes Care* 15:626-631, 1992.

81. Kostraba JN and others: Nitrate levels in community drinking waters and risk of IDDM, *Diabetes Care* 15:1505-1508, 1992.

82. Kostraba JN, Gay EC, Cai Y: Incidence of insulin-dependent diabetes mellitus in Colorado, *Epidemiology* 3:232-238, 1992.

83. Lai MS and others: Ingested inorganic arsenic and prevalence of diabetes mellitus, *Am J Epidemiol* 139:484-492, 1994.

84. LaPorte RE, Diabetes Epidemiology Research International: Preventing insulin dependent diabetes mellitus: the environmental challenge, *Br Med J* 295:479-481, 1987.

85. LaPorte RE and others: The Pittsburgh insulin-dependent diabetes mellitus (IDDM) registry: the incidence of insulin-dependent diabetes mellitus in Allegheny County, Pennsylvania (1965-1976), *Diabetes* 10:279-283, 1981.

86. LaPorte RE and others: The Pittsburgh insulin dependent diabetes mellitus registry: the relationship of insulin dependent diabetes mellitus to social class, *Am J Epidemiol* 114:379-384, 1981.

87. LaPorte RE and others: Geographic differences in the risk of insulin-dependent diabetes mellitus: the importance of registries, *Diabetes Care* 8(suppl. 1):101-107, 1985.

88. Lipman TH: The epidemiology of type I diabetes in children 0-14 yr of age in Philadelphia, *Diabetes Care* 16:922-925, 1993.

89. Littlefield CH and others: Influence of functional impairment and social support on depressive symptoms in persons with diabetes, *Health Psychol* 9:737-749, 1990.

90. Lloyd CE and others: Psychosocial factors and complications of IDDM: the Pittsburgh epidemiology of diabetes complications study. VIII, *Diabetes Care* 15:166-172, 1992.

91. Lorenzi M, Cagliero E, Schmidt NJ: Racial differences in incidence of juvenile-onset type I diabetes: epidemiologic studies in southern California, *Diabetologia* 28:734-738, 1985.

92. Lustman PJ: Anxiety disorders in adults with diabetes mellitus, *Psychiatr Clinics North Am* 11:419-431, 1988.

93. Lustman PJ and others: Psychiatric illness in diabetes: relationship to symptoms and glucose control, *J Nerv Ment Dis* 174:736-742, 1986.

94. Mayer EJ and others: Reduced risk of IDDM among breast-fed children: the Colorado IDDM registry, *Diabetes* 37:1625-1632, 1988.

95. Mayou R and others: Psychiatric morbidity in young adults with insulin-dependent diabetes mellitus, *J Psychol Med* 21:639-645, 1991.

96. McLarty DG and others: The incidence of youth-onset diabetes in the African population of Dar es Salaam, Tanzania, *Diabetic Med* 9(suppl.):43A, 1992.

97. Menser MA, Forrest JM, Honeyman MC: Diabetes, HLA antigens, and congenital rubella (Letter), *Lancet* 2:1508-1509, 1974.

98. Metcalfe MA, Baum JD: Incidence of insulin dependent diabetes in children aged under 15 years in the British Isles during 1988, *Br Med J* 302:443-447, 1991.

99. Monif GR: Rubella virus and the pancreas, *Med Chir Dig* 3:195-197, 1974.

100. Morel PA and others: Aspartic acid at position 57 of the HLA-DQ beta chain protects against type I diabetes: a family study, *Proc Natl Acad Sci USA* 85:8111-8115, 1988.

101. Muntoni S, Songini M: High incidence rate of IDDM in Sardinia, *Diabetes Care* 15:1317-1322, 1992.

102. Murawski BJ and others: Personality patterns in patients with diabetes mellitus of long duration, *Diabetes* 19:259-263, 1970.

103. Murrell SA, Himmelfarb S, Wright K: Prevalence of depression and its correlates in older adults, *Am J Epidemiol* 117:173-185, 1983.

104. Nathanson N, Martin JR: The epidemiology of poliomyelitis: enigmas surrounding its appearance, epidemicity, and disappearance, *Am J Epidemiol* 110:672-692, 1979.

105. Nerup J and others: HLA antigens and diabetes mellitus, *Lancet* 2:864-866, 1974.

106. Norden CW, Kuller LH: Identifying infectious etiologies of chronic disease, *Rev Inf Dis* 6:200-213, 1984.

107. Nystrom L and others: The Swedish childhood diabetes study. An analysis of the temporal variation in diabetes incidence 1978-1987, *Int J Epidemiol* 19:141-146, 1990.

108. Olmos P and others: The significance of concordance rate of type I (insulin-dependent) diabetes mellitus in identical twins, *Diabetologia* 31:747-750, 1988.

109. Onodera T and others: Virus-induced diabetes mellitus: autoimmunity and polyendocrine disease prevented by immunosuppression, *Nature* 297:66-68, 1982.

110. Onodera T and others: Virus-induced diabetes mellitus. XX. Polyendocrinopathy and autoimmunity, *J Exp Med* 153:1457-1473, 1981.

111. Orchard TJ and others: The development of type I (insulin-dependent) diabetes mellitus: two contrasting presentations, *Diabetologia* 25:89-92, 1983.

112. Pagano G and others: An In vivo and in vitro study of the mechanism of prednisone-induced insulin resistance in healthy subjects, *J Clin Invest* 72:1814-1820, 1983.

113. Pak CY and others: Association of cytomegalovirus genome with autoimmune insulin-dependent diabetes mellitus (Abstract), *Diabetes* 36(suppl. 1): 82a, 1987.

114. Palmer JP and others: Antibodies to viruses and to pancreatic islets in nondiabetic and insulin-dependent diabetic patients, *Diabetes Care* 4:525-528, 1981.

115. Patterson CC and others: Epidemiology of type I (insulin-dependent) diabetes in Scotland 1968-1976: evidence of an increasing incidence, *Diabetologia* 24:238-243, 1983.

116. Patterson K, Chandra RS, Jenson AB: Congenital rubella, insulitis, and diabetes mellitus in an infant, *Lancet* 1:1048-1049, 1981.

117. Platz P and others: HLA-D and DR antigens in genetic analysis of insulin dependent diabetes mellitus, *Diabetologia* 21:108-115, 1981.

118. Podar T and others: Insulin-dependent diabetes mellitus in native Estonians and immigrants to Estonia, *Am J Epidemiol* 135:1231-1236, 1992.

119. Popkin MK and others: Prevalence of major depression, simple phobia, and other psychiatric disorders in patients with longstanding type I diabetes mellitus, *Arch Gen Psychiatry* 45:64-68, 1988.

120. Powers PS and others: Insulin-dependent diabetes mellitus and eating disorders: a prevalence study, *Compre Psychiatry* 31:205-210, 1990.

121. Prosser PR, Karam JH: Diabetes mellitus following rodenticide ingestion in man, *JAMA* 239:1148-1150, 1979.

122. Pyke DA, Nelson PG: Diabetes mellitus in identical twins. In Creutzfeldt W, Kobberling J, Neel JV, editors: *The genetics of diabetes mellitus,* Berlin, 1976, Springer-Verlag.

123. Raffel LJ, Rotter JI: The genetics of diabetes, *Clinical Diabetes* 3:47-50, 1985.

124. Ratzmann KP: Autoimmunity and the development of diabetes mellitus in relation to mumps infection (Letter), *Diabetologia* 29:673-674, 1986.

125. Reunanen A, Akerblom HK, Karr ML: Prevalence and ten-year (1970-1979) incidence of insulin-dependent diabetes mellitus in children and adolescents in Finland, *Acta Paediatr Scand* 71:893-899, 1982.

126. Rewers M and others: Trends in the prevalence and incidence of diabetes: insulin-dependent diabetes mellitus in childhood, *World Health Stat* 41:179-189, 1988.

127. Rewers M and others: Apparent epidemic of insulin-dependent diabetes mellitus in midwestern Poland, *Diabetes* 36:106-113, 1987.

128. Rewers M and others: Poisson regression modeling of temporal variation in incidence of childhood insulin-dependent diabetes mellitus in Allegheny County, Pennsylvania, and Wielkopolska, Poland, 1970-1985, *Am J Epidemiol* 129:569-581, 1989.

129. Robertson P, Rosenvinge JH: Insulin-dependent diabetes mellitus: a risk factor in anorexia nervosa or bulimia nervosa: an empirical study of 116 women, *J Psychosom Res* 34:535-541, 1990.

130. Robinson N, Fuller JH: Role of life events and difficulties in the onset of diabetes mellitus, *J Psychosom Res* 29:583-591, 1985.

131. Robinson N, Fuller JH, Edmeades SP: Depression and diabetes, *Diabetic Med* 5:268-274, 1988.

132. Rosmark B and others: Eating disorders in patients with insulin-dependent diabetes mellitus, *J Clin Psychiatry* 47:547-550, 1986.

133. Rotter JI, Anderson CE, Rimoin DL: Genetics of diabetes mellitus. In Ellenberg M, Refkin H, editors: *Diabetes mellitus: theory and practice,* New York, 1983, Medical Examination Publication Co.

134. Rubenstein P and others: The HLA system in congenital rubella patients with and without diabetes, *Diabetes* 31:1088-1091, 1982.

135. Ruwaard D and others: Increasing incidence of type I diabetes in the Netherlands: the second nationwide study among children under 20 years of age, *Diabetes Care* 17:599-601, 1994.

136. Savilahti E and others: Children with newly diagnosed insulin dependent diabetes mellitus have increased levels of cow's milk antibodies, *Diabetes Res* 7:137-140, 1988.

137. Schmidt WAK and others: Course of Coxsackie B antibodies during juvenile diabetes, *Med Microbiol Immunol* 164:291-298, 1978.

138. Schoenle EJ and others: Epidemiology of IDDM in Switzerland: increasing incidence rate and rural-urban differences in Swiss men born 1948-1972, *Diabetes Care* 17:955-960, 1994.

139. Schranz AG, Prikatsky V: Type I diabetes in the Maltese Islands, *Diabetic Med* 6:228-231, 1989.

140. Schulz B and others: Islet cell antibodies in individuals at increased risk for IDDM, *Exp Clin Endocrinol* 83:192-198, 1984.

141. Scott RS and others: Temporal variation in incidence of IDDM in Canterbury, New Zealand, *Diabetes Care* 15:895-899, 1992.

142. Sereday MS and others: Establishment of a registry and incidence of IDDM in Avellaneda, Argentina, *Diabetes Care* 17:1022-1025, 1994.

143. Serrano Rios M, Moy CS, Martin Serrano R: Incidence of type I (insulin-dependent) diabetes mellitus in subjects 0-14 years of age in the Comunidad of Madrid, Spain, *Diabetologia* 33:422-424, 1990.

144. Shaltout AA and others: High incidence of childhood-onset IDDM in Kuwait, *Diabetes Care* 18:923-927, 1995.

145. Shubnikov E and others: Low incidence of childhood IDDM in district of Novosibirsk (Russia), *Diabetes Care* 15:915-917, 1992.

146. Siemiatycki J and others: Incidence of IDDM in Montreal by ethnic group and by social class and comparisons with ethnic groups living elsewhere, *Diabetes* 37:1096-1102, 1988.

147. Singal DP, Blajchman MA: Histocompatibility (HLA) antigens, lymphocytotoxic antibodies, and tissue antibodies in patients with diabetes mellitus, *Diabetes* 22:429-432, 1973.

148. Slawson PF, Flynn WR, Kollar EJ: Psychological factors associated with the onset of diabetes mellitus, *JAMA* 185:166-170, 1963.

149. Stancin T, Link DL, Reuter JM: Binge eating and purging in young women with IDDM, *Diabetes Care* 12:601-603, 1989.

150. Steel JM and others: Clinically apparent eating disorders in young diabetic women: associations with painful neuropathy and other complications, *Br Med J* 294:859-862, 1987.

151. Stein SP, Charles E: Emotional factors in juvenile diabetes mellitus: a study of early life experiences of adolescent diabetics, *Am J Psychiat* 128:56-60, 1971.

152. Svejgaard A, Platz P, Ryder LP: Insulin-dependent diabetes mellitus. In Terasaki PI, editor: *Histocompatibility testing,* Los Angeles, 1980, UCLA.

153. Szmukler GI: Anorexia nervosa and bulimia in diabetics, *J Psychosom Res* 28:365-369, 1984.

154. Tattersall RB, Pyke DA: Diabetes in identical twins, *Lancet* 2:1120-1124, 1972.

155. Tenconi MT and others: IDDM in the province of Pavia, Italy, from a population-based registry, *Diabetes Care* 18:1017-1019, 1995.

156. The Association for the Study of Infectious Diseases: A retrospective survey of the complications of mumps, *J R Coll Gen Pract* 24:552-556, 1974.

157. Tull ES, Roseman JM, Christian CLE: Epidemiology of childhood IDDM in U.S. Virgin Islands from 1979 to 1988: evidence of an epidemic in early 1980's and variation by degree of racial admixture, *Diabetes Care* 14:558-564, 1991.

158. Tuomilehto J: The classification of mortality in IDDM: the DERI experience. In Laron Z, Karp M, editors: *Prognosis of diabetes in children,* 1989, Basel Karger.

159. Tuomilehto J and others: Incidence of IDDM in Mauritian children and adolescents from 1986 to 1990, *Diabetes Care* 16:1588-1591, 1993.

160. Tuomilehto J and others: Epidemiology of childhood diabetes mellitus in Finland—background of a nationwide study of type I (insulin-dependent) diabetes mellitus, *Diabetologia* 35:70-76, 1992.

161. Tuomilehto J and others: Comparison of the incidence of insulin-dependent diabetes mellitus in childhood among five Baltic populations during 1983-1988, *Int J Epidemiol* 21:518-527, 1992.

162. Tuomilehto J and others: Comparison of incidence of IDDM in childhood between Estonia and Finland, 1980-1988, *Diabetes Care* 14:982-988, 1991.

163. Tuomilehto J and others: Increasing trend in type I (insulin-dependent) diabetes mellitus in childhood in Finland: analysis of age, calendar time, and birth cohort effects during 1965 to 1984, *Diabetologia* 34:282-287, 1991.

164. Verge CF, Silink M, Howard NJ: The incidence of childhood IDDM in New South Wales, Australia, *Diabetes Care* 17:693-696, 1994.

165. Virtanen SM and others: Infant feeding in Finnish children <7 yr of age with newly diagnosed IDDM, *Diabetes Care* 14:415-417, 1991.

166. Virtanen SM and others: Feeding in infancy and risk of type I diabetes mellitus in Finnish children, *Diabetic Med* 9:815-819, 1992.

167. Virtanen SM and others: Early introduction of dairy products associated with increased risk of IDDM in Finnish children, *Diabetes* 42:1786-1790, 1993.

168. Wagenknecht LE, Roseman JM, Alexander WJ: Epidemiology of IDDM in black and white children in Jefferson County, Alabama, 1979-1985, *Diabetes* 38:629-633, 1989.

169. Wagenknecht LE, Roseman JM, Herman WH: Increased prevalence of insulin-dependent diabetes mellitus following an epidemic of Coxsackievirus B5, *Am J Epidemiol* 133:1024-1030, 1991.

170. Warram JH and others: Differences in risk of insulin-dependent diabetes in offspring of diabetic mothers and diabetic fathers, *N Engl J Med* 311:149-152, 1984.

171. Warram JH, Krolewski AS, Kahn CR: Determinants of IDDM and perinatal mortality in children of diabetic mothers, *Diabetes* 37:1328-1334, 1988.

172. Wells KB, Golding JM, Burnam MA: Affective, substance use, and anxiety disorders in persons with arthritis, diabetes, heart disease, high blood pressure, or chronic lung conditions, *Gen Hosp Psychiatry* 11:320-327, 1989.

173. West R and others: Epidemiologic survey of juvenile onset diabetes in Montreal, *Diabetes* 28:690-693, 1979.

174. WHO DIAMOND Project: WHO Multinational project for childhood diabetes, *Diabetes Care* 13:1062-1068, 1990.

175. Wilkinson G and others: Psychiatric morbidity and social problems in patients with insulin-dependent diabetes mellitus, *Br J Psychiatry* 153:38-43, 1988.

176. Wolf E, Spencer KM, Cudworth AG: The genetic susceptibility to Type I (insulin-dependent) diabetes: analysis of the HLA-DR association, *Diabetologia* 24:224-230, 1983.

177. Wong GWK, Leung SSF, Oppenheimer SJ: Epidemiology of IDDM in southern Chinese children in Hong Kong, *Diabetes Care* 16:926-928, 1993.

178. Yoon JW: Role of viruses in the pathogenesis of IDDM, *Ann Med* 23:437-445, 1991.

179. Yoon JW and others: Virus-induced diabetes mellitus: inhibition by a non-diabetogenic variant of encephalomyocarditis virus, *J Exp Med* 152:878-892, 1980.

179a. Yoon JW and others: Virus-induced diabetes mellitus: isolation of a virus from the pancreas of a child with diabetic ketoacidosis, *N Engl J Med* 300:1173-1179, 1979.

180. Yoon JW, Bachurski CJ, McArthur RG: Concept of a virus as an etiological agent in the development of insulin-dependent diabetes mellitus (Letter), *Diabetes Res Clin Prac* 2: 365-366, 1986.

181. Yoon JW, Cha CY, Jordan GW: The role of interferon in virus-induced diabetes, *J Infect Dis* 147:155-159, 1983.

182. Yoon JW, Ihm SH, Kim KW: Viruses as a triggering factor of type I diabetes and genetic markers related to the susceptibility to the virus-associated diabetes, *Diabetes Res Clin Prac* 7:47-58, 1989.

183. Yoon JW, Notkins AL: Virus-induced diabetes mellitus, VI. Genetically determined host differences in the replication of encephalomyocarditis virus in pancreatic beta cells, *J Exp Med* 143:1170-1185, 1976.

184. Yoon JW, Notkins AL: Virus-induced diabetes in mice prevented by a live attenuated vaccine. *N Engl J Med* 306:486, 1982.

3 Epidemiology of Non-Insulin-Dependent Diabetes Mellitus

Jill M. Norris

INTRODUCTION

The purpose of this chapter is to describe non-insulin-dependent diabetes mellitus (NIDDM) as it occurs in the population and how these patterns can provide clues into the etiology of the disease. Population studies have uncovered several potential determinants of NIDDM. These determinants are discussed, along with the strengths and weaknesses of the epidemiologic tools employed to evaluate them.

NIDDM is the most common form of diabetes and accounts for 90% to 95% of all diabetes in the United States. However, many cases of diabetes go undiagnosed. Even in countries that have a high level of medical care, there is typically one undiagnosed case of NIDDM for every one that is known.[11] The high proportion of undiagnosed diabetes complicates population studies of NIDDM and suggests that epidemiologists cannot rely on patient self-reporting of diabetes status or medical records to identify NIDDM. Only studies testing for diabetes through standardized methods can provide an accurate population assessment of the disease. The World Health Organization's (WHO's) and National Diabetes Data Group's (NDDG's) adoption of specific criteria for diagnosis of NIDDM has created a new environment for the conduction of epidemiologic studies, because now comparisons

---

CHAPTER OBJECTIVES

- Discuss the descriptive epidemiology of NIDDM.
- Describe the analytic epidemiology of NIDDM.
- Report indirect evidence for environmental risk factors.
- Describe behavioral and life-style factors of NIDDM.
- Present evidence for genetic factors associated with NIDDM.

---

of the descriptive epidemiology of NIDDM can be made across studies, nationally and internationally.[35] Every effort has been made in this chapter to discuss only data from studies that have confirmed the presence or absence of NIDDM through testing using WHO criteria.

NIDDM is not a single disease. Rare forms are associated with type A insulin resistance, occurrence of mutant insulins, acromegaly, Cushing syndrome, and leprachaunism. In addition, the more common "garden-variety" form of NIDDM may also have variations in its etiopathogenesis. Complicated models of the etiology of NIDDM have been proposed[11,86] and have been clearly explained in a previous review.[33] Briefly, it appears that the first step toward development of diabetes is from normoglycemia to *impaired glucose tolerance* (IGT), and the second step is from IGT to NIDDM. IGT is defined as a glycemic response to the standard 75 g oral glucose tolerance test (GTT) that is intermediate between normal and diabetic.[108] Limited studies have examined the epidemiology and etiology of IGT,[46,112] but a review of these is beyond the scope of this chapter. However, the IGT group is important because individuals with IGT have a sixfold to tenfold excess risk of developing NIDDM in the future. The investigation of risk factors related to the progression from IGT to NIDDM may reveal areas in which an effective intervention can be implemented to prevent NIDDM in this high-risk group.

The progression from normoglycemia to NIDDM appears to involve two separate pathologies, beta-cell failure and insulin resistance/hyperinsulinemia. The beta cell of the pancreas is responsible for insulin secretion, and *beta-cell failure* in the pathogenesis of NIDDM is suggested through the observed falling insulin secretory response.[34] *Insulin resistance* is defined as a subnormal biologic response to a given concentration of insulin[71] and is suggested by the observed *hyperinsulinemia* before the development of IGT.[86] Insulin resistance may also impact obesity. Longitudinal studies suggest that insulin resistance develops as a result of weight gain, perhaps as a mechanism to prevent further obesity.[13,25,98]

This chapter is divided into two major sections, descriptive epidemiology and analytic epidemiology of NIDDM. The descriptive epidemiology section presents the distribution of NIDDM in populations in terms of person, place, and time. These observations provide important clues as to the genetic and environmental determinants of NIDDM. The analytic epidemiology section explores specific factors that place individuals or populations at risk for NIDDM. Included in this section is a brief discussion of evidence for genetic factors in the etiology of NIDDM, particularly how these genetic factors may interact with the environment to produce the epidemiologic patterns described. Box 3-1 summarizes potential environmental and familial risk factors for NIDDM.

DESCRIPTIVE EPIDEMIOLOGY OF NIDDM

Descriptive epidemiology is typically presented in terms of the prevalence and incidence of a disease. The *prevalence* of a disease refers to the number of cases present in a population at a specified moment in time. This measure is important because it describes the amount of

---

BOX 3-1
_____

POTENTIAL RISK FACTORS FOR NIDDM

- Obesity
- Physical inactivity
- High-fat diet
- High or no alcohol intake
- Gestational diabetes
- Multiple pregnancies
- Offspring of diabetic pregnancy
- Thinness at birth
- Urban residence
- Initial westernization of life-style
- Native American, Hispanic American, African American, Asian American, or Pacific Islander
- Positive family history of diabetes

---

disease in the community and the load on health care services. Prevalence, however, represents the balance between the rate of development of new cases and the effect of any excessive mortality among those with the disease. Thus interpretation of comparisons of prevalence may be limited, since mortality may differ by country, ethnic group, and gender. The *incidence* of a disease refers to the number of individuals developing the disease in the population in a specified time. Minimal good incidence data are available for NIDDM, mainly because of the cost and time involved in data collection. Because of the unreliability of self-reported diabetes status and medical records, the incidence of diabetes can best be determined by first screening the population so that diabetes status can be established in every person and then, some number of years later, rescreening the previously nondiabetic population to ascertain all new cases of diabetes occurring during that interval.

Geography

One striking characteristic of NIDDM is that its prevalence varies greatly around the world. Fig. 3-1 displays the prevalence of NIDDM in selected countries.[2,46,57,90] The prevalence in Nauru, an island in the South Pacific, is extremely high compared with all other countries.[46] In addition, the incidence of NIDDM in Nauru is one of the highest in the world, second only to the Pima Indians of Arizona[4,49] (Table 3-1). In comparison, the prevalence and incidence of NIDDM in Caucasians in the United States and in other European populations are relatively low.[6,31,46,68] The prevalence of NIDDM is not entirely consistent throughout Asia, where the prevalence in China is substantially lower than in Japan[46,90] (Fig. 3-1).

Table 3-1   Incidence of NIDDM in Studies Using WHO or NDDG Criteria to Diagnose NIDDM

Population	Age-group	Incidence/1000 population/year	
		Male	Female
Nauru[4]	Adult	16.0	
Rochester, Minn[68]	0+	1.49*	1.08
San Luis Valley, Colo (Caucasian)[6]	20-74	1.91*	1.30
San Antonio, Texas (Caucasian)[30]	25-64	1.00	3.55
San Luis Valley, Colo (Hispanic)[6]	20-74	4.20	5.24
San Antonio, Texas (Hispanic)[31]	25-64	7.60*	8.94
Pima Indians, Ariz[49]	5-84	23.60*	29.0

Data from Balkau B and others: *Am J Epidemiol* 122:594-605, 1985; Baxter J and others: *Ethnic Dis* 3:11-21, 1993; Haffner SM and others: *Diabetes Care* 14:102-108, 1991; Knowler WC and others: *Am J Epidemiol* 108:497-505, 1978; and Melton LJ, Palumbo PJ, Chu C: *Diabetes Care* 6:75-86, 1983.
WHO, World Health Organization; *NDDG,* National Diabetes Data Group.
*Rates are age-adjusted to 1970 U.S. Caucasian population.

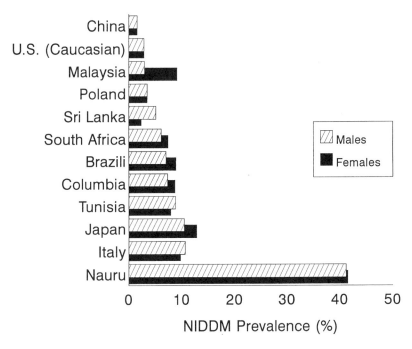

Fig. 3-1   National prevalences of NIDDM by gender. (Data from Aschner P and others: *Diabetes Care* 16(1):90-93, 1993; King H, Rewers M, WHO Ad Hoc Diabetes Reporting Group: *Diabetes Care* 16:157-177, 1993; Levitt NS and others: *Diabetes Care* 16:601-607, 1993; and Sekikawa A and others: *Diabetes Care* 16:570-574, 1993.)

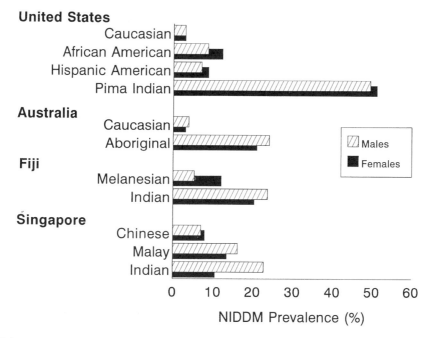

Fig. 3-2   Prevalence of NIDDM in ethnic and racial groups living in the same country. (Data from Bennett PH and others: In Alberti KGMM and others, editors: *International textbook of diabetes,* New York, 1992, Wiley; and King H, Rewers M, WHO Ad Hoc Diabetes Reporting Group: *Diabetes Care* 16:157-177, 1993.)

Ethnicity and Race

Geographic differences in the prevalence of NIDDM may result from differences in the ethnic and racial makeup of the populations inhabiting the countries listed in Fig. 3-1 and Table 3-1. These differences are evidenced by the observation that large variations exist in the prevalence of NIDDM in different groups living within countries. Fig. 3-2 shows the prevalence of NIDDM in ethnic and racial groups living in the United States, Australia, Fiji, and Singapore, using WHO criteria for the diagnosis.[1,6,11,46] In the United States, NIDDM prevalence is lowest in Caucasians (non-Hispanic whites), elevated in the African-American and Hispanic-American communities, and highest in the Native-American population. Likewise, Australian Caucasians have a lower prevalence of NIDDM than Australian aboriginals. This suggests that standard of living may determine prevalence of NIDDM, since the previous comparisons indicate that groups with a lower standard of living have higher rates of diabetes. In Fiji and Singapore, however, the Indian ethnic population has a higher prevalence of NIDDM compared with other ethnic and racial groups (i.e., Melanesian, Malay, Chinese), but Indian ethnic groups have a relatively high standard of living. In terms of annual incidence data, Caucasian rates range from one to four new cases per 1000 population.* Hispanic

*References 6, 7, 31, 69, 111.

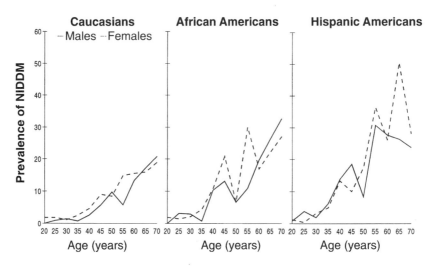

Fig. 3-3 Age-specific prevalence of NIDDM in Caucasians, African Americans, and Hispanic Americans living in the United States. (Data from King H, Rewers M, WHO Ad Hoc Diabetes Reporting Group: *Diabetes Care* 16:157-177, 1993.)

Americans have two to seven times greater incidence rates than non-Hispanic white Americans.[6,31] These data suggest that the differences by ethnic and racial groups in NIDDM prevalence and incidence are caused by differences in genetic makeup and behavioral practices of these ethnic and racial groups, which should be further explored using analytic epidemiologic tools.

Age

Fig. 3-3 displays the age-specific prevalence of NIDDM for Caucasians, African Americans and Hispanic Americans.[46] The prevalence of NIDDM is highest in individuals over age 50. African Americans and Hispanic Americans have a higher prevalence at all ages, but particularly in the earlier ages (before age 50) when compared with U.S. Caucasians, suggesting these groups may have an earlier age at onset of the disease. In most populations, NIDDM incidence is low before age 30 and increases rapidly with older age. In high-risk populations, however, incidence of NIDDM is substantially higher in younger persons when compared with lower-risk populations. Limited incidence data suggest that U.S. ethnic minority groups have a higher incidence of NIDDM at younger ages when compared with U.S. (non-Hispanic) whites.[6,31,58] Incidence data from Colorado[6] and Texas[31] demonstrate that NIDDM risk in Hispanics ages 20 to 39 is equal to, if not higher than, that in Caucasians who are 20 years older (Fig. 3-4).

Gender

Figs. 3-1 to 3-3 demonstrate the prevalence of NIDDM by gender varies in all countries, by ethnic groups, and possibly in different age-groups. In many populations, including the U.S.

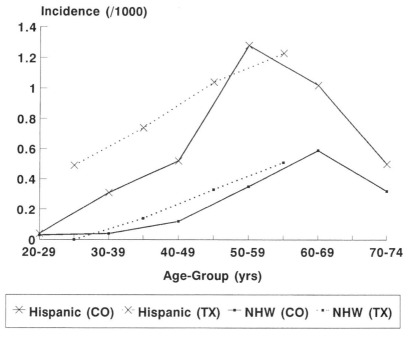

Fig. 3-4 Age-specific incidence of NIDDM in Hispanics and non-Hispanic whites *(NHW)* in Colorado and Texas. (Data from Baxter J and others: *Ethnic Dis* 3:11-21, 1993; and Haffner SM and others: *Diabetes Care* 14:102-108, 1991.)

minority populations and those in Malaysia, Brazil, Columbia, South Africa, and Japan, females have a slightly higher prevalence and incidence of NIDDM than males* (see Figs. 3-1 and 3-2 and Table 3-1). Alternatively, in the populations of Sri Lanka, Tunisia, Italy, India, and Australia, NIDDM is more predominant in males.[11,46] The reported gender differences in prevalence and incidence of NIDDM are small and inconsistent. These differences are most likely the result of known gender differences in exposure to other risk factors, such as physical activity and diet, as described under analytic epidemiology.

Time

The prevalence and incidence of NIDDM has increased rapidly over time in some but not all populations,[8,106,113] including Pima Indians[52] and even in Eskimos,[88] who were once thought to be largely immune to NIDDM.[107] The prevalence in Pima Indians has increased steadily since regular measurements were started in 1965, and the incidence has also increased except for a slight reduction in females between 1982 and 1990.[53] The lowest prevalence among the Native-American population has been found in the Eskimos, who nonetheless have experienced an increase in prevalence in recent years.[89] The increase in prevalence of NIDDM has been noted in all Native-American communities studied, but most of these studies have

*References 2, 6, 31, 46, 57, 90.

used Indian Health Service data rather than comprehensive surveys. Several studies have been published describing an increase in the prevalence of NIDDM in Chinese populations. The Singapore National Health Survey of 1992[73] showed that the prevalence of NIDDM in the Chinese population had doubled since 1984, from 4% to 8%.

The descriptive epidemiology of NIDDM suggests that both genetic and behavioral and life-style factors play a role in the etiology of NIDDM. Specific factors are explored in the next section.

ANALYTIC EPIDEMIOLOGY OF NIDDM
Study Designs

Analytic epidemiology employs several different study designs to evaluate risk factors for disease, with each design having varying levels of strength. *Cross-sectional studies* survey a single group and collect information about disease and the potential risk factor at the same time. This type of epidemiologic study is limited because one cannot use these data to establish causality, since disease and risk factor are measured at the same time without indication of which appeared first. In *case-control,* or *retrospective, studies,* individuals with and without disease are asked questions about their past, particularly their exposure to the risk factor in question. This type of study is valuable in situations where the disease outcome is rare. However, when data collection relies on a subject's memory, as it often does, the data are vulnerable to *recall bias,* in which the diseased individual remembers or recalls past events differently than the nondiseased individual. The primary measure of association in retrospective studies is the *odds ratio* (OR), which depicts the likelihood of exposure in the diseased individuals (cases) compared with that in the nondiseased individuals (controls). An OR of 1.0 indicates that no difference exists in exposure between cases and controls, whereas an OR of 2.0, for example, indicates that cases were twice as likely to have been exposed than controls.

A more powerful observational study design is the *prospective,* or *longitudinal, study.* This design identifies and follows individuals initially free of the disease and seeks to establish whether exposure to a particular factor differentiates those who do or do not subsequently develop the disease. Prospective studies require large sample sizes and a substantial amount of follow-up time, which make them costly and sometimes prohibitive to conduct. The common measure of association of a prospective study is the *relative risk* (RR), which is the ratio of the risk of disease in exposed persons over the risk of disease in unexposed persons. An RR of 1.0 indicates that exposed individuals have the same risk of disease as unexposed individuals, and an elevated RR indicates that the exposed individuals had a greater risk of disease than the unexposed individuals.

The most powerful and by far the most labor-intensive epidemiologic study design is the *intervention trial,* in which efforts are made to prevent or delay the onset of the disease by manipulating risk factors. In this design an initially healthy cohort is randomly assigned to receive either the intervention or no intervention. Follow-up of the two groups over time determines whether the groups differ in the development of disease.

To reduce the cost of prospective observational and interventional studies, investigators may choose to follow a high-risk population rather than the general population. For example, individuals with IGT have a high risk of developing NIDDM[112] in the future. This means that fewer of them need to be followed and that they do not need to be followed as long to obtain enough cases of disease to analyze study results properly, thus substantially reducing the cost.

Indirect Evidence for Environmental Risk Factors

A classic epidemiologic study design is the *migration study,* which compares disease rates in populations who remain in their homeland with populations who have migrated to a region with different exposure and disease rates. This is an attempt to determine how much influence a change in environment (and behavior) has on genetically similar populations. Migrants to a different environment invariably change their life-styles. Many examples now indicate that migrants show a marked difference in the prevalence of NIDDM compared with the native population.[100] Migration studies found that individuals who left their homeland and migrated to a more westernized environment developed more NIDDM than those who remained in their traditional environment.[45,54,84] For example, a migration study by Kawate and others[45] compared Japanese living in Hiroshima with those who migrated to Hawaii. Despite the similar genetic background, the prevalence of diabetes was almost two times higher in Japanese Hawaiians than in those in Hiroshima.

Secular changes in the prevalence and incidence of diabetes have occurred over a short time, as discussed previously. These are well documented among the Pima Indians and have almost certainly been experienced by other populations, such as Micronesians and Polynesians as well as other Native-American peoples.[9,87] In addition, less dramatic but persuasive changes have occurred in the frequency of NIDDM in countries as diverse as the United States and Japan over the course of a few decades. Such changes over a short time cannot be explained by changes in genetic susceptibility. Both these lines of evidence point to the importance of environmental factors or changes in life-style as important determinants of the appearance of NIDDM.

Behavioral and Life-style Factors
Obesity

NIDDM occurs more frequently among obese persons, but not all obese persons, even very obese ones, develop NIDDM. The development of obesity most likely is one of the factors responsible for the high prevalence of NIDDM in populations who have migrated from low- to high-NIDDM-risk areas. In addition, the increasing incidence of NIDDM over time in some populations is accompanied by increasing frequency of obesity. In epidemiologic studies, body mass index (BMI) is used as a marker of obesity and is calculated in the following manner: weight (kg)/height (m)^2. Based on cross-sectional studies of diabetes prevalence in several populations, West[107] showed that obesity was closely correlated with the prevalence of diabetes. Since that time, numerous cross-sectional and retrospective studies have shown that obesity, as measured by BMI, is associated with NIDDM prevalence.[1,11,57] However, the evaluation of the relationship between NIDDM and obesity is confounded because NIDDM, when untreated, results in weight loss. Furthermore, because diet treatment to achieve weight loss is a major therapeutic modality, assessment of associations between obesity and NIDDM using known cases of NIDDM, as is done in cross-sectional and retrospective studies, is fraught with difficulty. Therefore the most rigorous study design to evaluate these associations is the prospective study, which measures obesity before the development of NIDDM.

All prospective studies that have examined the question of whether obesity is associated with NIDDM risk have shown consistently higher incidence rates among obese compared with nonobese persons. A positive association between obesity, as measured by BMI, and future NIDDM has been found in studies of diverse populations, such as female nurses in the United States,[16] Israeli civil servants,[67] Swedish men,[77] Nauruans,[4] Pima Indians,[50] U.S. Hispanics,[32,34] male health professionals,[14] National Health And Nutrition Examination Survey-1 (NHANES-1) population (United States),[58] and U.S. veterans.[112] The risk of NIDDM in persons with a BMI of 35 or higher was 42 to 58 times greater than that of persons with a BMI less than 23.[14,16] Colditz and colleagues[16] calculated that within their cohort, 90.4% of all diagnoses of diabetes could be attributed to a BMI greater than 22, showing that obesity could be an important factor for which to intervene to prevent NIDDM.

The duration of obesity and the age at which one becomes obese may also be important risk factors for NIDDM. Several studies have found a weak positive association between BMI in early adulthood and subsequent NIDDM.[14,16,70] In addition, the Israeli study found a significant relationship between maximum lifetime weight/height ratio and NIDDM prevalence independent of current BMI.[70] In Pima Indians, for subjects who attained a BMI of at least 30, the duration of obesity increased NIDDM risk from 24.8:1000 person-years for 0 to 5 years of obesity to 35.2 for 5 to 10 years and to 59.8 for 10 or more years of obesity, adjusted for age, gender, and current BMI. It appears that the incidence of NIDDM in the group with the highest degree of obesity in early adulthood is much higher than in those who were less obese in early adulthood.[23] Interestingly, Lipton and co-workers[58] found that at nearly every level of BMI, African Americans had a higher risk of diabetes than whites, suggesting that factors other than obesity contributed to risk.[8] This was also seen in a comparative study of Japanese in Hiroshima, Japan, and Hawaii. Although the Hawaiian Japanese were more obese than their counterparts in Hiroshima, the prevalence of NIDDM in the Hawaiian Japanese was greater at all degrees of obesity.[45] Furthermore, differences in the prevalence of NIDDM in some Pacific Islanders are only partially explained by differences in the current degree of obesity.[11] Thus factors other than obesity, as measured by BMI, apparently play a role in determining the risk of developing NIDDM.

Measures of *fat patterning* that describe the distribution of obesity are also thought to be important in predicting NIDDM. Examples of measures of fat patterning used in epidemiologic studies are waist/hip ratios (i.e., the ratio of the abdominal circumference to hip circumference) and subscapular/triceps ratios (i.e., the ratio of the subscapular skinfold thickness [mm] to that of the triceps), and these are used to determine upper versus lower body obesity (i.e., apple versus pear shape). Associations between upper body obesity and NIDDM were found in both cross-sectional[1,36,57,105] and prospective* studies. Studies have investigated whether body composition (i.e., where the fat is distributed) is a more powerful predictor of NIDDM than BMI. In a cross-sectional study, Dowse and others[21] found that

*References 12, 14, 32, 58, 76.

although BMI and waist/hip ratio were independent risk factors for NIDDM, waist/hip ratio conveyed relatively stronger risks for NIDDM than BMI in women. Prospectively, individuals in the highest tertile of the waist/hip ratio had a 2.4-fold greater risk of NIDDM compared with those in the lower two tertiles of waist/hip ratio, independent of their BMI.[12] Lipton and co-workers[58] found that as the subscapular/triceps ratio increased, NIDDM risk increased, independent of BMI. Longitudinal studies have shown that as persons age, both weight gain and increased waist circumference occur, and among older persons who lose weight over time, waist circumference continues to increase.[96] Such trends may partially account for the increased NIDDM seen with aging.

Obesity and fat patterning therefore may be frequent precipitants of NIDDM in persons who are otherwise susceptible to its development. Although NIDDM clearly develops in persons who are not obese, obesity definitely is a major risk factor and perhaps the most important factor amenable to change. However, the mechanism by which obesity increases the risk of NIDDM is not certain. Several models are possible for the relationship of NIDDM and obesity: (1) obesity precedes NIDDM and is in the etiologic pathway; (2) a similar genetic predisposition leads to both obesity and NIDDM, and these two factors play no role in each other's etiology; and (3) a similar genetic predisposition leads to both, and additional factors (genetic or environmental) differentiate between NIDDM and obesity. Finally, it is unclear whether obesity itself or whether factors that lead to obesity (e.g., physical activity, diet) are more important risk factors for NIDDM.

Diet

Diet has long been believed to play a role in the development of diabetes, particularly since obesity is so closely associated with NIDDM. Most of the studied populations who have migrated from a traditional environment (e.g., Polynesians and Micronesians in the Pacific) and who have higher prevalences of diabetes than found in their countries of origin consume diets that contain much higher quantities of refined carbohydrates than in the traditional environment. In studies comparing Mexican Americans in San Antonio with Mexicans in Mexico City and comparing the Pima Indians of Arizona with a population of Pima ancestry living in Mexico, each found differences in NIDDM prevalence in their genetically similar populations living in different environments.[84,95] Both studies found that the low-prevalence population was consuming less fat and more carbohydrates than the high-prevalence population, suggesting a role for diet in the etiology of NIDDM. Cross-sectional and retrospective studies have been inconsistent in documenting a convincing relationship between dietary intake and NIDDM. In a cross-sectional study, Marshall and colleagues[64] reported an OR of 1.5 for a 40 g/day increase of dietary fat intake among persons with NIDDM compared with nondiabetic individuals, suggesting a 50% increase in NIDDM risk in persons with higher fat intake. Two case-control studies have observed similar associations between dietary fat intake and NIDDM status.[40,103]

Few attempts have been made to perform prospective studies on the relationship between the risk of developing NIDDM and dietary intake. Over a 5-year period, the Israeli heart study found no effect of diet or its components on the incidence of diabetes among men.[43] During a 12-year follow-up in Sweden, no association between dietary fat/low carbohydrate intake and incidence of NIDDM was seen in 1462 women.[60] Likewise, no association between dietary fat intake and NIDDM was found for the incidence of NIDDM in 841 men in the Netherlands in a 25-year follow-up.[24] Marshall and others[66] followed 134 persons with IGT for the development of NIDDM over 2 years. In these individuals a 40 g/day increase in dietary fat intake was associated with a sixfold increased risk of NIDDM, independent of energy intake. A study of Japanese Americans has reported similar associations with a 5-year follow-up of 66 persons with IGT.[104] Among 187 Pima Indian women, who were initially ages 25 to 44 and without diabetes, an increased total and complex carbohydrate intake, but not fat intake, was found among the 87 who subsequently developed the disease.[10] Unfortunately, these analyses of the Pima population were not adjusted for obesity, total caloric intake, weight gain, and other factors, making it impossible to determine whether this is an independent association. Because total and complex carbohydrate intake is highly negatively correlated with fat intake, it would be unwise to conclude that carbohydrate intake is more important to NIDDM risk than dietary fat intake.

Only one study has examined the effects of dietary intervention on the incidence of diabetes among subjects with IGT.[87] This Swedish study showed that the incidence of diabetes among those given dietary advice (reduction of total caloric and carbohydrate intake) was significantly lower over a 10-year period. Although methodologic inconsistencies limit the interpretation of this study, the findings suggest that advice to moderate diet may have an effect on the incidence of diabetes in this high-risk population.

Recent studies have examined the relationship between alcohol intake and NIDDM.[41,42,57,93] Prevalence studies from South Africa, Mauritius, Kiribati, and Nauru have shown that alcohol consumption was similar in individuals with and without NIDDM.[41,57] In Rancho Bernardo in southern California, males who reported high use (176 g/week or more) of alcohol had double the incidence of NIDDM compared with men who drank less alcohol after adjustment for other risk factors, although men who drank no alcohol had higher rates than drinkers of small amounts of alcohol. Among women in this study, nondrinkers had the highest rates of NIDDM.[42] Consistent findings were reported from a 4-year follow-up study of 85,000 female nurses, in which a decreased risk of developing diabetes with increased alcohol intake was found, independent of obesity.[93] The risk of developing diabetes was reduced by 50% among those whose alcohol intake exceeded 15 g/day compared with that in nondrinkers. This apparent protective effect of alcohol intake on NIDDM risk should be explored further because it is a behavior most likely amenable to modification. However, encouraging alcohol consumption, particularly in populations at high risk for alcohol abuse, has obvious ethical problems.

Physical activity

Ecologic studies from the South Pacific[109,114,115] and from Mexico City and San Antonio, Texas,[95] suggest that population differences in NIDDM prevalence may be explained by differences in physical activity, since those populations with higher levels of habitual physical activity consistently had lower levels of NIDDM. Cross-sectional and retrospective studies have generally found that groups of individuals with NIDDM are currently less active than those without the disease.* A study in Fiji examined the prevalence of diabetes among those performing moderate or heavy activity compared with those considered sedentary or undertaking only light activities. The prevalence of diabetes was twice as high in those with the lower degrees of physical activity.[102] Pima Indians with diabetes reported less physical activity over their lifetime than those without diabetes.[55] Using the NHANES-1 baseline data, significantly less physical activity was detected in persons with NIDDM compared with nondiabetic individuals.[15] In these studies, however, physical activity was reported after the known onset of NIDDM, and activity level could have been the result of diabetes rather than the cause. The prevalence of diabetes among women who had participated in athletic programs while in college was half that of women who had not.[26] This association could also be related to the fact that the women who had been athletes in college also tended to remain more active in later years, so the effect of current physical activity on NIDDM outcome cannot be discounted.

The most informative studies are prospective in design, with measurement of activity levels before NIDDM onset. Manson and others[61] followed 87,253 women of the Nurses's Health Study cohort for 8 years, using self-reported NIDDM as the end point. They found a relative risk of 0.83 for women who reported at least weekly physical activity versus those with less activity. In addition, a dose-response relationship, in which levels of a factor differentially influence the risk of disease, was not observed with different amounts of exercise and NIDDM risk.[61] A study of male physicians found that after 5 years of follow-up, those who reported engaging in vigorous exercise at least once a week were found to have a lower incidence of self-reported NIDDM (RR = 0.7). This study indicated evidence of a dose-response relationship, and the greatest effect was seen in men who were more overweight.[63] The NHANES Epidemiologic Follow-up Study found that persons reporting a high physical activity level had a decreased risk of NIDDM compared with those reporting a low physical activity level (RR = 0.78).[58] In a study with 15 years of follow-up of male college alumni, leisure-time physical activity, expressed in kilocalories (kcal), was inversely related to the development of NIDDM.[39] With each 2000 kcal increase in energy expenditure, the risk of NIDDM was reduced by 24% (RR = 0.76). Similar to a previous study,[63] this effect was greatest in the more obese men, and no effect was noted among lean men.[39]

Although the results of these prospective epidemiologic studies suggest a causal relationship between physical inactivity and NIDDM, the strength of their findings is weakened because diabetes is determined by self-reporting. Nonetheless, the consistent findings of the prospective studies suggest that physical activity is a good candidate for modification in the prevention of NIDDM.

Parity and pregnancy

During pregnancy, glucose tolerance is decreased. Some women who have not previously had glucose intolerance develop it and are diagnosed with diabetes, or in this case, gestational

---

*References 1, 15, 26, 27, 54, 55, 101, 102.

diabetes. In the postpartum period, glucose tolerance frequently reverts to normal, but many of these women will develop diabetes in later years.[79] Thus previously diagnosed gestational diabetes is considered a strong predictor of NIDDM.

Retrospective studies have found both positive[9,97] and no[92,114] associations between increasing parity and risk of NIDDM in women. A positive association between increased parity and NIDDM was found in the prospective Rancho Bernardo study.[56] This association was independent of current BMI, suggesting that parity may have an effect on diabetes risk beyond that of increasing the risk of obesity in these women. In contrast, a large prospective study of nurses found that the association between parity and NIDDM risk was not independent of BMI.[62] An examination of data from four Pacific and Indian Ocean island populations showed inconsistent relationships between number of full-term pregnancies and the prevalence of NIDDM. In each population a higher prevalence of NIDDM was found in women with 10 or more pregnancies compared with women with one to three pregnancies, but this was not independent of BMI.[17]

The intrauterine environment may influence subsequent development of NIDDM.[80,81] In Pima Indians, NIDDM occurs much more frequently in persons whose mothers were diabetic during the pregnancy compared with persons whose mothers were nondiabetic during pregnancy but who subsequently developed the disease.[81]

Birth size

It has been proposed that persons who are thin at birth are at an increased lifetime risk of NIDDM.[32] This association exists independent of other risk factors for NIDDM. The initial interpretation of this association was that poor fetal nutrition led to poor development of the insulin-producing beta cells and their dysfunction later in life.[32,82,83] An alternative explanation is that low birth weight and low ponderal index at birth reflect an intrauterine infection affecting pancreatic beta cells, and that the increased incidence of NIDDM in persons with low birth weight reflects a latent beta-cell defect. Another possibility is that low-birth-weight infants may be overfed after birth, thus increasing their risk of NIDDM.

Socioeconomic status

In India, NIDDM prevalence was strongly related to per capita income and was highest in those with professional occupations.[9] In contrast, in the United States the prevalence of diabetes, as ascertained by questionnaires in the National Health Interview Survey, is greater in those with lower income levels and less education.[22] One or more years of college education was associated with a 30% reduction in risk of NIDDM compared with less than a high-school education, independent of other risk factors of NIDDM.[18] Similarly, Lipton and colleagues[58] found that having less than 9 years of education increased risk of NIDDM by more than 60% compared with those with at least a college education. Obesity is more common among less affluent persons in the United States, and obesity may be driving the association observed between socioeconomic status and NIDDM. In rural San Luis Valley, Colorado, however, lower income was associated with higher prevalence of NIDDM, independent of measures of obesity and fat patterning.[65] In addition, an interaction occurred between the effects of education and ethnicity; Hispanics with less than a high-school education had 3.6 times the diabetes prevalence of non-Hispanic whites, whereas Hispanics with a high-school education or greater had no excess risk compared with non-Hispanic whites, independent of obesity and other relevant risk factors.[65] Differences in physical activity and diet might also be responsible for the association between socioeconomic status and NIDDM. Other related factors, including urbanization and acculturation, are discussed next.

Urbanization

Studies of the consequences of habitation in a rural compared with an urban environment also support the hypothesis of an environmental factor for NIDDM.[19,48,54,115] In general, urban residents have higher NIDDM rates than rural dwellers.[11] In Kiribati, a Central Pacific nation, the age-standardized prevalence of diabetes in urban residents was more than twice that of rural residents.[54] In South Africa, spending greater than 40% of one's life in the city was significantly associated with the prevalence of NIDDM, independent of age and measures of obesity.[57] A number of life-style factors implicated in the etiology of NIDDM (e.g., sedentary life-style, high-fat diet, obesity) are associated with urban life.

Acculturation

It has been postulated that as persons from a very traditional society become westernized, NIDDM risk increases. This is suggested by ecologic data comparing an area of Mexico City with San Antonio, Texas.[94] Prevalence and incidence of NIDDM have increased quickly in populations undergoing rapid westernization.[8,106,113] Such changes were also documented in Native Americans,[52] including Eskimos,[88] who were once thought to be largely immune to NIDDM.[107] The westernization transition is usually accompanied by increases in obesity, decreases in physical activity, and alterations in dietary intake toward more calories and fat and less complex carbohydrates. However, with further cultural assimilation, increased leisure-time physical activity and decreased dietary fat intake begin to be adopted, leading to inversion of the relationship between westernization and NIDDM. This transition has been observed in San Antonio, where the most acculturated Hispanics have the lowest NIDDM risk, and the least acculturated barrio Hispanics have the highest NIDDM risk, even higher than that found in their native Mexico.[38,94,95]

Evidence for Genetic Factors

A strong genetic predisposition to NIDDM was suggested by evidence from three areas of investigation: (1) race/ethnicity studies, (2) family history studies, and (3) twin studies. Box 3-2 summarizes the lifetime risk of NIDDM by degree of relatedness to someone with NIDDM.

Racial admixture

Studies of populations that are derived from racial groups who differ in NIDDM risk provide indirect evidence for the genetic factors in NIDDM. For instance, Hispanics in the southwestern United States share genes of Native Americans, who have one of the highest NIDDM rates in the world,[8,107] and genes of European Caucasians, who are at a much lower

---

BOX 3-2

LIFETIME RISK OF NIDDM BY DEGREE OF RELATEDNESS TO SOMEONE WITH NIDDM

- 70%-90% for a monozygotic twin
- 15% for a first-degree relative
- 5% for a second-degree relative
- 3% for a third-degree relative

Data from Rich SS: *Diabetes* 39:1315-1319, 1990.

---

risk. If one plots NIDDM risk by level of Native-American genetic admixture in Hispanic Americans, an almost linear positive association appears.[28,51] Similar findings are seen in South Pacific populations[47,91] and in Australian aborigines with Caucasian-aboriginal admixture.[110] At the population level these studies provide support for the hypothesis that genes present in high-risk populations are associated with NIDDM risk and that their effects are also seen in admixed populations.

Family history

Presence of NIDDM in a family member is an established risk factor for NIDDM. Pima Indians[51] and Caucasians[3,78] with at least one diabetic parent have a much higher incidence of NIDDM than those who are equally obese but do not have a diabetic parent. However, family history data are limited because they may be subject to biased or inaccurate reporting by the person who has diabetes. Ideally, all family members should be tested to confirm diabetes status to obtain an accurate measure of family history.

Twin studies

Studies of twins suggest that NIDDM is highly concordant among monozygous (MZ) twins and less so among dizygous (DZ) twins. Studies have found a diabetes concordance in MZ twins ranging from 34% to 100%.* A twin study of U.S. veterans[75] reported concordance rates of 58% for MZ twins and 17% for DZ twins. Similar rates were reported in a Danish study.[37] Twin studies indicate that genetic factors play a major role in the etiology of NIDDM. These studies also support a role for nongenetic factors, since the concordance is less than 100%.

Thrifty genotype hypothesis

The thrifty genotype hypothesis was developed primarily to explain the rapid increase in diabetes in certain populations undergoing westernization. It is hypothesized that in populations regularly subjected to cycles of feast and famine, the presence of the "thrifty

---

*References 5, 20, 29, 37, 44, 59, 75, 99.

genotype," which causes rapid deposition of fat, would have conferred a survival advantage during the famines.[74] Genetic mixing, as would have continuously occurred in Europe and the Middle East, would have ameliorated the genetic effects of feast and famine by diluting the thrifty genotype, but in isolated areas, such as the Pacific islands (particularly Nauru, which is very isolated), the potential for famines to promote the prevalence of the thrifty genotype is high. As populations still possessing the thrifty genotype underwent westernization and experienced a state of virtually continuous "feast," obesity would rise as the thrifty genotype rapidly deposited fat. This situation is worsened because these populations are decreasing their physical activity at the same time. Thus populations with the thrifty genotype are likely to experience excess obesity and NIDDM as a result of westernization.

Gene-environment interaction

Although it has been postulated for some time that diet, physical activity, and other environmental factors operate on a susceptible genotype, few studies have explored this directly. Twin studies found that male MZ twins who were discordant for NIDDM had no differences in diet composition,[75] suggesting that differences in dietary intake did not explain why one twin had NIDDM and the other did not.

A crude way to examine gene-environment interaction is to stratify risk factor analysis by whether or not individuals have a family history of NIDDM. The theory is that those with a family history are more genetically susceptible to the disease compared with those without a family history of NIDDM. Manson and colleagues[63] stratified their large prospective study of physical activity and incidence of NIDDM in U.S. male physicians by presence of family history of diabetes and found no differences in effects. In addition, the San Luis Valley Diabetes Study cohort was also stratified in this manner, and no difference was found in the effect of fat intake among persons with and without a family history of diabetes.[64] In a large cross-sectional study of 32,662 white women, however, obesity and family history of diabetes had a positive synergistic (multiplicative) effect.[72]

With the recent advances in molecular biology, definitions of genetic susceptibility are rapidly being refined, which will assist in the analysis of gene-environment interactions. Given the observed effect of both genetic and environmental factors in the risk of NIDDM, future epidemiologic studies should take into account genetic makeup when assessing the importance of a particular environmental factor, and vice versa.

SUMMARY

This chapter has addressed only those aspects of NIDDM related to its prevalence, incidence, and risk factors. The descriptive and analytic epidemiology of NIDDM suggests that it is a heterogeneous disorder caused by behavioral and genetic factors. The role of physical inactivity, dietary fat intake, and obesity in the etiology of NIDDM is established, and these factors are likely candidates for use in intervention studies. It remains to be elucidated how these behavioral factors interact with genetic factors to produce diabetes at the individual and population levels. In the future, based on knowledge of the determinants of the disease and of the risk factors, it may be possible to prevent or delay the development of NIDDM.

REFERENCES

1. Ali O and others: Prevalence of NIDDM and impaired glucose tolerance in aborigines and Malays in Malaysia and their relationship to sociodemographic, health, and nutritional factors, *Diabetes Care* 16:68-75, 1993.

2. Aschner P and others: Glucose intolerance in Colombia, *Diabetes Care* 16(1):90-93, 1993.

3. Baird JD: Diabetes mellitus and obesity, *Proc Nutr Soc* 32:199-204, 1973.

4. Balkau B and others: Factors associated with the development of diabetes in the Micronesian population of Nauru, *Am J Epidemiol* 122:594-605, 1985.

5. Barnett AH and others: Diabetes in identical twins: a study of 200 pairs, *Diabetologia* 20:87-93, 1981.

6. Baxter J and others: Excess incidence of known non-insulin-dependent diabetes mellitus (NIDDM) in Hispanics compared with non-Hispanic whites in the San Luis Valley, Colorado, *Ethnic Dis* 3:11-21, 1993.

7. Bender AP and others: Incidence, prevalence, and mortality of diabetes mellitus in Wadena, Marshall and Grand Rapids, Minnesota: the three city study, *Diabetes Care* 9:343-350, 1986.

8. Bennett PH: Diabetes in developing countries and unusual populations. In Mann JI, Pyorala K, Teuscher A, editors: *Diabetes in epidemiologic perspective,* Edinburgh, 1983, Churchill-Livingstone.

9. Bennett PH, Knowler WC: Increasing prevalence of diabetes in the Pima (American) Indians over a ten-year period. In *International Congress Series No 500: diabetes 1979,* Amsterdam, 1979, Excerpta Medica.

10. Bennett PH and others: Diet and development of diabetes mellitus: An epidemiological perspective. In Pozza B, editor: *Diet, diabetes, and atherosclerosis,* New York, 1984, Raven.

11. Bennett PH and others: Epidemiology and natural history of NIDDM: non-obese and obese. In Alberti KGMM and other editors: *International textbook of diabetes,* New York, 1992, Wiley.

12. Cassano PA and others: Obesity and body fat distribution in relation to the incidence of non-insulin-dependent diabetes mellitus: a prospective cohort study of men in the Normative Aging Study, *Am J Epidemiol* 136:1474-1486, 1992.

13. Catalano PM and others: Longitudinal changes in insulin release and insulin resistance in nonobese pregnant women, *Am J Obstet Gynecol* 165:1667-1672, 1991.

14. Chan JM and others: Obesity, fat distribution, and weight gain as risk factors for clinical diabetes in men, *Diabetes Care* 17:961-969, 1994.

15. Chen MK, Lowenstein FW: Epidemiology of factors related to self-reported diabetes among adults, *Am J Prev Med* 2:14-19, 1986.

16. Colditz GA and others: Weight as a risk factor for clinical diabetes in women, *Am J Epidemiol* 132:501-513, 1990.

17. Collins VR, Dowse GK, Zimmet PZ: Evidence against association between parity and NIDDM from five population groups, *Diabetes Care* 14(11):975-981, 1991.

18. Cowie CC and others: Effect of multiple risk factors on differences between blacks and whites in the prevalence of non-insulin-dependent diabetes mellitus in the United States, *Am J Epidemiol* 137:719-732, 1993.

19. Cruz-Vidal M and others: Factors related to diabetes mellitus in Puerto Rican men, *Diabetes* 28:300-307, 1979.

20. Diabetes mellitus in twins: a cooperative study in Japan, Committee on Diabetic Twins, Japan Diabetes Society, *Diabetes Res Clin Pract* 5:271-280, 1988.

21. Dowse GK and others: Abdominal obesity and physical inactivity as risk factors for NIDDM and impaired glucose tolerance in Indian, Creole, and Chinese Mauritians, *Diabetes Care* 14:271-282, 1991.

22. Drury TF, Powell AL: Prevalence of known diabetes among black Americans, *Vital Health Stat* 130:1-13, 1987.

23. Everhart JE and others: Duration of obesity increases the incidence of NIDDM, *Diabetes* 41:235-240, 1992.

24. Feskens EJM, Kromhout D: Cardiovascular risk factors and the 25-year incidence of diabetes mellitus in middle-aged men, *Am J Epidemiol* 130:1101-1108, 1989.

25. Friedman CI, Richards S, Kim MH: Familial acanthosis nigricans: a longitudinal study, *J Reprod Med* 32:531-536, 1987.

26. Frisch RE and others: Lower prevalence of diabetes in female former college athletes compared with nonathletes, *Diabetes* 35:1101-1105, 1986.

27. Fulton-Kehoe D and others: Physical activity and the risk of non-insulin dependent diabetes mellitus (NIDDM): the San Luis Valley Diabetes Study, *Ann Epidemiol,* 1995 (in press).

28. Gardner LI and others: Prevalence of diabetes in Mexican Americans: relationship to percent of gene pool derived from Native American genetic admixture, *Diabetes* 33:86-92, 1984.

29. Gottlieb MS, Root HF: Diabetes mellitus in twins, *Diabetes* 17:693-704, 1968.

30. Haffner SM and others: Incidence of type II diabetes in Mexican Americans predicted by fasting insulin and glucose levels, obesity, and body-fat distribution, *Diabetes* 39:283-288, 1990.

31. Haffner SM and others: Increased incidence of type II diabetes mellitus in Mexican-Americans, *Diabetes Care* 14:102-108, 1991.

32. Hales CN, Barker DJ: Type 2 (non-insulin-dependent) diabetes mellitus: the thrifty phenotype hypothesis, *Diabetologia* 35:595-601, 1992.

33. Hamman RF: Genetic and environmental determinants of non-insulin-dependent diabetes mellitus (NIDDM), *Diabetes Metab Rev* 8:287-338, 1992.

34. Hamman RF and others: Non-insulin-dependent diabetes (NIDDM) risk in persons with impaired glucose tolerance (IGT): role of insulin, obesity, and fat patterning: the San Luis Valley Diabetes Study, *Diabetes* 39(75A):297, 1990 (abstract).

35. Harris MI and others: International criteria for the diagnosis of diabetes mellitus and impaired glucose tolerance, *Diabetes Care* 8:562-567, 1985.

36. Hartz AJ, Rupley DC, Rimm AA: The association of girth measurements with disease in 32,856 women, *Am J Epidemiol* 119:71-80, 1984.

37. Harvald B, Hauge M: Selection in diabetes in modern society, *Acta Med Scand* 173:459-465, 1963.

38. Hazuda HP and others: Effects of acculturation and socioeconomic status on obesity and diabetes in Mexican-Americans: the San Antonio Heart Study, *Am J Epidemiol* 128:1289-1301, 1988.

39. Helmrich SP, Ragland DR, Paffenbarger RS Jr: Prevention of non-insulin-dependent diabetes mellitus with physical activity, *Med Sci Sports Exerc* 26:824-830, 1994.

40. Himsworth HP, Marshall EM: The diet of diabetics prior to the onset of the disease, *Clin Sci* 2:95-115, 1935.

41. Hodge AM and others: Abnormal glucose tolerance and alcohol consumption in three populations at high risk of non-insulin-dependent diabetes mellitus, (published erratum appears in *Am J Epidemiol* 138[4]:279) *Am J Epidemiol* 137:178-189, 1993.

42. Holbrook TL, Barrett-Connor E, Wingard DL: A prospective population-based study of alcohol use and non-insulin-dependent diabetes mellitus, *Am J Epidemiol* 132:902-909, 1990.

43. Kahn HA and others: Factors related to diabetes incidence: a multivariate analysis of two years observation on 10,000 men: the Israel Ischemic Heart Disease Study, *J Chronic Dis* 23:617-629, 1971.

44. Kaprio J and others: Incidence of diabetes in the nationwide panel of 13,888 twin pairs in Finland, *Diabetologia* 33(suppl A):57, 1990 (abstract).

45. Kawate R and others: Diabetes mellitus and its vascular complications in Japanese migrants and on the island of Hawaii, *Diabetes Care* 2:161-170, 1979.

46. King H, Rewers M, WHO Ad Hoc Diabetes Reporting Group: Global estimates for prevalence of diabetes mellitus and impaired glucose tolerance in adults, *Diabetes Care* 16:157-177, 1993.

47. King H and others: Glucose tolerance and ancestral genetic admixture in six semitraditional Pacific populations, *Genet Epidemiol* 1:315-328, 1984.

48. King H and others: Risk factors for diabetes in three Pacific populations, *Am J Epidemiol* 119:396-409, 1984.

49. Knowler WC and others: Diabetes incidence and prevalence in Pima Indians: a 19-fold greater incidence than in Rochester, Minnesota, *Am J Epidemiol* 108:497-505, 1978.

50. Knowler WC and others: Diabetes in Pima Indians: contributions of obesity and parental diabetes, *Am J Epidemiol* 113:144-156, 1981.

51. Knowler WC and others: Gm 3, 5, 13, 14 and type 2 diabetes mellitus: an association in American Indians with genetic admixture, *Am J Hum Genet* 43:520-526, 1988.

52. Knowler WC and others: Determinants of diabetes mellitus in the Pima Indians, *Diabtes Care* 16:216-227, 1993.

53. Kriska AM, Blair SN, Periera MA: The potential role of physical activity in the prevention of non-insulin-dependent diabetes mellitus: the epidemiological evidence, *Exerc Sport Sci Rev* 22:121-143, 1994.

54. Kriska AM and others: The association of physical activity with obesity, fat distribution and glucose intolerance in Pima Indians, *Diabetologia* 36:863-869, 1993.

55. Kritz-Silverstein D, Barrett-Connor E, Wingard DL: The effect of parity on the later development of non-insulin-dependent diabetes mellitus or impaired glucose tolerance, *N Engl J Med* 321:1214-1219, 1989.

56. Levitt NS and others: The prevalence and identification of risk factors for NIDDM in urban Africans in Cape Town, South Africa, *Diabetes Care* 16:601-607, 1993.

57. Lipton RB and others: Determinants of incident non-insulin-dependent diabetes mellitus among blacks and whites in a national sample: the NHANES I follow-up study, *Am J Epidemiol* 138:826-839, 1993.

58. Lo SS and others: Studies of diabetic twins, *Diabetes Metab Rev* 7:223-238, 1991.

59. Lundgren H and others: Dietary habits and incidence of noninsulin-dependent diabetes mellitus in

a population study of women in Gothenburg, Sweden, *Am J Clin Nutr* 49:708-712, 1989.

60. Manson JE and others: Physical activity and incidence of non-insulin-dependent diabetes mellitus in women, *Lancet* 338:774-778, 1991.

61. Manson JE and others: Parity and incidence of non-insulin-dependent diabetes mellitus, *Am J Med* 93:13-18, 1992.

62. Manson JE and others: A prospective study of exercise and incidence of diabetes among US male physicians, *JAMA* 268:63-67, 1992.

63. Marshall JA, Hamman RF, Baxter J: High fat, low carbohydrate diet and the etiology of non-insulin-dependent diabetes mellitus: the San Luis Valley Diabetes Study, *Am J Epidemiol* 134:590-603, 1991.

64. Marshall JA and others: Ethnic differences in risk factors associated with the prevalence of non-insulin-dependent diabetes mellitus: the San Luis Valley Diabetes Study, *Am J Epidemiol* 137:706-718, 1993.

65. Marshall JA and others: Dietary fat predicts conversion from impaired glucose tolerance to NIDDM: the San Luis Valley Diabetes Study, *Diabetes Care* 17:50-56, 1994.

66. Medalie JH and others: Diabetes mellitus among 10,000 adult men. I. Five-year incidence and associated variables, *Isr J Med Sci* 10:681-697, 1974.

67. Melton LJ, Palumbo PJ, Chu C: Incidence of diabetes by clinical type, *Diabetes Care* 6:75-86, 1983.

68. Michaelis D, Jutzi E, Albrecht G: Prevalence and incidence trends of non-insulin-dependent diabetes mellitus (NIDDM) in the population of the GDR, *Dtsch Z Verdau Stoffwechselkr* 47:301-310, 1987.

69. Modan M and others: Effect of past and concurrent body mass index on prevalence of glucose intolerance and type 2 (non-insulin-dependent) diabetes and on insulin response: the Israel study of glucose intolerance, obesity and hypertension, *Diabetologia* 29:82-89, 1986.

70. Moller DE, Flier JS: Insulin resistance: mechanisms, syndromes, and implications, *N Engl J Med* 325:938-948, 1991.

71. Morris RD and others: Obesity and heredity in the etiology of non-insulin-dependent diabetes mellitus in 32,662 adult white women, *Am J Epidemiol* 130:112-121, 1989.

72. *National Health Survey 1992,* Research and Evaluation Department, Singapore, 1992, Ministry of Health.

73. Neel JV: The thrifty genotype revisited. In Kobberling J, Tattersall R, editors: *The genetics of diabetes mellitus,* London, 1982, Academic Press.

74. Newman B and others: Concordance for type 2 (non-insulin-dependent) diabetes mellitus in male twins, *Diabetologia* 30:763-768, 1987.

75. Ohlson LO and others: The influence of body fat distribution on the incidence of diabetes mellitus: 13.5 years of follow-up of the participants in the study of men born in 1913, *Diabetes* 34:1055-1058, 1985.

76. Ohlson LO and others: Diabetes mellitus in Swedish middle-aged men, *Diabetologia* 30:386-393, 1987.

77. O'Sullivan JB, Mahan CM: Blood sugar levels, glycosuria, and body weight related to development of diabetes mellitus, *J Am Med Assoc* 194:117-122, 1965.

78. O'Sullivan JB, Mahan CM: Prospective study of 352 young patients with chemical diabetes, *N Engl J Med* 278:1038, 1968.

79. Pettitt DJ and others: Congenital susceptibility to NIDDM: role of intrauterine environment, *Diabetes* 37:622-628, 1988.

80. Pettitt DJ and others: Diabetes and obesity in the offspring of Pima Indian women with diabetes during pregnancy, *Diabetes Care* 16:310-314, 1993.

81. Phillips DI and others: Thinness at birth and insulin resistance in adult life, *Diabetologia* 37:150-154, 1994.

82. Phipps K and others: Fetal growth and impaired glucose tolerance in men and women, *Diabetologia* 36:225-228, 1993.

83. Ravussin E and others: Effects of a traditional lifestyle on obesity in Pima Indians, *Diabetes Care* 17:1067, 1994.

84. Rich SS: Mapping genes in diabetes: genetic epidemiological perspective, *Diabetes* 39:1315-1319, 1990.

85. Saad MF and others: A two-step model for development of non-insulin-dependent diabetes, *Am J Med* 90:229-235, 1991.

86. Sartor G and others: Ten-year follow-up of subjects with impaired glucose tolerance: prevention of diabetes by tolbutamide and diet regulation, *Diabetes* 29:41-49, 1980.

87. Schraer CD and others: Prevalence of diabetes mellitus in Alaskan Eskimos, Indians, and Aleuts, *Diabetes Care* 11:693-700, 1988.

88. Schraer CD and others: Diabetes prevalence, incidence, and complications among Alaska Natives, 1987, *Diabetes Care* 16:257-259, 1993.

89. Sekikawa A and others: Prevalence of diabetes and impaired glucose tolerance in Funagata area, Japan, *Diabetes Care* 16:570-574, 1993.

90. Serjeantson SW and others: Genetics of diabetes in Nauru: effects of foreign admixture, HLA antigens,

and the insulin-gene-linked polymorphism, *Diabetologia* 25:13-17, 1983.

91. Sicree RA and others: The association of non-insulin-dependent diabetes with parity and stillbirth occurrence amongst five Pacific populations, *Diabetes Res Clin Pract* 2:113-122, 1986.

92. Stampfer MJ and others: A prospective study of moderate alcohol drinking and risk of diabetes in women, *Am J Epidemiol* 128:549-558, 1988.

93. Stern MP and others: Genetic and environmental determinants of type II diabetes in Mexican Americans: is there a "descending limb" to the modernization/diabetes relationship? *Diabetes Care* 14:649-654, 1991.

94. Stern MP and others: Genetic and environmental determinants of type II diabetes in Mexico City and San Antonio, *Diabetes* 41:484-492, 1992.

95. Stevens J and others: Changes in body weight and girths in black and white adults studied over a 25 year interval, *Int J Obes* 15:803-808, 1991.

96. Swai ABM and others: Diabetes and impaired glucose tolerance in an Asian community in Tanzania, *Diabetes Res Clin Pract* 8:227-234, 1990.

97. Swinburn BA and others: Insulin resistance associated with lower rates of weight gain in Pima Indians, *J Clin Invest* 88:168-173, 1991.

98. Tattersall RB, Pyke DA: Diabetes in identical twins, *Lancet* II:1120-1125, 1972.

99. Taylor R, Zimmet P: Migrant studies in diabetes. In Mann JI, Pyorala K, Teuscher A, editors: *Diabetes in Epidemiological Perspective,* Edinburgh, 1983, Churchill-Livingstone.

100. Taylor RJ and others: The prevalence of diabetes mellitus in a traditional-living Polynesian population: the Wallis Island Survey, *Diabetes Care* 6:334-340, 1983.

101. Taylor R and others: Physical activity and prevalence of diabetes in Melanesian and Indian men in Fiji, *Diabetologia* 27:578-582, 1984.

102. Tsunehara CH, Leonetti DL, Fujimoto WY: Diet of second-generation Japanese-American men with and without non-insulin-dependent diabetes, *Am J Clin Nutr* 52:731-738, 1990.

103. Tsunehara CH, Leonetti DL, Fujimoto WY: Animal fat and cholesterol intake is high in men with IGT progressing to NIDDM, *Diabetes* 40:427A, 1991 (abstract).

104. Van Noord PAH and others: The relationship between fat distribution and some chronic diseases in 11,825 women participating in the DOM project, *Int J Epidemiol* 19:564-570, 1990.

105. Weiss KM, Ferrell RE, Hanis CL: A New World syndrome of metabolic disease with a genetic and evolutionary basis, *Yearbook Phys Anthropol* 27: 153-178, 1984.

106. West KM: *Epidemiology of diabetes and its vascular lesions,* New York, 1978, Elsevier.

107. WHO Study Group: *Diabetes mellitus—technical report series 727,* Geneva, 1985, World Health Organization.

108. Wicking J and others: Nutrient intake in a partly westernized isolated Polynesian population: the Funafuti survey, *Diabetes Care* 4:92-95, 1981.

109. Williams DRR and others: Diabetes and glucose tolerance in New South Wales coastal Aborigines: possible effects of non-Aboriginal genetic admixture, *Diabetologia* 30:72-77, 1987.

110. Wilson PWF, Anderson KM, Kannel WB: Epidemiology of diabetes mellitus in the elderly, *Am J Med* 80(suppl 5A):3-9, 1986.

111. Yudkin JS and others: Impaired glucose tolerance: is it a risk factor for diabetes or a diagnostic ragbag? *Br Med J* 301:397-401, 1990.

112. Zimmet PZ: Kelly West Lecture 1991: challenges in diabetes epidemiology—from West to the rest, *Diabetes Care* 15:232-252, 1992.

113. Zimmet P and others: Diabetes mellitus in an urbanized, isolated Polynesian population: the Funafuti Survey, *Diabetes* 26:1101-1108, 1977.

114. Zimmet P and others: The prevalence of diabetes in the rural and urban Polynesian population of Western Samoa, *Diabetes* 30:45-51, 1981.

4   Nutritional Management of Diabetes Mellitus

Joan M. Heins and Christine A. Beebe

Food is more than a source of nutrition. Food holds cultural significance, binds social customs, and satisfies individual appetite and senses of taste and smell. Although diets are prescribed as nutrients to meet metabolic requirements, they are consumed as food selected in kitchens, restaurants, vending machines, and diverse social settings. Adherence to a prescribed diet requires knowledge of correct food choices but is strongly influenced by societal demands and personal preferences.

In addition to promoting overall good health, diets prescribed for diabetes must compensate for an abnormal metabolic response to food. Size, composition, and timing of meals need to be designed to maximize insulin efficiency and promote as near normal energy metabolism as is possible. The value of good metabolic control was confirmed by the Diabetes Control and Complications Trial (DCCT), which showed that tight glycemic control reduces the onset and progression of long-term complications associated with diabetes.[45] The DCCT also demonstrated the key role of nutrition therapy in metabolic control. Intensively treated subjects reporting excellent adherence to meal plans (>90% of the time) had significantly lower glycated hemoglobin levels than those who were less adherent.[48]

Although the importance of nutrition therapy is well established, individuals with diabetes say that dietary compliance is the most difficult part of their treatment regimen.[8] Dietary regimens must be planned in consultation with the person with diabetes so that nutrient and metabolic requirements are incorporated into meal patterns that reflect the individual's life-style and personal goals. Because of the magnitude of information, physiologic ramifications, and psychosocial implications, it is not possible to provide adequate nutrition therapy for diabetes through a preprinted diet pamphlet.

DIETARY RECOMMENDATIONS

Nutritional requirements for individuals with diabetes are fundamentally the same as those for healthy individuals without diabetes.[12] While restoration of optimal blood glucose and lipid

CHAPTER OBJECTIVES

- Review principles of nutrition in diabetes management.
- Describe the goals of medical nutrition therapy.
- Summarize the American Diabetes Association nutritional recommendations for dietary modifications for individuals with diabetes.
- Present the goals for nutritional management of IDDM.
- Discuss goals and strategies to promote achievement of nutritional goals for individuals with IDDM and NIDDM.
- Discuss goals and strategies for nutritional management of women with gestational or overt diabetes.
- Discuss nutritional recommendations for children and older adults with diabetes.
- Summarize Nutrition Practice Guidelines.
- Describe approaches and resources for nutrition education.
- Discuss approaches to nutrition counseling.
- Review dietary modifications necessary for the treatment of problems with metabolic control.

levels is a primary goal,[8] medical nutrition therapy for diabetes starts with principles of good nutrition and adds modifications to accommodate abnormalities of glucose metabolism. These two goals are integrated in the dietary prescription to assure adequate nutrient intake while promoting normoglycemia. Recognizing the dual roles of nutrition therapy for diabetes provides insight into the processes involved in developing individual meal plans.

Guidelines for Good Nutrition

Several approaches to defining good nutrition have gained wide acceptance in the United States. The Recommended Dietary Allowances (RDAs) are a quantitative method developed by the Food and Nutrition Board of the National Research Council (Appendix 4a). The RDAs are described as "the levels of intake of essential nutrients that, on the basis of scientific knowledge, are judged by the Food and Nutrition Board to be adequate to meet the known nutrient needs of practically all healthy persons."[57] The RDAs should not be interpreted as minimal or optimal standards but as guidelines for adequate levels of essential nutrients to be consumed as part of a normal diet. As nutrients required for growth, development, and maintenance of a healthy body vary across the life span and to some degree by gender, the RDAs are defined for females and males in age groupings that reflect major stages of development. Individual nutrient requirements will vary by body size, energy requirements, and health status. Currently, the RDAs do not specify upper limits of nutrient intake—a change that may be included in future editions.

The RDAs give information on nutrients but not on food. Guidelines translating the RDAs into practical information for the average person include The *Guide to Good Eating, Dietary Guidelines for Americans,* and the *Food Guide Pyramid.* Each of these approaches provides the fundamentals of good nutrition and can be used as a basis for nutrition counseling in diabetes.

The National Dairy Council's *Guide to Good Eating* is an adaptation of the *Basic Four Food Groups* introduced by the U.S. Department of Agriculture in 1954. This teaching tool was developed to help individuals select foods that will provide an adequate daily intake of vitamins and minerals to meet the RDAs. Foods are grouped by their nutrient content into four categories: milk, meat, fruit and vegetable, and grain. Serving sizes are adjusted to make the nutrient composition comparable; however, the caloric content may differ. Recommendations are given on the minimum number of servings from each group needed to meet nutritional requirements at various stages of the life span.

The *Dietary Guidelines For Americans* give advice on how to (1) choose a diet that provides sufficient nutrition to promote health and (2) limit excessive intakes of nutrients associated with chronic disease. The *Dietary Guidelines* are published by the U.S. Department of Agriculture (USDA) and Department of Health and Human Services (DHHS) and reflect up-to-date advice from nutrition specialists that is the basis of federal nutrition policy. First released in 1980, the *Guidelines* were revised in 1985 and 1990; a fourth revision is in process.

To help people implement the *Dietary Guidelines,* the USDA and DHHS introduced the *Food Guide Pyramid* in the early 1990s (Fig. 4-1). The pyramid shape illustrates the proportion of foods to be selected from different sources. Grains (breads, pasta, and rice) are highlighted by their position at the base of the pyramid; fruits and vegetables share the next level, followed by dairy and other protein-rich foods; fats and sugars are placed at the tip to emphasize that they should be used sparingly. The agencies publish a pamphlet to guide use of the pyramid. Details are given on portion sizes for servings, number of servings that would constitute three levels of caloric intake, and discussion of fat, cholesterol, sodium, and sugar contents of food. The pamphlet also includes a simple method for individuals to use to rate the nutritional adequacy of their diet and to determine if they are eating too much sugar or fat.

Nutritional Recommendations for Individuals With Diabetes

Recommendations on dietary modifications have changed throughout the history of diabetes to reflect new knowledge of the underlying disease processes and advances in treatment modalities. The American Diabetes Association (ADA) published its first nutritional recommendations in 1950 as precalculated meal plans that accompanied the newly introduced *Exchange Lists.*[32] The 40% carbohydrate, 20% protein, and 40% fat distribution of calories used in these meal plans became the standard dietary prescription for diabetes. In 1971 emerging information on the effect of diet on blood glucose and cholesterol levels prompted the ADA to publish a special report: "Principles of Nutrition and Dietary Recommendations

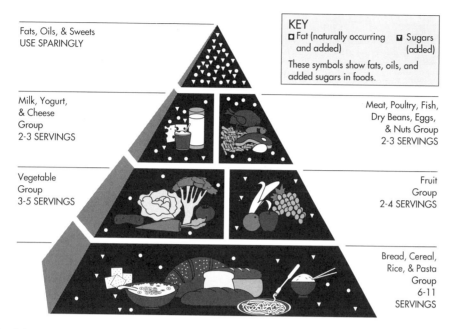

Fats, Oils, & Sweets
USE SPARINGLY

KEY
◻ Fat (naturally occurring   ▨ Sugars
  and added)   (added)
These symbols show fats, oils, and
added sugars in foods.

Milk, Yogurt,
& Cheese
Group
2-3 SERVINGS

Meat, Poultry, Fish,
Dry Beans, Eggs,
& Nuts Group
2-3 SERVINGS

Vegetable
Group
3-5 SERVINGS

Fruit
Group
2-4 SERVINGS

Bread, Cereal,
Rice, & Pasta
Group
6-11
SERVINGS

Fig. 4-1   The Food Guide Pyramid is an outline of what to eat on a daily basis. The pyramid calls for eating a variety foods to get the necessary nutrients and the right amount of calories. Each of the food groups provide some but not all of the nutrients needed. (Courtesy U.S. Department of Agriculture and the U.S. Department of Health and Human Services; from Schlenker ED: *Nutrition in aging,* ed 2, St Louis, 1993, Mosby.)

for Patients With Diabetes Mellitus,"[11] which, when updated in 1979, provided specific recommendations to liberalize the carbohydrate content of the diet to 50% to 60% of calories and to restrict saturated and polyunsaturated fats each to 10% of total calories.[12] The 1979 update also stressed that every person with diabetes should have the opportunity to meet with a diet counselor to set personal goals and plan an individualized diet. Preprinted handout diets were discouraged, and the ADA discontinued publication of their series of precalculated *Exchange Diets.* A 1986 update of the "Dietary Recommendations" maintained the high-carbohydrate/low-fat distribution of calories and introduced a limitation on protein to the 0.8 g/kg recommended by the RDAs.[10] The concern over protein intakes in excess of nutritional requirements was stimulated by research showing restriction of dietary protein deterred progression of diabetic nephropathy.[37,54] Although there were no studies demonstrating that excess protein intake caused diabetic nephropathy, a limitation to normal requirements was considered prudent. The 1986 "Recommendations" also set intake levels for dietary fiber and several micronutrients and gave specific guidelines for insulin-dependent diabetes mellitus (IDDM) and non-insulin-dependent diabetes mellitus (NIDDM).

In 1994 the American Diabetes Association nutrition recommendations were revised extensively to reflect changes in philosophy and terminology, as well as scientific knowledge.[137] The task force writing the revisions sought to base the 1994 "Recommendations" on definitive scientific data.[8] An extensive technical review of the literature guided the revisions and was published along with the new guidelines.[58]

Table 4-1   1994 American Diabetes Association Nutrition Goals, Principles, and Recommendations

Calories	Sufficient to maintain reasonable body weight in adults Sufficient to allow normal growth/development in children Sufficient to provide adequate nutrition for pregnancy/lactation
Protein	10%-20% of daily calories No less than adult RDA (0.8 g/kg/day)
Fat	Total amount varies with treatment goals Saturated fat <10% of calories; <7% with high LDL Polyunsaturated fat up to 10% of calories Monounsaturated fats preferred
Cholesterol	<300 mg/day
Carbohydrate	Difference after protein and fat Total amount varies with treatment goals/preferences
Sweeteners	Sucrose—not restricted in context of healthy diet; substitute as carbohydrate Nutritive sweeteners—no advantage over sucrose; substitute as carbohydrate Nonnutritive sweeteners—can be useful
Fiber	20-35 g/day; same as general population
Sodium	<3000 mg/day for overall health <2400 mg/day if hypertensive
Alcohol	No more than 2 alcoholic beverages/day
Vitamins/Minerals	Same as general population; individualize if at high risk

Modified from American Diabetes Association.

One shift in philosophy that emerged from this rigorous review process is the conclusion that no "one" diet can be recommended as treatment for all types of diabetes. Metabolic variations in the presentation of diabetes require different nutrition interventions. The 1994 "Recommendations" (Table 4-1) discontinue using macronutrient composition as the basis for defining the diet for diabetes and introduce the concept of individual diet prescriptions based on nutrition assessment and treatment goals. A second philosophic change is found in the guidelines for nutritional management of NIDDM. Glucose, lipid, and blood pressure goals are emphasized. Weight loss, a primary focus of past recommendations for NIDDM, is listed as one of several strategies to achieve metabolic control. This change in emphasis recognizes the difficulty that people have in sustaining weight loss and underscores the potential to achieve metabolic goals by strategies other than weight loss. The section of this chapter on nutritional management of NIDDM will discuss this new philosophy.

New terms introduced in the 1994 "Recommendations" included *medical nutrition therapy* and *diabetes self-management training*. Medical nutrition therapy is a comprehensive approach to nutritional care that includes assessment, goal setting, intervention, and evaluation. A description of the process of medical nutrition therapy is provided in the final section of this chapter. Diabetes self-management training is the expanded term for diabetes patient education that emphasizes the critical role of the person with diabetes in implementing therapy.

The 1994 "Recommendations" are based on an evaluation of scientific data to determine when nutrition recommendations for people with diabetes should differ from guidelines for the general population. Revisions reflect new information or a lack of data to support a prior recommendation. For example, the review of studies examining the effect of sucrose and of fiber on glycemia showed blood glucose control does not deteriorate with sucrose ingestion or improve substantially with increased fiber intake; therefore recommendations for use of these two carbohydrates are similar to the *Dietary Guidelines for Americans.* Dietary protein needs of persons with diabetes were found to be no more or less than for the general population so the previous recommendation to limit protein intake to 0.8 g/kg/day was modified to 10% to 20% of calories, a level that parallels general consumption. The recommendation to limit fat intake to 30% or less of calories was replaced with guidelines to adjust the carbohydrate/fat ratio of the diet to reflect individual therapeutic goals. This variation from nutrition guidelines for the general population was guided by data demonstrating that lipid abnormalities in insulin-resistant diabetes can be aggravated by a high-carbohydrate diet.[58]

The goals of medical nutrition therapy in the 1994 "Recommendations" (Box 4-1) underscore the shift from an "ADA" diet prescription that is *tailored to* the individual, to a unique diet prescription *developed for* the individual based on nutrition assessment and treatment goals. This new approach to dietary management requires a thorough understanding of nutrition, metabolism, and diabetes. A registered dietitian has the professional expertise to implement medical nutrition therapy; however, all members of the diabetes treatment team should have a fundamental understanding of underlying principles and of the process.

BOX 4-1

GOALS OF MEDICAL NUTRITION THERAPY FOR DIABETES

Overall goal

To assist persons with diabetes in making changes in nutrition and exercise habits leading to improved metabolic control.

Specific goals

1. Maintain near-normal blood glucose levels
2. Achieve optimal serum lipid levels
3. Provide adequate calories to
   - promote reasonable weight for adults
   - allow normal growth and development for children and adolescents
   - meet increased needs of pregnancy, lactation, or recovery from catabolic illnesses
4. Prevent, delay, or treat nutrition-related risk factors or complications
5. Improve overall health through optimal nutrition

Nutrition

Food provides fuel for energy, substrates for building bones and tissue, and an array of other nutrients that support metabolism. Energy is derived from the carbohydrate, protein, and fat content of food and from ethanol in alcoholic beverages. Dietary protein contributes an exogenous source of amino acids needed for tissue replacement including eight amino acids not adequately synthesized by humans (a ninth amino acid is required for growth in children). Humans rely on dietary sources for essential elements including protein, vitamins, minerals, fiber, two fatty acids, and water. The abnormalities of metabolism that present with diabetes impact most areas of nutrition.

Carbohydrate

Carbohydrates are naturally occurring compounds constructed of carbon, hydrogen, and oxygen and are found in a variety of forms in food. Simple carbohydrates (i.e., sugars) include monosaccharides, such as glucose, fructose, and galactose, and disaccharides, such as sucrose and lactose. Sucrose (table sugar) is composed of glucose and fructose, whereas lactose (milk sugar) is made up of glucose and galactose. Complex carbohydrates (starches) contain a large number of glucose molecules in either straight chains (amylose) or branched chains (amylopectin).

Metabolism of carbohydrates. Digestion of carbohydrates begins in the mouth, continues in the stomach, and is completed in the small intestine where the end-product monosaccharides are absorbed into the portal blood.[16] The concentration of blood glucose achieved and the rate at which it rises depend on the amount of carbohydrate consumed and factors that affect how quickly food is digested and absorbed, such as form of the food, presence of other nutrients, and gastric motility.[110] The normal pancreas senses rising glucose levels and releases insulin in appropriate amounts.

The liver plays a key role in glucose homeostasis. Nearly 60% of ingested glucose is taken up by the liver, where it is converted to glycogen and stored.[69] Some glucose is assimilated by muscle tissue, converted to glycogen, and stored. The amount of glucose retained as glycogen in the muscle depends on the amount already stored. If exercise has occurred recently and muscle glycogen stores are low, glucose uptake and conversion to glycogen are rapid. Excess glucose is converted to fat and stored in adipose tissue. This process is facilitated by lipoprotein lipase—an insulin-sensitive enzyme.

The assumption that molecular structures of carbohydrates (complex versus simple) directed the rate of digestion and predicted glycemic response supported the belief that starches digested slowly because they needed to be broken down into individual glucose molecules. Thus starches were considered the preferred carbohydrate in the diabetic meal plan. Simple sugars were to be avoided because it was assumed that they digested rapidly. In the 1970s this concept was challenged when Crapo and colleagues[44] found wide variations in glucose responses to four starchy foods, selected for their similarity in macronutrient content. Subsequent studies demonstrated that the chemical distinction of complex versus simple structure did not differentiate the rate of carbohydrate metabolism nor did it predict subsequent physiologic response of blood glucose.[79,80]

Recommended amount in diet. The 1994 American Diabetes Association "Nutrition

Recommendations" suggest that after protein requirements are met, decisions on the proportion of carbohydrate and fat in the diet be directed by individual treatment goals (see Table 4-1). Guidelines for the general population recommending a high-carbohydrate/low-fat diet may not be therapeutic for all individuals with diabetes. In particular, lipid abnormalities in NIDDM frequently include hypertriglyceridemia and can differ from other forms of hypercholesterolemia. The usual therapeutic approach of a low-fat diet with the accompanying higher carbohydrate content may exacerbate rather than improve the hyperlipidemia. Therefore the recommendations on carbohydrate in diets for diabetes are to (1) use individual metabolic goals to set the percent of calories and (2) consider the total amount of carbohydrate in a food versus the type (sugar or starch) or glycemic effect.

Glycemic index. Attempts to reclassify carbohydrates by their impact on blood glucose led to development of the "glycemic index" by Jenkins and colleagues in 1981.[80] Some common starchy foods, such as cornflakes and potatoes, were found to raise blood glucose quickly and to a greater degree than sucrose (table sugar), whereas others, including oatmeal and spaghetti, showed much lower effects.[80] Table 4-2 shows glycemic values for selected foods based on data from multiple studies.[79] The somewhat moderate glycemic effect of sucrose (GI = 89) may be explained by the rankings of its component monosaccharides (i.e., the high value of glucose [GI = 138] is offset by the low score of fructose [GI = 31]).

Clinical application of the "glycemic index" is limited by differences in individual response. Self-monitoring of blood glucose (SMBG) can help persons with diabetes measure their own glycemic response to different carbohydrate foods and meal combinations. Multiple factors, however, influence a food's effect on blood glucose. Variety, ripeness, form, method of processing, and cooking methods can alter the impact of a single food. Coingested fat, protein, liquid, and salt influence the glycemic response, as does the rate at which the meal is consumed.[43] It is important to recognize that the nutrient value of a food is independent of its "glycemic effect." Table sugar may produce a lower rise in blood glucose than potatoes, but it lacks the essential vitamins and minerals provided by the potatoes. Decisions on foods must be made on the basis of contribution to overall nutrition, as well as on the impact on glucose homeostasis.

Dietary fiber. Dietary fibers are predominantly nonstarch carbohydrate polysaccharides and lignin that are not digested within the human small intestine. Although not absorbed, fibers play an important role in human nutrition. Dietary fibers increase satiety, alter transit time through the gastrointestinal (GI) tract, increase colonic bulking, and bind or absorb organic materials. Fibers that are water insoluble (e.g., cellulose) seem to have their greatest effect in the lower GI track. As a fecal bulking agent they improve bowel regularity, decrease constipation and diverticular disease, and may bind and dilute carcinogens, thus reducing the risk of colon cancer.[14a,138]

Water-soluble fibers (e.g., pectins, gums) affect the upper GI track by delaying stomach emptying and by altering transit and absorption in the small intestine.[14a,138] The therapeutic benefits of water-souble dietary fiber is thought to be on lipid and glucose metabolism and has been studied in normal and diabetic individuals. A decrease in total and LDL cholesterol with consumption of >20 g/day of soluble dietary fiber has been reported in several studies;

Table 4-2 Glycemic Index: Values for Selected Foods

Mean glycemic index (GI) values of foods adjusted proportionately so that GI of white bread = 100*

Food	GI
Glucose	138
Russet potato, baked	128
Honey	126
Instant potatoes	118
Cornflakes	115
White bread	100
Sucrose	89
Porridge oats	87
Banana	84
New potato, boiled	80
Sweet corn	80
Polished brown rice, boiled 15 minutes	79
Potato chips	77
All bran	74
Parboiled brown rice, boiled 25 minutes	65
Green peas, frozen	65
Spaghetti, boiled 15 minutes	61
Orange	59
Ice cream	52
Whole milk	49
Skim milk	46
Kidney beans	45
Red lentils	37
Fructose	31

Modified from GI values from Jenkins DJA, Wolever TMS, Jenkins AL: Starchy food and glycemic index, *Diabetes Care* 11:149-159, 1988.
*Mean GI values from studies using normal, NIDDM, or IDDM subjects.

however, the extent of reduction may be limited (about 5 mg/dl).[123] Importantly, HDL cholesterol levels are maintained. Data examining the influence of fiber on triglycerides are not conclusive, in part because of a number of confounding variables such as body weight and caloric intake. These same problems interfere with interpretation of studies of dietary fiber and glucose metabolism. Although certain soluble fibers can reduce glucose absorption in the small intestine, the overall impact of high-fiber diets on blood glucose control appears minimal.[108] Use of concentrated fiber supplements as a method for improving glycemic control is therefore of no value and not recommended.

Although glucose lowering may not be a primary property of dietary fiber, the benefits in bowel health and on lipid levels are the same for individuals with or without diabetes. Nutrition guidelines encourage a daily intake of 20 to 35 g of dietary fiber from a variety of foods including fruits, vegetables, grains, and legumes.[14a] Individuals can easily increase fiber intake by selecting fiber-rich choices of foods they commonly consume. For example, switching from white to whole grain bread, from cornflakes to 40% bran flakes, and from orange juice to orange slices provides three to four times more dietary fiber per serving. Consuming recommended servings of fruits and vegetables in the food pyramid plus a high-fiber diet as in cereal or legumes daily is about the only way to achieve the recommended 20 to 35g of fiber per day. Although most individuals with diabetes can increase the fiber content of their diet without side effects, some general guidelines are important. A gradual increase in consumption of high-fiber foods and an increase in fluid intake should be recommended to avoid GI discomfort. Although data do not support prescribing high-fiber diets for glycemic control, some individuals may experience lower glucose levels when they comsume a high-fiber diet or eat a very-high-fiber meal. Individuals treated with insulin should use SMBG to monitor their response to high-fiber intakes and to guide adjustment of insulin dose.

Sugars. Sugars occur naturally in fruits and vegetables (glucose, fructose, and sucrose) and in milk (lactose); however, these sources generally are not included in evaluations of sugar in the diet. It is sugars used as sweeteners that are targeted in recommendations on consumption. For all individuals, the nutritionally "empty" (i.e., low nutrient) calories of sugar should be evaluated. For persons with diabetes, the effect of sugars on blood glucose has been an additional consideration.

The determination by Crapo and colleagues[44] that glycemic effect is not associated with carbohydrate structure and the "glycemic index" studies by Jenkins and colleagues[79,80] have stimulated research on the effect of adding sucrose to the diet of individuals with diabetes. Ten studies comparing the glycemic effects of isocaloric amounts of sucrose and starch were included in the technical review accompanying the 1994 "Recommendations."[58] No adverse effect on blood glucose was found when 12% to 35% of carbohydrate calories was replaced with sucrose either in single-meal feedings or in meal plans consumed for as long as 4 weeks. These studies support the conclusion that restriction of sucrose because of glycemic concern is not warranted. The possibility that adding sucrose to the diet may exacerbate lipemia in type II diabetes was raised by the findings of one study; however, two other studies did not see a deleterious effect.

The 1994 "Recommendations" advise that the total amount versus type of carbohydrate is the important consideration in diabetes. This recommendation, although well grounded in scientific data, represents a major paradigm shift. Accepting the fact that sugar is allowed in the diet for diabetes can be difficult for diabetic individuals, health professionals, and the community at large. Permitting sugar in the diet for diabetes is not new. The original version of the *Exchange Lists* included sugar-containing options such as angel cake, ice cream, and graham crackers. The *Family Cookbook Series,* introduced in 1980 by The American Diabetes Association and The American Dietetic Association, contains recipes using limited amounts of sugar. The 1994 "Recommendations" confirmed these applications and extended them with a careful review of data demonstrating no difference in the glycemic response to sugars versus starches.[58]

The concept of total carbohydrate is not as simple to communicate to the general public as the long-held good-versus-bad classification of starch and sugar. Education is required to understand the trade-off of eating food sweetened with regular sugar versus a non-caloric sweetener. For example, portion size may need to be smaller to keep the carbohydrate content equal when an item sweetened with sucrose is used instead of one sweetened with aspartame. Many sucrose-containing foods have a high concentration of fat, as well as carbohydrate. Selecting apple pie versus an apple for dessert requires adjustments in the carbohydrate and fat content of the meal. Most important, the concept of a healthy diet should guide use of sucrose by *all* individuals, independent of diabetes.

Protein

Metabolism of protein. Metabolism of protein to amino acids begins in the stomach and continues through the lumen and brush border of the small intestine. Once absorbed into the bloodstream, amino acids circulate through the portal vein to the liver and then to the rest of the body. Entry of amino acids into muscle cells is facilitated by insulin released from the pancreas. Certain amino acids are known to stimulate insulin secretion, whereas others stimulate the secretion of glucagon.

Amino acids are used for muscle protein synthesis, as well as the production of enzymes, hormones, and other constituents of cells. Any amino acids consumed in excess of those required to build tissue will be converted to carbohydrate or lipids and used for energy. As much as 50% to 58% of protein ingested may be metabolized to glucose. This gluconeogenic tendency of many of the amino acids has led some clinicians to conclude that protein should be considered when counting the total amount of glucose available from a given food or meal. Others surmise that the presence of protein-rich foods stabilizes blood glucose levels by providing substrate for gluconeogenesis after carbohydrate itself has been absorbed and metabolized. Peters and Davidson[115] found that increased protein intake at a mixed meal does not affect glycemic response unless consumption exceeds 6 ounces at one time. Those large servings of protein influence postprandial blood glucose by increasing the response 2½ to 4 hours after consumption.

Because protein breakdown and synthesis occur continuously and concurrently, it is not clear whether amino acids ingested at the most recent meal are specifically earmarked for gluconeogenesis after that meal. In reality, amino acids are not truly stored in the body but circulate and turn over constantly. As much as 300 to 400 g of protein/day is recycled through synthesis and breakdown.[105] This represents three to five times the amount of protein consumed by an average 70 kg adult.

Nine of the twenty amino acids found in the diet are considered essential in that they cannot be made by the body. Protein requirements are based on meeting the need for these nine amino acids. Animal protein is considered to be of higher biologic value than vegetable protein, since all of the essential amino acids are present. Yet vegetable proteins can be combined to provide all of the essential amino acids.

Recommended amount in diet. The 1994 American Diabetes Association "Nutrition Recommendation" for protein is 10% to 20% of calories (see Table 4-1). This is similar to recommendations for individuals without diabetes. The RDA for protein is currently 0.8 g/kg/day. More research is needed to substantiate whether persons with diabetes need more or less protein than the general population.

Young children require greater amounts of protein to promote normal growth and development. Infants require approximately 1.6 to 2.2 g/kg/day; 1.1 to 1.2 g/kg/day is required by children ages 1 to 6; and approximately 1.0 g/kg/day is required by children ages 7 to 14.[57] Adolescent males require 0.9 g/kg/day to age 18. The requirement for adolescent females is the same as the RDA for adults.

Pregnant and lactating women have increased protein needs to promote fetal development and milk production. The RDA for protein in pregnant women is 60 g/day. This represents an increase of 10 g/day above requirements for nonpregnant women.[57]

Older adults may also have increased protein needs. The rate of protein synthesis decreases with age, requiring more protein to originate from the diet. Thus at least 12% to 14% of calories should come from protein in the person older than 51 years.[62] This represents an intake of 0.8 to 1.0 g/kg/day. Even higher levels of protein may be necessary after periods of undernutrition or increased protein loss, such as after surgery, prolonged illness, or during wound healing.[74]

Diabetic nephropathy is a serious complication of long-term poor glycemic control and hypertension. Genetic predisposition may also influence its development. Dietary protein intake has not been directly linked to development of nephropathy but does play a role in the progression of established renal disease. High protein intake increases kidney work load and increases glomerular filtration rate and renal plasma flow. Studies restricting protein intake in nondiabetic individuals in renal failure fail to show a significant alteration in the rate of decline of renal function.[84] However, individuals with diabetes and established proteinuria respond to a reduced protein intake with a corresponding decrease in proteinuria and improvement in glomerular filtration rate and renal plasma flow.[37,140,145] It appears logical to reduce protein at the first evidence of microalbuminuria. Severe restriction to less than the RDA of 0.8 g/kg/day is not recommended. Not only is compliance difficult, but malnutrition has been reported at a level of 0.6 g/kg.[30]

Increasing data suggest that specific amino acids, particularly those from animal proteins, are more detrimental to renal function than those from vegetable proteins.[49,87] Egg, tofu, cheese, and vegetable proteins may not require restriction if these data prove to be true. Long-term adherence to a protein-restricted meal plan would be enhanced if vegetable proteins turn out to be less nephrotoxic.

As a rule, most experts agree that the majority of Americans consume too much protein. It is not uncommon for an American man to consume 100 to 150 g/day, or as much as 17% to 29% of total calories. Frequently the person with diabetes has a rather high protein intake for various reasons. Most clinicians are well aware of the diabetic diet history that includes eggs, cheese, or peanut butter at every breakfast or snack. Whether the original intent was to diminish the blood glucose response or satisfy the "meat group" requirement, the current trend is to decrease these high-fat protein sources.

Modifying protein intake. Usual protein intake should be assessed in individuals with diabetes and be modified as necessary to meet the nutrition goals. A realistic amount of protein is the amount recommended in the USDA nutrition guidelines *(Food Guide Pyramid)* of 5 to 7 ounces from the meat group daily. If nephropathy is evident, a more restricted intake may be necessary, such as 3 to 4 ounces/day. Evaluation parameters, such as 24-hour urine protein and creatinine levels, can be used to assess progress and provide feedback on the efficacy of dietary modifications.

The question of whether protein should be included at every meal and snack is controversial and needs to be individualized. Protein ingested with carbohydrate has been found to increase insulin secretion response in type II diabetes.[63] However, over 50 g doses (7 oz) were needed to produce significant results. It is not clear if all proteins (i.e., vegetable and animal) produce this result and would therefore be required at particular meals. Many people insist that protein is needed in snacks to maintain blood glucose levels because protein in large amounts elevates BG 2½ to 5 hours postprandial.[115] Insulin doses may need to be adjusted when large servings of protein are consumed at one time. This seems to be an individualized response and requires SMBG data to determine for each person. Fat will shift the glycemic response curve to the right by slowing digestion of food, and since many protein foods also contain fat, this may contribute to a longer blood glucose response as well.[115]

Fat

Dietary fat is digested predominantly in the intestine to its component parts. Before fat can be absorbed across the intestinal wall, it must be combined with proteins to form chylomicrons. These chylomicrons then carry fat into lymph and from there to the blood.

Chylomicrons are one of several lipoproteins that function as transport vehicles for fats. Because of the hydrophobic nature of fat, it must be combined with protein to be soluble in the aqueous blood system. Lipoproteins consist of a combination of triglyceride, cholesterol, phospholipids, and apoproteins. Phospholipid surrounds a core layer of cholesterol, cholesterol esters, and triglyceride. Phospholipids serve to suspend fat by having the hydrophobic ends facing toward the fat and the hydrophilic ends facing outward toward blood. Apoproteins are present on the surface of the particle to strengthen its structure, guide the lipoprotein particle to its receptor, and serve as cofactors for enzymes involved in cholesterol and triglyceride metabolism.

Lipoproteins are classified by their density. Each class of lipoprotein varies in the amount of triglyceride, cholesterol, phopholipid, and protein present (Fig. 4-2). Chylomicrons are the least dense lipoprotein because they are made up almost entirely of exogenous triglyceride.

More than 90% of chylomicrons are taken up by the liver where they are catabolized to free fatty acids (FFA), glycerol, cholesterol, and phospholipids. Before these products reenter the bloodstream, they are recombined into very-low-density lipoproteins (VLDL). The major component of VLDL is triglyceride. The rate of VLDL production and secretion by the liver is influenced by factors such as the diet, degree of obesity, and glucagon and insulin levels. Insulin stimulates VLDL production by the liver; thus the hyperinsulinemia and insulin resistance found so often in obesity and NIDDM can lead to an overproduction of VLDL and hypertriglyceridemia.[51,144] Excessive caloric consumption increases the level of FFA in the blood and increases hepatic production of VLDL. Hypertriglyceridemia is a hallmark of the obese person with NIDDM.

The VLDL particle is normally catabolized to low-density lipoprotein (LDL) through intermediate-density lipoprotein (IDL). LDL transports cholesterol from the liver to peripheral tissues. The LDL particle is nearly 43% cholesterol; the remainder of the particle is

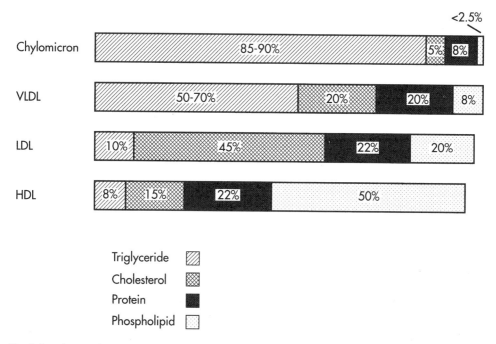

Fig. 4-2   Approximate content of plasma lipoproteins. (Modified from Silver EN: *Heart disease,* ed 2, New York, 1987, Miller.)

phospholipid and protein. Measurement of serum LDL cholesterol is generally described as "bad cholesterol" because it represents the majority of circulating cholesterol. Normally, LDL particles are taken up and metabolized by receptor-mediated pathways on the liver and the peripheral tissues. These receptors, located on the surface of cells, recognize and bind the apoproteins attached to LDL particles. More than 30% of daily LDL production is metabolized this way.[33,68]

Hypercholesterolemia occurs in diabetes, although to a much lesser extent than hypertriglyceridemia. The cause of elevated cholesterol in diabetes may be hypertriglyceridemia, since LDL is derived from VLDL, but is also thought to result from altered receptor pathways.[51,118,124] It appears that LDL particles may be glycosylated during poor diabetes control.[143] This glycosylation interferes with LDL uptake, and cholesterol accumulates in the bloodstream.

High-density lipoprotein (HDL) is often referred to as the "good cholesterol" because of its primary function in transporting cholesterol from peripheral tissues back to the liver where it is metabolized. HDL cholesterol is composed primarily of protein and phospholipid, with less than 18% of the particle containing cholesterol. Studies have found an inverse relationship between HDL concentration and atherosclerosis. It has been observed that HDL levels may be low in many individuals with diabetes but are increased with improvements in glycemic control.[23,83] Because HDL is inversely related to triglyceride levels, it is not unusual to find low HDL levels in NIDDM patients.

Recommended amount in diet. A desire to reduce the increased cardiovascular disease risk in diabetes is the rationale for the American Diabetes Association's guidelines for modifying dietary fat intake. Before 1994 the American Diabetes Association recommendation for total dietary fat was identical to that of the American Heart Association and the USDA *Dietary Guidelines for Americans,* that is, less than 30% of total calories from fat, less than 10% saturated fat, and less than 300 mg cholesterol. The 1994 "Recommendations" retain the guidelines for saturated fat and cholesterol but do not recommend a specific percentage of calories from fat (see Table 4-1). The total amount of fat in the daily nutrition plan needs to be individualized, since metabolic responses to fat and carbohydrate differ among individuals, depending on type of diabetes and degree of insulin resistance.

Epidemiologic data clearly associate elevated serum cholesterol levels with increased risk of cardiovascular disease. The Lipid Research Clinics Coronary Prevention Trial has indicated that for every 1% reduction in serum cholesterol there is an estimated 2% reduction in risk for a cardiovascular event.[93] Metabolic studies suggest that a high-fat diet raises serum cholesterol levels.[39] For most persons with diabetes, reducing the total fat intake, modifying the type of fat, reducing obesity, and improving blood glucose control will reduce serum lipid levels. However, some persons with insulin-resistant type II diabetes may respond to a low-fat, high-carbohydrate intake with an increase in triglycerides.[41,42,64]

Cholesterol. There is no dietary requirement for cholesterol, since cholesterol is made by the liver, intestinal cells, and several other tissues. In fact, the majority of plasma cholesterol is derived from endogenous sources. Cholesterol entering through the diet comes only from foods of animal origin and should be limited to less than 300 mg/day. Approximately 40% of dietary cholesterol is absorbed, and the rest is excreted. The concern is that excess cholesterol from the diet will be stored in tissues such as the coronary arteries. Connor and Connor[39] have found that consuming dietary cholesterol in excess of 100 mg/day can produce a rapid rise in plasma cholesterol. It is currently estimated that the average American diet contains nearly 400 to 500 mg/day.

Reducing dietary cholesterol by 100 mg/day results in a 7 mg/dl reduction in plasma cholesterol.[39] Individuals with cholesterol intakes above 400 mg/day are most likely to benefit from dietary cholesterol restriction. Egg yolks remain one of the largest sources of cholesterol in the diet, containing approximately 200 mg/yolk. Current recommendations suggest that egg yolk consumption be limited to four per week. Liver, kidney, and brains contain large amounts of cholesterol (up to 1500 mg/serving) but are consumed less frequently than eggs. They should be severely limited in a low-cholesterol diet. A common misconception is that beef and pork contain more cholesterol than chicken or turkey. In reality, each contains about 75 mg in a 3-ounce serving. Poultry, however, contains less total fat and much less saturated fat than either beef or pork.

Total fat intake. The total amount of fat consumed daily can have an impact on serum lipid levels, since the quantity of chylomicrons circulating in the bloodstream is directly proportional to the amount of fat consumed. The average American consumes approximately 36% of his or her calories from fat. Reducing fat to 20% to 30% of calories decreases chylomicron production and reduces atherogenic risk in most individuals.

Restricting fat to 20% to 30% of calories in turn requires a corresponding increase in carbohydrate to 50% of calories or more. Although such a high-carbohydrate intake is preferred for individuals with type I diabetes, it may be detrimental to metabolic control in insulin-resistant type II diabetes. Serum glucose and triglyceride levels may worsen under a high-carbohydrate regimen.[41,42,64] The increased postprandial hyperglycemia resulting from increased carbohydrate intake in turn increases insulin response, which stimulates liver production of triglycerides. A modest reduction in dietary carbohydrate to approximately 40% of calories can reduce both the hyperglycemia and hypertriglyceridemia so characteristic of insulin-resistant type II diabetes. However, restricting carbohydrate necessitates an increase in dietary fat to nearly 40%. Because saturated fat must be limited to less than 10% of calories and polyunsaturated fat is best limited to 7% to 10% of calories, the majority of fat calories need to come from monounsaturated fatty acids.

In addition to its lipemic effects, dietary fat may have an impact on the development and maintenance of obesity. Fat provides 9 cal/g—more than twice the amount of calories provided by either protein or carbohydrate. Although excess calories from protein and carbohydrate are stored as fat in the adipocyte, dietary fat appears to be more readily available for storage as body fat. In fact, the body utilizes 23% of energy to convert every gram of carbohydrate to fat, but only 3% of energy for every gram of fat converted to fat.[128] Thus by controlling total fat intake, fewer calories may be converted to fat. It has been shown that as much as 200 to 300 more calories/day are required for weight maintenance in subjects consuming diets that contain 20% of calories as fat.[50]

Saturated fat. Saturated fat (stearic and palmitic acid) has been shown to be highly atherogenic and has an even greater impact on serum cholesterol than does dietary cholesterol or total dietary fat.[20] Saturated fatty acids increase chylomicrons and LDL cholesterol concentration. The American Diabetes Association agrees with the American Heart Association in reducing saturated fat intake to less than 10% of calories. It is estimated that the American diet may contain as much as 17% to 20% as saturated fat.

Nearly all saturated fat comes from animal sources such as whole-milk dairy products and high-fat meats. Saturated fats by nature have all carbon atoms in the fatty acid chain saturated with hydrogen. As a result, these fats are generally solid at room temperature. Some plant fats are also saturated. Coconut, palm oil, palm kernel and cocoa butter, for example, are highly saturated. They have been routinely used in commercial baked products because of their stability and long shelf life, as well as low price. Recent concern over their atherogenicity has prompted many baked goods and snack manufacturers to replace them with less saturated fats such as soy, cottonseed, and corn oils. Table 4-3 shows the fatty acid composition of common fats consumed in the American diet.

Monounsaturated fat. The majority of fat in the diet of persons with diabetes should come from monounsaturated fatty acids (MUFA). Traditionally, MUFAs (oleic acid) were thought to have a neutral effect on plasma cholesterol levels. Recent research suggests that they may not be as innocuous as once thought. Studies with normal subjects[70,100] and persons with hyperlipidemia[64] have found that substituting MUFAs for saturated fatty acids in the diet reduces triglycerides and LDL cholesterol while maintaining or increasing HDL cholesterol. A criticism of substituting polyunsaturated fat for saturated fat in the diet is that polyunsaturated fatty acids lower HDL, as well as LDL, cholesterol.

Several studies have shown that hypertriglyceridemia in NIDDM is exaggerated by high-carbohydrate diets regardless of the carbohydrate source (i.e., complex or simple).[42,64,98]

Table 4-3 Fatty Acid Composition of Selected Fats (Percentage of Total Lipid)*

Type of fat	Saturated fat (SFA)	MUFA	PUFA
Animal			
Beef†	39	44	4
Butter	66	30	4
Chicken	28	36	21
Lamb†	33	42	7
Pork†	34	45	12
Turkey	29	41	26
Veal†	24	31	9
Vegetable			
Canola	7	55	33
Coconut	86	6	2
Corn	13	25	62
Olive	14	72	9
Palm	49	37	9
Peanut	19	46	30
Safflower	9	12	74
Soybean	15	23	58

*Pennington J: *Bowes and Church: Food values of portions commonly used,* ed 15, Philadelphia, 1989, Lippincott.
†Source: National Livestock and Meat Board, Food and Nutrition News 59:2, 1989.

Garg and associates[64] suggest that partial replacement of complex carbohydrates with monounsaturated fats may improve the hypertriglyceridemia of NIDDM without raising LDL cholesterol or compromising diabetes control. Ginsberg and others[65] demonstrated that a diet containing 38% fat—predominantly from MUFA (18%)—reduced serum lipid values to the same extent as the American Heart Association step-one diet.

The major sources of MUFA in the diet are peanut, canola, and olive oils (see Table 4-3). Poultry, beef, lamb, and pork each contain 40% to 45% of fatty acids from the monounsaturated variety. In general, increasing the MUFA content of the diet can be accomplished by substituting olive or canola oil in salads and cooking and using small amounts of nuts as a snack and avocado or olives in salads and sandwiches.

Polyunsaturated fat. Polyunsaturated fatty acids (PUFAs) are found predominantly in plant sources but are also found in marine life. The most common PUFAs are linoleic, linolenic, and arachidonic. PUFAs can be divided into two types—omega-6 or omega-3 fatty acids—meaning they have a double bond on either the sixth carbon or the third from the methyl end of the fatty acid chain. PUFAs maintain the function and integrity of cells and are precursors to prostaglandin synthesis. Because the body does not synthesize polyunsaturated fatty acids, they are considered essential.

Studies have shown that substituting polyunsaturated fatty acids for saturated fat lowers plasma cholesterol levels, particularly LDL cholesterol. Concern has been raised that excessive consumption may have unfavorable effects.[133] Moderate consumption of polyunsaturated fats is considered safe and acceptable. (7% to 10%).

Because of the nature of their chemical structure (i.e., containing more than one double bond), PUFAs are liquid at room temperature (corn, safflower, soy, and sunflower oils). However, these oils are often hydrogenated to produce margarine. This process produces trans fatty acids that have the same atherogenic properties as saturated fatty acids.[99] Thus the softer tub varieties of margarine or the liquid oil itself is a better dietary choice.

The major source of omega-3 polyunsaturated fatty acids is fish oils. Eicosapentaenoic acid (EPA) and docosahexaenoic acid (DHA) are the major fatty acids in this class. Epidemiologic studies suggest that these omega-3 fish oils may be beneficial to individuals with NIDDM because of their ability to reduce serum triglycerides and decrease platelet aggregation.[89,118] Clinical trials with supplementation of omega-3 fatty acids are inconclusive, however, because large doses of fish oil are needed to produce an effect. Studies in individuals with diabetes have found that supplementation with large amounts of fish oil can elevate blood glucose levels and increase insulin requirements.[66,75]

Dietary supplementation with fish oil capsules is not generally recommended. The practice of consuming a tablespoon of cod liver oil daily also is discouraged because of the high vitamin A content and the high caloric value. Older adults are most vulnerable to such claims and practices. Instead, individuals should be encouraged to consume about 6 to 8 ounces of fish per week. Usually this is done by choosing two to three fish meals per week. Although salmon, mackerel, and herring are the best sources of omega-3 fatty acids, consumption of all fish should be encouraged because of its low fat content and proportion of polyunsaturated fatty acids. Previous limitations on shellfish consumption (because of cholesterol content) are no longer encouraged, since fish has very low levels of total and saturated fat.

Sweeteners

Advice on the use of sweeteners by persons with diabetes has varied over the years as new information and new items become available. The term *sweeteners* includes a variety of products that traditionally have been classified by their caloric value. The introduction of new products with properties of intense sweetness or of volume and texture has expanded the number of ways to evaluate sweeteners; however, for individuals with diabetes, calories and glycemic effect are the important considerations.

Caloric sweeteners. Sucrose, fructose, and polyols (sugar alcohols) are the most frequently used caloric sweeteners. Sucrose and fructose contribute 4 calories/g to the diet. The caloric yield of polyols varies by the form ingested and individual digestive factors. The standard in Europe is 2.6 calories/g; in the United States it is 4 calories/g—the same as carbohydrate. In 1994 the Food and Drug Administration began to recognize individually determined energy values for polyols (Table 4-4).

Sucrose (cane sugar) is a disaccharide composed of a glucose and a fructose molecule. It enhances the color, texture, and stability of manufactured and baked products and is the most widely used sweetener. Although sugar is not banned from the diet for diabetes, use should be guided by certain considerations. Because the total amount versus type of carbohydrate is the best predictor of glycemic effect, sucrose and sucrose-containing foods must be substituted for other carbohydrate foods rather than added to the usual intake. When making such

Table 4-4   Caloric Values of Selected Sweeteners

Sweetener	Caloric value
Sucrose	4 calories/g
Fructose	4 calories/g
Hydrogenated starch hydrolysates	3 calories/g
Maltitol	3 calories/g
Sorbitol	2.6 calories/g
Xylitol	2.4 calories/g
Isomalt	2 calories/g
Lactitol	2 calories/g
Mannitol	1.6 calories/g

Data from Calorie Control Council: *Questions and answers about polyols,* Atlanta, Author.

substitutions, the nutrient composition, as well as glycemic effect, should be considered. A piece of fruit and a cookie may contain equal amounts of carbohydrate, but the latter has fewer vitamins, may have more dietary fat, and a greater number of calories.

Fructose is a monosaccharide found primarily in fruits and honey. It is available in a crystalline form, which is 100% fructose, or as high-fructose corn syrup, which includes from 10% to 58% glucose. Fructose has been rated 1.2 to 1.8 times sweeter than sucrose and is most effective in cold and high-acid foods. Fructose produces a lower rise in blood sugar than sucrose in nondiabetic individuals and in diabetic individuals who have adequate available insulin.[18,43] However, the effect of fructose on serum lipids is not conclusive. Also, an intake of more than 50 g/day has been shown to cause osmotic diarrhea.[14b] Because of these potential problems, fructose does not offer a distinct advantage over other sweeteners for the person with diabetes but can be used as one of several options.

Polyols are a group of sweeteners that are found naturally in a variety of plants or are produced commercially from carbohydrates. These sweeteners offer advantages of bulk and texture not found in noncaloric sweeteners and a lower caloric value than sucrose or fructose. Until recently, sorbitol, mannitol and xylitol were the polyols used by food processors in the United States. New technologies and recognition of the reduced caloric values of these sweeteners have stimulated development of a wide range of products. Studies of the glycemic effect of these sweeteners show no significant impact on blood glucose or insulin levels.[127] For individuals with diabetes, these sweeteners can be considered a source of calories that has little direct effect on blood glucose; therefore polyols should not be considered as treatment for hypoglycemia or included when counting carbohydrate content of foods as a meal-planning strategy. The safety of polyol sweeteners has been evaluated by the World Health Organization's Joint Committee on Food Additives and by the U.S. Food and Drug Administration, with conclusions that the products are safe and a limitation on intake does not need to be specified. Some individuals consuming large amounts of these sweeteners may experience gastrointestinal disturbance, and in the United States the label statement "Excess consumption may have a laxative effect" is required on food products where ingestion of 50 g/day of sorbitol is foreseeable.

Noncaloric sweeteners. Saccharin is a white powder synthesized from toluene that is up to 400 times sweeter than sucrose. The oldest of the nonnutritive sweeteners, it was initially marketed to the food canning industry as an economic alternative to sugar. Saccharin gained wider use during wartime sugar shortages. Saccharin can be used in cooking but does not act as a sugar in providing texture or color. Many people complain that it leaves a bitter aftertaste. When the FDA banned cyclamates in 1970, saccharin was the only nonnutritive sweetener approved for use in the United States. In 1977 an FDA ban on saccharin was proposed after a study showing a high incidence of bladder cancer in rats fed very large quantities in relationship to their body weight.[96] The relative risk to humans was debated by the scientific community, and Congress responded with a moratorium on the ban to allow time for further study. The proposed ban was lifted by the FDA in December 1991. Suggested limits for saccharin intake are given in a 1955 GRAS (Generally Recognized as Safe) list published by the FDA. Recommended limits are as follows: 500 mg/day in children and 1000 mg/day for a 70 kg adult.[14b] Although saccharin contains no calories, it may be packaged with a nutritive compound. The product Sweet and Low, for example, includes dextrose, which provides 4 calories per packet.

Aspartame is an amino acid compound that contains 4 calories/g. Because it is approximately 200 times sweeter than sucrose, the amount used as a substitute for table sugar is calorically insignificant. Aspartame is marketed under the brand name NutraSweet and as the tabletop sweetener Equal. Equal includes a nutritive buffer that provides 4 calories/ teaspoon. High consumer satisfaction has made it one of the most popular low-calorie sweeteners. Although it is stable in dry foods, when combined with liquids or subjected to high temperatures, aspartame can be degraded. An encapsalated form is now approved for use in baked goods. Aspartame does not affect blood glucose control in diabetes; however, there are questions on safety that are applicable to the general population including people with diabetes. The normal metabolic breakdown of aspartame yields aspartic acid, phenylalanine, and methanol. Phenylalanine is restricted in diets of people with phenylketonuria; therefore aspartame consumption is contraindicated. About 10% by weight of aspartame is converted to methanol—an amount that is less than levels naturally occurring in many common fruits and vegetables. The FDA has established the acceptable daily intake (ADI) of aspartame at 50 mg/kg/day.[14b]

Acesulfame potassium (K), a synthetic sweetener that received FDA approval in 1988, is marketed by Hoechst under the name Sunnette. Acesulfame-K is 130 to 200 times sweeter than sugar and has a synergistic effect with other sweeteners that increases this value. For example, when combined in a 1→1 ratio with aspartame, the mixture can be four to six times sweeter. It is heat stable and therefore suitable for baking. Acesulfame-K resembles saccharin in chemical structure. Some people say that it leaves a saccharin-like aftertaste when used in large concentrations. After FDA approval, the safety of acesulfame-K was contested by a consumer affairs group who claimed a study showed tumor formation in rats fed large amounts of the compound. The FDA reviewed the study data and found the tumors were not related to acesulfame-K consumption.[24,141] Acesulfame-K is packaged for retail sale as a tabletop sweetener under the label Sweet One. Each packet contains 1 g of dextrose, which contributes 4 calories. The ADI for acesulfame-K is 15 mg/kg/day.[141]

Sucralose, a noncaloric sweetener derived from sucrose, is rated 600 times sweeter than table sugar. It is not metabolized by the body and therefore yields no calories and has no effect on blood glucose. Sucralose is stable in a wide range of foods, is acceptable for baking, and has a synergistic effect when combined with other sweeteners. Application for FDA approval was filed by McNeil Specialty Products Company in 1987. The sweetener is approved for use in Canada, where it is marketed as Splenda. For retail market packaging, Sucralose is combined with a maltodextrin to provide volume so that it can be measured like table sugar. The maltodextrin contributes 4 calories/teaspoon.

Alitame is a protein consisting of the amino acids L-aspartic acid, d-alanine, and a new amine (2,2,3,3-tetramethylthietanyl amine).[24,141] It is 2000 times sweeter than sucrose; therefore calories are negligible. Alitame also has a synergistic effect with other sweeteners. It is stable at high temperatures except in an acidic condition, when it can give an "off" taste. Approval by FDA, petitioned by The Pfizer Company in 1986, is still pending.

Cyclamate, a derivative of cyclohexylsulfamic acid, is only 30 times sweeter than sucrose but is stable in heat and cold, has a long shelf life, and leaves almost no aftertaste. It was used in the United States from 1950 until 1970 when it was banned based on evidence of bladder tumors in rats. The carcinogenic effect may be related to the conversion of cyclamates to cyclohexylamine by rats and some humans.[38] Not all humans convert cyclamates, however, and cyclamate use is not banned in some countries, including Canada. Application for reapproval by the FDA was submitted by Abbot Laboratories in 1984. A National Academy of Sciences committee reviewed cyclamate at the FDA's request and concluded that cyclamate alone is not a carcinogen but may be a cocarcinogen in that it may enhance the effect of other cancer-causing substances.[24,38,141] The FDA has no policy for cocarcinogens; therefore reapproval of cyclamates may be delayed for an extended period.[24]

Considerations for use of sweeteners. Several points must be emphasized in discussing the use of sweeteners by individuals with diabetes. The caloric content and glycemic effect of caloric sweeteners need to be evaluated. Sucrose contributes the same number of calories and has a similar glycemic effect as most starches. Fructose has the same number of calories as starch but less effect on blood glucose. Sweeteners in the polyol family have lower caloric values and little glycemic effect. Noncaloric sweeteners, although not contributing calories of their own, may be associated with caloric nutrients either in the packaging (e.g., dextrose or lactose buffers in tabletop sweeteners) or in the food product they are sweetening. Terms on labels such as "sugar-free" often lead individuals to ignore other ingredients in the product that may exacerbate blood glucose, as well as promote undesirable weight gain.

The increasing number of sweeteners available offers consumers the opportunity to use a variety of products in their diet. Selections can be made based on the advantages of a sweetener in enhancing a particular food (e.g., baked product, canned beverage). New products offer a synergistic quality that, when combined with other sweetening agents, gives more sweetness for less sweetener. The advantages of diverse intake and synergistic effect are that amounts ingested of any one sweetener are reduced and overall consumption of sweeteners can be moderated.

Use of sweeteners by children must be evaluated by body weight and maturation. The advisability of pregnant women using sweeteners is often questioned. No evidence of fetal distress has been found for any of the products currently approved by the FDA. Saccharin, acesulfame-K, and phenylalanine (a by-product of aspartame) cross the placenta. Although there is no demonstrated effect on the fetus, avoiding heavy use appears prudent.[14b] For pregnant women seeking guidelines, use of a variety of sweeteners, in moderation, can be advised.

Alcohol

Drinking alcoholic beverages is neither encouraged nor discouraged for individuals with diabetes. Cautions on alcohol intake, made for reasons of safety and health, apply to people independent of diabetes status. For the person with diabetes, alcohol consumption has an added risk of causing hypoglycemia and/or potentiating medication- or exercise-induced hypoglycemia. Alcohol inhibits hepatic gluconeogenesis, a source of glucose that can be critical in the fasted state or when glycogen stores are depleted, such as after exercise.[60] A major concern for persons with diabetes is the similarity of signs of hypoglycemia and of intoxication. Symptoms of a severe insulin reaction may be ignored by observers who could offer assistance but assume they are dealing with an inebriated individual.

Some studies have examined alcohol's influence on hyperglycemia. Moderate consumption with a meal showed no adverse effect on glucose control in one study with IDDM and NIDDM subjects.[86] Another study examined the effect of moderate alcohol intake on overnight glucose levels of IDDM subjects and found hyperglycemia followed by a drop below fasting levels several hours later.[101] Chronic alcohol intake was associated with poor metabolic control in a study of NIDDM subjects, and withdrawal from alcohol improved lipid and blood glucose control after a few days.[22] Individuals with diabetes should be counseled to use SMBG to determine their metabolic response to alcohol.

Alcohol may induce side effects other than hypoglycemia or hyperglycemia with some diabetes medications. Two of the first-generation oral hypoglycemic agents—chlorpropamide and, to a lesser extent, tolbutamide—can interact with alcohol and cause headache, flushing, and nausea. These reactions have not been observed with the second-generation sulfonylureas.[14] Alcohol can potentiate the effect of metformin on lactate metabolism. Patients treated with metformin should be counseled to avoid excessive alcohol consumption.[28]

Guidelines for alcohol consumption by individuals with diabetes follow the *Dietary Guidelines for Americans:* if alcohol is used, women should consume no more than one drink a day and men no more than two drinks a day. Some alcoholic beverages, such as liqueurs, sweet wines, wine coolers, and sweet mixes contain large amounts of carbohydrate. Regular beer also contains carbohydrate—about as much as a slice of bread. Light beer offers the advantage of less carbohydrate, alcohol, and calories. Table 4-5 provides information on the composition of common alcoholic beverages.

The way that alcohol should be incorporated into the meal plan varies by the type of diabetes therapy and treatment goals. Alcohol contributes 7 calories per gram to the diet but does not require insulin for metabolism. Individuals treated with insulin or sulfonylurea who consume alcohol should do so with a meal. Alcohol should be used sparingly if weight loss is a goal or if triglycerides are elevated. Adjustments in food intake can be made to compensate for calories. The similarity in caloric value (7 kcal/g in alcohol; 9 kcal/g in fat) and in

Table 4-5   Composition of Alcoholic Beverages and Mixes

Beverage	Serving (oz)*	Alcohol (g)	Carbohydrates (g)	Calories
Beer				
Regular	12	13	13	150
Light	12	11	5	100
Near beer	12	1.5	12	60
Distilled spirits				
80 proof (gin, rum, vodka, rye, whiskey, scotch)	1.5	14	Trace	100
Dry brandy, cognac	1	11	Trace	75
Table wine				
Dry white	4	11	Trace	80
Red or rose	4	12	2	85
Sweet wine	4	12	5	105
Light wine	4	6	1	50
Wine cooler	12	13	30	215
Dealcoholized wines	4	Trace	6-7	25-35
Sparkling wines				
Champagne	4	12	4	100
Sweet kosher wine	4	12	12	132
Appetizer/dessert wines				
Sherry	2	9	2	74
(Sweet sherry, port, muscatel)	2	9	7	90
Cordials, liquers	1.5	13	18	160
Vermouth				
Dry	3	13	4	105
Sweet	3	13	14	140
Cocktails				
Bloody Mary	5	14	5	116
Daiquiri	2	14	2	111
Manhattan	2	17	2	178
Martini	2.5	22	Trace	156
Old fashioned	4	26	Trace	180
Tom Collins	7.5	16	3	120

Modified from Franz MJ: *Diabetes Spectrum,* 3:210-216, 1990.
*One alcohol equivalent is equal to the amount of alcohol in the following: 1½ ounces of distilled spirits, 4 ounces of dry wine, 2 ounces of dry sherry, 12 ounces of beer.

metabolic pathway suggests substituting alcohol for fat in the diet. One drink (1 oz alcohol) is equivalent to 2 fat exchanges.

Sodium

The general American diet contains large amounts of sodium (4000-5800 mg/day) primarily from salt in processed foods. The association between dietary sodium intakes and blood pressure is not clear. Some people appear more sensitive to sodium and at greater risk for hypertension from high sodium intakes. For the population with diabetes, with an independent risk for hypertension, moderation in sodium intake is prudent.[109] The American Heart Association recommends no more than 3000 mg/day of sodium,[15] and the National High Blood Pressure Education Programs uses a more conservative limit of 2400 mg/day.[106] The 1994 "Nutrition Recommendations" follow these guidelines suggesting an upper limit of 3000 mg/day for normotensive individuals and 2400 mg/day or less for individuals with mild to moderate hypertension.[8] For individuals with diagnosed hypertension, particularly associated with renal disease, sodium restriction is critical. In certain clinical conditions such as severe metabolic derangement, fluid imbalance, or postural hypotension, an increase in salt intake may be prescribed.

Vitamins and minerals

Vitamins and minerals are utilized in small quantities by the human body, yet they play a highly specific role in facilitating energy transfer and tissue synthesis. The reciprocal nature of the micronutrient issue in diabetes is that many of these substances can directly affect blood glucose homeostasis and in turn, poor blood glucose control can significantly alter status of the micronutrients.[103] Poorly controlled diabetes can result in excessive loss of water-soluble vitamins and minerals. Serum magnesium levels, for example, may be low during and after diabetic ketoacidosis (DKA) because of excessive urinary losses of magnesium.[97] This hypomagnesemia can potentially cause insulin resistance.[78] A study of children with diabetes found magnesium levels decrease with increasing duration of diabetes.[55]

Increased urinary excretion of the B vitamins also occurs in poorly controlled diabetes.[103] Each of these B vitamins plays a role in homeostasis, and a deficiency can affect glucose tolerance. Chromium is part of glucose tolerance factor and is important in insulin action. Chromium-deficient animals develop hyperglycemia and hypertriglyceridemia. Deficiency in humans is rare despite popular concensus to the contrary. Chromium supplementation is not considered beneficial in persons with diabetes.[1]

Chronic complications of diabetes may be influenced by micronutrient status. Antioxidant vitamins C, E, and beta-carotene have been studied in nondiabetic populations with favorable, although controversial, results. Epidemiologic data and clinical studies associate high levels of antioxidant consumption, particularly vitamin E, with reduced cardiovascular risk.[122,131] Vitamin E, the antioxidant linked most strongly to reduced risk, is thought to function by reducing LDL oxidation and reducing lipid deposits in the arteries. Plasma vitamin E levels are found to be elevated in persons with diabetes;[139] however, supplementation has been found to normalize platelet aggregation[90] and reduce glycosylated hemoglobin.[34]

Table 4-6 Selected Micronutrient Sources and Recommendations

	Food sources	Adult RDA	Potential role in diabetes	Supplementation
Chromium	Brewers yeast, liver, wheat germ	50-200 mg	Part of GTF	No effect unless deficient; 20 μg
Zinc	Meat, whole grains	Men: 15 mg Women: 12 mg	Insulin secretion Insulin action	No effect; 250 mg in wound healing
Copper	Organ meats, seafood, nuts, seeds	1.5 mg	None in humans	
Magnesium	Nuts, legumes, grains	Men: 350 mg Women: 280 mg	Glucose oxidation and transport	Poor control; dose unclear
Selenium	Seafood, organ meats, grains	Men: 70 μg Women: 55 μg	Antioxidant	18 mg
Iron	Meat, eggs, cereals	Men: 10 mg Women: 15 mg	Minor	Toxic
Beta-carotene	Carrots, sweet potatoes, cantaloupe	None	Antioxidant	6-15 mg
Vitamin C	Citrus fruits, strawberries, tomatoes, potatoes	60 mg	Antioxidant	250-500 mg
Vitamin E	Vegetable oils, nuts, wheat germ	Men: 15 IU Women: 12 IU	Antioxidant	200-800 IU
Thiamine (B$_1$)	Grains, beans, meats, nuts	Men: 1.5 mg Women: 1.0 mg	Carbohydrate metabolism	Not recommended

Deficiencies in the antioxidant vitamins do not generally exist in the United States, yet their role in reducing free radical formation is considered valuable in potentially preventing heart disease, cataracts, and cancer. Evidence suggesting that diabetes is a state of increased free radical formation suggests that vitamin supplementation may be therapeutic.[103] More studies involving individuals with diabetes are necessary to draw conclusions regarding the efficacy of supplemental antioxidant therapy in diabetes.

Individuals at greatest risk for vitamin and mineral deficiency include those on weight-reducing diets where fewer than 1200 to 1500 kcal/day are consumed, strict vegetarians, older adults, pregnant or lactating women, persons taking medications that affect vitamin and mineral status, persons in critical care environments, and persons in poor metabolic control. A nutrition assessment that includes a food frequency evaluation can assist in evaluating intake.

In general, individuals who consume a healthy, well-balanced diet that mimics the USDA *Food Guide Pyramid* should ingest the RDA for vitamins and minerals without taking supplements. The recommendation for five to nine servings of fruit and vegetables each day is targeted at providing ample amounts of the antioxidants vitamin C and beta-carotene. Whole-grain breads and cereals, as well as nuts and legumes, are good sources of many of the vitamins (especially E) and minerals (Table 4-6). Vitamin E intake of 200 IU/day is thought to be necessary to obtain cardiovascular risk-reduction benefits. Unfortunately, this is unattainable by natural foods. Although supplementation with vitamin E is thought to be benign, long-term effects have not been studied.

Nutritional supplements may be necessary in cases where deficiencies are identified or a therapeutic trial is considered potentially beneficial. Elemental zinc has been reported to aid wound healing in patients with leg ulcers.[73] Calcium and iron supplementation may be necessary in many women. Persons with type I diabetes may be at risk for significant changes in vitamin D and calcium metabolism associated with reduced bone mass, yet epidemiologic studies fail to show a higher incidence of fractures in individuals with diabetes.[76]

CLASSIFICATION OF DIABETES AND NUTRITIONAL GUIDELINES

Although principles of nutrition are the same for all individuals with diabetes, dietary approaches to normalizing blood glucose levels can differ by type of diabetes. Priorities vary according to insulin defect and metabolic goals. This chapter presents strategies for nutritional management of IDDM and NIDDM and for pregnancy in gestational and overt diabetes.

Nutritional Management of IDDM

IDDM represents an absolute dependence on exogenous insulin for survival. Diet and insulin prescriptions need to be integrated to achieve optimum energy metabolism and avoid hyperglycemia or hypoglycemia. Fortunately, modern insulin regimens and blood glucose monitoring allow increased flexibility in meal planning to accommodate individual life-styles. IDDM is generally associated with youth because most people are diagnosed before age 30. People with IDDM, however, are of all ages and require dietary modifications appropriate for their chronologic age. Adjustments for metabolic changes resulting from the duration of diabetes may also be required.

Goals for nutritional management

Nutritional management of IDDM requires micromanagement on a daily basis. Close attention must be given to the postprandial glycemic effect of food, bioavailability of injected insulin, time from or to a meal, activity level, and other variables that influence glucose homeostasis. In addition, nutritional care of IDDM must address long-term issues of normal growth and development, optimal health, and prevention of cardiovascular and other nutrition-related diseases.

Nutritional strategies

Specific strategies that will help achieve nutritional goals for individuals with IDDM are to (1) emphasize consistency in day-to-day food intake, (2) determine a meal plan from a nutrition assessment that is appropriate for the individual's life-style and integrates insulin therapy, and (3) modify the composition of the diet as needed to achieve specific goals, provide optimal nutrition, promote growth and development, and maintain desirable body weight.

Consistency in food intake. Flexible insulin regimens and SMBG now allow great latitude in meal planning for IDDM. Dietitians in the DCCT used a variety of nutrition interventions to enable participants to attain excellent glycemic control.[46] The most sophisticated insulin regimen, however, still cannot mimic the exquisite secretory response of the pancreas and must rely on estimates of the amount of insulin required for metabolic balance. Therefore day-to-day *consistency*—in meal times, in meal composition, and in caloric intake—is an important strategy in nutritional management of IDDM. Evaluation of diet behaviors of DCCT participants in the intensive therapy group showed a significant association between lower glycated hemoglobin levels and greater consistency in food intake.[48]

Consistency in eating patterns helps to moderate the multiple factors that can influence glucose homeostasis. The greatest demand for insulin is during postprandial metabolism. In the postabsorptive state, insulin requirements are minimal. When erratic eating patterns result in widely varying insulin demands, it is increasingly difficult to match insulin doses with metabolic needs. Changes in activity, emotional status, and other factors also affect insulin requirements; therefore consistency in the diet helps reduce the number of variables that can interfere with glucose regulation.

Coordinating diet and insulin therapy. Meals, snacks, and the insulin regimen should be planned based on an assessment of the person's life-style. A child who is bused to and from school, a nurse who works the evening shift, or a trial lawyer has a very different schedule that directs when he or she injects insulin and eats meals. SMBG provides valuable information that individuals with diabetes can use to integrate diet, exercise, and insulin therapy into their daily routines and adjust for planned or unplanned changes in their usual activities.

Intensive management regimens use adjustments in food and in insulin dosage as strategies to attain optimal blood glucose control. These techniques are used to correct for hyperglycemia or hypoglycemia and to fine-tune the insulin/food ratio for a meal. Methods for measuring the total glucose available from a meal, for estimating the glycemic impact from carbohydrate and protein, or for counting carbohydrate alone are in use. Of these, carbohydrate counting is the most popular. A ratio of 1 unit of insulin per 10 to 15 g of carbohydrate is a commonly used formula for adjusting meals and snacks. Insulin sensitivity varies from individual to individual and even during the day for any one individual; therefore it is important to determine a carbohydrate/insulin ratio for each person managed with intensive therapy.

When developing individualized meal plans, certain fundamentals must be considered. First, the time and composition of a meal and the time, type, and amount of injected insulin must be coordinated. Second, availability of food varies and often dictates what and when people eat. Third, the ability and willingness of the individual to cooperate in the treatment regimen has a direct effect on the therapeutic outcome.

Timing and composition of meals. Meal planning varies with the insulin regimen. When two injections of mixed short- and intermediate-acting insulins are prescribed, meals and snacks need to correspond to four periods of insulin activity. On a daytime schedule using Regular and NPH insulins, the pharmacokinetics of the Regular and NPH in the morning injection cover breakfast and lunch, respectively, whereas the evening dose of Regular insulin covers dinner. A bedtime snack is needed to compensate for the hypoglycemic potential of the evening NPH insulin. Additional snacks may be required to provide readily available glucose at insulin activity peaks of midmorning and midafternoon.

Intensive insulin therapy, by multidose insulin injections, continuous subcutaneous insulin infusion, or implanted pump provides low levels of insulin to mimic basal secretion and uses boluses of short-acting insulin before meals. Between-meal snacks usually are not required on these regimens.[112] The need for a bedtime snack varies by type of basal insulin and by individual metabolic differences. If a bedtime snack is indicated, or requested by personal preference, the need to bolus Regular insulin also must be evaluated.

Snacks, to offset the caloric expenditure and hypoglycemic effect of exercise, are an important consideration in meal planning for IDDM. The frequency, intensity, time, and duration of exercise, individual weight, insulin regimen, and other food intake should be taken into consideration when planning exercise snacks. Guidelines for snacks are provided in Chapter 5.

Availability of food. To facilitate adherence to the planned diet, practical consideration must be given to the availability of food.[77] Access to food can be restricted by job and school schedules, living conditions, travel, and other factors. The type of food available is limited when meals are prepared by others or eaten away from home and by economic, social, religious, or ethnic constraints. The feasibility of making changes in food access or food type can be discussed with the individual during the diet assessment. Meal planning and insulin therapy should be guided by realistic decisions on what modifications in food availability can, or will, be made.

Involvement of the person with diabetes. The willingness and ability of the individual to carry out the treatment plan are prime considerations. Nutrition and insulin therapies should be based on the goals of the person with diabetes, even when they appear in conflict with good diabetes management. The trial lawyer who may miss meals during court days, the teenager who is going to consume alcoholic beverages with peers, or the person with limited skills or limited desire to monitor self-care behaviors needs a diet and insulin regimen that will help him or her stay out of metabolic crises. Guidelines on modifications that can be made in the diet plan based on SMBG values enable the person with diabetes to adjust for expected and unexpected changes in routine.[112] The importance of making appropriate adjustments was underscored in analysis of dietary behaviors of subjects in the intensive treatment group of the DCCT. In addition to adherence to the prescribed meal plan, adjusting food and/or insulin in response to hyperglycemia was a diet behavior significantly associated with lower HbA_{1c} levels.[48] Use of SMBG in nutrition counseling is discussed later in this chapter.

Calories and nutrients to promote health. Caloric requirements increase from birth through the growth years and then stabilize and depend more on activity levels. Monitoring developmental growth and adjusting the diet plan to accommodate changing nutrient requirements are very important for the child with IDDM. Estimating the right number of calories is challenging, since requirements vary dramatically with day-to-day activities, from season to season, and during growth spurts. Advocates for a nonstructured approach to the diet argue that an individual's appetite is more sensitive to caloric requirements than professional estimates.[35,85] However, some dietary guidelines, whether in a structured or unstructured teaching format, are needed to assure adequate nutrition and to assist in glucose control.

Excess weight gain can occur in individuals of all ages with IDDM but is most common in teenage women and in adults. Weight gain has been found to be an undesired side effect of improved metabolic control and has been most evident when a person is changed to intensive insulin therapy.[47,112,142] This phenomenon has been attributed to improved utilization of glucose calories, increased experimentation with foods and meal patterns, and overtreatment of insulin reactions. Planning a weight-loss program for an individual with IDDM includes reducing food intake, increasing exercise, and decreasing the insulin dose. Information from SMBG can guide adjustments and help maintain stable diabetes control during the period of weight loss.

Eating disorders including anorexia nervosa and bulimia nervosa occur in diabetic individuals as they do in nondiabetic individuals. Some authors suggest that adolescents with diabetes are at increased risk because of the intense focus on diet;[132] however, several studies of women with IDDM have found rates of anorexia and bulimia within the range identified for the general population.[25,134,120] A "purging" method unique to diabetes—glycosuria induced by insulin manipulation—has been identified in 5% to 15% of subjects in these studies. This technique was used by participants both with and without evidence of clinical eating disorders.[117] The combination of IDDM and an eating disorder intensifies management problems associated with either diagnosis and requires a team effort to provide psychologic, nutritional, and metabolic counseling.

Nutritional Management of NIDDM

Nearly 90% of individuals with diabetes have type II, or non-insulin-dependent diabetes (NIDDM). Because NIDDM generally manifests itself after age 40, nutritional issues are those of the adult individual. Yet, there are an increasing number of individuals who develop the disease in their 20s and 30s. Obesity, a sedentary life-style, and a family history of diabetes are risk factors for developing type II diabetes.

Goals and strategies for nutritional management

Overall dietary treatment goals in type II diabetes do not differ from those for individuals with type I diabetes (see Table 4-1). Strategies or methods used to achieve these goals, however, are unique to each individual and can be influenced by the type of diabetes, body weight, and other factors.

Type II diabetes is characterized by varying degrees of insulin resistance and insulin secretion (normal, less than normal, or greater than normal). Metabolic response to dietary fat, cholesterol, carbohydrate, and sodium is also different among individuals. In turn, the nutrition approach necessary to achieve desired medical outcomes varies. Life-style, eating habits, food preferences, medical condition, medications (including insulin and oral agents), attitude toward health, and support systems each influence selection of the approach as well.

Glucose intolerance and the incidence of diabetes rise with increasing body weight; thus the primary treatment strategy for at least 80% of individuals with NIDDM is weight reduction. Indeed, losing weight generally improves all aspects of metabolic control including hyperglycemia, hyperlipidemia, and hypertension.[107] For the remaining 10% to 20% of type II individuals who are already at a reasonable body weight, other strategies can be used to achieve metabolic control. As a rule, the diet in NIDDM can be manipulated to improve metabolic control in the following ways:

1. Altering the composition of the diet (i.e., macronutrients)
2. Altering meal timing
3. Altering the distribution of calories at meals and snacks
4. Reducing calories to reduce body weight

Composition of the diet. An appreciation for the heterogeneity of type II diabetes is necessary to develop an effective nutrition plan. Nutrition priorities need to be developed based on medical goals. Clearly, achieving and maintaining optimal blood glucose values are priorities, as are normalizing the hypercholesterolemia and hypertriglyceridemia. In contrast, not every person with type II diabetes has hypertension and/or responds to salt restriction. Multiple restrictions only lead to nonadherance, particularly in persons with NIDDM who are older and bring with them years of dietary habits.

The appropriate distribution of carbohydrate, protein, and fat in a person with type II diabetes is the one that achieves desired medical outcomes for that individual. The process to determine this begins with a nutritional assessment of current food intake. Obvious sources of excess nutrients should be modified first, for example, regular pop or juice ad lib, large amounts of carbohydrate at a particular meal or snack, large quantities of fat (particularly from animal products), or excessive protein consumption. A discussion of the *Food Pyramid Guidelines* is useful when illustrating desired changes.

Actual percentages of calories contributed by carbohydrate, protein, or fat are not as important as the medical outcome. Decreased medical outcomes include improved preprandial and postprandial blood glucose values, and HbA_{1c} and improved LDL cholesterol and improved triglyceride levels. Indeed, most individuals will achieve desired outcomes with modest dietary modifications.

Carbohydrate, regardless of its source, may be tolerated to different degrees depending on insulin availability. Persons using insulin can adjust insulin dose to accommodate more carbohydrate at a meal or snack than can a person on oral agents or diet and exercise alone. Weight loss in obese individuals usually improves insulin sensitivity, and carbohydrate tolerance can return to near normal. If elevated lipids and poor blood glucose control persist despite weight loss or if weight-reduction efforts are unsuccessful, the composition of the diet needs more intensive manipulation.

A practical approach to most obese individuals with type II diabetes is to begin with a focus on restricting fat to near 30% and restricting calories. The resulting diet is then composed of 10% to 20% protein and 50% to 60% carbohydrate. If blood glucose control and lipid levels remain less than desired after a 3- to 6-month evaluation period, an alternative approach is warranted. Decreasing carbohydrate to 40% to 45% and increasing fat to 30% to 40% (predominately MUFA) is an alternative approach that should be considered and evaluated.

Calorie and carbohydrate distribution. Because the pancreas of the person with NIDDM cannot secrete enough insulin after a meal to maintain normal glycemia, it has traditionally been considered best to distribute calories and carbohydrate evenly throughout the day. Three equal meals with one or two snacks has been considered ideal. The most common food intake pattern for an obese person is one of a small or nonexistent breakfast, a small lunch, and a large evening meal and snack in which the majority of the day's calories are consumed.[26] Because the majority of patients with NIDDM are obese, this pattern is not uncommon in this population.

It remains to be seen whether the pattern in which food is consumed has an impact on blood glucose control or obesity in NIDDM. Body weight may not be influenced by what time calories are consumed as long as calorie requirements are not exceeded. When calories are held constant, mean blood glucose levels are similar in moderately well-controlled NIDDM subjects whether they consume their daily calories as three equal meals or with 70% of calories consumed at the evening meal.[21] If this is true, long-standing eating habits of the older NIDDM patients may not need to be altered to improve control. Daily blood glucose testing and close follow-up are required to evaluate the best way to distribute calories and carbohydrate.

Carbohydrate should be distributed among three meals. The size of meals varies with individual preferences and life-style but is also influenced by preprandial and postprandial blood glucose values. Most individuals are least carbohydrate tolerant in the morning hours. As a result, the breakfast meal contains the least amount of carbohydrate of the day. One- to two-hour postprandial blood glucose values are useful to evaluate the amount of carbohydrate that can be tolerated at each meal or snack. Once this value has been established, consistency in CHO intake can be achieved by carbohydrate counting or an exchange type plan.

Whereas snacks are often valuable in IDDM to prevent hypoglycemia between meals, this habit may not be of any value to the person with NIDDM. In type II diabetes, postprandial glucose responses are influenced by endogenous insulin production as well as peripheral glucose uptake. Snacking has been shown to delay or prevent blood glucose from returning to baseline values,[22] thus prolonging hyperglycemia throughout the day. Some individuals may prefer a small snack between meals to reduce hunger or reduce the fear of an insulin reaction. Because individual responses may vary, blood glucose monitoring is necessary to evaluate whether snacks are necessary or how large they should be.

Meal timing. Because of a delayed and sluggish insulin response in NIDDM, generally 4 to 5 hours is required for enough insulin to be secreted to bring blood glucose down to baseline levels. As a result, it has been postulated that meals should be spaced 4 to 5 hours apart.[129] In theory this should allow blood glucose to fall to baseline before another glucose challenge from another meal or snack. This again is another theory that requires additional research.

Strict attention to consuming meals at specific times is not an issue for NIDDM patients who do not take insulin or oral agents. Consistency is required in those NIDDM individuals who take exogenous insulin just as in IDDM. As a rule, however, NIDDM patients have a better counterregulatory response and do not have problems with very severe hypoglycemic reactions. Planning ahead and not delaying or skipping meals are still important in NIDDM patients taking insulin, particularly in older adults. It has been suggested that cognitive functioning decreases in older adults. Hypoglycemia also alters cognitive functioning. Forgetting or delaying a meal may have serious implications in the elderly NIDDM patient.

Promoting reasonable body weight. Maintaining normal body weight is important to maintaining normoglycemia. As body weight increases, insulin resistance, glucose intolerance, and the propensity to develop diabetes increase. Because nearly 90% of patients with NIDDM are overweight, a hypocaloric diet to facilitate weight loss is the primary treatment goal for the majority of NIDDMs. Yet some 5% to 10% of NIDDM patients are normal weight at the time of diagnosis. For these individuals, consuming an appropriate calorie level to *maintain* their normal body weight is important. Frequently, improved glycemic control can result in weight gain because glucose calories are no longer lost in the urine. As a rule, a specific calorie prescription is unnecessary in a normal weight individual who is successfully regulating body weight. Carbohydrate counting and guidelines to reduce saturated and total fat are effective techniques in such cases.

Obesity is defined as an excess of body fat. Normal body fat content is approximately 15% to 17% in men and 22% to 25% in women.[96] Overfatness is defined as body fat in excess of 20% for men and 30% for women. Body fat content has a tendency to increase with advancing age. It is not clear if this is normal or merely reflects a decrease in muscle mass from inactivity and lack of use.

Development of the bioelectrical impedance technique for measuring body fatness has made it easier to determine actual percentage of body fat. This technique measures total body water and, in turn, lean body mass (LBM) by measuring resistance to a slight electrical current passed through the body. Because water is a good conductor of electricity, less resistance is present when more water is present—indicating more LBM. Use of this technique is increasing in frequency because it is painless, relatively accurate, and easy to perform.

Most health professionals, however, continue to rely on body mass index (BMI) or relative body weight to determine degree of obesity. BMI is an expression of weight where the effect of height is minimized (wt [kg] $\div$ ht [m^2]). It is considered more accurate than height-weight values. A BMI above 27 is generally indicative of obesity because it is equivalent to 20% above desirable weight. This term is not easily translated to the patient; therefore relative body weight is often used.

Relative body weight is the percentage of actual weight compared with ideal. Individuals above 20% of desirable body weight are considered obese. Controversy exists as to what is ideal body weight. Height and weight tables published by the Metropolitan Life Insurance Company are generally used as guides for desirable weight. Some clinicians are concerned over the fact that weights in the 1983 tables are higher than weights in the 1959 tables. The question often asked is "Are we accepting a heavier weight as normal when it is merely just reflecting a national trend toward obesity?"

Whenever body weight is being assessed, it is important to be realistic about what is a reasonable weight goal. This must be established with each individual patient based on age, degree of obesity, activity level, medical condition, and ability to restrict intake and alter life-style. Because most patients with NIDDM are older, realistic target weight goals are even more important.

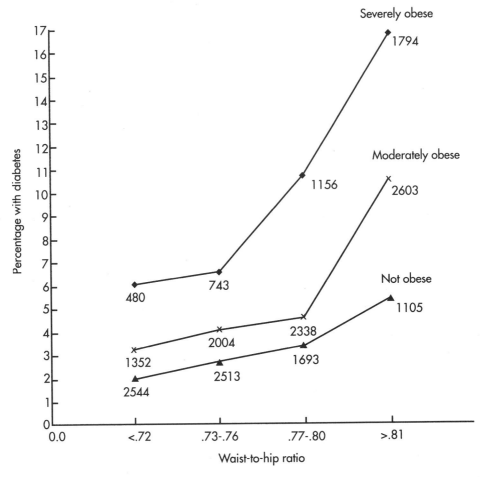

Fig. 4-3 The prevalence of diabetes according to relative weight and body fat distribution in 20,325 women. (From Hartz AJ and others: *Am J Epidemiol* 119:76, 1984.)

Not only is the degree of obesity and body fatness significant in determining glucose intolerance, so is body fat distribution.[71] Individuals with body fat located above the waist generally have higher insulin, blood glucose, and serum lipid levels than individuals in whom body fat is located predominantly in the hips and thighs.[111,130] Such upper body obesity increases risk of cardiovascular disease, hypertension, and diabetes. Interestingly, upper body fat increases risk even at modest or slight levels of obesity (Fig. 4-3). Risk becomes greater as the degree of obesity increases.

Promoting weight loss. An effective weight reduction diet for the obese person with NIDDM should have several components. It should be safe, should be hypocaloric enough to promote a reasonable weight loss of 1/2 to 2 pounds/week, should focus on developing healthy eating behaviors, should enhance self-esteem, and should promote increased physical activity. Many weight loss approaches are available that can in most instances be used in

NIDDM patients. The most frequently used approach is the "exchange" plan in its many variations. This is an excellent approach, since it promotes healthy eating choices and the consistency in calories and nutrient intake that is needed for individuals on hypoglycemic medication.

Not all patients with NIDDM can be treated the same way when it comes to diet. Many individuals may have trouble with the exchange diet because of the rigidity and complex nature of the exchange system. Some individuals would prefer fewer choices and a less complicated approach such as individualized menus. Many older individuals in particular are less apt to experiment with new foods and prefer eating similar foods on a regular rotation.

Counting calories or counting grams of fat may be preferred by many NIDDM patients who are not on medication, because these methods are simple to use. Patients can be taught to limit fat intake to 50 g/day or 25% to 30% of calories. Grams of fat can be determined using the exchange lists, nutrition labeling, and various other sources. This is often a good place to start with a newly diagnosed obese patient who may be easily overwhelmed by the many required diabetes self-care behaviors in addition to the diet.

Counting calories may be most effective when the patient is given guidelines for calorie distribution at meals, (e.g., breakfast, 300 kcal; lunch, 400; dinner, 500; and snacks, 300). A major drawback to this method of weight loss is the lack of control regarding sources of calories. There is no guarantee that food choices will be healthy. Using the *Food Guide Pyramid* as a guide for daily food choices is helpful.

The popularity of prepackaged and liquid diet regimens has had an impact on the approach to managing obesity in diabetes. These "no choices" approaches can be used in NIDDM patients under close medical and dietary supervision. Studies have demonstrated that very-low-calorie diets (VLCDs) of less than 800 calories/day can be used successfully with obese diabetic patients.[17] These diets can produce rapid weight loss, dramatically improve blood glucose levels, and improve hypertension. Sustaining improved blood glucose responses with refeeding appears to depend largely on duration of diabetes and pancreatic insulin reserve.

Because of the drastic caloric restriction of these approaches, they should be limited to individuals who are at least 50 pounds overweight. Risks involved with use, such as cholecystitis, pancreatitis, and dysrhythmias, are minimized by careful patient screening and close medical supervision.

The protein-sparing modified fast (PSMF) is a VLCD approach that has been used for years by many clinicians and involves real food in the form of lean meat, fish, and poultry. These high-protein foods are distributed as two to three meals per day in amounts to provide 1.2 to 1.5 g protein/kg ideal body weight. Fruits and vegetables may be incorporated to a level of 50 g carbohydrate/day. The result is similar to liquid regimens with the advantage of using real food. This allows the clinician and patient to focus on eating behaviors during the diet process. A major drawback to this approach is that supplements of vitamins and minerals are required and can sometimes be forgotten by even the most well-intending patient.

Pharmacologic therapy is emerging as an adjunct to core weight reduction therapies of low-fat eating, exercise, and behavior modification. Phentermine and fenfluramine are two popular appetite suppressants that are generally used in combination. They can produce good weight loss results with few side effects.[67] To be effective, individuals must use these medications for life, just as in therapy for hypertension and other medical disorders.

Careful monitoring of blood glucose is a must in patients who are taking insulin and on a calorie-restricted diet. Blood glucose levels generally decrease as soon as caloric restriction is initiated. If insulin doses are not tapered accordingly, the patient may develop hypoglycemia. To many individuals, including older adults, this is a very unpleasant and fearful experience. As a result, they may often "feed" the insulin to prevent hypoglycemia. The patients' comfort level and trust can be enhanced if the insulin dose is reduced at the onset of a hypocaloric diet. Patients using VLCDs should have their insulin dose reduced by one-third to one-half on initiating the diet. Patients on oral hypoglycemic agents will need the dose reduced or discontinued. Failure to lose expected weight may be the result of frequent reactions that are overtreated with high-calorie foods.

One of the greatest concerns with any weight loss regimen (most recently the VLCDs) is the poor weight maintenance results. All successful weight loss regimens must focus on helping the patient develop permanent changes in eating and activity behaviors. Cognitive restructuring of self-defeating thoughts is a concept receiving considerable attention in weight loss therapy. Obese patients with NIDDM can often have a poor self-image not only because of obesity but also because of the stigma of a chronic disease. Helping patients develop positive attitudes toward life in general can help weight loss efforts immensely.

Setting reasonable weight loss goals is one way to promote confidence and improve self-image in the obese persons with NIDDM. Generally, even small losses such as 10 to 20 pounds can substantially improve blood glucose levels. This improvement can be considered an important marker of success for the obese patient with NIDDM and can be used by the clinician to instill a sense of achievement in the patient. This is particularly true in the older individual in whom weight loss is frequently more difficult.

Weight goals should be kept reasonable in older persons who may have additional factors impacting their health. Clinicians differ as to their philosophy regarding weight goals in older adults. Some believe that a few pounds over desirable weight may be better because it may act as a nutritional reserve in the event of illness, infection, or surgery. Current health status, degree of overweight, body fat distribution, and activity level should all be considered when determining the impact that individual body weight is having on the older adult's health.

Nutritional Management of Pregnancy in Gestational and Overt Diabetes

Goals for nutritional management

Healthy babies and healthy mothers are the goals for nutritional management of diabetes during pregnancy. These goals are the same for pregnant women with previously diagnosed diabetes (IDDM and NIDDM) and women who develop gestational diabetes (GDM). In nondiabetic individuals, glucose levels are lower during pregnancy than in the nonpregnant state.[6,121] In pregnancies complicated by diabetes, the outcome of a healthy baby appears associated with achieving and maintaining these lower norms for blood glucose control. The risk for fetal abnormalities to occur during embryogenesis (gestational weeks 3 to 7) and for macrosomia to develop in the third trimester can be reduced with tight diabetes control.[6,121] The need for excellent blood glucose control during the first weeks of pregnancy mandates that nutritional counseling actually begins before conception.

Nutritional strategies

Goals for nutrition therapy for the pregnant woman are to provide adequate nutrition for fetal and maternal health, to promote appropriate weight gain, and to maintain blood glucose levels in a near normal range. The RDAs show increased requirements for most nutrients during pregnancy.[57] Protein needs increase by 10 g/day and during the second and third trimesters, caloric requirements by 300 cal/day. Women who are well nourished can achieve adequate intakes of most vitamins and minerals by selecting appropriate foods; however, supplementation is required to meet the requirements for iron and folate.[6] A ferrous sulfate supplement is recommended for the second and third trimesters. Folate supplementation (400 mg/day) should be given before conception as well as during pregnancy to reduce the risk of neural tube defects. Undernourished women, those with special problems, and women whose nutrient intake does not meet the recommendations for pregnancy should receive a vitamin/mineral supplement containing iron, zinc, copper, calcium, vitamin B_6, folate, vitamin C, and vitamin D. Because caffeine may retard fetal growth, intake should be limited to <300 mg/day (2 ½ cups regular coffee).

Recommendations on caloric intake are related to pregestational weight and the desired weight gain for the pregnancy (Table 4-7). Fetal caloric requirements are minimal during the first trimester; therefore women entering pregnancy in the desirable weight range do not need to increase their caloric intake until the fourth month. An intake of 30 cal/kg of prepregnancy body weight is recommended.[6] Women in the low-weight category should eat sufficient calories (36-40 kcal/kg/day) throughout pregnancy to replenish depleted nutrient and energy stores and reduce the risk of a low-birth-weight baby. Women in the overweight category have a reserve of adipose tissue—thus a lower weight-gain goal and a lower caloric need (18-22 kcal/kg/day). Caloric intake should be monitored to prevent large weight gains. At all weight levels, calories should be sufficient to prevent starvation ketosis. For individuals with diabetes the changes in metabolism associated with each trimester and more stringent goals for blood glucose levels require adjustments in meal patterns throughout pregnancy.

It is important to recognize that pregnancy is marked by hormonal changes that foster hypoglycemia in the first trimester and hyperglycemia in the latter trimester. Adjustments

Table 4-7   Recommended Weight Gain for Pregnant Women Based on Prepregnancy Body Mass Index (BMI)

Weight-for-height category	Recommended weight gain	
	kg	lb
Low (BMI <19.8)	12.5-18	28-40
Normal (BMI 19.8-26)	11.5-16	25-35
High (BMI 26-29)	7.0-11.5	15-25
Obese (BMI >29)	≥6	≥15

Modified from Subcommittee on Nutritional Status and Weight Gain During Pregnancy, Food and Nutrition Board, National Academy of Science: *Nutrition During Pregnancy,* Washington, DC, 1990, National Academy Press.
BMI, wt(kg)/ht(m^2).

in the meal pattern from trimester to trimester should be made to accommodate the changing hormonal effects. Whereas SMBG is essential for women on insulin therapy, it is a valuable tool for all pregnant women with diabetes to use to adjust food intake to attain glycemic goals.

Composition and distribution. As just noted, protein needs increase during pregnancy by 10 g/day. Protein will provide approximately 20% of the caloric intake. The amount of carbohydrate in the diet should be adjusted to promote optimal postprandial blood glucose values. Several studies suggest that normoglycemia will be attained only if carbohydrate is limited to approximately 40% of total calories.[2,81] Individual tolerance of carbohydrate should be assessed with frequent blood glucose monitoring. With 60% of calories coming from protein and carbohydrate sources, the remaining 40% is fat calories. This level is higher than general recommendations for American adults but illustrates the 1994 "Nutrition Recommendations" to select the macronutrient composition of the diet to achieve metabolic goals—not predetermined algorithms.

Achieving "tight glycemic control" while meeting maternal and fetal nutrient needs requires careful meal planning by the registered dietitian and diligence on the part of the pregnant woman. Whether the woman is taking exogenous insulin or relying on her endogenous supply, the need to minimize postprandial glycemic excursions is so critical that the glycemic effect of each meal and snack must be considered. Self-monitoring of blood glucose should be used to evaluate the current meal plan and insulin doses (when applicable), and modifications should be made in one or both therapies to achieve targeted blood glucose goals.

A plan of three meals and three snacks is a recommended guideline.[6] Carbohydrate counting as a meal-planning strategy and a sliding scale for insulin adjustment provide the pregnant woman with tools to fine tune her diabetes management and better achieve blood glucose goals. Morning insulin resistance, caused by growth hormone and cortisol, is greater during pregnancy, resulting in increased carbohydrate intolerance at breakfast. For this reason, a juice, cereal, and skim milk breakfast may raise blood glucose levels above the targeted postprandial range. A meal pattern more typical of lunch (i.e., higher in protein and complex carbohydrate and with some fat) may be a better choice for breakfast. Fruit and skim milk can be eaten at meals or snacks later in the day. SMBG should be used throughout pregnancy to adjust the carbohydrate content of meals and the insulin dose for women on insulin therapy.

Special considerations

Morning sickness usually occurs during the first trimester—the period marked by hypoglycemia in pregnant women with diabetes. Morning sickness can contribute to hypoglycemia, and hypoglycemia can cause nausea. Dietary strategies include small, frequent feedings of easily digested foods spread throughout the day and at night. Crackers, melba toast, rice cakes, and similar carbohydrate foods are easy to keep available at bedside, work, or in the car and are well tolerated by many women, although nausea is idiosyncratic and food tolerances vary. Some aspects of good nutrition, such as milk consumption, may be poorly tolerated and require adjustments in the diet during the period of nausea. If morning sickness persists and compromises nutrition, a vitamin-mineral supplement should be prescribed with the advice to take the pills in the evening rather than in the morning.[6] Again, careful SMBG and use of carbohydrate counting to make decisions on food selection can help avoid hypoglycemia.

The tendency for ketosis, a common result of fetal demands on maternal fuel sources, requires routine monitoring of ketone as well as glucose levels to evaluate optimum energy metabolism. A positive test for ketones in the morning is a common result of the long period between the evening snack and breakfast. Adjustment of composition, size, and time of the evening snack may reduce morning ketonuria, but as adjustments are made, the effect on evening blood glucose values must be monitored. A 3 AM snack may give optimal therapy and, with the nocturia of pregnancy, may not be too inconvenient for the expectant mother.

Postpartum

The postpartum diet will reflect the status of diabetes, the mother's plans to breast feed, and the mother's desire to lose weight. Most women with gestational diabetes will return to normal glucose metabolism after pregnancy. These women can resume their usual eating patterns without concern for the effect of food on blood glucose levels; however, they should be aware of their risk for developing NIDDM and that weight control can reduce this risk. Women with IDDM will need to decrease their insulin dosage and their caloric intake (if not nursing). Blood glucose values from self-monitoring can guide adjustments in therapy as the body returns to a nonpregnant status. The mother with diagnosed NIDDM before pregnancy will need careful evaluation to determine optimal postpartum diabetes therapy.

Breastfeeding is feasible for women with pregestational and gestational diabetes. For women on insulin, the effect of breastfeeding on blood glucose needs to be added to the usual list of factors influencing glycemia. Blood glucose levels may vary widely during lactation, possibly in relation to the amount of milk produced and the frequency of feedings. Caloric requirements also vary by the amount of milk produced and activity levels. The RDAs recommend an increase of 500 calories a day for lactation to include an additional 15 g/day of protein during the first 6 months of lactation and 12 g/day thereafter.[57] The calories should be distributed throughout the day. Adding between-meal snacks can help prevent hypoglycemia and may avert the need for increasing the insulin dose to cover larger meals.

Return to a normal weight is a postpartum goal for most women. For women with IDDM, the calories of the prepregnancy diet may need to be adjusted to allow for weight loss. Calorie restriction and exercise, coupled with careful monitoring of blood glucose, facilitate return to a desirable weight. For the woman with gestational diabetes, the tendency to be overweight and the potential for later development of NIDDM indicate that postpartum weight control counseling is very important. Nutritional counseling routinely should be provided to postpartum GDM women.

Nutrition Recommendations for Children

Nutrition therapy for children with diabetes needs to be individualized and directed to "maintain health and a sense of normalcy for the child and his/her family."[58] A nutrition assessment of the child's eating patterns, activity level, and weight history provides information on food habits that can be maintained and areas to suggest modifications. Food intake records are the best tool for determining caloric requirements. If the child has lost weight or is underweight, calories can be increased to achieve a "goal" weight gain.

Children's caloric requirements will need ongoing assessment to provide sufficient calories for growth and development.

Children with diabetes have an increased risk for heart disease. The American Diabetes Association recommends that children over the age of 2 years have a full lipid profile upon diagnosis, after blood glucose is stabilized, with results evaluated by National Cholesterol Education Program guidelines.[9] Diets for children with diabetes should follow adult guidelines for healthy eating to limit total fat intake to 30% or less of calories with no more than 10% of calories from saturated fat. Rigorous restriction of dietary fat or cholesterol is not recommended for children under 2 years, in whom metabolic processes are in developmental phases.[27]

Early exposure to cow's milk has been investigated as a risk factor for IDDM. A case control study of children with IDDM in a diabetes registry matched with nondiabetic subjects found a combined effect of genetic and environmental factors.[88] The risk for IDDM was associated with early exposure (before 3 months) to cow's milk or solid foods and a genetic susceptibility to IDDM measured by an HLA marker. The hypothesis is that a cow's milk protein, bovine serum albumin (BSA), triggers an autoimmune reaction resulting in circulating antibodies that attack a pancreatic beta cell protein with a molecular structure that mimics BSA.[82] The importance of early exposure appears related to maturation of the digestive system. The immature digestive system has difficulty breaking down proteins, and intact molecules can be absorbed into the bloodstream before "gut closure," which occurs between 3 and 12 months of age. Thus BSA can enter the bloodstream and initiate antibody formation.

BSA is found in most dairy products including whey, which is an ingredient in a number of nondairy foods (e.g., canned soups). Beef and foods containing beef products also contain BSA. Because BSA can cross mammary glands, breast milk may contain BSA. At present, more studies are needed to clarify the BSA theory and determine appropriate interventions, including any recommendations on manipulation of infant diets. Current guidelines from the American Academy of Pediatrics Committee on Nutrition are that babies be breastfed for the first 6 to 12 months of life and only iron-fortified formula be used to supplement; cow's milk should not be given during the first year.[3]

Nutrition Recommendations for Older Adults with Diabetes

The prevalence of non-insulin-dependent diabetes increases with age, with an estimated 20% of the U.S. population over age 65 having diabetes.[104] It is uncertain if the increase in diabetes in this age-group is related to aging, to changes in life-style, or to adiposity. Age does impose several challenges for nutritional management of the older adult with diabetes.

At present, little information is available on the nutritional requirements of older adults with or without diabetes. The RDAs use age categories to define variations in nutrient requirements across the life span but use 51+ years as the upper age category.[57] The increased number of people living into their 80s and 90s raises questions about differences in nutrient requirements for the "elderly," often defined as 75 years and older.

Although different nutrient requirements for older adults have not been demonstrated, the disproportion of nutrition problems among older Americans has been documented.[52] Many factors contribute to the decline in health status in older adults. Changes of aging such as decreased sensory function, limitations in mobility, loss of vision and hearing, and alterations in mental status and in life-style can impact eating behaviors and compromise nutritional status.

Adequate nutrient intake is a primary goal for many older persons. Those with diabetes have the added goal of glycemic control. Older individuals living alone may find it difficult to buy and prepare foods required for their meal plan. Many older adults do not eat three meals a day, choosing to eat a late breakfast and early dinner. Others eat on a random schedule driven by sleep/wake patterns, socialization, or diverse other triggers. The range of foods consumed often is limited by practical constraints such as size available for purchase and the potential for spoilage before items are used. Home-delivered meals have been shown to improve eating regularity and the range of foods eaten by older diabetic persons living at home.[53] Nursing home residents do not have difficulty acquiring food but have little choice in meal time or type of food. Residents with diabetes often are placed on a special diet, which imposes an additional restriction on their food choices. The 1994 "Nutrition Recommendations" make prescription of "a diabetic diet" obsolete; however, individual diet counseling is not readily available to all nursing home residents. One study has shown that the regular menu of a nursing home can be fed to residents with NIDDM without significant deterioration of glycemic control.[40] Helping an older adult with diabetes develop an eating pattern of routine meals consisting of foods that provide adequate nutrition should be the first strategy for nutritional management.

Blood glucose control is important in older adults, but the risk of hypoglycemia needs to be carefully weighed with the benefits of optimal glycemia. Target blood glucose levels should be individualized. Assessment of usual eating patterns allows identification of nutritional deficiencies and problems contributing to hyperglycemia. A meal pattern based on general guidelines for healthy eating may be sufficient to achieve goals of good nutrition and glycemic control for many elderly persons with diabetes.

INDIVIDUALIZATION OF DIET THERAPY

The "Principles of Nutrition" and the guidelines for nutritional management of IDDM, NIDDM, and GDM are generalizations. The true diet for diabetes is the nutrition regimen developed to meet physical, metabolic, and life-style requirements of an individual. The success of the nutrition intervention in diabetes depends on how well the diet fits the unique metabolic needs of the individual and how well the individual incorporates the diet plan into his or her life-style. Therefore each diet prescription must be based on nutrition assessment and treatment goals identified by the person with diabetes and other members of the health care team.[8] The process of medical nutrition therapy includes (1) assessment to identify nutrition and metabolic problems, (2) collaboration of the person with diabetes and the health care team in setting goals of therapy, (3) design and implementation of the nutrition intervention, and (4) evaluation of the treatment plan using clinical data and input from the person with diabetes (Fig. 4-4).

Assessment

Development of the nutrition regimen starts with an assessment of the individual with diabetes (Box 4-2). Clinical data will identify specific goals for nutrition therapy. For example, if blood

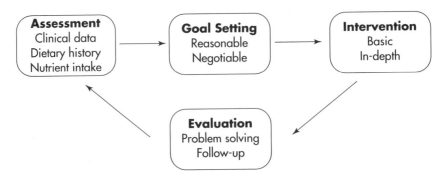

Fig. 4-4   The four-step model for medical nutrition therapy for diabetes. (From Tinker LF and others: *J Am Dietetic Assoc* 94:507-511, 1994.)

BOX 4-2

NUTRITION ASSESSMENT

Clinical data	Dietary history	Nutrient intake	Social history
Height and weight	Usual food intake	Overall nutritional	Daily schedule
Body frame	Attitudes toward	adequacy	Family relation-
Reasonable weight	nutrition and	Caloric intake	ships
Blood pressure	health	Nutrient distribution	Friends—social
Insulin regimen	Previous dietary	Type of carbohy-	support
Family history	education and	drate, protein, and	Finances and living
Laboratory data	outcomes	fat	environment
• Blood glucose	Cultural food prac-		Education—learning
and lipids	tices		style
• Glycated hemo-			
globin			
• Abnormal			
laboratory			
findings			

Modified from Tinker LF, Heins JM, Holler HJ: Commentary and translation: 1994 nutrition recommendations for diabetes, *J Am Diet Assoc* 94:507-511, 1994; and American Diabetes Association: *Medical management of insulin-dependent (type I) diabetes* (ed 2), Alexandria, VA, 1995, The Association.

---

lipid levels are abnormal, the nutrition intervention will focus aggressively on lowering lipids rather than on a more general plan of preventing hyperlipidemia. Current eating patterns should form the basis for the treatment plan with decisions on modifications made in consultation with the person with diabetes. Evaluation of nutrient intake will uncover deficiencies that can be corrected by food or supplements and show excesses in caloric or macronutrient intake or distribution that need to be modified to promote treatment goals. Collecting these data can be time consuming, but the information is essential for providing medical nutrition therapy. A diet for diabetes no longer can be planned simply from information on height, weight, gender, and age. Registered dietitians need to request clinical data before meeting with the person with diabetes. Questionnaires, SMBG logs, and food records, completed by the diabetic individual or by a family member, can save time and may elicit more accurate information than verbal reporting.[91]

There are several common methods for obtaining information on food intake. Retrospective approaches include recall of all food consumed in a 24-hour period or the frequency in which a food is consumed in a specified time period (e.g., per day, week, or month). Prospective assessment, using food diaries kept for 3, 7, or more days, provides greater accuracy in information on eating patterns but is still subject to the bias of self-report or seasonal variation. Size of portion and method of preparation must be delineated to be able to determine caloric and macronutrient intake. Meal times and their relationship to medication, work, social and physical activity, and sleep patterns provide very useful information. This information can be obtained by inquiring about daily schedules for weekdays and weekends. Open-ended questions, such as, "When do you start your day? What is the first thing that you eat? What time is your first meal?" will provide valuable information that may not be elicited if the first question is "What do you usually eat for breakfast?" For individuals on diabetes medication, a question asking when they take their medicine should be included. The value of learning that the person is injecting the morning insulin dose at home, driving the 45-minute commute to work, and then eating breakfast is obvious.

Goal Setting

The goal-setting process actively engages the person with diabetes in his or her care and focuses the health care team on the desired outcomes of therapy. Information from the nutrition assessment, along with options in dietary modifications, should be discussed with the diabetic individual and with other members of the team. Goal setting is a negotiation process in which the expert advice of clinicians and the individual's concerns about diabetes management guide development of the dietary intervention.

Goals for nutrition therapy are behavioral and are directed to help the diabetic individual make changes in diet and exercise that will result in the desired outcomes.[137] It is important that goals be achievable. Small, incremental goals promote success and allow clinicians and the diabetic individual to identify strategies that are successful.

Nutrition Intervention

The nutrition intervention is based on information obtained in the assessment and modified through the goal-setting process. The diet prescription is designed as therapy for specific metabolic abnormalities and tailored to facilitate eating habits that will promote the desired outcomes. Traditionally, the diet prescription has been qualitative—calculated in terms of total calories and macronutrient distribution and then translated into a meal plan using teaching materials such as the exchange lists. A qualitative or behavioral approach that has grown in popularity targets one or two changes in eating behaviors that are identified through review of the diet history. This approach is effective with newly diagnosed individuals or when those with a prior diagnosis are motivated to achieve better diabetes control.

Evaluation

The effectiveness of the nutrition intervention is evaluated by clinical outcomes and feedback from the person with diabetes. Were metabolic goals met? Does the meal plan fit the person's life-style? Evaluation can indicate a need for different strategies to attain metabolic goals or affirm that the nutrition prescription is effective. Adjustments in meal plans are needed for maintenance of some goals, such as weight loss. Medical nutrition therapy is ongoing with evaluation indicating need to change because of life-style, altered diabetes status, or the availability of new therapies.

Caloric Prescription

An individual's caloric needs vary by body size, activity, and the demands for growth. For adults, caloric requirement is estimated to be the number of calories that would maintain weight given the activity pattern of the individual. Adjustments in the estimated requirement would be made to promote weight gain or loss, for the maternal needs of pregnancy and lactation, and to compensate for a catabolic condition caused by illness. Caloric requirements of children include energy to support growth and development, as well as daily energy needs.

An accurate food intake record is the best method for determining caloric requirements. Formulas for calculating energy requirements are available and widely used; however even the most complicated formulas have been shown to underpredict caloric needs in children and overestimate caloric requirements of obese adults.[56] Because accuracy in food records can be difficult to achieve, a combination of caloric estimates obtained from food records and calculated by formula can be used to estimate caloric requirements.

Some formulas calculate the calories for basal or resting energy expenditure (BEE or REE) and then add calories for physical activity. Harris-Benedict equations calculate REE using factors of gender, weight, height, and age:

$$\text{Males: REE} = 66.47 + (13.75 \times \text{wt}) + (5.03 \times \text{ht}) - (6.75 \times \text{age})$$
$$\text{Females: REE} = 655.1 + (9.56 \times \text{wt}) + (1.85 \times \text{ht}) - (4.68 \times \text{age})$$

Weight is measured in kilograms, height in centimeters, and age in years. In contrast, using ideal body weight underestimates requirements by as much as 38%. The RDAs use equations published by WHO that calculate REE by weight, gender, and age in categories.[57] Both the Harris-Benedict equations and the WHO equations can be used in children. The Harris-Benedict equation for males should be used for both genders in children younger than 10 years.[114]

Table 4-8   Estimating Energy Requirements for Adults

Daily activity	Activity factor × REE	kcal/kg*	kcal/pound*
Sedentary	1.3	25-30	11-13
Moderate	1.6	31-38	14-17
Strenuous	2.0	39-47	18-21

*Calculation based on method of Pellet PL: Food energy requirements in humans, *Am J Clin Nutr* 51:717, 1990.
Sedentary: majority of day seated or standing ≤2 hours walking or other light activity. *Moderate:* approximately 8 hours of day walking, gardening, house cleaning, exercising, carpentry, restaurant trades, electrical trades. *Strenuous:* approximately 8 hours a day walking, digging, carrying load, manual labor, climbing, skiing, cycling.

Energy requirements for activity must be added to the REE or basal rate. Factors have been developed to calculate energy requirements based on average daily activity. Table 4-8 gives factors for calculating calorie requirements for adults.

Energy requirements for children are more difficult to estimate. For children ages 1 to 8 years, an activity factor of 2.0 × REE estimates allowances consistent with intake.[114] After age 8, a steady decline in factors from 1.8 to 1.6 (adult level) at age 17 is suggested, with adolescent males having higher energy requirements than females. Another method for calculating calorie requirements of children is to allow 1000 calories for the first year and add 100 calories for girls and 125 calories for boys for each additional year. Up to 20% more calories may be needed to compensate for activity levels. Independent of the method of calculation, the pediatric norms in height-weight grids should guide evaluation of caloric requirements of children.

Providing sufficient calories to promote growth has always been a primary concern when planning diets for diabetic children. Recently, being overweight has become a pediatric problem. More sedentary life-styles are common in children as well as adults, with television and computer games competing with sports and active play for recreational activities. For children with diabetes, overweight also can be attributed to improved blood glucose control and curtailment of the loss of calories in the urine. Careful monitoring of actual calories consumed and of exercise patterns will provide valuable information for a weight management strategy and is a better approach than arbitrary reduction of calories. A child may be eating more calories than planned because of selection of high-fat snacks.[125]

To facilitate weight gain or weight loss, the calories estimated for maintaining weight are increased or decreased. A pound of body fat represents about 3500 calories; therefore adjustments of 500 calories a day should achieve a 1 pound/week change in weight. A greater reduction in calories would allow a faster rate of weight loss; however, minimum daily intakes of 1200 calories for women and 1500 for men are recommended. Diets with calorie levels below the recommended minimum may be nutritionally inadequate, may require supplementation, and should be medically monitored. When weight loss is desired, caloric restriction should be combined with an exercise prescription to increase daily energy expenditure. The combined effect of a reduction in caloric intake and an increase in caloric expenditure is more effective in promoting weight loss than either approach independently.

Distribution of calories among the macronutrients (i.e., carbohydrate, protein, and fat) is guided by dietary habits and target metabolic goals. When developing a diet prescription, the caloric and macronutrient values of current food intake should be calculated first and then modified in consultation with the patient. The effectiveness of these modifications needs to be evaluated through SMBG and laboratory assessment of glycated hemoglobin and lipids and changes made if goals of therapy are not being achieved.

Nutrition Practice Guidelines

Throughout health care a growing trend exists to define good care by guidelines or standards. Interest in having a definition of quality care comes from health professionals, patient/consumers, government, and agencies paying for services. The American Dietetic Association is developing nutrition practice guidelines for diabetes. The first guidelines—for nutrition care for outpatients with NIDDM—were developed, field tested, and analyzed for cost-effectiveness by the International Diabetes Center under a contract from the American Dietetic Association.[59] Guidelines for IDDM are being developed and field tested by the Diabetes Care and Education practice group of the American Dietetic Association. Nutrition guidelines can be used to justify the process of medical nutrition therapy to administrators of health care services, to reimbursement agencies, and to legislators.

TRANSLATING THE NUTRITION PRESCRIPTION INTO MEAL PATTERNS

The best-designed diet prescription is only as effective as the individual's ability and/or willingness to follow instructions. Adhering to a diet requires knowledge to make correct food choices and motivation to alter eating behaviors. Teaching materials and methods should be carefully selected for each person after an educational assessment to identify current knowledge, learning preferences, motivation to learn, reading level, visual acuity, and cultural eating patterns. More than one approach may be used with a single person. For example, initial diet instruction may be limited to survival skills taught with general guidelines, followed by a more detailed meal-planning method introduced in subsequent counseling sessions to increase both precision and flexibility in nutrition therapy. The American Diabetes Association and the American Dietetic Association, recognizing the need for a variety of diabetes nutrition education materials, appointed a task force in 1993 to evaluate current materials and identify and design new ones. Based on an assessment of available materials and input from a number of health professionals, priority was given to development of five publications: four new ones plus a revision of the existing Meal Planning and Exchange Lists. The five tools were developed, field tested, and introduced in 1995. They include a simple guideline based on the *Food Guide Pyramid,* a series on carbohydrate counting, a set of 21 single topic sheets (10 related to food and nutrition, 6 addressing diabetes in general, and 5 discussing diabetes and the life cycle), a resource manual for health professionals to use in helping people with diabetes make behavior changes, and the revised *Exchange Lists.* The range of materials reflects the philosophy of the 1994 "Nutrition Recommendations"—that one single approach is not effective to treat the many metabolic abnormalities found in diabetes.

Teaching Materials

A variety of meal-planning approaches and teaching tools are available in a range of options including general guidelines on healthy eating, targeted approaches focused on one macronutrient or eating behavior, and complex programs providing detailed information on food and techniques for self-evaluation. An extensive review of available teaching materials for diabetes is provided in *Diabetes Medical Nutrition Therapy: A Guide for Professionals,*[4] scheduled for publication in 1996 by the American Diabetes Association and the American Dietetic Association. The handbook combines two popular resources for diabetes nutritional management—*Nutrition Guide for Professionals: Diabetes Education and Meal Planning*[14] and *Meal Planning Approaches for Diabetes Management*[113]—offering health professionals a comprehensive handbook for nutritional management of diabetes. This chapter describes the types of tools available; however, the valuable information contained in *Diabetes Medical Nutrition Therapy* is not replicated. Health professionals involved in diabetes nutrition education should refer to this handbook to guide selection of teaching materials.

Basic Nutrition Guidelines

The first step in nutritional management of diabetes often is simply to establish healthy eating patterns. General guidelines for good eating described in the beginning of this chapter can be used, or simple teaching tools developed for diabetes are available. *First Step in Diabetes Meal Planning,* introduced in 1995 by the American Diabetes Association and the American Dietetic Association, is a simple teaching tool that applies the general guidelines of the *Food Guide Pyramid* to nutritional management of diabetes. The pamphlet was designed to be used as an initial intervention with newly diagnosed individuals. Other basic guidelines developed for diabetes include *Healthy Food Choices* and *Eating Healthy Foods,* available from the ADAs, and *Healthy Eating,* developed by the International Diabetes Center. For some individuals, basic nutrition guidelines are sufficient to promote diet behaviors that achieve metabolic goals. Other individuals require and/or desire more detailed information available in other teaching materials.

Menu Approaches

Several instructional methods using menus have been developed to assist diabetic individuals in translating nutrition guidelines into meals. They include individualized menus for several days detailing specific foods to be eaten at each meal and snack. These menus should be written in collaboration with the person with diabetes to assure that familiar foods are included and to initiate training for independent menu planning. Personalized menus can be designed by computer using software programs such as Computer Planned Menus available from the American Diabetes Association. A collection of menus is provided in the Month of Meals series published by the American Diabetes Association. A 1500-calorie meal plan is used with instructions on how to adjust calories to a higher or lower level. The menus are designed to be flexible; a breakfast from one day can be combined with a lunch from another and a dinner from a third. Although these menus are not individualized, they are popular with persons who do not have the time or interest to do meal planning for themselves.

The Exchange Lists for Meal Planning is a well-established method for menu planning that groups foods into six categories: starch/bread, meat, vegetable, fruit, milk, and fat. Each category lists foods with portion sizes of approximately the same nutritional value. One food portion can be substituted or "exchanged" for another on the list with minimum difference in calories or the amount of carbohydrate, protein, and fat it contains.[61] The *Exchange Lists* were initially published in 1950 and revised in 1976, 1986, and 1995. The 1995 edition maintains the six categories but groups the starch/bread, fruit, and milk exchanges into a carbohydrate class with the option to substitute foods across these three exchanges. Another change in the 1995 edition is the expansion of the meat list to 4 levels of calories and fat with the addition of a very lean group providing 0 to 1 g of fat and 35 calories. To use this teaching method, the dietary prescription of calories, carbohydrate, protein, and fat is calculated into servings from each of the lists. Selection of exchanges and distribution into meal patterns is guided by patient preference, life-style, nutrient composition, and glycemic effect. Individualization allows the same diet prescription to result in very different meal patterns. This flexibility creates confusion when patients perceive that all 1800 calorie diets for diabetes should be the same and interchangeable. The *Exchange Lists* are available in large print and in Spanish translation. Cultural differences are addressed in the *Ethnic and Regional Food Practices* series, which provides professional guides for nutrition counseling of individuals from selected ethnic backgrounds. An adaptation of the *Exchange Lists* for high-fiber diets has been developed by James Anderson, MD, and is available from the HCF Nutrition Research Foundation in Lexington, Ky.

Counting Approaches

Several methods focus on counting calories or a macronutrient. Many of these methods need to be used in conjunction with guidelines on selecting a healthy diet. The Point System, developed in 1944 by Virginia Stuckey, RD, is a structured meal-planning approach that provides a simple method of counting daily intake of calories and/or selected other nutrients. Fat-gram counting gained popularity with the heightened concern over cholesterol and heart disease. Many fat-gram counting tools are available, and although not specific to diabetes, they can be very effective for many people with NIDDM. Carbohydrate counting is a very old approach in diabetes nutritional management that has experienced a renaissance with the growth of intensive diabetes therapy. One of the nutrition publications introduced by the ADAs in 1995 is a three-part series of instructional materials, *Carbohydrate Counting: Getting Started, Moving On, Intensive Diabetes Management.* Booklets on carbohydrate counting also have been published by some diabetes centers and insulin pump manufacturers.

Expanding Nutrition Education

Persons following a diet for diabetes will most often eat a variety of foods in diverse settings. In addition to instructional materials used to teach the principles of diet, multiple forms of information exist that can help individuals follow their diets and enjoy favorite foods. A wealth of supplemental material can be used to expand culinary options within the guidelines of the diet plan. Cookbooks, tips on dining out, suggestions for bagged lunches, and steps for converting recipes or nutritional label information into dietary measures (e.g., calories or exchanges) are available from many sources. A resource list is provided in Appendix A.

Nutrition Counseling Strategies

Staged education

Nutrition education and counseling for diabetes is a continuous process. As individuals adjust to the diagnosis of diabetes and begin to master self-management skills, their needs for nutrition information will change and their interest in learning more about their diet usually will increase. Educators and experienced clinicians advocate a staged approach to diabetes nutrition counseling. Initial diet instruction should teach survival skills. The goal should be to provide knowledge and skills that enable the individual to participate in self-management of diabetes.[5] This would include (1) information on how to eat to achieve nutrition goals and avoid hyperglycemia or hypoglycemia and (2) steps to take during illness. In-depth education on ways to enhance the diet regimen with a wider variety of foods, to increase flexibility for variations in daily schedules, or to intensify diabetes management can be provided in follow-up sessions. Goals for initial and in-depth nutrition education for IDDM, NIDDM, GDM, and pregnancy in overt diabetes are outlined in *Diabetes Education Goals,* published by the American Diabetes Association (see resource in Appendix A).

Behavior modification

The literature on diabetes contains a large number of articles written about adherence to treatment regimens. Health beliefs, social learning, motivation, family and societal influences, regimen complexity, and patient-provider relationships are among the many factors that have been studied as they relate to diabetes regimen adherence.[91]

Eating is a behavior that occurs frequently, has emotional, cultural, and social ties, and must be modified rather than extinguished. These factors contribute to the difficulty many individuals have in adopting and maintaining changes in eating habits required for diabetes management. It is important to acknowledge that changing eating habits is difficult for most individuals and that assistance in making changes in eating patterns is as important to nutritional counseling as guidelines on what to eat. *Facilitating Lifestyle Change: A Resource Manual* was introduced by the ADAs in 1995 to provide registered dietitians and diabetes educators with methods and tools to use in helping their clients make changes in eating and exercise behaviors. The manual includes tools such as an eating behavior diary, a life-style questionnaire, and life-style change plan and provides evaluation resources. People with diabetes vary psychologically just as they vary metabolically; therefore no single approach

Table 4-9 Options for Regimen Adjustments Based on Self-Monitoring Glucose Blood Tests

SMBG values	Regimen adjustments to consider
Hyperglycemia	
Fasting	Increase PM intermediate-acting or long-acting insulin dose or time injection later*
	Reduce calorie intake to promote weight reduction and decrease insulin resistance and hepatic glucose secretion
	Decrease PM snack
Pre-lunch	Increase AM dose of short-acting insulin*
	Alter breakfast meal plan by:
	Decreasing size
	Adjusting composition†
	Dividing into meal and AM snack
	Increase activity level in morning
Pre-dinner	Increase dose of AM intermediate-acting or pre-lunch short-acting insulin*
	Alter meal plan by:
	Decreasing or omitting afternoon snack
	Decreasing size of lunch
	Adjusting composition of lunch†
	Increase activity level in afternoon
Bedtime	Increase dose of PM short-acting insulin*
	Alter dinner meal plan by:
	Decreasing size
	Adjusting composition†
	Increase activity level after dinner
Hypoglycemia	
Fasting	Decrease PM intermediate-acting or long-acting insulin*
Pre-lunch	Decrease AM dose of short-acting insulin*
	Alter meal plan by:
	Increasing size of breakfast
	Adjusting composition of breakfast†
	Adding mid-morning snack
Pre-dinner	Decrease AM dose of intermediate-acting or pre-lunch short-acting insulin*
	Alter meal plan by:
	Increasing size of lunch
	Adjusting composition of lunch†
	Adding afternoon snack
	Adjust time of lunch
Bedtime	Decrease PM short-acting insulin dose*
	Alter meal plan by:
	Increasing size of dinner
	Adjusting composition of dinner†
	Increasing size of evening snack

Note: Oral hypoglycemia agents are not included in this table. The choice of an oral agent should be guided by the patient's eating pattern. SMBG patterns of hyperglycemia or hypoglycemia can direct change to an oral agent with a different pharmacokinetic time frame.

*Options for insulin adjustments vary by regimens.

†Changes can be made in the amount or type of carbohydrate or the amount of protein or fat, or fiber can be increased.

will be effective in changing eating behaviors. More detailed information on educational and behavioral theories that can be used in nutrition counseling is provided in other chapters of this text.

Self-monitoring of blood glucose

SMBG provides feedback on the success of the diabetes treatment plan. In nutrition counseling, test results can be used to evaluate the mix of foods in a meal or a snack, distribution of foods throughout the day, meal spacing, the effect of specific foods on an individual's blood glucose levels, and the relationship of meals with other therapeutic agents (i.e., medications and exercise). It is an essential component of nutrition therapy in intensive diabetes management where insulin and dietary adjustments are used to maintain optimal blood glucose control.[48] SMBG also is critical to successful nutrition management of pregnancy complicated by diabetes.

When evaluating SMBG tests, patterns of blood glucose values should be determined before an adjustment is made. Common problems and optional regimen changes to consider are presented in Table 4-9. Changes in therapy generally are made after review of records from several days and are not based on a blood glucose value from a single test.[14]

SMBG can be used to evaluate the glycemic effect of a specific food or to compare two meal patterns, such as two breakfast menus. Premeal blood glucose values need to be similar if a comparison is to be made. To test the glycemic effect of particular foods in mixed meals, equivalent portions of all foods must be included in the meal on each occasion. Only one food should be changed at a time. To test the glycemic effect of a single food, such as a snack option, the portion size should be reasonable. In evaluating the adequacy of an evening snack, the morning fasting blood glucose value and ideally a 3 AM value should be considered.

PROBLEMS WITH METABOLIC CONTROL: DIET MODIFICATIONS
Sick-Day Management

During periods of illness and surgery, blood glucose levels become elevated and diabetes may get out of control. Counterregulatory hormones such as epinephrine, glucagon, norepinephrine, and cortisol increase in response to the stress of infection, illness, or injury. Hepatic glucose production increases dramatically and in turn raises insulin requirements. Thus the person with diabetes who normally takes insulin may need to increase the insulin dose while ill. Likewise, the person not normally using insulin may need insulin coverage at least temporarily to control blood glucose well during illness.

Because food intake generally decreases during illness, it is not uncommon for individuals with diabetes to reduce or stop insulin under the false assumption that they do not need it because they are not eating as much as usual. All patients with diabetes should be taught to identify the signs and symptoms of hyperglycemia and be given personalized guidelines for managing diabetes during times of illness. This should increase their comfort level and skills needed to prevent serious problems with hyperglycemia during illness.

The goal of nutritional management during times of illness is to prevent dehydration and provide adequate nutrition to promote recovery. Carbohydrate intake is the most important

Table 4-10 Food and Beverage Suggestions for Illness

Item	Measure	CHO/g	Calories
Liquids			
Apple juice (unsweetened)	1/2 c	15	58
Beef broth	1 c	0.1	16
Cola drink	1/2 c	14	53
Cranberry juice cocktail	1/2 c	19	74
Eggnog	1/2 c	17	171
Ginger ale	3/4 c	15	62
Grape juice	1/3 c	13	51
Instant breakfast + skim milk	1/2 c	17	101
Gatorade	1 c	15	50
Skim milk	1 c	12	90
Orange juice	1/2 c	13	56
Tomato juice	1 1/2 c	15	64
Semisolids			
Applesauce (unsweetened)	1/2 c	14	53
Cream of Wheat	1/2 c	15	76
Cream soup	1 c	15	153
Custard	1/2 c	15	153
Frozen juice bar (DOLE)	1	16	70
Honey	1 T	16	64
Ice cream (vanilla)	1/2 c	16	135
Gelatin (regular)	1/2 c	16	80
Popsicle	1	10	40
Popsicle (sugar-free)	1	5	18
Pudding	1/2 c	30	180
Pudding (sugar-free)	1/2 c	16	103
Saltines	6	15	80
Graham crackers	3	16	80
Sherbet	1/4 c	15	68
Sugar	1 T	12	48
Yogurt (plain, low-fat)	1 c	12	120
Yogurt (fruited, low-fat)	1/2 c	20	112
Frozen yogurt	1/2 c	16	118
Frozen yogurt (sugar-free)	1/2 c	8	70

From Pennington J, Church H: *Bowes and Church food values of portions commonly used,* ed 15, Philadelphia, 1989, Lippincott.

concern during brief illness. In general, most diabetic patients should be taught to do the following[14,92]:

- Monitor blood glucose at least 4 times/day at the onset and throughout illness.
- Test urine for ketones when blood glucose is above 240 mg/dl.
- Continue to take their usual dose of insulin or oral hypoglycemic agent.
- Substitute easily digested liquids or semiliquid foods when solid foods are not tolerated. Replacing 15 g of carbohydrate from solids (starches, breads, or fruit) with 15 g of carbohydrate from liquids every 1 to 2 hours is usually sufficient (Table 4-10).

- Sip 8 to 12 ounces of fluid every hour; this may include a carbohydrate source, as well as water, tea, broth, and diet soda.
- Call a physician if unable to eat normally for more than 24 hours or if diarrhea and vomiting persist for more than 6 hours.

Treating Hypoglycemia

Hypoglycemia, or low blood glucose, is usually defined as a blood glucose concentration below 70 mg/dl. Hypoglycemia associated with diabetes is a man-made, or treatment-induced, phenomenon because it is produced from either exogenous insulin or oral hypoglycemic agents—thus the more common term *insulin reaction*. To produce an insulin reaction, circulating insulin levels must be elevated in relation to blood glucose levels. The primary causes are either too much insulin, too much exercise, or too little food. Occasionally, insulin dosage may be increased inadvertently. During exercise, blood glucose is used rapidly and hepatic glucose production is suppressed. Children and young adults are more susceptible to hypoglycemic reactions caused by variable and sporadic activity levels.

The most common cause of an insulin reaction is skipping or delaying meals or eating less than normal amounts of carbohydrate at a meal. In general, meals cannot be delayed more than 30 to 60 minutes without a drop in blood glucose when exogenous insulin is being administered. The tighter the blood glucose control, the greater the risk. A snack should be consumed at the regular meal time if a meal is delayed more than 30 to 60 minutes.

Overweight NIDDM patients may experience hypoglycemia during weight-reduction diets in which food intake is reduced. If oral agent or insulin dosages are not reduced accordingly, frequent hypoglycemia may result. This is counterproductive to weight loss efforts, since extra food must be eaten to treat a hypoglycemic reaction. Most insulin-requiring NIDDM patients benefit from a reduction in insulin dose at the onset of dieting. It provides the peace of mind they often need to suppress fears of hypoglycemic reactions and can motivate them to stay with their diet plan.

If hypoglycemia is suspected, it should be identified by SMBG and treated quickly and appropriately. Most patients have learned to identify the "feeling" or symptoms of hypoglycemia specific to them. Identifying a reaction in small children, however, may be difficult because of their inability to describe or recognize symptoms. Family members can be taught to look for changes in behavior that are often the only clue to impending hypoglycemia. Severe hunger is one behavior. Good-natured children may suddenly become irritable and cranky. High-strung children may become quiet and lethargic. Whenever a reaction is suspected, a blood glucose test should be done quickly to confirm.

Most older individuals rely on symptoms to forewarn a reaction. Yet some individuals do not become symptomatic until blood glucose levels become dangerously low (i.e., neurologic changes occur). Because of the unpleasantness of the experience, low blood glucose reactions are often overtreated with too much food to obtain quick relief. Although the treatment goal is to raise blood glucose quickly, rebound hyperglycemia frequently follows a low blood glucose reaction.

Because food used to treat hypoglycemia should be in addition to regular daily intake, weight gain can result if reactions are too frequent or treated inappropriately. An astute clinician will look at SMBG records and frequency of reactions if weight gain is a problem for a person in normally good control.

Overtreating reactions can be avoided by teaching patients to use the 15/15 rule when blood glucose falls below 70 mg/dl[29]:

- Eat 15 g of carbohydrate (Table 4-11).
- Wait 15 minutes; then retest blood glucose—if still less than 70 mg/dl, repeat 15/15 rule; do this until blood glucose returns to normal range.
- If there is more than 1 hour to next meal, eat another 15 g of carbohydrate.

Special "treat" foods such as ice cream, cake, and cookies should not be reserved only to treat reactions. A low blood glucose reaction can then be used to justify consuming sweets. These treats should be incorporated into the meal plan appropriately as they would be in any healthy diet plan.

Readily portable foods such as raisins, regular soft drinks, juice boxes, and low-fat candies are common foods used to treat reactions. Skim milk is preferred by some individuals but is not always accessible. Some health professionals choose to recommend pure glucose in the form of tablets, liquid, or gel. These products provide a rapid rise in glucose that is considered ideal. Studies suggest that it is the amount of available glucose in a food that

Table 4-11   Glucose Sources of Treating Hypoglycemia

Source	Measure	CHO/g
Glucose products		
Glucose tablets	3	15
Glutose	1-25 g tube	10
Insta glucose	1-31 g tube	30
Monoject gel	1-25 g packet	10
Dextro tabs	9 tablets	15
Foods/drinks		
Hard candy (Life Savers)	5	15
Jelly beans	6	15
Junior Mints	7	15
Marshmallows	3 large	15
Raisins	2 T	14
Honey	1 T	17
Sugar	1 T	16
Gelatin (regular)	1/2 c	17
Juice (apple, orange)	1/2 c	14
Milk (skim)	1 c	12
Soft drinks (cola, lemon-lime)	1/2 c	13
Ginger ale	3/4 c	16
Gatorade	1 c	15

From Pennington J, Church H: *Bowes and Church food values of portions commonly used,* ed 15, Philadelphia, 1989, Lippincott.

determines its usefulness in treating a reaction. Carbohydrate sources that contain more glucose are preferred.

Patients should be taught to be prepared to treat a reaction at all times but that preventing a reaction is probably the best form of preparation. A regular eating schedule plus anticipating extra exercise with extra food or reduced insulin dose are the best ways to prevent reactions. If hypoglycemia occurs too frequently (two to three times/week), the meal plan and medication regimen need to be evaluated and adjusted if necessary.

A hypoglycemic reaction that leads to unconsciousness must be treated with glucagon or IV glucose. Individuals with IDDM and their families should be taught the use of a glucagon kit.

Nutrition Problems Related to Autonomic Neuropathy

A small number of people with diabetes may develop autonomic neuropathy that progresses to the point that nutritional health is compromised. Gastrointestinal motility can be either slowed or enhanced. Symptoms include heartburn, increased satiety and feeling of fullness, nausea, vomiting, anorexia, and constipation. Some individuals may experience severe diarrhea. Because absorption of nutrients may be delayed or altered by changes in motility, blood glucose control becomes erratic. Blood glucose may peak or drop at unexpected times after eating (i.e., 3 to 4 hours) instead of the expected 2 hours. Careful SMBG and insulin adjustment are necessary to compensate.

Severe nausea, swallowing disorders, vomiting, and diarrhea can lead to fluid, electrolyte, and nutrition imbalances that must be treated appropriately. Nutrition intervention is limited to dividing food intake into frequent smaller meals of easily digested foods that are low in fat. Occasionally, pureed foods or tube feedings need to be used. Drugs such as metoclopramide and antidiarrheals are frequently prescribed.

THE TEAM APPROACH TO DIABETES NUTRITIONAL MANAGEMENT

Diabetes is a team disease. Therapy requires integration of expertise from a variety of health care disciplines. Standards of medical care, published by the American Diabetes Association, specify that individuals with diabetes should receive care from a health care team that includes, but is not limited to, a physician, nurse, dietitian, and mental health worker with expertise and interest in diabetes.[9] Ideally, the health care team and the person with diabetes collaborate to develop a diabetes management plan that is tailored to his or her abilities, goals, and life-style. Although all members of the team have specific roles, the interrelated nature of diabetes therapy requires each health care member to be knowledgeable about all treatment modalities.

Role of the Person with Diabetes

Diabetes requires patient self-management. Persons with diabetes must assume an active role in the desig as well as in the implementation of their diabetes treatment regimen. Personal involvement has a special significance in planning nutrition therapy. Medications and monitoring are new skills that the person needs to learn from health professionals. By contrast, the health professionals must learn from diabetic individuals about established dietary practices and changes they are willing or able to make. When individuals select the changes in their diet, they are more likely to assume responsibility for the diet plan and may be more motivated to adhere to the regimen.[72]

Role of the Dietitian

The registered dietitian provides the professional expertise to design the nutrition regimen, to translate it into a practical and flexible meal plan, and to counsel the patient in making dietary modifications. The importance of nutrition therapy to diabetes management has been demonstrated in studies showing dietary adherence is highly correlated with metabolic control.[36] Acquiring knowledge and skills to correctly follow a meal plan for diabetes requires time with a registered dietitian. Initial nutrition consultations are frequently scheduled to last an hour. Follow-up visits are planned according to needs of the individual and generally require from 15 to 30 minutes. Availability of registered dietitians varies. Hospitals are providing both inpatient and outpatient nutrition counseling services. Many diabetes treatment centers include a registered dietitian on their staff. A growing number of dietitians are specializing in diabetes and are members of the Diabetes Care and Education Practice Group of the American Dietetic Association. The American Dietetic Association's Nutrition Network provides a listing of registered dietitians who counsel persons with diabetes (see resource list in Appendix A for information.)

Role of the Health Care Team

Although other members of the health care team contribute their own expertise to diabetes management of the diabetic patient, they need to support the nutrition education process as well. Questions on diet relate to insulin therapy, exercise, illness, and other aspects of diabetes management. Questions on diet are asked when individuals think of them, which may be when they are being instructed on SMBG by the nurse or having their feet examined by the podiatrist. Although technical questions can be referred to the dietitian as the authoritative member of the team, patients will benefit if their dietary education can be reinforced as often as possible by as many members of their health care team as possible.

REFERENCES

1. Abraham HS, Brooks BA, Eylate U: The effects of chromium supplementation on serum glucose and lipids in patients with and without non-insulin dependent diabetes, *Metab Clin Exp* 41:768-771, 1992.
2. Abrams RS, Coustan DR: Gestational diabetes update, *Clin Diabetes* 8:17-24, 1990.
3. American Academy of Pediatrics Committee on Nutrition: The use of whole cow's milk in infancy, *Pediatrics* 89:1105-1109, 1992.
4. American Diabetes Association/American Dietetic Association: *Diabetes medical nutrition therapy: a guide for professionals,* Alexandria, Va and Chicago, (expected 1996), The Associations.
5. American Diabetes Association: *Diabetes education goals, 1995,* Alexandria, Va, The Association.

6. American Diabetes Association: *Medical management of pregnancy complicated by diabetes,* ed 2, Alexandria, Va, 1995, The Association.

7. American Diabetes Association/Diabetes Care and Education Practice Group—American Dietetic Association: Maximizing the role of nutrition in diabetes management, 1994, Alexandria, Va, The Associations.

8. American Diabetes Association: Nutrition recommendations and principles for people with diabetes mellitus, *Diabetes Care* 17:519-522, 1994.

9. American Diabetes Association: Standards of medical care for patients with diabetes mellitus, *Diabetes Care* 17:616-623, 1994.

10. American Diabetes Association: Nutritional recommendations and principles for individuals with diabetes mellitus: 1986, *Diabetes Care* 10:126-132, 1987.

11. American Diabetes Association: Principles of nutrition and dietary recommendations for patients with diabetes mellitus: 1971, *Diabetes Care* 20: 633-634, 1971.

12. American Diabetes Association: Principles of nutrition and dietary recommendations for individuals with diabetes mellitus: 1979, *Diabetes Care* 28:1027-1030, 1979.

13. American Diabetes Association: Glycemic effects of carbohydrates, *Diabetes Care* 7:607-608, 1984.

14. American Diabetes Association/American Dietetic Association: *Nutrition guide for professionals,* Alexandria, Va and Chicago, 1988, The Associations.

14a. The American Dietetic Association: Position of the American Dietetic Association: health implications of dietary fiber, *J Am Diet Assoc* 93:1446-1447, 1993.

14b. The American Dietetic Association: Position of the American Dietetic Association: Use of nutritive and non-nutritive sweeteners, *J Am Diet Assoc* 93:816-821, 1993.

15. American Heart Association Nutrition Committee: Rationale of the diet heart statement of the American Heart Association, *Circulation* 88:3009-3029, 1993.

16. Anderson CE: Energy metabolism. In Schneider HA, Anderson CE, Coursin DB, editors: *Nutritional support of medical practices,* ed 2, Philadelphia, 1983, Harper & Row.

17. Armatruda JM and others: The safety and efficacy of a controlled low-energy (very low calorie) diet in the treatment of NIDDM and obesity, *Arch Intern Med* 148:873-877, 1988.

18. Bantle JP: Clinical aspects of sucrose and fructose metabolism, *Diabetes Care* 12:56-61, 1989.

19. Bantle JP, Laine DC, Thomas JW: Metabolic effects of dietary fructose and sucrose in type I and II diabetic subjects, *JAMA* 256:3241-3246, 1986.

20. Barr SL and others: Reducing total dietary fat without reducing saturated fatty acids does not significantly lower total plasma cholesterol concentration in normal values, *Am J Clin Nutr* 55:675, 1992.

21. Beebe CA and others: Effects of temporal distribution of calories on diurnal patterns of glucose levels and insulin secretion in NIDDM, *Diabetes Care* 13:748-755, 1990.

22. Ben G and others: Effects of chronic alcohol intake on carbohydrate and lipid metabolism in subjects with type II (non-insulin-dependent) diabetes, *Am J Med* 90:70-76, 1991.

23. Bergman M, Gidez LI, Eder HA: High-density lipoprotein subclasses in diabetes, *Am J Med* 81:488-492, 1986.

24. Bertorelli AM, Czarnowski-Hill JV: Review of present and future use of nonnutritive sweeteners, *Diabetes Educ* 16:415-420, 1990.

25. Birk R, Spencer ML: The prevalence of anorexia nervosa, bulimia, and induced glycosuria in IDDM females, *Diabetes Educ* 15:336-341, 1989.

26. Bray GA and others: Eating patterns of massively obese individuals, *J Am Diet Assoc* 70:94-97, 1980.

27. Brink SJ: Pediatric, adolescent and young adult nutrition issues in IDDM, *Diabetes Care* 11:192-200, 1988.

28. Bristol-Myers Squibb: Glucophage package insert, Princeton, NJ, 1995, Bristol-Myers Squibb.

29. Brodows RG, Williams C, Arakuda JM: Treatment of insulin reactions in diabetes, *JAMA* 252:3378-3381, 1984.

30. Brodsky IG and others: Effects of low protein diets on protein metabolism in insulin-dependent diabetes mellitus patients with early nephropathy, *J Clin Endocrinol Metab* 75:351, 1992.

31. Calorie Control Council: Questions and answers about polyols, Atlanta, Ga, Calorie Control Council.

32. Caso EK: Calculation of diabetic diets: report of the committee on diabetic diet calculations, *J Am Diet Assoc* 26:575-583, 1950.

33. Deleted in proofs

34. Ceriello A and others: Vitamin E reduction of protein glycosylation in diabetes: new prospect for prevention of diabetic complications? *Diabetes Care* 14:68, 1991.

35. Chantelau E and others: Diet liberalization and metabolic control in Type I diabetic outpatients created by continuous subcutaneous insulin infusion, *Diabetes Care* 5:612-616, 1982.

36. Christensen NK and others: Quantitative assessment of dietary adherence in patients with insulin-

dependent diabetes mellitus, *Diabetes Care* 6:245-250, 1983.

37. Ciavarella A and others: Reduced albuminuria after dietary protein restriction in IDDM patients with clinical nephropathy, *Diabetes Care* 10:407-413, 1987.

38. Collings AJ: Metabolism of cyclamate and its conversion to cyclohexylamine, *Diabetes Care* 12:50-55, 1989.

39. Connor W, Connor S: The dietary prevention and treatment of coronary heart disease. In Connor W, Bristow JD, editors: *Coronary heart disease: prevention, complications and treatment,* Philadelphia, 1985, Lippincott.

40. Coulston AM, Mandelbaum D, Reaven GM: Dietary management of nursing home residents with non-insulin-dependent diabetes mellitus, *Am J Clin Nutr* 51:67-71, 1990.

41. Coulston AM and others: Persistence of hypertriglyceridemic effect of low-fat high-carbohydrate diets in NIDDM patients, *Diabetes Care* 12:94-101, 1989.

42. Coulston AM and others: Deleterious metabolic effects of high-carbohydrate, sucrose-containing diets in patient with non-insulin-dependent diabetes mellitus, *Am J Med* 82:213-220, 1987.

43. Crapo PA: Carbohydrate. In Powers MA, editor: *Handbook of diabetes nutritional management,* Rockville, Md, 1987, Aspen.

44. Crapo PA, Reaven G, Olefsky JM: Postprandial glucose and insulin responses to different complex carbohydrates, *Diabetes* 26:1723-1728, 1977.

45. Diabetes Control and Complications Trial Research Group: The effect of intensive treatment of diabetes on the development and progression of long-term complications in insulin-dependent diabetes mellitus, *N Engl J Med* 329:977-986, 1993.

46. DCCT Research Group: Nutrition interventions for intensive therapy in the Diabetes Control and Complications Trial, *J Am Diet Assoc* 93:768-772, 1993.

47. DCCT Research Group: Weight gain associated with intensive therapy in the Diabetes Control and Complications Trial, *Diabetes Care* 11:567-573, 1988.

48. Delehanty LM, Halford BN: The role of diet behaviors in achieving improved glycemic control in intensively treated patients in the Diabetes Control and Complications Trial, *Diabetes Care* 16:1453-1458.

49. Dheene M and others: Effects of acute protein loads of different sources on glomerular filtration rate, *Kidney Int* 32:S25, 1987.

50. Dreon DM and others: Dietary fat: carbohydrate ratio and obesity in middle-aged men, *Am J Clin Nutr* 47:995-1000, 1988.

51. Ducimetiere P and others: Relationship of plasma insulin levels to the incidence of myocardial infarction and coronary heart disease mortality in a middle-aged population, *Diabetologia* 19:205-210, 1980.

52. Dwyer JR: Screening older Americans' nutrition health: current practices and future possibilities, Washington, DC, 1991, Nutrition Screening Initiative.

53. Edwards DL and others: Home delivered meals benefit the diabetic elderly, *J Am Diet Assoc* 93:585-587, 1993.

54. Evanoff GV and others: The effect of dietary protein restriction on the progression of diabetic nephropathy, *Arch Intern Med* 147:492-495, 1987.

55. Ewald U, Gebre-Medhin M, Luvemo T: Hypomagnesemia in diabetic children, *Acta Paediatr Scand* 72:367, 1983.

56. Feurer ID and others: Resting energy expenditure in morbid obesity, *Ann Surg* 197:17-21, 1983.

57. Food and Nutrition Board, National Academy of Sciences–National Research Council: Recommended Dietary Allowances, ed 10, 1989.

58. Franz MJ and others: Nutrition principles for the management of diabetes and related complications (Technical Review), *Diabetes Care* 17:490-518, 1994.

59. Franz M: Practice guidelines for nutrition care by dietetics practitioners for outpatients with non-insulin-dependent diabetes mellitus: consensus statement, *J Am Diet Assoc* 92:1136-1138, 1992.

60. Franz MJ: Alcohol and diabetes. I. Metabolism and guidelines, *Diabetes Spectrum* 3:136-144, 1990.

61. Franz MJ and others: Exchange lists: revised 1986, *J Am Diet Assoc* 87:28-34, 1987.

62. Fukargawa NK, Young VR: Protein and amino acid metabolism and requirements in older persons, *Clin Geriatr Med* 3:329-337, 1987.

63. Gannon MC and others: The insulin and glucose responses to meals of glucose plus various proteins in type II diabetic subjects, *Metabolism: Clinical and Experimental* 37:1081-1088, 1988.

64. Garg A and others: Comparison of a high-carbohydrate diet with a high-monounsaturated-fat diet in patients with non-insulin-dependent diabetes mellitus, *N Engl J Med* 319:829-834, 1988.

65. Ginsberg HN and others: Reduction of plasma cholesterol levels in normal men on an American Heart Association step 1 diet or a step 1 diet with added monounsaturated fat, *N Engl J Med* 322:574-579, 1990.

66. Glauber H and others: Adverse metabolic effect of omega-3 fatty acids in non-insulin-dependent diabetes mellitus, *Ann Intern Med* 108:663-668, 1988.

67. Goldstein DJ, Potvin JH: Longterm weight loss: the effect of pharmacologic agents, *Am J Clin Nutr* 60:647-657, 1994.

68. Gordon T and others: High density lipoprotein as a protective factor against coronary heart disease: the Framingham Study, *Am J Med* 62:707-714, 1977.
69. Gore GP, Huff TA, Stachuro ME: Pathophysiology. In Powers MS, editor: *Handbook of diabetes nutritional management,* Rockville, Md, 1987, Aspen.
70. Grundy SM: Comparison of monounsaturated fatty acids and carbohydrates for lowering plasma cholesterol, *N Engl J Med* 314:745-748, 1986.
71. Haffner SM and others: Do upper-body and centralized adiposity measure different aspects of regional body-fat distribution? Relationship to NIDDM, lipids and lipoproteins, *Diabetes* 36:43-51, 1987.
72. Haire-Joshu D: Motivation and diabetes self-care: an educational challenge, *Diabetes Spectrum* 1:279-282, 1988.
73. Hallbook T, Lanner E: Serum-zinc and healing of venous leg ulcers, *Lancet* 2:780, 1972.
74. Heber D: Macronutrient nutrition for aging. In Morley JE, moderator: Nutrition in the elderly, *Ann Intern Med* 109:890-904, 1988.
75. Hendra TJ and others: Effects of fish oil supplements in NIDDM subjects, *Diabetes Care* 13:821-829, 1990.
76. Hui S, Epstein S, Johnston C: A prospective study of bone mass in patients with type I diabetes, *J Clin Endocrinol Met* 60:74, 1985.
77. Irvine AA and others: Validation of scale measuring environmental barriers to diabetes regimen adherence, *Diabetes Care* 13:705-711, 1990.
78. Jain A, Gupta N, Kumar A: Some metabolic effects of magnesium in diabetes mellitus, *J Assoc Physicians India* 24:827, 1976.
79. Jenkins DJA, Wolever TMS, Jenkins AL: Starchy food and glycemic index, *Diabetes Care* 11:149-159, 1988.
80. Jenkins DJA and others: Glycemic index of foods: a physiological basis for carbohydrate exchange, *Am J Clin Nutr* 34:362-366, 1981.
81. Jovanovic-Peterson L, Peterson C: Dietary manipulation as a primary treatment strategy for pregnancies complicated by diabetes, *J Am Col of Nutrition* 9:320-325, 1990.
82. Karjalainen J and others: A bovine albumin peptide as a possible trigger of insulin-dependent diabetes mellitus, *N Engl J Med* 327:302-307, 1992.
83. Kennedy AL and others: Relation of high-density lipoprotein cholesterol concentration to type of diabetes and its control, *BMJ* 2:1191-1194, 1978.
84. Klahr S and others: The effects of dietary protein restriction and blood pressure control on the progression of chronic renal disease, *N Engl J Med* 330:877, 1994.
85. Knowles H and others: The course of juvenile diabetes treated with unmeasured diets, *Diabetes* 14:239-273, 1965.
86. Koivisto VA and others: Alcohol with a meal has no adverse effects on portprandial glucose homeostatis in diabetic patients, *Diabetes Care* 16:1612-1614, 1993.
87. Kontessis P and others: Renal, metabolic and hormonal responses to ingestion of animal and vegetable proteins, *Kidney Int* 38:136, 1990.
88. Kostraba JN and others: Early exposure to cow's milk and solid foods in infancy, genetic predisposition, and risk of IDDM, *Diabetes* 42:288-295, 1993.
89. Kromhout D, Bosschieter EB, Caulander C: The inverse relation between fish consumption and 20-year mortality from coronary heart disease, *N Engl J Med* 312:1205-1209, 1985.
90. Kunisaki M and others: Effects of vitamin E administration of platelet function in diabetes mellitus, *Diabetes Res* 14:37, 1990.
91. Kurtz MS: Adherence to diabetes regimens: emperical status and clinical applications, *Diabetes Educ* 16:50-56, 1990.
92. Ley B, Goldman D: Sick-day management: a partnership in preparation for the expected, *Clin Diabetes* 8:25-30, 1990.
93. Lipid Research Clinics Program: The lipid research clinics coronary primary prevention trial results. II. The relationship of reduction in incidence of coronary heart disease to cholesterol lowering, *JAMA* 251:365-374, 1984.
94. Marcus MD and others: Eating disorders symptomatology in a registry-based sample of women with insulin-dependent diabetes mellitus, *Int J E Disord* 12:425-430, 1992.
95. Marshall RE: Infant of the diabetic mother: a neonatologist's view, *Clin Diabetes* 8:51-57, 1990.
96. McArdle WD, Katch FI, Katch VL: Obesity and weight control: exercise physiology, energy, nutrition and human performance, Philadelphia, 1986, Lea & Febiger.
97. McNair P and others: Renal hypomagnesemia in human diabetes mellitus: its relation to glucose homeostasis, *Eur J Clin Invest* 12:81, 1982.
98. Mensick RD and others: Effects of monounsaturated fatty acids versus complex carbohydrates on serum lipoproteins and apoproteins in healthy men and women, *Metabolism* 38:172-178, 1989.
99. Mensink RP, Katan MB: Effect of dietary trans fatty acids on high-density and low-density lipoprotein cholesterol levels in healthy subjects, *N Engl J Med* 323:439, 1990.
100. Mensink RP, Katan MB: Effect of monounsaturated fatty acids versus complex carbohydrates on

high-density lipoproteins in healthy men and women, *Lancet* 1:122-125, 1987.

101. Menzel R and others: Effect of moderate ethanol ingestion on overnight diabetes control and hormone secretion in type I diabetic patients (Abstract), *Diabetologia* 34:188, 1991.

102. Miller SA, Frattali VP: Saccharin, *Diabetes Care* 12:75-80, 1989.

103. Mooradian A and others: Selected vitamins and minerals in diabetes, *Diabetes Care* 17:464, 1994.

104. Mooradian AD: Diabetes in the elderly, *Diabetes Spectrum* 7:357-381, 1994.

105. Munro HN, Crim MC: The proteins and amino acids. In Goodhart RS, editor: *Modern nutrition in health and disease,* Philadelphia, 1980, Lea & Febiger.

106. National High Blood Pressure Education Program: Working group report on primary prevention of hypertension, Bethesda, Md, 1993, U.S. Department of Health and Human Services, National Institutes of Health.

107. National Institutes of Health: Consensus development conference on diet and exercise in NIDDM, *Diabetes Care* 10:639-644, 1987.

108. Nuttal FQ: Dietary fiber in the management of diabetes, *Diabetes* 43:503-508, 1993.

109. Nuttall FQ, Hollenbeck CB: Current issues in nutrition and metabolism, Part I, *Diabetes Spectrum* 2:123-128, 1989.

110. O'Dea K, Snow P, Nestel P: Rate of starch hydrolysis in vitro as a predictor of metabolic responses to complex carbohydrate in vivo, *Am J Clin Nutr* 34:1991-1993, 1981.

111. Ostlund RE and others: The ratio of waist-to-hip circumference, plasma insulin level, and glucose intolerance as independent predictors of the HDL2 cholesterol level in older adults, *N Engl J Med* 322:229-234, 1990.

112. Paige MS, Heins JM: Nutritional management of diabetic patients during intensive insulin therapy, *Diabetes Educ* 14:505-509, 1988.

113. Pastors JM, Holler HJ, Editors: *Meal planning approaches for diabetes management,* ed 2, 1994, Chicago, The American Dietetic Association.

114. Pellett PL: Food energy requirements in humans, *Am J Clin Nutr* 51:711-722, 1990.

115. Peters AL, Davidson MB: Protein and fat effects on glucose responses and insulin requirements in subjects with insulin-dependent diabetes mellitus, *Am J Clin Nutr* 58:555, 1993.

116. Peters AL, Davidson MD, Eisenberg K: Effect of isocaloric substitution of chocolate cake for potato in type I diabetic patients, *Diabetes Care* 13:888-892, 1990.

117. Peveler RC and others: Eating disorders in adolescents with IDDM: a controlled study, *Diabetes Care* 15:1356-1360, 1992.

118. Phillipson BE and others: Reduction of plasma lipids, lipoproteins, and apoproteins by dietary fish oils in patients with hypertriglyceridemia, *N Engl J Med* 312:1210-1216, 1985.

119. Pietri AO and others: The effect of continuous subcutaneous insulin infusion on very-low-density lipoprotein triglyceride metabolism in type I diabetes mellitus, *Diabetes* 32:75-81, 1983.

120. Polonsky WH and others: Insulin omission in women with IDDM, *Diabetes Care* 17:1178-1185, 1994.

121. Powers MA, Metzger BE, Freinkel N: Pregnancy and diabetes. In Powers MS, editor: *Handbook of diabetes nutritional management,* Rockville, Md, 1987, Aspen.

122. Rim E and others: Vitamin E consumption and the risk of coronary heart disease in men, *N Engl J Med* 328:1450, 1993.

123. Ripsin CM and others: Oat products and lipid lowering: a meta-analysis, *JAMA* 267:3317-3325, 1992.

124. Rosenstock J and others: Reduction in cardiovascular risk factors with intensive diabetes treatment in insulin-dependent diabetes mellitus, *Diabetes Care* 10:729-734, 1987.

125. Schmidt LE and others: The relationship between eating patterns and metabolic control in patients with non-insulin-dependent diabetes mellitus (NIDDM), *Diabetes Educ* 20:317-321, 1994.

126. Schmidt LE, Klover RV, Arfken CL: Compliance with dietary prescriptions in children and adolescents with insulin-dependent diabetes mellitus, *J Am Diet Assoc* 92:567-570, 1992.

127. Siebert G, Grupp U, Heinkel K: Studies on isomaltitol, *Nutrition and Metabolism* 18:191-196, 1975.

128. Sims EAH, Danforth E: Expenditure and shortage of energy in man, *J Clin Invest* 79:1019-1025, 1987.

129. Skyler JS: Non–insulin-dependent diabetes mellitus: a clinical strategy, *Diabetes Care* 7(suppl 1):118-129, 1984.

130. Sparrow D and others: Relationship of fat distribution to glucose tolerance, *Diabetes* 35:411-415, 1986.

131. Stampfer MJ and others: Vitamin E consumption and the risk of coronary heart disease in women, *N Engl J Med* 328:1444-1449, 1993.

132. Stancin T, Link DL, Reuter JM: Binge eating and purging in young women with IDDM, *Diabetes Care* 12:601-603, 1989.

133. Stone JN: Diet, blood cholesterol levels and coronary heart disease, *Coron Artery Dis* 4:871, 1993.

134. Striegel-Moore RH, Nicholson TJ, Tamborlane WV: Prevalence of eating disorder symptoms in preadolescent and adolescent girls with IDDM, *Diabetes Care* 15:1361-1368, 1992.

135. Deleted in proofs

136. Deleted in proofs

137. Tinker LF, Heins JM, Holler HJ: Commentary and translation: 1994 nutrition recommendations for diabetes, *J Am Diet Assoc* 94:507-511, 1994.

138. Tinker LF: Dietary fiber: variables that affect its nutritional impact, *Diabetes Spectrum* 3:191-196, 1990.

139. Vatassery G, Morley H, Kuskowski M: Vitamin E in plasma and platelets of human diabetic patients and control subjects, *Am J Clin Nutr* 37:641, 1983.

140. Walker JD and others: Restriction of dietary protein and progression of renal failure in diabetic nephropathy, *Lancet* ii:1411, 1989.

141. Warshaw HS: Alternative sweeteners: past, present, pending and potential, *Diabetes Spectrum* 3:335-343, 1990.

142. Wing RR, Klein R, Mars SE: Weight gain associated with improved glycemic control in population-based sample of subjects with type I diabetes, *Diabetes Care* 13:1106-1109, 1990.

143. Witztum JL and others: Nonenzymatic glycosylation of low-density lipoprotein alters its biologic activity, *Diabetes* 31:283-291, 1982.

144. Zavaroni I and others: Risk factors for coronary artery disease in healthy persons with hyperinsulinemia and normal glucose tolerance, *N Engl J Med* 320:702-706, 1989.

145. Zeller K and others: Effect of restricting dietary protein on the insulin-dependent diabetes mellitus, *N Engl J Med* 324:78, 1991.

CASE STUDY

Sam Jones is a 45-year-old man diagnosed 5 years ago with NIDDM. He had been treated successfully with diet and maximum dosage of an oral hypoglycemic agent; however, blood glucose control has deteriorated over the past year. Sam's physician decides to initiate insulin therapy using a regimen of 2 injections a day of premixed 70/30 insulin and refers him to a registered dietitian, Chris Nelson, RD, for nutrition counseling. Chris uses the four-step process of medical nutrition therapy to develop meal plans for Sam.

NUTRITION ASSESSMENT

Clinical Data

Height: 5 feet 9 inches (172.5 cm)*
Weight: 162 pounds (73.6 kg)*
Frame: medium
Reasonable weight: 129-169 lbs (Dietary Guidelines)
                        160 lbs (patient's goal)
Blood pressure: normal
Activity: sedentary—business requires out-of-town travel by car
Medication: OTC for allergy; has just received instruction on insulin administration and self-monitoring of blood glucose
Health: good—reports no other medical problems; father has NIDDM
Education: college degree
Life-style: married with two children; hobbies include fishing and reading

Laboratory Data

Hemoglobin A_{1c}: 10.6%
Total serum cholesterol: 243 mg/dl
LDL cholesterol: 162 mg/dl
HDL cholesterol: 45 mg/dl
Triglycerides: 335 mg/dl
All other values are within normal range

Diet History

Sam reports receiving a printed diet sheet when first diagnosed with diabetes. He found it did not reflect his life-style so decided to "just cut out sweets." Eats many meals away from home because of travel (Table 4A-1).

---

*Conversion table: inches × 2.5 = centimeters; pounds ÷ 2.2 = kilograms.

156

Table 4A-1   24-Hour Dietary Recall: (See Table 4A-2 for Exchange Lists System Used to Quantify Caloric Content

	Exchanges	Calories
Breakfast		
1 egg, fried	1 medium-fat meat	75
	1 fat	45
2 slices toast	2 starch	160
2 pats butter	2 fat	90
2% low-fat milk, 8 oz.	1 low-fat milk	120
Lunch (fast food chain)		
Hamburger, quarter pound	3 medium-fat meat	225
	1 fat	45
Bun	2 starch	160
French fries, large	2 starch	160
	2 fat	90
Soft-serve cone	2 carbohydrates	170
	1 fat	45
Dinner		
Roast beef, 2 slices (4 oz)	4 medium-fat meat	300
Mashed potatoes with gravy	1 starch	80
	1 fat	45
Roll with butter	1 starch	80
	1 fat	45
Green beans	1 vegetable	25
Salad with ranch dressing	free food	
	2 fat	90
Iced tea with sweetener	free	
Snack		
Ice cream, 1 c.	2 carbohydrates	170
	2 fat	90
	TOTAL: 2310 calories	

Summary of Assessment

Sam's weight is at a reasonable level. Laboratory data show hyperglycemia and hyperlipidemia. Dietary history indicates a high-fat intake from meat and dairy products, as well as fat added in food preparation and while eating. Life-style modifications in diet and exercise will improve blood glucose and lipid levels.

Goal Setting

Sam is eager to improve his diabetes management but concerned about the potential of hypoglycemia while he is traveling. He also is concerned about his hyperlipidemia. Sam and Chris agree on a diet and exercise program to improve blood glucose and lipid levels but prevent hypoglycemia.

INTERVENTION
Nutrition Prescription

Chris calculates Sam's energy requirement to maintain a body weight of 160 lbs. based on the Harris-Benedict equation:

$$REE = 66.5 + (13.75 \times 73 \text{ kg}) + (5.03 \times 172.5 \text{ cm}) - (6.75 \times 45) = 1634.18$$
$$REE \times \text{Activity factor} = \text{Estimate of daily calorie requirement: } 1634 \times 1.3 = 2124 \text{ calories/day}$$

The diet history is evaluated to determine Sam's current caloric intake and to identify modifications that would facilitate achieving the identified goals.

Calorie level: current intake is close to estimate of caloric requirement to maintain reasonable weight.

Modifications to achieve metabolic goals: reduce total fat intake (particularly saturated fat) and increase exercise to lower lipid levels; glucose levels will improve with therapy that integrates food intake and insulin bioavailability.

Distribution of food among meals: good; however, initiation of insulin therapy requires close evaluation of meal pattern to prevent hypoglycemia.

Overall good nutrition: diet is low in servings from the base of the food pyramid (i.e., grains, fruits, and vegetables).

NUTRITION TEACHING TOOL

Sam's life is not routine. He will need information that will enable him to make wise food selections in a variety of settings and make dietary adjustments to accommodate his erratic schedule and prevent hypoglycemia. The fixed-ratio insulin does not accommodate meal-by-meal insulin adjustments but provides options of convenience and dependability that are attractive to Sam. Self monitoring of blood glucose is an essential component of Sam's therapy to evaluate blood glucose levels throughout the day and adjust food intake to prevent hypoglycemia. Sam also needs information to help him lower his fat intake—particularly saturated fat—while maintaining his current caloric intake. Chris selects the Exchange Lists (Table 4A-2) as a teaching tool because it provides detailed information on both the fat and carbohydrate composition of foods. Also, a wealth of supplemental information is available for restaurant eating, particularly the fast food chains that Sam frequents when he is traveling. A meal pattern is developed that accommodates Sam's life-style and provides the nutrients to support achieving the goals of nutrition therapy. Chris provides ideas for foods that can be selected when traveling or at home.

Table 4A-2   Exchange Lists

Groups/lists	Carbohydrate (grams)	Protein (grams)	Fat (grams)	Calories
Carbohydrate groups				
Starch	15	3	1 or less	80
Fruit	15	—	—	60
Milk				
Skim	12	8	0-3	90
Low-fat	12	8	5	120
Whole	12	8	8	150
Other carbohydrates	15	Varies	Varies	Varies
Vegetables	5	2	—	25
Meat and meat substitute group				
Very lean	—	7	0-1	35
Lean	—	7	3	55
Medium-fat	—	7	5	75
High-fat	—	7	8	100
Fat group	—	—	5	45

MEAL PLAN

Chris reviews the meal plan (Table 4A-3) with Sam and identifies adjustments that can be made to accommodate special situations, such as delayed meals. They discuss target blood glucose values and adjustments in food intake that Sam can make to prevent hypoglycemia. The benefits of exercise are reviewed, but they agree to wait to initiate a program until after the next visit to allow time to evaluate the insulin and diet therapies. In the interim, Sam will examine the feasibility of different ways to fit exercise into his schedule. Chris encourages Sam to call when questions arise and sets an appointment for a return visit in 6 weeks. He is instructed to write down his food intake and activity on any days when he has low blood glucose levels and to bring this information and his blood glucose monitoring records with him.

EVALUATION

At the 6-week visit, Sam reports that he has not experienced the symptoms of hypoglycemia but has checked his blood glucose levels on days when lunch was delayed. He found that on some days his blood glucose levels were low and preventive measures were needed and that on other days they were in the normal range. A review of the food and activity levels of different days showed greater than usual activity (e.g., raking leaves) or less food intake (partial breakfast) on days when blood glucose levels were low. A review of the blood glucose monitoring records showed fasting levels in recent weeks generally were between 150 and 200 mg/dl and predinner values were between 70 and 260 mg/dl but most values were between

Table 4A-3 Meal Plan

Meal Plan for: _Sue Jones_ Date: _6-15-95_

Dietitian: _Chris Nestor RD_ Phone: _327-7654_

	Grams	Percent
Carbohydrate	284	53
Protein	99	18
Fat	68	29
Calories	2144	

Time	Number of exchanges/choices	Menu ideas — Travel	Menu ideas — Home
	5 Carbohydrate group 3 Starch 1 Fruit 1 Milk _Skim_ — Meat group 1 Fat group	3/4 c. dry cereal 1 c. skim milk 1 bagel 1/2 c. orange juice 1 T. cream cheese	2 reduced-fat waffles 2 T. sugar-free syrup 1 T. reduced-fat margarine 1 c. low-fat yogurt 1/4 c. Grape Nuts 2 T. raisins
	5 Carbohydrate group 3 Starch 2 Fruit 1 Milk _Skim_ ✓ Vegetables 3 Meat group 2 Fat group	Large hamburger on Bun—lettuce, tomato and mustard Salad with 1 T. reduced-fat dressing 1 c. Apple juice 1 c. fat & sugar-free frozen yogurt	1/2 c. split-pea soup 1/2 c. Ham on Rye w/ mustard Celery sticks stuffed w/ peanut butter Large nectarine 2 small cookies
	6 Carbohydrate group 3 Starch 2 Fruit 1 Milk _Skim_ ✓ Vegetables 3 Meat group 2 Fat group	Broiled Beef Kebob Large Baked Potato 2 T. sour cream Steamed Broccoli w/ lemon Salad w/ 1 T. Italian dressing Slice Angel food cake 1 c. fresh peaches 1 c. skim milk	Char-grilled Chicken breast Medium corn-on-the-cob 1/3 c. Baked Beans Sliced tomatoes Small roll 2 T. reduced-fat margarine 1 c. lemon low-fat yogurt 1 1/2 c. blueberries
	2 Carbohydrate group 1 Fat	1 medium soft-serve cone	Frozen fruit juice bar 3 c. microwave popcorn

100 and 175 mg/dl. The effect that exercise would have on Sam's blood glucose levels was discussed and an exercise program developed with guidelines for monitoring and food adjustments to prevent hypoglycemia. Sam had several questions about foods he would like to order in restaurants but did not know how to fit into his meal plan. Chris gave him supplemental teaching materials on eating out. A follow-up visit was scheduled at 6 months to evaluate the meal plan with laboratory data on Sam's blood glucose and lipid levels, to determine if an increase in calories is needed because of increased energy expenditure through exercise, and to assess in general the insulin and diet therapies.

5 Exercise and Diabetes

Marion J. Franz

INTRODUCTION

For persons with diabetes, exercise has both benefits and risks. Today with more research available, health care providers have been better able to prepare guidelines to assist persons with diabetes to exercise safely. However, for individuals with diabetes, the response to exercise is still highly variable and requires a participant who is willing and able to monitor

---

CHAPTER OBJECTIVES

- Identify three sources of fuel substrate used by exercising muscle.
- List hormones involved with exercise and discuss their role in maintaining glucose balance.
- Discuss the metabolic and hormonal responses to exercise in persons with diabetes.
- Explain five factors related to the effects of exercise in persons with insulin-dependent diabetes mellitus (IDDM).
- Compare five strategies that can be used to assist persons with IDDM to exercise safely.
- Assess five strategies that can be used by athletes with diabetes to exercise safely
- Discuss the benefits and risks of exercise for persons with non-insulin-dependent diabetes mellitus (NIDDM).
- Summarize five strategies that can be used to assist persons with NIDDM to exercise safely.
- Describe precautions women with diabetes should take if exercising during pregnancy.
- Describe precautions during exercise for older adults with diabetes and others with complications of diabetes.
- Identify the components of an exercise program.

BOX 5-1

EXERCISE EDUCATIONAL OBJECTIVES FOR SELF-MANAGEMENT OF DIABETES

Upon completion of an exercise educational session, participants with diabetes will be able to do the following:
1. List three benefits from exercise.
2. Discuss risks of exercise.
3. List guidelines that will assist in exercising safely.
4. List components of an exercise program.
5. Monitor and evaluate the effects of exercise on blood glucose control.

---

the individualized effects of exercise on metabolic parameters. The goal is to assure that the benefits of exercise outweigh the risks.

As in other areas of diabetes management, a team approach to exercise is essential, beginning with the physician, who needs to provide medical clearance for the person with diabetes to begin or continue an exercise program and who provides support for the educational recommendations. Diabetes educators, including dietitians and nurses, can provide the guidelines necessary to integrate exercise into overall diabetes self-management. Furthermore, nutrition is a vital adjunct to exercise programs for all individuals and takes on added importance for the person with diabetes. Exercise physiologists or specialists are vital team members. Their expertise in testing and prescribing appropriate exercise programs ensures that the recommended exercise program is safe for the individual with diabetes. They also need to be knowledgeable about diabetes management and the demands having diabetes places on individuals in regard to exercise. Box 5-1 lists educational objectives for individuals with diabetes.

This chapter begins by reviewing the metabolic and hormonal adaptations of exercise in nondiabetic persons and the alterations that occur in persons with diabetes mellitus. Research related to strategies recommended to help persons with diabetes exercise safely is reviewed next. Special situations, such as exercise recommendations for pregnant women, for older adults, for persons with long-term complications of diabetes, and for athletes with diabetes, are also discussed.

In persons with IDDM, treated with conventional therapy of two injections of a short- and intermediate-acting insulin, metabolic control is best achieved by a regular or consistent life-style that includes regular meals and snacks covered by the appropriate amount of insulin. Adding exercise to this equation often increases the difficulty of maintaining metabolic control, since exercise, especially acute exercise bouts, can drastically alter the delicate balance of glucose. However, this does not mean that persons with IDDM should be discouraged from exercising. Instead, assistance from the health care team may be necessary for individuals to be able to exercise safely and thus receive the same benefits and enjoyment from exercise that persons without diabetes receive.

In contrast, in the majority of persons with NIDDM, exercise has been shown to be a useful adjunct to nutrition therapy for improved metabolic and weight control and to lessen the risk for cardiovascular disease. The beneficial effects of exercise on blood glucose levels are, however, of short duration and appear to result primarily from the overlapping acute effects.[77] This emphasizes the importance of regular exercise. For exercise to be beneficial, it must be performed regularly (a minimum of three to four times a week) and on a long-term basis. If exercise is to be performed correctly and safely, persons with NIDDM will also require assistance from professionals.

FUEL METABOLISM DURING AND AFTER EXERCISE

During exercise it is necessary to ensure the delivery of oxygen and metabolic fuels to working muscles, as well as the removal of metabolic end-products. Increased oxygen delivery and carbon dioxide removal are accomplished by increased respiration, increased cardiac output, redistribution of blood flow, and increased capillary perfusion of working muscles. Changes in the use of metabolic fuels is a more complex process.

For example, blood glucose during exercise of long duration in nondiabetic persons is maintained at a fairly stable level despite what can be a twentyfold increase in whole body oxygen, a fivefold to sixfold increase in cardiac output, and an even greater increase in blood flow and oxygen consumption in the working muscles.[68]

Muscle Metabolism During Exercise

In the resting state, skeletal muscle accounts for 35% to 40% of total oxygen consumption. During exercise, consumption of oxygen and metabolic fuels in muscle increases dramatically to provide adenosine triphosphate (ATP), the energy necessary for muscle contractions. At the start of exercise the muscle cells use fuel stored locally in the form of glycogen and triglycerides (Fig. 5-1) because these substances are readily available as sources of fuel for the glycolytic pathway and the citric acid cycle.

The rapid breakdown of glycogen stores in working muscles is stimulated by increasing work intensities and in working muscles that have been inactive before exercise by catecholamines, more specifically epinephrine,[55] and by a high preexercise glycogen contribution.[70] It may be inhibited by high concentrations of nonesterfied fatty acids (NEFA).[21] The regulation of muscle triglyceride use during exercise has not been studied thoroughly. Because intracellular fuel sources are limited, muscle cells soon depend on fuel sources from circulating blood and from tissue stores.

After an overnight fast, the major fuel of resting muscle is NEFA released from adipose tissue.[1] During exercise, use of carbohydrate as fuel increases, and the increase is greater as the intensity of exercise increases.[86] As shown in Fig. 5-1, glycogen breakdown and glucose uptake into the muscle cell are increased, as are the flux of glucose through the glycolytic pathway, the conversion of pyruvate to acetyl coenzyme A (CoA), and the oxidation of acetyl CoA in the citric acid cycle. Some of the glucose not oxidized by muscle is released into the circulation as lactate, which may be used for glucose synthesis by the liver (Cori cycle).

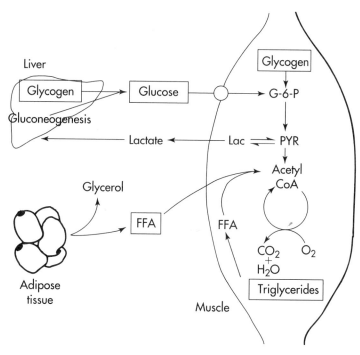

Fig. 5-1 Muscle cell fuel sources. A schematic diagram of the muscle cell and its intracellular and extracellular fuel sources. During exercise the use of both carbohydrate and lipid fuels increases, and nearly all steps in the pathway of glucose metabolism are enhanced. Some of the glucose not oxidized by muscle is released into the circulation as lactate, which, in turn, may be used for glucose synthesis by the liver (Cori cycle). Glycerol derived from the hydrolysis of adipose tissue triglyceride may also be used by the liver for gluconeogenesis. (Modified from Richter EA, Ruderman NB, Schneider SH: *Am J Med* 70:202, 1981.)

During exercise the use of lipid fuels also increases, and glycerol derived from the hydrolysis of adipose tissue triglycerides may also be used by the liver for gluconeogenesis.[63,69]

The mechanism that accounts for the increase in glucose uptake in contracting muscle is thought to involve both an increase in membrane permeability for glucose[67] and an increase in the activity of the enzymes involved in glucose disposal.[47] The transport of glucose into the muscle cell is almost exclusively by facilitated diffusion, brought about by a process involving membrane-associated glucose-transporter units that facilitate hexose transport through the membrane.[91] The rate of glucose transport increases in response to both insulin and muscle contractions.[90]

It was thought that muscle contractions would increase this glucose transport and uptake only with the availability of some small but necessary amount of insulin. However, research in isolated perfused rat muscle has shown that muscles contracting in the absence of insulin can increase transport and uptake of glucose into muscle cells, although this effect is short-lived.[63] Despite this, in persons with diabetes, insulin-deficient ketotic states impair peripheral glucose use. This has been ascribed to the exaggerated counterregulatory hormone response that acts to further augment hepatic glucose production.[94] In addition, a rise in the concentration of NEFA and ketone bodies seen during ketosis decreases glucose uptake.[65] These responses, rather than impairment of membrane permeability for glucose per se, produce a progressive hyperglycemia and can lead to ketoacidosis in ketoacidosis-prone diabetic patients.[10]

Blood Glucose Use During Exercise

Blood glucose concentrations change little during mild to moderate exercise but may increase 1.1 to 1.7 mM (20 to 30 mg/dl) with more intense exercise. However, if exercise continues 90 minutes or more, blood glucose levels may decrease 0.5 to 2.2 mM (10 to 40 mg). Hypoglycemia (blood glucose <2.2 mM [<40 mg/dl]) is rare, however, in nondiabetic persons.[29]

If exercise continues for 10 to 40 minutes, glucose uptake by muscle rises to 7 to 20 times the basal level and accounts for 30% to 40% of total oxygen consumed by muscle.[85] This is comparable to the need for blood-borne NEFA, which provides an additional 40% of oxidizable fuel. The remainder continues to be from non-blood-borne fuels (muscle glycogen and intramuscular lipids). After 40 minutes of exercise, glucose use increases until it peaks at 90 to 180 minutes and then declines slightly.[1] NEFA use continues to increase during 1 to 4 hours of exercise as the uptake of NEFA by muscles rises to approximately 70%. Thus after 4 hours of continuous mild exercise, NEFA contribute twice the fuel as does glucose.[29]

Exercise leads to a work rate–dependent increase in muscle glucose utilization. Moderate-intensity exercise (<50% maximum oxygen uptake) increases whole-body glucose uptake by 2 to 3 mg/kg/min. This means that in a 70-kg individual, an added 140 to 210 mg of blood-borne glucose is required for every minute of moderate exercise and that an added 8.4 to 12.6 g is required for every hour. During high-intensity exercise (80% to 100% of maximum oxygen uptake), the rate of whole-body glucose uptake may increase by 5 to 6 mg/kg/min. In this circumstance, an added 350 to 420 mg of glucose will be extracted from the blood and used every minute. Despite the increased rate of glucose utilization during high-intensity exercise, the demand on glucose stores and the risk of hypoglycemia is less since exercise of this intensity cannot be sustained for long intervals.[93]

Liver Metabolism During Exercise

To maintain euglycemia and to prevent hypoglycemia during exercise, the increase in glucose use at the cellular level must be counterbalanced by an increase in hepatic glucose output (see Fig. 5-1). The increase in glucose production at the beginning of exercise mainly results from glycogenolysis, but as exercise continues, gluconeogenesis plays an increasingly important role.[1]

At rest, approximately 75% of the hepatic glucose output comes from glycogenolysis, with the remaining 25% to 30% coming from gluconeogenesis. During short-term exercise, liver glucose output increases two to five times and keeps pace with the use of glucose by muscle tissue. This is primarily as a result of additional glycogenolysis.[85] The liver usually contains no more than 50 to 100 g of glycogen, and if exercise is prolonged and intense, it will be completely expended. (During 4 hours of exercise, 50 to 60 g of liver glycogen can be mobilized—a 75% or more depletion of total liver glycogen stores.) When this occurs, glucose can be derived only from gluconeogenesis. Therefore gluconeogenesis becomes more important during prolonged exercise and may account for 40% to 50% of hepatic glucose output. The principal gluconeogenic precursor during exercise is lactate released by the contracting, and also by the resting, muscles in heavy exercise.[2] However, alanine and glycerol may also be used, especially during the later stages of prolonged exercise.[28]

Fat Mobilization for Fuel

An orderly sequence of fuel use takes place during prolonged exercise. During the first 5 to 10 minutes of exercise, muscle glycogen is the major fuel consumed.[45] As exercise continues, the blood-borne fuels of glucose and eventually NEFA become increasingly important (Fig. 5-2). As exercise progresses, circulating substrates are also limited, requiring mobilization of substrates from tissue stores, that is, glycogen from the liver and fat in the form of triglycerides stored in adipose tissue. (See Table 5-1 for a summary of sources of fuel for exercise.) This switch from local to circulating fuels and from carbohydrates to lipid is important for endurance capacity, since extramuscular fat stores are the most abundant energy source. Ketone bodies can be used, but they do not normally make a substantial contribution to the overall energy supply.[38]

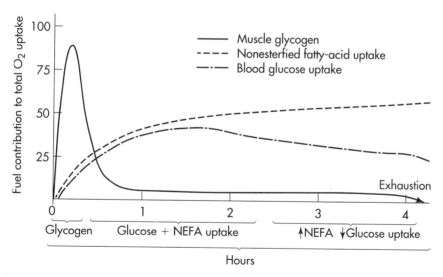

Fig. 5-2   Stages of fuel utilization by muscle in prolonged exercise. The relative contribution of muscle glycogen and blood glucose and nonesterfied fatty acids to oxidative energy during various time periods of exercise. (From Felig P, Koivisto VA: Metabolic response to exercise: implications for diabetes. In Lowenthal DT, Bhradwaja K, Oaks WW, editors: *Therapeutics through exercise,* New York, 1979, Grune & Stratton.)

Table 5-1 Sources of Fuel for Exercise

Exercise duration	Source of fuel	Substrate
First 5-10 minutes	Intramuscular	Glycogen (triglycerides)
10-40 minutes	Circulating substrates	Glucose and NEFA
~40 minutes and longer	Tissue store	
	Liver	Glucose from glycogenolysis and gluconeogenesis
	Adipose tissue	Triglyceride
		NEFA

From Franz MJ: Exercise and diabetes mellitus. In Powers MA, editor: *Handbook of diabetes nutritional management,* Rockville, Md, 1995, Aspen.

In a nonobese man, fat accounts for 80% to 85% of body fuel stores (approximately 140,000 kcal in a 70-kg man).[29] Metabolizing this fat requires a substantial amount of oxygen, which means exercise intensity must be reduced and some carbohydrate made available. To the endurance athlete, an important function of fat metabolism is glycogen sparing. With training, the body develops the ability to sustain long periods of muscle contractions by using fat for 50% to 85% of energy needs. Glycogen stores are thereby conserved.

However, the oxidation of fat-derived fuels cannot fully replace the use of glucose, even during prolonged exercise. When the supply of carbohydrate is limited, the oxidation of fat is incomplete, resulting in the production of ketone bodies. These ketone bodies can later be reused in the fatty acid oxidation cycle of skeletal musculature, but they may also be excreted in the urine, resulting in a net energy loss.

Blood NEFA levels are increased gradually during exercise. This increase is regulated by insulin and the catecholamines. The increase in ketogenesis that occurs with prolonged exercise requires increased NEFA mobilization from adipose tissue and delivery to the liver. In addition to hepatic NEFA delivery, the exercise-induced rise in glucagon stimulates hepatic fat oxidation and is necessary for the full ketogenic response to exercise.[92]

Hormonal Response to Exercise

In the resting state, glucose production is modulated by the balance between insulin and the counterregulatory hormones. Increases in plasma insulin and glucose inhibit hepatic glucose production, whereas increases in glucagon, glucocorticoids, and catecholamines and decreases in insulin and glucose promote it. These factors also influence hepatic glucose output during exercise.[34]

The plasma concentration of insulin decreases during exercise of an intensity above approximately 50% Vo_{2max}, 66% of which is the result of alpha-adrenergic inhibition of insulin secretion, and 33% of which is the result of an enhanced insulin removal rate.[35,94] This, in combination with the increase in counterregulatory hormones, induces an impressive increase of glucose output from the liver and may also contribute to the increase in adipose tissue lipolysis, as well as act as a restraint on glucose use by nonexercising muscle.

The fall in insulin and rise in glucagon are the major determinants of glucose production during moderate exercise. The fall in insulin is necessary for the full increase in hepatic glycogenolysis, and the rise in glucagon is necessary for the full increase in both hepatic glycogenolysis and gluconeogenesis.[93] In contrast to the importance of glucagon and insulin during moderate-intensity exercise, epinephrine plays only a minor role in regulating hepatic glucose production and appears to occur only during the latter stage of prolonged exercise.

The hormonal response to high-intensity exercise differs, however. In this type of activity, glucose production no longer matches but, in fact, exceeds the rise in glucose utilization.[18,51] It has been hypothesized that during exercise of high intensity, there may be a shift in the control of glucose production away from the pancreatic hormones to the catecholamines.[93] This is based on the observation that norepinephrine and epinephrine can increase by tenfold to twentyfold, whereas the increase in the glucagon-to-insulin ratio is considerably less.

Fuel Sources for Exercise

Carbohydrate is the main fuel for short-duration, high-intensity exercise. Its glucose structure contains more oxygen than do other nutrients. This allows for rapid oxidation and release of energy. Glucose is the only substrate that can be used in anaerobic glycolysis and is the main substrate serving the energy needs of the brain and nervous system. The major problem with glucose as the primary fuel source is its limited storage capacity. In contrast to stored fat, stored carbohydrate accounts for approximately 1500 kcal—300 to 400 g of muscle glycogen (approximately 15 g/kg muscle), 50 to 100 g of liver glycogen, and 20 g of glucose in extracellular water.[87] Muscle glycogen can be used to meet the energy needs of only the muscle in which it is contained. Liver glycogen, however, can be used gradually during periods of starvation or rapidly mobilized in response to exercise or hypoglycemia.

Physical training enhances the body's ability to store and use carbohydrate; however, even trained athletes store only approximately 2000 kcal in the body as blood glucose and liver and muscle glycogen. If carbohydrates were the only fuel used during exercise, sports activities lasting more than 2 hours would be impossible because overwhelming fatigue and exhaustion occur when muscle glycogen becomes depleted. Why glycogen depletion coincides with fatigue is not clear, since large amounts of circulating substrate in the form of NEFA are still available.[29]

Protein combustion during exercise is generally believed to be insignificant, provided the exercise is not excessively heavy or prolonged. Protein accounts for 15% to 20% of body fuel stores (30,000 to 40,000 kcal). Its usefulness as a fuel is limited because its consumption would necessitate the breakdown of muscle or other tissue.[29]

Postexercise Response

After exercise of an intensity that depletes muscle glycogen stores, replenishment becomes a high metabolic priority. This happens by a non-insulin-dependent increase in muscle glucose uptake and by an increase in insulin sensitivity of the exercised muscles. Whole-body insulin sensitivity has been found to be increased for at least 48 hours after 1 hour of bicycling at a moderately intense rate.[57] This increase in insulin sensitivity after exercise may contribute to hypoglycemia in persons with IDDM.

Exercise appears to simply accelerate the transition of the body into a more fasting state. Liver and muscle glycogen stores are progressively depleted, and hepatic gluconeogenesis is accelerated, dependent on the work intensity and duration. Muscle glycogen depletion is a potent stimulus for glycogen synthesis and facilitates the initial repletion of stores after exercise.[46] Glycogen resynthesis after exercise is greatly influenced by the supply of substrate. In subjects on a carbohydrate-free diet, muscle glycogen storage is slow and hepatic glycogen stores will decrease further or remain the same unless carbohydrate is ingested.

The repletion of muscle glycogen after exercise has been shown to occur in two phases. In phase one, which occurs immediately after exercise, there is increased cell permeability to glucose and elevated glycogen synthetase activity, leading to muscle glycogen being rapidly restored. This phase does not require insulin. In the second phase, muscle glycogen has returned to near-normal levels and glucose uptake is no longer elevated in the absence of insulin. Instead there is a marked and persistent increase in insulin action. The added insulin-stimulated glucose disposal after exercise is attributable solely to an increase in nonoxidative glucose metabolism.[46]

ALTERATIONS IN FUEL METABOLISM DURING AND AFTER EXERCISE IN PERSONS WITH IDDM

During exercise, the working muscles use their own store of glycogen and triglycerides, as well as glucose released by the liver and NEFA derived from adipose tissue lipolysis. Changes in the use of these metabolic fuels can occur in persons with diabetes, especially persons with IDDM.

Muscle Glycogen Use

Direct measurements of muscle glycogen content in acutely insulin-deprived persons with diabetes indicate that the rate of glycogen use is the same as in nondiabetic persons. However, resynthesis is an insulin-dependent process. Thus in the absence of insulin therapy, muscle glycogen repletion is minimal in persons with diabetes, whereas with insulin the rate of repletion is the same.[87]

Blood Glucose Levels During Exercise

Before the advent of insulin, accumulated evidence showed that in insulin-deficient persons with diabetes, exercise resulted in a more pronounced hyperglycemia, hyperketonemia, and glycosuria; in fact, strenuous exertion occasionally led to coma.[87] After the introduction of insulin, it soon became apparent that in persons treated with insulin, blood glucose levels fell during exercise and that regular insulin reduced the exogenous insulin requirement.

The metabolic and hormonal response to exercise varies depending on the degree of metabolic control at the start of exercise, more specifically the availability of insulin. In nonketotic persons with diabetes with mild-to-moderate hyperglycemia (>15 mM [270 mg/dl]), moderately heavy exercise 24 hours after insulin withdrawal causes the blood glucose level to fall. In contrast, in persons with more severe hyperglycemia and mild ketonemia (blood ketones 2 to 3 mM), exercise causes a significant rise in blood glucose concentration.[10] This may reflect either an overproduction of glucose from the liver or underuse by the working muscles, or both. Furthermore, because lipolysis is also enhanced during insulin deficiency, NEFA and ketone body concentrations rise in the blood, resulting in an inhibition of glucose uptake by muscle, which counterbalances the effect of exercise in the glucose transport process.[30,65]

Liver Metabolism During Exercise

The rise of hepatic glucose output in response to exercise is similar in persons with and without diabetes.[88] However, in persons with diabetes, the use of gluconeogenic precursors during short-term exercise rises two to three times the basal level; in persons without diabetes, it remains the same. Thus gluconeogenesis was estimated to account for 30% of the liver glucose output in persons with diabetes compared with no more than 11% for those without diabetes. As a result, the influence of brief (40 minutes) exercise on hepatic glucose metabolism in persons with diabetes is comparable to that of prolonged (4 hours) exercise in nondiabetic subjects.[87]

Nonesterfied Fatty Acid (NEFA) Levels

Plasma concentrations of NEFA increase at low insulin levels, such as during exercise or with uncontrolled diabetes, and the use of NEFA in muscles increases during these two conditions. In general, the importance of NEFA as a fuel relative to carbohydrate increases with the duration of exercise and decreases as exercise intensity increases.[38] During prolonged exercise of low intensity (40% of maximal aerobic capacity [$V_{O_{2max}}$]), NEFA oxidation accounts for approximately 60% of muscle oxygen consumption.[1] The uptake of NEFA is not insulin-dependent but is proportional to the concentration of NEFA in plasma. Thus in poorly controlled diabetes with elevated levels of NEFA, the uptake and oxidation of NEFA during exercise are increased relative to those of glucose.[38]

In nonketotic diabetic persons with mild hyperglycemia, as well as in nondiabetics, an initial decline in NEFA concentration is followed by a modest gradual rise as exercise continues.[10] In contrast, persons with diabetes with marked hyperglycemia and ketosis already show an elevated NEFA level at rest, and the rise during exercise is more marked.[88] As a result of this greater availability of NEFA, uptake of NEFA by working muscle is increased. In mildly ketotic persons with diabetes, a sevenfold increase in NEFA uptake by muscles was shown, as compared with a threefold to fourfold increment in nondiabetics.[88]

Ketone Body Use

The short-chain fatty acids, 3-hydroxybutyric acid, and acetoacetic acid are present in plasma in low amounts normally, and during exercise ketone bodies make no net contribution to the fuel supply of muscles.[67] However, mildly ketotic persons with diabetes use ketone bodies during exercise. In severely insulin-deficient persons with diabetes with marked hyperketonemia, strenuous exercise causes a further rise in blood ketone body levels.[10,88]

The mechanism for this rapid development of ketosis is not altogether clear. Studies suggest that a defect in peripheral clearance of ketones rather than a marked increase in ketogenesis during exercise in insulin-deprived individuals is the major factor.[31]

Hormonal Changes with Exercise

Plasma insulin levels may be much higher in persons with diabetes than in those without diabetes. In such a setting hepatic glucose production is inhibited and glucose clearance is enhanced by peripheral glucose uptake and stimulated glucose oxidation by the exercising muscle. As a result, plasma glucose falls. The major effect of the high insulin levels is inhibition of glucose production; both glycogenolysis and gluconeogenesis are inhibited. Although counterregulatory hormone response may be excessive, the hepatic glucose production cannot match the rate of peripheral glucose use and blood glucose falls. This fall in blood glucose with mild-to-moderate exercise may be beneficial to some persons with diabetes but, with more prolonged exercise, hypoglycemia may result. This is a problem particularly in persons who are also glucagon deficient.

Persons who exercise when in moderately poor control of their diabetes induce an abnormally increased secretion of the glucoregulatory hormones. Insulin deficiency plus a high concentration of counterregulatory hormones enhances gluconeogenesis at levels two to three times those seen in nondiabetic persons, resulting in an exaggerated increase in hepatic glucose production and circulating plasma glucose concentrations.[87]

Whether the decrease in plasma glucose with exercise is large enough to produce signs of neuroglucopenia depends on factors such as initial plasma glucose levels, intensity and duration of exercise, actual plasma insulin concentrations, and relation of exercise to the last meal. Furthermore, the setpoint of the glucoregulatory system may be higher in persons with diabetes. As a result they may have symptoms of neuroglucopenia when their plasma glucose concentration is normal or even in the hyperglycemic range.[24] However, some persons with diabetes have poor counterregulatory defense mechanisms, possibly as a result of autonomic neuropathy; these persons are especially prone to develop frank hypoglycemia.[22]

Exercise and Hyperglycemia

The metabolic and hormonal responses to exercise vary with degree of metabolic control at the onset of exercise and more specifically the availability of insulin. A minimal level of insulin is necessary for glucose uptake by the muscles, as well as for the regulation of glucose production by the liver. With insulin deficiency there is also an abnormal increase in the secretion of the glucoregulatory hormones—catecholamines, glucagon, cortisol, and growth

---

BOX 5-2

CAUSES FOR POST EXERCISE, LATE-ONSET HYPGLYCEMIA

1. Muscle and/or liver glycogen depletion from unusually intense or long exercise
2. Increased insulin sensitivity in those making a transition from the untrained to a trained state
3. Ongoing glucose use after exercise for replacement of glycogen stones
4. Defective counterregulatory response
5. Inappropriate adjustments in insulin or food before or after exercise
6. Lack of blood glucose monitoring after exercise, which might allow for preventive intervention (e.g., increased caloric intake or subsequent decreased insulin)
7. A combination of all of the above

---

hormone. Exercise is not always effective in decreasing elevated blood glucose levels and is not a complete replacement for insulin.

High-intensity exercise can be more deleterious to metabolic control than moderate exercise of the same duration. Even persons with well-controlled diabetes may have an increase in blood glucose and NEFA levels after high-intensity exercise. This may be a result of the increase in counterregulatory hormones during this type of exercise or because insulin fails to rise as it would normally with heavy exercise in persons without diabetes.[59,64]

Postexercise Hypoglycemia

Campaigne and associates[19] investigated the effects of different diets and insulin adjustments in nine persons with IDDM. When hypoglycemia occurred, it was noted 5 hours after exercise five of eight times. MacDonald[50] selected 300 young people with IDDM for study. Postexercise, late-onset (PEL) hypoglycemia occurred in 48 of the subjects during the 2-year study period. The incidence of hypoglycemia varied from 3 to 31 hours after exercise but was most common 6 to 15 hours after exercise. Hypoglycemia during exercise, or 1 to 2 hours after exercise, was relatively uncommon. Furthermore, persons who experienced hypoglycemia did not appear to be in "tighter" control than those who did not. Exercise was usually vigorous or prolonged and often occurred after a period of relative inactivity. Box 5-2 lists causes for PEL.

EXERCISE AND IDDM

Considering the complexity of fuel flux during exercise and the important regulatory role played by insulin and the counterregulatory hormones, it is not surprising that persons with diabetes, especially IDDM, can run into management problems when exercising. Because of the increased risks of exercise, experts have debated whether exercise should be recommended for all persons with IDDM. However, the current consensus is that persons with IDDM should be encouraged to participate in regular exercise for the same reasons that persons without diabetes should be encouraged to exercise.[93]

Benefits of Exercise

Persons with diabetes gain the same benefits that persons without diabetes gain from a regular exercise program—namely, improved fitness and psychologic state, increased lean body mass, decreased adipose tissue stores, weight control, and improved physical work capacity. For persons with diabetes, exercise has additional benefits; for example, increased insulin sensitivity results in a potential reduction in insulin dosage,[87] as well as in a reduction of risk factors for atherosclerosis.[43]

Short-Term Effects of Exercise

Insulin taken by injection does not duplicate the normal secretion of insulin from the pancreas, which can vary acutely depending on food intake and the performance of physical activity. Sporadic exercise can exert acute or short-term effects on fuel metabolism in persons with IDDM as a result of variable states of insulin excess and insulin deficiency. When insulin deficiency and ketosis are present, exercise can cause an increase in plasma glucose and accelerated ketone body formation. In contrast, with a relative excess of insulin in the circulation, blood glucose levels decrease during and after exercise and exercise-induced hypoglycemia occurs.

   During exercise of high intensity, hepatic glucose production may exceed the increase in glucose utilization. This process can result in an increase in blood glucose levels that extends into the postexercise state.

Training Effects of Exercise

With training, clinical observations suggest that the risk of hypoglycemia with exercise is reduced. Several factors may contribute to this decreased risk: (1) the meal plan is adjusted so that snacks are planned to coincide with usual exercise times; (2) insulin dosages are reduced to compensate for the decreased need for insulin with exercise; (3) higher levels of counterregulatory hormones exist in trained persons[56]; or (4) a combination of the above. Furthermore, postexercise hypoglycemia is also reduced with training.[50]

   A limited number of studies have been done on the effect of exercise training on long-term metabolic control in IDDM. Most studies focus on the short-term effects of exercise and suggest that physical training can increase insulin sensitivity and glucose storage and improve lipoprotein concentrations. Long-term effects of exercise, such as improved blood glucose control as measured by glycated hemoglobin, have not been demonstrated.

   The lack of a long-term beneficial effect of exercise in persons with IDDM, as measured by glycohemoglobin, is somewhat unexpected because of the acute glucose-lowering effect that can occur with each exercise session. It was hoped that this acute response would have a summation effect on overall control. Zinman and others[97] reported that although 45 minutes of supervised exercise was undertaken three times a week for 12 weeks in 13 persons with IDDM, fasting blood glucose and HbA_{1c} values remained unchanged with training. This lack of improvement was attributed to the increased intake of approximately 300 kcal on exercising days.

Wallberg-Henriksson and others[89] reported a similar lack of unchanged glucose control related to exercise. They studied nine men with IDDM who participated in a training program consisting of 1 hour of exercise 2 to 3 times a week for 16 weeks. Despite increased peripheral insulin sensitivity, decreased total cholesterol, and increased high-density lipoprotein cholesterol, there was no improvement in glycated hemoglobin, glycosuria, or 24-hour urinary glucose excretion. Subjects also consumed a snack of approximately 400 kcal after exercise. They concluded that, although other benefits from exercise were noted, in the absence of efforts to alter food intake and insulin administration, physical training by itself does not improve blood glucose control in persons with IDDM.

The long-term effect of physical activity among persons with IDDM on other risks from diabetes is not known. LaPorte and others[48a] studied the relationship of physical activity and diabetes complications in 696 persons with IDDM. They reported that the long-term effect of physical activity does not appear to accelerate development of severe eye disease, coronary heart disease, or death. On the contrary, it may be beneficial. Because persons with IDDM have at least a sevenfold increased risk of these complications, any factor associated positively with prevention has important implications.

FACTORS RELATED TO THE EFFECTS OF EXERCISE IN PERSONS WITH IDDM

The metabolic response to exercise is highly variable, even in the same individual, because of the many variables related to exercise and to metabolic homeostasis. Exercise variables include exercise intensity, type, and duration, timing of exercise in relation to meals, the time of day exercise is performed, and time of exercise in relation to insulin injections.

Metabolic Control

A major determinant of the response to exercise is related to insulin availability. Aside from the effects of this on metabolic control at the start of exercise, which have already been discussed, diabetes also influences the size of the body fuel reserves, primarily the carbohydrate store. The amount of carbohydrate stored is related to the degree of glycemic control. Insulin availability determines the extent of glycogen storage and depletion in both liver and muscles; therefore a person experiencing frequent bouts of hypoglycemia or hyperglycemia may have inadequate hepatic and muscle glycogen stores available for exercise. The degree of glycogen depletion is intimately related to the extent of insulin deprivation.[10,87] These persons can be more susceptible to fluctuations in blood glucose levels, especially hypoglycemia, and they should be advised to avoid prolonged exercise until diabetes control is improved.

Duration and Intensity of Exercise

Brief, intense exercise tends to induce mild hyperglycemia, whereas prolonged exercise can result in hypoglycemia, both in persons with diabetes and in those persons without diabetes, in whom circulating insulin levels can change.

Mitchell and others[59] found that periods of intense exercise (80% Vo_{2max}) in nondiabetic subjects produce sustained postexercise hyperglycemia, 20% above basal, with a 100% increase in plasma insulin. In persons with IDDM incapable of generating that rise in insulin by increased secretion, postexercise hyperglycemia was greater and sustained longer. Thus in the recovery period after intense exercise, glycemia may be raised rather than improved. In persons with IDDM exercising to exhaustion at 80% Vo_{2max}, when preexercise plasma glucose was normal (4.8 ± 0.2 mM [86 ± 4 mg/dl]), hyperglycemia rose to 7.0 ± 1.5 mM (127 ± 7 mg/dl) and was sustained for 2 hours after exhaustion. When plasma glucose was 8.3 ± mM (149 ± 9 mg/dl), it rose progressively throughout the 2 hours to 12.7 ± 1.5 mM (229 ± 28 mg/dl). The type of sport that most closely resembles exercise of the intensity used in this study would involve sprints or repeated bouts of exercise, such as in hockey or basketball.

Food Intake

Stratton and others[83] studied adolescents with IDDM who entered a structured 8-week exercise program held after their usual afternoon snack. Food intake was not increased on exercise days. Although glycohemoglobin values did not improve, glycated serum albumin, which is a more sensitive index of glycemic changes over a shorter period, showed a significant decline. Blood glucose concentrations before exercise were also significantly lower in the last 3 weeks of the program than in the first 3 weeks. Stratton and colleagues attributed this improvement to better control of food intake.

Timing of Exercise

Free-insulin levels in persons with IDDM tend to be lower before breakfast than before subsequent meals or bedtime. As a result, less hypoglycemia in response to exercise before breakfast, as opposed to late afternoon exercise, might be expected. Ruegemer and others[72] studied persons with IDDM at rest and when exercising before breakfast and at 1600 hours. Plasma glucose increased from 6.7 ± 0.4 to 9.1 ± 0.4 mM (121 ± 7 to 164 ± 7 mg/dl) during morning exercise as compared with no change in plasma glucose during afternoon exercise. However, there was a 0.3 to 1.0 mM (5 to 18 mg/dl) decrease with afternoon exercise in *half* of the individuals. They concluded that the risk of exercise-induced hypoglycemia is lowest before breakfast. The hyperglycemia induced by prebreakfast exercise is mild and short-lived and thus would likely have a minimal impact on overall glucose control.

Type of Exercise

Recommendations for exercise programs for persons with diabetes should emphasize a complete exercise program. Aerobic exercises for cardiovascular conditioning; warm-up and cool-down exercises designed to increase flexibility (persons with diabetes may lose flexibility because of glycation of collagen); and muscle strengthening exercises. Durak and others[26] reported that a supervised strength-training program 3 days a week for 10 weeks for men with IDDM was associated with no morbidity, increased strength, reduced blood glucose and glycated hemoglobin with no change in insulin dose, and lower cholesterol levels. Caution is recommended with high levels of resistance training because of the acute response associated with high-intensity-type training (e.g., hyperglycemia[64] and increased blood pressure).

Amount of Insulin Injected

Schiffrin and Parikh[76] studied persons with near-normal glycated hemoglobins who exercised moderately $1\frac{1}{2}$ hours after breakfast (2 hours after insulin injections). They reported that a 30% to 50% reduction of premeal insulin dose appeared to accommodate 45 minutes of exercise without hypoglycemia. When adjustments in insulin are not feasible, they suggested that 15 g of glucose before each 45 minutes of unplanned exercise and 15 to 30 g of glucose after physical activity would be appropriate to prevent hypoglycemia.

Injection Sites

In persons with IDDM, plasma insulin concentrations do not decrease during exercise and may even increase substantially if exercise is undertaken within 1 hour or so after an insulin injection. This is caused by increased absorption of insulin from the subcutaneous tissue, particularly if regular insulin is used and the injection site is in an exercising part of the body. However, when 40 minutes have elapsed after injection of regular insulin and before exercise has begun, more than half the administered insulin has been mobilized. In addition, intermediate insulins are also unaffected when exercise is begun $2\frac{1}{2}$ hours after injection.[11] Because in reality exercise rarely occurs immediately after an insulin injection, it appears to be unnecessary to recommend rotating insulin sites to parts of the body that are not involved in physical activity to prevent exercise-induced hypoglycemia. However, exercising at peak action times of any insulin can still lead to hypoglycemia.

Physical Fitness

Inactivity has long been shown to be a cause of glucose intolerance and insulin resistance. Arslanian and others[7] studied adolescents with IDDM and adolescents without diabetes and reported that insulin-mediated glucose disposal was positively related to the state of physical fitness as assessed by Vo_{2max} and negatively related to diabetes control as assessed by HbA_1. However, for similar degrees of physical fitness, adolescents with diabetes had lower total-body insulin-mediated glucose metabolism than did control group members. They concluded that adolescents with IDDM are insulin-resistant as compared with nondiabetics, and this resistance is attributable to the state of diabetes control. However, the level of physical fitness explains a major part of the interindividual variations in insulin action in adolescents both with and without IDDM.

Meinders and others[56] also studied trained athletes with diabetes performing activities of long duration and compared them with well-trained nondiabetics during a 3-hour marathon-training run. Insulin was withheld the morning of the run, but a normal breakfast was eaten 2½ hours before the start of the run. All subjects ate a banana after 90 minutes and a 3-g dextrose tablet after 150 minutes of running. Blood glucose dropped from 17 mM to 5 mM (306 to 90 mg/dl) after 150 minutes of running. However, the runners with diabetes had higher peripheral serum concentrations of counterregulatory hormones than did the control group, which presumably helped to prevent hypoglycemia. This may help explain why well-trained persons with diabetes are less prone to hypoglycemia than athletes with diabetes who are not well trained.

PRECAUTIONS WITH EXERCISE FOR PERSONS WITH IDDM

It is important that persons with diabetes who want to exercise be encouraged to participate in either recreational or competitive activities or both. However, physical exercise is not without risks to individuals with IDDM. Hypoglycemia, hyperglycemia, ketosis, cardiovascular ischemia and dysrhythmia, exacerbation of proliferative retinopathy, and lower-extremity injury are potential complications of exercise.[43]

Participants should undergo a thorough medical evaluation before undertaking unusual or particularly vigorous exercise programs. This is especially important for persons who are over age 35 and/or those who have had diabetes for more than 10 years.[5] Individuals should be screened carefully for the presence of cardiovascular disease, proliferative retinopathy, and nephropathy, all of which present risks for exercise. Some types of exercise should be avoided if specific risks are present. With exercise, blood pressure may rise higher in persons with IDDM than in nondiabetic individuals, placing the patient with retinopathy at risk. Furthermore, those with proliferative retinopathy should not participate in heavy lifting or straining and should avoid head-low positions or excessive jarring of the head, all of which may precipitate a vitreous hemorrhage. Those with peripheral neuropathy should be particularly careful to avoid cuts, blisters, and pounding exercises of the lower extremities, and those with autonomic neuropathy should be careful to maintain appropriate fluid and electrolyte balance during exercise in a warm climate.[5] Exercise has also been shown to result in proteinuria in persons with diabetes;[60] this is probably a transient hemodynamic response, and it is unknown if exercise has any deleterious effect on the progression of renal disease.[43]

STRATEGIES TO ASSIST PERSONS WITH IDDM TO EXERCISE SAFELY

Although each individual responds differently to exercise, general guidelines are important so persons can begin to exercise safely. As individuals gain experience with exercise, they can adapt specific issues to meet their needs. Ideally, exercise should be performed at about the same time each day, but for practical reasons, this is often not possible. Therefore the goal is to assist persons to exercise safely at times of the day that are convenient for them. Persons who are trained will also find they have fewer problems when exercising.

A good general rule of thumb regarding exercise concerns blood glucose levels, food intake, and insulin adjustment. If blood glucose is <5.5 mM (<100 mg/dl) before exercise, the person should eat a pre-exercise snack. If blood glucose is 5.5 to 8.3 mM (100 to 150 mg/dl), the person can go ahead and exercise and, if necessary, eat a snack afterwards. If fasting blood glucose is >14 mM (>250 mg/dl) and ketone bodies are present in the urine or if fasting blood glucose is >16.6 mM (>300 mg/dl), irrespective of whether ketones are present, it is generally advisable for the person to take insulin according to supplemental insulin guidelines and delay exercising.[93]

Self-monitoring of blood glucose levels is essential. Blood glucose monitoring before, during (if exercise is of long duration), and after exercise is essential if persons are to determine their response to exercise. Monitoring records are the most effective tool for determining a particular pattern of response to exercise. Patterns can then be used to adapt food or insulin to the time and amount of exercise planned. Carefully determining how exercise affects blood glucose levels will decrease the risk of hypoglycemia.

When monitoring blood glucose, it is important to consider not only the absolute glycemic levels but also the rate at which any change in glycemia may occur. For example, a glucose level that is stable at 5.5 mM (100 mg/dl) may reflect a safe situation but a glucose level of 5.5 mM (100 mg/dl) is indicative of an imbalance between glucose production and utilization if the preceding glucose measurement was 8.3 mM (150 mg/dl). In this case, extra carbohydrate may be needed before exercise.[93]

Food intake may need to be increased to accommodate activity or exercise. The individual's meal plan should take into consideration the person's exercise pattern. If exercise is done regularly, the snacks should be a part of the usual meal plan. In general, persons with IDDM tend to overeat before exercise. Well-trained individuals who regularly exercise at about the same time each day need less additional food than persons who exercise only occasionally. (See Table 5-2 for suggestions for preexercise and postexercise snacks.)

Guidelines for increasing food intake for exercise need to be based on blood glucose levels before and after exercise, the duration of the exercise, the proximity of unscheduled exercise to scheduled meals, the times of day, and the regularity of exercise sessions. It may be best to delay consumption of extra food until after exercise, when testing of blood glucose can help determine how many (if any) calories are needed. In general, 15 g of carbohydrate—one fruit or starch exchange—should be eaten before (or after) 1 hour of moderate exercise, such as tennis, swimming, jogging, cycling, or gardening. For more strenuous activity of a 1- to 2-hour duration, such as football, hockey, racquetball, basketball, strenuous cycling, or swimming, 30 to 50 g of carbohydrate—half a meat sandwich with one milk or fruit exchange—may be needed. Mild exercise, such as walking a half mile, probably will not require any extra food.[33] (See Table 5-3 for general guidelines on increasing food intake for exercise that is not done regularly.)

Persons with IDDM should not overeat with exercise. Many persons use exercise as an opportunity to liberalize their usual food intake with foods they might normally avoid, such as desserts, candy bars, or regular soft drinks.

Table 5-2 Preexercise and Postexercise Snacks

Food	Amount	Carbohydrate content	Exchanges
Bagel or English muffin	½	14 g	1 starch
Graham cracker squares	3	15 g	1 starch
Snack crackers	4-5	15 g	1 starch
Muffin	1	17 g	1 starch, 1 fat
Pretzels	6 3-ring	14 g	1 starch
Soup (not cream)	1 cup	15 g	1 starch
Yogurt (plain or sweetened with aspartame)	1 cup	16 g	1 milk
Apple	1 medium	22 g	1½ fruit
Banana	1 small	22 g	1½ fruit
Dried fruit	¼ cup	15 g	1 fruit
Orange	1 medium	18 g	1 fruit
Raisins	2 Tbsp	15 g	1 fruit
Fruit juice	½ cup	15 g	1 fruit
Gatorade	1 8-oz. cup	12 g	1 fruit
Exceed (fluid replacement and energy drink)	1 8-oz. cup	17 g	1 fruit

Modified from Franz MJ, Barry B: *Diabetes and exercise: guidelines for safe and enjoyable activity,* Minneapolis, Minn, 1993, International Diabetes Center.

Strenuous exercise over an extended time may require a decrease in insulin dosage. A conservative recommendation is to begin decreasing the insulin acting during the time of the activity (morning or afternoon) by 10% of the total insulin dose per day. If the person is active during the entire day, both the short-acting and intermediate-acting insulin can be decreased by 10%, for a total of 20%.[33]

Because blood glucose continues to decrease after exercise, it is important to continue testing blood glucose after exercise is completed. Blood glucose levels can continue to decrease for up to 30 hours after exercise, especially after vigorous or prolonged exercise or exercise that is not done regularly. The most frequently reported time for hypoglycemia is 4 to 10 hours after exercise. Hypoglycemia during exercise, or even 2 hours after exercise, is not as common as hypoglycemia later. Replacing stored liver and muscle carbohydrate used during exercise can take from 24 to 48 hours. Blood glucose testing is essential for a person to determine whether to eat extra food and/or decrease insulin dosage after exercise.

Timing is also a factor in making decisions about exercise. Depending on the time of day that exercise is done and the blood glucose level before exercise, various changes in blood glucose can occur. For example, exercising late in the afternoon may cause a greater drop in blood glucose values than exercising before or after breakfast. When possible, exercise should be scheduled so it will improve postprandial hyperglycemia. Ideally, exercise should occur 1 to 2 hours after a meal, when blood glucose is >5.5 mM (>100 mg/dl). An excellent time to exercise may be before or after breakfast because blood glucose levels are often elevated during this time.

Table 5-3   Suggested General Guidelines for Making Food Adjustments for Exercise for Individuals With IDDM

Type of exercise and examples	If blood glucose is:	Increase food intake by:	Suggestions of food to use:
Exercise of short duration and of low to moderate intensity (walking a half mile or leisurely bicycling for less than 30 min)	Less than 100 mg/dl	10 to 15 g of carbohydrate per hour	1 fruit or 1 starch exchange
	100 mg/dl or above	Not necessary to increase food	
Exercise of moderate intensity (1 hr of tennis, swimming, jogging, leisurely bicycling, golfing)	Less than 100 mg/dl	25 to 50 g of carbohydrate before exercise, then 10 to 15 g per hour of exercise	½ meat sandwich with a milk or fruit exchange
	100 to 180 mg/dl	10 to 15 g of carbohydrate	1 fruit or 1 starch exchange
	180 to 300 mg/dl	Not necessary to increase	
	300 mg/dl or above	Do not begin exercise until blood glucose is under better control	
Strenuous activity or exercise (about 1-2 hr of football, hockey, racquetball, or basketball; strenuous bicycling or swimming; shoveling heavy snow)	Less than 100 mg/dl	50 g of carbohydrate, monitor blood glucose carefully	1 meat sandwich (2 slices of bread) with a milk and fruit exchange
	100 to 180 mg/dl	25 to 50 g of carbohydrate, depending on intensity and duration	½ meat sandwich with a milk or fruit exchange
	180 to 300 mg/dl	10 to 15 g of carbohydrate	1 fruit or 1 starch exchange
	300 mg/dl or above	Do not begin exercise until blood glucose is under better control	

Modified from Franz MJ, Barry B: *Diabetes and exercise guidelines for safe and enjoyable activity,* Minneapolis, Minn, 1993, International Diabetes Center.

Peak times of injected insulin and the excessive lowering of blood glucose levels that exercise may produce at these times must be considered. Exercising when insulin is at peak effect can result in a precipitous fall in blood glucose, and additional carbohydrate may be needed to prevent hypoglycemia.

Fluid intake is important. Persons with IDDM often become so preoccupied with replacing carbohydrate that they forget that the most important nutrient needed during exercise is water. Individuals whose diabetes is not well controlled are particularly prone to dehydration when exercising, especially on warm days. Cool water, sports drinks, or diluted fruit juices are good choices. A half cup of fruit juice (15 g of carbohydrate) diluted with a half cup of water, for a total of 1 cup/hour, or as often as needed, is an excellent way to take in both carbohydrate and fluid when exercising. For every pound of weight lost during exercise, 2 cups of fluid are needed for replacement.

Persons should have adequate metabolic control. When an insulin deficiency results in poor metabolic control (BG >13.8 to 16.6 mM [>250 to 300 mg/dl]), especially with ketonuria, the production of glucose and the breakdown of fat to ketones exceed the ability of the muscles to use them. This is of particular concern when diabetes control has been suboptimal over several days or more.

Injection sites are not a major concern, unless the injection is given in a part of the body that will be exercising immediately. If it has been more than 40 minutes between the injection of regular insulin and the start of exercise, more than half of the injected insulin will be mobilized from the injection site. Likewise, absorption of intermediate-acting insulin remains unaffected when exercise is begun 1½ hours after an injection. If exercise is performed immediately after an insulin injection, the injection should be given in an area that is not involved in the exercise, such as the abdomen.

All individuals should carry adequate identification and a source of readily available carbohydrate. (See Table 5-4 for a summary of strategies to assist persons with IDDM to exercise safely.)

Table 5-4   Strategies to Assist Persons With IDDM to Exercise Safely

1. Adequate metabolic control should be established before an exercise program is initiated.
2. Self-monitoring of blood glucose levels is essential.
3. Food intake may need to be increased to accommodate exercise. In general, 15 g of carbohydrate should be eaten before or after 1 hour of moderate activity.
4. Strenuous exercise over an extended time period may require a decrease in insulin doses.
5. Testing of blood glucose after exercise is important to prevent postexercise hypoglycemia.
6. Timing of exercise can be a factor in making decisions about additional food intake.
7. Peak times of injected insulin and the possible decrease in blood glucose levels with exercise at that time should be considered.
8. Fluid intake is important.
9. Injection sites are not a major concern unless the injection is given in a part of the body that will be exercising immediately.
10. All persons should carry adequate identification and a source of readily available carbohydrate.

STRATEGIES FOR ATHLETES WITH IDDM

Athletes with IDDM find that if they begin training gradually and extend it over a period of time, their bodies adapt physically and metabolically. As a result, there can be gradual adjustments (usually decreases) in insulin and adaptations in food intake. When training for more than 1 hour at a time, insulin dosage may need to be reduced even further.

An exercising body uses carbohydrate as its main fuel source. In athletes who do not have diabetes, blood glucose reaches a point at which noticeable fatigue sets in after about 90 to 180 minutes of exercise. At that point they also will perform better with a carbohydrate replacement. This can delay the onset of fatigue by slowing depletion of muscle glycogen stores. For athletes with IDDM, a carbohydrate replacement may be needed after approximately 60 minutes of exercise to prevent hypoglycemia, especially if blood glucose levels were in the normal range before exercise.[32]

Drinks containing 5% to 10% carbohydrate are absorbed best. Concentrated drinks that exceed 10% carbohydrate can cause gastrointestinal upset such as cramps, nausea, diarrhea, or bloating.[20] Fruit juices and most regular soft drinks contain about 12% carbohydrate, so they need to be diluted. The advantage of sports drinks or glucose polymer drinks is that they average 6% to 7% carbohydrate. In events lasting less than 60 minutes, plain cold water is usually the beverage of choice. In events lasting longer than 60 minutes, athletes with diabetes should try to consume 15 to 30 g of carbohydrate every hour.[93] The athlete should not wait for symptoms of hypoglycemia to develop. Loss of consciousness is not only embarrassing but also may go unnoticed or be misunderstood in the excitement of an athletic event.

Hypoglycemia can be prevented if some of the carbohydrate is eaten during rather than before exercise. This may result in increased use of blood glucose with a proportionate slowing of muscle glycogen use.[20] For events of long duration, such as cross-country skiing or marathons, the limited stores of liver and muscle glycogen, even after supercompensation, are not sufficient to complete the event. Carbohydrate ingestion is essential for the successful completion of the event.

Combining carbohydrate before and during events increases performance ability, but of equal importance is carbohydrate after exercise. Carbohydrate should be consumed as soon as possible after exercise. Eating carbohydrate immediately compared with waiting 2 hours has been shown to replete carbohydrate stores more efficiently. To optimize repletion of muscle glycogen after exhaustive exercise, 1.5 g/kg of carbohydrate should be consumed immediately after cessation of exercise and a second 1.5 g/kg dose 1 to 2 hours later.[48]

To prevent hypoglycemia, especially PEL hypoglycemia, athletes with IDDM may need to take longer and make a more gradual progression to a higher level of training than is generally prescribed. This may allow the athlete to tolerate more intense and longer duration activities than usual. This higher level of fitness may offer some protection from PEL hypoglycemia, or at least may lower the individual's sensitivity to unusual increases in intensity or duration of exercise. A more gradual progression from the untrained to the trained state may also offer some protection for athletes in the training progression who may be more likely to experience PEL hypoglycemia.[50] (See Table 5-5 for a summary of strategies that can be used to assist athletes with diabetes to exercise safely.)

Table 5-5   Strategies to Assist Athletes With IDDM to Exercise Safely

1. Begin training gradually and over an extended period of time.
2. To prevent hypoglycemia during exercise of a long duration, carbohydrate is usually needed after about 60 minutes of exercise. Drinks containing 5% to 10% carbohydrate (such as diluted fruit juices or sports drinks) are absorbed better than a more concentrated carbohydrate drink (such as regular soft drinks or undiluted fruit juice).
3. Adjustments in insulin doses may also be needed for events of a long duration.
4. Athletes with IDDM may need to take longer and have a more gradual progression to a higher level of training than is generally recommended. The higher level of fitness may allow the athlete to tolerate more intense and longer duration activities than usual and may offer protection from postexercise, late-onset hypoglycemia as well.

EXERCISE AND NIDDM

Hyperglycemia in IDDM is primarily the result of an absolute insulin deficiency, whereas in NIDDM hyperglycemia is the result of insulin resistance and impaired insulin secretion. Many persons with NIDDM are hyperinsulinemic, and many are obese. Therefore any form of therapy that reverses or lessens insulin resistance and assists in weight loss has potential benefit. Furthermore, the prevention of NIDDM in genetically predisposed persons and the prevention of cardiovascular disease are also desirable goals. Increased activity levels or exercise has the potential to assist in any or all of the above.

Most studies[41,66,79,84] suggest that exercise is most effective in persons with impaired glucose tolerance or mild-to-moderate diabetes (i.e., fasting glucose levels <11.1 mM [<200 mg/dl]). Hyperinsulinemic patients also respond best to exercise, which is consistent with the observation that exercise acts by reversing insulin resistance.

Benefits of Exercise

Exercise and insulin resistance

Regularly performed vigorous exercise can result in significant improvement in glucose tolerance within a relatively short time (fewer than 7 days) in some persons with NIDDM.[58,79] The improvement in glucose tolerance appears to be caused by a decrease in insulin resistance—that is, to a greater susceptibility to the action of insulin. This can occur even without changes in body weight, body fat content, or Vo_{2max}. Regular exercise has been shown to result in decreased insulin levels in nondiabetic, obese persons and in persons with impaired glucose tolerance (IGT).[12]

Improvements in glycemic control and glucose tolerance associated with exercise in persons with NIDDM occur *without* a decrease in elevated insulin levels, consistent with improved insulin sensitivity in trained persons.[13,75] It has been shown that in persons with NIDDM, training improves glucose tolerance but the effect is short-lived.[17]

In studies on obese, insulin-resistant men and in persons with NIDDM, Devlin and others[25] have shown that a single bout of glycogen-depleting exercise can significantly increase insulin sensitivity and increase the rate of glucose disposal. In studies by Schneider and others,[77] 6 weeks of training, 3 times a week at 60% Vo_{2max} for 30 minutes, diminished fasting glucose levels and improved glucose tolerance for 12 hours but not for 72 hours after the last exercise session. Glycohemoglobin levels were also slightly reduced by training. Similar results have been obtained in several other studies.[23,66,84]

Exercise and weight loss

Exercise can be an effective adjunct to weight loss and weight control regimens. Wing and others[96] have shown that a combination of diet and exercise improves weight loss in persons with NIDDM and allows for greater reduction in hypoglycemic medication. Exercise may affect weight loss in several different ways. First, exercise increases calorie expenditure during the exercise bout. Second, it may offset the effect of calorie restriction on energy expenditure. Another possibility is that moderate levels of exercise may decrease appetite. Exercise may also promote dietary adherence and may improve mood and self-esteem, leading to more control over dietary intake. Although the mechanism is still unclear, exercise seems to be effective in promoting long-term weight loss and has consistently been one of the strongest predictors of long-term weight control.[95]

Prevention of NIDDM

Physical training may be of significant value in preventing or delaying the development of overt NIDDM in genetically predisposed persons. Exercise may be a means of delaying the onset of insulin-resistance cardiovascular disease and NIDDM in persons at high risk[79] including those with a positive family history of NIDDM or hypertriglyceridemia, women who have had gestational diabetes, and persons with android-type obesity.[6]

Regular exercise can reverse insulin resistance, thereby preventing the sequence of events that can result in clinical disease. Three large studies, two in men and one in women, have shown that individuals at increased risk of developing NIDDM who maintain high levels of physical activity significantly decreased their risk of developing diabetes. Helmrich and associates, in a study of 5990 males over a 14-year-period, reported the risk of developing NIDDM fell by 6% for every 500 kcal of exercise done each week.[39] In the Nurses Health Study, 8 years of information from 87,253 women, ages 34 to 59, showed risk for developing NIDDM was 33% lower among women who did vigorous physical activity at least once a week compared with women less active.[53] The same group reported that in 22,271 male physicians between 1982 and 1988 regular exercise decreased the incidence of NIDDM. Men who exercised more than five times per week had a 42% reduction in risk compared with a 23% drop in men who exercised only once a week.[54]

Prevention of cardiovascular disease

Diabetes is a major risk factor for macrovascular disease (see Chapter 8). Cerebrovascular, coronary, and peripheral artery disease are more common in diabetes and occur at an earlier age.[71] In addition, diabetes eliminates the relative protection from coronary problems possessed by premenopausal women. The incidence of coronary heart disease is approximately doubled for persons with IGT. Hyperinsulinemia and insulin resistance have been implicated as risk factors for atherosclerosis. Glucose intolerance may also contribute to atherosclerotic risk by the nonenzymatic glycosylation of lipoproteins, both low-density lipoprotein (LDL) and high-density lipoprotein (HDL).[78]

Epidemiologic studies suggest that endurance-type exercise diminishes the mortality and morbidity from macrovascular disease in nondiabetic populations.[49,62] In persons with diabetes, it is not known whether physical training is associated with decreased cardiovascular disease, but the cardiovascular risk factors can be reduced, making physical training especially beneficial for persons with diabetes. By enhancing body sensitivity to insulin, plasma insulin levels are reduced. If hyperinsulinemia is indeed a risk factor for macrovascular disease, as has been postulated, lower insulin levels may help prevent macrovascular complications.

Most studies of persons with NIDDM undergoing physical training report a significant decrease in plasma triglyceride levels and very low–density lipoproteins (VLDL). Plasma cholesterol and HDL-cholesterol levels appear not to change significantly. In a clinical study by Schneider and Kanj[78] of 108 patients followed in a diabetes exercise program, an average fall in plasma triglyceride levels of 15% from the basal level was found over 3 months with no change in cholesterol and HDL-cholesterol levels. The time course of changes in plasma triglyceride levels suggests that, as with glucose, many of the benefits of exercise training are caused by the summed effects of individual bouts of exercise. In Schneider's studies, a significant decrease in plasma triglyceride was consistently noted 12 hours after a typical exercise training bout, but 72 hours later the improvement was no longer measurable.

The fact that exercise training has not been consistently found to result in elevated HDL cholesterol in persons with NIDDM may be because the exercise required to elevate plasma HDL levels in persons with NIDDM is of a longer duration and greater intensity than is usually recommended, or current studies may not have been conducted long enough to realize this benefit.[78]

Lowering blood pressure

Exercise and nutrition therapy have been shown to be effective in reducing blood pressure of hypertensive persons with NIDDM, resulting in a mean reduction of 10 to 15 mm Hg of diastolic blood pressure.[78] The mechanism by which exercise reduces blood pressure is poorly understood at present.

Psychologic benefits

As noted, exercise training and improved cardiorespiratory fitness are associated with decreased anxiety, improved mood and self-esteem, an increased sense of well-being, and an enhanced quality of life.[6] These and other benefits suggest the need for careful incorporation of exercise into the therapeutic regimen of persons with NIDDM.

Short-Term Effects of Exercise

The effect of a single exercise session in persons with NIDDM is to lower blood glucose concentrations. The acute decrease in plasma glucose levels leading to improvements in glucose metabolism may persist for hours to days, possibly related to an increase in insulin sensitivity in muscles and other tissues that persists for several hours after the exercise. This is related to (1) the need for replenishment of decreased muscle and liver glycogen stores and (2) increased glucose metabolism in muscle. Minuk and others[58] determined that 45 minutes of moderately intense exercise (60% Vo_{2max}) resulted in a significant decrease in plasma glucose concentration during glucose turnover determinations in persons who were being treated with diet and oral hypoglycemic agents. The reduction in plasma glucose level was about 1.9 mM (35 mg/dl) and persisted during the recovery study period of 60 minutes.

Devlin and others[25] studied the effects of exercise until muscle fatigue, at 1900 hours, compared with no exercise in persons with NIDDM, and reported that on the mornings after exercise, endogenous glucose production rates were 20% lower than on days with no exercise the preceding evening. Because increased endogenous glucose production that occurs overnight is believed to be a primary cause of fasting hyperglycemia in NIDDM, a single bout of evening exercise can have clinical significance 12 to 16 hours later.

Blake and others[14] compared blood pressure changes during mild-to-moderate exercise in persons with NIDDM and nondiabetic persons. Both groups were sedentary and usually normotensive. A greater exercise-induced systolic blood pressure (mean maximum 208 ± 6 versus 177 ± 3 mm Hg) occurred in the NIDDM group. Neither pulse rate nor diastolic pressure differed between the groups before or during exercise. Return to basal pulse and blood pressure was also similar. They suggest that in investigations of exercise as a therapeutic modality in diabetes, intraexercise blood pressure should be considered in assessing the safety of this form of treatment.

Training Effects of Exercise

Several factors may contribute to the lack of improvement in glucose tolerance after endurance exercise training. In the studies with NIDDM patients in whom there was little improvement in glucose tolerance, the exercise stimulus in terms of intensity and duration of exercise training was relatively low. Furthermore, glucose tolerance was also measured 4 to 7 days after the last bout of exercise. More recently Holloszy[41] determined that 12 months of vigorous exercise training resulted in normalization of oral glucose tolerance and reduced insulin resistance in a group of patients with NIDDM and a group with impaired glucose tolerance (IGT). The data are consistent with the concept that improved glycemic control is the result of the summed effects of the individual bouts and not the state of aerobic fitness per se. Improved aerobic fitness may potentiate and prolong the metabolic effects of an acute exercise bout. Thus physical training may play an indirect role in enhancing glucose tolerance.

Bogardus and others[15] elucidated the mechanism for improved insulin sensitivity with exercise. The major effect of training, compared with the effect of diet alone, was to increase the peripheral use of glucose during hyperinsulinemia. The improved glucose disposal was caused primarily by an increase in the nonoxidative pathways of glucose metabolism, presumed to represent predominantly glycogen synthesis. This is important because the body's capacity to increase carbohydrate storage in response to insulin is greater than its capacity to increase carbohydrate oxidation rates.[42,73]

Physical endurance training results in not only an increased capacity for aerobic exercise but also an improved cardiovascular system. From studies in persons with NIDDM it appears their response to physical training is qualitatively similar to that in nondiabetic persons.[74,89]

PRECAUTIONS WITH EXERCISE FOR PERSONS WITH NIDDM

Persons with NIDDM should be examined thoroughly for diabetic complications before starting an exercise program. Those who are about to start an exercise program should have a preexercise evaluation specifically designed to uncover previously undiagnosed hypertension, neuropathy, retinopathy, nephropathy, and, particularly, silent ischemic heart disease.[5] Further evaluation is essential for diabetic persons with a history of angina or for those who develop marked fatigue or dyspnea with exercise.[61] An evaluation of peripheral sensitivity and circulation should be done, and individuals with peripheral neuropathy or decreased circulation should avoid forms of exercise that involve trauma to the feet.

Myocardial ischemia can be present during exercise without chest pain in a substantial number of persons with diabetes. Therefore it may be prudent to consider whether cardiovascular autonomic neuropathy is present when advising individuals about exercise goals to avoid too great a stress during routine exercise. Because of this higher prevalence of silent ischemic heart disease, an exercise stress electrocardiogram is recommended in all subjects over 35 years of age.[5] This test is also helpful for identifying persons who have an exaggerated hypertensive response to exercise and/or who develop postexercise orthostatic hypertension.[6]

Persons with NIDDM have been shown to have unexpectedly low Vo_{2max} both before and after 6 weeks of training.[79] Whether this is secondary to metabolic abnormalities or is independent of and precedes them remains to be established. This may also be caused by subtle autonomic dysfunction in persons with NIDDM.

Schneider and others[79] also report that standard tables of maximal heart rates based on nondiabetic populations correlate poorly with maximal heart rate in individuals with NIDDM. They report a maximal heart rate 15% to 20% lower than in age-matched controls in the absence of clinically evident neuropathy or coronary heart disease. Autonomic neuropathy or beta-blocker drugs may further impair maximal heart rate and aerobic exercise performance. Exercise programs should be initiated at the lower target pulse and gradually increased to the desired pulse rate over 2 to 3 weeks.

People taking oral medications or insulin should self-monitor their glycemic response to exercise. Those treated with sulfonylureas are at some increased risk of developing hypoglycemia during or after exercise, although this is less of a problem than the hypoglycemia that occurs with insulin treatment. Individuals using insulin or oral medications have higher than normal insulin concentrations during exercise that may inhibit hepatic glucose production sufficiently and result in hypoglycemia. They must follow the same precautions as persons with IDDM; however, because they are still producing endogenous insulin, their blood glucose levels are not as unstable as those of the person who produces no endogenous insulin.

Special precautions should be taken if individuals use drugs that can produce hypoglycemia, such as alcohol. The recognition of hypoglycemia may also be retarded or obscured by beta-adrenergic receptor-blocking drugs, such as propranolol and nadolol, that may prevent glycogenolytic responses that normally correct hypoglycemia.[52]

Blood glucose regulation during exercise in persons with NIDDM controlled by diet alone is not significantly different from that in persons without diabetes. During mild-to-moderate exercise, elevated blood glucose concentrations fall toward normal but do not reach hypoglycemic levels. There is no need for supplementary food before, during, or after exercise, except when exercise is exceptionally vigorous and of long duration. In this case, extra food may be beneficial just as it is in persons who do not have diabetes.

STRATEGIES FOR SAFE EXERCISE FOR PERSONS WITH NIDDM

Because many individuals with NIDDM may have been sedentary for many years, they are frequently deconditioned and unable to exercise continuously for any period of time. It is important that these individuals be encouraged to start with a mild exercise program, such as walking or riding a stationary bicycle, and be urged to rest if they feel out of breath. A program of gradually increasing exercise sessions, beginning with sessions of 5 to 10 minutes, is most successful and safest for this group. It is important to encourage any increase in activity and to help the individual continue exercising during the sometimes lengthy period before improvement is actually evident.

Available evidence suggests that to improve insulin sensitivity and glycemic control, individuals should exercise at least 3 days per week or every other day. When no exercise is performed for 24 hours, glucose tolerance declines significantly. *Exercise should therefore be performed more than three times a week to achieve continuous improvement in glucose control.* Muscle-strengthening exercises may also lead to improved glucose disposal and lipid levels.

If weight reduction is a major goal, exercise 5 to 6 days per week is probably necessary. The goal is to burn 250 to 300 kcal per exercise session. Rhythmic aerobic exercises recommended for weight loss include brisk walking, jogging, swimming, bicycling, and aerobic dance. It is important that exercise be low impact in nature, thus avoiding injury to bones and joints.

The most efficient way to burn fat with exercise is to exercise at a level that results in no shortness of breath and to exercise continuously for a minimum of 20 to 30 minutes. Exercise of low intensity and long duration (for more than 20 to 30 minutes) uses stored fat as its major energy source. Exercise of short duration (for less than 2 to 3 minutes) and high intensity uses glycogen as the major energy source.

However, it is important for health professionals to guard against giving unrealistic expectations of quick or easy weight loss to individuals beginning an exercise program. Although exercise appears to be at least partially protective of lean body mass when energy restriction is implemented, it does not significantly increase the resting metabolic rate nor the rate of weight loss seen with the intensities of exercise possible in individuals at the initiation of exercise programs.[16,44] (See Table 5-6 for a summary of strategies to assist persons with NIDDM to exercise safely.)

Table 5-6   Strategies for Safe Exercise for Persons With NIDDM

1. Start with mild and gradually increasing exercise sessions such as walking or riding a stationary bike.
2. To improve insulin sensitivity and glycemic control, exercise should be done at least 4 days a week or every other day.
3. For weight control, persons should exercise 5 to 6 days a week.
4. Exercise should not result in shortness of breath. Perceived exertion may be a better indicator of exercise intensity than pulse rate. Pulse rate may not increase normally in persons with NIDDM because of autonomic neuropathy.
5. Intensity of exercise should be limited so that blood pressure does not exceed 180 mm Hg.
6. Fitness can be achieved by exercising 4 to 7 days/week at 50% to 70% predicted maximum heart rate for a minimum of 20 minutes/exercise session or by physical activity every day (walking, taking the stairs, housework, programmed activity) at moderate intensity (equivalent to a brisk walk) for an accumulated 30 minutes or more over each day.
7. If aerobic exercise is performed, it should be of low impact (one foot on the floor at all times).
8. Muscle strengthening exercises may also lead to improved glucose disposal.
9. Warm up and cool down exercises are important to increase flexibility, which is frequently lost with glycation of collagen, and to prevent exercise-related injuries.

EXERCISE IN SPECIAL CIRCUMSTANCES
Pregnancy, Diabetes, and Exercise

Pregnant women with IDDM have traditionally been denied the option of exercising during pregnancy primarily because of fear of affecting the fetus. However, women who are doing regular exercise before becoming pregnant can usually continue their exercise program during pregnancy, with appropriate timing of exercise to balance insulin action and food intake. It has been suggested that exercise may be another tool to facilitate the maintenance of optimal blood glucose levels during pregnancy.[8] However, Hollingsworth and Moore,[40] in a study of 42 pregnant women with IDDM and 28 nondiabetic controls who participated in a postprandial walking exercise program, reported no significant improvement in glycemic control in women with IDDM. Exercise patients were instructed to walk 20 minutes (1 mile) after each meal. Exercise was associated with lower fasting cholesterol and triglyceride values in both groups and with significantly lower fasting plasma triglyceride levels in the diabetic exercise group. There were no adverse effects of postprandial walking exercise in mothers or infants.

It would seem prudent to advise women who wish to exercise during pregnancy to exercise at a lower intensity than nonpregnant diabetic women. Target heart rates for exercise prescription are not available for pregnancy; however, heart rates at 50% of target rate are believed to be of adequate intensity.[8] Guidelines published by the American College of Obstetricians and Gynecologists[4] also caution about exercise with ballistic movements (jerky, bouncy movements) and deep flexion or extension of joints because of connective tissue laxity during pregnancy.

Exercise appears to be effective in normalizing glucose tolerance only in patients who still have an adequate capacity to secrete insulin and in whom insulin resistance is the major cause for abnormal glucose tolerance. Thus it is perhaps reasonable to suggest that exercise in pregnancy might be more beneficial for pregnant women with NIDDM (but "insulin requiring" during pregnancy) and for women with gestational diabetes mellitus (GDM).[40]

Because most women with GDM are diagnosed at approximately 28 weeks, they probably have not undergone any supervised training program. Although exercise should not be so vigorous as to cause maternal or fetal complications (such as increased core temperature, excessive fatigue, fetal heart rate dysrhythmias), it should be of adequate intensity to cause some change in blood glucose levels independent of other metabolic factors, such as calorie intake and time of day of exercise.[27]

The safest form of exercise would be the type that does not cause fetal bradycardia or uterine contractions, or produce maternal hypertension. Exercises that do not cause uterine activity are those using the upper body muscles or placing little mechanical stress on the trunk region during exercise.[27]

For women with GDM, mild aerobic exercise does not seem to have an adverse effect on the pregnant woman or her fetus. An exercise program done three or four times weekly could be used to attain improved glucose control and reduce the need for exogenous insulin. Because it is often difficult to maintain blood glucose levels in the desired range after breakfast, a mild exercise program, such as a brisk walk, may be especially beneficial at this time.

Exercise for the Older Person with Diabetes

In his review, Schwartz[80] states that guidelines for exercise training for the older patient with diabetes are difficult because no published data pertain directly or specifically to this issue. Extrapolation from information on the effects of exercise on older adults in general, as well as the effects of exercise on persons with diabetes, must be used. Because most older adults with diabetes have NIDDM, the data from this group are of particular interest.

Maximal aerobic capacity (Vo_{2max}) declines with age in all persons, but evidence suggests that the slope of the decline can be significantly reduced with exercise training.[37] This can be extremely important in older adults because symptoms of fatigue, weakness, and breathlessness as related to percent Vo_{2max} limit task performances. In training studies of older adults (over 65 years of age), researchers have usually demonstrated significant training effects with improvements of Vo_{2max} of up to 30%.[9]

Improvements in risk factors for atherosclerosis are potentially even more important than the increase in Vo_{2max} after training for the older adult with diabetes, who is already at increased risk for atherosclerosis because of diabetes.[82]

Lean body mass declines with age, and a reduction in adipose tissue and an accompanying increase in lean body mass occur after exercise training. Of equal importance may be the change in the distribution of adiposity. Abdominal obesity is associated with an increased risk for cardiovascular disease. A decrease in the waist/hip ratio and a greater than 20% decline in central fat areas after an intensive exercise training program in older adults has been reported.[81]

Because of the potential risks of exercise in persons with diabetes, especially an older adult, a thorough evaluation by a physician should be performed before an exercise training program is begun. Diabetes treatment, complications, and glucose control should be evaluated. An exercise stress test (with blood pressure and 12-lead electrocardiogram monitoring) should be done to uncover any unknown coronary artery disease. The stress test can also be used to obtain a maximal heart rate measure that can then be used as the basis of a specific exercise prescription. It is recommended that exercise begin at 50% to 60% of target heart rate, with a gradual increase in exercise every 2 to 4 weeks, as tolerated, to 70% to 80% of target heart rate. Appropriate stretching, warm-up, and cool-down periods should accompany all exercise.[80]

Long-Term Complications of Diabetes and Exercise

Disuse syndrome results from disruption of the normal balance between rest and physical activity, thereby decreasing the optimal functioning capacity of an individual. Disuse syndrome can develop within as few as 3 days of immobilization and glucose intolerance in nondiabetic persons begins within 72 hours of absolute bedrest. Disuse combined with diabetes generally yields more disability than would be predicted by diabetes alone, increasing the cost of medical care and home health programs.

Exercise can assist in preventing or reversing disuse syndrome and can be provided for persons with diabetes, even those with severe complications. Unfortunately, disuse syndrome is easier to prevent than to correct. Graham and Lasko-McCarthey[36] have reviewed the role of exercise for persons with diabetic complications. The following is a summary of their recommendations.

Peripheral vascular disease/claudication

Assessment of the arterial circulation of a diabetic patient with peripheral vascular disease (PVD) should be conducted before engaging in a physical activity program. Interval training (e.g., 2-minute walk, 1-minute rest, 2-minute walk), swimming, stationary cycling, walking on a slow treadmill at 1 mile/hr, and chair exercises are all options for diabetic persons with PVD. Chair exercises or upper body exercises can be performed by those unable to use the lower extremities because of PVD and claudication. Exercise that provokes intense pain should be discontinued immediately.

Retinopathy

Before diabetic persons with proliferative retinopathy begin an exercise program, submaximal testing should be conducted under the guidance of trained personnel to establish a training heart rate according to blood pressure response.

Aerobic exercise for patients with retinopathy includes stationary cycling, low-intensity rowing on a rowing machine, swimming, and walking. A guide wire or guide person may be needed for assistance with walking or jogging if vision is lost or badly impaired. Resistive exercise using standard weight-lifting equipment is not recommended. Exercise is contraindicated if the person has recently undergone retinal photocoagulation or eye surgery.

Nephropathy

The elevated risk factors for cardiovascular disease in patients with nephropathy indicate a role for exercise. However, goals need to be established on the basis of the patient's limitations, because exercise capacity is usually exceptionally low.

Low hemoglobin and hematocrit values and abnormal cardiac function are characteristic for this population and contribute to a low physical work capacity. Exercise must be done at mild-to-moderate levels. Renal osteodystrophy begins very early when renal function begins to decline. Thus weight-bearing exercises, done with dynamic physical activity, may result in improvements in bone volume.

Hemodialysis patients may benefit from aerobic-type activities such as brisk walking, cycling, and swimming; however, anemia, cardiovascular dysfunction, and low physical working capacity underscore the importance of a gradual, progressive training program. No exercise training should begin until the patient is stabilized on a program of medication, dialysis, and diet. Exercises that involve fluid changes, damage weakened bones, or cause sustained elevations in blood pressure should be avoided.

Sensorimotor neuropathy

Although exercise cannot reverse symptoms of sensorimotor neuropathy, it can prevent the loss of physical fitness associated with disuse syndrome. Adaptive shortening of connective tissue can be caused by disuse and immobilization. Daily range-of-motion exercises for the major joints, such as the ankle, knee, hip, shoulder, wrist, and trunk area, are essential for preventing or minimizing contractures. Loss of sensation to the extremities can create a greater susceptibility to overstretching in muscles and connective tissue. Stretching exercises should be performed gently through the pain-free range of motion at all times.

The frequent incidence of blisters, stress fractures, red and hot spots, and muscle strains requires inspection of the feet after every workout session and frequent observations of the feet as part of the daily hygiene routine.

Autonomic neuropathy

Exercise tolerance with autonomic neuropathy may be severely limited because of impairment of the sympathetic and parasympathetic nervous systems that normally augment cardiac output and redirect peripheral blood flow to the working muscles. Commonly the person becomes easily fatigued with little exertion.

Cardiac denervation syndrome (sudden death, silent myocardial infarction) has been attributed to the neuropathic diabetic syndrome in which the heart becomes unresponsive to nerve impulses. In autonomic neuropathy, the counterregulatory response may also be impaired, putting the individual at increased risk with exercise. Clinically, this state is recognized by a fixed heart rate of 80 to 90 beats/minute while the patient rests or exercises.

Activities to be avoided are those that cause rapid changes in body position or elicit and require rapid and significant changes in heart rate or blood pressure. As exercise tachycardia is often blunted, high-intensity exercise should be avoided.

Table 5-7 American College of Sports Medicine Revised Scale for Rating
Perceived Exertion

Rating	Description
0	Nothing at all
0.5	Very, very weak (just noticeable)
1	Very weak
2	Weak (light)
3	Moderate
4	Somewhat strong
5	Strong (heavy)
6	
7	Very strong
8	
9	
10	Very, very strong (almost max)
•	Maximal

From Borg G: Subjective effort in relation to physical performance and working capacity. In Pick HL,
editor: *Psychology: from research to practice,* New York, 1978, Plenum.

EXERCISE PRESCRIPTION

The goal of exercise training is to achieve optimal cardiovascular, muscular, and metabolic
adaptations to aerobic stimulus. Cardiovascular fitness to prevent or minimize the long-term
complications related to diabetes is of obvious importance for persons with diabetes. Flexibility in persons with diabetes can be impaired if muscle collagen becomes glycated. Warm-up
and cool-down components, which increase flexibility, therefore take on added significance.
Muscle strength may deteriorate as a result of neuropathy; muscle-strengthening exercise can
improve muscle strength. Furthermore, increased muscle mass resulting from strength training
may also result in a reduction of plasma insulin concentrations; but despite the lower insulin
concentrations, glucose tolerance improves and peripheral glucose disposal increases.

Each exercise session should begin with a warm-up and end with a cool-down period.
A warm-up period of at least 5 minutes is adequate for circulatory adjustment to exercise and
to minimize potential dysrhythmias; 5 to 7 minutes of stretching and cardiovascular warm-up
are added to this initial period. This is followed by aerobic activity. Aerobic activities require
large amounts of oxygen and usually involve movement of many large muscles. An exercise
prescription clearly specifies type, intensity, duration, and frequency of the activity in days
per week.

Heart rate (pulse rate) and perceived exertion (PE) are two methods used to determine
the intensity of exercise. PE involves having individuals rate how hard (strong) they
"perceive" they are exercising and how tired they are. The original scale, developed by
psychologist Gunnar Borg, allows persons to rate their activity on a scale from 6 to 20. In 1986
the American College of Sports Medicine released a revised scale from 0 (nothing at all) to
10 (very, very strong).[3] See Table 5-7 for the scale and the written description for rating the

Table 5-8 Target Heart Rates During Exercise: Heartbeats Per 10 Seconds

Intensity	Age											
	15	20	25	30	35	40	45	50	55	60	65	70
50%	17	17	16	16	15	15	15	14	14	13	13	12
60%	20	20	19	19	18	18	17	17	16	16	15	15
75%	25	25	24	23	23	22	22	21	20	20	19	19
85%	29	28	27	27	26	25	25	24	23	22	22	21

Modified from Franz MJ, Barry B: *Diabetes and exercise: guidelines for safe and enjoyable activity,* Minneapolis 1993, International Diabetes Center.

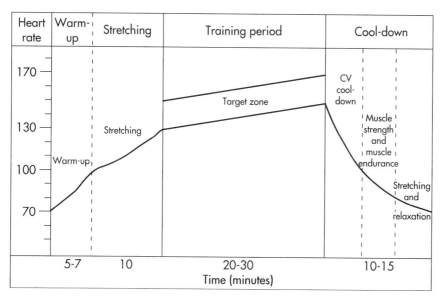

Fig. 5-3 Training pattern for an exercise session. (From Franz MJ, Barry B: *Diabetes and exercise guidelines for safe and enjoyable activity,* Minneapolis, Minn, 1993, International Diabetes Center.)

degree of perceived exertion. Table 5-8 lists target heart rates for exercise related to the desired exercise intensity.

Muscle-strengthening exercises are usually performed after the aerobic portion of exercise and take on added importance for persons with diabetes. The exercise session should end with a cool-down period of 10 to 12 minutes, consisting of cardiovascular cool down, specific muscle strengthening exercises, and exercises for flexibility and relaxation. Fig. 5-3 details a typical exercise session.

Adherence to a regular exercise program, like most other life-style changes, is difficult to maintain. Approximately 50% of enrolled persons drop out within the first few months.[52]

BOX 5-3

SUGGESTIONS TO IMPROVE ADHERENCE TO AN EXERCISE PROGRAM

1. Make the exercise program an enjoyable social experience.
2. Provide enthusiastic leadership.
3. Give personalized feedback and praise.
4. Promote spouse and family support.
5. Set flexible goals.
6. Prepare attendance contracts.
7. Use distraction techniques (music).

It may also be helpful to provide persons with a set of strategies to cope with the problem of relapse at the beginning of the program, thus minimizing the likelihood of a complete relapse. See Box 5-3.

SUMMARY

Persons with diabetes get the same benefits from exercise that persons without diabetes gain from a regular exercise program, namely, improved fitness and psychologic state, improved body composition, weight control, and improved physical work capacity. For persons with diabetes, exercise has additional benefits, for example, increased insulin sensitivity and improved glucose tolerance, potential reduction in insulin dosage, reversal of resistance to insulin, reduction of risk factors for atherosclerosis, and a potential lowering of blood pressure.

The goals of an exercise program are (1) to allow individuals with diabetes to have the same benefits and enjoyment that people without diabetes gain from a regular exercise program, (2) to maintain or improve cardiovascular fitness, (3) to improve flexibility and muscle strength, (4) to allow persons with IDDM to safely participate in and enjoy physical and/or sporting activities, and (5) to assist in blood glucose and weight control and overall diabetes management in people with NIDDM.

Above all, exercise should be fun. It should be presented as part of a reasonable health care plan. Regular exercisers stick with it because they enjoy it. It may take time to develop this attitude toward exercise, but eventually the rewards are worth it.

CASE PRESENTATION

T.E. is a 30-year-old man with a 5-year history of insulin-dependent diabetes mellitus (IDDM) for which he takes 5 U Regular and 10 U NPH insulin before breakfast, 6 U Regular at supper and 7 U NPH at bedtime. He generally monitors his blood glucose 2 to 3 times daily. His most recent glycated hemoglobin was 7.8% (normal 4.1% to 5.9%). T.E. plays sports on a sporadic basis (softball during the summer and basketball during the winter) but does not exercise on a regular basis. He eats about 2900 calories daily. He has enrolled in an education program, with one of his goals being to begin a regular exercise program.

T.E. is 71 in. tall and weighs 173 lb. He has no evidence of complications related to diabetes. He has a job in sales, and his work schedule varies on a daily basis. Breakfast and lunch times are fairly consistent, and he eats dinner between 6 and 7:30 PM. He either prepares his own meals in his apartment or eats at a family-type restaurant.

DISCUSSION

The health care team, including the physician, dietitian, nurse educator, and exercise physiologist, all spent time with T.E. during the education program. The overall goal was to assist T.E. to self-manage his diabetes and, more specifically, to help him begin an exercise program.

Assessment. T.E. plans to exercise 4 or 5 days a week, but some days it will be before breakfast and work and other days after work and before dinner or after dinner. He can walk or run in his neighborhood and has also joined a local health club where he can exercise on days when the weather is inclement and can do weight lifting.

Plan. The educators and physician will review with T.E. time actions of insulin and how to make adjustments in his insulin doses based on blood glucose patterns. As he masters that concept, insulin algorithms will be added. He will use the algorithms to make adjustments in his basic insulin doses based on his exercise plans or changes in his usual food intake. The dietitian and nurse educators will review with T.E. general guidelines for exercise and changes in diabetes management based on the timing of his exercise and blood glucose monitoring results. The exercise physiologist will outline an exercise program for T.E. including suggestions for warm-up and cool-down exercises, a gradually increasing walk/run program, and a weight-lifting program T.E. plans to do 3 times a week. Target heart rates and monitoring of intensity of exercise will also be reviewed.

Education. The following guidelines were discussed with T.E.
1. Exercise can both lower and increase blood glucose levels.
   - Exercise is more likely to lower blood glucose levels after exercise than during exercise, especially in persons who are untrained or do sporadic exercise.
   - Exercise of a high intensity can cause blood glucose levels to be higher after exercise than at the start because of the effects of "stress" hormones.
   - If blood glucose measures higher than 250 to 300 mg/dl with urine ketones, exercise may also cause blood glucose levels to remain elevated; control should be improved before continuing to exercise.
2. The following are general guidelines for moderate exercise of about 1 hour:
   - If blood glucose is less than 100 mg/dl before exercise, eat a preexercise snack of 25 to 50 g of carbohydrate.
   - If blood glucose is 100 to 180 mg/dl, go ahead and exercise, and eat a snack of 10 to 15 g of carbohydrate either before or after exercise. If blood glucose is 180 to 300 mg/dl, if necessary, eat a snack afterward.
   - If blood glucose is greater than 250 mg/dl with ketones or greater than 300 mg/dl, do not exercise until control is improved.

3. General guidelines based on timing of exercise:
   - To exercise before breakfast: Test blood glucose level; if 100 mg/dl or higher, eat or drink 15 g of carbohydrate. Exercise, do another blood glucose test, take morning insulin, eat breakfast, and enjoy the rest of the day. If blood glucose is less than 100 mg/dl, eat or drink 30 g of carbohydrate instead of 15, wait 10 to 15 minutes, and test again. When above 100 mg/dl, go ahead and exercise.
   - To exercise after breakfast: Monitor blood glucose, eat usual breakfast, exercise, and have usual morning snack. Because blood glucose levels are often higher after breakfast, no extra food may be needed. Occasionally, monitoring blood glucose levels after exercise can provide useful information.
   - To exercise later in the afternoon: Do a blood glucose test. If blood glucose is 100 to 180 mg/dl, eat or drink an extra 15 g of carbohydrate and exercise. If it is less than 100 mg/dl, eat or drink 30 to 50 g of carbohydrate before exercise. If blood glucose is 180 to 300 mg/dl, it may not be necessary to eat any extra carbohydrate; eat or drink usual afternoon snack.
   - To exercise after dinner: Take your evening injection of insulin and eat dinner and exercise. Test your blood glucose before evening snack. You may need to add some extra food to your evening snack, depending on the type and amount of exercise done and the blood glucose level.
4. When exercising for an extended period of time, consider also decreasing insulin. Reduce the dose of insulin acting during the time of activity by 10% of daily insulin dose. For activity lasting an entire day, decrease both short and intermediate insulins by 10%. Evening insulin may also need to be decreased to prevent hypoglycemia from occurring after exercise.

Monitoring. After a week of exercise T.E. will call one of the team members to discuss the effects of the exercise program on his blood glucose levels. At that time, additional changes in T.E.'s diabetes management may need to be made.

REFERENCES

1. Ahlborg G and others: Substrate turnover during prolonged exercise, *J Clin Invest* 53:1080-1090, 1974.
2. Ahlborg G, Felig P: Lactate and glucose exchange across the forearm, legs, and splanchnic bed during and after prolonged leg exercise, *J Clin Invest* 69:45-54, 1982.
3. American College of Sports Medicine: *Guidelines for exercise testing and prescription,* Philadelphia, 1986, Lea & Febiger.
4. American College of Obstetricians and Gynecologists: *Exercise during pregnancy and the postnatal period* (ACOG home exercise program), Washington, DC, 1985, ACOG.
5. American Diabetes Association: Diabetes mellitus and exercise (position statement), *Diabetes Care* 18(suppl 1): 28, 1995.
6. American Diabetes Association: Exercise and NIDDM, (technical review), *Diabetes Care* 13:785-789, 1990.
7. Arslanian S and others: Impact of physical fitness and glycemic control on in vivo insulin action in adolescents with IDDM, *Diabetes Care* 13:9-15, 1990.
8. Artal R, Wiswell R, Romen Y: Hormonal response to exercise in diabetic and nondiabetic pregnant patients, *Diabetes* 34 (suppl 2):78-80, 1985.
9. Barenhop DT and others: Physiologic adjustments to higher- or lower-intensity exercise in elders, *Med Sci Sports Exerc* 15:496-502, 1983.
10. Berger M and others: Metabolic and hormonal effects of muscular exercise in juvenile type diabetics, *Diabetologia* 13:355-365, 1977.
11. Berger M and others: Absorption kinetics and biological effects of subcutaneously injected insulin preparations, *Diabetes Care* 5:77-91, 1982.
12. Bjorntorp P and others: Effects of physical training on glucose tolerance, plasma insulin and lipids and body composition in men after myocardial infarction, *Acta Med Scand* 192:439-443, 1972.

13. Bjorntorp P, daJounge K, Sjostrom L: The effect of physical training on insulin production in obesity, *Metabolism* 19:631-637, 1970.

14. Blake GA, Levin SR, Koyal SN: Exercise-induced hypertension in normotensive patients with NIDDM, *Diabetes Care* 13:799-801, 1990.

15. Bogardus C and others: Effects of physical training and diet therapy on carbohydrate metabolism in patients with glucose intolerance and non–insulin-dependent diabetes mellitus, *Diabetes* 33:311-318, 1984.

16. Broeder CE and others: The effects of aerobic fitness on resting metabolic rate, *Am J Clin Nutr* 55:795-801, 1992.

17. Burstein R and others: Acute reversal of the enhanced insulin action in trained athletes: associate with insulin receptor changes, *Diabetes* 34:756-760, 1985.

18. Calles J and others: Glucose turnover during recovery from intensive exercise, *Diabetes* 32:734-738, 1983.

19. Campaigne BN, Wallberg-Henrikssen H, Gunnarsson R: 12-hour glycemic response following acute physical exercise in type I diabetes in relation to insulin dose and caloric intake, *Diabetes Care* 10:716-721, 1987.

20. Costill DL: Carbohydrate nutrition before, during and after exercise, *Fed Proc* 44:364-368, 1985.

21. Costill DL and others: Effects of elevated plasma FFA and insulin on muscle glycogen usage during exercise, *J Appl Physiol* 43:695-699, 1977.

22. Cryer PE: Hypoglycemic glucose counterregulation in patients with insulin-dependent diabetes mellitus, *J Lab Clin Med* 99:451-456, 1982.

23. DeFronzo RA, Ferrannini E, Koivisto V: New concepts in the pathogenesis and treatment of NIDDM, *Am J Med* 74:52-81, 1983.

24. DeFronzo RA, Hendler R, Christensen NJ: Stimulation of counterregulatory hormonal responses in diabetic man by a fall in glucose concentration, *Diabetes* 29:125-131, 1980.

25. Devlin JT and others: Enhanced peripheral and splanchnic insulin sensitivity in NIDDM after single bout of exercise, *Diabetes* 36:434-439, 1987.

26. Durak E, Jovanovic-Peterson L, Peterson CM: Randomized crossover study of effect of resistance traning on glycemic control, muscular strength, and cholesterol in type I diabetic men, *Diabetes Care* 13:1039-1043, 1990.

27. Durak EP, Jovanovic-Peterson L, Peterson CM: Physical and glycemic response of women with gestational diabetes to a moderately intense exercise program, *Diabetes Educator* 16:309-312, 1990.

28. Felig P: The glucose-alanine cycle, *Metabolism* 22:179-207, 1973.

29. Felig P, Wahren J: Fuel homeostasis in exercise, *N Engl J Med* 293:1078-1084, 1975.

30. Ferrannini E and others: Effect of fatty acids on glucose production and utilization in man, *J Clin Invest* 72:1737-1747, 1983.

31. Fery F, deMaertelaer V, Balasse EO: Mechanism of hyperketonaemic effect of prolonged exercise in insulin-deprived Type I (insulin-dependent) diabetic patients, *Diabetologia* 30:298-304, 1987.

32. Franz MJ: Nutrition: can it give athletes with diabetes a boost? *The Diabetes Educator* 17(3):163-172, 1991.

33. Franz MJ, Barry B: *Diabetes and exercise: guidelines for safe and enjoyable activity.* Minneapolis, Minn, 1993, CHRONIMED.

34. Franz MJ: Exercise and diabetes mellitus. In Powers MA, editor: *Handbook of diabetes nutritional management,* Rockville, Md, 1995, Aspen.

35. Galbo H: Hormonal and metabolic adaptations to exercise, Stuttgart, New York 1983, Georg Thieme Verlag.

36. Graham C, Lasko-McCarthey P: Exercise options for persons with diabetic complications, *Diabetes Educator* 16:212-219, 1990.

37. Hagberg JM: Effect of training on the decline of $V_{O_{2max}}$ with aging, *Fed Proc* 46:1830-1833, 1987.

38. Hagenfeldt L: Metabolism of free fatty acids and ketone bodies during exercise in normal and diabetic man, *Diabetes* 28 (suppl 1):66-70, 1979.

39. Helmrich SP and others: Physical activity and reduced occurrence of non-insulin-dependent diabetes mellitus, *N Eng J Med* 325:147-152, 1991.

40. Hollingsworth DR, Moore TR: Postprandial walking exercise in pregnant insulin-dependent (type I) diabetic women: reduction of plasma lipid levels but absence of a significant effect on glycemic control, *Am J Obstet Gynecol* 157:1359-1363, 1987.

41. Holloszy JO and others: Effects of exercise on glucose tolerance and insulin resistance, *Acta Med Scand Suppl* 711:55-65, 1986.

42. Holloszy JO, Coyle EF: Adaptation of skeletal muscle to endurance exercise and their metabolic consequences, *J Appl Physiol* 56:831-838, 1984.

43. Horton ES: Exercise and diabetes mellitus, *Med Clin North Am* 72:1301-1321, 1988.

44. Horton TJ, Geissler CA: Effect of habitual exercise on daily energy expenditure and metabolic rate during standardized activity, *Am J Clin Nutr* 59:13-19, 1994.

45. Hultman E: Studies on muscle metabolism of glycogen and active phosphate in man with special reference to exercise and diet, *Scand J Clin Lab Invest* 19:1-63, 1967.

46. Garetto LP and others: Enhanced muscle glucose metabolism after exercise in the rat: the two phases, *Am J Physiol* 246:E471-E475, 1984.

47. Issekutz B: Clearance rate of metabolizable and nonmetabolizable sugar in insulin-infused dogs and in exercising dogs, *Diabetes* 29:348-354, 1980.

48. Ivy JL and others: Muscle glycogen synthesis after exercise: effects of time of carbohydrate ingestion, *J Appl Physiol* 64:1480-1485, 1988.

48a. LaPorte RE and others: Pittsburgh insulin-dependent diabetes mellitus morbidity and mortality study: physical activity and diabetes complications, *Pediatrics* 78:1027-1033, 1986.

49. Leon AS and others: Leisure-time physical activity levels and risk of coronary heart disease and death: the multiple risk factor intervention trial, *JAMA* 258:2388-2395, 1987.

50. MacDonald MJ: Postexercise late-onset hypoglycemia in insulin-dependent diabetic patients, *Diabetes Care* 10:584-588, 1987.

51. Marliss EB and others: Glucoregulatory and hormonal responses to repeated bouts of intense exercise in normal male subjects, *J Appl Physiol* 71:924-933, 1991.

52. Martin JE, Dubbert PM: Adherence to exercise, *Exerc Sport Sci Rev* 13:137-167, 1985.

53. Manson JE and others: Physical activity and incidence of non-insulin-dependent diabetes mellitus in women, *Lancet* 338:774-778, 1991.

54. Manson JE and others: A prospective study of exercise and incidence of diabetes among US male physicians, *JAMA* 268:63-67, 1992.

55. McDermott SC, Elder GC, Boren AC: Adrenal hormones enhance glycogenolysis in nonexercising muscle, *J Appl Physiol* 63:1275-1283, 1987.

56. Meinders AE, Willekens FLA, and Heere LP: Metabolic and hormonal changes in IDDM during long-distance run, *Diabetes Care* 11:1-7, 1988.

57. Mikines KJ and others: Insulin sensitivity and responsiveness after acute exercise in man, *Clin Physiol* 5 (suppl 4):A67, 1985.

58. Minuk HL and others: Glucoregulatory and metabolic response to exercise in obese noninsulin-dependent diabetes, *Am J Physiol* 240:E458-E464, 1981.

59. Mitchell TH and others: Hyperglycemia after intense exercise in IDDM subjects during continuous subcutaneous insulin infusion, *Diabetes Care* 11:311-317, 1988.

60. Morgensen CE, Vittinghus E: Urinary albumin excretion during exercise in juvenile diabetes, *Scand J Clin Lab Invest* 35:295-300, 1975.

61. Nesto RW and others: Angina and exertional myocardial ischemia in diabetic and nondiabetic patients: assessment by exercise thallium scintigraphy, *Ann Intern Med* 108:170-175, 1988.

62. Paffenbarger RS and others: Physical activity, all-cause mortality and longevity of college alumni, *N Engl J Med* 314:605-613, 1986.

63. Plough T, Galbo H, Richter EA: Increased muscle glucose uptake during contractions: no need for insulin, *Am J Physiol* 247:E726-E731, 1984.

64. Purdon C and others: The roles of insulin and catecholamines in the glueoregulatory response during intense exercise and early recovery in insulin-dependent diabetic and control subjects, *J Clin Endocrinol Metab* 76:566-573, 1993.

65. Randall PJ, Newsholme EA, Garland PB: Regulation of glucose uptake by muscle. 8. Effects of fatty acids and ketone bodies and pyruvate acid of alloxan-diabetes and starvation on the uptake and metabolic fate of glucose in rat heart and diaphragm muscle, *Biochem J* 93:652-655, 1964.

66. Reitman JS and others: Improvement of glucose homeostasis after exercise in NIDDM, *Diabetes Care* 7:434-441, 1984.

67. Rennie MJ, Paik DM, Salaiman WR: Uptake and release of hormones and metabolites by tissues of exercising leg in man, *Am J Physiol* 231:967-973, 1976.

68. Richter EA, Galbo H: Diabetes, insulin and exercise, *Sports Med* 3:275-288, 1986.

69. Richter EA, Ruderman NB: Diabetes and exercise, *Am J Med* 70:201-209, 1981.

70. Richter EA, Galbo H: Rate of glycogen breakdown and lactate release in contracting isolated skeletal muscle is dependent on glycogen concentration, *Clin Physiol* 5 (suppl 4):82, 1985.

71. Ruderman NB, Haudenschild C: Diabetes as an atherogenic factor, *Prog Cardiovasc Dis* 16:373-412, 1984.

72. Ruegemer JJ and others: Differences between prebreakfast and late afternoon glycemic responses to exercise in IDDM patients, *Diabetes Care* 13:104-110, 1990.

73. Saltin B: Physiologic adaptation to physical conditioning: old problems revisited, *Acta Med Scand* (Suppl) 711:11-24, 1986.

74. Saltin B and others: Physical training and glucose tolerance in middle-aged men with chemical diabetes, *Diabetes* 28(Suppl 1):30-32, 1979.

75. Sato Y, Igudi A, Sakamoto N: Biochemical determination of training effects using insulin clamp technique, *Horm Metab Res* 16:483-486, 1984.

76. Schiffrin A, Parikh S: Accommodating planned exercise in type I diabetic patients on intensive treatment, *Diabetes Care* 8:337-342, 1985.

77. Schneider SH and others: Studies on the mechanism of improved glucose control during regular exercise in type 2 (noninsulin-dependent) diabetes, *Diabetologia* 26:355-360, 1984.

78. Schneider SH, Kanj H: Clinical aspects of exercise and diabetes mellitus, *Curr Concepts Nutr* 15:145-182, 1986.

79. Schneider SH and others: Abnormal glucoregulation during exercising in type II (noninsulin-dependent) diabetes, *Metabolism* 36:1161-1167, 1986.

80. Schwartz RS: Exercise training in treatment of diabetes mellitus in elderly patients, *Diabetes Care* 13 (suppl 2):77-85, 1990.

81. Schwartz RS and others: Intensive exercise training in the elderly decreases body fat and controls fat distribution, *Clin Res* 37:149A, 1989 (Abstract).

82. Seals DR and others: Effects of endurance training on glucose tolerance and plasma lipid levels in older men and women, *JAMA* 252:645-649, 1984.

83. Stratton R and others: Improved glycemic control after supervised 8-wk exercise program in insulin-dependent diabetic adolescents, *Diabetes Care* 10:589-593, 1987.

84. Trovati M and others: Influence of physical training on blood glucose control, glucose tolerance, insulin secretion and insulin action in NIDDM, *Diabetes Care* 7:416-420, 1984.

85. Wahren J and others: Glucose metabolism during leg exercise in man, *J Clin Invest* 50:2715-2725, 1971.

86. Wahren J and others: Glucose and amino acid metabolism during recovery after exercise, *J Appl Physiol* 34:838-845, 1973.

87. Wahren J, Felig P, Hagenfeldt L: Physical exercise and fuel homeostasis in diabetes mellitus, *Diabetologia* 14:213-222, 1978.

88. Wahren J, Hagenfeldt L, Felig P: Splanchnic and leg exchange of glucose, amino acids, and free fatty acids during exercise in diabetes mellitus, *J Clin Invest* 55:1303-1314, 1975.

89. Wallberg-Henriksson H and others: Increased peripheral sensitivity and muscle mitochondrial enzymes but unchanged blood glucose control in type I diabetics after physical training, *Diabetes* 31:1044-1050, 1982.

90. Wallberg-Henriksson H and others: Glucose transport into rat skeletal: interaction between exercise and insulin, *J Appl Physiol* 65:909-913, 1988.

91. Wardzala LJ, Cushman SW, Salans LB: Mechanisms of insulin action on glucose transport in the isolated rat adipose cell, *J Biol Chem* 253:8002-8005, 1978.

92. Wasserman DH and others: Exercise-induced rise in glucagon and the increase in ketogenesis during prolonged exercise, *Diabetes* 38:799-807, 1989.

93. Wasserman DH, Zinman B: Exercise in individuals with IDDM (American Diabetes Association technical review), *Diabetes Care* 17:924-937, 1994.

94. Wasserman DH, Vranic M: Interaction between insulin and counterregulatory hormones in control of substrate utilization in health and diabetes during exercise, *Diabetes Metab Rev* 1:359-384, 1986.

95. Wing RR: Behavioral strategies for weight reduction in obese type II diabetes patients, *Diabetes Care* 12:139-144, 1989.

96. Wing RR and others: Behavior change, weight loss, and physiological improvements in type II diabetic patients, *J Consult Clin Psychol* 53:111-122, 1985.

97. Zinman B, Zuniga-Guajardo S, Kelly D: Comparison of the acute and long-term effects of exercise on glucose control in type I diabetes, *Diabetes Care* 7:515-519, 1984.

6 Pharmacologic Therapies in the Management of Diabetes Mellitus

John R. White, Jr. and R. Keith Campbell

Effective pharmacologic management of diabetes mellitus is a relatively recent development. Before the 1920s a diagnosis of insulin-dependent diabetes mellitus (IDDM) (also type I diabetes mellitus) carried with it the grave prognosis of a rapid downhill course. The first effective treatment was realized, and research into the prevention and treatment of diabetes burgeoned with Banting and Best's discovery in 1922[7] of insulin and its hypoglycemic properties. In the early 1920s a patient requiring insulin therapy was subjected to multiple daily injections of a crude animal insulin extract with reusable and often dull needles. Today a patient may use a myriad of various highly purified animal or human insulins with a choice of time action profile injected with disposable microfine needles and disposable syringes or delivered via internal or external insulin pump. The first oral agent, Synthalin, was synthesized

---

CHAPTER OBJECTIVES

- Discuss the normal physiologic effects of insulin.
- List the clinical indications for exogenous insulin use.
- Differentiate sources and the adverse effect profiles for various insulin sources.
- Counsel a patient about the appropriate procedure for insulin storage, dose preparation, and administration.
- Discuss the pros and cons of the various insulin regimens.
- List the various complications of insulin, and state the treatments of the complications.
- Discuss the physiologic effects of the sulfonylureas.
- Choose an oral hypoglycemic agent and regimen for a given patient.
- List the complications associated with sulfonylureas.
- Discuss the potential drug interaction types associated with oral hypoglycemic agents.

---

in the 1920s by Frank and others.[11] Synthalin has long since been replaced by the less toxic sulfonylurea agents. Currently in the United States two generations of sulfonylurea agents are in use. Outside the United States two biguanide compounds (buformin and metformin) are being used as well. Recently the biguanide metformin was approved by the Food and Drug Administration for use in the United States. Although significant advances have been made, unfortunately there is still no cure for diabetes. It is important to note, however, that the Diabetes Control and Complications Trial (DCCT) proved conclusively that improved glycemic control is associated with a reduction in the appearance and progression of chronic complications in patients with type I diabetes.[10] Insulin and the sulfonylurea agents can decrease morbidity and mortality when used appropriately but are far from the wanted panacea.

This chapter reviews the pharmacology, clinical dosing, and monitoring of insulin and the oral hypoglycemic agents available to the clinician in the United States.

INSULIN

Structure and Production

Preproinsulin is produced in the beta cells of the islets of Langerhans in the pancreas. It is a large molecular weight (mw ~ 12,000) protein with a half-life of approximately 1 minute. Preproinsulin is cleaved to form proinsulin (mw ~ 9000). Proinsulin is in turn cleaved to form equimolar amounts of insulin and C-peptide.[38] Insulin is a protein composed of 51 amino acids arranged in two polypeptide chains (A and B) that are connected via disulfide bonds. The plasma half-lives of insulin and C-peptide are ~4 and ~30 minutes, respectively.[38,39,43]

Approximately 200 units (U) of insulin are stored in the normal human pancreas, whereas virtually none is found in the pancreas of the patient with IDDM after approximately 7 years of disease.[14] The normal human pancreas has a basal insulin secretory rate of 1 to 2 U per hour, with postprandial rates increasing to 4 to 6 U per hour (Fig. 6-1). Normal daily total amounts of secreted insulin range from 40 to 60 U. Clearance of insulin takes place in the periphery, the liver, and the kidneys. Patients who suffer diabetic nephropathy may require downward adjustments in their insulin regimens caused by decreases in renal insulin metabolism that parallel renal failure.

C-peptide measurement is useful in both the clinical and the research setting. The measurement of C-peptide may be utilized in the differential diagnosis of hypoglycemia when factitious insulin administration is a possibility. Factitious insulin administration is confirmed when elevated levels of insulin are present with decreased C-peptide concentrations and hypoglycemia. C-peptide measurement is also useful as an indicator of residual beta-cell function in patients receiving exogenous insulin and in the evaluation of pancreatectomy status.

Physiologic Effects of Insulin

Insulin exerts an effect on carbohydrate, fat, and protein metabolism. Therefore disruption of insulin secretion or disposition or action such as encountered with diabetes mellitus results

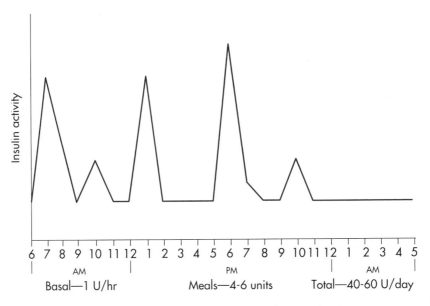

Fig. 6-1 Normal physiologic insulin secretion.

in abnormal carbohydrate, fat, and protein disposition and utilization. These metabolic abnormalities are closely linked to the acute and chronic complications encountered in the patient with diabetes.[20]

The effects of insulin on carbohydrate metabolism include (1) enhanced rate of glycogen synthesis and storage in the liver, skeletal muscle, and other tissue and (2) increased facilitated transport of glucose from the systemic circulation into skeletal muscle, adipose tissue, and some smooth muscle organs. Insulin is not required for glucose transport in the central nervous system, intestinal mucosa, ocular lens, and renal tubular epithelium. Therefore when hyperglycemia is present, these tissues are subjected to high intracellular glucose concentrations. Lack of insulin or insulin activity results in hyperglycemia caused by impaired glucose transport and glycogen storage. A relative intracellular deficiency of glucose in insulin-dependent tissue triggers the liberation of hepatic glucose (glycogenolysis), thus escalating the systemic hyperglycemia.[17,20,43]

Insulin affects protein synthesis and storage in a variety of ways: (1) insulin suppresses the formation of glucose from amino acids (gluconeogenesis); (2) insulin depresses the rate of protein catabolism; (3) the presence of insulin favors the transport of amino acids into cells; and (4) insulin affects mRNA to increase the rate of protein production. Lack of insulin results in an increase in protein catabolism coupled with a decreased ability to form new proteins from constituent amino acids. Hyperglycemia is again escalated, but in this case it is secondary to increased rates of gluconeogenesis.[17,20,43]

Insulin also affects fat metabolism. Lipase enzymes are inhibited by insulin. Lipase is responsible for the breakdown of triglycerides into free fatty acids. Insulin also promotes the transport of glucose into fat cells. A fraction of this glucose is utilized to synthesize free fatty acids, while another fraction eventually is converted to glycerol. Glycerol is essential in the

Table 6-1   Amino-Acid Sequences of Various Insulins

Source	A chain	B chain
	Position 8/10	**Position 30**
Human	Threonine/isoleucine	Threonine
Beef	Alanine/valine	Alanine
Pork	Threonine/isoleucine	Alanine

formation of triglycerides from free fatty acids. Therefore insulin is lipogenic and promotes fat storage. Lack of insulin results in depletion of fat stores and high concentrations of circulating free fatty acids.[17,20,43]

Indications for the Clinical Use of Exogenous Insulin

Insulin is indicated for use in the following situations:

1. All persons with IDDM.
2. Women with gestational diabetes, if diet alone does not adequately control blood glucose levels (see Chapter 11).
3. Persons with non-insulin-dependent diabetes (NIDDM) whose conditions are not controlled by diet or oral hypoglycemic agents.
4. Persons with NIDDM who are undergoing stress such as infection or surgery or who require corticosteroid therapy.
5. Treatment of diabetic ketoacidosis (see Chapter 10).
6. Treatment of hyperosmolar nonketotic syndrome.
7. Some individuals who are receiving parenteral nutrition or who require high caloric supplementation to meet increased intermittent energy needs.[4,5]
8. Low-dose insulin is being evaluated experimentally for the prevention of type I diabetes in predisposed patients.[32]

Sources of Insulin

The three species sources of insulin that are currently clinically used are beef, pork, and human. The six product types include beef, pork, beef/pork combination, biosynthetic recombinant human derived from bacteria, biosynthetic recombinant human derived from yeast (available in Europe), and semisynthetic human insulin derived from pork. Structurally, pork and beef insulin differ from human insulin by one and three amino acids, respectively (Table 6-1).[43,44]

Human insulin is currently produced by three different methods in the United States. Human insulin of recombinant DNA origin (Eli Lilly and Company) is produced by *Escherichia coli* into which plasmids bearing the sequencing information for human proinsulin have been inserted. The bacteria are then placed into an appropriate medium under conditions conducive to multiplication and proinsulin production. The proinsulin is harvested and enzymatically cleaved, and the resultant insulin purified.[13] Similarly, human insulin of recombinant DNA origin (Novo-Nordisk) is produced by insertion of the appropriate human DNA into brewers yeast.[35] In the past, semisynthetic human insulin was produced by enzymatic transpeptidation of pork insulin at position 30 of the B chain with the substitution of threonine for alanine; however, this process is no longer utilized.[31] Last, human insulin (Velosulin Human Regular) is produced by chemical conversion of pork insulin to human insulin.

Clinically, human insulins differ from animal source insulins with respect to antigenicity and solubility. Human insulins are less antigenic than pork insulins; in turn, pork insulins are less antigenic than beef insulins. Theoretically, decreased antigenicity parallels a decreased incidence of lipoatrophy, local and systemic allergic reactions, and antibody production. Although it is clear that persons treated with human insulin produce lower titers of insulin antibodies, the clinical significance is uncertain. Insulin antibodies, when present in high titers, may cause insulin resistance. Some clinicians believe that insulin antibodies may bind and subsequently release insulin, resulting in erratic time action profiles. Human insulin is more soluble than animal source insulins and thus displays a slightly different pharmacokinetic pattern.[25,28,37] A higher rate of subcutaneous absorption and a shorter duration of action have been observed with human insulin as compared with animal source insulins. Thus the individual with diabetes switching from one species source to another must be closely monitored and subsequently have doses adjusted appropriately. Insulin requirements may decline as antibody titers wane in persons switched from animal source insulin to human insulin because of immunologically mediated insulin resistance.

There is a great deal of discussion about which insulin source is the most efficacious. Insulins from all sources are apparently equally effective in normalizing blood glucose levels. Human insulin, however, has the most acceptable side-effect profile of all the insulins. Lower titers of antibodies and resolution of lipoatrophy may be seen in the individual who is switched from animal source to human insulin. At this time no evidence supports an across-the-board switch to human insulin; thus persons who are maintained without problems on animal source insulins should probably remain on those insulins. Human insulin is indicated in the following situations.

1. Persons who use insulin temporarily (e.g., individual with type II [NIDDM] disease undergoing surgery).
2. Persons who have a history of drug allergies.
3. Persons with an active allergic response to animal source insulin (including lipoatrophy and insulin resistance).
4. Persons with religious or ethical aversion to animal source products.
5. Newly diagnosed persons with type I diabetes or persons with type II diabetes being placed on insulin therapy.
6. Pregnant women with diabetes or those planning pregnancy.

It should be noted that human insulin was produced in part as a response to the U.S. Diabetes Advisory Board's findings in 1978. An insulin shortage in the 1990s was predicted by this group, based on figures of expected population growth and anticipated decreases in red meat consumption in the Western world.[1] With the continued population expansion, decreases in red meat consumption, advances in biotechnology, and side-effect profile of human insulin, and the recent trend to discontinue some forms of animal source insulin, it is reasonable to predict that animal source insulins will eventually be completely phased out.

Preparations

Insulins are available in short-, intermediate-, and long-acting preparations (Table 6-2). The time action profile of each of these categories is obviously different (Fig. 6-2). In addition, the time action profile of the various preparations in each category will vary slightly. Last, the time action profile of each particular insulin preparation varies with different injection sites, changes in ambient temperature, among individuals, and with source. These three categories are used for ease of classification and should not imply that insulins within a given category are interchangeable without proper monitoring and dosage adjustment. Clinicians are cautioned against relying too heavily on chart descriptions of time action profiles of insulin; they should base dosage adjustments on the person's self-monitoring of blood glucose (SMBG).

The short-acting insulins include Regular, buffered Regular, and Semilente. When administered subcutaneously, the onset of action of these insulins is ~ ½ to 1 hour, peak activity is ~ 2 to 4 hours, and duration is ~ 6 to 8 hours (see Fig. 6-2). Regular and buffered Regular are formulations containing solubilized crystalline insulin. These formulations are solutions; their appearance should thus be clear. *Regular insulin is the* **only** *insulin that may be administered intravenously, since all other insulin formulations are suspensions.* Velosulin Human Regular (Novo-Nordisk) is the insulin of choice for continuous subcutaneous insulin infusion (CSII) devices. Semilente is a suspension containing an amorphous precipitate of insulin and zinc. Semilente insulin has a slightly delayed onset and peak and a longer duration than Regular insulin.[16,17]

The intermediate-acting insulins include Lente and Neutral Protamine Hagedorn (NPH), also known as *isophane*. The intermediate-acting insulins have an onset of ~ 1 to 4 hours, a peak effect at ~ 6 to 8 hours, and a duration of ~ 10 to 16 hours (see Fig. 6-2). Some clinicians consider human Ultralente to be an intermediate-acting preparation because its time action profile falls between the "classic" intermediate-acting preparations and traditional long-acting preparations of beef Ultralente. This difference in time action profile is secondary to the greater solubility and enhanced absorption of human insulin.[16,17]

NPH insulin was introduced in 1946 by researchers at Nordisk laboratories in Denmark.[27] NPH insulin contains a combination of zinc-insulin crystals and protamine sulfate in a ratio such that the solid phase is composed of insulin, zinc, and protamine. Protamine is a protein derived from fish sperm. This foreign protein, which causes an allergic response in a small fraction of patients, helped prompt researchers to develop Lente insulins.[21] Lente insulin is a 70 $\rightarrow$ 30 combination of Ultralente and Semilente. Lente insulin is a useful intermediate-acting formulation, particularly in those patients sensitive to protamine. Both NPH and Lente display time action profiles that favor their use in twice-daily injection regimens.

Table 6-2 Insulins Available in the United States

Product	Manufacturer	Strength
Short-acting		
Beef		
Iletin II Regular	Lilly	U-100
Semilente	Novo-Nordisk	U-100
Pork		
Iletin II Regular	Lilly	U-100, -500
Regular	Novo-Nordisk	U-100
Purified pork Regular	Novo-Nordisk	U-100
Velosulin	Novo-Nordisk	U-100
Beef/pork		
Iletin I Regular	Lilly	U-40, -100
Iletin I Semilente	Lilly	U-40, -100
Human		
Humulin Regular	Lilly	U-100
Humulin BR	Lilly	U-100
Novolin R	Novo-Nordisk	U-100
Velosulin human R	Novo-Nordisk	U-100
Intermediate-acting		
Beef		
Iletin II Lente	Lilly	U-100
Iletin II NPH	Lilly	U-100
Lente	Novo-Nordisk	U-100
NPH	Novo-Nordisk	U-100
Pork		
Iletin II Lente	Lilly	U-100
Iletin II NPH	Lilly	U-100
Purified pork Lente	Novo-Nordisk	U-100
Purified pork NPH	Novo-Nordisk	U-100
Insulatard NPH	Novo-Nordisk	U-100
Beef/pork		
Iletin I NPH	Lilly	U-40, -100
Iletin I Lente	Lilly	U-40, -100
Human		
Humulin L (Lente)	Lilly	U-100
Humulin N (NPH)	Lilly	U-100
Novulin L (Lente)	Novo-Nordisk	U-100

Table 6-2   Insulins Available in the United States—cont'd

Product	Manufacturer	Strength
Human—cont'd		
Novulin N (NPH)	Novo-Nordisk	U-100
Insulatard NPH human	Novo-Nordisk	U-100
Long-acting		
Beef		
Iletin II PZI	Lilly	U-100
Ultralente	Novo-Nordisk	U-100
Pork		
Iletin II PZI	Lilly	U-100
Beef/pork		
Iletin I PZI	Lilly	U-40, -100
Iletin I Ultralente	Lilly	U-40, -100
Human		
Humulin U (Ultralente)	Lilly	U-100
Fixed combinations (all are U-100 insulins)		
		NPH/REG
Pork		
Mixtard	Novo-Nordisk	70/30
Human		
Humulin 70/30	Lilly	70/30
Novolin 70/30	Novo-Nordisk	70/30
Mixtard human 70/30	Novo-Nordisk	70/30

Long-acting insulins include Protamine Zinc Insulin (PZI) and Ultralente. These insulins have an onset of between 6 and 14 hours and a duration that may range from 18 to 36 hours (see Fig. 6-2). The long-acting insulins are not usually associated with a peak effect but instead provide a sustained, relatively consistent insulin effect to mimic basal insulin secretion. Protamine Zinc Insulin is no longer available.

Strength and Purity

Insulin is available in the United States in two strengths: (1) U-100 and (2) U-500 (by special order from Eli Lilly and Company). The strength correlates to the number of units of insulin per milliliter of product. In the past, U-80 and U-40 insulins were available; these insulins are no longer available in the United States. However, the clinician should be aware that these

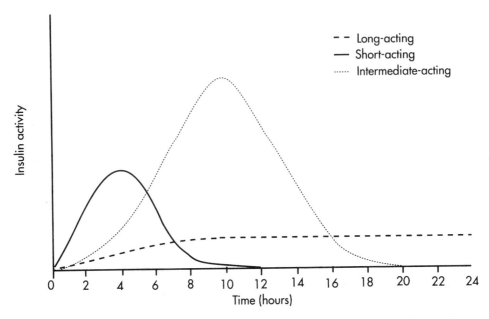

Fig. 6-2 Insulin time action profiles: short- versus intermediate- versus long-acting.

insulins do still exist in other countries and may present special problems to those traveling abroad.

Persons traveling abroad should be cautioned that in many countries only U-40 insulin is available, and sometimes specific insulin types are limited. In this situation, it is advised that the individual carry sufficient quantities of insulin and syringes for the entire trip, continue to wear a Med-Alert bracelet, and carry prescriptions for both extra insulin and syringes.

Persons resistant to insulin who require greater than 100 units of insulin per injection may be treated with U-500 insulin. U-500 insulin is a legend medication and therefore requires a prescription. Also, U-500 is not routinely stocked in pharmacies and must be specially ordered from the manufacturer, Eli Lilly and Company.

Insulin purity is measured in terms of parts per million (ppm) of proinsulin. Contamination by proinsulin is considered representative of non-insulin contaminants; since precise measurement of proinsulin is possible, it is utilized as the standard of purity.[34]

Insulin was purified by means of crystallization before the 1960s. Currently insulin products undergo extensive purification by chromatographic processes that yield highly purified products. Standard insulins today contain less than 10 ppm proinsulin, while most insulin products contain ≤1 ppm and are associated with a reduced incidence of allergic responses. Many allergic responses associated with insulin today are probably caused by differences in species or exogenous components such as protamine. However, some persons experience lipoatrophy while using standard insulin (<10 ppm proinsulin) that resolves with the use of highly purified products such as human insulin or purified pork (≤1 ppm proinsulin).[34]

Stability and Storage

Insulin must be refrigerated by the manufacturer, the distributor, and the dispenser. Insulins are stable at room temperature (68° to 75° F) for several months. Higher temperatures will cause an accelerated degradation of the insulin product and may induce flocculation. Persons living in areas subjected to high temperatures should be warned against leaving their insulin in automobiles or in any location where extreme temperatures may occur. Freezing insulin will alter the physical suspension characteristics of modified insulins and is not recommended. Refrigeration at ~ 40° F is the best method for insulin storage, although persons may keep bottles of insulin they are using at room temperature for as long as 1 month.[17] Individuals who refrigerate their insulin should be instructed to roll the insulin syringe between their palms after the appropriate dose has been withdrawn, to warm the insulin, making the injection more comfortable.

Flocculation and frosting of various intermediate-acting insulins has been reported with recombinant human insulin, semisynthetic human insulin, and purified pork insulin. When flocculation occurs, the insulin loses its homogeneous characteristics and appears as large clumped particles. Frosting is characterized by a frosted or crystallized appearance on the inner wall of the vial. Flocculation and frosting usually occur in vials that are less than half full and that have been in use for 3 to 6 weeks. Factors that may contribute to flocculation and frosting include excessive agitation of the insulin vial, temperature extremes, and inappropriate zinc/insulin ratios. Persons should be instructed to examine insulin products before use and not use insulin products with a flocculated or frosted appearance. The expiration date, stamped on each bottle, should be examined carefully before use. A slight loss in potency may occur if the bottle has been used for more than 30 days and if it has been stored at room temperature. Unexplained fluctuations in blood glucose may be related to reduced insulin potency.[3]

Mixing Insulins

Many intensive insulin regimens are based on multiple daily injections of various types of insulin. Mixing of two insulin types in one syringe or vial is a simple procedure that sometimes circumvents the need for an excessive number of injections. This technique is not without risk, because any combination may result in physical or chemical changes in the components, which may in turn alter the predicted physiologic response. The questions concerning the appropriateness of insulin mixtures have been difficult to answer because of problems associated with measuring free insulin and its effects. The recent introduction of improved assay techniques, coupled with a number of well-designed clinical studies, have answered some previously unresolved questions.

The Lente insulins (Semilente, Lente, Ultralente) may be mixed in any ratio, with the clinical response of each of the constituents preserved. Mixtures of Lente insulins remain stable for as long as 18 months.[45]

Regular insulins may be mixed with NPH in any ratio while retaining the time action profiles of the components. This is probably the combination of choice when a mixture of short-acting and intermediate-acting insulins is required. In the United States premixed

---

BOX 6-1

GUIDELINES FOR MIXING INSULIN

According to the American Diabetes Association,[3] the following guidelines for mixing insulin should be followed:

- Individuals with diabetes who are well controlled on a particular mixed-insulin regimen should maintain their standard procedure for preparing their insulin doses.
- No other medication or diluent should be mixed with any insulin product unless approved by the physician.
- Use of commercially available premixed insulins is preferred to extemporaneously mixing by the individual with diabetes if the insulin ratio is appropriate to the individual's insulin requirements.
- Currently available NPH and regular insulin formulations may interact when mixed.
- Lente insulins do not interact with each other.
- Mixing of Regular and Lente insulin is not recommended except for patients already adequately controlled on such a mixture. This is caused by the binding of Lente insulins with Regular insulin, delaying onset of action.
- Phosphate buffered insulins should not be mixed with Lente insulins.
- There is no rationale for mixing animal with human insulin.
- Insulin formulation may change; therefore the manufacturer should be consulted in cases in which recommendations appear to conflict with the American Diabetes Association guidelines.

---

insulins currently are available in a ratio of 70% NPH with 30% Regular and 50% NPH with 50% Regular. In addition to the 70/30 and 50/50, mixtures in the ratios of 90/10, 80/20, and 60/40 NPH/Regular are available in Europe.[45]

When Regular insulins are mixed with Lente insulins, a binding phenomenon occurs between the excess zinc in the Lente and the free insulin from the Regular insulin, causing a blunting of the Regular insulin's effect.[8,16,33] The binding begins within 15 minutes after injection and continues for as long as 24 hours. The amount of attenuated Regular insulin is dependent on the ratio of Regular to Lente. The greater the Lente concentration, the greater the amount of binding. If this type of mixture is to be used, it is recommended that mixtures be allowed to stand for 24 hours before injection to ensure consistency between the Regular → Lente interaction from injection to injection. In the past, it has been recommended that as an alternative to the 24-hour waiting period, this type of mixture be injected immediately. This immediate injection method is not currently recommended because when human insulins are used, the interaction begins immediately,[36] and with all source insulins, the interaction may continue once the mixture is in the subcutaneous reservoir, resulting in inconsistent time action profiles. This interaction also occurs when Ultralente is mixed with Regular. One solution to the problem is to have the patient inject the two types separately. This solution obviates binding interactions but does not always meet with acceptance by the individual.

*Buffered insulins such as NPH, premixed NPH/Regular, and buffered Regular insulins (Velosulin) should **never** be mixed with Lente insulins.* Precipitation of zinc from the suspension by phosphorus will result in an increase in Regular insulin in the mixture. This shift may cause hypoglycemia in the patient. See Box 6-1 for guidelines for mixing insulin.

INSULIN REGIMENS
Initiation of Treatment

Initial insulinization of the person with diabetes should be aimed at eliminating hyperglycemic symptoms and reestablishing metabolic and fluid balance without causing hypoglycemia. In the past, most persons were hospitalized during initial treatment. Today many individuals begin insulin therapy on an outpatient basis unless they have been initially diagnosed with diabetic ketoacidosis (DKA). Education at this point is extremely important because these individuals are establishing habits that affect their long-term outcome. Unfortnately, approximately 10% to 20% of newly diagnosed persons do not receive even rudimentary education about insulin dose preparation or injection, but are simply handed a prescription. It is probably best to begin a person on a twice-daily regimen and to immediately teach self-monitoring of blood glucose. Some clinicians prefer to stabilize the individual by initiating therapy with twice-daily injections of NPH, switching later to a split mixed regimen; others prefer to begin therapy with an intensive insulin regimen (three or more injections per day).

Initial diabetes education should include cursory information about the disease, its complications, and the importance of treatment and monitoring. Education should also include teaching of insulin injection technique, preparation of insulin doses, information about storage of insulin, and recognition and treatment of hypoglycemia. Individuals who have access to comprehensive diabetes education programs offered by health care organizations should be strongly encouraged to enroll in such programs.

Insulin should be initiated at a dose of 0.5 U/kg/day. Based on this recommendation, a person weighing 70 kg would begin therapy with a total daily dose of 35 U of insulin. A person receiving this amount of insulin in two divided doses is less likely to become hypoglycemic than the individual who receives the entire amount as a single injection. Two thirds of the total daily dose should be given in the morning, and one third of the dose should be given around the evening meal. The ratio of AM/PM doses may be adjusted, based on blood glucose monitoring. It should be anticipated that this dose will eventually need to be titrated upward toward the 1 U/kg/day range, especially for persons with NIDDM. Some persons (20% to 30%) often experience a ''honeymoon'' or remission phase within weeks after their diagnosis; this phase is characterized by a temporary recovery of beta-cell function.[2] During this time insulin requirements may decline to the point at which no exogenous insulin is needed. Most clinicians prefer to continue insulin at very small doses rather than discontinue insulin altogether. Total discontinuance of insulin may give the individual a false impression of cure and may also result in immunologic problems associated with intermittent insulin administration. Individuals who do not monitor blood glucose levels and do not have insulin doses adjusted accordingly during the honeymoon period run a high risk of hypoglycemia.

BOX 6-2

INSULIN ADMINISTRATION GUIDELINES

Wash hands.

Insulin vials should be checked for flocculation or frosting and expiration date.

Intermediate-acting and long-acting insulins should be resuspended by gently rolling the vial between the palms—DO NOT SHAKE.

Clean the tops of the insulin vials with an alcohol swab.

After the alcohol has dried, an amount of air equal to the dose of insulin required should be drawn up and injected into the vial. When mixing insulins, put sufficient amount of air into both bottles.

Insert the needle into the vial, invert the vial, and pull back the plunger until the appropriate amount has been withdrawn. Withdraw appropriate amount of intermediate-acting insulin. When mixing insulins, the clear short-acting insulin should be drawn into the syringe first.

If bubbles appear, tap the side of the syringe and inject the bubbles back into the vial; then withdraw the needed amount of insulin.

Carefully recap needle.

Cleanse injection site with alcohol and allow alcohol to dry.

Pinch a fold of skin at the injection site with one hand (pinching lifts fat off of muscle and circumvents intramuscular or intravenous injection that may cause hypoglycemia). Hold the syringe like a pencil in the other hand. Insert the needle with the beveled edge pointed up at a 45-degree to 90-degree angle (the angle will depend on the level of subcutaneous fat—the greater the fat, the more perpendicular the injection may be).

Smoothly and continuously press plunger in as far as it will go; routine aspiration is not necessary.

Withdraw needle, and gently apply pressure with cotton swab.

Record dose, time, and injection site.

Discard syringe in an appropriate manner.

Administration of Insulin

Insulin may be administered with traditional syringes, jet injectors, pumps, or modified syringes (pen injectors). The vast majority of persons administer insulin via subcutaneous injection with disposable plastic syringes with small-gauge lubricated needles. Dosage preparation and administration should be explained to the individual; he or she should then be asked to explain the procedure to the health care provider. This will ensure that the individual understands what is being taught and will allow the clinician to detect problems. See Box 6-2 for insulin administration guidelines to stress with patients.

Syringe Reuse

Manufacturers of disposable syringes recommend that they be used only once because the sterility of the syringe cannot be guaranteed. However, some individuals prefer to reuse syringes several times. If reuse is planned, the needle must be recapped after each use, by means of a technique that supports the syringe in the hand and replaces the cap with a straight motion of the thumb and forefinger. The individual should be instructed to discard the syringe if the needle becomes dull or bent or has contact with any surface other than the skin. Syringe reuse is not recommended for persons exhibiting poor personal hygiene, acute concurrent illness, open wounds, or decreased resistance to infection for any reason.[3]

Selection of Sites

Insulin absorption is affected by a number of factors:

1. Injection site—the predictability and completeness and rate of absorption is > abdomen > deltoid > thigh > hip.
2. Ambient temperature—the greater the temperature, the greater the rate of absorption.
3. Exercise or massage—may increase absorption.

All the above-mentioned factors must be considered when designing a patient regimen. In the past, most clinicians agreed that injection sites should be routinely rotated from one area to another because rotation of sites is important to the prevention of lipohypertrophy or lipoatrophy. However, since an injection in the abdominal area may elicit a different time action profile than an injection in the hip, dosage response observations may be difficult to interpret. Therefore some clinicians now recommend that individuals with IDDM inject in a given area (e.g., abdominal area) and systematically rotate sites within the area before moving to a different area (e.g., the individual would systematically use abdominal sites before moving on to using sites identified in the deltoid). Persons who exercise should avoid injecting into subcutaneous tissue adjacent to the muscles to be used. Rapid absorption can lead to hypoglycemia.

In the newly diagnosed individual, one method of teaching injection technique is for the instructor to self-inject using sterile water. This graphically demonstrates to the individual that the technique is virtually painless, and with the use of sterile water the patient can practice a few injections, thus lowering his or her apprehension in a less than pleasant situation.

Insulin Regimens and Dosage Adjustments in Patients with Type I Disease

Normal insulin secretion is depicted in Fig. 6-1 and is best described as a continuous basal release with superimposed bolus doses triggered by food intake or blood glucose concentration changes. Insulin replacement regimens should seek to mimic this secretory pattern. The most effective method of achieving this goal will probably be via a closed loop pump system that constantly monitors blood glucose levels and adjusts insulin infusion rates accordingly. Unfortunately, at this time a closed loop system of this nature is much too large and expensive to be considered pragmatic. The regimen that most closely resembles physiologic secretion and is used to any great degree is the external insulin pump in combination with frequent (usually at least 4 times per day) blood glucose monitoring.

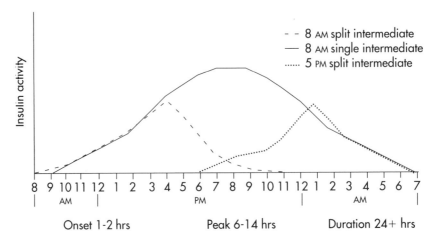

Fig. 6-3 Insulin time action profile: intermediate-split versus single.

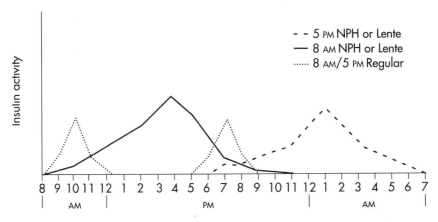

Fig. 6-4 Insulin time action profile: split and mixed Regular/NPH or Lente.

One-injection regimens

Unfortunately, one of the most frequently encountered insulin regimens is the once-daily intermediate-acting insulin regimen. Many clinicians learned this method during their initial training and continue to make use of it today even in light of new evidence that strongly suggests that it is suboptimal. Persons with diabetes who have not been educated about the long-term implications usually resist changing to more complex but much more efficacious regimens. To understand the shortcomings of such a regimen, one simply needs to examine the time action profile for intermediate-acting insulins (Figs. 6-2 and 6-3). The individual taking an injection in the early morning upon arising has no insulin coverage until around the midday meal and no coverage the following morning before the next injection. Because the entire insulin dosage is given as one dose, a large peak effect that may cause severe hypoglycemia will occur 8 to 12 hours after the dose. In persons with IDDM, a single injection per day of an intermediate-acting insulin is predictably almost always insufficient. In individuals with an active insulin reserve, the single-injection regimen may at times prove beneficial.

Two-injection regimens

Two injections per day is probably the minimum number to adequately cover the patient with type I disease. The total daily insulin dose (0.5 to 1.0 U/kg) is typically divided into a morning dose of two thirds to one half of the total daily dose and an evening dose of the remaining one third to one half of the total daily dose. The two injections may consist of intermediate-acting insulin alone (see Fig. 6-3) but are much more effective if given as a mixture of intermediate- and short-acting insulins (Fig. 6-4). Mixtures of intermediate- and short-acting insulins usually provide two thirds of the daily dose as intermediate acting and one third of the daily dose as rapid-acting insulin. This ratio and the total daily dose must be adjusted based on blood glucose monitoring. If Lente is used in place of NPH, the ratio may need to be adjusted to increase the activity of the fast-acting insulin. Doses should be adjusted based on information obtained under stable exercise and diet conditions, in the absence of other stressors. Preprandial blood glucose determinations are more consistent than postprandial blood glucose determinations and are probably the routine test of choice. Refer to Table 6-3 for dosage adjustment guidelines.

Currently, premixed formulations of NPH and Regular insulin are available in the United States in a ratio of 70/30 and 50/50 NPH/Regular. Although these mixtures are an improvement over twice-daily injections of NPH alone, they do not offer the needed flexibility

Table 6-3 Split and Mixed Regimen Dose Adjustment

	Test time				
	Fasting	Prelunch	Predinner	Prebedtime	Early morning
Insulin dose	Evening NPH If elevated, check early AM blood glucose	Morning Regular	Morning NPH	Evening Regular	Evening NPH
Meal or snack	Late-night snack	Breakfast	Lunch Snack	Dinner	Dinner Late snack

Insulin doses and meals or snacks that may affect blood glucose levels at the above mentioned times are listed.

This table assumes the patient is on a normal 8-to-5 schedule, with regular meals and snacks.

If fasting blood glucose levels are elevated, consider Somogyi effect and dawn phenomenon (see Chapter 8); evaluate with the early AM levels. The clinician should usually attempt to correct one unacceptable level at a time. Goals should be approached slowly. Increase or decrease insulin dose 1 to 2 U for every 40 to 50 mg/dl desired change in blood glucose level.

to adjust doses on an as-needed basis. These mixtures may be appropriate for the individual who cannot or will not use the split and mix approach. In the future, a variety of mixed ratios may be available in the United States. In Europe, ratios of 50/50, 60/40, 70/30, 80/20, and 90/10 NPH/Regular are available.

Three-injection regimens

In some individuals on the mixed dose two-injection regimen, the intermediate-acting insulin administered with the evening meal is not sufficient to control the individual's blood glucose throughout the following night. The resulting fasting hyperglycemia can be countered by further splitting the regimen into an evening meal short-acting insulin dose and a bedtime intermediate-acting dose. When early morning hyperglycemia is encountered, the Somogyi effect should first be ruled out before regimen changes are made. When this regimen is used, persons with diabetes usually take two thirds of their total daily insulin in their morning dose, one sixth with their evening meal, and one sixth at bedtime.

Multidose regimens

Basically, two multidose regimens may be used. The first is a regimen of four daily doses of rapid-acting insulin given before each meal and at bedtime. Initially the daily dose is divided into four equal doses. Doses are then adjusted from this baseline. One of the problems with this regimen is that the evening dose Regular insulin (especially human Regular) may not provide sufficient coverage throughout the night, particularly if the dose is taken early. If larger doses are given, the individual may experience early morning (2 to 3 AM) hypoglycemia during the peak effect of the short-acting insulin. An alternative is to give injections of short-acting insulin before each meal with a single morning injection of long-acting insulin such as PZI or Ultralente. The long-acting insulin dose should initially comprise two fifths of the total daily dose and will provide a basal amount of insulin. Most clinicians recommend using Ultralente with this regimen. Each short-acting insulin dose in this regimen comprises approximately one fifth of the total daily dose. Inasmuch as individuals with diabetes can adjust doses of regular insulin to compensate for various meals, this regimen offers good glycemia control and flexibility of life-style. It does, however, require multiple injections and frequent blood glucose monitoring, which some individuals find burdensome. Refer to Fig. 6-5 for a graphic description of this regimen.

Continuous subcutaneous insulin infusion

Continuous subcutaneous insulin infusion (CSII) devices, both internal (experimental) and external, can be programmed to release a basal amount of insulin and bolus doses on an as-needed basis. Most available pumps can be programmed with about the same amount of difficulty as a programmable wristwatch and can contain alarms for malfunctions (such as low batteries) and dosage ceilings to prevent accidental overdose. Subcutaneous access may be achieved by a small needlelike catheter or a flexible plastic catheter (inserted with a needle). The catheters may be used for 2 to 3 days before they are replaced. Only Regular insulin should be used in a pump, preferably human buffered Regular insulin. Pumps offer tight control and great flexibility of life-style for those health care providers and patients motivated enough to learn about the functioning and maintenance of CSII.

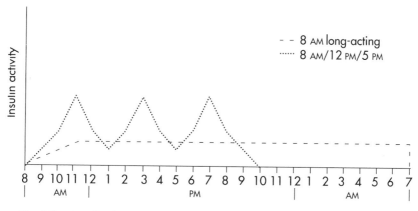

Fig. 6-5   Insulin time action profile: split Regular with long-acting insulin.

Goals

The short-term goals for insulin therapy can be divided into four categories: blood glucose levels, glycosylated hemoglobin levels, urine test results, and symptoms. Symptoms of hyperglycemia such as polydipsia, polyphagia, and polyuria should completely resolve with near normalization of blood glucose levels. This resolution of hyperglycemic symptoms should be attained without the induction of hypoglycemia. Three degrees of acceptability have been delineated for blood glucose levels measured at various times for the different types of regimens. Simplistically, the more intensive the regimen, the closer to normal ranges the blood glucose levels and glycosylated hemoglobin levels should be. The three levels of treatment and/or expected short-term outcomes are minimal, average, and intensive. An example of minimal treatment would be the use of a single injection of intermediate-acting insulin in an individual with IDDM. Given this common situation, one could expect that the person's glycosylated hemoglobin would measure between 11% and 13%, urine glucose loss would be common, and blood glucose measurements would often be in the 300 mg/dl range. The individual would at times be symptomatic and, if still growing, may do so at a slower rate than an age-, weight-, and genetically matched counterpart. Under normal circumstances (e.g., without infection, surgery), this individual would not develop diabetic ketoacidosis.

With average treatment (possibly two injections of intermediate-acting insulin), the same person would have average preprandial blood glucose levels in the range of 160 to 200 mg/dl with glycosylated hemoglobin levels of 8% to 10%. The individual would not usually be symptomatic, would experience self-treatable hypoglycemia every week or so, and would grow at a normal rate. If treated in an intensive manner, this same person would be seen with a blood glucose diary that reveals preprandial glucose concentrations in the range of 80 to 120 mg/dl and with a hemoglobin A_{1c} in the range of 6% to 8%. The patient would note a sense of increased energy and well-being but would probably have an increased incidence of hypoglycemic episodes.

Setting goals for the individual with diabetes is much more meaningful for all involved if the person is educated about various levels of treatment, the consequences, and the costs (in money, time, and commitment) and has an input into their formulation. Overall, the goal should be to maintain all measurable parameters as close to the euglycemic values as possible while maintaining the individual's quality of life and not running too great a risk of hypoglycemia. The benefits of strict glycemic control as elucidated by the DCCT are described in several chapters of this text.

Dose Adjustments

When evaluating an individual's blood glucose levels, several questions must be answered:
1. Are these concentrations taken from the individual's normal situation? (For instance, is infection, a large meal or snack, or a missed insulin dose a factor?)
2. Were the insulin dose, time administered, and time of glucose concentration measurement recorded accurately?
3. Is the person's SMBG technique acceptable?
4. Are the presented values believable? Do they generally correspond to glycosylated hemoglobin concentration?

Persons with diabetes should routinely monitor blood glucose levels at least four times per day when therapy is being adjusted: at fasting in the morning, before lunch, before dinner, and before bedtime. They should also check their early morning (2 to 3 AM) blood glucose levels when beginning treatment and adjust evening insulin doses to rule out early morning hypoglycemia. Postprandial glucose levels are more difficult to interpret but may be beneficial occasionally, particularly in persons undergoing intensive therapy.

In a two-injection split and mixed regimen, the individual's SMBG diary should be evaluated and the adjustment of insulin doses should then be made based on observed trends. When possible, persons with diabetes may also be taught to adjust their own insulin doses as needed. Goals should be approached carefully, and in most cases only one dose should be altered at a time. A patient-specific algorithm should be established. An insulin dose change of two units may affect two different persons in dramatically different degrees. A change of one to two units of insulin will usually cause a difference of 40 to 50 mg/dl of glucose.

Complications of Insulin Therapy

Complications associated with insulin therapy can be divided into two categories—immunologically mediated and nonimmunologically mediated. The nonimmunologically mediated complications include hypoglycemia, insulin edema, and lipohypertrophy, which are effects directly attributable to the pharmacologic effects of insulin. Immunologically mediated side effects of insulin include local dermatologic reactions, systemic immunologic response, and antibody-induced insulin resistance and lipotrophy. With the introduction of better purification methods and the use of human insulin, the incidence of immunologically mediated problems would be expected to decrease.

Hypoglycemia

The most significant and common adverse effect of insulin therapy is hypoglycemia. Almost all persons with diabetes who undergo exogenous insulin therapy will experience hypoglycemia at some time in their therapeutic course. Approximately 1 of 10 persons with diabetes will have, on a yearly basis, at least one episode of hypoglycemia severe enough to require the assistance of another person for recovery. As many as 59% of insulin-treated patients who were evaluated had nocturnal hypoglycemia; many of these patients were asymptomatic.[15] About 3% of the deaths in patients with IDDM are attributed to hypoglycemic reactions. The DCCT reported a threefold increase in the incidence of severe hypoglycemia in patients who were treated with intensive insulin therapy compared with those who were treated with conventional therapy.

Signs and symptoms of hypoglycemia include mental confusion, nervousness, sweaty palms, dizziness, blurred vision, anxiety, hunger, and tingling and numbness around the mouth. Nocturnal hypoglycemia sometimes presents with nightmares, a feeling of "hangover" in the morning upon awakening, morning headache, night sweats, or restless sleep. Signs and symptoms of hypoglycemia may be very predictable in a given individual (based on history) or may be quite erratic. A person is usually considered to be hypoglycemic when his or her blood glucose drops below 60 mg/dl. Symptoms sometimes are not noted until the concentration falls below 40 mg/dl, with coma and seizures resulting from levels of less than 20 mg/dl. Hypoglycemia may result in permanent brain damage or may induce cardiac dysrhythmias or even myocardial infarction. Central nervous system impairment secondary to hypoglycemia can result in injury or accident. The hyperglycemic response to hypoglycemia (Somogyi effect) may be a cause of prebreakfast hyperglycemia and ketonuria. Fear of development of hypoglycemia may deter the person from achieving good glycemia control.

Normally, glucose counterregulatory hormones work to maintain glucose homeostasis in the plasma. Counterregulatory hormones include glucagon, epinephrine, growth hormone, and cortisol. Under normal conditions, the secretion of these hormones prevents the development of hypoglycemia. Glucagon and epinephrine are the dominant hormones in the counterregulatory system, having rapid onsets of action and being activated as soon as blood glucose levels begin to decline. The effects of growth hormone and cortisol are not noticed until approximately 2 hours after the hypoglycemic event.

In addition to the potential hypoglycemic problems caused by injections of exogenous insulin, the person with diabetes may also have impaired counterregulatory responses to insulin-induced hypoglycemia. Deficits in counterregulatory response are common in the IDDM population and have been well documented.[18] Reduction or loss of glucagon response is usually present in patients who have had diabetes for 5 years or more. Attenuation of the sympathetic response also frequently occurs in persons who have been treated with insulin for a number of years. The individual who has a blunted counterregulatory response will have "hypoglycemic unawareness" and may undergo periods of prolonged hypoglycemia. Persons who are treated with intensive management regimens have a higher incidence of hypoglycemia. See Box 6-3 for possible causes of hypoglycemia.

Hypoglycemia in the conscious person may be treated by the administration of 10 to 15 g of oral carbohydrate (see Chapter 4). Examples of food sources providing 10 g of carbohydrate include ½ cup of orange juice or 5 Life Saver candies. Resolution of symptoms usually occurs in 15 to 20 minutes. If the patient remains hypoglycemic after 15 minutes, he or she should be instructed to ingest another 15 g of oral carbohydrate, and, if a mealtime is 2 hours or more away, the person should also consume a small complex carbohydrate/protein snack.

BOX 6-3

POSSIBLE CAUSES OF HYPOGLYCEMIA

1. Skipping or delaying meals
2. Excessive or incorrect insulin dose.
3. Altered sensitivity to insulin (e.g., an individual switched to less antigenic insulin with resulting decrease in antibodies).
4. Insulin clearance decreased (e.g., renal-failure patients may require dose reductions as renal failure progresses).
5. Glucose intake decreased.
6. Hepatic glucose production decreased.
7. Injection inadvertently given IM or IV.
8. Drug interactions.
9. Increased physical exertion.
10. Ethanol ingestion.

The unconscious person with diabetes may be treated with either intravenous 25 g glucose or 1 mg glucagon subcutaneously, intramuscularly, or intravenously. Because glucose administration requires intravenous access, glucagon is the drug of choice for the unconscious hypoglycemic patient in the home setting. All individuals utilizing exogenous insulin who have a teachable significant other or a home caretaker should have a glucagon kit. Unfortunately, only 1 of 90 persons who receives insulin therapy owns a glucagon kit. The procedure for preparing and administering glucagon is simple and can be taught in minutes. The individual receiving the medication must always be placed in a position to prevent aspiration, since glucagon may induce emesis. Because of the relatively short duration of action of glucagon, the individual should be fed immediately upon awakening.

Lipodystrophies

Lipodystrophies can be divided into two categories: lipoatrophy and lipohypertrophy. Lipohypertrophy, or hypertrophic lipodystrophy, is nonimmunologically mediated; it is discussed first.

Lipohypertrophy is characterized by a fatty, tumorlike growth at or around the injection site. In advanced cases, the skin around the hypertrophied area becomes anesthetized. These spongy growths are thought to be caused by the lipogenic properties of insulin when it has been repeatedly injected into a single area. No evidence uncovered thus far implicates an immunologic cause for this problem. Apparently, persons who focus their injections in a single area eventually develop lipohypertrophy and then magnify the problem by continuing to inject into this area because of the loss of pain sensation. The treatment of lipohypertrophy consists of systematically rotating injection sites. Switching to human insulin should have no effect on this condition.

Lipoatrophy, or a loss of fatty tissue, at or distant from the site of insulin injection, is a problem that is probably of immunologic origin. Persons treated with unchromatographed insulins have a much higher incidence of this problem than patients treated with highly purified pork insulins or human insulins. A high percentage of individuals who have insulin allergy also experience lipoatrophy. Locally injected steroids sometimes will result in the resolution of lipoatrophy. Histologic studies also indicate that an active immunologic process is taking place with lipoatrophy.

Lipoatrophy is more common in females than males and is most often reported in young females. The treatment of choice is human insulin injected at the borders of the lipoatrophic area. Use of the least antigenic insulin will theoretically attenuate the immunologic response and allow the lipogenic properties of insulin to be elicited. Resolution sometimes begins after 2 weeks of therapy but usually requires 4 to 6 months of therapy for complete resolution. After complete resolution, the individual should be instructed to continue to inject into the area every 2 to 3 weeks to avoid recurrence. A small percentage of persons will not respond to human insulin therapy. Unfortunately, these individuals do not show favorable outcomes when treated with local steroids.

Antibodies, allergy, and resistance

Insulin allergy may reveal itself as a small, local, subdermal nodule or may, on rare occasions, present as a full-blown anaphylactic reaction. Allergies to alcohol (or any skin preparation), protamine, and zinc may sometimes be mistaken for insulin allergy. The most common type of allergic response is a local cutaneous reaction to insulin at the injection site that is evident 4 to 8 hours after the injection, is erythematous and indurated, and resolves in a few days. Other forms of dermatologic reactions to insulin include late-phase and Arthus reactions. On rare occasions, a person with diabetes may present with an anaphylactic reaction to insulin. This type of reaction is mediated by IgE antibodies and is treated with epinephrine, antihistamines, and corticosteroids. Desensitization is almost always required in these patients, even if they are switched to human insulin.

Persons who require greater than 200 U of insulin per day for more than several days in the absence of ketoacidosis, infection, or coma are said to be insulin resistant. Insulin resistance is caused by insulin-binding antibodies (IgG) but may also be observed secondary to obesity, glucocorticoid administration, Cushing's syndrome, acromegaly, and several other rare causes. Immunologically mediated insulin resistance is typically observed in persons who have been treated intermittently with insulin or who have had other allergic problems. The treatment of choice of immunologically mediated insulin resistance is treatment with either human insulin or purified pork insulin. Immunologically mediated insulin resistance usually resolves soon after the person begins treatment with a less antigenic insulin. Persons who require large doses of insulin may be treated with a special U-500 insulin available by special order from Eli Lilly and Company. In some cases the individual may be treated with a short course of corticosteroids (40 to 80 mg of prednisone or equivalent daily for 1 to 3 weeks), with improvement observed in about 75% of reported cases. Nonimmunologically mediated insulin resistance such as is observed with obesity does not respond to alterations in insulin types but may be managed by caloric restriction.

Table 6-4 Potential Pharmacokinetic and Pharmacodynamic Interactions Altering Blood Glucose Levels

Intrinsic hyperglycemic effect	Beta-blockers
	Caffeine (with large doses)
	Corticosteroids
	Diazoxide
	Diuretics (thiazide > loop > K^+ sparing)
	Epinephrine-like compounds (decongestants)
	Glucagon
	Niacin
	Oral contraceptives
	Pentamidine (beta cell toxic—see also hypoglycemia)
	Phenytoin
	Sugar-containing syrups
Intrinsic hypoglycemic effect	Beta-blockers noncardioselective > cardioselective
	Chloroquine
	Disopyramide
	Ethanol
	MAO inhibitors
	Pentamidine
Displacement of sulfonylureas from binding sites (hypoglycemia)	Clofibrate
	Phenylbutazone
	Salicylates (large doses)
	Sulfonamides
Decreased hepatic metabolism of sulfonylureas	Chloramphenicol
	Dicumerol
	Phenylbutazone
Increased hepatic metabolism of sulfonylureas	Ethanol (chronic use)
	Thyroid
Decreased renal excretion of sulfonylureas	Allopurinol
	Probenecid
	Phenylbutazone
	Salicylates
	Sulfonamides
Decreased insulin absorption	Nicotine

Drug interactions

Many compounds may alter the effects of insulin. Unexpected alterations in glucose levels, either positive or negative, may adversely affect diabetes care. Nonselective beta-blockers may cause prolonged hypoglycemia, while masking some of the signs and symptoms of hypoglycemia. Ethanol ingestion, particularly large quantities taken without food, may accentuate the effects of insulin, resulting in profound hypoglycemia. Corticosteroids and diuretics are among the list of agents that may increase blood glucose levels.

Complete medication histories should be taken on all persons being screened for potential reactions (Table 6-4).

ORAL HYPOGLYCEMIC AGENTS

There are two types of oral hypoglycemic agents—biguanides and sulfonylureas. In the United States, sulfonylurea agents are the only oral hypoglycemic medications available. Phenformin, a biguanide, was removed from the U.S. market in 1977 because of its association with lactic acidosis. The biguanide metformin was recently approved for use in the United States. Sulfonylureas can be divided into two categories—first generation and second generation. The second-generation agents were introduced later (1984) than the first-generation agents and display about 100 times the potency of the first-generation agents. However, no evidence suggests that the second-generation agents are more effective than the first-generation agents. All of the agents differ by dose, dosing interval, route of metabolism and excretion, and activity of metabolites.

Pharmacologic Effects

The exact mechanism of action of each of the sulfonylurea agents is still controversial. Sulfonylureas may work by several mechanisms of action including (1) stimulation of insulin release, (2) reduction of glucagon concentration, (3) increased sensitivity of tissue to insulin action, and (4) by a reduction in insulin extraction by the liver.[18,19] Increased insulin secretion is probably the most significant of these mechanisms of action. Because sulfonylurea agents work in concert with existing beta-cells and insulin, they are of no use in the individual with IDDM or those who have undergone a pancreatectomy.

Indications

Sulfonylurea agents are indicated in the person with NIDDM who has not responded to a reasonable course of exercise and diet therapy. Older persons, obese persons, and those with lower plasma glucose levels should be subjected to longer trials of diet and exercise than the individual who is close to ideal body weight or who has very high plasma glucose levels. Those with NIDDM who have fasting plasma glucose levels of greater than 250 mg/dl should have their glucose levels brought under control with a few weeks of insulin therapy. Once plasma glucose levels are controlled, the individual may be switched to an oral agent.

Contraindications

Individuals who meet the following criteria should not be treated with oral agents but, instead, should use insulin:
• Women with gestational diabetes
• Persons with IDDM
• Pregnant or lactating women

- Ketosis-prone individuals
- Persons in whom rapid glucose control is desired
- Persons with severe infections or surgery
- NOTE: Sulfonylureas should be used only with extreme caution in individuals with a history of allergic response to sulfa or sulfonylurea compounds.

Predictors of Outcome

Several factors have been shown to be predictive of a positive or negative response to sulfonylureas. These include age, weight, duration of disease, prior treatment with insulin, and fasting blood glucose levels.[22,29,30] Persons are more likely to respond to sulfonylurea therapy if their diagnosis of NIDDM is recent (within 5 years). Age of the individual being treated is sometimes predictive of response, with persons older than 40 years of age responding better than younger patients. Body weights of between 110% and 160% of ideal body weight and fasting blood glucose levels of less than 200 mg/dl are predictive of a positive outcome. Individuals who have in the past required insulin and were stabilized with doses of less than 40 U per day tend to respond more favorably than those who require more than 40 U per day. Physically active persons who follow a meal plan respond more favorably than sedentary persons who do not adhere to a meal plan.

Of all individuals treated with sulfonylureas, approximately 60% to 75% will respond favorably. When persons are chosen according to the criteria just described, the rate of successful treatments rises to 85%.[30] Primary treatment failures are those individuals not responding to a 1-month trial of oral sulfonylurea given at maximum doses. Of the persons who respond favorably in the initial months of treatment, 5% to 10% per year will have secondary treatment failures. After 10 years of treatment with oral sulfonylureas, 50% of the initial positive responders will become secondary treatment failures. Secondary treatment failure may be a result of the natural progression of diabetes or may be induced by other treatable causes, such as drug interactions, infection, weight gain, or surgery. For the person with secondary treatment failure without an explainable underlying cause, a different oral agent may be substituted or a small evening dose of intermediate-acting insulin may be added. Persons who do not respond initially or who have secondary treatment failure when being treated with tolazamide, tolbutamide, or acetohexamide may respond to glyburide, glipizide, or chlorpropamide. Substitution will probably not affect persons already being treated with maximum doses of glyburide, glipizide, or chlorpropamide.

Specific Agents

No evidence suggests that one sulfonylurea is the most efficacious, and, indeed, all of the agents seem to be equally effective when given in equipotent doses. The differences in the agents arise from the various pharmacokinetic and side effect profiles. Care must be taken when choosing a sulfonylurea for a particular person (Table 6-5).

Acetohexamide (Dymelor) should be dosed two times daily with total daily doses ranging from 250 to 1500 mg. It is metabolized to hydroxyhexamide, the activity of which is equal

Table 6-5   Sulfonylurea Comparison

Drug	Total daily dose	Number of doses per day	Considerations
Acetahexamide (Dymelor)	250-1500 mg	1-2	Renally excreted metabolite may have greater activity than parent compound; adjust dose for renal failure
Chlorpropamide (Diabenese)	100-500 mg	1	Highest incidence of side effects; longest duration; adjust dose in presence of renal failure
Glipizide (Glucotrol)	2.5-40 mg	1-2	Metabolized to inactive metabolites that are excreted renally
Glucotrol XL	5-20 mg	1	
Glyburide (Diabeta, Micronase)	1.25-20 mg	1-2	Metabolized to less active forms; 50% excreted renally, 50% via feces
Glynase (PresTAB)	0.75-12 mg	1-2	
Tolbutamide (Orinase)	500-3000 mg	2-3	Shortest acting; metabolites inactive
Tolazamide (Tolinase)	100-1000 mg	1-2	Converted to inactive metabolites

to or greater than the parent compound.[12,22] This active metabolite is excreted via the kidney; therefore dosage adjustment is necessary with renal failure.

Chlorpropamide (Diabenese) has the longest duration of action (24 to 72 hours) of all the sulfonylureas and is dosed once daily.[22] Daily dosage range is from 100 to 500 mg. Average elimination half-lives of chlorpropamide are ~ 33 hours; therefore time required to reach steady state is 7 to 10 days. Chlorpropamide is both metabolized to slightly active metabolites and excreted unchanged by the kidneys. Dosage adjustment is required in older individuals and in patients with renal failure. When compared with other sulfonylureas, chlorpropamide is associated with the highest incidence of severe hypoglycemic reactions (4% to 6% of patients treated). Approximately 50% of all reported cases of sulfonylurea-induced hypoglycemia can be attributed to chlorpropamide. Chlorpropamide is also noted for its disulfiram-like effect in 33% of patients treated.[26] Last, chlorpropamide has also been associated with syndrome of inappropriate antidiuretic hormone secretion (SIADH) that can result in severe hyponatremia.

Glipizide (Glucotrol, Glucotrol XL), a second-generation sulfonylurea, is normally given in daily doses of 2.5 to 40 mg. Persons receiving less than 15 mg per day may take their medication as a single dose, whereas persons taking more than 15 mg per day should take two divided doses. Glucotrol XL is available in 5- and 10-mg tablets. Normal daily doses range from 5 to 20 mg administered once daily. Glipizide is completely metabolized by the liver to inactive metabolites that are renally excreted. Twelve percent of the dose is excreted via the feces.[6]

Glyburide (Diabeta, Micronase, Glynase PresTab) is also a second-generation sulfonylurea. Its normal daily dosage range is from 1.25 to 20 mg (note a different dose range for Glynase PresTab secondary to improved bioavailability, 0.75-12 mg). Because it has an effective duration of action of up to 24 hours, glyburide may be dosed on a once-daily basis. If doses of greater than 10 mg per day are required, the dose should be divided. Glyburide is metabolized by the liver to three metabolites, one retaining about 15% activity; the metabolites are excreted by both the renal and biliary routes in a ratio of 1:1. Accumulation of the partially active metabolite may cause hypoglycemia in the patient with renal failure.[11,37]

Tolazamide (Tolinase) is administered one to two times daily with a total daily dose of 100 to 1000 mg. It is metabolized to three metabolites with varying degrees of activity that are renally excreted.[18] Tolazamide has a slower absorption rate than the other sulfonylureas and therefore displays a delayed onset of action.

Tolbutamide (Orinase) is the least potent and shortest acting of all the sulfonylureas. It must be administered two to three times daily with a total daily dose of between 500 and 3000 mg.[12,22] Tolbutamide is metabolized to less active forms that are excreted renally. Tolbutamide may be a reasonable choice for the person in whom prolonged hypoglycemia is likely.

Side Effects

Overall, sulfonylureas are very well tolerated, with only 2% of patients experiencing side effects sufficient to warrant discontinuance of the medication.[22] The most common side effects associated with the sulfonylurea agents include hypoglycemia, a diuretic effect (sometimes leading to hyponatremia), gastrointestinal disturbances, and a disulfiram-like effect. Less common adverse effects include rashes, pruritus, and, rarely, hematologic reactions (hemolytic anemia and bone marrow aplasia).

The disulfiram-like activity of chlorpropamide has been well documented and occurs in approximately one third of individuals who ingest ethanol while being treated with chlorpropamide. This reaction occurs in fewer than 5% of patients taking tolbutamide and at an even lower frequency in those being treated with the second-generation agents.

The complete mechanism for this reaction is still the subject of research, but most agree that chlorpropamide inhibits acetaldehyde dehydrogenase, with a resultant build up of acetaldehyde (Fig. 6-6). The reaction is elicited about 15 minutes after the ingestion of ethanol and is associated with a flushed and tingling sensation in the neck that may extend to the arms. Occasionally the flush will be accompanied by headache, nausea, and breathlessness. The reaction, which is not dose dependent, rarely progresses to vomiting and hypotension; tolerance does not usually develop.[24]

Hypoglycemia is the most common, severe reaction associated with sulfonylurea administration. In one study it was estimated that 20% of treated persons experienced a minimum of one severe episode of hypoglycemia during a 6-month evaluation period.[23] Chlorpropamide, the sulfonylurea with the longest history of use and the longest duration of action, is responsible for 50% of recorded cases of hypoglycemia.[26] Risk factors for the

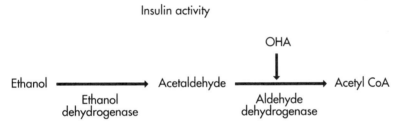

Fig. 6-6   Oral hypoglycemic agent–induced disulfiram-like reaction.

development of hypoglycemia include advanced age (greater than 60 years), poor nutrition, alcohol use, multidrug regimens, hepatic dysfunction, and renal dysfunction. Sulfonylurea-induced hypoglycemia can be severe and prolonged, requiring treatment with intravenous glucose.[18]

Chlorpropamide and tolbutamide have been associated with an increased release and increased activity of antidiuretic hormone. Chlorpropamide has been linked to syndrome of inappropriate secretion of antidiuretic hormone (SIADH) and may cause hyponatremia severe enough to elicit weakness, headache, nausea, vomiting, confusion, and even coma. Risk factors for the development of SIADH include age (greater than 60 years), gender (female > male), and diuretic use. Tolazamide, acetohexamide, glyburide, and glipizide all exert a mild diuretic effect.

Drug Interactions

Several varieties of drug interactions are possible with the sulfonylurea agents. Pharmaco-dynamic interactions are possible with any medication that may increase or decrease blood glucose levels. Pharmacokinetic interactions can occur with agents that cause displacement of sulfonylureas from plasma protein-binding sites (which is less problematic with second-generation agents), compounds that alter hepatic enzyme activity (either ↑ or ↓), or medications that alter renal elimination (see Table 6-4).

Combination Therapy

Multiple studies have evaluated the use of combination therapy with insulin and sulfonylureas. Insulin requirements may be reduced in the person who receives both insulin and sulfonylureas. In the majority of sulfonylurea treatment failures, cost-effective treatment that achieves better glycemic control is possible with the use of insulin alone when appropriate doses of insulin are administered. Combination therapy is probably indicated only in persons who fail optimal regimens of oral agents and insulin given independently. A metaanalysis of combination therapy studies recently concluded, "Combination insulin-sulfonylurea therapy leads to modest improvement in glycemic control compared with insulin therapy alone. With combined therapy, lower insulin doses may achieve similar control. Obese patients with higher fasting C-peptides may be more likely to respond than others."

CASE PRESENTATION
Case Study I

A.H. is a 57-year-old white man referred by a primary care physician to a diabetes clinic for evaluation. He was diagnosed as obese and a non-insulin-dependent diabetic about 15 months ago. Despite numerous attempts with diet control, A.H. failed to have satisfactory weight reduction. His fasting blood glucose concentrations have risen lately and ranged from 180 to 195 mg/dl over the past few weeks. His glycohemoglobin is 10% (normal, 4% to 8%). He complains of weakness, fatigue, increased urination, and increased thirst.

The patient has a past medical history of hypertension for 10 years and type II diabetes mellitus for 16 months. The patient has no remarkable past surgical history. The patient's family history is positive for diabetes and hypertension. The patient smokes one pack of cigarettes per day ($\times$ 30 years) and consumes 2 to 3 beers per day.

Current medications are hydrochlorothiazide 50 mg per day and propranolol 40 mg four times a day.

The physical examination of the patient reveals an obese man in no apparent distress who weighs 90 kg (ideal body weight 68 kg). The patient's blood pressure sitting is 154/94 (previous BP ranged from 150/92 to 160/96), with a pulse rate of 88, and a respiratory rate of 14.

The patient's current laboratory findings are within normal limits except for serum creatinine 1.9 mg/dl (normal, 0.6 to 1.3), BUN 21 mg/dl (normal, 10 to 20), and total cholesterol 279 mg/dl (normal, <200).

DISCUSSION

The patient in this case has several problems that should be considered: hyperglycemia, hypertension, weight control, hypercholesterolemia, impaired renal function, and alcohol and cigarette use.

Hyperglycemia and hypertension. The patient's blood glucose is not being reasonably controlled with diet and exercise. Overt symptoms, which include weakness, fatigue, polyuria, and polydipsia, are present. A review of the patient's medication list reveals that he is currently being treated with two drugs, hydrochlorothiazide and propranolol, both of which may cause problems in this patient. Hydrochlorothiazide may cause hyperglycemia, hypercholesterolemia, hypertriglyceridemia, and sexual dysfunction in this patient. Propranolol may cause hyperglycemia, hypertriglyceridemia, reductions in HDL cholesterol, a reduction in the symptoms accompanying hypoglycemia, an impairment in the counteregulatory response to hypoglycemia, and sexual dysfunction. In this case it would probably be prudent to discontinue both drugs. The hydrochlorothiazide could be discontinued at once, whereas the propranolol should be tapered slowly over several days. During this period, hypertensive therapy with an ACE inhibitor, a calcium channel blocker, or an $alpha_1$-antagonist could be initiated and appropriately titrated. Although the ACE inhibitors are usually the drugs of choice in this instance, and may be in this case as well, one should rule out bilateral renal artery stenosis before initiation of therapy or follow the patient's progress after initiation of a small dose. These changes in therapy will probably result in a downward reduction of glucose concentrations (possibly 5% to 15%) but in all likelihood will not result in normalization of blood sugar levels. It would be appropriate to start administration of sulfonylurea at this time. Chlorpropamide and acetohexamide should not be considered because of the patient's reduced renal function. Glipizide (2.5 mg), glyburide (1.25 mg), tolazamide (100 mg), or tolbutamide (500 mg) daily could be used initially. Tolbutamide should probably be avoided because of its need for administration two or three times daily. The dose of the sulfonylurea should be titrated over the next 2 weeks until a reasonable fasting blood sugar is obtained.

Weight control. The patient should receive counseling from a dietitian. The patient should understand that oral medication does not replace the need to follow a diet and exercise program. Appropriate goals for weight loss, diet, and exercise should be set for the patient.

Hypercholesterolemia. The patient's elevated cholesterol should be further worked up with an appropriate lipid panel. The patient's cholesterol level may drop some as blood glucose levels are reduced but more than likely will not drop into the normal range. If pharmacotherapy for dyslipidemia is indicated, one should avoid the use of niacin since it may worsen the patient's level of glycemic control. Choice of medication will be based on the patient's specific lipid profile and metabolic parameters.

Impaired renal function. The patient displays evidence of impaired renal function as evidenced by his elevated creatinine and blood urea nitrogen. The serum creatinine of 1.9 mg/dl suggests a creatinine clearance of about 50 to 60 ml/min—well below what would be expected for a patient of this age. A careful workup of this problem should be carried out. If the diagnostic workup suggests diabetic nephropathy (as evidenced by proteinuria), the patient may benefit from ACE inhibitor therapy and may benefit from improved glycemic control. The initiation of ACE inhibitors in patients with renal dysfunction should be closely monitored.

Alcohol and cigarette use. Alcohol use, although not absolutely contraindicated in patients with diabetes, should be very controlled. Concurrent use of ethanol and hypoglycemic drugs may result in profound hypoglycemia. The patient should be counseled that if he is going to consume ethanol, he should do so only in small quantities (1 to 2 oz) per setting, should do so only once or twice a week, and should never drink alcohol in a fasting state. The caloric intake should also be considered. In addition, ethanol use may result in a flushing reaction when taken in the presence of sulfonylureas (particularly chlorpropamide). Cigarette smoking should be discouraged, and the patient should be offered support by any possible means if he elects to attempt cessation. This man carries virtually every cardiovascular risk factor known (hyperglycemia, hyperlipidemia, hypertension, male, cigarette smoker, obesity, family history) and would probably benefit greatly from cigarette cessation.

Case Study 2

A.B. is a 23-year-old woman with a 10-year history of type I diabetes. Prior to 1 year ago she had received no formal diabetes education and had not been evaluated by a specialist. One year ago after a hospitalization for DKA she completed a week-long diabetes education program and began seeing an endocrinologist.

The patient returns to the clinic for follow-up of her diabetes. She is currently testing her blood sugar four times daily (fasting, preprandial, and at bedtime) and is being treated with injections of NPH/Regular insulin two times daily.

Physical examination reveals that all vital signs are within normal limits. Urine dipstick shows no ketones but 2+ proteinuria. Her glycohemoglobin is 9.5% (normal, 4% to 8%). The patient's current laboratory findings are within normal limits (including serum creatinine and BUN).

The patient is currently taking the following: insulin (human) NPH/Regular 16/8 U every morning and 14/6 U every evening; 1 multivitamin orally daily.

She has self-monitored her blood glucose for the past 3 days:

	Fasting	Prelunch	Predinner	Bedtime
Monday	257 mg/dl	120 mg/dl	105 mg/dl	98 mg/dl
Tuesday	171 mg/dl	99 mg/dl	92 mg/dl	101 mg/dl
Wednesday	188 mg/dl	110 mg/dl	115 mg/dl	91 mg/dl

DISCUSSION

This patient has several problems that warrant further workup, including fasting hyperglycemia and probable microvascular disease.

Hyperglycemia. The patient's blood sugar levels are elevated in the morning; however, blood sugar levels during the remainder of the day are acceptable. The early morning hyperglycemia could be caused by high caloric intake in the evening, inadequate intermediate-acting insulin dose in the evening, or the Somogyi effect (posthypoglycemic hyperglycemia). It would be appropriate to question the patient about possible signs of early morning hypoglycemia and have her check her blood sugar between 2 and 3 AM for 1 or 2 nights. If the patient is hypoglycemic at 3 AM, several options could be considered. First, one could lower her evening NPH dose by one to two units. Second, her evening dose of NPH could be taken at bedtime rather than at dinner. This shifts the peak activity of the dose from between 2 and 3 AM to between 6 and 7AM, when the patient is awake and consuming breakfast. Third, the patient could eat a snack at bedtime and not change the insulin regimen. If, on the other hand, the patient's blood sugar levels were normal or elevated between 2 and 3AM, one could either reduce caloric intake in the evening, add some exercise to the evening, or increase the insulin dose 1 to 2 units.

Microvascular disease. Dipstick testing showed that the patient has significant proteinuria. This finding should be followed up by a 24-hour urine collection. If the patient has significant proteinuria and etiologic factors other than diabetes are ruled out, therapy with an ACE inhibitor should be considered. ACE inhibitors have been shown to slow down the progression of diabetic nephropathy, but increase the time to end-stage renal disease (ESRD) and death. In addition to ACE-inhibition therapy, strict glycemic control also reduces the risk of rapid escalation of this problem.

In addition, this patient should be evaluated by an ophthalmologist on an annual basis.

REFERENCES

1. *A study of insulin supply and demand.* A Report of the National Diabetes Advisory Board, publication No. 78-1588, Washington, DC, 1978, US Dept of Health, Education, and Welfare.
2. Agner T and others: Remission in IDDM: prospective study of basal C-peptide and insulin dose in 268 consecutive patients, *Diabetes Care* 10:164, 1987.
3. American Diabetes Association: Clinical practice recommendations, *Diabetes Care* (suppl 1) 13:28-31, 1990.
4. American Diabetes Association: *Physicians guide to insulin-dependent (type I) diabetes,* Alexandria, Va, 1988, The Association.
5. American Diabetes Association: *Physicians guide to insulin-dependent (type II) diabetes,* Alexandria, Va, 1988, The Association.
6. Balant L and others: Behaviour of glibenclamide on repeated administration to diabetic patients, *Eur J Clin Pharmacol* 11:19-25, 1977.
7. Banting FG and others: Pancreatic extracts in the treatment of diabetes mellitus: a preliminary report, *Can Med Assoc J* 12:141-146, 1922.
8. Binder C and others: Insulin pharmacokinetics, *Diabetes Care* 7:188-199, 1984.
9. Campbell RK: Why you've got to become involved in diabetes patient care, *US Pharm Guide Diabetes Manage* Nov. suppl:36-47, 1988.
10. The Diabetes Control and Complications Trial Research Group: The effect of intensive treatment of diabetes on the development and progression of long-term complications in insulin-dependent diabetes mellitus, *N Engl J Med* 14:977-986, 1993.
11. Fabre J and others: Hypoglycemic activity of the main metabolite of glibenclamide: influence of renal insufficiency, *Kidney Int* 13:435, 1978 (abstract).
12. Ferner RE, Chaplin S: The relationship between the pharmacokinetics and the pharmacodynamic effects of oral hypoglycaemic drugs, *Clin Pharmacokinet* 12:379-401, 1987.
13. Frank BH and others: The production of human proinsulin and its transformation to human insulin and C-peptide. In Rich DH, Gross R, editors: Peptides: synthesis-structure-function. Proceedings of the Seventh American Peptide Symposium, Rockford, Ill, 1981.
14. Fredichs H, Creutzfeldt W: Hypoglycemia: insulin secreting tumors, *Clin Endocrinol Metab* 5:747, 1976.
15. Gale E, Tattersall R: Unrecognized hypoglycemia in insulin-treated diabetes, *Lancet* 1:1049-1052, 1979.
16. Galloway JA and others: Mixtures of intermediate-acting insulin (NPH and Lente) with regular insulin: an update. In Skyler JS, editor: *Insulin Update: 1982, Proceedings of a symposium,* Key Biscayne, Fla, December 7-9, 1981.
17. Galloway JA, Potvin JH, Shuman CR, editors: *Diabetes mellitus,* ed 9, Indianapolis, Ind, 1988, Eli Lilly.
18. Gerich JE: Oral hypoglycemic agents, *N Engl J Med* 321:1231-1245, 1989.
19. Groop LC: Sulfonylureas in NIDDM, *Diabetes Care* 15(6):737-754, 1992.
20. Guyton AC: *Textbook of medical physiology,* Philadelphia, 1986, WB Saunders.
21. Hallas-Moller K: The Lente insulins, *Diabetes* 5:7-14, 1956.
22. Jackson JE, Bressler R: Clinical pharmacology of sulfonylurea hypoglycaemic agents, *Drugs* 22:211-245; 295-320, 1981.
23. Jennings AM, Wilson RM, Ward JD: Symptomatic hypoglycemia in NIDDM patients treated with oral

hypoglycemic agents, *Diabetes Care* 12:203-208, 1989.

24. Johnston C and others: Chlorpropamide-alcohol flush: the case in favor, *Diabetologia* 26:1, 1984.

25. Kemmer FW and others: Absorption kinetics of semisynthetic human insulin and biosynthetic (recombinant DNA) human insulin, *Diabetes Care* 5(suppl 2):23, 1982.

26. Koda-Kimble MA, Rotblatt MD: Diabetes mellitus. In Young LYY, Koda-Kimble MA, editors: *Applied therapeutics, the clinical use of drugs,* ed 4, Vancouver, Wash, 1988, Applied Therapeutics.

27. Krayenbuhl C, Rosenberg T: Crystalline protamine insulin, *Rep Steno Mem Hosp* 1:60-73, 1946.

28. Krosnick A: Newer insulins, insulin allergies and the clinical uses of insulins. In Bergman M, editor: *Principles of diabetes management,* New Hyde Park, NY, 1986, Medical Examination Publishing.

29. Leahy JL and others: Chronic hyperglycemia is associated with impaired glucose influence on insulin secretion: a study of normal rats using chronic in vivo glucose infusions, *J Clin Invest* 77:908-915, 1986.

30. Lebovitz H: Clinical utility of oral hypoglycemic agents in the management of patients with noninsulin–dependent diabetes mellitus, *Am J Med* 75 (suppl 5B):94-99, 1983.

31. Markussen J and others: Human insulin (Novo): chemistry and characteristics, *Diabetes Care* 6(suppl 1):4-8, 1983.

32. National Institutes of Health, National Institute of Diabetes and Digestive and Kidney Diseases: *Diabetes Prevention Trial—Type I (DPT-1) Protocol,* Bethesda, Md, 1993.

33. Nolte MS and others: Reduced solubility of short-acting soluble insulins when mixed with longer-acting insulins, *Diabetes* 32:1177-1181, 1983.

34. Notes from the Meeting of the Medical Advisory Board of the Food and Drug Administration Concerning Standards for Insulin Purity, Washington, DC, December 1979.

35. Novo-Nordisk Product Information, Princeton, NJ.

36. Olsson PO, Arnqvist H, Von Schenck H: Miscibility of human semisynthetic regular and Lente insulin and human biosynthetic regular and NPH insulin, *Diabetes Care* 10:473-477, 1987.

37. Pearson JG and others: Pharmacokinetic disposition of 14C-Glyburide in patients with varying renal function, *Clin Pharmacol Ther* 39:318-324, 1986.

38. Permutt MA, Kipnis DM: Insulin biosynthesis. I. On the mechanism of glucose stimulation, *J Biol Chem* 247:1194, 1972.

39. Polonsky K, Rubenstein A: C-peptide as a measure of the secretion and hepatic extraction of insulin: pitfalls and limitations, *Diabetes* 33:486, 1984.

40. Pramming S and others: Absorption of soluble and isophane semisynthetic human and porcine insulin in insulin-dependent diabetic subjects, *Acta Endocrinol* 105:215, 1984.

41. Pugh J and others: Is combination sulfonylurea and insulin therapy useful in NIDDM patients? *Diabetes Care* 15(8):953-959, 1992.

42. Robbins D, Tager H, Rubenstein A: Biologic and clinical importance of proinsulin, *N Engl J Med* 310:1165, 1984.

43. Schade DS, Santigo JV, Skyler J: Intensive insulin therapy, Princeton, NJ, 1983, Excerpta Medica.

44. Steil CF: Drug therapy for diabetes mellitus, *US Pharm Guide Diabetes Manage* Nov Suppl:36-47, 1988.

45. White J, Campbell K: Guide to mixing insulins, *Hosp Pharm* 26(12):1046, 1991.

7 Microvascular Complications of Diabetes

William H. Herman and Douglas A. Greene

INTRODUCTION

Microvascular complications have a far-reaching impact on the individual with diabetes. Research in this area has been critical to defining the course of these complications and identifying avenues for preventive care and education, diagnosis, and treatment.

GLYCEMIC CONTROL AND DIABETIC MICROVASCULAR AND NEUROPATHIC COMPLICATIONS

For many decades, cross-sectional and observational studies demonstrated an association between hyperglycemia and microvascular and neuropathic complications. Unfortunately, because of their design, these studies could not determine whether this relationship was causal and they could not weigh the relative benefits and risks of treatment to improve glycemic control. In the early 1980s the methods to achieve improved glycemic control (self-monitoring of blood glucose, intensive insulin therapy) and the methods to assess the impact of therapy (glycohemoglobin, stereo retinal photography) became available and allowed for the conduct of prospective clinical trials.

The early randomized clinical trials of glycemic control involved too few patients and were too brief to determine whether the different treatments changed the rates of development of complications. The most consistent findings were that patients who initiated tight control had an early worsening of their retinopathy. There was some suggestion of decreased long-term progression of retinopathy and a more clear-cut decrease in the risk for the development of microalbuminuria. A recent metaanalysis of these and other small, short-term trials estimated the impact of intensive blood glucose control on the progression of diabetic retinopathy and nephropathy in insulin-dependent diabetes mellitus (IDDM).[123a] In the intensive therapy group the risk of retinopathy progression was insignificantly higher after 6 to 12 months of intensive therapy but approximately 50% lower after more than

---

CHAPTER OBJECTIVES

- Review the relationship between glycemic control and the development of microvascular complications.
- Summarize the current state of research with regard to the occurrence and treatment of microvascular complications.
- Describe the clinical manifestations of microvascular complications.
- Discuss the pathogenesis of microvascular complications.
- Describe the diagnostic criteria for complications.
- Summarize the management and treatment of microvascular complications.
- Review the goals of preventive education and care.

---

2 years of intensive therapy. The risk of nephropathy progression was decreased by more than 60%.

The Stockholm Diabetes Intervention Study was initiated in 1982 to compare the effects of intensified insulin treatment and standard treatment on the progression of the microvascular and neuropathic complications of IDDM.[108a] Forty-eight patients were assigned to receive intensified insulin treatment, and 54 patients were assigned to receive standard insulin treatment. At entry, glycohemoglobin (normal range 3.9% to 5.7%) was approximately 9.5% in both treatment groups. During the study, the mean value was 7.1 ± 0.7 in the intensified treatment group and 8.5 ± 0.7 in the standard treatment group. After 8 years, serious retinopathy developed in 27% of patients in the intensified treatment group and in 52% of those in the standard treatment group. Nephropathy developed in 2% of the patients in the intensified treatment group and 18% of those in the standard treatment group. None of the patients in the intensified treatment group and 12% in the standard treatment group developed glomerular filtration rates below the normal range. Changes in symptoms of neuropathy and sensory thresholds did not differ between groups, but deterioration of nerve conduction velocities was greater in the standard treatment group than in the intensified treatment group. This was the first prospective study to demonstrate that intensified insulin therapy slowed the progression of microvascular complications in IDDM.

The Diabetes Control and Complications Trial (DCCT)[28a] was a multicenter, randomized clinical trial designed to compare the impact of intensive and conventional diabetes therapy on the development and progression of the early microvascular and neuropathic complications of IDDM. It was designed to be of sufficient size and duration to answer two separate but related questions: (1) Will intensive therapy prevent the development of diabetic retinopathy in patients with no retinopathy (primary prevention)? (2) Will intensive therapy slow the progression of early retinopathy (secondary intervention)?

Subjects eligible for participation in the DCCT had IDDM, were between the ages of 13 and 39 years, and had no evidence of severe diabetic complications, hypertension, or dyslipidemia. Subjects eligible for the primary prevention cohort had IDDM for 1 to 5 years, no evidence of diabetic retinopathy, and no microalbuminuria (urinary albumin excretion [UAE] <40 mg/24 hrs). Subjects eligible for the secondary intervention cohort had IDDM for 1 to 15 years, very-mild-to-moderate nonproliferative retinopathy, and no evidence of clinical nephropathy (UAE <200 mg/24 hrs).

In the DCCT, therapy was carried out by expert teams of nurses, dietitians, behavioral specialists, and diabetologists; and the time, effort, and costs required were considerable. Conventional therapy consisted of one or two daily injections of insulin, daily self-monitoring of urine or blood glucose, clinic visits every 3 months, and a comprehensive program of education about diabetes. Conventional therapy did not include or encourage daily adjustments in the insulin dose in response to self-monitoring data. Intensive therapy involved the administration of insulin by three or more injections daily, or by external pump, self-monitoring of blood glucose four times daily, weekly telephone calls, and monthly clinic visits. The insulin dosage was adjusted according to the results of self-monitoring, dietary intake, and anticipated exercise to achieve preprandial blood glucose concentrations between 70 and 120 mg/dl, 90-minute postprandial concentrations less than 180 mg/dl, a weekly 3 AM measurement greater than 65 mg/dl, and a hemoglobin A_{1c} measured monthly, within the normal range (<6.05%).

A total of 1441 patients were recruited at 29 centers between 1983 and 1989. At baseline the mean age of the subjects was 26 years. The mean duration of IDDM was 2.6 years in the primary prevention cohort and approximately 8.8 years in the secondary intervention cohort. In June 1993, after an average follow-up of 6.5 years (range, 3 to 9 years), the trial was terminated. Ninety-nine percent of patients completed the study. Treatment group crossover was uncommon, and follow-up was complete. Patients received their assigned treatment more than 97% of the time, and more than 95% of scheduled examinations were completed.

At baseline, mean HbA_{1c} was approximately 8.9% (normal <6.05%). HbA_{1c} reached a nadir at 6 months in patients receiving intensive therapy. A statistically significant difference in average HbA_{1c} was maintained between the intensive therapy and conventional therapy groups in both cohorts. Almost one half of the patients receiving intensive therapy achieved the goal of a HbA_{1c} value of 6.05% or less at least once during the study, but fewer than 5% maintained an average value in the target range.

In the primary prevention cohort, the cumulative incidence of retinopathy, defined as a three-step change or more on fundus photography that was sustained over a 6-month period, was similar in the two treatment groups until approximately 3 years, when the cumulative incidence curves began to separate (Fig. 7-1, *A*). From 5 years onward, the cumulative incidence of retinopathy was approximately 50% less in the intensive therapy group than in the conventional therapy group. Intensive therapy reduced the adjusted mean risk of retinopathy by 76%, and the reduction in risk increased with time.

In the secondary intervention cohort, patients in the intensive therapy group had a higher cumulative incidence of retinopathy during the first year than did those in the conventional therapy group, but they had a lower cumulative incidence beginning at 3 years and continuing for the rest of the study (Fig. 7-1, *B*). Intensive therapy reduced

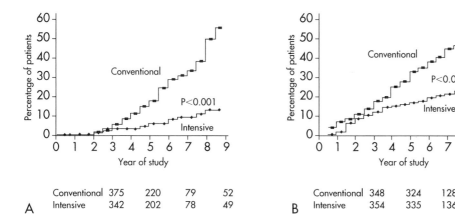

Fig. 7-1 Cumulative incidence of sustained change in retinopathy in patients with IDDM receiving intensive or conventional therapy. **A,** In the primary prevention cohort, intensive therapy reduced the adjusted mean risk of the onset of retinopathy by 76% during the course of the study, as compared with conventional therapy (P <0.001). **B,** In the secondary intervention cohort, intensive therapy reduced the adjusted mean risk of progression of retinopathy by 54% as compared with conventional therapy (P <0.001). The numbers of patients in each therapy group who were evaluated at years 3, 5, 7, and 9 are shown below the graphs. (Modified from Nathan DM and others: *N Engl J Med* 329:981, 1993.)

the average risk of progression by 54%. Intensive therapy reduced the adjusted risk of severe nonproliferative and proliferative retinopathy by 47% and the risk of treatment with photocoagulation by 56%. The reduction in risk of retinopathy with intensive therapy was evident in all subgroups of patients, in all clinics, and in both the primary prevention and secondary intervention cohorts.

In the primary prevention cohort, intensive therapy reduced the mean adjusted risk of microalbuminuria by 34%. In the secondary intervention cohort, intensive therapy reduced the risk of microalbuminuria by 43% and the risk of albuminuria by 56%.

In patients in the primary prevention cohort who did not have neuropathy (defined as peripheral sensorimotor neuropathy on physical examination by a study neurologist plus either abnormal nerve conduction in two different peripheral nerves or unequivocally abnormal autonomic test results) at baseline, intensive therapy reduced the appearance of neuropathy at 5 years by 69% (to 3% versus 10% in the conventional therapy group). Similarly, in the secondary intervention cohort, intensive therapy reduced the appearance of clinical neuropathy at 5 years by 57% (to 7% versus 16%).

The DCCT was not designed to assess impact of therapy on macrovascular disease. The relative youth of the patients made the detection of treatment-related differences in macrovascular events unlikely. When all major macrovascular events were combined, intensive therapy reduced the risk of macrovascular disease by 41% (to 0.5 events per 100 patient-years versus 0.8 events per patient-year), but the difference was not significant. Intensive therapy was, however, associated with a 34% reduction in the develoment of hypercholesterolemia, defined as a serum concentraton of low-density lipoprotein cholesterol greater than 160 mg/dl, and small but insignificant reductions in the development of hypertriglyceridemia and hypertension.

Intensive therapy was not without side effects. In the intensive therapy group, there were 62 hypoglycemic episodes per 100 patient-years in which assistance was required in the provision of treatment. This compared with 19 such episodes per 100 patient-years in the conventional therapy group. Despite the higher risk of hypoglycemia with intensive therapy, there was no difference between groups in the occurrence of clinically important changes in neuropsychologic function or quality of life. Weight gain was also a problem with intensive therapy. The incidence of overweight, defined as a body weight more than 120% above the ideal, was 12.7 cases per 100 patient-years in the intensive therapy group and 9.3 per 100 patient-years in the conventional therapy group. The event rates for diabetic ketoacidosis did not differ between groups.

The results of the DCCT prove that in IDDM, hyperglycemia causes microvascular and neuropathic complications and that intensive therapy both delays the onset and slows the progression of clinically important retinopathy, nephropathy, and neuropathy. The DCCT confirmed that implementation of intensive therapy is associated with an early worsening of retinopathy, especially in those with existing retinopathy, but confirmed the long-term benefits of such treatment. The DCCT also demonstrated that the risk of severe hypoglycemia is three times higher with intensive therapy but did not suggest that this risk outweighed the benefits of reduced microvascular and neurologic complications in this population of patients.

The DCCT Research Group has recommended that most patients with IDDM be treated with closely monitored intensive regimens, with the goal of maintaining glycemic control as close to the nondiabetic range as safely possible. This therapy should be carried out by an expert multidisciplinary team. Because of early worsening of retinopathy, patients with nonproliferative retinopathy beginning intensive therapy should be followed closely by their ophthalmologists. Because of the risk of hypoglycemia, intensive therapy should be implemented with caution in patients with repeated severe hypoglycemia or unawareness of hypoglycemia. The DCCT research group also cautioned that the benefit/risk ratio of intensive therapy might be less favorable in patients younger than 13 years and in those with advanced complications. Suboptimal glycemic control before puberty may be associated with less risk of microvascular complications than is suboptimal glycemic control after puberty. Likewise, the long-term sequelae of severe hypoglycemia may be more severe in young children than in older children and adults. Patients with blindness caused by diabetes and end-stage renal disease are less likely to benefit from intensive therapy than those with less advanced microvascular complications. Likewise, those with unstable cerebrovascular or cardiovascular disease are more likely to have serious sequelae of hypoglycemia when compared with those without macrovascular disease. The DCCT research group took a rather narrow view of the implications of the DCCT for NIDDM. The American Diabetes Association (ADA) has taken a broader perspective on the implications of the DCCT for diabetes management.[4]

Unfortunately, no convincing prospective data support a beneficial effect of intensive therapy on long-term complications in NIDDM. The United Kingdom Prospective Diabetes Study (UKPDS) is an ongoing multicenter, prospective, randomized clinical trial designed to determine whether improved blood glucose control will prevent complications and reduce morbidity and mortality in patients with newly diagnosed NIDDM. The trial was started in 1977 and by March 1991 had recruited a complement of 5100 patients. All were treated initially by diet, and those who remained hyperglycemic were randomly allocated to diet, sulfonylurea, or insulin. Obese patients were also randomized to metformin. Patients who failed monotherapy with sulfonylurea were further randomized to combination therapy, those who failed monotherapy with metformin also received sulfonylurea, and those who developed hyperglycemic symptoms or fasting hyperglycemia on maximal oral therapy were transferred to insulin therapy.[120a] Although originally planned to terminate in 1994, with a median follow-up of 9 years (range 3 to 16 years), the trial has recently been extended until 1997.

In the absence of definitive clinical trials, practitioners have been somewhat reluctant to take an aggressive approach to the treatment of hyperglycemia in NIDDM. Some of this reluctance is clearly fueled by concern about the risks of intensive insulin therapy. In both IDDM and NIDDM, the potential risks of intensive insulin therapy include hypoglycemia, weight gain, hypertension, hyperlipidemia, and accelerated atherogenesis. Data from clinical trials suggest that hypoglycemia is less often associated with intensive therapy in NIDDM than in IDDM, and although weight gain is a problem in NIDDM, it is not unique to insulin treatment. In NIDDM, weight gain occurs with either insulin or sulfonylurea therapy in proportion to the degree of improvement in glycemic control.[45a] Epidemiologic studies have shown associations between hyperinsulinemia and hypertension, hyperlipidemia, and cardiovascular disease.[44c,106b,109a,125a] This has led some to question the appropriateness of insulin administration to patients with NIDDM, since the resulting iatrogenic hyperinsulinemia may exacerbate atherosclerosis, the major cause of morbidity and mortality in NIDDM. Other epidemiologic studies have not found this association and have suggested that hyperglycemia itself and closely associated risk factors including obesity, hypertension, and lipid abnormalities, may be more important CVD risk factors than insulin level.[44a,82b,125b]

In summary, it is now clearly established that intensive therapy of patients with IDDM delays the onset and slows the progression of clinically important retinopathy, nephropathy, and neuropathy by 35% to more than 70%. The risk of severe hypoglycemia is approximately three times higher with such therapy, and such therapy is associated with weight gain. In IDDM, the reduction in microvascular and neurologic complications outweighs the risk of these adverse effects.

Although no convincing prospective data support a beneficial effect of intensive therapy on long-term complications in NIDDM, treatment of NIDDM should be comprehensive and address glycemic control and other important cardiovascular risk factors including hypertension, hyperlipidemia, and cigarette smoking. The therapeutic approach to hyperglycemia may include diet, physical activity, sulfonylureas, biguanides, and insulin. Physical activity is especially important because it provides specific treatment for many of the major physiologic abnormalities associated with NIDDM. Current evidence does not warrant withholding insulin therapy or compromising on dosage when it is needed.

DIABETIC RETINOPATHY

Diabetic eye disease is the leading cause of new cases of legal blindness in American adults. Sight-threatening retinopathy may exist even when a patient has good vision. Better

---

BOX 7-1

CLINICAL MANIFESTATIONS OF DIABETIC RETINOPATHY

Nonproliferative diabetic retinopathy

Microaneurysms
Blot hemorrhages
Hard exudates
Occasional soft exudates

Preproliferative diabetic retinopathy

Multiple large blot hemorrhages
Multiple soft exudates
Venous beading and venous duplications
Multiple intraretinal microvascular abnormalities

Proliferative diabetic retinopathy

New vessels on the disc (NVD)
New vessels elsewhere (NVE)
Fibrous tissue proliferation
Preretinal or vitreous hemorrhage

---

understanding of the risk factors for retinopathy and recent advances in treatment have provided the rationale for developing an approach to prevent visual loss. This approach requires that patients with diabetes who are at risk for visual loss be systematically examined, referred, and treated.[53]

Clinical Manifestations

The clinical manifestations of diabetic retinopathy are outlined in Box 7-1. The earliest clinical sign of diabetic retinopathy seen with the ophthalmoscope is the retinal microaneurysm, a small out-pouching of a retinal capillary that appears as a small red dot in the retina. Retinal microaneurysms are usually not a threat to vision. Retinal blot hemorrhages and hard exudates may also occur early in the course of diabetic retinopathy. Both may occur in other types of retinal disease, especially hypertension, and neither is specific for diabetes. Retinal blot hemorrhages, which are larger than microaneurysms, are round with blurred edges. They represent hemorrhagic infarcts secondary to retinal ischemia and result from extravasation of blood from retinal capillaries into the retina. Retinal hard exudates or waxy exudates are variable in size, usually yellow in color, and may be scattered, aggregated, or ringlike (circinate) in their distribution. Hard exudates are thought to arise from leakage of lipoprotein material from retinal capillaries into the outer retinal layer.

In more advanced retinopathy, closure of retinal capillaries and arterioles may occur. These changes cause ischemic swelling of the nerve fiber layer of the retina. These appear as white or grayish white areas with ill-defined borders and are termed soft exudates or cotton wool spots. Other manifestations of advanced nonproliferative diabetic retinopathy include intraretinal microvascular abnormalities (IRMA), venous beading, and venous duplications.

Proliferative diabetic retinopathy is a more advanced form of retinopathy characterized by proliferation of new vessels and fibrous tissue. Contraction of fibrous tissue may be associated with hemorrhage or retinal detachment as a result of traction. Proliferative retinopathy is thought to be associated with retinal hypoxia. The appearance of cotton wool spots and other manifestations of retinal ischemia should thus be considered warning signs of impending proliferative diabetic retinopathy.[66-68]

Pathogenesis

The primary effect of diabetes on the retina appears to be on its capillaries. Functional changes in the retinal circulation precede structural changes. These include alterations in retinal blood flow and breakdown in the blood retinal barrier. The mechanisms responsible for the structural changes associated with diabetic retinopathy are not well understood. Pericyte dropout has been suggested as a cause of microaneurysm formation. Alterations in aldose reductase activity in vascular endothelial cells, nonenzymatic glycosylation of retinal proteins, defects in vascular autoregulation, and hemodynamic factors including increased red blood cell and platelet aggregation, have been suggested as possible pathophysiologic mechanisms leading to retinal ischemia.

Diagnostic Criteria

Nonproliferative diabetic retinopathy may be diagnosed when retinal microaneurysms, hard exudates, blot hemorrhages, soft exudates, or intraretinal microvascular abnormalities are present.

Preproliferative retinopathy is a more advanced form of nonproliferative diabetic retinopathy. Preproliferative retinopathy may be diagnosed when multiple soft exudates, venous caliber abnormalities, and intraretinal microvascular abnormalities are present. Eyes with preproliferative changes have an increased risk of progressing to proliferative retinopathy.[53]

Proliferative retinopathy may be diagnosed when new vessels develop on the surface layer of the retina. Prospective studies have defined characteristics associated with proliferative diabetic retinopathy that increase the risk of severe visual loss. These characteristics, termed *high-risk characteristics,* are as follows: (1) the development of new vessels and preretinal or vitreous hemorrhage, and (2) the development of new vessels on or within one disc diameter of the optic disc equaling or exceeding one-fourth to one-third disc area in extent, even in the absence of preretinal or vitreous hemorrhage.[32]

Any of the pathologic processes associated with diabetic retinopathy may affect the macula, the parafoveal region of the retina responsible for sharp central vision. This condition is referred to as *diabetic maculopathy.* The diabetic maculopathies have been classified into two groups: intraretinal maculopathies and vitreoretinal maculopathies. The intraretinal maculopathies may occur in the presence of nonproliferative or proliferative retinopathy. They are associated with leakage or occlusion of the retinal capillaries and arterioles in the macula and appear clinically as macular edema, hard exudate deposition, and macular ischemia. The vitreoretinal maculopathies occur in the presence of proliferative retinopathy. They arise when fibrovascular proliferation and contraction cause macular distortion or detachment. Diabetic maculopathy is designated as being "clinically significant" if any of the following characteristics apply: (1) thickening of the retina at or within 500 microns of the center of the macula, (2) hard exudates at or within 500 microns of the center of the macula, if associated with thickening of adjacent retina, or (3) a zone or zones of retinal thickening one disc area or larger, any part of which is within one disc diameter of the center of the macula.[37]

Occurrence

In IDDM, the prevalence of nonproliferative diabetic retinopathy varies from 17% in persons with diabetes for less than 5 years to 98% in those with diabetes for 15 or more years.[66] The prevalence of proliferative retinopathy varies from 1% in persons with IDDM for less than 10 years to 67% in those with IDDM for 35 or more years.[66] The prevalence of macular edema varies from 0% in those with IDDM for less than 5 years to 29% in those with IDDM for 20 or more years.[68] In IDDM, both retinopathy and macular edema are associated with longer duration of diabetes, higher glycosylated hemoglobin levels, higher blood pressure, presence of proteinuria, and male gender.[66,68]

In NIDDM, the prevalence of nonproliferative diabetic retinopathy varies from 29% in those with diabetes for less than 5 years to 78% in those with diabetes for 15 or more years.[67] The prevalence of proliferative diabetic retinopathy varies from 2% in those with NIDDM for less than 5 years to 16% in those with diabetes for 15 or more years.[67] The prevalence of macular edema varies from 3% in those who have had NIDDM for less than 5 years to 28% in those with diabetes for 20 or more years.[68] Nonproliferative and proliferative diabetic retinopathy and diabetic macular edema are more common in insulin-treated than in non-insulin-treated subjects with NIDDM.[67,68] In NIDDM, retinopathy is associated with longer duration of diabetes, younger age at diagnosis, higher glycosylated hemglobin levels, higher systolic blood pressure, and presence of proteinuria.[67] In NIDDM, presence of macular edema is associated with longer duration of diabetes, higher glycosylated hemoglobin levels, higher systolic blood pressure, and presence of proteinuria.[68]

It is estimated that in IDDM, 1.4% of subjects have moderate visual impairment (best corrected visual acuity in the better eye of 20/80 to 20/160) and 3.6% are legally blind (visual acuity in the better eye of 20/200 or worse).[72] In IDDM, visual impairment and legal blindness are associated with older age, longer duration of diabetes, presence of proliferative retinopathy, and presence of senile cataracts.[72] In NIDDM, approximately 3% of subjects have moderate visual impairment and 1.6% are legally blind.[72] In NIDDM, visual impairment and legal blindness are associated with older age, longer duration of diabetes, presence of senile cataracts, presence of macular edema, and proliferative diabetic retinopathy.[72] When assigning causes of legal blindness, diabetic retinopathy is the sole or contributing cause in about 86% of subjects with IDDM and in about 33% of subjects with NIDDM.[72] In subjects with

NIDDM, macular edema, cataracts, glaucoma, and macular degeneration are more important contributors to legal blindness.[72]

Progression of Retinopathy

In a population-based study of the incidence and progression of diabetic retinopathy, 59% of subjects with IDDM who were initially free of retinopathy developed it in 4 years, and 11% of those initially free of proliferative retinopathy developed it in 4 years.[69] Overall, worsening of retinopathy occurred in 41% of the population in 4 years and improvement occurred in 7%.[69] Among insulin-using subjects with NIDDM, 47% of those who did not have any retinopathy developed it in 4 years and 7% of those initially free from proliferative retinopathy developed it.[70] Worsening of retinopathy occurred in 34% over 4 years.[70] Among non-insulin-using subjects, 34% of those who did not have any retinopathy developed it in 4 years, whereas 2% of those initially free from proliferative retinopathy developed it in 4 years, and 25% had worsening of retinopathy over 4 years.[70] The 4-year incidence of macular edema in subjects with IDDM was 8.2%; in subjects with insulin-treated NIDDM, 8.4%; and in non-insulin-treated subjects, 2.9%.[71] Controlled clinical trials have now demonstrated that intensive therapy prevents the development and slows the progression of retinopathy in IDDM (see earlier discussion).

Prospective follow-up studies have demonstrated that the risk of progression of retinopathy is higher in those with the highest glycosylated hemoglobin levels compared with those persons with the lowest glycosylated hemoglobin levels.[69-71] The association between progression of retinopathy and glycosylated hemoglobin persists after controlling for duration of diabetes, age, gender, and baseline retinopathy status. Other studies have shown associations between proliferative diabetic retinopathy, difficulty in managing diabetes, and less effort expended in managing diabetes. Hypertension is associated with progression of background retinopathy in both IDDM and NIDDM.[75,99] Pregnancy has been prospectively determined to be a progression of diabetic retinopathy,[63] as has nephropathy.[27,65] In IDDM, proliferative retinopathy has also been associated with the HLA-DR phenotypes 4/0, 3/0, or X/X. These results support a multifactorial model for the development of proliferative diabetic retinopathy, which includes both metabolic and genetic risk factors.

Management and Treatment

The Diabetes Control and Complications Trial demonstrated that near normoglycemia can prevent the development and slow the progression of diabetic retinopathy. Health care providers should work with their patients to achieve blood glucose levels as near normal as possible. Blood pressure control is also important. Efforts to control blood pressure should be intensified in patients with evidence of diabetic retinopathy. Although intensive therapy can prevent the development and slow the progression of diabetic retinopathy, it should not be forgotten that therapies exist that can prevent visual loss and restore vision in diabetic patients with proliferative diabetic retinopathy, vitreous hemorrhage, and diabetic macular edema.

The Diabetic Retinopathy Study (DRS) Research Group demonstrated that panretinal laser photocoagulation reduces the 5-year incidence of severe visual loss (visual acuity, 5/200 or worse) by more than 50%, and from 49% to 22% in persons with proliferative diabetic retinopathy and high-risk characteristics (see earlier).[32] Side effects of treatment are relatively mild. Panretinal photocoagulation may lead to some long-term loss of peripheral and night vision; about 10% of treated patients have minor reductions in visual acuity. This reduction in visual acuity is especially prominent in eyes with preexisting macular edema and is more common in intensively treated eyes than in less intensively treated eyes.

The Early Treatment Diabetic Retinopathy Study (ETDRS) Research Group demonstrated that focal photocoagulation of clinically significant diabetic macular edema substantially reduces the risk of visual loss even if visual acuity is not reduced.[37] At 3 years, 12% of eyes with clinically significant diabetic macular edema assigned to immediate focal photocoagulation had lost greater than or equal to three lines of visual acuity, and 24% of those in whom photocoagulation was deferred had lost greater than or equal to three lines. Focal treatment increases the chance of visual improvement, decreases the frequency of persistent macular edema, and causes only minor visual field losses.

Vitrectomy is performed in people with advanced proliferative diabetic retinopathy. The role of vitrectomy in the treatment of diabetic retinopathy has been defined by the Diabetic Retinopathy Vitrectomy Study (DRVS).[33] When eyes with advanced, active, proliferative diabetic retinopathy and visual acuity of 10/200 or better were randomly assigned to either early vitrectomy (vitrectomy 1 year from the onset of hemorrhage) or conventional management, the percentage of eyes with a visual acuity of 10/20 or better was 44% in the early vitrectomy group and 28% in the conventional management group. The proportion with very poor visual outcome was similar in the two groups. The advantage of early vitrectomy tended to increase with increasing severity of new vessels.

In persons with IDDM and vitreous hemorrhage with severe visual loss, there is a clear-cut advantage to early vitrectomy, as reflected in the percentage of eyes recovering visual acuity of 10/20 or better (36% in the early group versus 12% in the deferred group).[34] In persons with NIDDM, spontaneous clearing of vitreous hemorrhage occurs more frequently than in patients with IDDM (29% versus 16%), and there is no advantage to early vitrectomy (16% recovery of visual acuity of 10/20 or better in the early group versus 18% in the deferred group).[34]

A recent analysis of data from these trials (the DRS, the ETDRS, and the DRVS) suggests that currently recommended treatments are considerably more effective in preventing blindness from proliferative diabetic retinopathy than has been previously appreciated.[44b]

Guidelines for Preventive Care

As a rule, diabetic retinopathy is asymptomatic in its most treatable stages. Patient education is therefore critical to preventive care. Patients should be reminded to report ocular symptoms, since essentially any symptom may be associated with diabetic retinopathy. Blurred vision while reading may indicate changes in hydration of the lens associated with changes in blood glucose control, and it may also indicate macular edema. The presence of floaters may indicate hemorrhage, and flashing lights may indicate retinal detachment. Persons should also be informed of the relationship between glycemic control, hypertension, and diabetic retinopathy and of the importance of continuing treatment of hyperglycemia and hypertension. Most important, individuals should understand the natural history of diabetic retinopathy, the importance of regular eye examinations, and the benefits of timely therapy in reducing the risk of visual loss.[55]

Despite compelling evidence that treatment may prevent visual loss or restore vision in persons with eye disease caused by diabetes, many individuals with diabetes do not receive adequate eye care. In one large population-based survey, it was discovered that approximately one fourth of subjects with IDDM and one third of those with NIDDM had never had an ophthalmologic examination.[127] Risk factors for not having had an ophthalmologic examination included being older at time of diagnosis of diabetes, having a shorter duration of diabetes, having better visual acuity, having fewer years of education, receiving diabetes care from a family or general practitioner, and living in a nonmetropolitan county.[127] Barriers to care perceived by persons with diabetes in need of ophthalmic care include failure to be told of the benefits of care or needs for care, denial, dislike of the examination, cost, and distance.[73]

Because significant retinopathy may be present without symptoms, the responsibility to screen the patient with diabetes for retinopathy is substantial. Shortly after the initial publication of the results of the Diabetic Retinopathy Study, there was a lack of awareness of the study results among primary care physicians and a failure to incorporate the findings of the study into clinical practice.[117] More recently, there has been controversy about how best to diagnose diabetic retinopathy. Studies have examined the ability of ophthalmic opticians,[14] optometrists,[74] medical residents, internists, diabetologists, ophthalmologists,[118] nonmydriatic fundus photography,[64] and stereoscopic fundus photography[96] to diagnose diabetic retinopathy. Although difficult to compare, these studies suggest that either a thorough clinical examination performed by a well-trained examiner through dilated pupils or nonstereoscopic retinal photography through a pharmacologically undilated pupil provides a reasonable measure of the severity of retinopathy as assessed by stereoscopic fundus photography. In both cases, follow-up or referral for definitive diagnosis of patients with positive screen results is necessary.

Consensus Guidelines (including principles for patient education) now exist for ophthalmic care for persons with diabetes.[55] The National Eye Institute has sponsored the National Eye Health Education Program, which is designed to inform persons with diabetes about the need for dilated eye examinations to detect diabetic retinopathy. Patient education is critical to the promotion of eye care (Box 7-2). All patients with IDDM of more than 5 years' duration and all those with NIDDM should have a baseline eye examination. After the initial eye examination, persons with diabetes should receive complete eye examinations at least once a year. The examination should include a history of visual symptoms, measurement of visual acuity, measurement of intraocular pressure, dilation of the pupils, and a thorough retinal examination including stereoscopic examination of the macula. Because stereoscopic examination of the macula requires dilation of the pupils and binocular indirect ophthalmoscopy or other specialized techniques, referral to an ophthalmologist or optometrist skilled in the diagnosis and classification of diabetic retinopathy is preferred.

BOX 7-2

EYE CARE: EDUCATION PRINCIPLES

Inform persons with diabetes that sight-threatening eye disease is a common complication of diabetes and may be present even with good vision.

Remind them to report all ocular symptoms, since any symptoms may be diabetic in origin.

Blurred vision while reading may indicate macular edema.

Floaters may indicate hemorrhage.

Flashing lights may indicate retinal detachment.

Inform patients that early detection and appropriate treatment of diabetic eye disease greatly reduces the risk of visual loss.

Explain the causal relationship between glycemic control and the subsequent development and progression of ocular complications.

Tell persons with diabetes about the association between hypertension and diabetic retinopathy.

Stress the importance of the diagnosis and continuing treatment of hypertension.

Help persons with diabetes understand the natural course and treatment of diabetic retinopathy.

Stress the importance of yearly eye examinations.

Tell persons with diabetic retinopathy about the availability and benefits of early and timely laser photocoagulation therapy in reducing the risk of visual loss.

Inform individuals about their higher risks of cataract formation, open-angle glaucoma, and neovascular glaucoma.

Tell individuals with any visual impairment (including blindness) about the availability of visual, vocational, and psychosocial rehabilitation programs.

Modified from Herman WH, editor: *The prevention and treatment of complications of diabetes mellitus: a guide for primary care practitioners,* Atlanta, 1991, Dept of Health and Human Services, Public Health Services, Centers for Disease Control, Center for Chronic Disease Prevention and Health Promotion.

Children with nonproliferative retinopathy who are entering puberty and women with diabetes who are planning pregnancy should be examined by a practitioner who is experienced in the diagnosis and classification of diabetic retinopathy, since there is the tendency for retinopathy to progress more rapidly under these conditions. A woman with known diabetes who becomes pregnant should be examined for diabetic retinopathy in the first trimester and, at the discretion of the examiner, every 3 months until parturition. All individuals with preproliferative retinopathy, proliferative retinopathy without high-risk characteristics, and macular edema should be under the care of ophthalmologists and will require more frequent follow-up.

Persons with significant retinal disease or those who have lost vision from retinopathy should continue to receive regular eye care. Proper refraction, low vision evaluation, optical

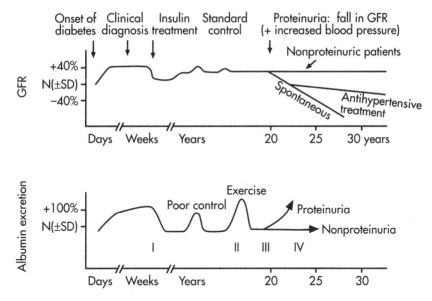

Fig. 7-2   Development of kidney function changes in juvenile diabetes mellitus: GFR and albumin excretion. (Modified from Morgenson CE, Christensen CK, Vittinghus E: *Diabetes* 32[suppl 2]:64-78, 1983.)

aids, and other techniques and devices are available to enable a person to use even severely limited vision. Referral to optometrists or ophthalmologists specializing in low vision may be appropriate. Support groups for the visually impaired and organizations providing vocational rehabilitation are available in most areas.

DIABETIC NEPHROPATHY

Diabetic nephropathy is a clinical syndrome characterized by albuminuria, hypertension, and progressive renal insufficiency. In the United States diabetic nephropathy is the leading cause of new cases of end-stage renal disease that requires dialysis or transplantation for survival. The number of new cases of diabetic end-stage renal disease has increased at an epidemic rate from approximately 2200 in 1980 to approximately 13,300 in 1989. Better understanding of the risk factors for nephropathy and the elucidation of treatments to slow the progression of nephropathy have provided the rationale for developing an approach to delay the onset of end-stage renal disease. This approach requires that patients with early diabetic nephropathy be identified, counseled, and treated.[55]

Clinical Manifestations

In IDDM, the natural history of diabetic nephropathy has been well characterized (Fig. 7-2).[92]

Stage I is the hyperfiltration-hyperfunction stage, found early after the diagnosis of IDDM. Glomerular size and kidney size are both increased. The glomerular filtration rate is high at this stage but returns toward normal with treatment. Slightly elevated urinary albumin excretion rates (microalbuminuria) may be present, but urinary albumin excretion is normalized by insulin treatment.

Stage II is an asymptomatic stage during which renal lesions may be present without clinical signs or symptoms. This stage is found as early as 2 years after the onset of IDDM. Glomerular basement membrane thickening and mesangial expansion are observed. The GFR remains high. Microalbuminuria may occur during poor metabolic control and exercise.

Stage III is the stage of high risk for diabetic nephropathy, also referred to as the *stage of incipient nephropathy*. It occurs 10 to 15 years after the diagnosis of IDDM in persons destined to develop overt diabetic nephropathy. GFR remains high, the blood pressure begins to rise, and urinary albumin excretion increases. Intervention at this stage is very important to slow the progression of the disease.

Stage IV is the stage of overt diabetic nephropathy. It develops 15 to 25 years after onset of diabetes in about 40% of people with IDDM. Hypertension almost invariably occurs. Clinical signs are now apparent. GFR steadily decreases. Levels of albuminuria greater than 300 mg per 24 hours are observed. Even at this stage, treatment can reduce the rate of decline in GFR and delay progression to stage V.

Stage V is end-stage renal disease (ESRD). Renal function is insufficient to sustain life, and to survive the patient must begin dialysis treatment or receive a renal transplant.

In IDDM, the course of diabetic nephropathy is quite consistent. About 80% of patients who progress to stage III (incipient nephropathy) progress to stage IV (overt nephropathy) over 10 years, and essentially all of those progress to stage V (ESRD) within 5 to 10 years.[89]

In NIDDM, some major differences have been described in the natural history of diabetic nephropathy. A population-based study of older subjects with diabetes, or with occult fasting hyperglycemia, and age- and sex-matched controls did not find evidence of hyperfiltration or hyperfunction early in the course of diabetes (stage I).[28] A light microscopy study of glomerular morphology found no evidence of increased glomerular volume early in the course of NIDDM (stage I).[114] In addition, in older persons with NIDDM, albuminuria appears to be a less specific marker for diabetic nephropathy. Elderly subjects who do not have diabetes have a wide range of urinary albumin excretion rates.[28] Only about 22% of patients with NIDDM and microalbuminuria (stage III) progress to overt nephropathy (stage IV) within 10 years,[89,93] and only 1 in 8 subjects with NIDDM and overt nephropathy (stage IV) have progressive renal insufficiency.[41] It appears that in NIDDM, the 20-year cumulative incidence of diabetic nephropathy is 25% to 50%.[9,80,128] However, the incidence of ESRD in NIDDM is significantly less than that observed in IDDM. In one study, the 10-year risk of ESRD was 5.8% for subjects with IDDM and 0.5% for subjects with NIDDM.[26] When ESRD is observed in persons with NIDDM, it generally develops at an older age but after a shorter duration of known diabetes than that seen in IDDM. These differences in the clinical course of nephropathy in IDDM and NIDDM may be partially explained by the frequently asymptomatic nature of NIDDM, which may result in its remaining undiagnosed for many years, and the increased risk of death of subjects with NIDDM and diabetic nephropathy.[58] Nevertheless, it is possible that real differences exist in the clinical course of nephropathy in IDDM and NIDDM.

Pathogenesis

The pathogenesis of diabetic nephropathy is multifactorial. Both metabolic and genetic factors are involved. One hypothesis has proposed that intrarenal hypertension is important in the initiation and progression of diabetic nephropathy.[57] Hyperfunction is stimulated by some of the features of the diabetic state such as extracellular fluid volume expansion (caused by hyperglycemia), renal hypertrophy, and increased levels of growth hormone and glucagon. Increases in the glomerular plasma flow rate and the glomerular transcapillary pressure gradient are responsible for hyperfiltration. Hyperfiltration leads to albuminuria and mesangial protein deposition. The latter effect promotes mesangial expansion and ultimately leads to glomerulosclerosis. The loss of functioning nephrons leads to further compensatory hyperfiltration in surviving glomeruli, contributing to their eventual destruction. Other metabolic hypotheses for the pathogenesis of diabetic nephropathy have focused on the altered polyol pathway metabolism and nonezymatic glycation of glomerular proteins.

None of these hypotheses can account for the observation that diabetic nephropathy develops in fewer than half of all patients with diabetes. As a result, studies have also focused on heredity as a possible risk factor for diabetic kidney disease. Some investigators have noted family clustering of nephropathy in IDDM, independent of duration of diabetes, glycemic control, and blood pressure.[115] Most studies have not, however, found associations between HLA type and the presence of nephropathy in IDDM.[10,106] A number of studies have found an association between family history of essential hypertension and nephropathy in IDDM.[78,83] In addition, increased rates of erythrocyte sodium-lithium countertransport, a marker for essential hypertension in Caucasian populations, have been found in patients with IDDM and increased glomerular filtration rates,[17] microalbuminuria,[62] and diabetic nephropathy.[78,83]

Despite these recent advances in current understanding of the pathogenesis of diabetic nephropathy in IDDM, the exact pathogenic factors responsible for the condition remain unknown. Less work has been done in NIDDM.[93]

Occurrence

In IDDM, overt diabetic nephropathy is unusual before 10 years' duration of diabetes but occurs in 30% to 50% of those with IDDM for 20 or more years. In IDDM, the cumulative incidence of overt nephropathy plateaus after about 25 years and the risk of ever developing nephropathy is low in patients with IDDM who have not developed nephropathy after 25 years' duration of diabetes.[7]

Three recent studies of nephropathy in NIDDM have found a cumulative incidence similar to that observed in IDDM. In a population-based study in Rochester, Minnesota, the 20-year cumulative incidence of persistent proteinuria in NIDDM was 25%.[9] In a clinic-based series from Michigan, the 20-year cumulative incidence of nephropathy in NIDDM was 34%.[128] Among the Pima Indians, the 20-year cumulative incidence of diabetic nephropathy was 50%.[80] Data in NIDDM suggest that the cumulative incidence of nephropathy may not plateau after 25 years' duration and that the risk of diabetic nephropathy may increase with increasing duration of diabetes to approximately 75% after 35 years.[128]

Population-based cross-sectional studies have found that in IDDM approximately 6% of patients with durations of diabetes less than 10 years have evidence of nephropathy compared with 34% of those with durations more than 15 years. In contrast, in NIDDM, about 12% of those with durations less than 10 years and 19% of those with durations more than 15 years have evidence of diabetic nephropathy.[65] Clinic-based studies of patients with IDDM and NIDDM[41,76,87,92] have reported similar findings. The apparent discrepancy between the high cumulative incidence of nephropathy in NIDDM and the low cross-sectional prevalence is probably related to selective mortality among subjects with NIDDM and nephropathy. A number of groups have now reported an association between microalbuminuria and mortality in NIDDM.[61,90] In these studies, patients with NIDDM and microalbuminuria have been found to have a twofold increased mortality as compared with subjects with NIDDM who did not have microalbuminuria. In all studies, cardiovascular disease appears to be the major cause of death. A study performed among the Pima Indians demonstrated that subjects with NIDDM and proteinuria had a death rate 3.5 times higher than those without proteinuria after controlling for age, gender, and duration of diabetes.[97,98] Mortality rates from uremia and cardiovascular disease were significantly higher in Pima Indians with diabetes with proteinuria than in those without.[97,98]

Data from the Medicare End-Stage Renal Disease System in the United States have shown that the number of incident cases of diabetic ESRD has increased since 1980.[35] Rates of diabetic ESRD are even higher among Native Americans and Hispanics. Two studies have compared the incidence of end-stage renal disease in IDDM and NIDDM. In these studies, the incidence of ESRD as a result of diabetic nephropathy was approximately twelvefold greater among patients with IDDM compared with those with NIDDM.[26,109] Most of the excess incidence of diabetic ESRD among blacks occurs among patients with NIDDM.[26] Blacks with NIDDM are approximately four times more likely to develop ESRD than are whites with NIDDM.[26] Blacks with IDDM are approximately 1.6 times more likely to develop ESRD than are whites with IDDM.[26]

Diagnosis

In monitoring persons with diabetes, the health care provider should maintain data on urinary protein or albumin excretion, serum creatinine, and blood pressure so that trends can be readily assessed.

A clinical diagnosis of diabetic nephropathy can be made when an individual who has had diabetes for more than 5 years and has evidence of diabetic retinopathy develops clinically apparent albuminuria or proteinuria. Because albuminuria and proteinuria may be caused by the presence of other complicating renal diseases, a person who does not meet these criteria or has evidence of other kidney disease may require a kidney biopsy. In general, however, a clinical diagnosis of diabetic nephropathy can be made without performing a kidney biopsy.[55]

Because early persistent subclinical increases in urinary albumin excretion can identify persons at risk for developing diabetic nephropathy and cardiovascular disease and because early intervention may slow or prevent the progression of diabetic nephropathy, there has been emphasis on the use of sensitive quantitative measures of urinary albumin excretion (microalbuminuria). Traditional urine dipstick methods are insensitive and only semiquantitative and therefore cannot be used to detect mild to moderate increases in urinary albumin excretion or to detect changes in urinary albumin excretion.[54]

Urinalysis should be performed at the time of diagnosis of diabetes. If infection is present, the urine should be cultured and the patient treated appropriately. When infection is not present, urinary albumin excretion (UAE) should be measured quantitatively. If UAE is normal, UAE and renal function (serum creatinine and/or glomerular filtration rate) should be measured yearly. If UAE is abnormal, it should be measured quantitatively on at least three occasions over 6 months. Clinical laboratories offer an array of sensitive quantitative techniques for measuring UAE, including radioimmunoassay, enzyme-linked immunosorbent assay (ELISA), and turbidimetry- or nephelometry-immunoassay. New semiquantitative techniques are also available.

UAE can be measured in a variety of different urine samples including first-morning urine samples, random urine samples, and timed collections. The results can be expressed as rates, as albumin/creatinine ratios, or as concentrations. All techniques have advantages and disadvantages, and the choice of technique and the selection of sample depend largely on local experience. Efforts must be made to ensure that different methods give comparable results and that the value chosen to define increased urinary albumin excretion should not misclassify healthy diabetic and nondiabetic subjects.[54] Table 7-1 summarizes criteria for the stages of diabetic nephropathy as defined by urinary protein and albumin concentrations, urinary protein and albumin excretion rates, and urinary protein to creatinine and albumin to creatinine ratios.

Management and Treatment

The results of the Diabetes Control and Complications Trial have clearly demonstrated that improved glycemic control can prevent the development and delay the progression of diabetic

Table 7-1   Criteria for the Diagnosis of Diabetic Nephropathy

	Urinary albumin (u albumin)			
	Concentration μg/ml	Rate μg/min	mg/24°	Ratio u albumin/ u creatinine
Normal	<20	<20	<30	<0.02
Microalbuminuria	20-199	20-199	30-299	0.02-0.19
Diabetic nephropathy	≥200	≥200	≥300	≥0.2

	Urinary protein (u protein)			
	Concentration μg/ml	Rate μg/min	mg/24°	Ratio u protein/ u creatinine
Normal	<30	<30	<50	<0.03
Microproteinuria	30-299	30-299	50-499	0.03-0.29
Diabetic nephropathy	≥300	≥300	≥500	≥0.3

nephropathy. It is also clear that blood pressure control and angiotensin-converting enzyme (ACE) inhibitors are critically important in slowing the progression of disease in patients with albuminuria. Other strategies that may slow the progression of renal disease include limiting dietary protein consumption, promptly treating urinary tract infections, and avoiding potentially nephrotoxic drugs and radiographic dyes.

Education

All persons with diabetes should be informed about the potential renal complications of diabetes and the relationship between poor glycemic control and the development and progression of diabetic kidney disease. Patients with diabetic kidney disease should know about the role of ACE inhibitors, the association between hypertension and accelerated kidney disease, and the critical importance of treating hypertension. They should be aware of the need for regular blood pressure monitoring and should be encouraged to measure their own blood pressures at home. In addition, they should know their target blood pressure levels. Patients with diabetic kidney disease should be informed about the role of excessive dietary protein in the progression of diabetic kidney disease and should be counseled to consume no more than the recommended daily allowance for protein. All persons with diabetes should know the symptoms and signs of urinary tract infections and pyelonephritis and should be instructed to contact their health care provider if such symptoms occur. Patients with diabetic kidney disease should also know which drugs are potentially nephrotoxic, and they should be made aware of the risks of radiographic dye studies. Persons with diabetic kidney disease should also be aware of the natural history of the condition and understand the therapeutic options for ESRD.

Metabolic control

Because of the well-established causal relationship between hyperglycemia and the development and progression of diabetic kidney disease, every effort should be made to optimize glycemic control. Improved glycemic control does not appear to affect the course of overt diabetic nephropathy.

Blood pressure

Hypertension is associated with nephropathy in IDDM and NIDDM and contributes to progressive deterioration in renal function in patients with diabetic nephropathy. Numerous studies have demonstrated that in diabetic nephropathy, the progressive decline in renal function may be slowed by antihypertensive drug treatment.

In patients with evidence of incipent nephropathy or overt diabetic nephropathy, blood pressure should be carefully monitored and hypertension should be aggressively treated. Blood pressure greater than 140/90 mm Hg should be treated, and treatment should be considered in patients with significant increments in blood pressure (20/10 mm Hg) on careful follow-up. Although controversial, the American Diabetic Association now states that the goal of blood pressure therapy for nonpregnant diabetic patients 18 years of age or older is to reduce and maintain blood pressure below 130 mm Hg systolic and below 85 mm Hg diastolic.[3a]

Angiotensin-converting enzyme inhibitors. Recently, increasing attention has been focused on the impact of different antihypertensive agents on proteinuria and glomerular filtration rate in diabetes.

A recent meta–regression analysis assessed the impact of different agents, treatment durations, patient characteristics, and study features on blood pressure and renal responses to antihypertensive therapy in patients with diabetes.[62a] In univariate analyses, the antihypertensive effect and renal responses of the different antihypertensive agents were similar. Antihypertensive agents of all classes lowered mean arterial pressure, reduced urine albumin and urine protein excretion, and tended to maintain glomerular filtration rate. In regression analysis, ACE inhibitors were uniquely associated with reductions in urine protein excretion and with increases in glomerular filtration rate independent of mean arterial pressure reduction, treatment duration, and other study variables. Reductions in proteinuria and improvements in GFR were seen whether or not patients had hypertension and whether they had microalbuminuria, clinical nephropathy, IDDM, or NIDDM. Reductions in proteinuria from other agents were entirely attributed to decreases in systemic blood pressure. When the analysis was restricted to randomized, controlled trials, ACE inhibitors were associated with a significant reduction in urine albumin excretion but no significant beneficial effect on glomerular filtration rate.

Three more recently published multicenter, controlled, clinical trials have confirmed and extended these findings. In the first trial, 92 patients with IDDM and persistent microalbuminuria but no hypertension were randomized to receive either captopril or a placebo twice per day.[120b] Captopril therapy significantly slowed progression to clinical nephropathy (UAE $\geq$200 µg/min). Over 2 years, 4 patients receiving captopril and 12 receiving the placebo developed clinical nephropathy.

In the second trial, 207 patients with IDDM who had urinary protein excretion greater than or equal to 500 mg/dl and serum creatinine less than or equal to 2.5 mg/dl were randomized to receive captopril and 202 were randomized to receive a placebo.[82a] Other antihypertensive agents were then used to achieve predetermined blood pressure goals. There was a small disparity in blood pressure between the groups (mean arterial pressure (MAP) 96±8 versus 100±8 mm Hg). Serum creatinine concentrations doubled in 25 patients in the captopril group and in 43 in the placebo group. The reduction in risk of a doubling of the serum creatinine concentration was 48% in the captopril group as a whole. The impact of captopril treatment was more apparent in subjects with more advanced baseline renal insufficiency. Captopril treatment was also associated with a 50% reduction in the risk of the combined end points of dialysis, transplantation, and death; this was independent of the small disparity in blood pressure between the groups.

The third study assessed the long-term effect of ACE inhibition on proteinuria and kidney function in patients with NIDDM.[107a] That study reported on 49 normotensive patients with NIDDM, microalbuminuria, and normal renal function who were randomized to receive enalapril and 45 who were randomized to receive placebos. Any increase in blood pressure was treated with long-acting nifedipine. Over 5 years of follow-up, the mean blood pressure remained stable in the enalapril group and tended to increase in the placebo group. In patients treated with enalapril, albuminuria decreased during the first year and then increased slowly.

Kidney function remained stable as assessed by reciprocal of serum creatinine. In the placebo group, albuminuria increased progressively and kidney function declined by 13%. At the 5-year follow-up, 12% of enalapril-treated patients and 42% of placebo-treated patients had developed clinical nephropathy (urinary albumin excretion greater than 300 mg/24 hours).

In summary, antihypertensive therapy slows the progression of diabetic nephropathy, reduces the likelihood of end-stage renal disease caused by diabetic nephropathy, and reduces mortality. ACE inhibitors have a beneficial impact independent of their antihypertensive effects and are superior to conventional antihypertensive drugs in reducing injury and in retarding the progression of diabetic nephropathy. ACE inhibitors appear to be a logical first-choice class of drugs for use in hypertensive diabetic patients with albuminuria greater than 30 mg/24 hours, when economically feasible and not contraindicated. ACE inhibitors may also be beneficial in normotensive patients with albuminuria. When ACE inhibitors are contraindicated or ineffective, other antihypertensive agents should be used.

Dietary measures

Since studies in small numbers of subjects with IDDM and NIDDM have suggested that dietary protein restriction may reduce the rate in rise of urinary albumin excretion and slow the rate of decline of renal function,[39,130] patients with incipient nephropathy or overt diabetic nephropathy should be encouraged to adhere to the recommended dietary allowance (RDA) for protein[4a,108] (see Chapter 4). For children ages 7 to 14 the RDA is 1.0 g of protein per kilogram of body weight per day, and for males ages 15 to 18 the RDA is 0.9 g of protein per kilogram of body weight per day. Females ages 15 and older require 0.8 g of protein per kilogram of body weight per day. Pregnant women require approximately 10 g more protein per day, and lactating women require approximately 15 g more protein per day. Adherence to these guidelines can be assessed by dietary history or by measurement of 24-hour urinary urea nitrogen. The grams of protein ingested per day can be estimated from the urinary urea nitrogen by the formula: protein intake (g/day) equals 24-hour urinary urea nitrogen (g/24 hours) times 6.25 and then divided by 0.80.

Risk reduction

Because of the associations among diabetic nephropathy, retinopathy, and cardiovascular disease, complete eye examinations should be performed at least yearly for subjects with nephropathy, and risk factors for coronary heart disease, including hypertension, dyslipidemia, and cigarette smoking, should be assessed and treated as needed.

Urinary tract infections should be treated promptly in patients with diabetes, and a urine culture should be repeated after treatment to ensure that the infection has resolved. In addition, potentially nephrotoxic drugs and radiographic dyes should be avoided when possible in patients with diabetes and especially in those with diabetic nephropathy. Persons with diabetes with preexisting renal insufficiency are at increased risk for exacerbation of renal failure following radiocontrast studies. Clinical series have demonstrated that 10% to 70% of diabetic persons with serum creatinine levels greater than or equal to 1.5 mg/dl will develop deterioration in renal failure following radiocontrast studies. As many as 95% of subjects with diabetes with serum creatine levels greater than 5 mg/dl may develop acute renal failure.[51,102,125]

Persons with renal disease

The management of diabetes in persons with renal disease requires special attention.[5] As renal insufficiency develops, many persons with diabetes require a reduction in their dose of insulin or sulfonylurea. Since approximately one third of insulin is metabolized and cleared by the renal parenchyma, it is generally prudent to reduce the insulin dose. Because the half-life of all sulfonylureas is prolonged with renal disease, use of a sulfonylurea that has a short half-life and is converted by the liver into inactive metabolites (Glipizide) as renal insufficiency supervenes is indicated. It is also important to recognize that uremia may be associated with anorexia, weight loss, and bowel dysmotility. Decreased calorie intake, erratic nutrient absorption, and decreased gluconeogenesis may also contribute to the risk of severe hypoglycemia.

Subjects with impending renal failure (serum creatine greater than 2 mg/dl and/or glomerular filtration rate less than 40 ml/min) should be referred for renal consultation. Patients with diabetes who have developed end-stage renal disease (ESRD) will require dialysis or kidney transplantation to prolong their lives. Because diabetic complications—especially retinopathy and neuropathy—progress more rapidly with the onset of renal failure, dialysis is instituted earlier for persons with diabetes than for those without diabetes. In general, treatment is initiated when the serum creatinine reaches about 6 mg/dl. Kidney transplantation is preferable to dialysis when a living relative of the patient is available as a donor. The ultimate choice of treatment will require input from the patient, the patient's family, and the health care team.

Compared with nondiabetic patients with ESRD, diabetic patients with ESRD have a significantly shorter 5-year survival rate (28% versus 40%). In general, survival decreases with increasing age at onset of ESRD. The difference in survival between nondiabetic patients and diabetic patients is greatest among older persons.[52] The higher mortality observed among diabetic patients with ESRD and the increasing age-specific mortality among diabetic ESRD patients are probably the result of a higher prevalence of comorbid conditions including cerebral vascular disease, atherosclerotic heart disease, and peripheral vascular disease.[23]

DIABETIC NEUROPATHY

Diabetic neuropathy can be defined as peripheral nerve dysfunction that occurs in persons with established diabetes; it is of a type known to be more prevalent among persons with diabetes than among persons without diabetes and cannot be attributed to any other disease process. Diabetes is probably the most common cause of neuropathy in the United States. Diabetic neuropathy is a major cause of suffering, disability, and lower extremity amputation. In the past, lack of consistency in the classification of diabetic neuropathy retarded efforts to define its occurrence, causes, prevention, and treatment. In recent years, there has been an emerging consensus about the classification of diabetic neuropathy. In addition, there have been improvements in current understanding of its biochemical and vascular bases.

Classification

Diabetic neuropathy can be best understood as a group of clinical syndromes. Each clinical syndrome of diabetic neuropathy has characteristic presentations, symptoms and signs, and courses. Although each syndrome is distinct, the syndromes may coexist in the same patient, making classification difficult. The classification of diabetic neuropathy is based on its presumed underlying pathophysiology.[36] Diabetic neuropathy may be classified as being either diffuse or focal (Box 7-3).

Distal symmetric sensorimotor polyneuropathy is a form of diffuse neuropathy. It is the most common type of neuropathy associated with diabetes. It is primarily a sensory neuropathy but may be associated with distal motor abnormalities and with autonomic dysfunction. Sensory deficits appear first in the toes and feet and progress proximally. Involvement of the fingers and hands is a relatively late finding. In advanced disease, distal portions of the truncal nerves may become involved, and sensory deficits may occur in a vertical band on the anterior chest. The symptoms and signs of distal symmetric sensorimotor

---

BOX 7-3

SYNDROMES OF DIABETIC NEUROPATHY

Diffuse neuropathy

Distal symmetric sensorimotor polyneuropathy
Acute painful neuropathy
Small fiber neuropathy
Large fiber neuropathy
Autonomic neuropathy
Sudomotor dysfunction
Abnormal pupillary function
Cardiovascular autonomic neuropathy
Gastrointestinal autonomic neuropathy
Genitourinary autonomic neuropathy
Hypoglycemia unawareness

Focal neuropathy

Cranial neuropathy
Radiculopathy
Plexopathy
Mononeuropathy multiplex
Mononeuropathy

polyneuropathy vary depending on the classes of nerve fibers involved. Three overlapping clinical syndromes have been described: (1) an acute painful neuropathy without evidence of significant neurologic deficits, (2) a small fiber neuropathy characterized by diminished pain and temperature sensation, and (3) a large fiber neuropathy characterized by loss of light touch, vibration, and position sensation.[120]

Diabetic autonomic neuropathy is a second form of diffuse neuropathy. It may involve virtually any sympathetic or parasympathetic autonomic function. Manifestations of diabetic autonomic neuropathy may include abnormal sweating, abnormal pupillary function, cardiovascular autonomic neuropathy, gastrointestinal autonomic neuropathy, genitourinary autonomic neuropathy, and hypoglycemia unawareness.[40]

Focal diabetic neuropathy is associated with deficits in the distribution of a single nerve (mononeuropathy), multiple peripheral nerves (mononeuropathy multiplex), the brachial or lumbosacral plexuses (plexopathy), or the nerve roots (radiculopathy). Individual cranial nerves may also be involved (cranial nerve palsies).[8]

Occurrence

In the past, the epidemiology of diabetic neuropathy was not well defined because of a lack of standardization of diagnostic methods and a lack of consensus on diagnostic criteria. In recent years, there has been increasing consensus on standardization of nomenclature and assessment of diabetic neuropathy including clinical measures, morphologic and biochemical measures, electrodiagnostic measures, quantitative sensory testing, and autonomic nervous system testing.[106a] In addition, a recent cross-sectional cohort study has, for the first time, provided population-based estimates of the frequency of diabetic neuropathy.[36a]

In a Rochester, Minnesota, study, Dyck and associates[36a] observed that 66% of patients with IDDM and 59% of patients with NIDDM have some form of neuropathy. The most common form of neuropathy was distal symmetric sensorimotor polyneuropathy. Fifteen percent of patients with IDDM and 13% of those with NIDDM had symptomatic distal symmetric sensorimotor polyneuropathy. In addition, 39% of those with IDDM and 32% of those with NIDDM had subclinical polyneuropathy. In general, the frequency and severity of diabetic polyneuropathy increased with duration of diabetes.

The next most frequently observed form of neuropathy was carpal tunnel syndrome. Two percent of both IDDM and NIDDM patients had symptoms of carpal tunnel syndrome with diagnostic electrophysiologic abnormalities. Nine percent of IDDM patients and 4% of NIDDM patients had symptoms of carpal tunnel syndrome with or without electrophysiologic abnormalities, and 22% of IDDM patients and 29% of NIDDM patients had electrophysiologic abnormalities without any symptoms. The frequency of electrophysiologic findings among diabetic patients was higher than in nondiabetic controls drawn from the same population (6%). Carpal tunnel syndrome was significantly associated with duration of diabetes.

After exclusion of other causes, the overall prevalence of symptomatic visceral autonomic neuropathy was 5%. Thirteen percent of men with IDDM and 8% of men with

NIDDM reported impotence. Fewer than 1% of persons with IDDM and NIDDM reported gastroparesis, nocturnal diarrhea, urinary incontinence, or postural fainting.

Proximal asymmetric neuropathy was present in 1% of patients with IDDM and NIDDM. Cranial neuropathy and truncal radiculopathy were not present in any patients at the time of examination, although a few had such neuropathies previously. Ulnar neuropathy occurred in 2% of patients. Peroneal neuropathy and lateral femoral cutaneous neuropathy (meralgia paresthetica) occurred in fewer than 1% of patients.

Pathogenesis

Distal symmetric sensorimotor polyneuropathy

Pathologic studies of diabetic distal symmetric sensorimotor polyneuropathy suggest that longer myelinated axons are preferentially involved. The diffuse nature and progressive course of distal symmetric sensorimotor polyneuropathy suggest a metabolic basis. A number of hypotheses have been proposed to explain the pathogenesis of the condition. Two leading hypotheses are the sorbitol-myo-inositol/sodium-potassium ATPase hypothesis and the nonenzymatic glycation hypothesis.[49] The sorbitol-myo-inositol/sodium-potassium ATPase hypothesis has linked acute hyperglycemia, metabolic abnormalities in peripheral nerve, nerve conduction slowing, and neuroanatomic defects in peripheral nerves.

Another metabolic process that has been proposed to explain the pathogenesis of diabetic neuropathy is nonenzymatic glycation. Nonenzymatic glycation occurs in various tissue proteins as a result of increased ambient glucose concentrations. Nonenzymatic glycation of peripheral nerve protein has been described, although its role in clinical diabetic neuropathy has not been critically examined.[49]

Autonomic neuropathy

Autopsy studies of people with diabetic autonomic neuropathy have demonstrated axonal degeneration and fiber loss in the sympathetic and parasympathetic systems. The intrinsic nerves of the gastrointestinal and genitourinary systems are also affected. The diffuse nature and chronic progressive course of autonomic neuropathy suggest a metabolic basis, and, as in distal symmetric sensorimotor polyneuropathy, alterations in sorbitol-myo-inositol/sodium-potassium ATPase and nonenzymatic glycation of nerve proteins have been hypothesized as pathogenetic mechanisms.[49] Complement-fixing antisympathetic ganglia antibodies and antivagus nerve antibodies have recently been described in subjects with IDDM and cardiovascular autonomic neuropathy. It has been postulated that autoimmunity may play a role in the pathogenesis of diabetic autonomic neuropathy.[107]

Focal neuropathy

The pathogenesis of the focal diabetic neuropathies has not been extensively studied but appears to be vascular. The natural history of the focal neuropathies, with sudden onset, gradual resolution, and confinement to a single nerve root, nerve, or plexus is consistent with a vascular etiology. Serial sections of the cranial nerves of two patients with diabetes who died after developing isolated third-nerve palsies revealed local thickening and occlusion of arterioles. Focal acute demyelinating lesions were also present. A second autopsy report of a patient with diabetes, who died shortly after developing femoral neuropathy, revealed multiple microinfarcts of the nerve, vessel wall thickening, and occlusion of the vasa nervora. Thus it appears that vascular pathologic factors in diabetic nerve and ischemic injury are critical in the pathogenesis of focal neuropathy.[49]

Clinical Manifestations, Diagnosis, and Treatment of Distal Symmetric Sensorimotor Polyneuropathy

Clinical manifestations

The symptoms and signs of distal symmetric sensorimotor polyneuropathy vary depending on the classes of nerve fibers involved.

Acute painful neuropathy is an uncommon and extremely unpleasant complication of diabetes. It may occur early in the course of diabetes with institution of insulin or sulfonylurea therapy. It is often associated with precipitous weight loss. Most commonly, persons have distal paresthesias (spontaneously occurring uncomfortable sensations), dysesthesias (uncomfortable sensations on contact), and pain. At times, the pain is described as superficial and burning, shooting or stabbing, or aching or tearing. Often the pain is worse at night, producing insomnia. Because damage is limited to the small myelinated fibers, objective signs of neuropathy may be minimal. Sensory loss may not be striking; vibration sensation may be intact; motor weakness may be absent; and conduction velocity may not be dramatically impaired. The presence of painful symptoms in the absence of striking neurologic deficits appears somewhat paradoxic. Pain may, however, reflect increased fiber regeneration. In general, pain subsides in months and is preceded by weight gain. Relapses are uncommon.[120]

Small-fiber neuropathy may appear after only a few years of diabetes. Pain may occur and is described as burning, shooting, or aching. Paresthesias may occur. Alternatively, patients with small-fiber neuropathy may present with subjective symptoms of numbness or feelings of "cold feet." The extent of peripheral nervous system damage is generally not severe. Objectively, patients have diminished pinprick and temperature sensation. Soft touch, vibration, and position sensation are generally spared. Motor weakness is usually not marked. If motor weakness occurs, it involves the most distal intrinsic muscles of the feet and hands as a rather late feature. Mild autonomic dysfunction may occur. If autonomic dysfunction occurs, it may be associated with abnormal sweating and dry skin on the feet. Patients with advanced small-fiber neuropathy may occasionally present with undetected trauma of the extremities such as burns or abrasions of the feet or with cigarette burns of the fingers. Neuropathic ulcers may occasionally occur at sites of trauma.[120]

Large-fiber neuropathy occurs insidiously or, at times, quite rapidly in the setting of small-fiber neuropathy. Subjective symptoms of paresthesias and pain are usually absent. Involvement of large fibers leads to impairment of touch, pressure, discriminative sense, vibration, and position sense. The ankle reflexes are depressed or lost. In more severe instances, there is sensory ataxia and a positive Romberg test. This condition is referred to as a "pseudotabetic" form of diabetic neuropathy. Large-fiber neuropathy is often associated with distal motor and autonomic abnormalities that manifest themselves as deformed feet with dry, thickened, and cracked skin. Since pain is generally not associated with large-fiber neuropathy, patients with large-fiber neuropathy are least likely to have complaints about their feet. Large-fiber neuropathy is, however, most strongly associated with the development of neuropathic foot ulcers and neuropathic arthropathy (Charcot's joint). Patients with large-fiber neuropathy are at greatest risk for amputation[120] (see Chapter 9).

Diagnosis

To detect distal symmetric sensorimotor polyneuropathy, the clinician should conduct an interview at each visit to determine whether the patient has pain, paresthesias, numbness, or weakness. Because patients with large-fiber neuropathy may have no symptoms, the clinician should remove the patient's shoes and socks and inspect the feet for deformities, dry skin, and ulcers. At least once a year, the clinician should perform a physical examination to assess sensation, muscle strength, and deep-tendon reflexes. Temperature sensation may be assessed by touching a cool piece of metal (such as a tuning fork) to the patient's foot and by asking the patient to describe the object's temperature. Pinprick sensation may be assessed by holding a clean straight pin lightly between the thumb and forefinger and touching it to the patient's foot. The patient is asked to say when a sensation is felt and whether it is sharp or dull. Vibration sensation may be assessed with a 128 HZ tuning fork applied to the distal first metatarsal head or the malleoli of the ankles. The patient is asked to report when the vibration ceases. Position sensation is assessed by having the patient describe the toe's position as it is alternately flexed and extended.[55]

The diagnosis of diabetic distal symmetric sensorimotor polyneuropathy requires that the patient have diabetes mellitus and have symptoms or signs of peripheral nerve dysfunction that are not attributable to any other cause. Since no features are unique to diabetic distal symmetric sensorimotor polyneuropathy, other causes of peripheral neuropathy must be excluded by careful history and physical examination and by appropriate diagnostic tests (Box 7-4).[49] Occasionally, nerve conduction studies with needle electromyography may help in the diagnosis.

Treatment

Current therapy for diabetic distal symmetric sensorimotor polyneuropathy is palliative and is directed at reducing pain. Troubling pain generally improves spontaneously within a number of months, although some patients have persistent disabling pain. Although a number of studies have shown that improved glycemic control is associated with improvement in nerve conduction velocity,[27,116] it is not clear that improved glycemic control reduces pain. The DCCT demonstrated that intensive therapy reduces the 5-year incidence of diabetic neuropathy by 60%. Every effort should be made to optimize glycemic control. Transcutaneous electrical nerve stimulation (TENS) is rarely effective in the treatment of painful neuropathy, but it deserves consideration because of its lack of systemic side effects. Various pharmacologic agents have been recommended for the treatment of painful neuropathy, including simple analgesics, antidepressants alone or with phenothiazines, mexiletine, capsaicin, and anticonvulsants.

Among simple analgesics, both ibuprofen (600 mg orally, 4 times daily) and sulindac (200 mg orally, twice daily) have been shown to be more effective than placebo in the treatment of painful diabetic neuropathy.[22] Numerous clinical trials have demonstrated the

---

BOX 7-4

DIFFERENTIAL DIAGNOSIS OF DISTAL SYMMETRIC SENSORIMOTOR POLYNEUROPATHY

Metabolic

Diabetes mellitus
Uremia
Hypothyroidism
Folic acid/cyanocobalamin deficiency
Acute intermittent porphyria

Toxic

Medications
Alcohol
Heavy metals (lead, mercury, arsenic)
Industrial hydrocarbons

Infectious or inflammatory

Human immunodeficiency virus (HIV/AIDS)
Sarcoidosis
Leprosy
Periarteritis nodosa
Other connective tissue diseases (e.g., systemic lupus erythematosus)

Other

Amyloidosis
Dysproteinemias
Leukemias and lymphomas
Psychophysiologic disorders (e.g., severe depression, hysteria)
Hereditary neuropathies

---

efficacy of tricyclic antidepressants in the treatment of painful diabetic neuropathy.* These medications appear to relieve the pain of diabetic neuropathy independent of any effect on mood.[84] Onset of analgesia is variable but may take days to several weeks. For this reason, a low dosage of medication should be started and the dosage increased in small steps until the patient's symptoms are relieved or the patient reaches the highest tolerable dose. Side effects common to all of the tricyclic antidepressants include drowsiness, dry mouth, orthostatic hypotension, constipation, and urinary retention. Studies have shown that the combination of a tricyclic antidepressant and a phenothiazine (nortriptyline and fluphenazine) are effective in the treatment of painful neuropathy[47] and that the addition of fluphenazine or clonazepam to a tricyclic antidepressant may provide relief of pain when a tricyclic antidepressant alone has not relieved pain.[129] More recently, mexiletine, an oral antidys-

---

*References 38, 47, 81, 84, 129.

rhythmic agent that is structurally similar to lidocaine, has been shown to be effective in the treatment of diabetic neuropathy.[29] Mexiletine is contraindicated in the presence of preexisting atrioventricular heart block (if no pacemaker is present) and is associated with reversible gastrointestinal and central nervous system side effects. Topical capsaicin applied to the affected areas four times daily[110] appears to be effective in the treatment of painful diabetic neuropathy, but there are concerns regarding possible neurotoxicity associated with its use.[82] Although anticonvulsant medications are used widely in the treatment of chronic pain[119] and although they have been found to be effective in uncontrolled studies of the treatment of diabetic neuropathy, they have not proved to be effective in controlled clinical trials.[18,113] Small, short-term trials of aldose reductase inhibitors and myo-inositol supplementation have yielded conflicting results.[12,46,100,112] Vitamins are not effective in the treatment of painful diabetic distal symmetric sensorimotor polyneuropathy.

Clinical Manifestations, Diagnosis, and Treatment of Diabetic Autonomic Neuropathy

The symptoms and signs of diabetic autonomic neuropathy are protean. The manifestations of diabetic autonomic neuropathy range from the annoying to the disabling and life-threatening.[49]

Sudomotor dysfunction

Autonomic sudomotor dysfunction may produce absence of sweating in a stocking-glove distribution and increased sweating in the face or trunk. Gustatory sweating—abnormal sweating associated with eating—is uncommon but may be quite bothersome to the patient. Distal anhydrosis is often associated with distal symmetric sensorimotor polyneuropathy. It is of clinical significance because it causes dry skin and diminished skin lubrication and may contribute to the development of plantar ulcers. Abnormal sweating may also contribute to decreased thermoregulation and may predispose to heat stroke or hyperthermia.[49] Unless the history is carefully elicited and the feet are examined, patients rarely report abnormal sweating. Diagnosis is important so that affected patients can be counseled to prevent foot lesions, heat stroke, and hyperthermia. Patients with dry, thickened skin should be instructed in foot care and the use of lubricating oils or creams. Patients with thermoregulatory dysfunction should be counseled to avoid intense heat and humidity.[49]

Abnormal pupillary function

The pupillary iris is innervated by both parasympathetic and sympathetic fibers. Parasympathetic fibers cause pupillary constriction, and sympathetic fibers cause pupillary dilation. Diabetic autonomic neuropathy of the eye is associated with abnormalities of both parasympathetic and sympathetic tone, but sympathetic tone is more severely affected. As a result, diabetic patients with autonomic dysfunction tend to have small pupils that dilate slowly in the dark. These changes may be apparent if the practitioner attempts to perform an undilated ophthalmoscopic examination in a darkened room and finds that the pupil dilates slowly. Patients themselves may note poor dark adaptation and should be counseled to allow themselves more time when entering poorly illuminated areas and to use lights when walking at night. Otherwise no specific therapy is required.[49]

Cardiovascular autonomic neuropathy

Cardiovascular autonomic neuropathy is associated with abnormalities of heart rate control and vascular dynamics. Parasympathetic tone slows the heart rate, and sympathetic tone speeds the heart rate and increases the force of cardiac contraction. Sympathetic tone also stimulates the vascular tree and increases blood pressure. The three syndromes of cardiovascular autonomic neuropathy are (1) cardiac denervation syndrome, (2) postural hypotension, and (3) abnormal exercise-induced cardiovascular performance.[49]

Cardiac denervation produces a fixed heart rate that does not change with stress, exercise, or sleep. Both parasympathetic and sympathetic tone are affected in cardiac denervation syndrome. Initially, parasympathetic tone decreases, resulting in a relative increase in sympathetic tone and an increase in the heart rate. Early in the course of cardiac denervation syndrome, patients have a fixed resting heart rate of 100 to 120 beats per minute. Progressive loss of sympathetic tone results in a gradual slowing of the heart rate. Finally, when both parasympathetic and sympathetic tone are impaired, cardiac denervation syndrome exists and patients have a fixed heart rate of 80 to 90 beats per minute.

Cardiac denervation can be diagnosed by checking the pulse during slow deep breathing (6 breaths per minute) or before and after exercise. Persons with cardiac denervation syndrome lack normal sinus arrhythmia, have no heart rate variation during deep breathing, and have no pulse change before or after exercise. Persons with cardiac denervation syndrome are at increased risk for cardiac dysrhythmias, sudden death, and painless myocardial ischemia.

Normally, blood pressure is maintained when a person stands by the "postural reflex," in which baroreceptors initiate a sympathetic reflex that increases heart rate and peripheral vascular resistance in association with an increase in the plasma norepinephrine level. Postural hypotension is defined as a fall of systolic blood pressure of more than 30 mm Hg or a fall of diastolic blood pressure of more than 10 mm Hg on changing from lying to standing position. Postural hypotension may or may not be associated with symptoms.

Symptoms of postural hypotension include postural faintness, weakness, visual impairment, or syncope in the absence of hypoglycemia or dysrhythmia. Measurement of the supine and standing blood pressure and pulse is critical in the evaluation of diabetic patients with postural symptoms. Postural hypotension as a result of cardiovascular autonomic neuropathy is a diagnosis of exclusion and requires a careful history and physical examination and appropriate laboratory testing to rule out other potential causes (Box 7-5). Volume depletion can be differentiated from cardiovascular autonomic neuropathy by evaluating the heart rate response and/or the plasma norepinephrine response to standing. In volume depletion, the heart rate and catecholamine levels increase in response to standing. In cardiovascular autonomic neuropathy, the heart rate and catecholamine levels are unchanged in response to standing.

The treatment of diabetic postural hypotension includes avoiding volume depletion by improving glycemic control to control glucosuria and by ensuring the intake of adequate

---

BOX 7-5

DIFFERENTIAL DIAGNOSIS OF AUTONOMIC NEUROPATHY

Orthostatic hypotension

Hypovolemia
Medications (diuretics, antihypertensives, tricyclic antidepressants)
Panhypopituitarism
Pheochromocytoma
Shy-Drager syndrome
Idiopathic orthostatic hypotension

Gastroparesis

Medications
Acute metabolic disturbances
Gastric or intestinal obstruction

Constipation

Medications
Dehydration
Intestinal obstruction

Diarrhea

Medications
Dietary sorbitol or lactose
Bacterial overgrowth
Pseudomembranous colitis
Enteric pathogens
Primary intestinal diseases
Pancreatic exocrine insufficiency

Impotence

Medications
Hormonal abnormalities
Vascular disease
Psychogenic disease

Hypoglycemia unawareness

Medications
Liver disease
Renal disease
Adrenocortical insufficiency
Lack of knowledge about hypoglycemia

dietary salt. Salt intake can be assessed by measuring 24-hour urinary sodium excretion. Mechanical measures such as waist-high elastic stockings, plasma volume expansion with salt supplementation and/or fludrocortisone,[15] and pharmacologic treatment with sympathetic agonists such as phenylephrine, ephedrine and Neo-Synephrine nasal spray may occasionally be necessary. Beta blockers,[11] clonidine,[1] metoclopramide,[79] and somatostatin analog[56] have been reported to be useful in the treatment of diabetic postural hypotension but have not been evaluated in large controlled clinical trials.

The cardiovascular response to exercise may be abnormal in patients with diabetes and cardiovascular autonomic neuropathy. Such patients may fail to increase their cardiac output or vascular tone with exercise and may develop hypotension in response to exercise. Persons with abnormal exercise-induced cardiac performance should be counseled not to attempt aerobic exercise.[49]

Gastrointestinal autonomic neuropathy

There are many gastrointestinal manifestations of diabetic autonomic neuropathy. Parasympathetic nervous system activity stimulates esophageal and gastric peristalsis. Dopaminergic innervation inhibits gastric peristalsis and sympathetic nervous system activity inhibits gastric emptying. Abnormalities in any of these pathways may result in abnormal gastrointestinal function.[49]

Upper gastrointestinal motility disorders may involve the esophagus, stomach, and proximal small intestine. Patients may complain of symptoms of dysphagia, heartburn, reflux, anorexia, bloating, early satiety, upper abdominal pain, nausea, and vomiting. Associated signs may include weight loss, gastric splash, and erratic glycemic control. The usual pattern of erratic glycemic control in insulin-treated patients with gastroparesis is one of postprandial hypoglycemia and late hyperglycemia reflecting normal insulin action but delayed nutrient absorption. Persons with gastroparesis are at risk for developing bezoars that may be associated with early satiety, gastric outlet obstruction, and vomiting.

Diabetic gastroparesis is a diagnosis of exclusion (see Box 7-5). Upper gastrointestinal (GI) endoscopy or a barium upper GI series may be necessary to rule out obstruction. Abnormal results of a barium upper GI series, which measures liquid-phase gastric emptying, almost always implies the existence of abnormal solid-phase emptying. Conversely, a normal liquid-phase emptying study does not exclude abnormal solid-phase emptying. A nuclear medicine solid-phase gastric emptying study, which uses a radiolabeled solid food (egg or chicken liver), is the most sensitive and specific way to diagnose delayed gastric emptying.

Treatment of gastroparesis includes improvement of glycemic control and correction of other metabolic abnormalities such as ketosis and hypokalemia. It also includes dietary modification with small, low-fat, low-fiber, and/or liquid meals.[45] Pharmacologic treatment with metoclopramide, domperidone, cisapride, and erythromycin has been shown to be effective in the treatment of diabetic gastroparesis.[19,60,85,124]

Constipation

Constipation is probably the most common gastrointestinal symptom associated with diabetes and has been reported by as many as 60% of patients with long-standing diabetes.

The pathogenesis of constipation is poorly understood. Measurement of distal colonic myoelectrical and motor activity has shown absent gastrocolic responses to feeding.[49] Other possible contributing factors must be excluded (see Box 7-5). Three stool specimens should be tested for occult blood, and patients should have careful digital examinations. Women should have pelvic examinations with careful bimanual examinations. If occult blood is detected, a complete blood count, iron, total iron-binding capacity (TIBC), and proctosig-moidscopy and barium enema or colonoscopy should be performed. Treatment of diabetic constipation includes improvement of glycemic control with correction of glycosuria, adequate hydration, high-fiber diet, psyllium, and stool softeners.

Diarrhea

Diabetic diarrhea is an uncommon but troubling complication of diabetes. Diabetic diarrhea may be preceded by abdominal cramps. It is severe and watery and may occasionally be associated with steatorrhea. It is generally not associated with weight loss, is often worse at night, and may fluctuate from season to season. It is intermittent, and during remissions the individual may experience constipation, which characteristically lasts from a few hours to several weeks. It may be associated with fecal incontinence (see below). Its pathogenesis appears to be multifactorial, as autonomic neuropathy, microangiopathy, and functional mucosal abnormalities may all contribute.[49] History, physical examination, and laboratory testing should rule out diarrhea resulting from other causes (see Box 7-5). The history should focus on ingestion of lactose, nonabsorbable artificial sweeteners such as sorbitol and mannitol, and antacids, all of which may be associated with diarrhea. When appropriate, history and laboratory studies should be obtained to rule out bacterial overgrowth, pseudomembranous colitis, enteric pathogens, primary intestinal disorders such as inflammatory bowel disease and celiac disease, and pancreatic exocrine insufficiency.

The diagnosis of diabetic diarrhea is established only by excluding other causes of diarrhea and by confirming the presence of autonomic neuropathy. The intermittent nature of diabetic diarrhea makes it difficult to assess the effectiveness of treatment. As a result, much of the treatment for diabetic diarrhea is empiric. Since afferent denervation may contribute to the problem, a bowel program that includes regular efforts to move the bowels should be tried. Fiber and psyllium may be used to increase stool bulk and consistency; codeine, loperamide, or diphenoxylate hydrochloride and atropine sulfate may be used to slow gastrointestinal motility. Use of broad-spectrum antibiotics with anaerobic coverage such as tetracycline or metronidazole hydrochloride have been reported to be beneficial.[48] If there is no improvement, bile salt binders such as cholestyramine and colestipol may be tried since patients with gallbladder atony have inappropriate spillage of bile salts into the gut between meals; this may result in diarrhea.[24] Clonidine, an alpha-2 adrenergic blocker, has been reported to increase intraluminal fluid absorption and to decrease diarrhea.[42] Finally, somatostatin analog has been used successfully in some cases.

Fecal incontinence is a devastating complication of diabetes. Patients with fecal incontinence will often become homebound and avoid social contact. Fecal incontinence is associated with a reduced threshold of conscious rectal sensation, low basal internal anal sphincter pressure, and reduced voluntary external anal sphincter squeeze pressure.[31] Patients do not generally volunteer a history of fecal incontinence, so the clinician must actively elicit a history of problems controlling the bowels. In patients with diarrhea and fecal incontinence, diarrhea should be assessed because treatment of diabetic diarrhea may reduce the severity of fecal incontinence. In addition, anorectal function may be evaluated by anorectal manometry, which quantitates maximal basal sphincter pressure and the rectal anal inhibitory reflex. Continence for solids and liquids may be assessed by simulating the stress of stools with a solid sphere or rectally infused saline. Patients with intact rectal sensation and good motivation may benefit from biofeedback training.[31]

Genitourinary autonomic neuropathy

Genitourinary autonomic neuropathy can affect bladder function and sexual function. Afferent autonomic fibers transmit sensation of bladder fullness. Efferent parasympathetic fibers promote bladder contraction during urination. Efferent sympathetic fibers maintain sphincter tone. Parasympathetic function mediates erections and vaginal lubrication. The sympathetic nervous system mediates both orgasm and ejaculation.[49]

Diabetic bladder dysfunction generally occurs in association with distal symmetric sensorimotor polyneuropathy and, in males, with impotence. Symptoms of diabetic bladder dysfunction develop insidiously and progress slowly. Initially, there may be lengthened intervals between voiding and increased urinary volume. Later, the urinary stream may become weak and prolonged. Evaluation for diabetic bladder dysfunction should be performed in any patient with diabetes and recurrent urinary tract infections, recurrent pyelonephritis, incontinence, or a palpable bladder. Evaluation should include assessment of renal function, urine culture, and measurement of a postvoiding residual. A postvoiding residual of greater than 150 ml is diagnostic of abnormal bladder function. It may be detected by postvoiding catheterization or a postvoiding sonogram. Postvoiding catheterization is invasive and may produce bacteriuria. Postvoiding sonograms can accurately and noninvasively evaluate the residual urine retained within the bladder.

The aim of treatment of diabetic bladder dysfunction is to improve bladder emptying and to reduce the risk of urinary tract infection. The patient with a grossly overdistended bladder should undergo an initial period of catheter drainage to improve bladder contractility. Care should be taken to avoid the introduction of infection. If infection exists, it should be treated. Thereafter, the person should be instructed to void by the clock rather than waiting for a conscious sensation of bladder distention. Pressure applied to the bladder (Credé's maneuver) will often facilitate emptying. Cholinergic agents (Bethanechol) and intermittent self-catheterization may be used to facilitate bladder emptying. Recurrent urinary tract infections may be treated with chronic suppressive antibiotic therapy.[49]

Sexual dysfunction in males

Sexual dysfunction is common in men with diabetes. In men, sexual dysfunction most often involves changes in libido, erectile ability, and ejaculation. Change in libido may result from chronic illness in patients with multiple diabetic complications. Impotence, defined as impairment or loss of penile erection sufficient for vaginal intercourse, may occur as a result of genitourinary autonomic neuropathy but is a diagnosis of exclusion (see Box 7-5). The history should focus on use of ethanol and medications associated with impotence such as antihypertensive and antidepressant medications. A history of pelvic surgery, especially prostate surgery, should be elicited.

Penile blood flow should be assessed by auscultating for bruits over the abdominal aorta and measuring the penile blood pressure with a Doppler probe. To rule out androgen deficiency, libido, virilization, and testicular size and consistency should be assessed. Prolactin, LH, and testosterone levels should be measured. In impotence associated with diabetic autonomic neuropathy, there is usually a gradual progression from partial to complete erectile failure over about 2 years. Impotence is not partner specific, and it is characterized by the absence of erections even during sleep. Impotence associated with diabetic autonomic neuropathy is often associated with diminished or absent testicular pain sensation to pressure, loss of perineal sensation (anal wink reflex and bulbocavernosus reflex), and neurogenic bladder dysfunction.

Therapy for impotence may include use of a suction apparatus, yohimbine, prostheses, and injections. Suction devices apply vacuum pressure to the penis, which draws blood into the penis and results in tumescence.[2] Yohimbine is an alpha-2 adrenergic blocker that increases vascular blood flow within the corpus of the penis and results in tumescence and rigidity. It is, however, associated with hypertension; use of this medication requires close monitoring of blood pressure.[94,95]

Several types of penile prostheses are currently available. These include semirigid, malleable, inflatable, and self-contained devices. Each has advantages and disadvantages, but each requires a surgical procedure for insertion. Injections of papaverine plus phentolamine into the corpus of the penis can be used to produce tumescence. This method has, however, been associated with priapism.[122] Ejaculatory failure caused by autonomic neuropathy is important if fertility is desired. Retrograde ejaculation is an unusual complication that results from damage to the efferent sympathetic nerves that normally coordinate the simultaneous closure of the internal vesicle sphincter and relaxation of the external vesicle sphincter during ejaculation. Retrograde ejaculation may be diagnosed by the presence of oligospermia or azospermia and the finding of sperm in the postcoitally voided urine. If retrograde ejaculation is incomplete or of recent onset, the patient should be instructed to have intercourse with his bladder distended. Sometimes ejaculation can be restored with use of an antihistamine or desipramine.[6,13]

Sexual dysfunction in females

Sexual dysfunction in women has not been investigated as extensively as it has been in men. Women with diabetes have been identified as having three basic sexual difficulties, including arousal, painful intercourse, and a nonorgasmic response. While it would seem unlikely that diabetes might affect orgasm in women, there is the possibility of related problems associated with lack of vasocongestion and clitoral engorgement. However, methodologies for assessing vaginal and clitoral circulation have not been developed substantially for the study of women with diabetes.[49]

Women with diabetes have an increased likelihood of dyspareunia from vaginal infections. Monilial infections are common in these women. Therapy for female sexual dysfunction may include the use of over-the-counter lubricants or estrogen creams. Estrogen creams have the advantage of providing lubrication and thickening the vaginal mucosa, which may decrease dyspareunia.[49]

Hypoglycemia unawareness

The metabolic response to hypoglycemia is mediated largely by the autonomic nervous system. The acute counterregulatory response to hypoglycemia consists of an increase in the secretion of glucagon, epinephrine, growth hormone, and corticol and an increase in glucose production by the liver. Patients with defective hypoglycemia counterregulation may present with hypoglycemia unawareness. Patients with hypoglycemia unawareness do not have typical adrenergic warning signs such as anxiety, nervousness, sweating, and palpitation. Instead, when hypoglycemic, they develop symptoms of neuroglycopenia, including irritability, mental dullness, lethargy, confusion, amnesia, loss of consciousness, and/or seizures. Patients with hypoglycemia unawareness are at increased risk of severe life-threatening hypoglycemia; patients with past histories of severe hypoglycemia are at increased risk for future occurrences.

Less is known about glucose counterregulation in NIDDM. In IDDM, the normal glucagon response to hypoglycemia deteriorates within approximately 5 years of the diagnosis of diabetes. The epinephrine response to hypoglycemia also declines with increasing duration of IDDM and in some patients is diminished or lost after 15 to 30 years. Absent glucagon and epinephrine responses to hypoglycemia greatly diminish glucose counterregulation and increase the risk for severe hypoglycemia.[49]

Hypoglycemia unawareness as a result of autonomic neuropathy is a diagnosis of exclusion (see Box 7-5). All persons who use oral hypoglycemic agents or insulin should understand the symptoms, signs, causes, and treatment of hypoglycemia (see Chapters 4 and 10). They should wear identification that identifies them as having diabetes and carry glucose or some other source of simple carbohydrate that can be used to promptly treat hypoglycemia. Patients with hypoglycemia unawareness should monitor their blood glucose levels at frequent intervals so that unexpected episodes of hypoglycemia can be recognized early and more severe hypoglycemia forestalled. Persons with hypoglycemia unawareness should have glucagon available, and family members and friends should know how and when to administer it. Adjustment of the goals for glycemic control should be considered for patients with hypoglycemia unawareness who have histories of severe hypoglycemia, for those who do not understand the educational details of avoiding or treating hypoglycemia, and for those whose life-styles make them vulnerable to life-threatening episodes of hypoglycemia.[55]

Clinical Manifestations and Diagnosis of Focal Neuropathies

A number of focal and multifocal neuropathies occur in association with diabetes mellitus.[104] The onset is typically acute and often heralded by pain. Most occur in middle-aged or older patients with NIDDM but do not seem to be correlated to the duration or control of diabetes. The neurophysiologic hallmark of focal neuropathy is the finding of abnormal nerve conduction in a distribution corresponding to the distribution of a single nerve, multiple peripheral nerves, the brachial or lumbosacral plexuses, or nerve roots. Focal neuropathies are often superimposed on diffuse symmetric sensorimotor polyneuropathy. Needle electromyography is a sensitive indicator of axonal degeneration and is very useful in documenting the presence of superimposed focal neuropathies. It can also be used to examine muscles inaccessible or poorly accessible to nerve conduction studies, including paraspinal, abdominal, and proximal extremities muscles. The subjective interpretation of the results of needle electromyography allows differentiation of acute, subacute, and chronic peripheral disorders.[49]

Cranial neuropathies

Third-nerve palsy, often termed "diabetic ophthalmoplegia," is the most common cranial mononeuropathy. Headache, eye pain, or prickling dysesthesias on the upper lid may precede a palsy by 1 or several days. Onset is usually abrupt. Ptosis is marked; the eye is deviated laterally by approximately 10 degrees, and the patient is unable to move the eye medially, up, or down. The pupil, however, is usually spared.

Progressive diminution of pain and return of oculomotor motor function is the rule, even in elderly patients. In general, findings persist for several weeks and then begin to improve gradually. Full resolution often takes 3 to 5 months. Differential diagnosis of isolated third-nerve palsy includes lesions of the midbrain, posterior circle of Willis, the cavernous sinus, the base of the brain, and the posterior orbit. Aneurysms and tumors must be considered (Box 7-6). High-resolution CT scanning or MRI is usually sufficient to rule out other potential causes.[8]

Radiculopathy

Diabetic radiculopathy presents with dermatomal pain and loss of cutaneous sensation. Although usually singular and unilateral, the syndrome may involve multiple dermatomal levels and may be bilateral in some cases. It may be associated with significant weight loss. Most often the pain is localized to the chest (truncal neuropathy) but may also affect the abdominal wall. Truncal neuropathy generally has an abrupt onset over days or weeks. Pain or dysethesia are heralding features. It is unusual to have sudden worsening with cough, sneezing, straining, or physical activity, but pain is almost universally worse at night. Since the clinical picture is that of pain, the issue of cardiopulmonary disease and visceral malignancy is usually raised. The condition resembles herpes zoster infection in the prevesicular phase. On examination, there may be hypesthesia to pinprick in the segments of greatest pain. The differential diagnosis of radiculopathy includes compressive lesions such as disk disease and cardiopulmonary and gastrointestinal disease, including pneumonia, pleurisy, myocardial infarction, cholecystitis, peptic ulcer disease, or appendicitis (see Box 7-6). Not uncommonly, multiple diagnostic procedures and even exploratory surgeries are performed before the correct diagnosis is made. Prognosis for recovery is generally good. Spontaneous resolution of both symptoms and signs is the rule and usually occurs within 6 to 24 months.[8,49]

BOX 7-6

DIFFERENTIAL DIAGNOSIS OF FOCAL NEUROPATHY

Cranial neuropathy

Increased intracranial pressure
Intracranial mass
Carotid aneurysm

Radiculopathy

Cardiopulmonary disease
Visceral malignancy
Acute abdomen
Degenerative spinal disk disease
Paget's disease

Plexopathy

Degenerative spinal disk disease
Paget's disease of the spine
Intrinsic spinal cord mass lesion
Cauda equina lesions
Coagulopathies

Mononeuropathy multiplex and mononeuropathy

Vasculitis
Amyloidosis
Hypothyroidism
Acromegaly
Coagulopathies

Plexopathy

In diabetes, the most commonly encountered plexopathy is that involving the lumbosacral plexus. The condition is relatively uncommon and of sudden onset. Patients are generally in older age-groups. The condition, also termed *femoral neuropathy,* often involves motor and sensory deficits at the level of the sacral plexus, as well as the femoral nerve. The relative excess of motor involvement differentiates diabetic femoral neuropathy from that seen in other conditions. The pain may develop insidiously or episodically and may be worse at night. Pain and sensory impairment occur in the anterior thigh and medial calf. This is associated with disabling weakness of thigh flexion and knee extension. The plantar response may be extensor, and areflexia is present. In general, pain is not present on straight leg raising, thus distinguishing diabetic femoral neuropathy from sciatica. Nevertheless, because of the similarities between diabetic femoral neuropathy and other conditions, diabetic femoral neuropathy remains a diagnosis of exclusion. Differential diagnosis includes space-occupying lesions, trauma, retroperitoneal hemorrhage, and nondiabetic vasculopathies (see Box 7-6). Nearly complete recovery is the rule, though not universal; the syndrome may persist for several years or recur.[49]

Mononeuropathy and mononeuropathy multiplex

Isolated peripheral neuropathies are more common in diabetes. It appears that diffuse diabetic neuropathy predisposes to focal nerve damage. This hypothesis is supported by the finding that 40% of unselected patients with clinically overt diffuse diabetic neuropathy have electrophysiologic or clinical evidence of superimposed focal nerve damage at common entrapment or compression sites. There is evidence that the risk of developing carpal tunnel syndrome is more than three times greater in patients with diabetes.[36a] Nerves not commonly exposed to compression or entrapment occasionally demonstrate focal impairment in patients with diabetes. This may simply reflect the coincidental occurrence of diabetes and mononeuropathy.[49]

The most common mononeuropathies associated with diabetes include those of the median nerve at the wrist (carpal tunnel syndrome associated with the pain and weakness in the hand), the ulnar nerve at the elbow (associated with weakness and loss of sensation over the palmar aspect of the fourth and fifth fingers), the radial nerve in the upper arm (associated with weakness of the upper arm, wrist drop, and loss of sensation on the back of the hand), the lateral cutaneous nerve of the thigh in the inguinal region (associated with pain in the thigh), and the peroneal nerve at the fibular head (associated with foot drop). Diagnosis of mononeuropathy or mononeuropathy multiplex should be confirmed by electrodiagnostic studies. Other nondiabetic causes should be excluded including hypothyroidism, vasculitis, and coagulopathy (see Box 7-6).[49]

Treatment of focal neuropathies

Diabetic cranial neuropathies, radiculopathies, and plexopathies generally resolve spontaneously. Reassurance often makes the pain more tolerable. If diabetic ophthalmoplegia causes diplopia, patching of the affected eye may help. Simple analgesics, antidepressants, and anticonvulsant medications can be used on a short-term basis for pain management. Physiotherapy is important to preserve range of motion and to prevent contractures for patients with femoral neuropathy. Compression and entrapment palsies in patients with diabetes respond to standard conservative or surgical management. Treatment of other mononeuropathies is essentially supportive. For example, patients with peroneal neuropathy should be fitted with ankle braces. Because diffuse diabetic neuropathy predisposes to focal nerve damage, protection against additional mechanical trauma is important.[49] For example, patients with carpal tunnel syndrome should wear neutral wrist splints, and patients with ulnar neuropathy should avoid applying pressure to their elbows and/or wear elbow pads.

General principles of preventive education

Were it not for a set of secondary complicating disorders, diabetic distal symmetric sensorimotor polyneuropathy would often be nothing more than an incidental finding on clinical examination. There are, however, a number of extremely serious consequences of sensory and/or motor denervation; many of these can be prevented through good self-care. For this reason, prophylaxis must be a major goal of diabetes patient education,[49] the principles of which are noted in Box 7-7.

Foot ulcers are a major complication of diabetic distal symmetric sensorimotor polyneuropathy (see Chapter 9). Diabetic foot ulcers arise as a result of traumatic damage to the skin and soft tissues of the feet. Insensitivity to pain is critical in the development of diabetic foot ulcers. Diminished proprioception and muscle strength, decreased sweating, and vascular factors also contribute.[49] In patients with distal symmetric sensorimotor polyneuropathy, neurogenic atrophy of the intrinsic muscles of the feet results in chronic flexion of the metatarsal-phalangeal joints, thereby drawing the toes into a cocked-up position. Autonomic dysfunction and distal anhydrosis result in decreased foot lubrication. Weight bearing is thus shifted to the metatarsal heads; and, in the absence of pain, thick calluses form over the bony prominences. With repeated trauma, the dry skin over these abnormal pressure points breaks down; the resulting ulcers may go unnoticed even when secondary infection develops.[49]

A second complication associated with distal symmetric sensorimotor polyneuropathy is neuroarthropathy, also called *Charcot's joint*. Neuroarthropathy occurs in any condition in which sensation is impaired but motor function is left relatively intact. Diabetic neuroarthropathy involves primarily the ankle, metatarsal, or metatarsal-phalangeal joints. Patients with neuroarthropathy often present with painless swelling and redness of the foot in the

---

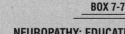

BOX 7-7

NEUROPATHY: EDUCATION PRINCIPLES

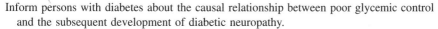

Inform persons with diabetes about the causal relationship between poor glycemic control and the subsequent development of diabetic neuropathy.

Explain possible risk factors (such as smoking, alcohol) and concomitant neural insults that may hasten the development or progression of diabetic neuropathy.

Stress that sensory or motor neuropathy may be asymptomatic.

Explain that routine evaluation is necessary even for patients who have no symptoms of neuropathy.

Explain that diabetic neuropathy can contribute to the development of other complications.

Inform patients who have lost sensation in their feet about the importance of caring for their feet and wearing proper shoes.

Stress the importance of proper exercise.

Discuss the signs and symptoms of autonomic neuropathy.

Explain the benefits of treatment to patients with autonomic neuropathy.

Modified from Herman WH, editor: *The prevention and treatment of complications of diabetes mellitus: a guide for primary care practitioners,* Atlanta, 1991, Dept of Health and Human Services, Public Health Services, Centers for Disease Control, Center for Chronic Disease Prevention and Health Promotions.

absence of fever or leukocytosis. Large-fiber neuropathy is almost universally present. Pedal pulses are generally intact and often quite strong. Unhealed fractures are often evident radiographically. In later stages, patients may present with gross architectural distortion of the foot. In the most advanced stages multiple fractures are accompanied by extensive bone demineralization and reabsorption. The pathogenetic mechanism is presumed to be multiple recurrent traumatic insults of the joint that are not noticed by the patient because of insensitivity to pain (see Chapter 9).[49,50]

Patient education

Persons with insensitive feet may not be aware of foot problems. Therefore, at each visit, the health care provider should inquire for symptoms of peripheral neuropathy. Shoes and socks must be removed at every visit—at least four times a year—and the feet inspected for dryness, calluses, deformities, ulcers, and evidence of neuroarthropathy. At least once a year, the health care provider should assess the patient's ability to sense temperature, pinprick, pressure, touch, and vibration and should test muscle strength and deep-tendon reflexes.[55]

Persons with diabetes and evidence of distal symmetric sensorimotor polyneuropathy must learn foot hygiene and foot protection. Patients who spend a lot of time on their feet, who do a great deal of walking, or who jog for exercise may need to change their activity. Patients with deformed feet almost always require specially molded, extra-depth shoes. Deformed feet will not fit into ordinary shoes, although the patient, because of loss of sensation, may think they fit. The wearing of ordinary shoes on deformed feet may result in abrasions, ulcerations, and infection, which can lead to gangrene and amputation.[55]

When patients present with foot ulcers, the ulcers should be vigorously debrided to establish the depth. Radiographs should be used to exclude the possibility of embedded foreign objects or osteomyelitis. If osteomyelitis is suspected, follow-up radiographs and appropriate scans should be used to help establish the diagnosis. Where there is significant infection, parenteral antibiotics should be used. Because anaerobes frequently occur in the foot ulcers of patients with diabetes, aerobic and anaerobic bacterial cultures should be obtained to select appropriate antibiotics.[55]

Patients with foot ulcers should not put weight on the affected foot. Those who do not feel pain will likely continue to walk; the resulting pressure on the foot will prevent healing. Total bedrest or the use of crutches may be required. Total-contact casts have been shown to help patients with foot ulcers ambulate while ulcers heal. The casts redistribute pressure so that the area of the ulcer bears much less weight than it would otherwise.[55]

Prophylactic measures to prevent neuroarthropathy include avoiding prolonged weight bearing, avoiding strenuous weight-bearing exercise or athletic activities, ambulating only over well-lighted, smooth terrain, and wearing cushioned shoes. Therapy is directed at removal of continued trauma by removing the involved extremity from weight bearing, either by decreasing ambulation or providing other means of weight bearing. The use of a bivalved ankle/foot orthosis and the use of a cane, crutches, or wheelchair are often necessary.[49]

All patients with diabetes should be informed about the relationship between poor glycemic control and diabetic neuropathy and the role of diabetic neuropathy in the development of other complications, including foot ulcers and amputation. Patients should be informed of the importance of routine clinical evaluations for diabetic neuropathy, even when they have no symptoms. Individuals with distal symmetric sensorimotor polyneuropathy should understand that other factors such as consumption of ethanol and exposure to chemical toxins may hasten the progression of neuropathy. Persons with insensitive feet should understand the importance of caring for their feet, of wearing proper shoes, and of getting appropriate exercise. They should be aware of the possible signs and symptoms of autonomic neuropathy and understand the availability and benefits of treatment for autonomic neuropathy.[55]

The prevalence of microvascular complications in diabetes makes the role of preventive education critical. The health care provider needs to carefully and regularly assess patient status with regard to the occurrence of complications and to provide frequent and regular patient and family education with regard to preventive or ongoing care. To ensure such systematic quality care, all members of the health care team need to carefully work with the person with diabetes and his or her family to ensure that principles of education and preventive guidelines of care are followed. The emphasis on education, leading to routine preventive follow-up care, is critical to assist the person with diabetes in achieving his or her optimal level of well-being.

REFERENCES

1. Abram DR: Decreased alpha-2 adrenergic receptors on platelet membranes from diabetic patients with autonomic neuropathy and orthostatic hypotension, *J Clin Endocrin Metab* 63:906-912, 1986.
2. Al-Juburi AZ, O'Donnell PD: Synergist erection system: clinical experience, *Urology* 35:304-306, 1990.
3. American Diabetes Association: Consensus statement—diabetic neuropathy, *Diabetes Care* 13(suppl 1):47-52, 1990.
3a. American Diabetes Association: Concensus statement: treatment of hypertension in diabetes, *Diabetes Care* 16:1394-1401, 1993.
4. American Diabetes Association: DCCT, diabetes control and complications trial: 1993, *Diabetes Care* 11:1517-1520, 1993.
4a. American Diabetes Association: Nutritional recommendations and principles for individuals with diabetes mellitus: 1986, *Diabetes Care* 10:126-132, 1987.
5. Amico JA, Klein I: Diabetic management in patients with renal failure, *Diabetes Care* 4:430-434, 1991.
6. Andaloro VA Jr, Dube A: Treatment of retrograde ejaculation with brompheniramine, *Urology* 5:520-522, 1975.
7. Andersen AR and others: Diabetic nephropathy in type I (insulin-dependent) diabetes: an epidemiologic study, *Diabetologia* 25:496-501, 1983.
8. Asbury AK: Focal and multifocal neuropathies of diabetes. In Dyck PJ and others, editors: *Diabetic neuropathy,* Philadelphia, 1987, WB Saunders.
9. Ballard DJ and others: Epidemiology of persistent proteinuria in type II diabetes mellitus: population-based study in Rochester, Minnesota, *Diabetes* 37:405-412, 1988.
10. Barbosa J: Is diabetic microangiopathy genetically heterogeneous? HLA and diabetic nephropathy, *Hormone Metab Res* 11:77-80, 1981.
11. Boesen F and others: Treatment of diabetic orthostatic hypotension with pindolol, *Acta Neurol Scan* 66:386-91, 1982.
12. Boulton AJ, Levin S, Comstock J: A multicentre trial of the aldose-reductase inhibitor, tolrestat, in patients with symptomatic diabetic neuropathy, *Diabetologia* 33:431-437, 1990.
13. Brooks ME, Berezin M, Braf Z: Treatment of retrograde ejaculation with imipramine, *Urology* 15:353-355, 1980.
14. Burns-Cox CJ, Hart JC: Screening of diabetics for retinopathy by ophthalmic opticians, *Br Med J* 290:1052-1054, 1985.
15. Campbell IW, Ewing DJ, Clarke BF: A-alpha-fluorohydrocortisone in the treatment of postural hypotension in diabetic autonomic neuropathy, *Diabetes* 24:381-384, 1975.
16. Campbell RK, Baker DE: New drug update: capsaicin, *Diabetes Educ* 16:313-316, 1990.
17. Carr S and others: Increase in glomerular filtration rate in patients with insulin-dependent di-

abetes and elevated erythrocyte sodium-lithium countertransport, *N Engl J Med* 322:500-505, 1990.

18. Chakrabarti AK, Samantaray SK: Diabetic peripheral neuropathy: nerve conduction studies before, during, and after carbamazepine therapy, *Aust NZ Med* 6:565-568, 1976.

19. Champion MC: Management of idiopathic, diabetic, and miscellaneous gastroparesis with cisapride, *Scand J Gastrointerol* 165(suppl):44-52, 1989.

20. Christensen CK, Mogensen CE: Antihypertensive treatment: long-term reversal of progression of albuminuria in incipient diabetic nephropathy. A longitudinal study of renal function, *J Diab Complic* 1:45-52, 1987.

21. Christensen CK, Mogensen CE: Effect of antihypertensive treatment on progression of disease in incipient diabetic nephropathy, *Hypertension* 7:109-114, 1985.

22. Cohen KL, Harris S: Efficacy and safety of nonsteroidal anti-inflammatory drugs in the therapy of diabetic neuropathy, *Arch Int Med* 147:1442-1444, 1987.

23. Collins AJ and others: Changing risk factors demographics in end-stage renal disease patients entering hemodialysis and the impact on long-term mortality, *Am J Kidney Dis* 25:422-432, 1990.

24. Condon JR and others: Cholestyramine and diabetic and post-vagotomy diarrhoea, *Br Med J* 4:423, 1973.

25. Constable IJ and others: Assessing the risk of diabetic retinopathy, *Am J Ophthalmol* 97:53-61, 1984.

26. Cowie CC and others: Disparities in incidence of diabetic end-stage renal disease according to race and type of diabetes, *N Engl J Med* 321:1074-1079, 1989.

27. Dahl-Jorgensen K and others: Effect of near normoglycemia for two years on progression of early diabetic retinopathy, nephropathy, and neuropathy: the Oslo study, *Br Med J* 293:1195-1199, 1986.

28. Damsgaard EM, Mogensen CE: Microalbuminuria in elderly hyperglycaemic patients and controls, *Diabetic Med* 3:430-435, 1986.

28a. DCCT Research Group: The effect of intensive treatment of diabetes on the development and progression of long-term complications in insulin-dependent diabetes mellitus, *N Engl J Med* 329:977-86, 1993.

29. Dejgard A, Petersen P, Kastrup J: Mexiletine for treatment of chronic painful diabetic neuropathy, *Lancet* 1:9-11, 1988.

30. Demarie BK, Bakris GL: Effects of different calcium antagonists on proteinuria associated with diabetes mellitus, *Ann Int Med* 113:987-988, 1990.

31. DePonti F, Fealey RD, Malagelada JR:Gastrointinal syndromes due to diabetes mellitus. In Dyck PJ and others, editors: *Diabetic neuropathy,* Philadelphia, 1987, WB Saunders.

32. Diabetic Retinopathy Study Research Group: Photocoagulation treatment of proliferative diabetic retinopathy: clinical application of Diabetic Retinopathy Study (DRS) findings, DRS Report Number 8, *Ophthalmology* 88:583-600, 1981.

33. Diabetic Retinopathy Vitrectomy Study Research Group: Early vitrectomy for severe proliferative diabetic retinopathy in eyes with useful vision, Diabetic Retinopathy Vitrectomy Study Report 3, *Ophthalmology* 95:1307-1320, 1988.

34. Diabetic Retinopathy Vitrectomy Study Research Group: Early vitrectomy for severe vitreous hemorrhage in diabetic retinopathy: two-year results of a randomized trial, Diabetic Retinopathy Vitrectomy Study Report 2, *Arch Ophthalmol* 103:1644-1652, 1985.

35. Division of Diabetes Translation: Diabetes surveillance, 1980-1987, Atlanta, 1990, US Department of Health and Human Services, Public Health Service, Centers for Disease Control.

36. Dyck PJ and others: *Diabetic neuropathy,* Philadelphia, 1987, WB Saunders.

36a. Dyck PJ and others: The prevalence by staged severity of various types of diabetic neuropathy, retinopathy, and nephropathy in a population-based cohort: the Rochester Diabetic Neuropathy Study, *Neurology* 43:817-24, 1993.

37. Early Treatment Diabetic Retinopathy Study Research Group: Photocoagulation for diabetic macular edema: Early Treatment Diabetic Retinopathy Study Report Number 1, *Arch Ophthalmol* 103:1796-1806, 1985.

38. Egbunike IG, Chaffee BJ: Antidepressants in the management of chronic pain syndromes, *Pharmacotherapy* 10:262-270, 1990.

39. Evanoff G and others: Prolonged dietary protein restriction in diabetic nephropathy, *Arch Intern Med* 149:1129-1133, 1989.

40. Ewing DJ, Clarke BF: Diabetic autonomic neuropathy: a clinical viewpoint. In Dyck PJ and others, editors: *Diabetic neuropathy,* Philadelphia, 1987, WB Saunders.

41. Fabre J and others: The kidney in maturity onset diabetes mellitus: a clinical study of 510 patients, *Kidney Int* 21:730-738, 1982.

42. Fedorak RN, Filed M, Chang BB: Treatment of diabetic diarrhea with clonidine, *Ann Intern Med* 102:197-199, 1985.

43. Feldman M, Schiller LR: Disorders of gastrointestinal motility associated with diabetes mellitus, *Ann Intern Med* 98:378-384, 1983.

44. Feldt-Rasmussen B, Mathiesen ER, Deckert T: Effect on the progression of diabetic renal disease during two years of strict metabolic control in insulin-dependent diabetes, *Lancet* 2:1300-1304, 1986.

44a. Ferrara A, Barrett-Connor EL, Edelstein SL: Hyperinsulinemia does not increase the risk of fatal cardiovascular disease in elderly men and women without diabetes: the Rancho Bernardo Study, 1984-1991, *Am J Epidemiol* 140:857-869, 1994.

44b. Ferris FL III: How effective are treatments for diabetic retinopathy? *JAMA* 269:1290-1291, 1993.

44c. Fontbonne A and others: Hyperinsulinaemia as a predictor of coronary heart disease mortality in a healthy population: the Paris Prospective Study, 15-year follow-up, *Diabetologia* 34:356-361, 1991.

45. Gentry P, Miller PF: Nutritional considerations in a patient with gastroparesis, *Diabetes Educ* 15:374-376, 1989.

45a. Genuth S: Insulin use in NIDDM, *Diabetes Care* 13:1240-64, 1990.

46. Gills JS and others: Effect of the aldose reductase inhibitor, ponalrestat, on diabetic neuropathy, *Diabetes Metab* 16:296-302, 1990.

47. Gomez-Perez FJ and others: Nortriptyline and fluphenazine in the symptomatic treatment of diabetic neuropathy. A double-blind cross-over study, *Pain* 23:395-400, 1985.

48. Green PA, Berge KG, Sprague RG: Control of diabetic diarrhea with antibiotic therapy, *Diabetes* 17:385-387, 1968.

49. Greene DA, and others: Diabetic neuropathy. In Rifkin H and Porte D, Jr, editors: *Ellenberg and Rifkin's diabetes mellitus, theory and practice,* ed 4, New York, 1990, Elsevier Publishing.

50. Deleted in proofs.

51. Harkonen S and Kjellstrand CM: Exacerbation of diabetic renal failure following intravenous pyelography, *Am J Med* 63:936-946, 1977.

52. Held PJ and others: Five-year survival for end-stage renal disease patients in the United States, Europe, and Japan, 1982-87, *Am J Kidney Dis* 15:451-457, 1990.

53. Herman WH and others: An approach to the prevention of blindness in diabetes, *Diabetes Care* 6:608-613, 1983.

54. Herman WH and others: Consensus statement. Proceedings from the International Symposium on Preventing the Kidney Disease of Diabetes Mellitus: public health perspectives, *Am J Kidney Dis* 13:2-6, 1989.

55. Herman WH, editor: The prevention and treatment of complications of diabetes mellitus: a guide for primary care practitioners, Atlanta, 1991, Department of Health and Human Services, Public Health Service, Centers for Disease Control, Center for Chronic Disease Prevention and Health Promotion.

56. Hoeldtke RD, Boden G, O'Dorisio TM: Treatment of postural hypotension with a somatostatin analogue (SMS 201-995), *Am J Med* 81(suppl 6B):83-87, 1986.

57. Hostetter TH, Rennke HG, Brenner BM: The case for intrarenal hypertension in the initiation and progression of diabetic and other glomerulopathies, *Am J Med* 72:375-380, 1982.

58. Humphrey LL and others: Chronic renal failure in non-insulin-dependent diabetes mellitus: a population based study in Rochester, Minnesota, *Ann Intern Med* 111:788-796, 1989.

59. Janka HU and others: Risk factors for progression of background retinopathy in long-standing IDDM, *Diabetes* 38:460-464, 1989.

60. Janssens J and others: Improvement of gastric emptying in diabetic gastroparesis by erythromycin: preliminary studies, *N Engl J Med* 332:1028-1031, 1990.

61. Jarrett RJ and others: Microalbuminuria predicts mortality in non-insulin-dependent diabetes, *Diabetes Med* 1:17-19, 1984.

62. Jones SL and others: Sodium-lithium countertransport in microalbuminuric insulin-dependent diabetic patients, *Hypertension* 15:570-575, 1990.

62a. Kasiske BL and others: Effect of antihypertensive therapy on the kidney in patients with diabetes: a meta-regression analysis, *Ann Int Med* 118:129-138, 1993.

63. Klein BEK, Moss SE, Klein R: Effect of pregnancy on progression of diabetic retinopathy, *Diabetes Care* 13:34-40, 1990.

64. Klein R and others: Diabetic retinopathy as detected using ophthalmoscopy, a nonmydriatic camera and a standard fundus camera, *Ophthalmology* 92:485-491, 1985.

65. Klein R and others: Proteinuria in diabetes, *Arch Intern Med* 148:181-186, 1988.

66. Klein R and others: The Wisconsin Epidemiologic Study of Diabetic Retinopathy. II. Prevalence and risk of diabetic retinopathy when age at diagnosis is less than 30 years, *Arch Ophthalmol* 102:520-526, 1984.

67. Klein R and others: The Wisconsin Epidemiologic Study of Diabetic Retinopathy. III. Prevalence and risk of diabetic retinopathy when age at diagnosis

is 30 or more years, *Arch Ophthalmol* 102:527-532, 1984.

68. Klein R and others: The Wisconsin Epidemiologic Study of Diabetic Retinopathy. IV. Diabetic macular edema, *Ophthalmology* 91:1464-1474, 1984.

69. Klein R and others: The Wisconsin Epidemiologic Study of Diabetic Retinopathy. IX. Four-year incidence and progression of diabetic retinopathy when age at diagnosis is less than 30 years, *Arch Ophthalmol* 107:237-243, 1989.

70. Klein R and others: The Wisconsin Epidemiologic Study of Diabetic Retinopathy. X. Four-year incidence and progression of diabetic retinopathy when age at diagnosis is 30 years or more, *Arch Ophthalmol* 107:244-249, 1989.

71. Klein R and others: The Wisconsin Epidemiologic Study of Diabetic Retinopathy. XI. The incidence of macular edema, *Ophthalmology* 96:1501-1510, 1989.

72. Klein R and others: Visual impairment in diabetes, *Ophthalmology* 91:1-9, 1984.

73. Klein R, Moss SE, Klein BEK: New management concepts for timely diagnosis of diabetic retinopathy treatable by photocoagulation, *Diabetes Care* 10:633-638, 1987.

74. Kleinstein RN and others: Detection of diabetic retinopathy by optometrists, *J Am Optom Assoc* 58:879-882, 1987.

75. Knowler WC, Bennett PH, Ballintine EJ: Increased incidence of retinopathy in diabetics with elevated blood pressure, *N Engl J Med* 302:645-650, 1980.

76. Knowles HC: Magnitude of the renal failure problem in diabetic patients, *Kidney Int* 1(suppl): 2-7, 1974.

77. The Kroc Collaborative Study Group: Blood glucose control and the evolution of diabetic retinopathy and albuminuria. A preliminary multicenter trial, *N Engl J Med* 311:365-372, 1984.

78. Krolewski AS and others: Predisposition to hypertension and susceptibility to renal disease in insulin-dependent diabetes mellitus, *N Engl J Med* 318:140-145, 1988.

79. Kuchel O and others: Treatment of severe orthostatic hypotension by metoclopramide, *Ann Intern Med* 93:841-843, 1980.

80. Kunzelman CL and others: Incidence of proteinuria in type 2 diabetes mellitus in Pima Indians, *Kidney Int* 35:681-687, 1989.

81. Kvinesdal B and others: Imipramine in treatment of painful diabetic neuropathy, *JAMA* 251:1727-1730, 1984.

82. Levy DM, Abraham RR, Tomlinson DR: Topical capsaicin in the treatment of painful diabetic neuropathy, *N Engl J Med* 324:776-777, 1991.

82a. Lewis EJ and others: The effect of angiotensin-converting-enzyme inhibition on diabetic nephropathy, *N Engl J Med* 329:1456-1462, 1993.

82b. Liu QZ and others: Insulin treatment, endogenous insulin concentration, and ECG abnormalities in diabetic Pima Indians. Cross-sectional and prospective analyses. *Diabetes* 41:1141-50, 1992.

83. Mangili R and others: Increased sodium-lithium countertransport activity in red cells of patients with insulin-dependent diabetes and nephropathy, *N Engl J Med* 318:146-150, 1988.

84. Max MD and others: Amitriptyline relieves diabetic neuropathy pain in patients with normal and depressed mood, *Neurology* 37:589-596, 1987.

85. McCallum RW and others: A multicenter placebo-controlled clinical trial of oral metaclopramide in diabetic gastroparesis, *Diabetes Care* 6:463-467, 1983.

86. Melton LJ III, Dyck PJ: Epidemiology. In Dyck PJ and others, editors: *Diabetic neuropathy,* Philadelphia, 1987, WB Saunders.

87. Mogensen CE: Complete screening of urinary albumin concentration in an unselected diabetic outpatient clinic population, *Diabetic Nephropathy* 2:11-18, 1983.

88. Mogenesen CE: Long-term antihypertensive treatment inhibiting progression of diabetic nephropathy, *Br Med J* 285:685-688, 1982.

89. Mogensen CE: Microalbuminuria as a predictor of clinical diabetic nephropathy, *Kidney Int* 31:673-689, 1987.

90. Mogensen CE: Microalbuminuria predicts clinical proteinuria and early mortality in maturity-onset diabetes, *N Engl J Med* 310:356-360, 1984.

91. Mogensen CE, Christensen CK: Predicting diabetic nephropathy in insulin-dependent patients, *N Engl J Med* 311:89-93, 1984.

92. Mogensen CE, Christensen CK, Vittinghus E: The stages in diabetic renal disease: with emphasis on the stage of incipient diabetic nephropathy, *Diabetes* 32(suppl):64-78, 1983.

93. Mogensen CE, Schmitz A, Christensen CK: Comparative renal pathophysiology relevant to IDDM and NIDDM patients, *Diabetes Metab Rev* 4:453-483, 1988.

94. Morales A, Surridge DH, Marshall PG: Yohimbine for treatment of impotence in diabetes, *N Engl J Med* 305:1221, 1981.

95. Morales A and others: Is yohimbine effective in the treatment of organic impotence? Results of a controlled trial, *J Urol* 137:1168-1172, 1987.

96. Moss SE and others: Comparison between ophthalmoscopy and fudus photography in determin-

ing severity of diabetic retinopathy, *Ophthalmology* 92:62-67, 1985.

97. Nelson RG and others: Effect of proteinuria on mortality in NIDDM, *Diabetes* 37:1499-1504, 1988.

98. Nelson RG and others: Incidence of end-stage renal disease in type 2 (non-insulin-dependent) diabetes mellitus in Pima Indians, *Diabetologia* 31:730-736, 1988.

99. Nelson RG and others: Proliferative retinopathy in NIDDM: incidence and risk factors in Pima Indians, *Diabetes* 38:435-440, 1989.

100. O'Hare JP and others: Aldose reductase inhibitor in diabetic neuropathy: clinical and neurophysiological studies of one year's treatment with sorbinil, *Diabetic Med* 5:537-542, 1988.

101. Palumbo PJ, Elveback LR, Whisnant JP: Neurologic complications of diabetes mellitus: transient ischemic attack, stroke, and peripheral neuropathy, *Adv Neurol* 19:593-601, 1978.

102. Parfrey PS and others: Contrast material induced renal failure in patients with diabetes mellitus, renal insufficiency, or both, *N Engl J Med* 320: 143-149, 1989.

103. Parving HH and others: Early aggressive antihypertension treatment reduces rate of decline in kidney function in diabetic nephropathy, *Lancet* 1:1175-1179, 1983.

104. Pfeifer MA, Greene DA: Diabetic neuropathy current concepts, Kalamazoo, Mich, 1985, The Upjohn Co.

105. Pirart J: Diabetes mellitus and its degenerative complications: a prospective study of 4,400 patients observed between 1947 and 1973, *Diabetes Care* 1:168-188, 1978.

106. Pitkanen E and others: HLA antigen distribution in juvenile diabetics with end-stage nephropathy, *Am Clin Res* 13:91-95, 1981.

106a. Proceedings of a consensus development conference on standardized measures in diabetic neuropathy, *Neurology* 42:1823-39, 1992.

106b. Pyorala K and others: Plasma insulin as coronary heart disease risk factor: relationship to other risk factors and predictive value during 9½-year follow-up of the Helsinki Policeman Study Population, *Acta Med Scand Suppl* 701:38-52, 1985.

107. Rabinowe SL and others: Complement-fixing antibodies to sympathetic and parasympathetic tissues in IDDM: autonomic brake index and heart-rate variation, *Diabetes Care* 13:1084-1088, 1990.

107a. Ravid M and others: Long-term stabilizing effect of angiotensin-converting enzyme inhibition on plasma creatinine and on proteinuria in normo-

tensive type II diabetic patients, *Ann Int Med* 118:577-81, 1993.

108. Recommended Dietary Allowances, ed 10, Washington, DC, 1989, National Research Council, National Academy Press.

108a. Reichard P, Nilsson B-Y, Rosenqvist U: The effect of long-term intensified insulin treatment on the development of microvascular complications of diabetes mellitus, *N Engl J Med* 329:304-9, 1993.

109. Rettig B, Teutsch SM: The incidence of end-stage renal disease in type I and type II diabetes mellitus, *Diabetic Nephropathy* 3:26-27, 1984.

109a. Ronnemaa T and others: High fasting plasma insulin is an indicator of coronary heart disease in non-insulin-dependent diabetic patients and non-diabetic subjects, *Arteriosclerosis Thrombosis* 11: 80-90, 1991.

110. Ross DR, Varipapa RJ: Treatment of painful diabetic neuropathy with capsaicin, *N Engl J Med* 321:474-475, 1989.

111. Saadoun AP: Diabetes and periodontal disease: a review and update, *Periodontal Abst* 28:116-139, 1980.

112. Salway JG and others: Effect of myo-inositol on peripheral-nerve function in diabetes, *Lancet* 2:1282-1284, 1978.

113. Saudek CD, Werns S, Reidenberg MM: Phenytoin in the treatment of diabetic symmetrical polyneuropathy, *Clin Pharmacol Ther* 22:196-199, 1977.

114. Schmitz A, Gundersen HJG, Osterby R: Glomerular morphology by light microscopy in non-insulin-dependent diabetes mellitus: lack of glomerular hypertrophy, *Diabetes* 37:38-43, 1988.

115. Seaquist ER and others: Familial clustering of diabetic kidney disease: evidence for genetic susceptibility to diabetic nephropathy, *N Engl J Med* 320:1161-1166, 1989.

116. Service FJ and others: Near normoglycemia: improved nerve conduction and vibration sensation in diabetic neuropathy, *Diabetologia* 28:722-727, 1985.

117. Stross JK, Harlan WR: The dissemination of new medical information, *JAMA* 241:2622-2624, 1979.

118. Sussman EJ, Tsiaras WG, Soper KA: Diagnosis of diabetic eye disease, *JAMA* 247:3231-3234, 1982.

119. Swerdlow M: Anticonvulsant drugs and chronic pain, *Clin Neuropharmacol* 7:51-82, 1984.

120. Thomas PK, Brown MJ: Diabetic polyneuropathy. In Dyck PJ and others, editors: *Diabetic neuropathy,* Philadelphia, 1987, WB Saunders.

120a. UK Prospective Diabetes Study Group. UK Prospective Diabetes Study (UKPDS). VIII. Study design, progress and performance, *Diabetologia* 34:877-90, 1991.

120b. Viberti G and others: *Effect of captopril on progression to clinical proteinuria in patients with insulin-dependent diabetes mellitus and microalbuminuria.* European Microalbuminaria Captopril Study Group (see comments) *JAMA* 271:275-79, 1994.

121. Vinik AI and others: Somatostatin analogue (SMS 201-995) in the management of gastroenteropancreatic tumors and diarrhea syndromes, *Am J Med* 81:23-29, 1986.

122. Virag R and others: Intracavernous self-injection of vasoactive drugs in the treatment of impotence: 8-year experience with 615 cases, *J Urol* 145:287-292, 1991.

123. Vlassara H, Brownlee M, Cerami A: Nonezymatic glycosylation peripheral nerve protein in diabetes mellitus, *Proc Natl Acad Sci* 78:5190-5192, 1981.

123a. Wang PH, Lau J, Chalmers TC: Meta-analysis of effects of intensive blood-glucose control on late complications of type I diabetes. *Lancet* 341: 1306-9, 1993.

124. Watts GF and others: Treatment of diabetic gastroparesis with oral domperidone, *Diabetic Med* 2:491-492, 1985.

125. Weinrauch LA and others: Coronary angiography and acute renal failure in diabetic azotemic nephropathy, *Ann Intern Med* 86:56-59, 1977.

125a. Welborn TA, Wearne K: Coronary heart disease incidence and cardiovascular mortality in Busselton with reference to glucose and insulin concentrations, *Diabetes Care* 2:154-60, 1979.

125b. Welin L and others: Hyperinsulinaemia is not a major coronary risk factor in elderly men. The study of men born in 1913, *Diabetologia* 35:766-70, 1992.

126. Wilson J: Periodontal diseases and diabetes, *Diabetes Educ* 15:342-345, 1989.

127. Witkin SR, Klein R: Ophthalmologic care for persons with diabetes, *JAMA* 251:2534-2537, 1984.

128. Yassine MD: Diabetic nephropathy in noninsulin dependent diabetes mellitus: natural history and risk factors, doctoral dissertation (Epidemiologic Science), Ann Arbor, 1990, University of Michigan.

129. Young RJ, Clarke BF: Pain relief in diabetic neuropathy: the effectiveness of imipramine and related drugs, *Diabetic Med* 2:363-366, 1985.

130. Zeller K and others: Effect of restricting dietary protein on the progression of renal failure in patients with insulin-dependent diabetes mellitus, *N Engl J Med* 324:78-84, 1991.

8 Features of Macrovascular Disease of Diabetes

Frank Vinicor

Although the availability of insulin since 1922 has resulted in a decrease in death as a result of acute complications such as diabetes ketoacidosis,[22] diabetes mellitus has not been cured. Thus patients with diabetes and their health care providers today face chronic complications associated with this disorder. It is traditional to consider these chronic conditions as microvascular disorders, such as retinopathy, nephropathy, metabolic conditions (e.g., peripheral neuropathy), and macrovascular disorders, such as coronary artery disease (CAD).[89] Chapter 7 focuses on microvascular disorders related to diabetes.

IMPACT OF MACROVASCULAR DISEASE
Definition

Macrovascular disease is defined as disorders of large vessels with resultant morbidity and mortality. Pathologically, macrovascular disease in diabetes mellitus reflects atherosclerosis, the deposit of material (e.g., lipids) within the inner layer—the intima—of vessel walls, discussed later in this chapter.[149]

Macrovascular disease clinically manifests as heart disease (e.g., myocardial infarction [MI]), central nervous system (CNS) conditions, cerebrovascular accident (CVA, stroke), and

---

CHAPTER OBJECTIVES

- Discuss the importance of diabetes-associated macrovascular disease.
- Describe why macrovascular disease is so common in persons with diabetes.
- Address the best clinical and public health strategies for reducing problems associated with macrovascular disease in diabetes.
- Discuss future therapeutic options and challenges.

---

lower extremity disease (vascular foot ulcers). At a cellular level, important pathophysiologic commonalities may exist between microvascular and macrovascular disease, but macrovascular disorders create a varied picture of a person with diabetes who exhibits exertion-associated chest pain, episodic symptoms of dizziness, and slurred speech, caused by transient ischemic attacks (TIAs) or exercise-related calf cramps (i.e., claudication).

This symptomatology can occur separately or concomitantly. Thus the quality and duration of life of the person with diabetes-related macrovascular disease can be greatly affected. This "burden of disease" has implications not only from an individual perspective, but also from a clinical and public health perspective.

Burden of Macrovascular Disease

The term *burden* refers to the extent to which a particular disease, or components of that disease, is important from a clinical and public health perspective. How does one decide if a disease is important? From a traditional clinical perspective, it is important that each individual under care for diabetes and its concomitant problems receive the best care possible to improve quality of life. Thus health care providers strive to reduce the individual clinical problems faced by each person with diabetes (e.g., hypoglycemia, visual loss, foot ulcers).

From a public health perspective, there are several other interrelated indicators of the impact, or burden, of a disease.[55,166] These are depicted in Fig. 8-1 and include the following:

1. Currently, the *prevalence* of diabetes indicates a significant problem for at least 8% to 10% of the population. This problem will become more significant in an aging, weight-gaining society.[44,74]

2. As previously noted, from an individual perspective, the extent to which a disease decreases *quality of life* certainly affects the person with diabetes. These same concerns affect the larger population and contribute to the definition of "burden" in terms of public health, with recognition of the extent to which a disease significantly impacts on national mortality, morbidity, or disability statistics. Problems associated with morbidity and disability, such as cardiovascular disease or amputations caused by vascular disease, indicate that diabetes-related complications weigh heavily on the public's health.[55,83]

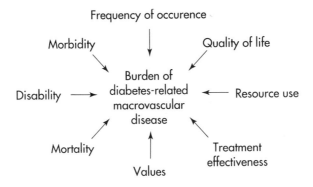

Fig. 8-1   The burden of diabetes-related macrovascular disease.

3. The extent to which persons with diabetes *use and "stress" health care resources* alters the public's perspective of the disease's degree of burden. This perception may impact the extent to which public health resources will be channeled to accommodate the needs of persons with diabetes. This issue, the use of health care system resources, has become particularly relevant with the conclusion of the Diabetes Control and Complications Trial (DCCT).[43,137] If extensive funding is needed to combat diabetes, it will be seen as a larger public health concern.[9,143]

4. The *effectiveness* of treatment might also influence the extent to which a disease is seen as a burden. From an individual perspective, diabetes may greatly impact daily life in terms of the therapeutic regimen and its requirements (e.g., blood glucose monitoring, dietary requirements). In terms of a public health burden, however, the advances associated with management of diabetes have enabled diabetic persons to engage in normal life activities and function as active members of society.

5. Finally, *individual or societal values* may impact the extent to which a disease is seen as a burden. For example, if the disease is a direct result of an individual's choice (e.g., sexually transmitted diseases, lung cancer from smoking cigarettes), the perception of a public health responsibility may be less, in contrast to a disease in which the individual is viewed as an innocent "victim."

Macrovascular Disease in Diabetic and Nondiabetic Populations

Impressive data exist to document the impact of diabetic macrovascular disease.* Macrovascular disease, especially CAD, is the most common cause of death in diabetic persons, accounting for 40% to 60% of all causes of mortality. More than one half of all nontraumatic lower extremity amputations, or approximately 56,000 per year,[44] in part caused by peripheral vascular disease, occur in persons with diabetes. These individuals are 15 to 20 times more likely to have a nontraumatic amputation than nondiabetic persons (see Chapter 9). Regrettably, about one half of these lower extremity amputations in persons with diabetes could have been prevented. The most common reasons for hospitalization among persons with diabetes are complications caused by macrovascular disease. Of the $105 billion estimated annual health care costs among persons with diabetes (nondiabetes plus diabetes costs) in the United States, primarily in non-insulin-dependent diabetes mellitus (NIDDM), macrovascular disorders are the major components of these costs, especially in patients over 65 years of age.[143]

However, it is not only epidemiologic and public health data that suggest diabetes-related macrovascular disease is important. Clinicians and practitioners frequently see patients with diabetes in the following situations: (1) in the coronary care unit with an MI, (2) with loss of cognitive and physical function as a result of a CVA, and (3) with a lower extremity amputation caused by peripheral vascular disease (see Chapter 9). These are all common health problems for persons with diabetes and familiar clinical issues that practitioners face daily.

---

*References 21, 44, 80, 111, 126, 155.

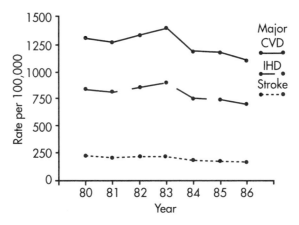

Fig. 8-2 Age-standardized mortality rates for major cardiovascular disease *(CVD)*, ischemic heart disease *(IHD)* and stroke (cerebrovascular accident, CVA) as underlying causes per 100,000 diabetic population, by year, United States, 1980 to 1986. (Modified from *Diabetes surveillance, policy, program, research: DHHS; PHS; Centers for Disease Control,* Center for Chronic Disease Prevention and Health Promotion, Division of Diabetes Translation, Atlanta, 1990, Centers for Disease Control.)

Features of Macrovascular Disease in Diabetes

Because only about 6% to 8% of persons in the United States have diabetes,[74] *most* people with MI or CVA, in terms of absolute numbers, do *not* have diabetes.[140] However, the *likelihood* or risk of experiencing an MI, stroke, or lower extremity amputation is substantially greater if one has diabetes.[82,84]

   Health care providers should focus on several special and important clinical characteristics about macrovascular disease in persons with diabetes, as follows:

1. The onset of the clinical syndromes of macrovascular disease typically occurs at a relatively young age in persons with diabetes.[83]
2. Mortality rates for major cardiovascular diseases in persons with diabetes appear to be declining slightly (Fig. 8-2).[44]
3. Although rates of hospital discharges for CAD are greatest in African-American and white females (Fig. 8-3), mortality rates are greatest for white males (Fig. 8-4).[44]
4. Nontraumatic lower extremity amputations appear to be more common in African Americans (Fig. 8-5).[44]
5. Although not supported by all studies, the general clinical experience is that with CAD or cerebrovascular disease, persons with diabetes are likely to experience complications of the initial clinical episode, as well as recurrence of coronary or cerebral attacks.[102,124]
6. Features that normally "protect" one from premature macrovascular disease (e.g., female gender) do not pertain to individuals with diabetes.[60,97]
7. The clinical manifestations of some macrovascular events such as CAD are often (although not usually) atypical,[1] such as "silent" myocardial or asymptomatic infarction,[81] gastrointestinal (GI) "indigestion," and unexplained congestive heart failure (CHF) as manifestations of atherosclerotic heart disease.[95]

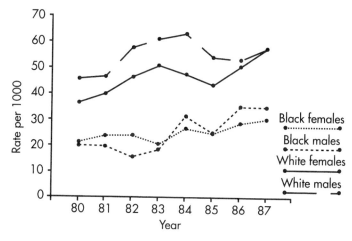

Fig. 8-3   Age-standardized rates of hospital discharges for ischemic heart disease as the primary diagnosis per 1000 diabetic population, by race, sex, and year, United States, 1980 to 1987. (Modified from *Diabetes surveillance, policy, program, research: DHHS; PHS; Centers for Disease Control,* Center for Chronic Disease Prevention and Health Promotion, Division of Diabetes Translation, Atlanta, 1990, Centers for Disease Control.)

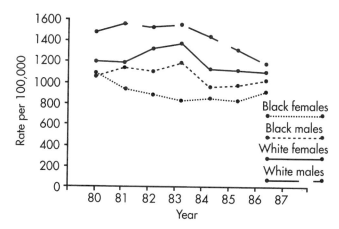

Fig. 8-4   Age-standardized mortality rates for major cardiovascular disease as the underlying cause per 100,000 diabetic population, by race, sex, and year, United States, 1980 to 1986. (Modified from *Diabetes surveillance, policy, program, research: DHHS; PHS; Centers for Disease Control,* Center for Chronic Disease Prevention and Health Promotion, Division of Diabetes Translation, Atlanta, 1990, Centers for Disease Control.)

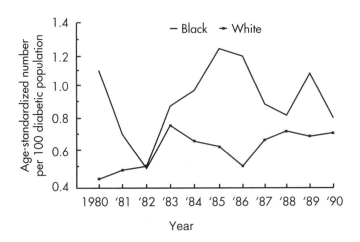

Fig. 8-5 Age-standardized number of hospital discharges listing diabetes and lower extremity amputation per 100 diabetic population by race, United States, 1980-1990. (Modified from Centers for Disease Control and Prevention, *Diabetes Surveillance, 1993,* Atlanta, Ga, US Department of Health and Human Services, 1993, pp. 87-93. National Diabetes Data Group, *Diabetes in America,* ed 2, National Institutes of Health, National Institute of Diabetes and Digestive and Kidney Diseases. NIH Publication No. 95-1468, 1995, p. 416.)

8. Treatment modalities for macrovascular episodes may be complicated by the presence of diabetes. For example, are symptoms such as weakness and dizziness a recurrent TIA or hypoglycemia? Should beta blockers be used to treat angina in patients with diabetes?

In summary, from a societal perspective, the burden of macrovascular disease in a disorder as common as diabetes mellitus is substantial. From a clinical perspective the challenge of preventing, recognizing, diagnosing, and treating macrovascular disease is great, since the various components of large vessel disease in diabetes are subtle and often atypical, complex, and devastating.

ETIOLOGY OF MACROVASCULAR DISEASE IN DIABETES

A single, clear, and convincing explanation does not yet exist to explain why macrovascular disease is so common in diabetes. Many interrelated factors most likely contribute to this problem.[40,58,134] It is useful to consider briefly these various pathogenetic factors to understand the rationale for present and future management strategies to prevent and treat macrovascular complications of diabetes. For purposes of this discussion, the reasons for macrovascular disease development can be categorized as follows: (1) factors associated with diabetes mellitus per se, (2) the treatment of diabetes, and (3) the presence of associated conditions (Table 8-1).

Diabetes-Specific Factors

Various factors may contribute to accelerated and premature macrovascular disease. As a result of hyperglycemia, protein glycosylation[31] and osmotic/metabolic sequelae of sorbitol

Table 8-1   Reasons for Diabetes-Associated Macrovascular Disease

Category	Examples
Diabetes	Hyperglycemia with glycoprotein formation and/or sorbitol accumulation
	Lipid abnormalities
	Microvascular abnormalities
	Neuropathy
	Clotting system dysfunction
	Genetics
	Insulin resistance/hyperinsulinemia
Diabetes treatment	Diet
	Exercise
	Oral hypoglycemic agents
	Insulin
Associated conditions	Hypertension
	Lipoprotein abnormalities
	Smoking
	Personality type

accumulation and myoinositol loss[67] may place the intima, the internal lining of large vessels, in a very vulnerable position.[30,112] Hyperlipidemia, whether primary or secondary to the hyperglycemia of diabetes, is common and most likely contributes to atherosclerosis.[19,28] Microvascular abnormalities, typical of diabetes, may occur and impede nutrient flow to the media and adventitia of large vessels, thus placing these vasculature layers at risk.[52]

The metabolic consequences of hyperglycemia include neuropathy, which could result in abnormal cell wall nutrition, and sympathetic/parasympathetic denervation.[109] Several components of the clotting system have been reported to be abnormal in persons with diabetes, including platelet function,[161] blood flow and viscosity,[107] and the fibrinolytic system.[148] For example, platelets appear unusually "sticky," blood flow is sluggish, and lysis of clots is impaired. Conceptually, those abnormalities could increase the likelihood of macrovascular disease in diabetic patients. The role of ethnicity and genetics in diabetes and macrovascular disease cannot be ignored, since both conditions may be influenced by this common genetic aberration.[80]

Finally, recent concepts of the pathogenesis of macrovascular disease in diabetes suggest a primary role for insulin resistance and thereby secondary hyperinsulinemia with an associated "atherosclerotic milieu." *Syndrome X,* or *insulin resistance syndrome,* is a condition in which insulin resistance, hyperinsulinemia, hyperglycemia, upper body obesity, hypertension, and lipid abnormalities occur with surprising frequency in the same individual, although in different combinations, and thus may be related to the development of arteriosclerosis.* This condition is interesting and perhaps controversial because it (1) predates the onset of hyperglycemia,[72,147] (2) may not occur in all racial/ethnic groups and

*References 14, 86, 135, 136, 170.

age-groups,[37] and (3) may be related to interuterine and neonatal nutrition and development.[157,169]

Treatment of Diabetes

Diet and Exercise

Since persons with diabetes are at increased risk for macrovascular disorders, one must consider the possibility that treatment modalities could minimize one aspect of diabetes (e.g., microvascular disorders through achievement of euglycemia) while increasing the risk for another important complication (e.g., large vessel disease). Diet has been and remains the cornerstone of therapy for diabetes; however, the recommended *content* of that diet has changed over the years (see Chapter 4). In the past, because of primary concern for glycemic excursions with varying carbohydrate ingestion, emphasis was placed on controlling the carbohydrate content of the diet, with relative inattention to fat ingestion.[92] Thus, to the degree that a relationship exists between fat consumption (amount and type) and atherosclerosis, it is theoretically possible that past high-fat diets may contribute to macrovascular disease. Although such a diet is not presently recommended,[8] one cannot ignore the possibility that previous recommendations may be a factor in the current prevalence of atherosclerosis.

Exercise therapy for persons with diabetes has also become an integral part of diabetes prevention and treatment regimens, and many guidelines exist.[6,144,154] Thus careful preexercise evaluation is recommended.[5]

Oral sulfonylurea agents

The use of oral sulfonylurea agents remains somewhat controversial,[62] particularly because of a putative association between tolbutamide and accelerated heart disease (see Chapter 6). Although the University Group Diabetes Program (UGDP) results have been repeatedly questioned,[90,100] and many experienced diabetologists do not support a strong link between sulfonylurea agents and macrovascular disorders in diabetic patients,[2] one should remain cognizant of the UGDP conclusions. The availability of metformin[153] and acarbose,[38] may make this issue moot.

Insulin

Many patients with diabetes take insulin.[7] Given the concepts of syndrome X and hyperinsulinism,* could the use of insulin actually contribute to macrovascular disorders? At present, although some epidemiologic studies relate insulin levels to the development of macrovascular disease[133,158,164] and concerns exist about insulin-antibody immune complexes,[45,71] such relationships must remain speculative but worthy of continued investigation.[64] Certainly, all the benefits of appropriate insulin use, such as lowering of glucose with decreased glycoprotein formation and sorbitol accumulation,[31,67] improved lipid parameters,[129] and reduced microvascular conditions,[43] should not be ignored or abandoned while such studies continue.

---

*References 14, 86, 135, 136, 170.

Associated Conditions

Several pathogenetic factors for macrovascular disease are not unique to the person with diabetes and also occur in the general population.[99,114,122]

Hypertension

Diabetes is a major risk factor for the development of hypertension. Specific hypotheses to explain abnormalities in blood pressure in the general population that apply as well to persons with diabetes include autoregulatory dysfunction, renal sodium retention, abnormal cellular sodium transport, increased intracellular calcium, or acquired mechanisms. Even with uncertainty about the exact pathogenesis of hypertension, several explanations can be deduced, including (1) an increased genetic sensitivity; (2) factors that increase the cardiac output, such as increased heart rate or fluid volume; and (3) neural stimulation, which may result in an increased activation of the autoregulatory process, increasing peripheral vascular resistance and thus blood pressure.[46,160]

Hypertension in diabetes seems to be volume dependent: increased insulin concentrations stimulate sodium reabsorption with resultant fluid retention. Other contributing factors may be related to abnormalities of the sympathetic and parasympathetic systems often seen in diabetic persons.

Elevated blood pressure may be more prevalent in a diabetic population and occurs at an earlier age because of the diabetes itself. Other nonmodifiable risk factors that may predispose the person with diabetes to concomitant development of hypertension include family history, with a particular genetic predisposition noted in African Americans. Males are at an increased risk to develop hypertension at a younger age than females and at a higher rate. Aging and obesity, risk factors for NIDDM, may also contribute to hypertension. Untreated hypertension can lead to severe cardiovascular occurrences, such as CVA or MI.[46]

Hyperlipidemia

Hyperlipidemia is frequently observed with diabetes and hypertension[86] and can contribute to the development of macrovascular disease in the general population as well.[150] This metabolic abnormality has a reported prevalence of 20% to 70% in patients with diabetes. The presence and severity of hyperlipidemia depend greatly on glycemic control, type and severity of diabetes, age, and nutritional habits. Hyperlipidemia is a major factor in atheroma formation, and persons with diabetes have higher triglyceride levels but lower high-density lipoprotein (HDL) levels than nondiabetic control subjects. Because HDL level is inversely related to coronary risk, the person with diabetes is at a heightened risk for cardiovascular events.[3]

Cigarette smoking

The prevalence of cigarette smoking in persons with diabetes is approximately the same as in the general population. Given all the other macrovascular risk factors present in diabetes, this is not good news! Further, a greater percentage of younger diabetic persons smoke compared with age-matched nondiabetic control subjects.[122] Cigarette smoking is a major contributor to cardiovascular disease in the nondiabetic population, a risk that increases several-fold in the presence of diabetes.[114,122] In diabetes, smoking is also associated with nephropathy, retinopathy, connective tissue changes, and neuropathy. Persons who already have vascular complications, pregnant women, or women using oral contraceptives are at particular risk. Smoking cessation reduces the risk of vascular morbidity and mortality in nondiabetic persons and, it is assumed, has the same beneficial effects in persons with diabetes.[73]

Other factors

Other factors related to macrovascular disease development in diabetes include *obesity, personality type, impaired glucose tolerance* (IGT), and *proteinuria*. Obesity complicated by the tendency for a sedentary life-style may contribute by itself to macrovascular disease. Reactions to stressful circumstances, such as seen in type A personality, are also associated with macrovascular disease. More recently, type E personality (the "hot reactor") has been described as characterizing a hypertensive, cardiovascular risk profile in the individual who is explosive when not achieving desired goals. Although this relationship between personality types and heart disease is controversial,[171] it is at least worth further exploration in terms of the potential stress imposed by the treatment regimen in the person with diabetes. IGT is an identified risk factor for macrovascular disease in several epidemiologic studies, perhaps related to the insulin resistance syndrome.[80] Proteinuria is also a finding that seems to predict the subsequent development of macrovascular disease, although a causal relationship remains uncertain.[120]

The essential feature underscoring the importance of these factors for macrovascular disease is that their impact is multiplicative, not additive, in diabetes.[3] Given the prevalence and potency of all these factors, they may contribute very significantly to the clinical and public health burden of a macrovascular disease in populations with diabetes.

TREATMENT OF MACROVASCULAR DISEASE IN DIABETES

What can be done *now* to reduce the burden of macrovascular disease in patients with diabetes, from both public health and clinical perspectives? To provide a framework, it is useful to consider three potential levels of prevention: primary, secondary, and tertiary[55] (Table 8-2).

Considering diabetes itself, one could reduce the societal and individual consequences of this condition by (1) decreasing the incidence of diabetes (e.g., *primary* prevention of new

Table 8-2 Prevention Strategies

Level	Concept	Example
Primary	Decrease incidence of disease.	Control weight to prevent NIDDM.
Secondary	Maintain normal metabolic state to prevent or delay complications.	Control glucose, blood pressure, and lipid levels.
Tertiary	Minimize extent of damage from complications associated with disease.	Administer beta blockers after myocardial infarction to decrease incidence of sudden death.

cases), (2) decreasing development and progression of complications of diabetes by aggressive treatment of basic metabolic abnormalities associated with diabetes (e.g., *secondary* prevention through therapy for hyperglycemia or hyperlipidemia), or (3) diminishing the consequences of the complications of diabetes (e.g., *tertiary* prevention through judicious use of beta blockers in the postinfarction period).

Primary Prevention

Primary prevention of diabetes, if effective, would presumedly reduce the burden of macrovascular disease in persons with diabetes to that of the nondiabetic population. In terms of primary prevention, (1) evidence supports a relationship between obesity and diabetes,[34,119] (2) reasons exist to consider prevention of NIDDM by weight control and obesity reduction,[127,174] and (3) sustained aerobic exercise may be beneficial.[94,108]

Obesity and diabetes mellitus

Several factors must be considered in the possible relationship between obesity and diabetes. First, although it is *logical* to relate obesity control to the prevention of NIDDM (and thereby the increased burden of macrovascular disease in this particular diabetic population), no large, long-term studies *at present* convincingly support the premise that weight loss or minimization of weight gain will prevent or even delay the onset of NIDDM and associated macrovascular disease.

Exercise and NIDDM

Several prospective observational studies indicate that sustained aerobic exercise is associated with a decreased likelihood of the development of NIDDM.[76,108] These investigations are encouraging, but other factors may account for the interesting results.[145]

Syndrome X and macrovascular disease

Recent data relevant to syndrome X, the insulin resistance syndrome,* suggest that the tendency for macrovascular disease may occur years before the onset of clinical diabetes or even unrecognized hyperglycemia.[72,147] Studies indicate that the likelihood of CAD (and perhaps cerebral and peripheral vascular disease) is similar in patients with IGT and those with established NIDDM.[79] If insulin resistance/hyperinsulinemia with associated atherogenic abnormalities do occur even *decades* before onset of clinical diabetes,[72,86,135,147] primary prevention effects for both NIDDM, and especially macrovascular disease, will need to occur well before obesity or hyperglycemia have established themselves.

The lack of firm scientific data to assist with issues related to primary prevention of diabetes should not necessarily limit the application of weight control and exercise programs on an individual, case-by-case basis, perhaps based on such other important factors as family history of vascular disorders and membership in certain ethnic groups. For example, if a strong family history for diabetes exist, weight control to prevent NIDDM seems reasonable. Such

---

*References 36, 56, 66, 104, 162.

an approach is logical, unlikely to do harm, and consistent with good general physical and emotional health. However, one must be somewhat guarded because of lack of clear data and established effective programs.[172] From a societal perspective, the science base regarding primary prevention of NIDDM and macrovascular disease needs to be expanded before national treatment programs should be implemented. Such studies are now in progress.[118]

Secondary Prevention

Treatment of hyperglycemia, hypertension, dyslipidemia, and tobacco use are the focus of secondary prevention efforts related to the development of macrovascular disease.

Limitation of studies in nondiabetic populations

It is important to note that most studies exploring risk factors for macrovascular disease used nondiabetic, white male subjects.* Thus entry criteria were restrictive to facilitate a well-defined, scientifically valid study. The ability to generalize the results is limited. For example, it is unclear whether the results of the extensive investigations conducted to date are relevant to females, older adults, minority populations, or persons with diabetes. However, to repeat all studies in all populations would be very demanding and certainly expensive. Thus one must use logic, inference, and reason.[3,27,77] Particularly when risk of therapy is low, it is appropriate to apply the general recommendations of studies on lipids, blood pressure, and tobacco use in the general population to persons with diabetes. Indeed, given the prevalence of macrovascular disease in diabetes[82,84] and the multiplicative interaction among the vascular risk factors and diabetes,[82] it may be *more* imperative to deal forcefully with these risk factors in persons with diabetes.

It is important that *all* strategies for risk reduction of macrovascular disease be used in persons with diabetes. Some risk exists, the goals of therapy may even be *more* rigorous than those in persons without diabetes, and the task is even more challenging given the complexity of a diabetic regimen itself, but the benefit may be substantial in persons with diabetes.[72,86,113,135]

Special considerations for secondary prevention

Special considerations and concerns exist regarding treatment recommendations in persons with diabetes mellitus. First, the goals for lipid and blood pressure levels may be different for the general public and for persons with diabetes, reflecting the need for more aggressive treatment in diabetes. For example, at all lipid levels, including ones considered to be "normal," persons with diabetes have a greater likelihood of having an adverse macrovascular event.[3,15,20,46] Similarly, although a blood pressure level of 140/90 is often stated as the goal of treatment in the general public,[159a] in persons with diabetes, therapeutic goals are set at considerably lower levels (e.g., 120/80) to minimize retinal and renal changes.[39,159] Even though the benefits of such blood pressure or lipid levels on macrovascular disease are not yet firmly established in diabetes, one would still treat abnormal lipid and blood

---

*References 36, 56, 66, 104, 162.

pressure levels in persons with diabetes earlier, more aggressively, and with more demanding goals in mind.

Treatment of risk factors

Hyperglycemia. Achieving *euglycemia* has remained a primary goal of therapy in diabetes care.[4] The results of the DCCT[43] and the Stockholm study[137] confirmed the benefits of euglycemia on microvascular and metabolic complications in persons with IDDM. Although it is logical to expect euglycemia also to result in a reduced atherogenic environment[29,53] and at present some suggestive evidence indicates that improved glucose regulation is associated with decreased morbidity and mortality caused by diabetic macrovascular disease,[35] one must recognize that as yet no rigorous evidence suggests that euglycemia will reduce the risk and incidence of macrovascular disease, including within the DCCT.[43] This reality does not mean that such a relationship does not exist, only that data from systematic investigations have not yet confirmed this relationship. Further, concern has been expressed about possible harmful effects of hyperinsulinemia with intensive therapy in persons with diabetes.[14,98,168]

Hypertension. The relationship between hypertension control and reduced risk for macrovascular events is less clear in the general public. The benefits and consequences of reducing blood pressure, especially on decreased risks for CHF, CVA, and renal failure, are well accepted.[113] Evidence that lowering blood pressure results in fewer acute coronary events and decreases the severity of acute coronary disease is less convincing,[115] but more recent reports suggest that controlling blood pressure does affect CAD.[117]

The treatment of hypertension, as previously noted, should therefore be an initial aim. Maintenance of ideal body weight is a primary means of achieving normal blood pressure. Nonpharmacologic measures should always be considered and discussed with the individual before drug therapy. Statistically, the most important treatment for more than 50% of hypertensive persons with diabetes is weight loss, which leads to improvement in not only blood pressure, but also diabetes and hyperlipidemia.

Antihypertensive drug treatment in persons with diabetes is begun early because of the deleterious interaction between diabetes and hypertension.[12,46] Adverse effects should be carefully monitored. In addition, the overall regimen should be as simple as possible in an effort to encourage adherence and perhaps limit burdensome drug costs.[12,115,117]

Four main groups of drugs are used to treat hypertension in persons with diabetes: diuretics, beta blockers, calcium antagonists, and angiotensin-converting enzyme (ACE) inhibitors. Table 8-3 summarizes the advantages and disadvantages of each of the four main groups of drugs used in the treatment of hypertension. Although each of these groups has proven effectiveness in control of blood pressure, untoward effects can pose serious problems for the person with diabetes. These problems must be monitored very carefully, with routine and frequent patient contact a major priority.[12,115,117]

As evidenced by several recent reviews,* the choice of medication in hypertensive diabetic persons is complicated, from the standpoints of both side effects and ability of certain

---

*References 12, 39, 86, 105, 173.

Table 8-3 Advantages and Drawbacks of Various Groups of Antihypertensive Drugs in the Treatment of Hypertension with Diabetes Mellitus

Advantages	Problems	Recommendations
Diuretics		
Monotherapy lowers high blood pressure effectively Once-daily regimen Inexpensive Pathophysiologically sound (elevated exchangeable sodium decreased; exaggerated norepinephrine (noradrenaline) reactivity reduced)	Impaired glucose homeostasis, depleted potassium, impaired insulin receptors(?) Serum lipid alterations Increased plasma uric acid Hyperosmolar coma Erectile impotence Orthostatic hypotension	Low dose Control potassium, glucose, lipids Potassium substitution if needed (diet, KCl, combination with potassium-sparing diuretic)
Beta blockers		
Monotherapy lowers high blood pressure effectively Once-daily regimen Cardiovascular protection Antianginal/antiarrhythmogenic properties	$Beta_2$ blockade impairs insulin output Hypoglycemia: prolonged by $beta_2$-blockers; altered perception of symptoms; hypertensive crisis ($beta_2$-blockers) Serum lipid alterations Decreased physical exercise performance	Cardioselective ($beta_1$) blocker (e.g., atenolol, metoprolol, acebutolol) Low to moderate dose Instruction: hypoglycemic problems Control: cardiac performance, atrioventricular (AV) conduction, serum lipoproteins
Calcium antagonists		
Monotherapy lowers high blood pressure effectively Once-daily regimen possible Antianginal effects Antiarrhythmic properties (verapamil, diltiazem) Metabolic "neutrality" (glucose, lipids, potassium) Cardioprotection (?) Antiarteriosclerotic (?) Preserved physical exercise performance Relative rarity of orthostatic and impotence problems (?)	Impaired insulin secretion in vitro; in high doses in vivo (?) Headache (often transient) Flushing, ankle edema, paradoxical angina (dihydropyridines) Constipation (verapamil)	Low to moderate dose Control: AV conduction (verapamil, diltiazem), glucose (at higher dosages)
ACE inhibitors		
Monotherapy lowers high blood pressure effectively Once-daily regimen possible Effective in heart failure Metabolic "neutrality" (glucose, lipids [?], no hypokalemia) Relative rarity of orthostatic and impotence problems (?)	Proteinuria (rare) Dose adjustment with declining renal function Renal failure (reversible) in renal artery stenoses Enhancement of hyperkalemia in hyporeninemic hypoaldosteronism (rare) False-positive test for acetone	Low to moderate dose Control: renal function, proteinuria, plasma potassium

Modified from Trost BH: *Drugs* 38(4):621-633, 1989.

hypertensive agents to minimize fully the risk for macrovascular disease. For example, thiazide diuretics have been and perhaps still are the foundation for hypertensive treatment because of cost, effectiveness, and apparent safety.[159a] Concern exists, however, regarding the attenuation of risk reduction efforts through decreased blood pressure by increased lipid values.[86] Similarly, other frequently used medications such as beta blockers or alpha antagonists may be associated with side effects (e.g., masking of hypoglycemia symptoms, impotence, postural hypertension) that are particularly problematic in persons with long-term diabetes.[105] The current movement is toward beginning therapy in hypertensive diabetic persons with calcium antagonists or ACE inhibitors. The latter, although expensive, are beneficial with concomitant diabetic renal disease.[26] Short-acting versions of the former, although effective in lowering blood pressure or controlling angina, have recently become controversial because of possible excess mortality.[57,93,125]

Hyperlipidemia. Definitive evidence is accumulating regarding the benefits of efforts to attenuate the morbidity and mortality of macrovascular disease associated with hyperlipidemia.* These data do support the view that individual clinical and public health efforts to control hyperlipidemia will result in a lower societal and individual burden from macrovascular disease. As noted in Chapter 4, dietary treatment of hyperlipidemia, including maintenance of ideal body weight, is critical to care from both a primary and a secondary prevention perspective.

The treatment for hyperlipidemia is challenging and is made more so by the presence of diabetes. Consider the demands of following the diet, exercise, and pharmacologic treatment program for diabetes itself. Add to that the challenge of *additional* dietary considerations because of hyperlipidemia (e.g., restriction in amount and type of dietary fat). Although one might logically think that the presence of these two serious conditions might result in *greater* effort and attention to the therapeutic regimen, the task may simply be too demanding. Further, it is often not clear how much of the hyperlipidemia is caused by poorly regulated diabetes itself (thus requiring even additional attention to blood glucose control) versus endogenous hyperlipidemia in someone who just happens to have diabetes. Finally, the questions of when antilipid agents should be begun and which one should be used are critical, especially since some (e.g., niacin) may be effective in lipid reduction but have adverse effects of special significance in persons with diabetes.[59,91] These are contributing factors to the challenge of treating hyperlipidemia in persons with diabetes.

Smoking cessation. Discontinuance of tobacco use is associated with improved health, especially a decreased likelihood of macrovascular events.[54,75,78] Considering the demands and complexities of a diabetic regimen, however, efforts to stop cigarette use may be problematic. For example, data indicate that persons younger than age 40 with diabetes smoke at a greater rate than nondiabetic persons, perhaps because cigarettes provide an opportunity for "rebelliousness" in one aspect of life to balance the rigidity in another (i.e., diabetes regimen).[78,114,121,122]

Prevention or cessation of smoking is critical to macrovascular disease prevention. The delivery of all routine diabetes education should therefore include content related to smoking from three perspectives: prevention information, cessation strategies, and maintenance and

---

*References 36, 49, 56, 104, 116, 130, 140, 162.

relapse prevention.[73] This information can be presented in several phases, including the following:

1. *Assess tobacco use.* The first step is to determine whether or not the individual smokes. This should be a routine part of care. If the answer is no, the health care provider should emphasize the importance of maintaining a smoke-free life-style, especially given a diagnosis of diabetes. If the individual reports smoking, a more detailed assessment, with information regarding smoking history, nicotine dependence, motivation to quit, and diabetes-specific concerns related to quitting, should be addressed.

2. *Determine readiness to quit.* Once a person with diabetes reports smoking, several steps should be initiated to further encourage cessation, including identifying cessation as a priority of diabetes care, building the smoker's confidence that quitting is possible, and addressing any concerns about quitting, particularly as they relate to diabetes care (e.g., weight concerns).

3. *Initiate cessation interventions.* The diabetes team should work together with the smoker to set a quit date within 3 weeks of the visit; review the diabetic regimen and discuss issues related to short-term nicotine withdrawal; identify smoking cessation strategies; assess the need for nicotine patches, nicotine gum, and so forth; determine a schedule for follow-up.

4. *Perform follow-up.* The focus of follow-up is to verify the status of patients and to assist those who may have relapsed and become smokers again. Those who are smoke free should be praised for their tremendous efforts. Those who have relapsed need to be encouraged not to feel badly but rather to try again, since cessation is a difficult process.

Tertiary Prevention

In the person with established diabetes *and* clinically apparent macrovascular disease (e.g., angina, recent MI, TIAs, or intermittent claudication), what should be the tertiary prevention strategies, that is, programs to reduce the consequences of existing macrovascular complication? In essence the same strategies that are applied to the nondiabetic patient population with macrovascular disease should be used in persons with diabetes. Thus medical approaches to anginal control (e.g., nitrates, calcium channel blockers), use of technologically based management strategies for coronary or cerebrovascular disorders[51,108a] (e.g., angioplasty, bypass grafting),[13] and very aggressive and innovative therapy for peripheral vascular disease (e.g., laser treatment)[42,132] are all tertiary treatment options that should be used in diabetic patients when clinically appropriate. However, in certain circumstances, i.e., persons on drug therapy for diabetes, bypass grafting should be utilized rather than angioplasty.[117a]

However, a few important issues must be considered when applying such tertiary strategies. First, is the overall prognosis in persons with diabetes and active macrovascular disease so limited that invasive and expensive procedures should not be considered? Some data suggest a very discouraging prognosis for persons with diabetes;[88,124,176] however, recent studies indicate that persons with diabetes can definitely benefit from tertiary treatment approaches,[146] including thrombolytic therapy after an acute MI.[16,63,106] Ensuring optimal metabolic control before tertiary interventions is essential[142,151] and often is the responsibility of a nonsurgical diabetes care team.

Second, two of the components of tertiary prevention need to be carefully considered in persons with diabetes. The first is the use of aspirin therapy.[17,33,128,156] Understandable concern exists, especially in persons with diabetic retinopathy, about possible problems with bleeding secondary to aspirin therapy.[17,33] Recent reports of the Early Treatment of Diabetic Retinopathy Study indicate no excessive tendencies for retinal hemorrhage with aspirin,[47] so if this therapy is otherwise clinically indicated, it should not be denied to persons with diabetes.

The second component is the use of beta blockers with a recent MI.[139] The use of beta blockers in persons with diabetes, particularly those at risk for hypoglycemia (see Table 8-3), may be problematic[41] because of possible masking of hypoglycemic symptoms. This risk must be balanced against the benefits associated with prevention of recurrent coronary events.

Future research

Assuming that the full burden of macrovascular disease in diabetes is recognized, three major areas of future research deserve attention. First, the possibility that macrovascular disease begin years before the onset of "clinical diabetes" (i.e., hyperglycemia)[72,147] and the relationships of these "early" macrovascular disease tendencies to insulin resistance syndrome[14,50,136,169,170] require intensive investigation. If certain high-risk individuals or groups could be reliably identified during the very early phases of diabetic macrovascular disease (well before the onset of hyperglycemia or even IGT), interventions could conceivably *prevent* macrovascular disease.

Women with diabetes lose their "gender protection" against macrovascular disease, even before menopause; this is the second area that must be aggressively studied and understood.[85] The risk of various manifestations of cardiovascular disease (e.g., CAD, CHF)[85] is (1) very similar in diabetic women and men and (2) *much* greater in women with diabetes compared with nondiabetic women. Further, mortality and morbidity rates for women with diabetes after an MI appear worse than in diabetic men.[65,106] The reason(s) for these devastating aspects of macrovascular disease in diabetic women must be understood and would expand our general knowledge about diabetic large vessel disease.

A third area of future research would examine the efficacy of risk factor reductions for diabetic macrovascular disease. As mentioned earlier, most investigations of macrovascular disease prevention and reduction intentionally exclude diabetic persons. One must learn if reduction of glucose, blood pressure, lipid, and so forth in persons with diabetes (or "prediabetes") will effectively reduce diabetic macrovascular disease without causing harm.

In the meantime, what can be expected from future secondary and tertiary prevention efforts in diabetes-associated macrovascular disease? For glycemia control itself, new classes and types of glucose-lowering agents are available, and others will most likely follow.[38,96,163] Manipulations of the insulin molecule itself may result in compounds that achieve comparable or even greater glucose-lowering effects without any undesirable consequences (e.g., putative accelerated atherosclerosis).[25] When euglycemia is not achieved, pharmacologic agents will block glycoprotein formation or sorbitol accumulation and myoinositol depletion.[24,32,152] Agents to reduce platelet abnormalities probably will also become part of the therapeutic armamentarium.

For hypertension and lipid abnormalities, one can anticipate many new varieties of existing classes of drugs, as well as new classes of pharmaceuticals. The availability of calcium channel blockers and ACE inhibitors has been a helpful step in managing hypertension in persons with diabetes.[39,103] Likewise, it is anticipated that newer and more effective antilipid agents (e.g., various 3-hydroxy-3-methylglutaryl (HMG) coenzyme A (CoA) reductase inhibitors)[70] will soon be available. This enlarging menu of agents will target specific macrovascular risks with precise, effective pharmacologic interventions.

What does the future hold regarding tertiary prevention efforts in persons who already have macrovascular disease? First, the early detection of clinically unrecognized macrovascular disease using sensitive (and initially expensive) procedures (e.g., angioscopes, ultrasonography) will most likely become available.[61,63,101] Pharmacologic agents other than those such as aspirin probably will be identified and could be useful in minimizing the extent or recurrence of macrovascular disease in persons with diabetes. Likewise, interventions such as laser therapy will become part of the therapeutic armamentarium. The development of these innovative approaches will continue with excitement and promise. Remaining issues amidst all the enthusiasm about new approaches will include documentation of usefulness when compared with other treatment modalities. Careful economic analyses will be required in these decisions.[68,69]

Goals of Education

Although the many etiologic factors provide numerous "intervention points" to reduce the consequences of coronary, cerebral, and peripheral vascular diseases, the very breadth and scope of the possibilities may not be fully useful to the *individual* practitioner responsible for the *individual* patient with diabetes. How can one use all the information in tailoring an individualized approach for a single patient?

First, it is important to remember that because diabetes is both a complex and a chronic disease, efforts over time involving many visits will be necessary to achieve lifelong changes. To this end, regular health care visits focusing on diabetes control and management, which allow for routine follow-up and preventive health care, are important.[141]

Second, these visits need to be structured to emphasize the importance of diabetes education that (1) allows the individual to become aware of the modifiable risks for macrovascular disease and (2) emphasizes the importance of preventive efforts (e.g., weight control, exercise, not smoking) to eliminate modifiable risk factors.

To summarize, the critical health facts that should be consistently reviewed with the diabetic individual include the following:

1. The major goals of management of diabetes include achieving near-normal metabolic biochemical control and prevention of vascular complications. Management of diabetes strives for achieving normal biochemical indices, as cited in Table 8-4.[10] To prevent accelerated development of macrovascular disease, achievement of normal blood pressure and body weight and elimination of modifiable risk factors, such as smoking, are stressed.

Table 8-4   Glycemic Control for People With Diabetes

Biochemical index	Nondiabetic	Goal	Action suggested
Preprandial glucose	<115	80-120	<80 >140
Bedtime glucose (mg/dl)	<120	100-140	<100 >160
Hemoglobin A$_{1c}$ (%)	<6	<7	>8

From *Diabetes Care* 18(suppl 1):9, Jan 1995.
These values are for nonpregnant individuals. "Action suggested" depends on individual patient circumstances. Hemoglobin A$_{1c}$ is referenced to a nondiabetic range of 4.0% to 6.0% (mean 5.0%, standard deviation 0.5%).

2. Diabetes is an independent risk factor for vascular disease. Women with diabetes may be at a particular risk, since they do not have the normal "protection" of the female gender that is noted in their nondiabetic counterparts.[85,116,117]
3. Lipid abnormalities occur often in persons with diabetes, from children to adults.[19,28,49]
4. Hypertension occurs frequently in diabetes and can have devastating consequences in terms of renal disease and macrovascular complications.[46]
5. Cigarette smoking is a major factor associated with cardiovascular disease and mortality. Prevention of smoking in those who have not started and elimination of this risk factor in those who smoke are crucial.[54,73,114]
6. Maintenance of ideal body weight, with an appropriate low-fat diet and adequate physical activity, can significantly reduce the likelihood of developing[5,6,114,154] concomitant risk factors of diabetes, including hyperlipidemia and hypertension.

Finally, at all three levels of prevention, the great challenge of *behavioral change* faces the provider, persons with diabetes, and the general public. Much has been learned, but although knowledge and skill alone are probably essential, it does not necessarily result in altered behavior.[110] Rather, other factors (e.g., beliefs, attitudes, barriers, circumstances)[18,141,160,170] and programs that recognize the complexities of personal behavior are being evaluated[165] and will become available in the near future. There is no simple single approach to the essential challenge of education, and multifaceted programs will be necessary. This will permit providers to reduce the risk of the development of macrovascular disease in persons with diabetes with greater effectiveness and compassion (Box 8-1).

SUMMARY

Diabetes is not a single disease, and macrovascular relationships in insulin-dependent diabetes mellitus (IDDM) may not necessarily pertain to non-insulin-dependent diabetes mellitus (NIDDM).[79,131] For example, in NIDDM, the onset of hypertension often coincides with recognition of hyperglycemia; in IDDM, hypertension usually follows diabetes by years in association with renal disease. Furthermore, epidemiologic data and clinical experience indicate that the three main vascular systems affected by atherosclerosis in diabetes may not be altered through the same mechanisms or to the same degree. Thus it should not be surprising

---

BOX 8-1

MACROVASCULAR DISEASE IN DIABETES: PATIENT EDUCATION

Primary prevention

Know your family. Be aware of any history of macrovascular disease, hypertension, or hyperlipidemia.
Do good. Follow a good diet; keep weight under control; exercise; have blood pressure and blood lipids checked.
Do no harm. Do not smoke.

Secondary prevention

Hypertension. Have blood pressure checked regularly; take medicine faithfully; keep weight under control and exercise.
Hyperlipidemia. Have blood lipid levels checked at least yearly; follow diet and, if necessary, take medicine faithfully; exercise; try to keep diabetes under control.
Cigarettes. Do not start; stop if using cigarettes and ask for help to do this.
Hyperglycemia. Try to keep diabetes under control, including monitoring of blood glucose, following diet and exercise program, and taking medicine faithfully.

Tertiary prevention

Keep track of how you feel. Be attuned to your symptoms; be sure to tell your physician how you are doing.
Keep trying to keep risk factors for macrovascular disease under control.
Work closely with your usual health team and new consultants.

---

to see persons with far-advanced peripheral vascular disease without any clinical evidence of CAD. The reason(s) for these differences is (are) not yet clear and will be the focus of important future research.

The major thrust of this discussion has been to emphasize that whether dealing with an individual patient or considering a larger diabetes community, macrovascular disease is *the* major burden of diabetes, regardless of how that burden is defined. Many factors account for the prevalence, morbidity, disability, mortality, and cost of macrovascular disease in diabetes. It is likely that an interaction among several of these factors will be of major pathogenetic importance. It is a remarkable challenge to apply the results of population, community, or cohort studies to the *individual* with diabetes who needs assistance.

Finally, the challenge is made more complex by (1) the important evolving role of nonphysician health professionals in the management of diabetes;[49,121] (2) the emerging responsibilities of primary care physicians in diabetes management, thereby requiring new relationships between specialty and primary care physicians;[11,166] and (3) an explosion in the "managed care" health system, wherein efficiency and cost have become important considerations (one hopes along with quality) in medical care decisions.[23,138] What is clear within all these changes is that given the complexity and seriousness of diabetes, *interdisciplinary care* is essential to maximize diabetic patient health.[167] Societal, community, and public health approaches to diabetes and macrovascular diabetes must be viewed as complementary to the clinical management of this complication. The huge burden of diabetes-associated macrovascular disease may be reduced through efforts at primary, secondary, and tertiary preventive education and care.

CASE PRESENTATIONS
Case Study 1

J.W., a 58-year-old male, was diagnosed with diabetes 17 years ago when he was evaluated for unexplained weight loss. He had been overweight, and both diabetes and hypertension ran in his family. Hypertension was also discovered 14 years ago, along with an elevated cholesterol level. He was treated by diet and a thiazide diuretic. His blood pressure improved, but his blood lipid and glucose levels remained abnormal. One year after diagnosis, he was begun on sulfonylurea treatment.

While on vacation, he cut the bottom of his foot while wading barefoot at the beach. Ten days after injuring his foot, he was seen in the emergency room, complaining of pain and discharge from his left foot. His blood pressure was 180/100; his temperature was 99.8°F. A necrotic, tender ulcer draining yellowish fluid was noted on the bottom of his left foot. His random glucose level was 280 mg/dl, and hemoglobin A_{1c} was 11.1%. After administration of fluids and antibiotics and diabetes/blood pressure control, he underwent a left below-the-knee (BK) amputation.

Four days postoperatively, he complained of severe substernal chest pain. An electrocardiogram (ECG) revealed an acute anterior MI. Despite cardiac treatment, he became hypotensive, developed frequent ventricular premature contractures (VPCs), and went into cardiac arrest and died despite resuscitative efforts.

DISCUSSION

Several health problems—diabetes, hypertension, hyperlipidemia, obesity—were present and are often seen together in persons with diabetes mellitus (DM). There is controversy whether a thiazide diuretic should be used in persons with DM because of the tendency for increases in lipid levels, and many would use ACE inhibitors.

Walking barefoot often leads to problems, and this individual developed an infected foot ulcer after cutting his foot. On admission, in addition to the evidence of the life-threatening foot lesion, evidence of poor diabetes and blood pressure control was apparent.

After the left BKA, the patient had signs and symptoms of acute cardiac ischemia and died despite appropriate resuscitative efforts.

Mortality in association with significant surgery in persons with long-standing (and poorly controlled) diabetes is not uncommon, even if the surgical procedure goes well from a technical standpoint. One wonders if the extensive macrovascular disease in this patient would have been present had preventative treatment of his various "risk factors" been initiated early during the course of his DM. And, of course, what would have been his future had he not walked barefoot at the beach?

Case Study 2

B.F., a 48-year-old woman with a 23-year history of IDDM, mentioned in a routine clinic visit that she was no longer able to participate in step aerobics. When asked why, she indicated that 5 to 10 minutes after beginning, she would experience severe indigestion. Cardiac evaluation revealed lowered ST segments on the ECG with controlled exercise.

DISCUSSION

This middle-age woman with long-standing IDDM apparently could no longer participate in step-aerobics. Of interest is that she would develop "indigestion" while exercising. Evidence of cardiac ischemia was present on a "stress-ECG."

Although non-diabetic women prior to menopause are usually protected against coronary artery disease (CAD), the long-standing IDDM removed her "gender protection" and in essence placed her at equal risk as men for clinically symptomatic CAD. Of special interest is the type of symptoms the patient described, certainly different from the more typical symptom complex displayed in case study 1 during the acute coronary event.

Given all the findings, one would pursue a careful assessment of cardiac risk factors and, if present, begin a vigorous "preventative program." Should revascular procedures be necessary if medical management of her cardiac symptoms is not based on very recent analyses of the Bypass Angioplasty Revascularization Investigation (BARI).

Case Study 3

C.L., a 46-year-old Hispanic woman in Los Angeles, had noted a 28 lb weight gain over the past 4 years and was worried about her health status because her mother had died from diabetes and her younger sister had recently been diagnosed with diabetes. Her screening blood glucose was normal, but she was concerned about further weight gain and her safety if she regularly walked for exercise.

After meetings with neighbors and church leaders, it was agreed to use the protected church grounds for a structured group exercise program. Further, nutritional counseling was made available each Sunday after church services.

C.L. began to lose approximately 2 lb every 2 weeks and continued to be screened annually for diabetes.

DISCUSSION

This middle-age Hispanic woman with a strong family history of diabetes mellitus was very worried about continuing weight gain and the possibility of developing DM in the near future.

Likely present would also be hypertension, hyperlipidemia, perhaps IGT, and hyperuricemia, i.e., evidence of Syndrome X or the Insulin Resistance Syndrome. Despite her interest in better nutrition and exercise programs, she was concerned about her safety if she walked in her own neighborhood. This is a good example of the impact of the "environment" on the individual, i.e., how the community, workplace, or neighborhood can limit the ability of a person to follow good health practices.

Utilizing the facilities and encouragement of her church, she was able to engage in "primary prevention" efforts for both DM and CAD.

Case Study 4

A.T., a farmer with 21 years of NIDDM, developed acute, pressing substernal chest pain, diaphoresis, and shortness of breath while lifting bales of hay. His wife rushed him to the hospital emergency room, where an acute inferior MI was diagnosed on ECG. He was stabilized and immediately taken to the intensive care unit, where he received thrombolytic treatment. His course was uneventful, without recurrent chest pain, dysrhythmias, or shortness of breath. Modified stress testing revealed no ECG changes. Because no coronary risk factors (e.g., cigarette use, elevated lipid levels) were noted, the patient was discharged and began aspirin and beta-blocker therapy.

DISCUSSION

This active and hard-working farmer with a long history of NIDDM displayed clinical and ECG evidence of an acute myocardial infarct. He was vigorously and appropriately treated in the coronary care unit and responded nicely without evidence of clinical complications. His modified "stress test" indicated that in spite of his long-standing DM, he would be considered in the "low risk" category for cardiac complications and was treated with medications to decrease the likelihood of a recurrent coronary event.

Although it is true that persons with DM are (1) much more likely to have a coronary event at an earlier age, (2) succumb from that MI, (3) have complications from the MI, and (4) experience another future coronary event than persons without diabetes, still the basic approach to assessment and treatment would be quite similar to that of non-diabetic individual.

REFERENCES

1. Airaksinen K, Koistinen M: Association between silent coronary artery disease, diabetes, and autonomic neuropathy: fact or fallacy? *Diabetes Care* 15:288-292, 1992.

2. American Diabetes Association: Policy statement: the UGDP controversy, *Diabetes Care* 2:1-3, 1979.

3. American Diabetes Association: Role of cardiovascular risk factors in prevention and treatment of macrovascular disease in diabetes: consensus statement, *Diabetes Care* 12:573-579, 1989.

4. American Diabetes Association: Blood glucose control in diabetes: position statement, *Diabetes Care* 13:16-17, 1990.

5. American Diabetes Association: Diabetes mellitus: position paper, *Diabetes Care* 13:804-805, 1990.

6. American Diabetes Association: Exercise and NIDDM, *Diabetes Care* 13:785-789, 1990.

7. American Diabetes Association: Insulin administration: position statement, *Diabetes Care* 13:28-31, 1990.

8. American Diabetes Association: Nutritional recommendations and principles for individuals with diabetes mellitus, *Diabetes Care* 13:18-25, 1990.

9. American Diabetes Association: *Direct and indirect costs of diabetes in the United States in 1992,* Alexandria, Va, 1993, The Association.

10. American Diabetes Association: Standards of medical care for patients with diabetes mellitus (position statement), *Diabetes Care* 17:616-623, 1994.

11. Anderson R: Subspecialization in internal medicine: a historical review, an analysis, and proposals for change, *Am J Med* 99:74-81, 1995.

12. Andrea L: General considerations in selecting antihypersensitive agents in patients with Type II diabetes mellitus and hypertension, *Am J Med* 87(suppl):6-39, 1987.

13. Antman E, Braunwald E: Acute MI management in the 1990s, *Hosp Pract* 25:65-82, 1990.

14. Arrants J: Hyperinsulinemia and cardiovascular risk, *Heart Lung* 23:118-124, 1994.

15. Austin M: Plasma triglycerides and coronary heart disease in men, *Arteriosclerosis,* 1995 (in press).

16. Barbash G and others: Significance of diabetes mellitus in patients with acute myocardial infarction receiving thrombolytic therapy, *J Am Coll Cardiol* 22:707-713, 1993.

17. Baudoein C and others: Secondary prevention of strokes: role of platelet antiaggregant drugs in diabetic and nondiabetic patients, *Diabetic Med* 2:145-146, 1985.

18. Becker MH: Understanding patient compliance: the contributions of attitudes and other psychosocial factors. In Cohen SJ, editor: *New directions in patient compliance,* Lexington, Mass, 1979, Heath.

19. Bierman E: Atherogenesis in diabetes, *Arterioscler Thromb* 12:647-656, 1992.

20. Bierman EB, Brunzell J: Diet low in saturated fat and cholesterol for diabetes, *Diabetes Care* 12:162-163, 1989.

21. Bild D and others: Lower-extremity amputation in people with diabetes: epidemiology and prevention, *Diabetes Care* 12:24-31, 1989.

22. Bliss M: *The discovery of insulin,* Toronto, 1982, McClelland and Stewart.

23. Bodenheimer T, Grumbach K: Reimbursing physicians and hospitals, *JAMA* 272:971-977, 1994.

24. Boulton A, Levin S, Comstock J: A multicentre trial of the aldose-reductase inhibitor, tolrestat, in patients with symptomatic diabetic neuropathy, *Diabetologia* 33:431-437, 1990.

25. Brange J and others: Monomeric insulins and their experimental and clinical implications, *Diabetes Care* 13:923-954, 1990.

26. Brown A, Feinglos M: Hypertension and diabetes, *Pract Diabetol* 14:14-19, 1995.

27. Brown E, Viscoli C, Horwitz R: Preventive health strategies and the policy makers' paradox, *Ann Intern Med* 116:593-597, 1992.

28. Brown W: Lipoprotein disorders in diabetes mellitus, *Med Clin North Am* 78:143-161, 1994.

29. Brownlee M, Cahill G: Diabetic control and vascular complications. In Pabletti R, Gotli A, editors: *Atherosclerosis reviews,* New York, 1979, Raven.

30. Brownlee M, Cerami E, Vlassara H: Advanced glycosylation end products in tissues: biochemical basis for a new therapeutic approach to the complications of diabetes, *N Engl J Med* 318:1315-1321, 1988.

31. Brownlee M, Vlassara H, Cerami A: Nonenzymatic glycosylation and the pathogenesis of diabetic complications, *Ann Intern Med* 101:527-537, 1984.

32. Bucala R, Cerami A, Vlassara H: Advanced glycosylation end products in diabetic complication, *Diabetes Rev* 3:258-268, 1995.

33. Buring J and others: Aspirin and stroke, *Arch Neurol* 47:1353-1354, 1990.

34. Burton B and others: Health implications of obesity: an NIH consensus development conference, *Int J Obes* 9:155-169, 1985.

35. Butler WJ and others: Mortality from coronary heart disease in the Tecumseh study: long-term effect of diabetes mellitus, glucose tolerance and other risk factors, *Am J Epidemiol* 125:541-547, 1985.

36. Casken-Hemphill L and others: Beneficial effects of colestepol-niacin on coronary atherosclerosis, *JAMA* 264:3013-3017, 1990.

37. Chaiken R and others: Do blacks with NIDDM have an insulin-resistance syndrome? *Diabetes* 42:444-449, 1993.

38. Chiasson J and others: The efficacy of acarbose in the treatment of non-insulin dependent diabetes mellitus, *Ann Intern Med* 121:928-935, 1993.

39. Christlieb AR: Treatment selection considerations for the hypertensive diabetic patient, *Arch Intern Med* 150:1167-1174, 1990.

40. Colwell J, Lopes-Virella M: A review of the development of large-vessel disease in diabetes mellitus: the genesis of atherosclerosis in diabetes mellitus, *Am J Med* 85:113-118, 1988.

41. Cryer P, White N, Santiago J: The relevance of glucose counterregulatory systems to patients with insulin-dependent diabetes mellitus, *Endocr Rev* 7:131-139, 1986.

42. DeFelice M, Gallo P, Masotti G: Current therapy of peripheral obstructive arterial disease, the non-surgical approach, *Angiology* 41:1-11, 1990.

43. The Diabetes Control and Complications Trial Research Group: The effect of intensive treatment of diabetes on the development and progression of long-term complications in insulin-dependent diabetes mellitus, *N Engl J Med* 329:977-986, 1993.

44. *Diabetes surveillance, policy, program, research: DHHS; PHS; Centers for Disease Control,* Center for Chronic Disease Prevention and Health Promotion, Division of Diabetes Translation, Atlanta, 1990, Centers for Disease Control.

45. DiMario V, Javicoli M, Andreani D: Circulating immune complexes in diabetes, *Diabetologia* 19:89-92, 1980.

46. Dunn FL: Hypertension in diabetes mellitus, *Diabetes Mellitus Rev* 6:47-61, 1990.

47. Early Treatment Diabetic Retinopathy Study Group: Aspirin, Paper presented at Annual Meeting of the American Academy of Ophthalmology, Atlanta, 1990.

48. Eddy D: Broadening the responsibilities of practitioners: the team approach, *JAMA* 269:1849-1855, 1993.

49. Edelman S, Henry R: Insulin therapy for normalizing glycosylated hemoglobin in type II diabetes, *Diabetes Rev* 3:308-334, 1995.

50. Elliott T, Viberti G: Relationship between insulin resistance and coronary heart disease in diabetes mellitus and the general population: a critical appraisal, *Baillieres Clin Endocrinol Metab* 7:1079-1103, 1993.

51. European Stroke Prevention Study Group: European Stroke Prevention Study, *Stroke* 21:1122, 1990.

52. Factor S, Okum E, Minase T: Capillary microaneurysms in the human diabetic heart, *N Engl J Med* 302:384-388, 1980.

53. Feingold KR: Preventing the vascular complications of diabetes. In *Current concepts series,* Kalamazoo, Mich, 1987, UpJohn.

54. Fiore M and others: Cigarette smoking: the clinician's role in cessation, prevention, and public health, *Dis Mon* 36:185-242, 1990.

55. Fletcher R, Fletcher S, Wagner E, editors: *Clinical epidemiology: the essentials,* Baltimore, 1988, Williams & Wilkins.

56. Frick M and others: Helsinki heart study: primary-prevention trial with gemfibrizole in middle-aged men with dyslipdemia: safety of treatment, changes in risk factors and incidence of coronary heart disease, *N Engl J Med* 317:1237-1245, 1987.

57. Furgerg C, Psaty B, Mayer J: Nifedipine: dose-related increase in mortality in patients with CAD, *Circulation* 92:1326-1331, 1995.

58. Ganda OP: Pathogenesis of macrovascular disease in the human diabetic, *Diabetes* 29:931-942, 1980.

59. Garber A: Diabetes and heart disease: a new strategy for managing lipid disorders, *Geriatrics* 48:34-36, 39-41, 1993.

60. Garcia M and others: Morbidity and mortality in diabetes in the Framingham population: 16-year follow-up study, *Diabetes* 23:105-111, 1974.

61. Gehani A and others: Experimental and clinical percutaneous angioscopy experience with dynamic angioplasty, *Angiology* 41:809-816, 1990.

62. Gerich J: Oral hypoglycemic agents, *N Engl J Med* 321:1231-1245, 1989.

63. Gianrossi R and others: Cardiac fluoroscopy for the diagnosis of coronary artery disease: a meta analytic review, *Am Heart J* 120:1179-1188, 1990.

64. Godsland I, Stevenson J: Insulin resistance: syndrome or tendency? *Lancet* 346:100-102, 1995.

65. Goff D and others: Greater case-fatality after myocardial infarction among Mexican Americans and women than among non-Hispanic whites and men: the Corpus Christi Heart Project, *Am J Epidemiol* 139:474-483, 1994.

66. Granger C and others: Outcome of patients with diabetes mellitus and acute myocardial infarction treated with thrombolytic agents, *J Am Coll Cardiol* 21:920-925, 1993.

67. Greene DA, Lattimer S, Sima A: Sorbitol, phosphoinositides and sodium-potassium-ATPase in the pathogenesis of diabetic complications, *N Engl J Med* 316:599-606, 1987.

68. Grumbach K, Bodenheimer T: Painful vs painless cost control, *JAMA* 272:1458-1464, 1994.

69. Grumbach K, Bodenheimer T: Mechanisms for controlling costs, *JAMA* 273:1223-1230, 1995.

70. Grundy SM: Cholesterol and coronary heart disease: future directions, *JAMA* 264:3053-3059, 1990.

71. Haeften TW: Clinical significance of insulin antibodies in insulin-treated diabetic patients, *Diabetes Care* 12:641-648, 1989.

72. Haffner S and others: Cardiovascular risk factors in confirmed prediabetic individuals, *JAMA* 263:2893-2898, 1990.

73. Haire-Joshu D: Smoking cessation and the diabetic health care team, *Diabetes Educ* 17:54-67, 1990.

74. Harris ML and others: Prevalence of diabetes and impaired glucose tolerance and plasma glucose levels in US population aged 20-74 years, *Diabetes* 36:523-534, 1987.

75. *The health benefits of smoking cessation: a report of the surgeon general,* DHHS, PHS, CDC, CCDPHP, OSN, Pub No 90-8416, Rockville, Md, 1990, US Department of Health and Human Services.

76. Helmrich S and others: Physical activity and reduced occurrence of non-insulin-dependent diabetes mellitus, *N Engl J Med* 325:147-152, 1991.

77. Hill AB: The environment and disease: association and causation, *Proc R Soc Med* 58:295-300, 1965.

78. Howard B, Howard W: The compelling case for smoking cessation in diabetes, *Circulation* 82:299-301, 1990.

79. Jarrett R: Type II (non–insulin-dependent diabetes mellitus) and coronary heart disease: chicken, egg, or neither? *Diabetologia* 26:99-102, 1984.

80. Jarrett RJ: Cardiovascular disease and hypertension in diabetes mellitus, *Diabetes Metab Rev* 5:547-558, 1989.

81. Kannel WB: Detection and management of patients with silent myocardial ischemia, *Am Heart J* 117:221, 1989.

82. Kannel WB: Coronary heart disease risk factors: Framingham study update, *Hosp Pract* 25:119-127, 1990.

83. Kannel WB, McGee DL: Diabetes and cardiovascular risk factors: the Framingham Study, *Circulation* 59:8-13, 1979.

84. Kannel WB, Sytkowski PA: Atherosclerosis risk factors, *Pharmacol Ther* 32:207-235, 1987.

85. Kannel W, Wilson P: Risk factors that attenuate the female coronary disease advantage, *Arch Intern Med* 155:57-61, 1995.

86. Kaplan N: The deadly quartet: upper-body obesity; glucose intolerance, hypertriglycerides, and hypertension, *Arch Intern Med* 149:1514-1520, 1989.

87. Kaplan N, Roserstock J, Raskin MP: A differing view of treatment of hypertension in patients with diabetes mellitus, *Arch Intern Med* 147:1160-1162, 1987.

88. Karlson B, Herlitz J, Hjalmarson A: Prognosis of acute myocardial infarction in diabetic and non-diabetic patients, *Diabetic Med* 10:449-454, 1993.

89. Keen H, Jarrett J, editors: *Complications of diabetes,* London, 1982, Arnold.

90. Kilo C, Miller J, Williamson J: The crux of UGDP: spurious results and biologically inappropriate data analysis, *Diabetologia* 18:179-185, 1980.

91. Kim D, Escalante D, Garber A: Prevention of atherosclerosis in diabetes: emphasis on treatment for the abnormal lipoprotein metabolism of diabetes, *Clin Ther* 15:766-768, 1993.

92. Kissebah A, Schectman G: Polyunsaturated and saturated fat, cholesterol, and fatty acid supplementation, *Diabetes Care* 11:129-142, 1988.

93. Kloner R: Nifedipine in ischemic heart disease, *Circulation* 92:1074-1078, 1995.

94. Knowler W and others: Preventing noninsulin-dependent diabetes, *Diabetes* 44:483-488, 1995.

95. Koistinen MJ: Prevalence of asymptomatic myocardial ischaemia in diabetic subjects, *Br Med J* 301:92-95, 1990.

96. Kolterman O, Gottlieb A, Moyses C: Amylin agonist, AC-137, reduced postprandial hyperglycemia in subjects with IDDM, *Diabetes* 43(S1):78A, 1994.

97. Kuhn F, Rackley C: Coronary artery disease in women: risk factors, evaluation, treatment, and prevention, *Arch Intern Med* 143:2626-2636, 1993.

98. Lasker R: The Diabetes Control and Complications Trial: implications for policy and practice, *N Engl J Med* 329:1035-1036, 1993.

99. Leaf A, Ryan T: Prevention of coronary artery disease: a medical imperative, *N Engl J Med* 323:1416-1419, 1990.

100. Lebovitz H, Melander A, editors: Sulfonylurea drugs: basic and clinical consideration, *Diabetes Care* 13(suppl 3):1, 1990.

101. Lefemine A, Broach J: Noninvasive imaging and frequency analysis for carotid artery diagnosis and surgical decisions, *Vas Surg* 24:161-166, 1990.

102. Lehto S and others: Myocardial infarct size and mortality in patients with non-insulin-dependent diabetes mellitus, *J Intern Med* 236:291-297, 1994.

103. Lewis E and others: The effect of angiotensin-converting enzyme inhibition on diabetic nephropathy, *N Engl J Med* 329:1456-1462, 1993.

104. Lipid Research Clinics Program: The Lipid Research Clinic Coronary Primary Prevention Trial results. I. Reduction in incidence of coronary heart disease, *JAMA* 251:351-364, 1984.

105. Lipson L: Special problems in treatment of hypertension in the patient with diabetes mellitus, *Arch Intern Med* 144:1829-1831, 1984.

106. Lynch M and others: Acute myocardial infarction in the thrombolytic era, *Diabetic Med* 11:162-165, 1994.

107. Macrury S, Lowe G: Blood rheology in diabetes mellitus, *Diabetic Med* 7:285-291, 1990.

108. Manson J and others: A prospective study of exercise and incidence of diabetes among US male physicians, *JAMA* 268:63-67, 1992.

108a. Maseri A: Medical therapy of chronic stable angina pectoris, *Circulation* 82:2258-2262, 1990.

109. Mason R and others: Diabetic astronomic neuropathy and cardiovascular risk, *Arch Intern Med* 150:1218-1222, 1990.

110. Mazzuca S: Does patient education in chronic disease have therapeutic value? *J Chron Dis* 35:521-529, 1982.

111. Morrish N and others: A prospective study of mortality among middle-aged diabetic patients (the London cohort of the WHO Multinational Study of Vascular Disease in Diabetics). I. Causes and death rates, *Diabetologia* 33:538-541, 1990.

112. Morrison A, Clements R, Winegrad A: Effects of elevated glucose concentrations on the metabolism of the aortic wall, *J Clin Invest* 51:3114-3123, 1972.

113. Moser M: Suppositions and speculations: their possible effects on treatment decisions in the management of hypertension, *Am Heart J* 118: 1362-1369, 1989.

114. Moy C and others: Insulin-dependent diabetes mellitus mortality: the risk of cigarette smoking, *Circulation* 82:37-43, 1990.

115. Multiple Risk Factor Intervention Trial: Risk factor changes and mortality results, *JAMA* 248:1465-1477, 1982.

116. Multiple Risk Factor Intervention Trial Research Group: Coronary heart disease death, non-fatal acute myocardial infarction and other clinical outcomes in the Multiple Risk Factor Intervention Trial, *Am J Cardiol* 58:1-13, 1986.

117. Multiple Risk Factor Intervention Trial Research Group: Mortality after 10½ years for hypertensive participants in the Multiple Risk Factor Intervention Trial, *Circulation* 82:1616-1627, 1990.

117a. National Heart, Lung, and Blood Institute: Bypass surgery results in lower death rates for diabetic patients than angiopathy (clinical alert to U.S. physicians), Sept. 21, 1995, National Institutes of Health, Public Health Services, U.S. Department of Health and Human Services.

118. National Institutes of Health: Noninsulin-dependent diabetes primary prevention trial, *NIH Guide Grants Contracts* 22:1-20, 1993.

119. National Institute of Health Consensus Development Conference: Health implications of obesity, *Ann Intern Med* 103:981-1077, 1985.

120. Nelson RG and others: Effect of protoviruses on mortality in NIDDM, *Diabetes* 37:1499, 1504, 1988.

121. Nettles A, Kreitzer M: Trends in advanced nursing practice and implication for care of diabetic patients, *Diabetes Spectrum* 7:344-349, 1994.

122. Newman J: Smoking in the diabetic population, *Diabetes* 39:208A, 1990.

123. Deleted in proofs.

124. Olsson T and others: Prognosis after stroke in diabetic patients: a controlled prospective study, *Diabetologia* 33:244-249, 1990.

125. Opie L, Messali F: Nifedipine and mortality: grave defects in the dossier, *Circulation* 92:1068-1073, 1995.

126. Pecoraro R, Reiber G, Burgess E: Pathways to diabetic limb amputation: basis for prevention, *Diabetes Care* 13:513-521, 1990.

127. Pederson O: The impact of obesity on the pathogenesis of non–insulin-dependent diabetes mellitus: a review of current hypothesis, *Diabetes Metab Rev* 5:494-509, 1989.

128. Peto R and others: Randomized trial of prophylactic daily aspirin in British male doctors, *Br Med J* 196:313-316, 1988.

129. Pietri A, Dunn F, Raskin P: The effect of improved diabetic control in plasma lipid and lipoprotein levels: a comparison of conventional therapy and continuous subcutaneous insulin infusion, *Diabetes* 29:1001-1005, 1980.

130. Pitt B and others: Pravastatin limitation of atherosclerosis in the coronary arteries (PRACT), *J Am Coll Cardiol*, 1995 (in press).

131. Pollet R, El-Kebbi I: The applicability and implications of the DCCT to NIDDM, *Diabetes Rev* 2:413-427, 1994.

132. Posevitz L, Greer S, Kovacs P: Laser-assisted balloon angioplasty: analysis of 132 clinical cases, *Vasc Surg* 24:377-381, 1990.

133. Pyorala K: Relationship of glucose tolerance and plasma insulin to the incidence of coronary artery disease: results from two population studies in Finland, *Diabetes Care* 2:131-141, 1976.

134. Pyorala K, Laakso M, Usitupa M: Diabetes and atherosclerosis: an epidemiologic view, *Diabetes Metab Rev* 3:463-524, 1987.

135. Reaven G: Role of insulin resistance in human disease, *Diabetes* 37:1595-1607, 1988.

136. Reaven G: Syndrome X: is one enough? *Am Heart J* 127:1439-1442, 1994.

137. Reichard P, Nilsson B-Y, Rosenquist U: The effect of long-term intensified insulin treatment on the development of microvascular complications of diabetes mellitus, *N Engl J Med* 329:304-309, 1993.

138. Relman A: Controlling costs by "managed competition": would it work? *N Engl J Med* 328:133-135, 1993.

139. Report of the National Cholesterol Education Program: Expert panel on detection, evaluation, and treatment of high blood cholesterol in adults, *Arch Intern Med* 148:36-69, 1988.

140. Rifkin B: Cholesterol redux, *JAMA* 264:3060-3061, 1990.

141. Rosenstock IM: Understanding and enhancing patient compliance with diabetic regimens, *Diabetes Care* 8:610-616, 1985.

142. Rosenstock J: Surgery: practical guidelines for diabetes management, *Clin Diabetes* 5:49-61, 1987.

143. Rubin R, Altman W, Mendelson D: Health care expenditures for people with diabetes mellitus, 1992, *J Clin Endocrinol Metab* 78:809A-809F, 1994.

144. Ruderman N, Schneider S: Exercise and the insulin-dependent diabetic, *Hosp Pract* 21:41-51, 1986.

145. Ruderman N, Schneider S: Diabetes, exercise and atherosclerosis, *Diabetes Care* 15:1787-1793, 1992.

146. Salomon M and others: Diabetes mellitus and coronary artery bypass: short-term and long-term prognosis, *J Thorac Cardiovasc Surg* 85:264-271, 1983.

147. Saudek C: When does diabetes start? *JAMA* 263:2934, 1990.

148. Schneider D, Nordt T, Sobel B: Attenuated fibrinolysis and accelerated atherogenesis in type II diabetic patients, *Diabetes* 42:1-7, 1993.

149. Schwartz C and others: Pathogenesis of the atherosclerotic lesion: implications for diabetes mellitus, *Diabetes Care* 15:1156-1167, 1992.

150. Sempos C and others: Prevalence of high blood cholesterol among US adults, *JAMA* 269:3009-3014, 1993.

151. Shuman C: Management of the diabetic patient undergoing surgery, *Cardiovasc Rev Rep* 3:1119-1124, 1982.

152. Sima A and others: Regeneration and repair of myelinated fibers in sural nerve biopsy specimens from patients with diabetic neuropathy treated with sorbinil, *N Engl J Med* 319:548-555, 1988.

153. Sirtori C, Pasik C: Reevaluation of a liguanide, metformin: mechanism of action and tolerability, *Pharm Res* 30:187-228, 1994.

154. Skarfors E, Weyerner T, Lithell H: Physical training as treatment for Type II (non-insulin-dependent) diabetes in elderly men: a feasibility study over 2 years, *Diabetologia* 30:930-933, 1987.

155. Smith J, Marcus F, Serokman R: Prognosis of patients with diabetes mellitus after acute myocardial infarction, *Am J Cardiol* 54:718-722, 1974.

156. Steering Committee of the Physicians' Health Study Research Group: Final report on the aspirin component of the Ongoing Physicians' Health Study, *N Engl J Med* 321:129-135, 1989.

157. Stern M: Diabetes and cardiovascular disease: the "common soil" hypothesis, *Diabetes* 44:369-374, 1995.

158. Stout R: Insulin and atheroma: 20 year perspective, *Diabetes Care* 13:631-654, 1990.

159. Surwit R: Of mice and men: behavioral medicine in the study of type II diabetes, *Ann Behav Med* 15:227-235, 1993.

159a. The 1984 report of the Joint National Committee of Detection, Evaluation, and Treatment of High Blood Pressure, *Arch Intern Med* 144:1045-1057, 1984.

160. Trost BH: Hypertension in the diabetic patient: selection and optimum use of antihypertensive drug, *Drugs* 38:621-633, 1989.

161. Tschoepe D and others: Platelets in diabetes: the role in the hemostatic regulation in atherosclerosis, *Semin Thromb Hemost* 19:122-128, 1993.

162. Tyroler H: Lowering plasma cholesterol levels decreases risk of coronary heart disease: an overview of clinical trials. In Steinberg D, Olefsky J, editors: *Hypercholesterolemia and atherosclerosis,* New York, 1987, Churchill-Livingstone.

163. UK Prospective Diabetes Study Group: UK Prospective Diabetes Study. VIII. Study design, progress and performance, *Diabetologica* 34:877-890, 1991.

164. Uusitupa M and others: Five year incidence of atherosclerotic vascular disease in relation to general risk factors, insulin levels, and abnormalities in lipoprotein composition in non–insulin-dependent diabetic and non-diabetic subjects, *Circulation* 82:27-36, 1990.

165. Vinicor F: Barriers to the translation of the Diabetes Control and Complications Trial, *Diabetes Rev* 2:371-383, 1994.

166. Vinicor F: Is diabetes a public health disorder? *Diabetes Care* 17(S1):22-27, 1994.

167. Vinicor F: Intersectoral and interdisciplinary care: a challenge in diabetes, *Int J Health Promot Educ,* 1995 (in press).

168. Whitcomb M: Correcting the oversupply of specialists by limiting residencies for graduates of foreign medical schools, *N Engl J Med* 333:454-456, 1995.

169. Wilden T: Early nutrition and diabetes mellitus, *Br Med J* 306:283-284, 1993.

170. Williams B: Insulin resistance: the shape of things to come, *Lancet* 344:521-524, 1994.
171. Williams RB and others: Type A behavior, hostility and coronary atherosclerosis, *Psychosom Med* 42:539-549, 1980.
172. Wing R: Behavioral strategies for weight reduction in obese Type II diabetic patients, *Diabetes Care* 12:139-144, 1989.
173. Working Group on Hypertension in Diabetes: Statement on hypertension in diabetes: final report, *Arch Intern Med* 127:830-842, 1987.
174. Zimmet P: Primary prevention of diabetes mellitus, *Diabetes Care* 11:258-262, 1988.
175. Zimmet P: Hyperinsulinemia—how innocent a bystander? *Diabetes Care* 16(S3):56-70, 1993.
176. Zuanetti G and others: Influence of diabetes on mortality in acute myocardial infarction: data from the GISSI-2 study, *J Am Coll Cardiol* 22:1788-1794, 1993.

9 Foot Care and Lower Extremity Problems of Diabetes Mellitus

William C. Coleman

Persons with diabetes are at significant risk for lower extremity amputation. Although persons with diabetes constitute 5% of the U.S. population, each year 50% of the 100,000 lower extremity amputations in the United States are performed on this segment of the population.[66] A person with diabetes is 15 times more likely to have a lower extremity removed than a nondiabetic individual.[75] About half of these amputees will develop a limb-threatening condition of the contralateral limb within 18 months and will require amputation in 3 to 5 years.[38,46] Pecoraro and colleagues[64] surveyed 80 consecutive diabetic foot amputations and found that an initial episode of minor trauma that resulted in cutaneous ulceration with subsequent failure to heal the wound preceded 72% of amputations.

Prevention of foot problems is therefore a primary consideration for diabetes care and practice. A goal of a 40% reduction in the rate of lower extremity amputations among patients with diabetes by the year 2000 has been set by the U.S. Department of Health and Human Services.[23] To achieve this objective, injury prevention programs must be established, specialized wound management programs instituted, and patient education enhanced.[17]

CHAPTER OBJECTIVES

- Describe the pathology of foot problems.
- Discuss causes of foot problems of a direct and concomitant nature.
- Summarize procedures for assessing foot care risk.
- Evaluate strategies for managing foot problems.
- Discuss the importance of preventing recurrence as it relates particularly to education and the diabetes health care team.

PATHOLOGY

Poorly controlled diabetes mellitus can produce pathologic changes resulting in lower extremity angiopathy and neuropathy. This process is highlighted in Fig. 9-1. Of these two secondary complications that affect the feet, three to five times as many patients are admitted as a result of painless foot trauma as for ischemic pain.[47]

Angiopathy

Persons with diabetes are more likely to develop arteriosclerosis and atheromatous occlusion in the lower extremities than persons without diabetes. In addition, when arteriosclerosis develops in a diabetic person, its progression is more rapid than in a nondiabetic person and occurs at a younger age and equally in women and men. The most frequently involved vessels in diabetes are located between the knee and the foot.[17] The result is that the normally

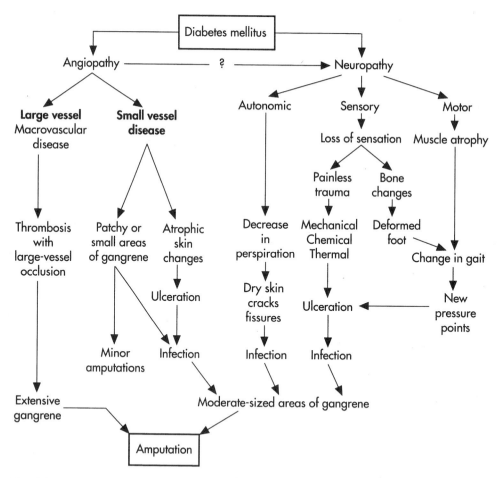

Fig. 9-1 Pathogenesis of diabetic foot lesions. (From Levin ME, O'Neal LW, editors: *The diabetic foot,* St Louis, 1988, Mosby.)

Table 9-1   Differences in Diabetes- and Nondiabetes-Related Peripheral Vascular Disease

	Persons with diabetes	Persons without diabetes
Clinical	More common	Less common
	Younger patient	Older patient
	More rapid	Less rapid
Male/female ratio	2:1	30:1
Occlusion	Multisegmental	Single segment
Vessels adjacent to occlusion	Involved	Not involved
Collateral vessels	Involved	Usually normal
Lower extremities	Both	Unilateral
Vessels involved	Tibial artery	Aortic artery
	Perineal artery	Iliac artery
	Small vessels	Femoral artery
	Arterioles	
Gangrene	Patchy areas of foot and toes	Extensive
In-hospital mortality with amputation	Approximately 3%	Significantly less

Modified from Levin ME, O'Neal LW, Bowker JH, editors: *The diabetic foot,* ed 5, St Louis, 1993, Mosby.

extensive collateral circulation in the foot is compromised by the multiple complete and partial arteriosclerotic blockages of large and medium-sized arteries. Occlusive microvascular lesions occur infrequently in the feet of patients with diabetes.[53] This results in a situation comparable to end arteries, such as in the heart or kidney, becoming blocked. In addition, the person with diabetes frequently has bilateral involvement, with multiple occlusions. This is different from the person without diabetes, in whom the lesions are thought to be localized and unilateral (Table 9-1).[26]

The primary signs of a decrease in blood flow include hair loss, shiny or atrophic skin changes, cold feet, feet and ankles that are darker in color than the leg, and dependent rubor. Box 9-1 summarizes symptoms that consistently result from decreased blood flow, including intermittent claudication or rest pain relieved by standing or walking.

Neuropathy

For several decades, health professionals have been observing the process of injury to the feet of individuals with diabetes and have been referring to it as a "trophic" change to the tissue. The term *neuropathic* may be more appropriate, since research has yet to document the exact mechanism of adverse tissue change resulting from diabetes.

Neuropathy can result in painful lower extremity symptoms or loss of the protective senses of touch and pain (Box 9-2). Touch and pain allow a person to quantify the levels of mechanical or thermal stress applied to the tissues by the environment. Without this protection, the insensate tissues can break down, in part because they are subjected to stresses greater than the tissues can withstand.[15] Most amputations ultimately result from this sensory loss, particularly related to pain and temperature sensation.[64] The nerve impairment and resulting

---

BOX 9-1

**SIGNS AND SYMPTOMS OF
PERIPHERAL VASCULAR DISEASE**

Intermittent claudication (pedal pulses
   usually absent)
Nocturnal and rest pain relieved with
   dependency
Shiny appearance of skin
Loss of hair on feet and toes
Failure of a wound to respond to
   appropriate treatment
Absent pulses

Blanching on elevation
Delayed venous filling after elevation
Dependent rubor
Thickened nails, often with fungal infections
Calcification of blood vessels
Gangrene
Miscellaneous
   Blue toe syndrome
   Acute vascular occlusion

---

continuous trauma lead to ulcer development and infection, further compromising an already stressed vascular system, as depicted in Fig. 9-1. Involvement of the autonomic nervous system also leads to foot lesions as a result of the absence of sweating, leading to dry, cracking, fissured skin and possibly infection.

In other forms of diabetic neuropathy, individuals often experience paresthesia or burning sensations in their feet. Persons with diabetes who develop neuropathic foot ulcers, however, rarely have such feelings.[73,74]

The prevalence of neuropathy increases with age and duration of diabetes. The Diabetes Control and Complications Trial (DCCT) found that intensive blood glucose control, which resulted in improved metabolic control, decreased the appearance of peripheral neuropathy at 5 years by 69%.[24]

Responses to touch and pain

To successfully manage the foot problems of most insensate patients, the diabetes team should understand how the psychology of sensory loss affects patients' behavior. At birth the senses of touch and pain are the most developed senses. As the other senses become more fully developed, touch and pain become more of a background means of monitoring the environment.

Hundreds of thousands of touch and pain receptors cover the entire surface of the body. These receptors form a protective boundary between the person and the environment. Persons mentally establish a body image. When they are touched or when a painful stimulus penetrates this boundary, persons are touched psychologically as well as physically. This effect has been demonstrated in work by Fisher and colleagues[31] that suggests even the slightest touch alters the individual's perception of other people and their surroundings. Other work has shown that touch not only affects perception but can be used to manipulate behavior as well.[42] For example, when touch accompanied a request for return of a missing coin, the likelihood of its return was almost 96%, compared with 63% when touch did not accompany the request.

BOX 9-2

**SIGNS AND SYMPTOMS OF
PERIPHERAL NEUROPATHY**

Paresthesia	Trophic ulcers
Hyperesthesia	Foot drop
Hypoesthesia	Changes in shape of foot
Loss of deep tendon reflexes	Muscle atrophy
Loss of vibratory, cutaneous pressure,	Changes in bone and joint
temperature, or position sense	Radiographic signs*
Anhidrosis	Demineralization
Heavy callus formation over	Osteolysis
pressure points	Neuropathic fracture

_____

*It may be difficult to distinguish these radiographic findings from those of osteomyelitis.

It is difficult to measure the degree to which levels of communication are lost when sensation is diminished. Portions of the body that have become insensitive appear to be perceived as somewhat "disassociated" from the body. Injury to the insensitive parts becomes less important and less personalized to the individual because painful sensation is lost. Health care providers unaccustomed to managing insensitivity often are surprised at insensate patients having an injury for several days or weeks before coming to a clinic for attention. Frequently this is because the first indication to the patient that an insensitive foot has been injured is an observed trail of blood on the floor. The patient becomes confused trying to remember when this injury could have occurred and usually will not be able to recall any particular incident.

CAUSES OF FOOT PROBLEMS

The ability to characterize, localize, and identify pain often begins the process of diagnosis for the clinician. *Pain* is an important mechanism whereby prognosis is evaluated. When the sense of pain is diminished, so is this mechanism of clinical evaluation. For example, a person in pain would be much more insistent on obtaining some form of treatment to eliminate the pain than would an individual without such a sensation. In addition, the physician is highly motivated in reducing the pain to improve the patient's sense of well-being.

Mechanical Causes of Injury

A direct correlation exists among the amount of mechanical stress, the time the stress is applied, and the breakdown of tissue being stressed. High pressures result in damage quickly, whereas lower pressures must be applied for a longer time to damage the tissues.[44,69]

In the sensate person the inflammatory process is a part of the healing process. First, the inflammation often causes discomfort that causes the sensate injured person to limit activity at the site of inflammation. In contrast, the insensate patient will continue to use the inflamed part without restriction, further amplifying the inflammation. Ultimately, the inflammatory process becomes destructive to the involved tissues in the insensate person.

Second, fluids accumulate in injured feet. These fluids can be localized, and infected areas can be surrounded by white blood cells (WBCs) as long as motion and pressure are kept to a minimum. One would expect limited motion in the sensate person, since it is the sense of pain that demands limited use of an injured foot.[55] Since the insensate person does not feel pain as readily, walking or other mechanical trauma continues causing pressure, forcing these fluids into previously uninvolved tissues. This movement of fluid is further complicated by the pull of the tendons when the foot is moved. Fluids and bacteria adjacent to the tendon can be carried to new areas within the foot. A person with an injured, sensate foot "splints" the tendons, holding the joint immobile. An insensate patient will not, which increases the possibility of infection.

Based on this mechanical process of injury, Brand[15] identified three distinct forms of injury to human soft tissues that result from mechanical stress. Discussion of these three forms follows.

High pressure (penetrating wounds)

The first form of insensate foot injury from mechanical stress is the result of a high-pressure penetrating wound. Any person might experience these injuries by stepping on a small object of sufficient height to break through the skin, such as a piece of glass, a thumbtack, or a nail. (A pressure of 600 to 900 pounds per square inch [lb/in^2] is required to break through the adult skin of the sole of the foot.[79])

In contrast to persons with normal sensation, those with insensitivity may not even feel the penetrating wound occur. They may continue to walk with the object imbedded in the bottom of the foot, resulting in repetitive crushing of the wound site. Each step thus results in a constant increase of inflammation and further injury.

Low pressure (ischemic necrosis)

Mechanical stress can cause injuries that result from low pressure applied for a long period. This form of ulcer may result because of unrelenting low pressure (2 to 8 lb/in^2) to the tissues for a long time (12 to 16 hours). The usual causes of this type of injury would include shoes that do not fit precisely.[12] Such footwear creates pressure that pushes blood from the capillaries as the skin is compressed between the leather of the shoe and a bony prominent area of the foot. The tissues break down in a manner similar to decubitus ulceration of immobilized patients. The low stress occludes the dermal capillaries.[25] The usual location for these ulcers are the toes, the metatarsal heads, and the styloid process at the base of the fifth metatarsal.

Moderate repetitive pressure (plantar ulceration)

The most common form of injury to insensitive feet comes as a result of the repetitive stress of walking.[13,14] Pressures generated under the foot by walking range from 20 to 80 lb/in[2]. Injury from the repetitive stress of walking usually develops when the tissues are subjected to a higher level of stress, either by walking faster or farther than the usual rate or distance to which the tissues are accustomed. When normal sensation is present, a person who walks longer than the accustomed time will have sore feet. To continue walking comfortably, this person will begin altering his or her gait and thus the way in which the foot meets the ground. The areas of the foot perceived as uncomfortable can then be "rested" as the person continues to walk.

In contrast, the person with insensate feet can develop foot ulcers, since a feeling of discomfort is not perceived in the insensitive foot. The person with insensate feet has no reason to alter the way the foot meets the ground. Thus the sore part of the foot is subjected to continuing stress which each step. The repetitive stress, the inflammatory process, and the associated accumulation of WBCs cause tissue breakdown.[12,13] Leukocytes release lytic enzymes into severely inflamed tissues, with the accumulation of these substances eventually serving to weaken the soft tissue structure.

Understanding the effects of repetitive stress is enhanced by the work of Manley and Darby,[54] who found that an increase in repetitions resulted in earlier ulcerations. They applied repetitive stress to the bottom of the feet of 45 neurectomized rats and 45 rats with nerves intact. When subjected to the same levels of repetitive stress, the neuropathic feet ulcerated more easily than the normal rat feet. Subsequent to each test, the temperature of the normal feet averaged 1.2° C warmer than the feet of the rats with neurectomy. The authors proposed that this observation may have indicated more capillary perfusion in the feet with intact neural pathways to dilate vessels of sympathetic innervation. With more perfusion, fewer metabolites, more cell debris, and less edema, fluid would remain in the tissues. In contrast, ulceration can be prevented by decreasing repetitive stress and allowing rest days.[15]

Locations of Ulcerations

Areas more likely to ulcerate are the forefoot areas of highest pressure.[5,11,55] The most frequent locations of ulcers formed as a result of repetitive walking stress are the first toe and the metatarsal heads.[27,72] Boulton and colleagues[11] found that patients with neuropathy develop significantly higher pressures under the metatarsal heads than normal sensate persons with or without diabetes. Calluses in these areas can increase the pressure by as much as 30%.[80] Neuropathic subjects with limited joint motion at the subtarsal joint and the first metatarsophalangeal joint may also have much higher focal pressures. Sixty-five percent of the insensate patients with limited joint motion had a history of plantar ulceration. Twenty percent of patients with neuropathy but normal subtalar and first metatarsophalangeal motion had previous plantar ulceration.[30] Thus limited joint mobility may predispose neuropathic feet to ulcers by concentrating pressure at susceptible sites.[22,52]

Infection and Diabetes

It is often reported that persons with diabetes mellitus are more susceptible to infection than cohorts without diabetes. The research on this topic is conflicting, without actual evidence of impaired immunologic competence in diabetic persons.[20] Despite the lack of specific epidemiologic evidence of increased infection or identification of a biochemical defect, many clinicians support the routine use of prophylactic antibiotics as important to the long-term health of the person with diabetes.

Although it is difficult to document overall increases in infection in diabetes, the diabetic person may be predisposed to certain organisms.[9] This predisposition may be mediated by alterations in host defenses, vascular insufficiency that limits infection fighting, and neurologic abnormalities that limit awareness of trauma or inflammation, as previously described.

Diabetic foot infections are one of the most frequent problems faced by the person with diabetes. Bacterial and fungal infections of the skin are the most common found in persons with diabetes. Mild foot infections are usually caused by aerobic, gram-positive cocci such as *Staphylococcus* or *Streptococcus*.[51] (Deeper infections usually involve multiple types of bacteria that may also include gram-negative and anaerobic organisms.[77] Identification of the infecting organism is greatly improved if a tissue sample from the base of the wound is taken with a cure after the wound has been débrided.[51])

Levin[46] characterizes patients most at risk for foot infections as older adults, patients with peripheral neuropathy, and those who have neglected the infection for longer than a month.

In addition to the neuropathic ulcers previously described, other common infections of the foot include those discussed next.

Infection of the nails

Various organisms can result in nail infections, a common finding in diabetes. Not all infections are caused by fungal organisms, although various types of fungi (e.g., *Candida albicans*) are frequently associated with nail infections. Depending on the extent of the infection, infected nails appear discolored and can thicken or become elevated. In final stages of infection the nail plate is separated from the nail bed by fluid or is traumatically avulsed.[16,46]

Osteomyelitis

Osteomyelitis is one of the most serious problems associated with care of the diabetic foot. It occurs frequently in diabetes, often beginning as a chronic perforating ulcer. Diagnosis of osteomyelitis is made difficult by the lack of a precise method of noninvasive detection. Plain radiographs are rarely conclusive for identifying bone infections.[61] Bone scans are expensive and nonspecific but are more sensitive.[61] Bone infections can easily be difficult to differentiate from soft tissue inflammation, particularly in insensitive feet, because the inflammation is enhanced by continued use of the insensitive limb.

If a probe can be inserted with light pressure deep enough to touch bone, treatment for osteomyelitis should be begun. If bone radiographs show no bone reaction and a probe does not touch the bone soft tissue, infection should be assumed.[17] Treatment focuses on antibiotic therapy, with surgery sometimes necessary to excise dead bone.

Plantar space abscess

Abscess of the plantar space is a lesion characterized by swelling and redness in the sole of the foot, which may or may not be tender.[16,46]

Infected vascular gangrene

Vascular insufficiency produces necrosis of distal tissue *(dry gangrene)* that may be secondarily infected *(wet gangrene).* Clinically the lesion is often black and produces a foul odor. Amputation is generally the form of treatment.[16,46]

Gas-forming infection

Gas gangrene is a fulminating, life-threatening infection caused by clostridia. The disease presents rapidly, generally within 3 days, and is characterized by necrotic, edematous skin. Antibiotics are supplemental to surgery.[16,46]

Skin Disorders

The condition of the skin provides clues to the presence of diabetes mellitus, such as frequency of infection, joint contractures, pruritus, and dryness.[26,47] The skin of the person with diabetes may have structural differences, including increased numbers of mast cells and increased capillary fragility. For this reason, diabetic persons are prone to various skin infections more frequently than nondiabetic persons. Discussion of the diabetic foot and leg would therefore be incomplete without inclusion of the skin lesions classically seen in the lower extremity of the person with diabetes. Although not intended to be all inclusive, Table 9-2 reviews some of the more common skin lesions found in persons with diabetes.

RISK ASSESSMENT

As reported earlier, programs that incorporate patient education and early identification of injury have a major impact on the reduction of diabetic foot amputations. Through the multidisciplinary approach, members of medical organizations have the best opportunity to develop comprehensive programs of injury prevention and early treatment.

Foot Care Protocol

The best approach to saving the diabetic foot involves several steps, including identification of the feet at risk, prevention of foot ulcers, treatment of foot ulcers, and prevention of recurrence of foot ulcers.[2,3]

The patient with peripheral vascular disease or distal symmetric polyneuropathy is at severe risk for foot problems. As noted in Box 9-2, signs and symptoms of vascular disease in the lower extremity should be carefully assessed at each patient visit. Examination of the feet should be routine and should include removal of shoes and socks. Thus a systematic foot care protocol should be followed. Although foot assessment should include observation of mobility, hydration, color, swelling or edema, temperature, sensation, and nail formation as a routine diabetes care practice, assessing for the presence of structural deformities or lesions is also necessary. Appendix 9 at the end of this chapter provides a sample foot assessment protocol (9a), including a teaching outline (9b).

Table 9-2   Common Skin Disorders in Diabetes Mellitus

Skin disorder	Symptoms
Primary skin disorders	
Diabetic dermopathy	Small, atrophic, red-brown, sharply circumscribed lesion that occurs on anterior skin in 50% of patients
Joint contractures	Thick, waxy skin overlying joints; noted in almost 30% of patients with insulin-dependent diabetes
	Increased dermal collagen yields waxy texture; increased risk for microvascular disease
Necrobiosis lipoidica	Asymptomatic, nonulcerated, yellowish, sclerotic plaque on unilateral or bilateral skin; affects women more than men
Lipodystrophy	Mass of scar and fatty tissue caused by hypertrophy of subcutaneous fatty tissue leading to muscle hyperdevelopment; found at site of insulin injections; incidence low with advent of purified insulins
Insulin resistance	
Acanthosis nigricans	Hyperpigmented, evenly thickened and folded skin of flexural body regions
Abnormal lipid levels	
Eruptive xanthomas	Multiple yellow-red and yellow-orange papules; located over joints, buttocks, and trunk; clears with good control
Xanthelasma	Irregular plaques over eyelids
	Most common type of xanthoma
	Begins as pinpoint yellow-orange spots that coalesce and become thicker
Xanthochromia	Yellowish skin discoloration accompanied by increase in carotene and blood cholesterol; rare condition, located on sole of foot

Modified from Haire-Joshu D: In Beare PG, Myers JL, editors: *Principles and practice of adult health nursing,* ed 2, St Louis, 1994, Mosby.

Sensory assessment

Fundamental to a prevention program is a quantifiable means of testing patients for the presence or absence of protective levels of sensation.[20] Protective levels of sensation are defined as adequate touch and pain sensation to prevent (1) injuries caused by sensory loss and (2) continued use of an injured part to a degree that causes further injury. The best means of achieving this involves a procedure that uses vibration, pressure, touch, and proprioception.[47]

Vibration. A 128-cycle tuning fork touched to each toe should result in a perception of vibration for not less than 15 seconds and usually for 20 to 25 seconds.

Pressure. Semmes-Weinstein monofilaments are a common form of quantifiable testing in use today. These are a set of nylon filaments similar to the bristles of a nylon brush. Each filament is the same length but varies in thickness; this difference in thickness requires a different force to bend them. Usually a thickness of 5.07 is used. The test is performed by

Table 9-3   Risk Categories and Associated Footwear Guidelines

Category	Clinical findings	Footwear changes
0	Has protective sensation	Provide education on proper footwear.
1	Has lost protective sensation	Add a soft insole to a shoe of proper contour and fit.
2	Has lost protective sensation and has a foot deformity	Prescribe depth footwear or a custom-made shoe for severe deformity; molded insoles.
3	Has lost protective sensation and has a history of foot ulcer	Inspect the type and condition of footwear and insoles at every visit.

applying a force to one end of the filament and pressing the other end against the patient's skin. The tester asks the patient to report when he or she feels the pressure from the filament. By not touching the patient with a filament every time, by varying the rate at which the filaments are applied, and by not following a regular pattern of sites to be tested, reliability can be increased.[71] An evaluation of sensory testing methods found monofilament testing to be as effective as and less time-consuming than vibration or thermal tests.[70]

Touch. This is a simple modification of the traditional pinprick test. The cotton end of a swab is used to evaluate sensitivity to the blunt touch, and the pointed end is used to assess "sharp" perception.

Proprioception. For this test the toes are moved up and down. Patients with significant neuropathy are unable to determine position in space. In addition, delayed venous or capillary filling time can be measured by having the patient lie supine with feet elevated at a 45-degree angle until one or both feet blanch. The patient then sits upright with the feet dependent until the color returns to normal, which should occur in 15 seconds or less. A filling time longer than this indicates moderate to severe ischemia.

Risk Categories

Once protective sensory loss is identified, diabetic patients can be categorized according to their risk of being injured. In this way, resources can be assigned to focus attention on the "at risk" patients. Such a program has been evolving at the Hansen's Disease Center in Carville, Louisiana, for almost 10 years.[20] The risk categories used by the Carville team are noted in Table 9-3 and described next.

Risk category 0

Patients assigned to risk category 0 have a disease process, such as diabetes, that has the potential to result in sensory loss. These patients have not yet lost protective sensation. They should have their sensory status evaluated each year and should be educated concerning sensory loss, footwear selection, smoking, diabetes control, and other possible risk factors. The need for proper footwear selection is discussed with these patients at every visit (e.g., for women, do not wear high heels). However, an overemphasis on proper footwear at this relatively low-risk time can also result in the person with diabetes resisting footwear changes later when the risk from shoe injuries is much greater. For example, when educating women who are in category 0, some of them may respond better to a gradual change from tapered toes and high heels.

Risk category 1

Patients in category 1 differ from category 0 patients by demonstrating loss of protective levels of sensation. With this higher risk, footwear is examined much more carefully. The shape of the shoe should be compared with the shape of the foot. If there is adequate room inside the shoe, a thin, soft insole can help protect the bottom of the foot. Category 1 patients should break in new shoes gradually until the upper leather parts conform to the shape of the foot. They are educated in foot inspection and early wound care. An appointment for foot examination is arranged every 6 months to assist the patient by assessing for skin temperature changes or changes in foot morphology.

Risk category 2

Category 2 patients not only have lost sensation but also have limited joint mobility or a deformity that creates focal points of pressure under the foot. Footwear and shoe inserts become even more important at this level of risk. Most of these patients require custom inserts and prescription footwear. Patients with severe foot deformity or partial foot amputation may need a custom-made shoe. Surgical correction of deformity may be considered to lower the patient's risk of injury. Clinical foot inspections with a footwear evaluation are performed every 3 months.

Risk category 3

Patients in category 3 are at highest risk of developing skin ulcers and have a history of previous ulceration. These patients should have molded inserts for their shoes and, if they also have a foot deformity, should wear prescription shoes. A health team member trained in footwear form and function must inspect the condition of the shoes and inserts at every visit. Often the shoes of insensate patients wear down and threaten the foot if not kept in repair. Return appointments should be arranged every 1 to 2 months to prevent recurrence of ulcers.

EDUCATION ON AND PREVENTION OF FOOT ULCERS
Guidelines for Teaching

Patients with diabetes must learn how to protect their feet. By identifying level of risk, education can be tailored to meet the particular needs of the diabetic person. These principles of education fall into three categories: general foot care principles, knowledge of types of footwear, and preventive care instructions, including involvement with the health care provider. Appendix 9a provides an example of a foot care assessment protocol, and Appendix 9b lists a teaching outline that addresses critical components to be included by the educator in any foot care program. Box 9-3 outlines specific care instructions for the patient.

Education programs specifically directed to teaching individuals with diabetes proper foot care practices have been the most effective methods for reducing amputation rates.

Amputations have been reduced by as much as 85% by institutions that focus on foot care education.[3] The time with the patient should be used to explore various methods of encouraging foot care as a diabetes management priority.[34,38,47] This includes the use of various educational methods, such as those addressed later in the text.

Footwear

As previously noted, insensate patients should always wear footwear with a sole thick enough to absorb the potential penetrating object. This means that footwear should be worn around the household, in the yard, or any time the patient is walking. *Depth footwear* has extra vertical space within the shoe. A wide variety of these types of footwear are now available "off the shelf" to make room for contracted toes or thicker insoles. However, neuropathy can result in loss of motor control as well as sensory pathology. The most common early sign of motor

---

BOX 9-3

PATIENT INSTRUCTIONS FOR DIABETIC FOOT CARE

Foot care

Do not use tobacco.

Inspect your feet daily for blisters, cuts, and scratches.

Use a mirror to see the bottom of the feet. Always check between the toes for dryness, redness, tenderness, and localized areas that rub (hot spots).

Inspect the inside of your shoes daily for foreign objects, nail points, torn linings, and rough areas.

Wash feet daily. Dry carefully, especially between the toes.

Avoid temperature extremes. Test water with elbow before bathing.

Soak feet only if specifically prescribed by your health care provider. For dry feet, use a very thin coat of lubricating cream or oil. Apply this after bathing and drying the feet. Do not put the oil or cream between the toes.

If feet are cold at night, wear socks to bed. Do not apply hot water bottles or heating pads or soak feet in hot water.

Cut nails in contour with the toes. Do not cut deep down the sides or corners.

Do not use chemical agents for the removal of corns and calluses. Do not use corn plasters.

Do not cut corns and calluses. These should be treated regularly by an experienced health care provider.

Do not use adhesive tape on your feet.

If your vision is impaired, have a family member or friend inspect your feet and shoes daily or assist with foot care.

Footwear

Avoid walking barefoot or in thongs or sandals if your feet are insensitive.

Avoid wearing open-toed shoes or sandals unless specifically prescribed by a health care provider.

Continued.

BOX 9-3

PATIENT INSTRUCTIONS FOR DIABETIC FOOT CARE—cont'd

Preventive care

Never walk barefoot on surfaces such as hot sandy beaches or on the cement or asphalt around swimming pools that are often hot; you may not be able to feel the increased temperature.

Wear clean and properly fitting socks or stocking at all times with your shoes. Avoid wearing mended socks or stockings with seams.

Avoid wearing garters, elastic bands on socks, and/or rolling hose.

Avoid crossing your legs; this can cause pressure on nerves and blood vessels.

Shoes should be properly measured and should fit at the time of purchase. Shoes should be made of material that breathes, such as leather.

Avoid pointed toes or high-heeled shoes.

If your feet have decreased sensation, rotate your shoes three or four times a day. Before putting on your shoes, check the insides of the shoes by hand to ensure that there are no rough surfaces (e.g., nail heads) and no small objects (e.g., pebbles, coins) in your shoes.

Wear appropriate shoes for the weather. In winter, take special precautions such as wearing wool socks and protective foot gear (e.g., fleece-lined boots).

Follow up with your health care provider

See your health care provider regularly and be sure that your feet are examined at each visit.

Notify your health care provider at once if you develop a blister, sore, or crack in the skin of your feet.

---

involvement is clawtoe deformity resulting from intrinsic muscle paralysis. This deformity requires extra room in the shoe to prevent toe ulcers.[6,7]

The option of therapeutic footwear should be explored with the general diabetic population and, more specifically, with those at high risk for foot problems. Footwear is one of the most critically important components of preventing injury to insensate feet. In a survey of previously ulcerated diabetic patients, Edmond and associates[28] found that among people who continued to wear special shoes, 26% had reulcerated their feet. Of those who reverted to using their former shoes, 83% had a reulceration.

Since plantar forefoot ulceration caused by repetitive stress is the most common form of insensate foot injury, outer shoe sole modifications such as a curved roller or single fulcrum rocker are being incorporated into the shoe design to reduce walking pressures under the forefoot. Inserts molded to the shape of the plantar aspect of the foot help to reduce focal pressures by increasing the areas of weight bearing over more of the foot. The need and availability of special footwear should be carefully examined with podiatrist, pedorthist, or physician. Box 9-4 summarizes criteria for therapeutic shoe design.

BOX 9-4

CRITERIA FOR THERAPEUTIC SHOE DESIGN

Critical conditions
Insensitivity
Multiple hammertoes, clawfoot, cocked-toe deformity
Charcot's feet
Bunions, calluses, and other deformities
Previously ulcerated or partially amputated feet
Accommodations
Shoe shape matching foot shape
Adequate shoe depth
Shock absorption
Adjustability by lace or straps
Breathability, softness, flexible material for uppers
Changes for gait and limb-length disorders
Ability to modify the shoe later

MANAGEMENT OF FOOT PROBLEMS

The identification of foot problems is a direct result of the assessment process. These data should then be used to identify treatment guidelines for the various foot problems typically associated with diabetes (see Appendix 9a). More specific aspects of treatment, especially related to ulcer care, are discussed next.

Grading Ulcers

Despite education, 15% of all persons with diabetes mellitus will develop foot ulcers.[62] Wagner[72] developed a system of classifying skin ulcers on the feet of persons with diabetes that is used worldwide[72] (Table 9-4). Grade 0 includes all feet that are not currently ulcerated. These feet may have skeletal deformity or other factors that could place the person at increased risk for skin ulceration. A grade 1 ulcer is a hole in the epidermis that exposes the underlying dermis. Grade 2 ulcers involve deeper tissue and penetrate to bone, tendons, or joint tissue. If an abscess or osteomyelitis is found, the wound is classified as grade 3. Some part of the toes or forefoot is gangrenous with grade 4. Grade 5 is used for feet with more extensive gangrene, usually requiring amputation.

When an ulcer is encountered, the wound is generally classified according to Wagner's criteria. The circumference and depth should be recorded, perhaps by tracing the ulcer on clear plastic film. One should look for evidence of purulence, necrosis, odor, edema, cellulitis, or abscess; assess the foot and leg for other signs of infection; and keep in mind that body temperature and WBC count can be normal in the presence of serious infection.[2] Radiographs may be required to rule out subcutaneous gas or foreign bodies and assess the possibility of

Table 9-4 Wagner's Grades of Foot Lesions

Grade	Criteria
0	Skin intact (all the risk categories are included here)
1	Localized superficial ulcer of the skin
2	Ulcer extending deeper to tendon, bone, ligament, or joint
3	Foot contains abscess or osteomyelitis
4	Gangrene present on or by one or more toes
5	Whole foot involved with gangrene

From Wagner FW: *AAOS Instr Course Lect* 27:143, 1979.

bone involvement. Changes in the bone structure would indicate the need for more extensive studies (e.g., bone scan or biopsy) to address the possibility of osteomyelitis.

Diagnosis and Treatment of Ulcers

Diabetic patients with infected ulcers should be hospitalized.[32] Most amputations are performed on patients with a history of infectious complications.[64] However, it is possible that some evaluations (e.g., bone scans) have recently been overemphasized in their ability to provide pure diagnostic information. Bone scans may be positive when no osteomyelitis is present and thus should not be used as an absolute diagnosis.[2,68] Three-phase bone scans may offer some increased specificity. Radioactive uptake in the entire bone may also be specific. Indium-labeled WBC scintigraphy has shown uptake at simple fracture sites. Scans can be helpful in showing the extent of osteomyelitis, but bone biopsy remains the only definitive means of diagnosing osteomyelitis.[1]

Débridement

All infected abscesses should be incised and drained.[2] Necrosis and calluses should be completely excised. Cultures should be taken at the time of débridement. Aerobic and anaerobic organisms must be cultured precisely. As cited earlier, surface débridement followed by some form of curettage most accurately represents the mixture of pathogens.[33] Infections are often polymicrobial, suggesting that broad-spectrum coverage may be needed initially. Antibiotic therapy should be carefully monitored and antibiotics changed as necessary.

Wound Care

There are no adequately controlled studies of topical agents for diabetic wound care.[2] Dry dressings are used in casts. Current preferred dressings are either wet-to-dry saline gauze changed two or three times a day or occlusive dressings.[39,78] The role of foot soaks and topical agents therefore remains controversial. Astringents, iodine agents, and hydrogen peroxide applied directly on an open wound disrupt the healing process.[49] The selection of a dressing depends on several factors. According to Christensen,[18] treatment options and dressing selections depend on type of tissue (red versus yellow or black), presence of infection or swelling, amount of drainage, size and depth of wound, location and whether bone or tendon is exposed, condition surrounding the skin, and the ease, frequency, and cost of dressing changes.

Flushing of the wounds is an important aspect of care because it allows for the loosening and removal of debris. A dry wound is not conducive to healing, since dehydration results in scab formation. This can become a mechanical barrier to epidermal cell migration.

Monitoring Mechanical Stress

When ulcers are found under forefoot or midfoot, the most successful forms of management address both the cause of the ulceration (repetitive stress or walking) and the mechanical factors that can exacerbate it. Denervation of the skin does not affect epithelialization of superficial wounds.[60] On insensate feet, healing is usually delayed by continuing injury and motion at the wound site; therefore, weight bearing should be restricted. Modification of weight bearing can include crutches, shoe insets, special shoes, bedrest with elevation of legs, and total-contact casting.

Recent studies indicate that total-contact casting is a very reliable means of healing these wounds in a timely manner.[37] The casting technique was first used and developed for healing ulcers on the feet of leprosy patients.[15] Mooney and Wagner[58] have called it the most effective means of controlling lower extremity edema. Total-contact coating casting prevents excessive compression of the wound site by weight bearing, controls edema, immobilizes the joints and tendons, and eliminates inflammation at the wound site. The technique of this form of casting has been described several times.[16,19,43] It is a weight-bearing, below-the-knee cast with little interior padding to shift and alter the support.

The results of the first controlled clinical trial on total-contact casting were published in 1989.[59] A group of physical therapists followed the wounds of 40 diabetic patients, 21 of whom were casted versus 19 who were given traditional wound dressings. These were wet-to-dry saline dressings changed two or three times a day. Ninety percent of the ulcers on casted feet healed in a mean time of 42 days. Thirty-two percent of the traditionally treated ulcers healed in a mean time of 65 days.

Metabolic Control

Attention to metabolic control is essential to the prevention of infection and the promotion of wound healing. Infection may result in fluctuations of blood glucose levels. Prompt, thorough treatment of foot ulcers or infections therefore encourages good blood glucose levels. In contrast, persons in poor control may be hindered in their recovery. Therefore attention to metabolic control is necessary.

Surgical Intervention

Persons with poor circulatory status may be candidates for surgical intervention. Referral to a vascular surgeon may yield positive results with regard to improved blood flow. However, careful evaluation by the diabetes team is needed before surgical intervention and requires thorough and comprehensive communication among the team members as well as thorough education of the patient and family.

PREVENTION OF RECURRENT FOOT ULCERS

Any patient with a history of diabetic foot ulcers is at high risk for future ulcers. An extensive education program emphasizing the principles listed in Box 9-3 is needed. In addition, frequent follow-up should be stressed, with referral to a specialist, such as a pedorthist, recommended as needed.

DIABETIC OSTEOARTHROPATHY

As previously noted, diabetic osteoarthropathy, often referred to as *Charcot's joint,* is a relatively painless, progressive, and destructive disorder found most often in the feet of persons with long-term diabetes. The term *osteoarthropathy* more appropriately attributes this joint disorder to an underlying neuropathic disease process. The terms *Charcot's joint* and *neuroarthropathy* are often misnomers in that the fractures often do not involve a joint at all.[35] A neuropathic fracture is unique from other forms of fracture mostly because the person has no feeling in the limb and thus continues to destroy the bone by walking on the unfelt fracture.[2] Denervation alone does not predispose the bone to fracture. In fact, most denervated joints function normally for a lifetime.

Diabetic osteoarthropathy has a high incidence in those patients who have had diabetes longer than 12 years, regardless of age. Usually only one foot is affected, although an 18% bilateral incidence has been reported in some studies. Two essential factors can be implicated in the development of neuropathic fracture: neuropathy and trauma. These result in further instability of the joint and degeneration, further perpetuating the destructive process (Fig. 9-2). Neuropathic fractures are also frequently seen after an inflammatory condition or casting that has resulted in demineralization. Increased blood flow has been implicated as a major factor in the development of neuropathic fractures.[10,81] The increased flow results in rarefaction of bone, making the area more prone to injury.[76]

In most patients a neuropathic fracture probably begins as an unfelt microtrauma.[35,41] A small fracture, sprain, or ligamentous tear occurs and goes unnoticed because of insensitivity. The insensate patient may notice instability, hear sounds of popping, or feel "rubbing" in the foot as an early symptom of fracture. There is no pain, however, and because the person is unaware of the injury, he or she continues to walk. With each step the inflammation increases. The inflammation creates hyperemia. The hyperemia results in local bone absorption that further weakens the structure. The characteristic destruction of neuropathic fracture develops as the insensitive patient continues to use the foot as though no injury were present.[63] Small fragments of bone are separated and spread through adjacent soft tissue by joint motion. The cartilage can become destroyed and, with the force of weight bearing and joint motion, the bones grind into one another. The redness created by the inflammatory process frequently leads to a diagnosis of infection.

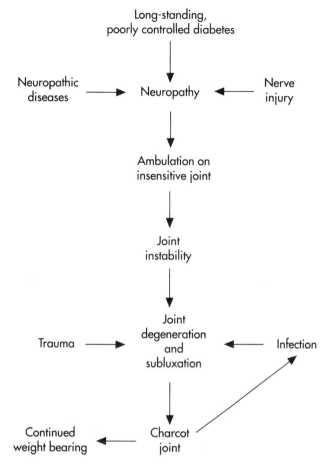

Fig. 9-2 Pathogenesis of the diabetic Charcot's joint. (From Frykberg RG, Kozak GP: *Am Fam Physician* 17:105-112, 1978.)

Diagnosis

Diabetic neuroarthropathy often eludes prompt diagnosis, despite increasing reports in the literature. This is most likely attributable to the clinician's lack of awareness or suspicion for the disorder. The possibility of fracture is not considered because of the absence of pain.

Differential diagnosis for neuropathic fracture is frequently necessary. Swelling, erythema, deformity, or symptoms may be absent. A history of injury or misstep is rarely encountered.[74] A patient with acute dislocation may have some pain or aching, but much less than might be expected. Usually the foot and ankle show a marked deformity, are grossly swollen, and may have a "fallen arch." The foot is very erythematous, warm, and anhidrotic with bounding pulses. These findings, in association with mild to absent pain, contribute significantly to a diagnosis of Charcot's joints.

As previously reviewed, much attention has been directed to various forms of bone scans to differentiate osteomyelitis from Charcot's joint.[1,56] Bone scans most reliably identify the presence of inflammation. Thermometry (temperature evaluation) will perform a similar task in less time and at much less expense. Virtually all structures in the foot are close to the surface. This makes thermometry an indispensable tool for early detection of injury on an insensate foot. Surface skin temperature is the key early sign that indicates the presence of fracture in an insensate foot.[8] With no skin ulcer present or with a recent history of ulceration, an area of skin on a foot 3° C warmer than the rest of the foot or at the same location on the other foot should be treated as a fracture until the temperature equalizes or another cause for the difference is identified.[35,40]

Treatment

For most neuropathic fractures the first form of treatment should arrest the possibility of continued use and breakdown. Progressive destruction can be halted if recognized early.[35,50] Hospitalization may be necessary to ensure that the individual's foot is kept absolutely non–weight bearing and elevated. During this time, diabetes control treatment for recurrent ulcerations and infections can occur. In addition, this allows time for the gross edema to subside.

Once the edema has subsided or is under control, below-the-knee casting remains the most effective form of immediate immobilization of the fracture sites. Surface skin temperatures can be measured at each cast change to monitor the inflammation. As the area of fracture cools to temperatures of those on the unfractured foot, less restrictive forms of support can be used to begin the rehabilitation back to footwear. The process of rehabilitation can take from 12 weeks to 1 year.[12,28]

If some fragmentation is present, reduction and surgical fusion may be indicated.[45] Surgery may also be useful when skin ulceration cannot be prevented by footwear or bracing.[36] With very flail ankle or midfoot fractures of long duration and cool surface skin temperature, amputation is the usual recourse.

Education

Many of the same principles for foot care education apply to the individual with osteoarthropathy. Emphasis on preventive education is critical. Frequent, regular follow-up needs to be emphasized. These individuals should be treated by the diabetes team as being at high risk for future foot care problems. As such, this aspect of diabetes care should assume a major focus. Daily foot assessments should be carefully stressed (see Box 9-3).

ROLE OF THE DIABETES HEALTH CARE TEAM IN FOOT CARE

The involvement of many disciplines from the diabetes health care team is necessary not only to promote optimal diabetes care in general but also to decrease the morbidity common among persons with diabetes. Models of the effectiveness of diabetes education with regard to impact on foot care are impressive. During the early 1970s, Grady Memorial Hospital in Atlanta developed a diabetes team that included nurses, clinicians, and a considerable amount of patient education in emphasizing the need for every health care professional to examine the feet of patients with diabetes. The protocol included utilizing the services of podiatrists when foot pathology was identified as well as the need for daily foot inspection by patients.[21]

Later in the 1970s the County Health Department of Memphis transferred 800 patients from the centrally located outpatient clinic to the patient's small neighborhood clinics, where nurse practitioners were specially trained in new conservative management and foot inspection protocols. Over 2 years a 68% reduction in hospital days and amputations was obtained.[67] At the University Hospital of Geneva a similar program of patient education and staff training in foot care resulted in an 85% reduction in below-the-knee amputations.[4]

Multidisciplinary members of the diabetes team can have particular impact regarding the care of the person with diabetes in the prevention or treatment of foot problems. These members range from the nurse as a primary source of education for the patient; the podiatrist, whose education spans functional biomechanics of the foot, recognition of early deformity, and management of foot problems; the pedorthist, a specialist in fitting, shaping, and molding shoes; the physical therapist, who can educate or aid in the development of exercise programs that minimize mechanical trauma to the foot; the neurologist, who can verify diagnosis of neuropathy; the vascular or orthopedic surgeon, who may be required to treat various deformities; and the social worker, who can assist in job-related problems that may occur as a result of foot problems. The involvement of all disciplines is critical to the care of the patient with diabetes in general, but in particular as it relates to foot problems.

CASE PRESENTATION

As this case study illustrates, foot specialists frequently encounter patients with diabetes who have had foot ulcers that have remained open, under medical care, for years. These patients rarely have significant vascular disease. The gangrene or wound necrosis would have resulted in professional intervention. This repeatedly underscores that the fundamental concepts of insensate foot management are not widely known or widely practiced.

A 59-year-old, 5 ft 11 in, 270-pound white male with a 15-year history of diabetes presents with an open ulcer 3 cm in diameter under the first metatarsal head of the left foot. The wound has been present for 4 years. He is employed as an appliance salesman. He does not know how the ulcer developed. For 18 months the ulcer was treated by his family physician. He was told to cleanse the wound two times a day with soap and water, apply full-strength Betadine solution to the wound site, and cover it with gauze pads. He continued to work in his leather oxford shoes without interruption. After that he sought care from several physicians. Many combinations of topical wound care, hyperbaric oxygen, and whirlpool were used. The wound would vary in size from 3 mm to 4 cm. The ulcer had become infected a year before and he was hospitalized, receiving intravenous antibiotics, for 3 weeks. The ulcer had been smallest after that admission.

DISCUSSION

Physical examination reveals a well-oriented, well-nourished obese male who appears his stated age and relates his own history clearly. Oral temperature is 98.7° F. A random blood glucose level is 147 mg/dl. Skin and skin appendages are within normal limits except for a 3 cm in diameter Wagner grade 1 ulceration plantar to the left first metatarsal head. The ulcer has a well-vascularized, red base. A 7 mm thick, 1 cm wide callus covers the edges of the wound. There is mild erythema around the immediate wound area. No streaking of erythema on the foot is present. No purulence or sign of abscess is noted. The patient has lost protective levels of sensation to the level of the ankle. Pedal pulses are 2/4+.

Treatment consists of removing the callus, cleansing the wound with hydrogen peroxide and normal saline, and applying Betadine solution to the surrounding skin only. A thin dressing is applied. A total-contact cast also is applied and changed weekly. Wound size is at 1 cm at 1 week, is 2 mm at 2 weeks, and heals in 3 weeks. The patient then receives custom-molded insoles and extra-depth shoes to control the pressures under the foot to prevent recurrence.

REFERENCES

1. Al-Sheikh W and others: Subacute and chronic bone infections: diagnosis using In-111, Ga-67 and Tc-99m MDP bone scintigraphy and radiology, *Radiology* 155:501, 1985.
2. American Diabetes Association: *Diabetic Foot Care,* Alexandria, Va, 1990, American Diabetes Association.
3. American Diabetes Association: Clinical practice recommendations, *Diabetes Care* 14(suppl 2):14, 1991.
4. Assal JP and others: Patient education as the basis for diabetic foot care in clinical practice, *Diabetologica* 28:602, 1985.
5. Barton AA, Barton M: Plantar ulcers occurring after neurectomy: light and electron microscope study, *Aust J Exp Biol Med Sci* 46:155, 1968.
6. Bauman JH, Brand PW: Measurement of pressure between foot and shoe, *Lancet* 1:629, 1963.
7. Bauman JH and others: Plantar pressures and trophic ulceration and evaluation of footwear, *J Bone Joint Surg* 45B:652, 1963.
8. Bergholdt HT: Thermography on insensitive limbs. In Uematsu S, editor: *Medical thermography: theory and clinical applications,* Los Angeles, 1976, Brentwood.
9. Bessman AN, Sapico FL: Infectious complications: a multifactorial problem, *Diabetes Spectrum* 4:68, 1991.
10. Boulton AJM, Scarpello JWB, Ward JD: Venous oxygenation in the diabetic neurotrophic foot: evidence of arteriovenous shunting? *Diabetologia* 22:6, 1982.
11. Boulton AJM and others: Dynamic foot pressure and other studies as diagnostic aids in diabetic neuropathy, *Diabetes Care* 6:26, 1983.
12. Brand PW: Pressure sores: the problem. In Kenedi RM, Cowden JM, Scales JT, editors: *Bedsore biomechanics,* London, 1976, Macmillan.
13. Brand PW: Management of the insensitive limb, *Phys Ther* 59:8, 1979.
14. Brand PW: The diabetic foot. In Ellenberg M, Rifkin H, editors: *Diabetes mellitus: theory and practice,* New Hyde Park, NY, 1983, Medical Examination Publishers.
15. Brand PW: The insensitive foot (including leprosy). In Jahss MH, editor: *Disorders of the foot,* ed 2, vol 3, Philadelphia, 1991, Saunders.
16. Burnett O: Total contact cast, *Clin Podiatr Med Surg* 4:471, 1987.
17. Caputo GM and others: Assessment and management of foot disease in patients with diabetes, *N Engl J Med* 331:854, 1994.
18. Christiansen MH: How to care for the diabetic foot, *Am J Nurs* 3:50, 1991.
19. Coleman WC, Brand PW, Birke J: The total contact cast: a therapy for plantar ulceration on insensitive feet, *J Am Podiatr Med Assoc* 11:548, 1987.
20. Cooper R: Infection and diabetes. In Marble A and others, editors: *Joslin's diabetes medicine,* ed 12, Philadelphia, 1986, Lea & Febiger.
21. Davidson JK and others: Assessment of program effectiveness at Grady Memorial Hospital—Atlanta. In Steiner G, Lawrence PA, editors: *Educating diabetic patients,* New York, 1981, Springer-Verlag.
22. Delbridge L and others: Limited joint mobility in the diabetic foot: relationship to neuropathic ulceration, *Diabetic Med* 5:333, 1988.
23. Department of Health and Human Services: *Healthy People 2000: national health promotion and disease prevention objectives,* DHHS Pub No 91-50213, Washington, DC, 1991, US Government Printing Office.
24. Diabetes Control and Complications Trial Research Group: The effect of intensive treatment of diabetes on the development and progression of long-term complications in insulin-dependent diabetes mellitus, *N Engl J Med* 329:977, 1993.
25. Dinsdale SM: Decubitus ulcers in swine: light and electron microscopy study of pathogenesis, *Arch Phys Med Rehabil* 54:51, 1973.

26. Donovan JC, Rowbotham JL: Foot lesions in diabetic patients: cause, prevention and treatment. In Marble A and others, editors: *Joslin's diabetes mellitus,* ed 12, Philadelphia, 1986, Lea & Febiger.

27. Duckworth T and others: Plantar pressure measurements and the prevention of ulceration in the diabetic foot, *J Bone Joint Surg* 67:79, 1985.

28. Edmonds ME and others: Improved survival of the diabetic foot: the role of a specialised foot clinic, *Q J Med* 232:763, 1986.

29. Deleted in proofs.

30. Fernando DJS and others: Relationship of limited joint mobility to abnormal foot pressures and diabetic foot ulceration, *Diabetes Care* 14:8, 1991.

31. Fisher JD, Rytting M, Heslin R: Hands touching hands: affective and evaluative effects of an interpersonal touch, *Sociometry* 39:416, 1976.

32. Gibbons GW, Eliopoulos GM: Infection of the diabetic feet. In Kozak GP and others, editors: *Management of diabetic foot problems,* Philadelphia, 1984, Saunders.

33. Goodson WH, Hunt TK: Wound healing and the diabetic patient, *Surg Gynecol Obstet* 149:600, 1979.

34. Haire-Joshu D: Endocrine system. In Beare PG, Myers J, editors: *Principles and practice of adult health nursing,* ed 2, St Louis, 1994, Mosby.

35. Harris JR, Brand PW: Patterns of disintegration of the tarsus in the anesthetic foot, *J Bone Joint Surg* 48B:4, 1966.

36. Heiple KG, Cammarn MR: Diabetic neuroarthropathy with spontaneous peritalar fracture dislocation, *J Bone Joint Surg* 48B:1177, 1966.

37. Helm PA, Walker SC, Pullium G: Total contact casting in diabetic patients with neuropathic foot ulcers, *Arch Phys Med Rehabil* 65:691, 1984.

38. Herman WM, editor: *The prevention and treatment of complications of diabetes mellitus: a guide for the primary care practitioner,* Atlanta, 1990, US Department of Health and Human Services.

39. Hutchinson JJ, McGuckin M: Occlusive dressings: a microbiologic and clinical review, *Am J Infect Control* 18:257, 1990.

40. Deleted in proofs.

41. Karat S, Karat ABA, Foster R: Radiological changes in bones of the limbs in leprosy, *Lepr Rev* 39:147, 1968.

42. Kleinke CL: Compliance to requests made by gazing and touching experimenters in field settings, *J Exp Soc Psychol* 13:218, 1977.

43. Kominsky SJ: The ambulatory total contact cast. In Frykberg RG, editor: *The high risk foot in diabetes mellitus,* New York, 1991, Churchill Livingstone.

44. Deleted in proofs.

45. Lesco P, Maurer RC: Talonavicular dislocations and midfoot arthropathy in neuropathic diabetic feet: natural course and principles of treatment, *Clin Orthop* 240:226, 1989.

46. Levin ME: Pathogenesis and management of diabetic foot lesions. In Levin ME, O'Neal LW, Bowker JH, editor: *The diabetic foot,* ed 5, St Louis, 1993, Mosby.

47. Levin ME, Poucher RL, Stavosky JW: Neuropathic ulcers and the diabetic foot. In *Treatment of chronic wounds,* No 1, 1991, Curative Technologies.

48. Deleted in proofs.

49. Lineaweaver W and others: Topical antimicrobial toxicity, *Arch Surg* 120:267, 1985.

50. Lippman HI, Perotto A, Farrar R: The neuropathic foot of the diabetic, *Bull NY Acad Med* 52:1159, 1976.

51. Lipsky BA and others: The diabetic foot: soft tissue and bone infection, *Infect Dis Clin North Am* 4:409, 1990.

52. Lithner F, Tornblom N: Gangrene localised to the lower limbs in diabetics, *Acta Med Scand* 208:315, 1980.

53. LoGerfo FW, Coffman JD: Vascular and microvascular disease of the foot in diabetes: implications for foot care, *N Engl J Med* 311:1615, 1984.

54. Manley MT, Darby T: Repetitive mechanical stress and denervation in plantar ulcer pathogenesis in rats, *Arch Phys Med Rehabil* 61:171, 1980.

55. Masson EA and others: Abnormal pressure alone does not cause foot ulceration, *Diabetic Med* 6:424, 1989.

56. Merkel K and others: Comparison of indium-labeled-leukocyte imaging with sequential technetium-gallium scanning in the diagnosis of low grade musculoskeletal sepsis, *J Bone Joint Surg* 67A:465, 1985.

57. Deleted in proofs.

58. Mooney V, Wagner FW: Neurocirculatory disorders of the foot, *Clin Orthop* 122:53, 1977.

59. Mueller MJ and others: Total contact casting in treatment of diabetic plantar ulcers, *Diabetes Care* 12:384, 1989.

60. Muren A, Zederfeldt B: Delayed effect of denervation on healing of superficial skin defects in rabbits, *Acta Chir Scand* 132:618, 1966.

61. Newman LG and others: Unsuspected osteomyelitis in diabetic foot ulcers: diagnosis and monitoring by leucocyte scanning with indium In-111 oxyquinoline, *JAMA* 266:1246, 1991.

62. Palumbo PJ, Melton LJ: Peripheral vascular disease in diabetes. In *Diabetes in America: diabetes data compiled in 1984,* NIH Pub No 85-1468, Washington, DC, 1985, US Government Printing Office.

63. Paterson DE, Job CK: Bone changes and absorption in leprosy. In Cochrane RG, Davey TF, editors: *Leprosy in theory and practice,* ed 2, Bristol, England, 1964, Wright and Sons.

64. Pecoraro RE, Reiber GE, Burgess EM: Pathways to diabetic limb amputation, *Diabetes Care* 13:513, 1990.

65. Deleted in proofs.

66. Reiber GE: Diabetic foot care: financial implications and practice guidelines, *Diabetes Care* 15(suppl 1):29, 1992.

67. Runyan JW: The Memphis Chronic Disease Program, *JAMA* 231:264, 1975.

68. Shih WJ and others: Malunion of a femoral fracture mimicking osteomyelitis in three phase bone imaging, *Clin Nucl Med* 13:38, 1988.

69. Soames RW and others: Measurement of pressure under the foot during function, *Med Biol Eng Comput* 20:489, 1982.

70. Sosenko JM and others: Comparison of quantitative sensory-threshold measures for their association with foot ulceration in diabetic patients, *Diabetes Care* 13:1057, 1990.

71. Visser HJ and others: The use of differential scintigraphy in the clinical diagnosis of osseous and soft tissue changes affecting the diabetic foot, *J Foot Surg* 23:74, 1984.

72. Wagner FW: A classification and treatment program for diabetic, neuropathic, and dysvascular foot problems, *AAOS Instr Course Lect* 27:143, 1979.

73. Ward JD and others: Pain in the diabetic leg, *Pharmatherapeutica* 2:642, 1981.

74. Warren G: Tarsal bone disintegration in leprosy, *J Bone Joint Surg* 53B:688, 1971.

75. Washington State Department of Health, Diabetes Control Program: *Lower extremity amputations among people with diabetes, Washington State 1985-1988,* Olympia, 1991, Washington State Department of Health.

76. Watkins PJ, Edmonds ME: Sympathetic nerve failure in diabetes, *Diabetologia* 25:73, 1983.

77. Wheat LJ and others: Diabetic foot infections: bacteriologic analysis, *Arch Intern Med* 146:1935, 1986.

78. Witkowski JA, Parish LC: Rational approach to wound care, *Int J Dermatol* 31:27, 1992.

79. Yamada H: *Strength of biological materials,* Baltimore, 1970, Williams & Wilkins.

80. Young MJ and others: The effect of callus removal on dynamic plantar foot pressures in diabetic patients, *Diabetic Med* 9:55, 1992.

81. Young RJ and others: Variable relationship between peripheral somatic and autonomic neuropathy in patients with different syndromes of diabetic polyneuropathy, *Diabetes* 35:192, 1986.

Foot care for the individual with diabetes requires a two-step process involving thorough assessment and treatment. This foot care protocol utilizes such a process. Section A requests information related to completing a foot assessment. Section B uses the responses from this information and suggests treatment recommendations based on these responses.

A. FOOT ASSESSMENT

1. Mobility *(circle one)*
   a. Walks without assistance
   b. Walks with help of equipment
   c. Does not walk; uses wheelchair
   d. Bedfast
   e. Amputation

	(Circle one)	
2. Ask, Does the condition of your feet or legs limit your activity in any way? _____	Yes	No
3. Ask to walk 10 feet. Any gait disturbance?	Yes	No
4. Are the feet clean?	Yes	No
5. Shoes and socks clean and in repair?	Yes	No
6. Shoes and socks well fitting?	Yes	No
7. Ask, Do you do anything special when you choose your shoes? _____	Yes	No

8. Hydration

a. Dry skin present on the feet?	Yes	No
b. Do the feet perspire excessively?	Yes	No
c. Ask, What do you do about the (dryness or perspiration)? _____		

9. Color

			If yes, which?	
a. Feet red or blue when dependent?	Yes	No	Rt.	Lt.
b. Feet blanched when elevated?	Yes	No	Rt.	Lt.
c. Do the feet have a brownish discoloration?	Yes	No	Rt.	Lt.

---

*Modified from King PA and others: *Diabetes foot care project,* Ann Arbor, 1990, University of Michigan Department of Public Health Foot Care Project.

10. Edema
    a. Is edema present?   Yes   No   Rt.   Lt.
    b. Ask, What do you do when your feet
       swell? _____

11. Temperature *(Check with the back of your*   If no, which
    hand.)   are cool?
    a. Feet warm to the touch bilaterally?   Yes   No   Rt.   Lt.
    b. Ask, What do you do to keep your feet
       warm? _____

12. Sensation   If no, not
                                                                                  intact in:

    a. Sense of touch intact?   Yes   No   Rt.   Lt.
    b. Pain?   Yes   No   Rt.   Lt.
    c. Position?   Yes   No   Rt.   Lt.
    d. Hot and cold?   Yes   No   Rt.   Lt.
    e. If no, ask, Do you take any special pre-
       cautions since your feet are not very
       sensi-
       tive? _____

13. Toenails   If yes,
                                                                                  which
                                                                                  foot?

    a. Ingrown   Yes   No   Rt.   Lt.
    b. Overgrown   Yes   No   Rt.   Lt.
    c. Thickened   Yes   No   Rt.   Lt.
    d. Discolored *(Describe.)* _____   Yes   No   Rt.   Lt.
    e. Ask, Who cuts your toenails? _____

14. Circulation   Not palpable
    a. Dorsalis pedis present bilaterally? *(Use*   Yes   No   Rt.   Lt.
       three fingers on dorsum of foot, usually
       just lateral to extensor tendon.)

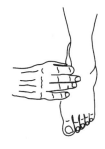

b. Posterior tibial present bilaterally? *(Curve your fingers behind and slightly below the medial malleolus.)*   Yes   No   Rt.   Lt.

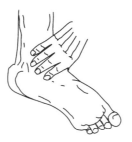

c. Capillary refill of great toe less than 2 seconds?   Yes   No   Rt.   Lt.

15. Structural deformities
    a. Hallux valgus (bunion)   Yes   No   Rt.   Lt.
    b. Hammer toes   Yes   No   Rt.   Lt.
    c. Overlapping digits   Yes   No   Rt.   Lt.
    d. Ask, What do you do to manage these conditions? _____

16. Lesions (Circle if present; mark picture with letter.)
    a. Fissures between toes
    b. Fissures on the heel
    c. Ulcers *(Describe.)*

    _____

    d. Corns
    e. Calloused areas
    f. Plantar wart
    g. Redness over pressure points

    h. Gangrene *(Describe.)*

    _____

    i. Cellulitis (local redness, warmth, swelling)
    j. Blisters
    k. Ask, what do you do to treat these problems? _____

    _____

Lateral right   Lateral left

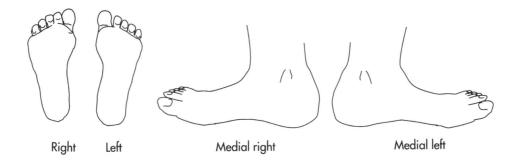

Right   Left   Medial right   Medial left

Summary of Risk Factors *(Circle if present)*

a. Previous amputations because of disease and/or circulation problem
b. Previous foot ulcers
c. Chronic illness for 10 years or more (e.g., diabetes mellitus, circulation problems, arthritis, heart disease, kidney disease, gout, hypertension, other)
d. Age 40 or over
e. Smokes
f. Poor compliance with diet or diabetes not well controlled
g. Reduced ability to care for own feet because of physical or cognitive impairment
h. Poor general hygiene of feet
i. Decreased circulation to feet (poor color, cold to touch, decreased palpable pulses)
j. Decreased sensation in feet
k. Existing lesions or structural deformities of the feet
l. Language/communication difficulty

Plan

a. Continued monitoring and assessing
b. Teaching by nurse/therapist/dietitian
c. Treatment by nurse/therapist
d. Referral to physician/podiatrist/pedorthist
e. Foot care prescription
f. Scheduled follow-up

B. GUIDELINES FOR TREATMENT OF FOOT PROBLEMS

Mobility	1.		
	2.	Yes	Refer to orthotic specialist or podiatrist for gait problems.
	3.	Yes	
Hygiene	4.	No	Wash feet daily with nondrying soap and water.

Shoes	5.	No	Teach regarding need to wear natural fiber shoes that protect the feet.
	6.	No	Wear shoes with ½- to ¾-inch toe room. Wear socks that allow feet to breathe. Avoid tight socks or those with holes or repairs.
	7.		Teach to buy new shoes in the afternoon when feet are a little swollen and to break in slowly (1 to 2 hours a day).
Hydration	8a.	Yes	Apply nondrying lotion one or two times a day.
	8b.	Yes	Apply powder or cornstarch and teach to wear absorbent socks.
	8c.		Teach that dry skin may lead to openings in the skin and that damp skin is prone to breakdown and fungal infections.
Color	9a.	Yes	Assist in maintaining a position that avoids dependent feet or obstructed blood flow.
	9b.	Yes	Teach to:
	9c.	Yes	• Avoid trauma and wear protective shoes as much as possible.
Edema	10a.	Yes	• Wear wool socks to keep feet warm.
			• Recognize signs of infection and that if a lesion develops, to wash with water, cover with bandage or
Temperature	11a.	No	sterile dressing, and notify a health care professional
	11b.		if it does not begin to heal within 3 days.
Edema	10b.		Teach to elevate feet as much as possible and to use powder or nylon stockings under support stockings to avoid skin trauma when putting on.
Sensation	12a.	No	Provide trauma-free environment. Teach to:
	12b.	No	• Avoid heating pads, sunlamps, and temperature extremes.
	12c.	No	• Wear wool socks to keep foot warm.
	12d.	No	• Avoid going barefoot when potential exists for foot injury.
	12e.		• Wear protective shoes as much as possible.
			• Inspect feet daily. If unable to see well, have another person do it.
			• Wear shoes that allow ½- to ¾-inch toe room.
			• Examine shoes for possible causes of injury before putting on. If feet are very insensitive, refer to orthotic specialist, podiatrist, or pedorthist for footwear.
Toenails	13a.	Yes	Pad edge with cotton or lamb's wool and refer to foot specialist for surgical removal.
	13b.	Yes	Reduce with pumice stone or other instrument and soften
	13c.	Yes	before cutting.
	13d.	Yes	Refer to physician for possible fungal infection.
	13e.		Demonstrate use of selected instrument until adequate skill is achieved. Trim nails to follow the natural curve of the toe. Refer to foot specialist for trimming if very thick.

Circulation	14a.	No	Teach to: • Avoid heating pads, sunlamps, and temperature extremes. • Wear wool socks to keep feet warm. • Avoid going barefoot when potential exists for foot injury. • Align extremities when sitting to avoid cutting off circulation (for those with very restricted blood flow). • Wear protective shoes as much as possible. • Inspect feet daily. If unable to see well, have another person do it. • Wear shoes that allow ½- to ¾-inch toe room. • Examine shoes for possible causes of injury before putting them on. • Recognize signs of infection. If a lesion develops, wash with water, cover with a bandage or sterile dressing, and notify a health care professional if it does not begin to heal within 3 days. Assist in maintaining position that avoids dependent feet or obstructed blood flow.
	14b.	No	
	14c.	No	
Structural deformities	15a.	Yes	Reduce pressure through use of pads or lamb's wool. If feet are very insensitive, refer to orthotic specialist, podiatrist, or pedorthist for footwear.
	15b.	Yes	
	15c.	Yes	
Fissures	16a.	Yes	Provide wound care.
	16b.	Yes	Clean open wounds. • Clean with normal saline or tap water (no soap). • Hydrotherapy to increase circulation and clean wound surfaces. • Maintain a moist environment (moist gauze, dressings, OpSite, Duoderm). • Apply Carrington gel to stimulate fibroblasts. Treat infected open or necrotic wounds. • Evaluate process for causative organism and extent of infection. • Débride necrotic tissue. • Clean with normal saline or tap water (no soap). • Administer hydrotherapy to increase circulation and clean wound surface. • Maintain a moist environment. Teach wound care as necessary.
Ulcers	16c.	Yes	
Corns	16d.	Yes	Perform mechanical reduction or remove with pumice stone or electric instrument. Refer to foot specialist if extensive treatment needed.
Calluses	16e.	Yes	
Plantar wart	16f.	Yes	
Redness from pressure	16g.	Yes	Teach regarding use of a pumice stone or similar device to débride calluses and corns; how to relieve pressure from bunions, corns, and calluses using various padding techniques; and the role of the foot specialist in diabetes foot care.

Gangrene	16h.	Yes	Treat dry gangrene.
			• Keep dry and clean.
			• Maintain activity as tolerated.
			Treat wet gangrene.
			• Administer intravenous antibiotics.
			• Consider surgery.
Cellulitis	16i.	Yes	Ensure bedrest and administer antibiotics.
Other	16j.	Yes	Teach regarding care of specific lesion and how to pre-
	16k.		vent further foot trauma.

Foot Care Teaching Outline for Health Care Providers*

Before beginning a foot care training program, the development of an education plan is essential. The plan needs to include both the information to be communicated and the mechanism to provide the information and the needed skills. An example of such a plan that includes the steps for skill acquisition is as follows:

- Explanation—includes the importance and steps for the skills
- Experience—includes observing and then practicing with the skills
- Debriefing—includes a discussion of the person's reactions to the skill and beliefs about his or her ability to carry it out
- Application—includes assisting the person to incorporate foot care into his or her life-style and care practices.

A. EXPLANATION

1. Explain benefits of carrying out the treatment program. This includes the patient being better able to recognize problems early when treatment can be most effective or to care for those problems at home as he or she is able.
2. Outline risk factors that put the patient at greater risk for foot problems and specific steps that the patient can take to reduce the risks.
3. Explain each step to take as demonstrated to the patients.

B. EXPERIENCE

1. Remove shoes and socks. The instructor should also remove shoes to demonstrate procedures.
2. Inspect shoes for proper fit. Shoes that allow for ½- to ¾-inch of toe room are generally best. Shoes should be fitted by a competent salesperson. For best results, buy shoes in the middle of the day, after feet have become somewhat swollen, but not as much as by the end of the day. Patients with loss of sensation caused by neuropathy can draw an outline of their feet on heavy paper and put that into the shoe as a test for fit.
3. Shoes should be made of natural fibers, either leather or canvas, that allow feet to breathe. Avoid thongs and plastic shoes. Use common sense about sandals and bare feet.
4. Feel inside shoes for foreign objects, wrinkled insoles, or breaks in the shoes that can cause lesions. Shake shoes out before putting them on each time.
5. Look at your socks. Socks should be made of natural fibers (wool or as much cotton as you can buy are best as these allow the feet to breathe). Socks do not have to be white.

*Modified from King PA and others: *Diabetes foot care project,* Ann Arbor, 1990, University of Michigan Diabetes Foot Care Project.

340

6. Socks should fit well and be free of darns or holes.

7. For women, stockings should also fit well and not decrease circulation. Knee-high stocking with a wider elastic band usually will decrease blood flow less than a narrow band. Avoid tight-fitting garters and rubber bands to hold up stockings.

8. Inspect feet. First look at the tops of the feet. Be sure to look at both feet every day. Is the skin dry or damp? If dry, use a lotion that does not contain alcohol. If damp, use talcum powder. Show samples of lotions and powders that are appropriate. Avoid soaking the feet as this can lead to dryness.

9. Look for areas of redness caused by shoes and corns, callouses, or lesions. If shoes are causing red areas, they do not fit correctly and may need to be replaced.

10. Corns should be treated by padding the area. Show samples of products that are widely available. Corns can also be débrided slowly with a pumice stone or similar deviced. Show examples. Avoid cutting the corn with a razor blade or other device. Avoid using caustic products to remove corns, since these can burn the skin.

11. Calluses can be débrided each day using a pumice stone or similar device. Show examples. Pumice stones should be used daily to gently rub the area. Avoid rubbing hard and damaging skin. After a bath, while feet are damp, is a good time to débride areas.

12. Look for any area of cracking or fissures in the skin. These can easily become infected. These are often caused by dry skin and can be treated with lotion.

13. Bunions can be padded to increase comfort. Demonstrate technique and products.

14. Look at the toenails. Nails should be cut to follow the curve of the toe and be even with the end of the toe. Nails that are split and cracked can be treated with oil. Nails should be clean. Nails that have fungal infections can be treated by a podiatrist.

15. Look at the bottoms of both feet. If you can't see the bottoms of your feet, use a full-length mirror on the wall or a mirror that you can place on the floor. Pass around a mirror, so that participants can look at their feet. This should also be done each day, looking for areas that have callouses, corns, or ulcers. Ulcers should be treated promptly.

10 Special Issues in Diabetes Management

Neil H. White and Douglas N. Henry

In this chapter special issues in the management of diabetes mellitus are reviewed. Many of these issues may affect diabetes and its treatment across the entire life span. Some can affect the control of diabetes at any age and stage of development, regardless of the type of diabetes or its underlying etiology. Other issues might be limited to subjects with one type of diabetes or only at certain times of life. These issues include management of diabetes during severe or persistent metabolic decompensation (diabetic ketoacidosis; hyperosmolar, nonketotic coma syndrome; hypoglycemia; "brittle diabetes") and during intercurrent events (surgery,

---

CHAPTER OBJECTIVES

- Review the management of DKA.
- Review the management of the HNKC.
- Discuss the recognition and the treatment of hypoglycemia.
- Review the role of glucose counterregulation hormones in persons with and without diabetes mellitus.
- Describe the syndrome of hypoglycemia unawareness.
- Define the dawn phenomenon and the Somogyi phenomenon in relation to diabetes management.
- Discuss the management of brittle diabetes.
- Explain Mauriac's syndrome.
- Summarize guidelines for sick day management.
- Contrast standard and intensive insulin therapies.

---

sick days). The inherent and external factors that contribute to ease of establishing diabetic control are also reviewed, along with alternative forms of insulin delivery that may help deal with some of these. The specifics of therapy at different stages of life are discussed in more detail elsewhere in this text.

DIABETIC KETOACIDOSIS

Diabetic ketoacidosis (DKA) is the most serious metabolic disturbance of insulin-dependent, or type I, diabetes mellitus (IDDM).[62,92] DKA is identified in approximately 40% of patients with newly diagnosed IDDM and is responsible for more than 160,000 hospital admissions each year.[58] The highest rates of DKA are found in teenagers and older adults. A precipitating cause can be identified in about 80% of cases of DKA. DKA should always be considered a medical emergency that requires immediate medical attention. The majority of the morbidity and mortality associated with DKA is preventable with appropriate treatment and careful monitoring. Prevention of DKA is a primary goal in the long-term management of IDDM, and many would consider the development of DKA in a person with known diabetes as a treatment failure.

Ketoacidosis is a state of severe metabolic decompensation manifested by the overproduction of ketone bodies and ketoacids resulting in metabolic acidosis.[62,92,104] Diabetic ketoacidosis (DKA) is the occurrence of ketoacidosis secondary to diabetes mellitus. During DKA, disturbances of protein, fat, and carbohydrate metabolism are all present. Although DKA is primarily a state of absolute or relative insulin deficiency, excess of counterregulatory hormones, particularly glucagon, appears to play an important role in the development of DKA (Fig. 10-1). In DKA, elevations of the counter-regulatory hormones (glucagon, catecholamines, cortisol, and growth hormone) antagonize the effects of insulin action. The elevated counterregulatory hormones increase lipolysis and ketogenesis. Inhibition of glucagon release by an infusion of somatostatin markedly slows the development of ketosis and DKA during acute insulin withdrawal from subjects with IDDM.[68] Ketoacidosis is best defined based on the presence of metabolic acidosis secondary to ketosis and not simply hyperglycemia. The hallmark features of DKA are ketosis and ketonuria, metabolic acidosis (low serum bicarbonate), and dehydration. In addition, since elevated counterregulatory hormones, accompanied by insulin deficiency, stimulate glucose production from glycogenolysis and gluconeogenesis, blood glucose is usually elevated (more than 250 mg/dl) in subjects with DKA. The ketosis and met-abolic acidosis result in electrolyte disturbances and vomiting. Hyperglycemia results in an osmotic diuresis, which together with reduced fluid intake and vomiting, results in dehydration.

Ketoacidosis can occur in association with conditions other than diabetes. If a person not known to have diabetes is seen with ketoacidosis without hyperglycemia, other diagnoses need to be considered. These include alcoholic ketoacidosis, starvation, and certain inborn errors of metabolism. However, diabetes is by far the most common cause of ketoacidosis. DKA is almost always associated with hyperglycemia (plasma glucose level higher than 250 mg/dl), although normoglycemia does not rule out DKA.[106] DKA without hyperglycemia can be seen

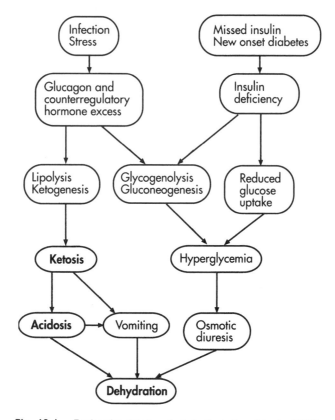

Fig. 10-1   Pathophysiology of diabetic ketoacidosis (DKA).

in pregnancy, partially treated cases, or in those with prolonged vomiting and little carbohydrate intake for many days before presentation.

The diagnosis of DKA should be considered in any person known to have diabetes who is seen with abdominal pain, vomiting, dehydration, rapid or deep breathing (Kussmaul breathing), or altered mental status. It should also be considered in any child with new onset of these symptoms, especially if classic diabetes symptoms (polyuria, polydipsia, nocturia, weight loss) have been present. DKA can be confused with many other medical conditions, including gastroenteritis, urinary tract infection or pyelonephritis, appendicitis, and pneumonitis. Precipitating factors in the development of DKA include the new diagnosis of IDDM, deliberate or inadvertent omission of insulin, infection (e.g., pneumonia, gastroenteritis, influenza, otitis media, meningitis, appendicitis), pancreatitis, trauma, psychologic and emotional stresses (especially in adolescents), and myocardial infarction or stroke in older persons. A search for precipitating factors should be initiated.

The classic signs and symptoms of DKA include polyuria, polydipsia, hyperventilation, and dehydration. Dehydration is usually apparent as dry mucus membranes, absent tearing, poor skin turgor, acute weight loss, and poor perfusion. A fruity odor to the breath, the result of exhaled ketone bodies, can often be detected. Abdominal pain, which can be severe enough to suggest an acute surgical abdomen, as well as tenderness to palpation, diminished or absent bowel sounds, and guarding, can be seen as a result of DKA alone. However, a surgical consultation may be indicated in some cases if appendicitis, bowel perforation, or infarction is suspected. Extreme thirst, tachycardia, nausea, vomiting, hypotension, weakness, anorexia, dehydration, warm, dry skin, visual disturbances, hyperventilation, somnolence, hypothermia, hyporeflexia, and impaired consciousness can all be present in DKA.

The common laboratory findings in DKA include metabolic acidosis, ketonemia and ketouria, elevated anion gap from ketoacids and lactate, hyperglycemia, leukocytosis, hyponatremia, hypophosphatemia, and, in some cases, hyperosmolarity and elevated amylase. Serum potassium can be high, low, or normal. In mild cases of DKA or simple ketosis, the serum bicarbonate and pH may be normal or only slightly reduced. In severe cases, arterial pH is usually less than 7.2, plasma bicarbonate is less than 15 mEq/L, and ketones are present in both blood and urine. Shock or coma can be present, although these are uncommon in children and in otherwise healthy young adults with uncomplicated diabetes. Although the blood glucose concentration is usually significantly elevated, a blood glucose level below 300 mg/dl (16.6 mM) and even one within the normal range does not exclude DKA.[106] In the presence of hyperglycemia, marked apparent hyponatremia can be seen; the serum sodium will be decreased by 1.6 mEq/L for each 100 mg/dl glucose increase above a plasma glucose concentration of 100 mg/dl. Serum potassium can be normal, elevated, or decreased. Regardless of the serum potassium, however, total body potassium depletion is nearly always present as a result of urinary and/or gastrointestinal losses. An elevation of the peripheral white blood cell count is often seen in DKA and is an unreliable indicator of infection. However, the white blood cell count normalizes quickly with treatment, and persistent elevations may indicate underlying infection. Underlying infection should be considered in any patient with DKA of unidentified etiology. An ECG should be performed in all adult patients to rule out myocardial infarction. The ECG can also be used as a rapid assessment of a critically low or high potassium. Hypokalemia results in flattened or inverted T waves, a depressed ST segment, a prolonged QT interval, and the presence of U waves. Hyperkalemia results in peaked T waves, a widened QRS interval, depressed P waves, or AV dissociation.

When the individual is brought to a hospital or clinic with known or suspected DKA, he or she should be considered a critically ill patient until proved otherwise. Sufficient support services must be available to deal with the patient's needs. Monitoring of vital signs, blood gas analysis, bedside blood glucose monitoring, skilled nursing care, and serum electrolyte analysis must all be readily and rapidly available. If adequate support is not available, the patient should be transferred as soon as possible to a facility where these services are available. Mild cases of DKA can sometimes be managed at home or with only very short stays in the emergency room setting (see "Sick Day Management" for discussion of managing mild DKA). In cases of severe DKA, hospitalization is necessary and access to a medical or pediatric intensive care unit is advisable.

Goals of Treatment

The general goals in the treatment of DKA are the following: (1) to correct the fluid and electrolyte imbalance, (2) to correct the metabolic acidosis, (3) to provide adequate insulin to prevent ketosis and lower plasma glucose, and (4) to prevent and monitor for complications of treatment. Initial therapy of severe DKA should be directed at correction of life-threatening abnormalities and stabilization of the patient. Adequate ventilation should be established, if necessary. Shock should be corrected with vigorous fluid resuscitation. Comatose patients should have nasogastric (NG) drainage to prevent aspiration. Intravenous access should be established as soon as possible and laboratory studies sent to confirm the diagnosis and the severity of the condition. A medical history, physical examination, and additional laboratory studies should be performed, as necessary, to rule out any precipitating causes and other underlying medical conditions. After initial stabilization and evaluation, the mainstays in the therapy of DKA are correction of dehydration and interruption of the metabolic imbalance (ketosis, acidosis, and hyperglycemia). The former is accomplished with intravenous fluid therapy; the latter is accomplished with insulin administration.

Basic Management Protocols

Insulin hormone replacement, fluid therapy, correction of electrolytes, and treatment of any underlying disorders will direct initial therapy.[98] A comprehensive flow sheet should be kept to follow intake and output, weight, fluids, insulin, ketones, and electrolytes. Patients with hyperglycemia and simple ketosis who are alert and not vomiting can often be rehydrated orally. Intravenous hydration is required in patients with vomiting, inability to drink, or severe acidosis. Good intravenous (IV) access with a relatively large catheter should be established. Initially, volume expansion should be given as 10 to 20 ml/kg of isotonic (0.9%) saline over 30 to 60 minutes. Subsequently, maintenance requirements, ongoing excessive fluid losses (vomiting, osmotic diuresis), and replacement of dehydration need to be considered in fluid therapy. If fluid deficits are not known, an estimated fluid deficit of 10% or greater should be assumed. Maintenance fluid needs can be calculated at 1500 to 2000 ml/M^2 per day or higher if fever is present. Ongoing losses can be minimized by keeping blood glucose below or near renal threshold (150 to 200 mg/dl). After the initial volume expansion, fluid replacement can usually be accomplished using 0.45% saline. If severe hyponatremia (serum sodium below what can be accounted for by hyperglycemia), extreme hyperosmolarity (serum sodium normal despite marked hyperglycemia), hypotension, or shock is present, it may be appropriate to continue hydration with 0.9% saline. It is essential to accurately monitor intake and output. Bladder catheterization may be indicated in very severe cases, especially if documentation of urine output is difficult and hydration status uncertain.

Potassium replacement

In nearly all cases of DKA, total body potassium depletion exists despite a normal or even elevated serum potassium level. Potassium depletion occurs secondary to urinary loss from polyuria, acidosis, catabolic state, and vomiting or diarrhea. Correction of potassium depletion requires cautious and timely intervention. Potassium replacement should begin immediately after the initial fluid bolus unless renal failure is suspected. If serum potassium is so low as to endanger the patient (generally serum potassium less than 2.5 mEq/L or ECG changes suggestive of hypokalemia), potassium should be started sooner. If renal failure (acute or chronic) is suspected and potassium is high (more than 5.5 mEq/L), potassium administration should be delayed until the serum potassium begins to fall. The potassium maintenance and replacement should be added to the IV fluid. Generally, the potassium concentration in the IV fluid is 30 to 40 mEq/L or 0.1 to 0.5 mEq/kg/hr. Potassium salts can be added as potassium chloride, potassium acetate, and/or potassium phosphate.

Phosphate replacement

Serum phosphate should be measured and if low, phosphate should be given. Some physicians routinely use some potassium phosphate in therapy. Without the use of any phosphate during the therapy of DKA, hypophosphatemia is common, although the clinical significance of this is unknown.[87,162] Administration of potassium phosphate should not exceed 1.5 mEq/kg/24 hours because of the danger of hypocalcemia. The exclusive use of potassium chloride can result in a hyperchloremic acidosis, especially in children, but the clinical significance of this is also unknown. Serum potassium levels should be monitored closely (at least every 2 hours) until stable, and then every 4 to 6 hours while intravenous fluid and insulin therapy continue. The rate of potassium administration can be adjusted accordingly, as necessary, based on the serum potassium concentrations. ECG monitoring can also serve as a guide to potassium status (see earlier discussion).

Insulin

All patients with DKA have an absolute or relative insulin deficiency.[62,92,104] Therefore exogenous insulin must be provided. Insulin suppresses ketone body and ketoacid formation and interrupts the production of excess acid and acidosis. Insulin also will reverse the catabolic state of protein breakdown and lipolysis. Once lipolysis, proteolysis, and ketogenesis are halted, IV fluids and rehydration will remove ketone bodies and ketoacids from the circulation and correct the acidosis. Insulin will lower blood glucose by inhibiting glycogenolysis and gluconeogenesis and stimulating glucose uptake and oxidation.

Insulin can be administered by different routes during the treatment of DKA. The choice of the route of insulin administration depends on the clinical picture. In mild DKA, especially that in which intravenous fluids may not be necessary, subcutaneous insulin can certainly be used (see "Sick Day Management" in this chapter for discussion of managing mild DKA). Preferably, these patients will seek medical assistance early in the course of their illness before severe DKA is present. In cases of severe DKA, intravenous insulin is usually the preferred route of administration, although subcutaneous or intramuscular insulin can be used. In cases complicated by shock, only intravenous insulin should be used, since, coupled with poor peripheral perfusion, absorption of insulin given subcutaneously or intramuscularly may be reduced or delayed. Regular (fast-acting) insulin is the primary insulin preparation used in the management of DKA and is the only insulin that should be given intravenously or intramuscularly.

Intravenous insulin therapy for DKA is most commonly given as a continuous low-dose insulin infusion.[56,150] This should begin with a bolus of regular insulin equivalent to 0.1 to 0.15 U/kg (rarely is more than 5 to 7 U necessary), followed by an infusion of regular insulin at 0.1 U/kg/hr (rarely is more than 5 to 7 U/hr necessary). Insulin should be mixed in normal saline, and the IV tubing should be flushed with about 50 ml of insulin solution to saturate binding sites on the IV tubing before administration. Failure to do this could result in diminished insulin delivery over the first few hours. The insulin infusion can be "piggy-backed" into the existing IV line and should be controlled by a pump. After initiation of IV insulin therapy, if no improvement in blood pH, anion gap, bicarbonate, or plasma glucose is seen in 2 to 3 hours, the insulin infusion rate can be doubled. If these measures fail to improve acidosis, other underlying problems should be considered, such as sepsis, meningitis, myocardial infarction, or pneumonia, and a diabetologist should be consulted.

Often the blood glucose will normalize more quickly than acidosis. After the initial volume expansion phase, adequate insulin administration should decrease the blood glucose concentration by about 1 to 2 mg/dl/min (60 to 120 mg/dl/hr). Attempts should be made to stabilize the plasma glucose near the renal threshold, that is, in the range of 150 to 200 mg/dl. This will minimize urinary fluid losses from osmotic diuresis and avoid the occurrence of hypoglycemia, which would trigger a counterregulatory hormone response. Therefore when blood glucose approaches 250 mg/dl, 5% dextrose should be added to the IV fluid. A 5% dextrose solution at the rate commonly used for rehydration in DKA delivers 3 to 5 mg/kg/min of dextrose. If this fails to stabilize the glucose, higher concentrations of dextrose infusion can be used or the insulin infusion rate can be reduced. However, the insulin infusion rate should not be reduced if acidosis is not correcting, and it should not be reduced to below 0.05 U/kg/hr. In general, IV insulin should be continued until the patient can take oral fluids well, electrolyte abnormalities are correcting, serum bicarbonate is greater than 15 mEq/L, and acidosis has resolved. Because of the short half-life of IV insulin (about 7 to 10 minutes), IV insulin infusion should not be discontinued until approximately 30 minutes after subcutaneous insulin has been given to allow time for subcutaneous insulin to start to work. In patients known to have IDDM, the usual insulin dose can be resumed. In patients with new onset of IDDM, subcutaneous insulin should be started as discussed elsewhere.

Following patients with DKA requires careful attention to every detail. Clinical status, including neurologic condition, should be assessed frequently (at least every 1 to 2 hours) for at least the first 6 to 12 hours. An accurate record of intake and output should be maintained, and blood glucose should be monitored hourly using bedside monitoring techniques. Serum electrolytes should be monitored at least every 2 to 6 hours, with serum potassium, bicarbonate, and pH monitored more frequently in severe cases. Unexpected changes in clinical status, mental status, or laboratory results should be promptly investigated and the therapy should be changed appropriately. The vast majority of subjects with DKA do quite well, unless the problem is complicated by a significant underlying medical or surgical condition. Most uncomplicated cases of DKA that do poorly are a result of a lack of appropriate evaluation, monitoring, and attention.

Complications of Treatment

Complications associated with the treatment of DKA include hypoglycemia, aspiration, fluid overload with congestive heart failure, and cerebral edema. The first three of these can usually be avoided by careful attention to all aspects of the therapy. Cerebral edema as a complication of DKA and its treatment occurs primarily in children.[91,121] Its cause is unclear but it may relate to too rapid correction of osmolality, acidosis, and/or hyperglycemia. Too rapid a rate of hydration should be avoided. Bolus doses of bicarbonate should be avoided, and when bicarbonate is used, it should be done only with great caution. A bicarbonate infusion of 1 to 2 mEq/kg over 2 hours can be given if the arterial pH is less than 7.0 to 7.1. This should rarely be continued beyond the first 2 to 3 hours. The benefits of bicarbonate infusion are not proven. Unexpected alteration in mental state or the development of neurologic signs, bradycardia, or hypertension could indicate developing cerebral edema. Although the incidence of clinically significant cerebral edema is low (probably about 1%), the outcome after its development is poor. Cerebral edema remains a leading cause of death in diabetic children, accounting for about 31% of deaths associated with DKA and 20% of the overall mortality in children with diabetes. Therefore cerebral edema warrants prompt and aggressive treatment with IV mannitol (0.5 to 1.0 g/kg), hyperventilation, and perhaps dexamethasone.

HYPEROSMOLAR NONKETOTIC COMA SYNDROME

Hyperosmolar nonketotic coma syndrome (HNKC) is the most common severe metabolic derangement in non-insulin-dependent type II diabetes mellitus. As is the case with DKA, HNKC is usually a life-threatening medical emergency with a high mortality rate. The mortality rate for HNKC is higher than that for DKA, primarily because these patients are older and frequently have significant other medical problems that either precipitate or are precipitated by HNKC. Factors associated with HNKC are shown in Table 10-1. Approximately half of those who are seen with HNKC are known to have type II diabetes, whereas the other half are newly diagnosed when they present with HNKC.

Table 10-1   Factors Associated with Hyperosmolar Nonketotic Coma Syndrome

Therapeutic agents	Therapeutic procedures	Chronic illness	Acute illness
Glucocorticoids	Peritoneal dialysis	Renal disease	Infection
Diuretics	Hemodialysis	Heart disease	Gangrene
Diphenylhydantoin	Hyperosmolar alimentation	Hypertension	Urinary tract infection
β-adrenergic blocking agents	Surgical stress	Previous stroke	Burns
L-asparaginase		Alcoholism	GI bleeding
Immunosuppressive agents		Psychiatric	Myocardial infarction
Chlorpromazine		Loss of thirst	Pancreatitis
Diazoxide			Stroke

Modified from *Physician's guide to non–insulin-dependent (type II) diabetes: diagnosis and treatment,* Alexandria, Va, 1988, American Diabetes Association, Inc.

Signs and Symptoms

Persons with HNKC present with markedly elevated blood glucose, extreme hyperosmolality, and severe dehydration without significant ketosis and often with minimal acidosis. They often present with neurologic manifestations such as severe obtundation, seizure, coma, or focal neurologic findings suggestive of a stroke. Plasma glucose is over 600 mg/dl and is usually between 1000 and 2000 mg/dl. Marked hyperosmolality is present with serum osmolality in excess of 340 mOsm/l of water and BUN over 60. Dehydration is usually 10% to 15%. Serum and urine ketones are absent or only slight.

Treatment

The general principles for the management of HNKC are similar to those for DKA: (1) to correct the fluid and electrolyte imbalance, (2) to provide adequate insulin to lower plasma glucose, (3) to prevent and monitor for complications of treatment, and (4) to treat any underlying medical conditions. Initial therapy of HNKC should be directed at correcting life-threatening abnormalities and stabilizing the patient. Adequate ventilation should be established if necessary. Shock should be corrected with vigorous fluid resuscitation. Comatose patients should have NG drainage to prevent aspiration. Intravenous access should be established as soon as possible and laboratory studies sent to confirm the diagnosis and the severity of the condition. A medical history, physical examination, and additional laboratory studies should be performed as necessary to rule out any precipitating causes and underlying other medical conditions. After initial stabilization and evaluation, the mainstays in the therapy of HNKC are correction of dehydration and interruption of the metabolic imbalance (hyperglycemia). The former is accomplished with intravenous fluid therapy, the latter with insulin administration.

After the initial volume expansion phase using isotonic saline, additional isotonic saline or colloid-containing solutions are used only if the patient is hypotensive or in shock. Subsequently, rehydration is usually accomplished using 0.45% saline with appropriate addition of potassium, phosphate, and other anions. Large amounts of potassium supplementation with ECG monitoring are usually necessary. Careful and frequent (at least every 1 to 2 hours) assessment of fluid and electrolyte status is essential, especially if acute or chronic renal failure complicates the course. Close monitoring of vital signs and neurologic status is also indicated. Therapy and monitoring should always be done in an ICU setting.

Although there have been reports of successful treatment of HNKC without insulin, insulin administration is certainly recommended as part of its therapy. The insulin regimen used is similar to that used in DKA (0.1 U regular insulin/kg/hr), except that the insulin can be stopped when the plasma glucose nears 200 to 250 mg/dl; there is no need to continue insulin therapy to interrupt ketosis and prevent recurrent acidosis. Because of the severe dehydration and marked volume depletion associated with HNKC, plasma glucose may fall rapidly even without insulin administration. Although cerebral edema is much less common in adults with HNKC than in children with DKA, it is probably advisable to limit the decline of plasma glucose to 1 to 2 mg/dl/min.

Identification and treatment of underlying illnesses or intercurrent events during the management of HNKC should be aggressive. Even though cerebral edema is less common than in DKA, the mortality associated with HNKC is greater and is probably in the range of 10% to 40%.

RECOGNITION AND TREATMENT OF HYPOGLYCEMIA

Hypoglycemia is a common feature of insulin-treated diabetes mellitus and can also be seen in subjects treated with oral agents. Hypoglycemia occurs as a result of an imbalance between the timing or amount of insulin in the circulation, physical activity, and exogenous availability of carbohydrate. Consumption of ethanol can also precipitate hypoglycemia. The signs and symptoms of hypoglycemia and the plasma glucose level at which they are noted will vary from person to person, but the hypoglycemic symptoms and signs are generally divided into two major categories: neurogenic (often also referred to as *adrenergic* or *autonomic*)[161a] and neuroglycopenic (Table 10-2).

The neurogenic symptoms and signs of hypoglycemia are those associated with triggering of the autonomic nervous system and the release of epinephrine and/or acetylcholine from autonomic neurons, or epinephrine from the adrenal medulla. These include shakiness, diaphoresis, irritability, nervousness, tachycardia, headache, hunger, and tremulousness. Paresthesias and pallor can also occur. These symptoms are usually present when the circulating plasma epinephrine concentration is above approximately 150 pg/ml.[35] Increments in plasma epinephrine to this level occur not only during hypoglycemia, but also during rapid decrements in blood glucose concentration from a hyperglycemic (200 mg/dl or 11.1 mM) to a nonhypoglycemic (100 mg/dl or 5.6 mM) level.[123] This occurs in the experimental setting and probably also occurs as a clinical event in some poorly controlled diabetic subjects with persistent hyperglycemia who report experiencing neurogenic symptoms of hypoglycemia even when blood glucose is not low.[29,133] Neurogenic symptoms can also occur during other stressful or anxiety-provoking events.

The neuroglycopenic signs of hypoglycemia are those associated with lack of glucose availability to the brain and the resultant cerebral dysfunction. The neuroglycopenic

Table 10-2   Symptoms and Signs of Hypoglycemia

Neurogenic	Neuroglycopenic
Shakiness	Headache
Irritability	Mental dullness
Nervousness	Inability to concentrate
Tachycardia/palpitations	Slurred speech
Tremor	Blurred vision
Hunger	Confusion
Diaphoresis	Irrational behavior
Pallor	Amnesia
Paresthesias	Severe lethargy
	Loss of consciousness
	Seizure
	Coma
	Death

manifestations of hypoglycemia include headache, inability to concentrate, slurred speech, blurred vision, confusion or irrational behavior, severe lethargy, seizure, coma, and rarely, death. Occasionally, transient focal neurologic findings can be seen in association with severe hypoglycemia.[149] Lesser degrees of neuroglycopenia can occur in the form of altered cognitive functioning,[17,50,80,116] as measured by increased reaction time and response time,[17] and increased latency of the P300 wave on auditory[50] or visual[17] evoked response testing. Neuroglycopenia occurs as a result of low plasma glucose concentration and diminished availability of glucose to the central nervous system and is rarely, if ever, observed during falling plasma glucose that is still within or above the normal range. Recognizable neuroglycopenia rarely occurs until the glucose concentrations is below about 45 mg/dl (2.5 mM).[29,133] However, subtle alterations in cerebral function (increased reaction time and P300 waves) can be documented in persons with diabetes with glucose levels only as low as about 60 mg/dl (2.2 mM)[17,50] and even at higher values in children or persons with poorly controlled diabetes. The ability to safely operate a motor vehicle is also impaired at glucose levels above those usually associated with neuroglycopenic symptoms.[36a]

Clinically, hypoglycemia in persons with diabetes is usually divided into mild and severe. Mild hypoglycemia is recognized and appropriately treated by the individual. The symptoms of mild hypoglycemia are usually primarily neurogenic (shaky, sweaty, hungry, tachycardia or palpitations, nervousness). The treatment of mild hypoglycemia should be with the oral ingestion of rapidly absorbed carbohydrate, either in the form of food or drink, or as glucose from one of the many commercially available sources to treat hypoglycemia (glucose tablets, Monojel, and others). The use of these preparations is convenient but not essential, because carbohydrate intake in the form of juice, milk, crackers, or hard candies is equally effective if taken in the appropriate quantity. Usually, 5 to 15 g of carbohydrate are adequate to treat mild hypoglycemia. This carbohydrate can be obtained from one to three glucose tablets, three to eight Life Savers candies, or 2 to 6 ounces of juice (see Chapter 4).

Severe hypoglycemia results in the inability of the subject to recognize the symptoms or treat himself or herself. Severe hypoglycemia usually appears with neuroglycopenic signs and can result in loss of consciousness, seizure, or coma. Severe hypoglycemia can occur as a complication of treatment in any subject treated with insulin or oral hypoglycemic agents but, fortunately, is uncommon according to most reports. Data in the literature suggest that severe hypoglycemia occurs in between 6.5% and 26% of adults with IDDM and between 4% and 9.8% of children.[12,72,105] The definition and documentation of severe hypoglycemia vary from study to study, and ascertainment bias is likely; therefore these estimates vary considerably and may be inaccurate. The frequency of severe hypoglycemia appears to be higher in those suffering from hypoglycemia unawareness, defective glucose counterregulation, or autonomic neuropathy, as well as in those using intensive insulin therapy (see appropriate sections that follow).

During severe hypoglycemia, the individual is unable to treat himself or herself. This can be the result of lack of recognition of symptoms, confusion, or inability to treat. Therefore treatment must be implemented by an outside party. If the individual is alert and awake, ingestion of oral carbohydrate (10 to 15 g) should be used. If the person will not allow oral carbohydrate to be used or is not fully alert and conscious (convulsing, postictal, unarousable, comatose), treatment should consist of either intravenous glucose or intramuscular or subcutaneous glucagon. Glucose should be given intravenously (either as 50% dextrose or 25% dextrose) if the setting allows, since this is the most rapid way to raise the blood glucose concentration. The usually recommended dose is 10 to 25 g of dextrose given over 1 to 2 minutes, followed by an infusion of a 5% dextrose solution at 5 to 10 g per hour (3 to 5 mg/kg/min in children). If intravenous dextrose is not immediately available for administration and the patient is unable to safely ingest oral carbohydrate, an injection of glucagon (1 mg for adults and children over 30 kg; 0.5 mg for children below 30 kg) should be given. Even though glucagon is effective in the majority of subjects, it is usually advisable to seek medical assistance after its administration in case hypoglycemia recurs (the effect of glucagon is relatively transient), vomiting occurs preventing oral intake of carbohydrate (vomiting is common after glucagon), or the subject's mental status does not improve. After glucagon administration, the patient should ingest oral carbohydrate or a meal to ensure that the blood glucose does not once again fall to the hypoglycemic range. After resolution of a severe hypoglycemic event, the patient and health care team should try to identify the cause and the patient should be educated about prevention.

Clinical hypoglycemia can occur at any time of day or night but seems to occur most commonly during exercise, 8 to 24 hours after strenuous exercise (late postexercise hypoglycemia),[100] and in the middle of the night (see later discussions of the dawn phenomenon and Somogyi phenomenon). Nocturnal hypoglycemia[78,96,135] has been reported to occur in 7% to 56% of adults with IDDM and in 10% to 26% of children. Reported percentages vary depending on the definition and the methods of ascertainment. Late postexercise hypoglycemia[100] refers to the occurrence of clinically significant, and sometimes severe, hypoglycemia 8 to 24 hours after strenuous exercise; usually this occurs overnight or early the following morning. The pathophysiology of late postexercise hypoglycemia is poorly understood. It does not occur in all subjects with diabetes, but it does represent a significant problem for some. Late postexercise hypoglycemia is best managed by monitoring blood glucose more frequently after strenuous exercise and using extra carbohydrate-containing snacks if the blood glucose is falling rapidly or falls to below the target range (see Chapter 5).

THE GLUCOSE COUNTERREGULATORY HORMONES

Insulin is the primary hormone resulting in lowering of blood glucose. However, there is a redundancy of the hormonal mechanisms for raising blood glucose.[37,39] The hormones that work to raise the blood glucose are generally referred to as the *glucose counterregulatory hormones*. Redundancy in the glucose counterregulatory hormone system seems appropriate because of the potential significant dangers associated with even brief periods of hypoglycemia. The central nervous system is the largest consumer of glucose. The brain utilizes glucose as its primary fuel, rarely using other substrates. Even brief periods of hypoglycemia can cause cerebral dysfunction,[17,50,80] brain damage, or death.

The glucose counterregulatory hormones include glucagon, catecholamines (epinephrine and norepinephrine), cortisol, and growth hormone. These hormones play an important role in regulating carbohydrate metabolism in subjects with, as well as those without, diabetes mellitus.[37,39] These hormones increase in the circulation during hypoglycemia and exercise and play an important role in bringing the blood glucose up to normal after hypoglycemia and preventing the occurrence of hypoglycemia during fasting and exercise.

Glucagon

Glucagon is a polypeptide hormone of molecular weight 3500 kD. It is synthesized in the α-cells of the pancreatic islets and is secreted into the portal venous circulation where it circulates directly to the liver. Glucagon acts on plasma membrane receptors of hepatic parenchymal cells to activate a G protein–dependent process resulting in stimulation of glycogenolysis, gluconeogenesis, and ketogenesis. The actions of glucagon are relatively transient, and it is thought that changes (increases) in glucagon concentration and the glucagon-to-insulin ratio in the portal vein may be more important determinants of its action than the absolute glucagon concentration. In nondiabetic individuals, plasma glucagon concentration increases in response to hypoglycemia or stress. However, subjects with type I diabetes mellitus develop α-cell dysfunction starting during the first few years of diabetes.[13,20] This α-cell dysfunction results in a failure of glucagon to be released in response to hypoglycemia or a rapidly falling glucose level despite normal or perhaps even an exaggerated glucagon response to stress and other stimuli. The etiology of this α-cell dysfunction is poorly understood. However, after the first few years of diabetes, it is clear that increments in endogenously released circulating glucagon play little, if any, role in hypoglycemic counterregulation, despite its important role in stress-induced hyperglycemia and ketosis.

Epinephrine

Epinephrine (also known as *adrenaline*) is synthesized in the adrenal medulla and norepinephrine in the preganglionic sympathetic and parasympathetic neurons. Together, epinephrine and norepinephrine are referred to as *catecholamines*. The catecholamines act on the α- and β-adrenergic receptors to cause peripheral vasoconstriction, tachycardia, and the typical neurogenic (adrenergic) symptoms of irritability, shakiness, tremor, hunger, and diaphoresis. It should be noted that, although diaphoresis is usually categorized as adrenergic, it is mediated by stimulation of cholinergic nerve fibers in the skin. In addition to producing these well-known adrenergic symptoms, the catecholamines serve as glucose counterregulatory hormones. By activation of β-adrenergic receptors, epinephrine and norepinephrine stimulate gluconeogenesis and lipolysis from muscle and perhaps liver resulting in an increase in glucose production and a rising blood glucose concentration.[49,115] Epinephrine also inhibits the release and action of insulin. This latter effect contributes to its glucose counterregulatory potential in diabetes. The catecholamines are released in both diabetic and nondiabetic individuals in response to stress, exercise, or hypoglycemia. However, some persons with diabetes develop a diminished or absent release of epinephrine in response to hypoglycemia or falling blood sugar. This blunted epinephrine response can be seen in subjects with neuropathy[81] and in those with the syndromes of defective glucose counterregulation,[20,40,128,158] hypoglycemia unawareness,[84] and hypoglycemia-associated autonomic failure (HAAF).[37a,40a]

Cortisol

Cortisol is the major steroid, glucocorticoid hormone of the human. Cortisol is synthesized in the adrenal cortex via a series of enzymatic reactions starting from the precursor cholesterol. Cortisol is released into the circulation in a diurnal pattern, with cortisol release and circulating cortisol concentration increasing during the early morning hours and in response to stress or hypoglycemia. Although cortisol acts as a glucose counterregulatory hormone, its effects are primarily long-term in the form of causing some resistance to insulin action. Although subjects with cortisol deficiency (Addison's disease, congenital adrenal hyperplasia, hypopituitarism, adrenalectomy) can be seen with hypoglycemia, cortisol seems to have little effect on raising blood glucose concentration quickly after insulin-induced hypoglycemia.[37]

Growth Hormone

Growth hormone is a 22,000 kD molecular weight polypeptide hormone produced and secreted by the anterior pituitary gland. Growth hormone exerts its effects on growth through modulation of growth factors, primarily insulin-like growth factor-1/ somatomedin-C (IGF-1). Growth hormone also exerts effects on carbohydrate metabolism that are not mediated through IGF-1. The effect of growth hormone on carbohydrate metabolism appears to be biphasic.[101] The initial response, which occurs within 1 to 2 hours after growth hormone administration or increments in endogenous growth hormone, is insulin-like; hepatic glucose production is diminished, and blood glucose concentration falls. This effect is short-lived, and after about 4 hours, growth hormone blunts insulin-mediated glucose uptake and oxidation. As with cortisol, growth hormone increases in response to hypoglycemia but probably has little effect on fluctuations in blood sugar over short periods.[37] Growth hormone is likely to play a role in the diurnal variation of blood glucose (see discussion of dawn phenomenon on p. 363).

Regulation of blood glucose within the narrow normal range depends on the rapid modulation of insulin and the counterregulatory hormones (glucagon, catecholamines, cortisol, growth hormone). In the nondiabetic individual, the fluctuations of these hormones are closely timed so that blood glucose remains in the narrow range of about 70 to 140 mg/dl (3.9 to 7.8 mM). Individuals with overproduction of insulin (hyperinsulinism) or underproduction of counterregulatory hormones (adrenalectomy, autonomic dysfunction, Addison's disease, hypopituitarism) can experience hypoglycemia as a manifestation of their disorder. Persons with diabetes have poorly timed insulin action either as a result of exogenous absorption (as in IDDM) or inappropriate secretion/action (as in NIDDM). This loss of glucose regulation by insulin makes glucose counterregulation by the counterregulatory hormones even more critical in maintaining a stable blood glucose.

GLUCOSE COUNTERREGULATION IN NONDIABETIC PERSONS

The works of Cryer and colleagues,[37,39] Gerich and associates,[20,49] and other investigators have clearly shown redundancy of the glucose counterregulatory mechanisms, with a hierarchical effect of the various hormones. Maintenance of euglycemia during fasting (in adults), exercise, and recovery from insulin-induced hypoglycemia all follow a similar pattern. Dissipation of insulin is a primary factor in preventing or recovering from hypoglycemia. Glucagon plays a primary role in the recovery from hypoglycemia. Epinephrine is not essential but can compensate for glucagon and becomes essential in its absence. Cortisol and growth hormone have counterregulatory effects, but these effects are not rapid and are not sufficiently potent to compensate for a diminished or absent glucagon and epinephrine response accompanied by mild hyperinsulinemia. Likewise, other substrate effects and hepatic glucose autoregulation,[24,75] though present, are weak.

In the absence of epinephrine release (such as after bilateral adrenalectomy) or action (such as during continuous α- and β-adrenergic blockade), glucose counterregulation during insulin-induced hypoglycemia occurs normally as a result of glucagon release.[37] In the absence of an incremental glucagon response during insulin-induced hypoglycemia, glucose counterregulation is essentially within normal limits, though slightly delayed. In the absence of a glucagon response and epinephrine secretion or action, glucose counterregulation fails to occur. Therefore epinephrine, though not essential for normal glucose counterregulation in the presence of normal glucagon secretion, becomes critical in the absence of glucagon. The combined effects of other glucose counterregulatory factors (cortisol, growth hormone, hepatic autoregulation) are insufficient to cause significant glucose counterregulation during insulin-induced hypoglycemia in the absence of glucagon and epinephrine secretion or action. These concepts are summarized in Fig. 10-2. In the presence of growth hormone deficiency *(panel C)* or epinephrine deficiency *(panel D)*, the glucose counterregulatory response is normal. Glucagon deficiency alone *(panel B)* and in combination with growth hormone deficiency blunts, but does not eliminate, the counterregulatory response. Combined glucagon and epinephrine deficiency *(panels E and F)* results in the absence of glucose counterregulation.

GLUCOSE COUNTERREGULATION IN PERSONS WITH IDDM

The physiologic and pathophysiologic concepts related to glucose counterregulation noted above are similar for subjects with diabetes mellitus.[39] However, as can be seen in Fig. 10-3, after 4 to 5 years of diabetes, subjects with type I diabetes fail to secrete glucagon in response to hypoglycemia or decrements of blood glucose.[13,20] Subsequently, they would depend on epinephrine as their primary counterregulatory hormone for defense against hypoglycemia. In the absence of an epinephrine response, subjects with diabetes would be essentially defenseless against the occurrence of significant hypoglycemia during even the slight hyperinsulinemia of day-to-day therapy; cortisol and growth hormone increments and hepatic autoregulation are not sufficiently potent to protect against the development of significant hypoglycemia. Individuals with diabetes who develop an absent or blunted epinephrine response to decrements in plasma glucose or absolute hypoglycemia are seen with the

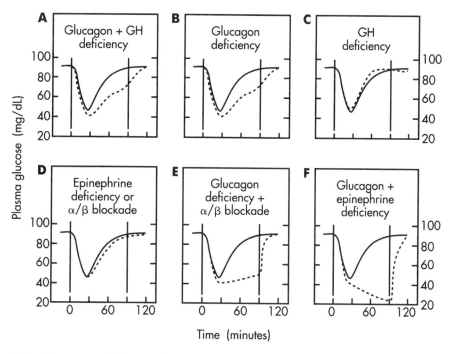

Fig. 10-2 Summary of the experimental evidence leading to the current views about the physiology of glucose counterregulation in a normal human. The plasma glucose following an IV injection of insulin without other intervention is shown in the solid lines, and that following insulin along with the indicated intervention is shown in the broken lines. **A,** Somatostatin infusion (glucagon + growth-hormone deficiency). **B,** Somatostatin infusion with growth-hormone replacement (glucagon deficiency). **C,** Somatostatin infusion with glucagon replacement (growth-hormone deficiency). **D,** Epinephrine deficiency or combined α/β-blockade with intact glucagon response. **E,** Glucagon deficiency and α/β-blockade. **F,** Glucagon and epinephrine deficiency. Note the complete absence of glucose counterregulation in **E** and **F.** (Modified from Cryer PE: *Diabetes* 30:261-264, 1981.)

syndromes referred to as *hypoglycemia unawareness*[84] or *defective glucose counterregula-tion*[39,40,128,158] (see discussion that follows). In such subjects, hypoglycemia often becomes the rate-limiting factor in maintaining good glycemic control.*

MANIFESTATIONS OF NORMAL OR ALTERED GLUCOSE COUNTERREGULATORY SYSTEMS IN DIABETES
Hypoglycemia Unawareness

Hypoglycemia unawareness refers to the syndrome in which persons with diabetes are unaware that they are hypoglycemic and therefore do not initiate treatment. Persons with hypoglycemia unawareness have a blunted epinephrine response to hypoglycemia[84] (Fig.

---

*References 23, 38, 39, 128, 158.

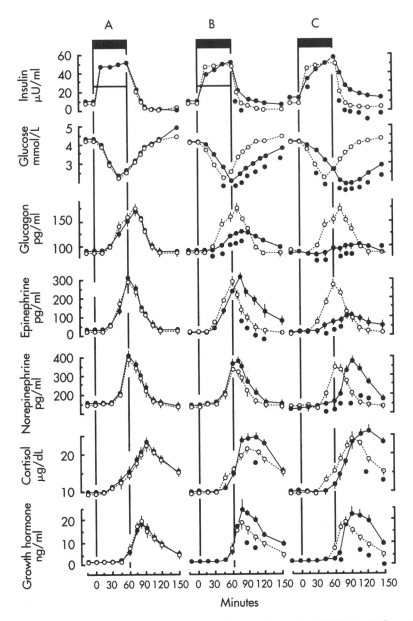

Fig. 10-3 Glucagon responses to insulin-induced hypoglycemia in IDDM. **Left,** Counterregulatory hormone response (mean ± SEM) to insulin-induced hypoglycemia in diabetic subjects *(closed circles/solid lines)* and 10 nondiabetic controls *(open circles/broken lines)*. Insulin infusion was 28 mU/m²/min from 0 to 60 minutes. **A,** IDDM less than 1 month; N = 5. **B,** IDDM 1 to 5 years; N = 11. **C,** IDDM 14 to 31 years; N = 5. **Right,** Correlation between the maximal incremental glucagon response to insulin-induced hypoglycemia and duration of IDDM. (Modified from Bolli G and others: *Diabetes* 32:134-141, 1983.)

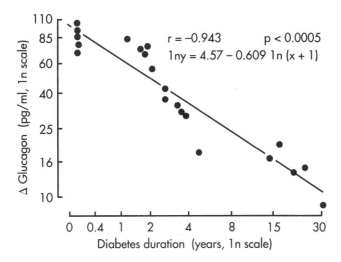

$r = -0.943$ $p < 0.0005$

$\ln y = 4.57 - 0.609 \ln (x + 1)$

Fig. 10-3 cont'd.   (For legend see opposite page.)

10-4, p. 360). Note that subjects with fewer recognizable symptoms of hypoglycemia (low hypoglycemic index) have reduced peak epinephrine response to hypoglycemia. As a result, they tend to lack the neurogenic symptoms of hypoglycemia and often develop neuroglycopenic symptoms and severe hypoglycemia without previous warning. Some subjects have neurogenic signs, which are observed by others but not recognized by the subjects themselves, preceding the development of neuroglycopenia. The etiology of this latter phenomenon is unclear, but individualized reeducation about the symptoms of hypoglycemia may diminish the frequency of severe hypoglycemia in these individuals.

There has been some concern that the use of β-adrenergic blockade medications, such as propranolol and metaprolol, could cause hypoglycemia unawareness and blunt the counterregulatory effects of the catecholamines in diabetic subjects, since neurogenic symptoms of hypoglycemia are primarily mediated via the β-adrenergic receptor.[49,88,115] Therefore many physicians recommend that these drugs not be used in subjects with diabetes unless absolutely necessary. Some consider intensive insulin therapy aimed at normalization of blood glucose to be contraindicated in subjects using β-adrenergic blockade medications.[51] Little in the literature, however, directly addresses this problem, and recent reports suggest that β-adrenergic blockade in individuals with diabetes may not present a significant clinical problem.

Persons with diabetes and hypoglycemia unawareness are more likely to have episodes of severe hypoglycemia.[84] Extensive discussion about the problem and reeducation about hypoglycemia, along with increased monitoring and vigilance, seems to be the best way to minimize severe hypoglycemia. In other persons, symptoms related to hypoglycemia may change (usually diminish) over time, and the patient or family may need guidance in recognizing subtle symptoms of hypoglycemia. In other persons with hypoglycemia unawareness, raising the glycemic target may be necessary to prevent repeated episodes of severe hypoglycemia.

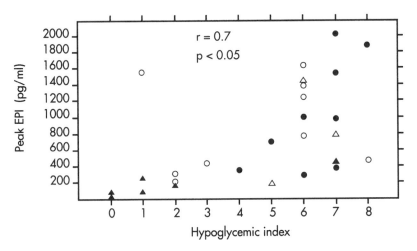

Fig. 10-4 Correlation between peak epinephrine (EPI) concentration during hypoglycemia and hypoglycemia symptom score. *Closed circles,* Healthy controls. *Open circles,* IDDM without autonomic neuropathy. *Closed triangles,* IDDM with autonomic neuropathy and hypoglycemia unawareness. *Open triangles,* IDDM without hypoglycemia unawareness. Note the low peak EPI response in those with hypoglycemia unawareness compared with those without hypoglycemia unawareness. (Modified from Hoeldke RD and others: *Ann Intern Med* 96:459-462, 1982.)

Defective Glucose Counterregulation

As discussed earlier, the rapid defense against insulin-induced hypoglycemia is primarily dependent on glucagon and epinephrine.[37,39] In persons with and without diabetes, cortisol, growth hormone, and hepatic autoregulation[24,75] are insufficiently potent to prevent significant hypoglycemia in the absence of decrements of insulin and increments of glucagon and epinephrine. Despite the fact that most persons with diabetes (after the first few years of diabetes) have a deficient glucagon response to hypoglycemia,[13,20] most have adequate glucose counterregulation because their epinephrine secretory response is normal or perhaps exaggerated. In association with mild overinsulinization, these persons will often maintain a stable plasma glucose in the mild hypoglycemia range for as long as 30 to 60 minutes.[158] This should give adequate time for the recognition of neurogenic symptoms and the treatment of hypoglycemia before it becomes severe.

Some individuals with diabetes, however, lose their incremental epinephrine response (mean peak epinephrine response, 115 pg/ml) to glucose decrements or hypoglycemia as compared with normal controls (mean peak epinephrine, 234 pg/ml) and responsive subjects with IDDM (mean peak epinephrine, 344 pg/ml)[128,158] (Fig. 10-5). This rarely occurs before 10 to 15 years of diabetes[20] and may be associated with the development of autonomic neuropathy. These subjects are said to have defective glucose counterregulation.[158] In subjects with defective glucose counterregulation, combined deficiencies of increments in both glucagon and epinephrine in response to hypoglycemia result in the inability to interrupt a falling plasma glucose during insulin infusion.

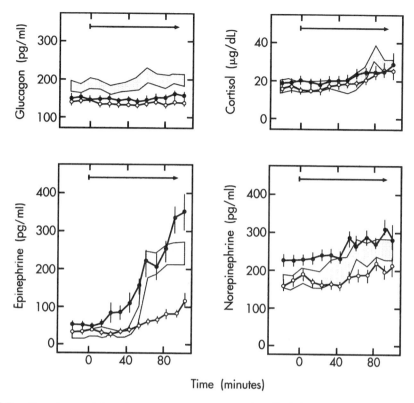

Fig. 10-5   Counterregulatory hormone responses to insulin infusion in controls and IDDM subjects with adequate or defective glucose counterregulation. Plasma glucagon, epinephrine, norepinephrine, and cortisol concentration (mean ± EM) during insulin infusion (40 mU/kg/hr) in 10 normal controls *(stippled area),* 13 IDDM subjects with adequate counterregulation *(closed circles),* and 9 IDDM subjects with defective counterregulation *(open circles).* Note the deficient glucagon response in both diabetic groups and the blunted epinephrine response in those with defective counterregulation. (Modified from White NH and others: *N Engl J Med* 308:485-491, 1983.)

   In addition, since the epinephrine response is blunted, defective glucose counterregulation is often accompanied by hypoglycemia unawareness. Therefore severe hypoglycemia can develop quickly and without warning. Persons with defective glucose counterregulation have a markedly increased risk of developing severe hypoglycemia, especially during the use of intensive insulin therapy, when the risk has been reported to be as high as 25 times that of subjects with adequate glucose counterregulation[23,38,158] (Table 10-3).
   Defective glucose counterregulation can occur in association with autonomic neuropathy,[81] but it can also occur in subjects without other signs or symptoms of peripheral or autonomic neuropathy. However, some investigators feel that defective glucose counterregulation that develops after 10 to 15 years of diabetes is a manifestation of autonomic neuropathy even when no other manifestations of neuropathic involvement are present.[61] This

Table 10-3 Incidence and Event Rate of Severe Hypoglycemia During Intensive Insulin Therapy in Patients With IDDM With Adequate (+CR) and Defective (−CR) Glucose Counterregulation as Determined by an Insulin Infusion Test

		Severe hypoglycemia	
	Number of subjects	Incidence (number of subjects)	Event rate (events/patient/year)
Cohort #1			
Total	22	9	1.2
+CR	13	1	0.1
−CR	9	8	2.5
Cohort #2 (includes Cohort #1)			
Total	37	14	—
+CR	24	2	—
−CR	13	12	—

Cohort #1 modified from White NH and others: *N Engl J Med* 308:485-491, 1983.

speculation is based on the observation that persons with defective glucose counterregulation have no pancreatic polypeptide response to hypoglycemia.* Because the pancreatic polypeptide response to insulin-induced hypoglycemia is generally thought to be a marker for parasympathetic function,[81,99] the epinephrine response, which correlates well with the pancreatic polypeptide response, seems likely to be a marker for sympathetic function.

In addition to occurring spontaneously as an isolated finding or in association with neuropathic complications, a form of defective glucose counterregulation has been reported to occur as a result of improving glycemic control using intensive insulin therapy (IIT).[4,6] In this form of defective glucose counterregulation, the hormonal response to hypoglycemia occurs in the same general pattern as in patients with normal counterregulation (epinephrine, cortisol, and growth hormone all rise). However, the threshold to trigger the counterregulatory hormone response (usually about 60 mg/dl or 3.3 mM) is lowered; neuroglycopenia may precede the appearance of significant neurogenic symptoms. These persons may be at increased risk for severe hypoglycemia during IIT despite having adequate counterregulation when beginning IIT. Improved glycemic control, or the use of IIT , does not normalize the counterregulatory hormone response in diabetic persons with defective glucose counterregulation.[13,21] Persons with defective glucose counterregulation may require similar educational interventions or adjustment of glycemic target to that of those with hypoglycemia unawareness.

Recently, increasing evidence has emerged suggesting a relationship between tight control and the occurrence of both hypoglycemia unawareness and defective glucose counterregulation. Antecedent hypoglycemia, even if asymptomatic, can induce subsequent hypoglycemia unawareness and defective glucose counterregulation.[40a,147a] This phenomenon

*References 61, 81, 99, 151, 152.

has been called *hypoglycemia-associated autonomic failure (HAAF)* by Cryer and his colleagues.[37a,40a] In the words of Cryer, "hypoglycemia begets hypoglycemia."[38b] In other words, tight control, which is associated with an increased rate of hypoglycemia, results in a blunted counterregulatory hormone response and hypoglycemia unawareness and defective glucose counterregulation. This, in turn, results in an increased risk of severe hypoglycemia during attempts at tight control. This phenomenon may partially explain the increased risk of severe hypoglycemia during intensive insulin therapy.[48a,48b,119a]

It has also been shown that meticulous avoidance of hypoglycemia for a 3-month period eliminates the blunted counterregulatory hormone response associated with HAAF.[59a] Minimizing all forms of hypoglycemia must be considered a key element of any diabetes management regimen.

The Dawn Phenomenon

For persons with IDDM, maintenance of good glycemic control presents as much of a problem overnight as at any other time of day. Hypoglycemia occurring between 1 and 4 AM is common,[78,96,135] and hyperglycemia before breakfast is also common. Diurnal variation in the counterregulatory hormones may play a significant role in glucose homeostasis overnight, especially in diabetic subjects. However, a cause-and-effect relationship between nocturnal hypoglycemia and morning hyperglycemia remains controversial. The controversy continues regarding relative importance of the *dawn phenomenon (DP)* and the *Somogyi phenomenon* in the development of morning hyperglycemia.[38] The dawn phenomenon refers to an early-morning (4 AM to 8 AM) rise in blood glucose concentration without antecedent nocturnal hypoglycemia. The Somogyi phenomenon refers to morning hyperglycemia occurring as a result of "rebound" from preceding nocturnal hypoglycemia.

The DP was first observed as early as the 1920s when it was described as a paradoxic rise in blood glucose, sometimes causing morning fasting hyperglycemia. The term *dawn phenomenon* was first used to describe this event by Schmidt and associates[132] in a 1981 paper reporting 24-hour glucose profiles in diabetic subjects. A prebreakfast, dawn-time rise of blood glucose was a common observation. This rise averaged 30 to 50 mg/dl (1.7 to 2.8 mM) between 5 AM and 8 AM before breakfast. The authors attributed this rise to the waning activity of the previous day's insulin, resulting in early morning insulin deficiency.

It soon became apparent, however, that the DP represented more than simply a waning of the previous day's insulin. Insulin deficiency alone appears not to be the sole cause of the rising blood glucose concentration during the dawn period. Even during continuous insulin infusions, blood glucose tended to rise during the dawn period. This was seen in studies using the Biostator,[34] as well as during continuous subcutaneous insulin infusion (CSII). Although the initial recognition and descriptions of the DP were in those persons with IDDM, it is now clear that this phenomenon is also present in those with NIDDM[25] and probably in nondiabetic subjects as well,[22] in whom insulin availability is not a problem.

The most concise definition of the DP is that of Bolli and Gerich[25] from their 1984 paper. They define the DP as "an abrupt increase in plasma glucose concentration or insulin requirements or both between 5 AM and 9 AM in the absence of antecedent hypoglycemia." For example, during constant insulin infusion, the DP is seen as a rising blood glucose between 5 AM and 8 AM after a stable period without hypoglycemia between about midnight and 5 AM. During variable-rate insulin delivery, the DP is seen as increasing doses of insulin required during the dawn period to maintain a stable, not rising, blood glucose concentration (Fig. 10-6).

A number of possible causes for the DP have been suggested. These include waning of the previous day's insulin,[132] diurnal variation of insulin clearance,[54,55,138,139] diurnal variation of insulin sensitivity,[22] and diurnal variation of counterregulatory hormones.[34] The latter could exert their effect through variations in either insulin clearance or insulin sensitivity, or both.

After the initial descriptions of the DP by Schmidt and associates[132] and Clarke and associates,[34] the diurnal variation of plasma cortisol seemed a likely candidate for its cause because of the temporal relationship between the rising insulin requirements and the early morning cortisol rise. However, Skor and associates[139] demonstrated that the rising cortisol appears not to be a significant factor in the etiology of the DP. During Skor's study,[139] it was also observed that despite a 30% to 50% higher insulin infusion rate during the dawn period, the plasma-free insulin concentrations were identical to those seen earlier in the night. This raised the possibility that some diurnal variation of insulin clearance may be a contributor to the DP.

Follow-up studies of Skor and associates[138] and Dux and colleagues[54,55] were able to show that insulin clearance was higher during the dawn period than during the earlier nighttime hours. This higher clearance is most pronounced at physiologic rates of insulin delivery. Despite some criticism of the methods used in some of these studies,[32] insulin clearance does appear to play some role in the etiology of the DP. However, other factors are probably also important.

Many glucose counterregulatory hormones have been studied as possibly contributing to the DP. There is general consensus, based on data in the literature, that cortisol,[139] glucagon,[40] and the catecholamines[35,40] play little or no role in the DP. Initial studies suggested that growth hormone played little role in the DP,[137] but subsequent investigations suggest that diurnal variation in growth-hormone secretion may be a key determinant of the DP.[30] Three lines of evidence support this hypothesis. First, somatostatin with glucagon replacement eliminates nocturnal growth-hormone spikes and blunts the DP.[31] Second, blunting growth-hormone spikes by cholinergic blockade blunted the DP in two separate studies.[7,43] Third, Boyle and associates[28] showed that the DP was absent in a group of five growth-hormone–deficient persons with IDDM.

In a report by Campbell and associates,[30] persons with IDDM were studied overnight on 3 nights—a control night, a growth-hormone–deficient night using somatostatin with glucagon replacement, and a growth-hormone–replacement night using somatostatin with replacement of both glucagon and growth hormone. The absence of growth hormone markedly blunted the overnight rise in blood glucose. The authors attributed this to blunting of the DP, but reduction of the nighttime insulin requirements without elimination of the DP might be another explanation.[10] Skor and others,[137] using a very similar study design but slightly higher rates of insulin replacement, came to different conclusions. Elimination of nocturnal growth-

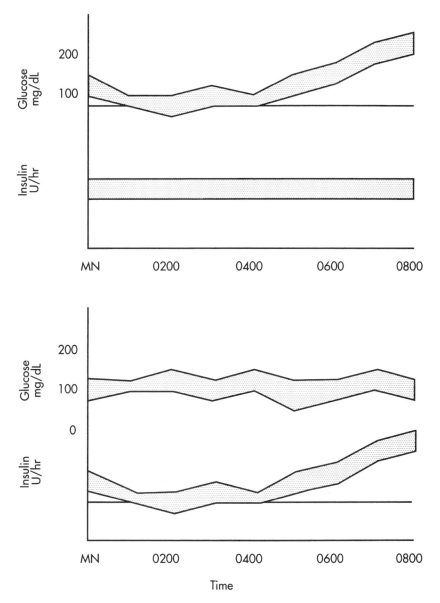

Fig. 10-6 Schematic representation of the dawn phenomenon. **Top,** During constant-rate overnight insulin infusion, blood glucose is stable from midnight to 0400 and rises during the dawn period (0400 to 0800). **Bottom,** During feedback-controlled overnight insulin infusion to maintain a stable blood glucose, insulin requirements increase during the dawn period.

hormone spikes with long-acting somatostatin analog[31] or anticholinergic agents[7,43] appeared to blunt the DP.

Data reported by Boyle and associates[28] appear to tie together the growth hormone hypothesis and the insulin clearance hypothesis for the DP. Boyle and colleagues[28] studied the DP and insulin clearance in five growth-hormone–deficient persons with IDDM and compared them with persons with IDDM but without growth hormone deficiency. The control subjects with IDDM demonstrated the DP as expected, whereas the growth-hormone–deficient subjects with IDDM did not. In addition, the control persons with diabetes showed a higher prebreakfast insulin clearance, whereas those with growth-hormone deficiency had a stable clearance throughout the night. This suggests that growth hormone does play a role in the DP and that its role may be, at least in part, causing changes in insulin clearance. Despite conflicting reports, it is the prevailing current opinion that growth hormone does play some role in the DP and is perhaps the primary determinant of the DP.

With growth hormone as a strong candidate for the etiology of the DP, questions related to mechanism have been asked. Growth-hormone spikes are known to occur during early hours of sleep. Growth hormone is known to have an insulin-like effect within the first few hours after a spike,[101] followed by an insulin-antagonistic effect subsequently. Blackard and associates[16] have suggested that the DP is not a "dawn phenomenon" at all, but rather a "sleep phenomenon." The observation of increasing early morning insulin requirements could indeed be explained by a lowering of basal insulin requirements earlier in the night, possibly as a result of the insulin-like effects of the sleep-related growth-hormone spikes, with a return to normal insulin sensitivity or clearance during the dawn period. This hypothesis appears to be consistent with all the previous observations related to the DP and warrants further study.

The Somogyi Phenomenon

The *Somogyi phenomenon (SP)* has been defined as a morning rise of blood glucose to hyperglycemic levels following an episode of nocturnal hypoglycemia and a counterregulatory hormone response (Fig. 10-7). The SP is named for Dr. Michael Somogyi, who, in 1938, stated[144]:

> We obtained evidence to the effect that the extreme fluctuations in the blood sugar level and the progressively increasing unstability of diabetic patients are the direct results of the administration of excessive amounts of insulin. . . . In the past, we failed to recognize the cause and effect relationship between hypoglycemia and hyperglycemia, and by administering insulin doses sufficiently large to cause hypoglycemias, we produced more severe hyperglycemias.

Dr. Somogyi's statement has been interpreted in various ways. The most widely used interpretation has been that of rebound hyperglycemia, or posthypoglycemic hyperglycemia.

The SP has been implicated as a common cause for fasting, morning hyperglycemia. The hypothesis is that nocturnal hypoglycemia is followed by a glucose counterregulatory hormone response, which, in turn, is followed by a rising plasma glucose and rebound hyperglycemia. This chain of events seems quite logical in theory and probably does occur in certain experimental settings.[26] However, in practice it appears to be a very rare occurrence during day-to-day management of diabetes. Numerous studies have now confirmed this fact.*

---

*References 67, 78, 83, 111, 118, 135, 146, 147.

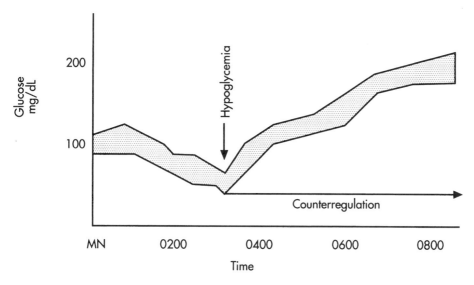

Fig. 10-7   Schematic representation of the Somogyi phenomenon. Nocturnal hypoglycemia causes stimulation of glucose counterregulation, which results in morning hyperglycemia (posthypoglycemic hyperglycemia, or rebound hyperglycemia).

Havlin and Cryer[78] evaluated 216 nighttime blood glucose profiles to determine if nocturnal hypoglycemia were followed by rebound morning hyperglycemia while patients with diabetes received their usual insulin therapy. They found that 2 AM blood glucose values below 100 mg/dl (5.5 mM) and below 50 mg/dl (2.8 mM) were associated with lower, not higher, glucose concentrations the following morning. In the 15 persons who experienced nocturnal hypoglycemia (2 AM blood glucose below 50 mg/dl), none had a fasting morning glucose concentration above 200 mg/dl (11.1 mM). In addition, following nocturnal hypoglycemia, a substantial rise in blood glucose between 2 AM and 7 AM was seen only in those 12 who had received carbohydrate treatment for their nocturnal hypoglycemia. The three persons whose nocturnal hypoglycemia was not treated had little or no rise in the blood glucose concentration between 2 AM and breakfast (Fig. 10-8). Lerman and Wolfsdorf[96] reported similar results and extended the findings to show that blood glucose concentrations later in the day on the day following nocturnal hypoglycemia were similar to those on days not following nocturnal hypoglycemia.

Shalwitz and associates,[135] studying children, found similar results. From 388 nights during 166 elective routine hospitalizations of 135 diabetic children ages 6 to 18 years, nocturnal hypoglycemia (blood glucose less than 60 mg/dl or 3.3 mM) occurred 70 times (18% of the nights). Only 3 of these, or 4.3%, were followed by a morning fasting glucose concentration above 200 mg/dl (11.1 mM). In addition, blood glucose concentrations throughout the remainder of the day following nocturnal hypoglycemia were no higher than they were in the same children on a day not following nocturnal hypoglycemia.

Three studies[83,111,147] in which nocturnal hypoglycemia was induced overnight and compared with nonhypoglycemic nights have likewise shown that morning fasting hyperglycemia does not necessarily follow insulin-induced nocturnal hypoglycemia. Tordj-

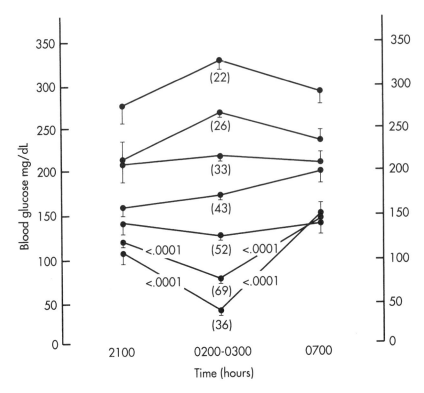

Fig. 10-8 Blood glucose concentrations from overnight profiles in patients with IDDM. Blood glucose concentration (mean ± SEM) at 2100 hours, 0200 to 0300 hours, and 0700 hours from 281 profiles in 66 IDDM patients. Profiles are separated based on 0200 to 0300 hours blood glucose into 50 mg/dl intervals. Numbers in parentheses refer to number of profiles in each group. Note that nocturnal hypoglycemia is not followed by morning fasting hyperglycemia. (Modified from Lerman IG, Wolfsdorf JI: *Diabetes Care* 11:639, 1988.)

man and colleagues[147] studied 10 persons with IDDM on three separate nights, one as a control, one in which hypoglycemia was prevented by IV dextrose, if necessary, and one in which nocturnal hypoglycemia was induced with IV insulin. Nocturnal hypoglycemia did not cause rebound hyperglycemia. Overall, morning plasma glucose concentration was not higher after the hypoglycemic nights than it was after the control or prevention nights. When a higher morning plasma glucose concentration was observed, these patients had been treated for their symptomatic nocturnal hypoglycemia.

Perriello and associates[111] reported the only study in which nocturnal hypoglycemia was followed by hyperglycemia in a predictable way. They found slightly higher morning glucose concentration following insulin-induced nocturnal hypoglycemia. However, the difference was only 13 mg/dl (0.7 mM)—of uncertain clinical significance. Perriello and colleagues[111] did, however, find substantially higher postbreakfast blood sugars following nocturnal hypoglycemia, suggesting rebound hyperglycemia as a cause of daytime postprandial hyperglycemia. Hirsch and associates,[83] however, were unable to confirm this finding and

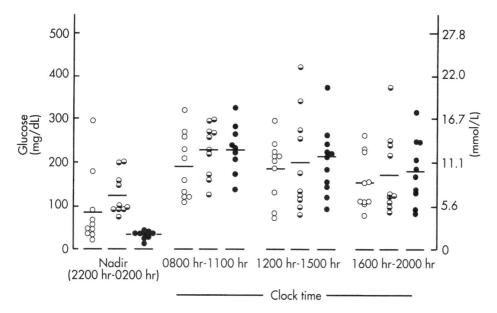

Fig. 10-9   Blood glucose concentration throughout the day following induction and prevention of nocturnal hypoglycemia. Blood glucose concentration during the morning (0800 to 1100 hours), afternoon (1200 to 1500 hours), and evening (1600 to 2000 hours) following a night of sampling only *(open circles)*, insulin-induced nocturnal hypoglycemia *(closed circles)*, and prevention of hypoglycemia with intravenous dextrose *(half-closed circles)*. Patients were maintained on their usual doses of insulin and dietary regimen. Note the similar blood glucose concentrations throughout the following day regardless of whether or not nocturnal hypoglycemia occurred. (Modified from Hirsch IB and others: *Diabetes Care* 13:133-142, 1990.)

found that blood glucose concentrations over the entire day following insulin-induced nocturnal hypoglycemia were similar to those following the control and prevention night (Fig. 10-9). They also found that the increment of glucose between 2 AM and 8 AM was directly, not inversely, correlated with the glucose nadir (i.e., the lower the nocturnal nadir glucose concentration, the lower the rebound observed). These data would be in good agreement with Gale's observation[67] that the morning glucose concentration following nocturnal hypoglycemia was inversely correlated with the free insulin concentration, not the nadir glucose concentration (Fig. 10-10). In other words, high morning sugars following nocturnal hypoglycemia are a result of absolute or relative insulin deficiency, or the dawn phenomenon, and not excessive glucose counterregulation, or the so-called Somogyi phenomenon. The recent studies of Stephenson and Schernthaner[146] would support this conclusion.

Taken together, these studies suggest that nocturnal hypoglycemia does not cause, or rarely causes, morning fasting hyperglycemia in patients with IDDM using their usual therapeutic regimens. Likewise, nocturnal hypoglycemia rarely causes postprandial hyperglycemia the following day. Morning hyperglycemia is more likely to be a result of absolute or relative underinsulinization during the dawn period than of excessive glucose counter-

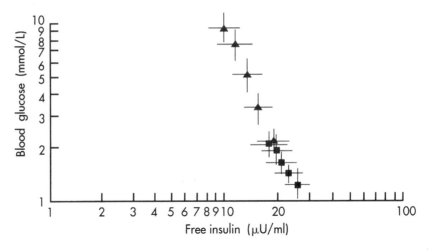

Fig. 10-10 Relationship between fasting blood glucose and plasma-free insulin after spontaneous nocturnal hypoglycemia. Correlation between fasting blood glucose and plasma-free insulin (mean ± SEM) following nocturnal hypoglycemia. Patients with fasting hyperglycemia had lower and falling free insulin concentrations, compared with those with lower morning glucose values. Fasting hyperglycemia after nocturnal hypoglycemia seemed to correlate with lower circulating insulin levels. (Modified from Gale E, Kurtz A, Tattersall R: *Lancet* 2:279, 1980.)

regulation earlier in the night. This is not to say that overinsulinization cannot lead to poor control through a mechanism of recurrent hypoglycemia, leading to sustained increases in counterregulatory hormone concentrations and insulin resistance. If poor control is associated with high doses of insulin and recurrent hypoglycemia, attempts at lowering or redistributing the insulin dose should be made. However, in the absence of recognized hypoglycemia and in the presence of morning hyperglycemia, lowering the insulin dose should not necessarily be the first course of action.

Implications of the Dawn and Somogyi Phenomena in the Management of Morning Fasting Hyperglycemia in Persons With Diabetes

The evaluation and management of morning hyperglycemia in persons with IDDM requires considerable monitoring, discussion, and patient education. First, it is important to be sure that an adequate bedtime snack is taken regularly. Too small or missed snacks are likely to result in nocturnal hypoglycemia; too large a snack could contribute to hyperglycemia throughout the night and into the next morning (see Chapter 4). Second, individuals and their family members should be carefully questioned for symptoms and signs of nocturnal hypoglycemia such as tremors, night sweats, nightmares, restlessness, nocturnal awakening, early morning headaches, or stomachaches. Third, whenever serious evaluation and management of morning hyperglycemia is being tried, blood glucose monitoring should be instituted at bedtime, morning, and, perhaps, at 2 to 3 AM. If the bedtime or 2 AM glucose level is low or if signs or symptoms of nocturnal hypoglycemia are present, the appropriate insulin dose should be reduced. Nocturnal hypoglycemia should be avoided even though it is not likely to be the primary cause of morning hyperglycemia. However, lowering the insulin dose is not likely to bring down the morning blood glucose concentration. If the 2 AM blood glucose concentration is normal or high, the appropriate dose of insulin should be increased. If satisfactory control of 2 AM and morning blood glucose concentration cannot be achieved using a split-mixed regimen of regular and NPH/Lente insulin twice daily, alternative regimens should be considered.

Recommended Regimens

A number of alternative therapeutic regimens have been suggested for dealing with unacceptable glycemic control as a result of either the DP or the SP. First, since normalization of the blood glucose may not be possible for all patients with IDDM, consideration should be given to tolerating some degree of morning hyperglycemia, especially in very young children or toddlers and especially if glucose control during the rest of the day is satisfactory and the glycosylated hemoglobin is in an acceptable range. Occasional monitoring of blood glucose at 2 to 3 AM may be necessary to guide therapy. If the 2 to 3 AM blood glucose is low, the suppertime dose of NPH should be reduced. If control is not considered acceptable and there is no evidence of nocturnal hypoglycemia, the first approach should be to increase the suppertime dose of NPH or Lente insulin in hopes of providing better insulin coverage throughout the entire night and bringing the morning blood glucose concentration down.

If both higher and lower doses of NPH fail or if nocturnal hypoglycemia becomes a problem after increasing the dose, the NPH or Lente dose can be moved to bedtime. Doing this causes its peak action to occur closer to the dawn period when there are increasing insulin requirements, and there is less insulin action between 2 and 4 AM when hypoglycemia is likely. A trial of IIT (see later discussion), especially CSII with multiple basal infusion rates, might be appropriate for some patients.

Finally, consideration should be given to similar approaches recently investigated by Johnson and associates[85] and Wolfsdorf and colleagues.[164a] Humulin Ultralente (Eli Lilly and Company) was substituted for NPH as part of a split-mixed insulin regimen in hopes of achieving more insulin action during the dawn period. The 31 patients studied by Johnson and associates[85] were between 5 and 18 years old with IDDM and an early morning blood glucose rise of at least 50 mg/dl (2.8 mM). They were randomized to either continue on their usual regimen of Regular and Lente insulin or be switched to Regular and Ultralente twice a day. In the group receiving Ultralente, the mean early morning rise of glucose was only 9 mg/dl (0.5 mM) as compared with 46 mg/dl (2.6 mM) for the control subjects remaining on Lente. Unexpectedly, the blood glucose values throughout the rest of the day, including the afternoon, were not higher on the Ultralente regimen than the Lente regimen, and the HbA_{1c} was similar. The fasting blood glucose concentration was lower (191 mg/dl or 10.6 mM versus 227 mg/dl or 12.6 mM) on the Ultralente regimen and blood glucose levels before lunch, supper, bedtime, and at 3 AM were similar. The study of Wolfsdorf and others[164a] gave similar results when

Ultralente was substituted for the NPH only in the presupper dose; NPH continued to be given before breakfast.

BRITTLE DIABETES

Most individuals with diabetes can be expected to successfully maintain a relatively normal life-style aside from the certain requirements and restrictions related to carrying out their complex medical regimen on a daily basis. Children with diabetes can be expected to attend and perform normally in school, to grow and develop normally, and to maintain a normal social life. Adults with diabetes can perform well at most careers, unless diabetes complications diminish their capabilities. Most subjects with diabetes rarely develop diabetic ketoacidosis or significant ketosis except during intercurrent medical illnesses. However, a minority of subjects with diabetes are unable to participate in the normal activities of daily living because of recurrent episodes of severe metabolic decompensation. These subjects are said to suffer from brittle diabetes.[113]

The term *brittle diabetes* should be reserved for those cases in which diabetic instability is manifest by recurrent episodes of ketosis or ketoacidosis or severe hypoglycemia, or both, and is significant enough to result in an inability to maintain a normal life-style or to endanger life.[113] It is not appropriate to use the term to describe patients with stable diabetes who maintain a relatively normal life-style despite less than optimal glycemic control with persistently elevated or widely fluctuating blood glucose. Rather, persons with brittle diabetes are frequently absent from school or the workplace and are often visiting emergency rooms or are hospitalized.

Brittle diabetes is almost exclusively limited to subjects with IDDM and is rarely seen in subjects with NIDDM. It occurs more commonly among females than males[69,114,156] and usually presents during the teenage or young adult years. It rarely presents before puberty and usually does not persist into adulthood. Brittle diabetes presents during this phase of life regardless of duration of diabetes.[156] For example, brittle diabetes will present after only 1 or 2 years of diabetes in a girl whose onset of diabetes occurred at age 10 to 12 years, whereas it may present after 8 to 10 years if the onset was during the preschool years (Fig. 10-11). The reason brittle diabetes presents primarily in teenage girls is not completely understood but probably relates to a combination of physiologic changes (insulin resistance, hormonal changes, menarche) and psychosocial and developmental events.

True brittle diabetes occurs in about 5% to 10% of the population seen in tertiary care subspecialty diabetes clinics.[69,114,156] Since it is presumed that the majority of persons with brittle diabetes are referred to specialists for care, whereas many stable persons with diabetes are not, the true prevalence of brittle diabetes is probably less than 5%. However, the greatest majority of emergency room visits and hospital admissions for patients with diabetes to pediatric or adolescent medical services, other than those for newly diagnosed subjects, are in this small group of patients. These persons consume a substantial portion of the time and effort of the staff at most pediatric diabetes units. It has been estimated that hospital bills for patients with brittle diabetes can be as high as $30,000 to $80,000 per patient per year.

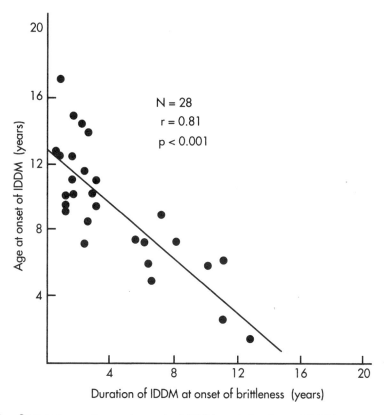

Fig. 10-11   Comparison of age at onset of IDDM and duration of IDDM at onset of brittle diabetes. Correlation between age at onset of IDDM and disease duration at onset of brittleness in 28 persons with brittle diabetes evaluated at St. Louis Children's Hospital from 1978 to 1985. Note that brittleness begins at the age of puberty, regardless of how long the patient has had IDDM. (Modified from White NH, Santiago JV: In Pickup JC, editor: *Brittle diabetes,* Oxford, 1985, Blackwell Scientific Publications.)

The causes of brittle, or unstable, diabetes are often difficult to sort out. Most patients have little, if any, endogenous insulin reserve. Brittle diabetes rarely occurs during the honeymoon period. However, in addition to a low endogenous insulin reserve, other factors are necessary to cause brittle diabetes. Cases of brittle diabetes have been described to be secondary to overinsulinization, underinsulinization, defective glucose counterregulation, erratic insulin absorption,[110] excessive insulin degradation,[64,110,126] recurrent or persistent infection or inflammation, insulin antibodies, and true insulin resistance. Multiple factors may contribute in one person. Underinsulinization is frequently one of the many factors contributing to recurrent episodes of DKA in teenagers, especially teenage girls. The dogma that total daily doses above 1.0 U/kg/day represent overinsulinization is incorrect. Puberty is associated with a degree of insulin resistance,[5,19] and teenagers will often require insulin doses of 1.0 to 1.5 U/kg/day, especially during their peak growth spurt and immediately preceding menarche.

However, the majority of cases of brittle diabetes are caused, at least in part, by psychologic or psychiatric problems.[69,156] Noncompliance with the prescribed regimen is common, including missed insulin doses,[70,108] surreptitious insulin administration,[107] failure of adequate monitoring, and even fabrication of monitoring results. Eating disorders[15] such as anorexia nervosa and bulimia, as well as the behavior known as *induced glycosuria,* which is considered to be a variation on an eating disorder, will precipitate brittle diabetes. Severe family problems, child abuse or neglect, school problems or phobias, and drug or alcohol abuse can also be associated with a picture of brittle diabetes. Certainly more than half,[156] and some believe nearly all,[70,130] of the cases of brittle diabetes are the result of emotional, family, or psychiatric disturbance, and cases that have an entirely physiologic basis are infrequent. Therefore whenever dealing with a case of brittle diabetes, aggressive psychosocial or psychiatric evaluation is essential.[73,76,131,153]

Management of Brittle Diabetes

When dealing with any case of brittle diabetes, a comprehensive multidisciplinary evaluation is required.[73,131] This often needs to take place over many visits, because all issues can rarely be addressed during one visit and it is necessary to establish a close working relationship with the patient and the family before all the issues can be openly and adequately addressed. Involvement of health care professionals, such as nurses, nutritionists, social workers, and psychologists or psychiatrists, is important.[79] During an initial visit, the goals of therapy should be reviewed and modified so that the primary goals are the avoidance of ketosis, ketoacidosis, and severe hypoglycemia, maintenance or establishment of normal growth, and the resumption of normal participation in school, employment, and day-to-day life. Initially, blood glucose targets should be loose or, perhaps, abandoned altogether. Realistic goals should be established. The entire diabetes care regimen should be reviewed by many members of the team to determine its appropriateness for the patient and the family in light of the established goals. Psychosocial parameters should be assessed, including compliance, behavior, school performance, family functioning, and cognitive function.[153] Health beliefs should be examined to determine their consistency with the established goals. The regimen should be modified as necessary to achieve these goals.

If brittle diabetes continues despite modification of the goals and the therapeutic regimen, more extensive evaluation and intensive intervention is required. It may be necessary to implement an increased amount of parental supervision, including in some cases parental responsibility for giving all insulin injections. This has proven to be helpful in some cases, even when missed injections cannot be documented. Reduced parental support has been associated with worsening of metabolic control in teenagers.[86] If increased parental responsibility for diabetes care–related events fails to correct the problem, in-hospital evaluation is indicated.

Inpatient evaluation for recurrent ketoacidosis or brittle diabetes should include a formal psychiatric evaluation.[76,131] All diabetes care (i.e., insulin injections, monitoring) should be performed, or at least very closely supervised, by the nursing staff. The regimen should be adjusted in the hospital to achieve the established goals. If control cannot be maintained despite all care being administered by the staff, physiologic causes of brittleness should be sought. This should include a search for persistent, recurrent, or occult infection or inflammation, erratic insulin absorption or degradation,[64,126] and insulin resistance. These are rarely found, however, and when they are not and brittle diabetes continues, admission to a psychiatric facility is often indicated.[70] This is also true if in-hospital care results in adequate control but outpatient management consistently fails. In some cases, management at home consistently fails to avoid DKA. In these cases, evidence of abuse or neglect should be sought and, if found, placement in a residential care facility or foster placement should be considered.

Steindel and others[144a] recently reported that the use of an insulin pump in six "brittle diabetic" teenagers resulted in a reduction in hospitalization and health care cost over the following year. Although we have not examined this in the form of a formal study, this has not been our experience. In our experience, persons with brittle diabetes rarely respond to intensification of the regimen using multiple daily injections or CSII unless erratic insulin absorption appears to be a major contributing factor. However, aggressive use of extra doses of regular insulin (a "sliding-scale" regimen), especially during ketosis or sick days, to prevent progression to diabetic ketoacidosis can be helpful. The addition of an extra 10% to 20% of the total daily dose given as Regular insulin every 4 to 6 hours when urine ketones are high will reduce the frequency of hospital visits, if implemented regularly. Because the overall daily insulin dose for many teenage girls needs to be 1.0 to 1.5 U/kg/day, an additional 5 to 15 U may be needed in some cases (see "Sick Day Management").

STABLE INSULIN-DEPENDENT DIABETES

Some persons with IDDM seem exceptionally easy to control and can achieve all the stated goals with minimal effort and often very little insulin. These individuals fall into three main categories, but endogenous insulin reserve is a common feature. The three situations likely to result in stable diabetes are the honeymoon period of IDDM, NIDDM of youth, and diabetes with a long duration of continued endogenous insulin release.

The honeymoon period occurs shortly after the diagnosis of IDDM. During the honeymoon period there is a temporary recrudescence of β-cell function, resulting in near normalization of blood glucose despite diminishing doses of exogenous insulin.[142] Some small children may appear to be insulin independent during the honeymoon phase, although most physicians elect to continue very low–dose insulin therapy during this time. The use of diluted insulin (U-10 or U-25) may be needed. The honeymoon usually starts during the first few weeks after diagnosis and can last anywhere from a few weeks to a year. The honeymoon rarely lasts beyond a year, although cases of an apparent prolonged honeymoon have been observed. Even if a true honeymoon does not occur, residual endogenous insulin reserve (measured as circulating C-peptide) will result in stable, easy-to-control diabetes. Adults tend to have a less rapid decline of C-peptide than do young children[47] and therefore may remain stable for longer periods.

Some cases of long-lasting stable diabetes in children could be the result of relatively rare causes of diabetes mellitus, which are not typical IDDM. These include maturity-onset diabetes of youth (MODY),[59] the diabetes unique to black Americans who present with DKA but subsequently respond similarly to NIDDM,[163] and genetic mutations of the insulin molecule, such as hereditary hyperproinsulinemia and biologically defective insulin.[145]

GROWTH FAILURE IN DIABETES AND MAURIAC'S SYNDROME

Most children with diabetes grow within the normal percentiles for age and gender, although some studies suggest that they are slightly shorter than expected. Our examination of a large cohort of children with diabetes,[154] for example, showed that the final adult height and the corrected height of diabetic children fall at about the fortieth percentile. This is about 1 to 2 cm below the median for the general population. Most of this reduced height is likely the result of poor glycemic control; subjects in good or fair glycemic control (HbA_{1c} is less than 11.0%) grow at an annualized growth velocity that was normal for age, whereas those in poor control (HbA_{1c} is more than 11.0%) grow approximately 0.5 cm per year less than expected.

However, despite these minor alterations in growth, major growth disturbance as a result of diabetes mellitus is unusual. Short stature or reduced growth velocity in children with diabetes should be investigated using the same guidelines and with the same vigor as in those without diabetes. Thyroid function tests and plasma cortisol should be measured, especially since hypothyroidism and Addison's disease are more common in subjects with IDDM. Celiac disease (gluten-sensitive enteropathy) may also be more common in type I subjects. Growth-hormone testing is rarely indicated, and measurement of somatomedin-C/IGF-1 may not be helpful since it is often low in poorly controlled diabetes.

Markedly diminished growth can be seen as a result of the Mauriac's syndrome.[95] Mauriac's syndrome is poor diabetic control in association with the combination of reduced growth, delayed sexual maturation, hepatomegaly, hypertriglyceridemia and, often, a cushingoid appearance of truncal obesity and peripheral muscle wasting. The etiology of the Mauriac's syndrome is unknown, but poor control is probably only one component, because not all children with poorly controlled diabetes will manifest this constellation of findings.

Whenever growth failure or Mauriac's syndrome occurs in a child with diabetes and no other etiology for growth failure is identified, aggressive efforts at establishing better diabetic control are indicated. Careful nutritional assessment is essential, and higher doses of insulin are usually needed. Teenagers may require 1.0 to 1.5 U/kg/day of insulin to maintain adequate control for the maintenance of normal growth and development. Increased parental involvement may be necessary, and an evaluation for possible psychosocial dwarfism should be considered. IIT should be utilized if other attempts to normalize growth fail. Improvement of glycemic control will usually result in a better growth velocity or even catch-up growth (Fig. 10-12). However, during the catch-up growth phase of treating Mauriac's syndrome, careful surveillance for diabetic microvascular complications should be performed because an apparent rapid progression of retinopathy and nephropathy[57] has been observed within the first few months of IIT in these subjects.

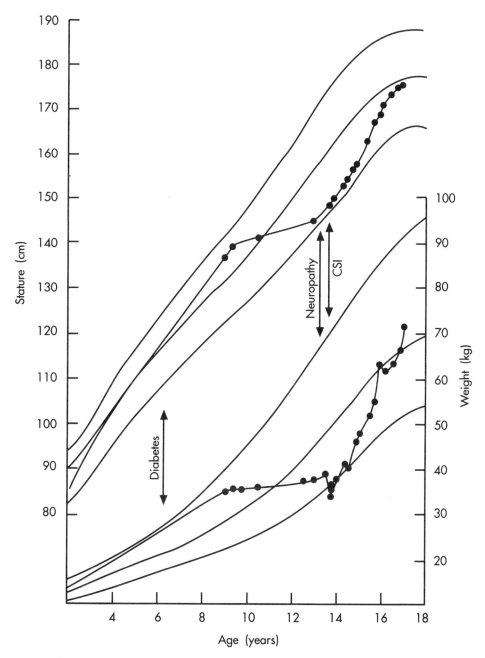

Fig. 10-12   Growth curve of a boy with IDDM and marked growth failure. IDDM was diagnosed at 6 years old. Growth failure started at about 9 years old and continued until aggressive insulin therapy and eventually CSII was started at 13 years old. Catch-up growth followed the initiation of intensive insulin therapy. Growth curve shows the fifth, fiftieth, and ninety-fifth percentile.

SICK DAY MANAGEMENT

The primary goal for the management of diabetes during any illness is to prevent the need for hospitalization. Of course individuals can and do develop other medical illnesses as well, and if these are serious enough to warrant hospitalization, the patient with diabetes will be hospitalized regardless of his or her ability to deal with diabetes. However, in most cases, early intervention in consultation with an experienced health care team can prevent the development of severe DKA, severe hypoglycemia, or dehydration requiring hospitalization. It is imperative that every person with diabetes and his or her family have an experienced health care team available to help during times of illness. Without rapid intervention, illnesses that might be relatively insignificant for the person without diabetes can develop into a major medical emergency in persons with diabetes, particularly IDDM. In addition, diabetes itself, or its complications, can mimic other serious health problems.

Common illnesses, even those as simple as a cold or the flu, can affect the control of diabetes in three ways. First, illness or stress raises the counterregulatory hormones (glucagon, catecholamines, growth hormone, cortisol), and these hormones will act to cause hyperglycemia (by stimulating gluconeogenesis and inhibiting insulin action) and ketosis (by stimulating lipolysis and ketogenesis). Second, since it may be difficult to eat during illness, hypoglycemia can occur. Third, illness, especially gastrointestinal illness, can cause vomiting and an inability to take fluids, resulting in dehydration. The problem of dehydration is worsened by the glucose-induced osmotic diuresis and acidosis accompanying DKA. Dehydration and acidosis combine to cause significant electrolyte imbalance. During the management of any sick day, the combination of ketosis and dehydration requires immediate and aggressive action. Likewise, the presence of hypoglycemia in a subject who is unable to eat or drink requires immediate and aggressive action.

Home management of sick days is best accomplished by a well-informed and highly motivated patient. If the patient is too young to care for himself or herself or is temporarily incapacitated by the illness, it is important that the assistance and supervision from a family member or friend is available at times of intercurrent illness. Occasionally, hospitalization may become necessary for a relatively mild illness because of the lack of family support and motivation. However, if this happens repeatedly, other action needs to be taken, including the possibility of obtaining outside help for the family (see discussion, "Brittle Diabetes").

Guidelines for Management of Sick Days

Guidelines for the management of sick days[97] should be established and discussed early in the relationship between the patient and health care team. Whenever possible, specific individualized guidelines should be discussed with each patient and should be reviewed and updated regularly. General guidelines that all persons with diabetes should follow as a part of sick day management, as discussed in Chapter 4, include (1) never omitting insulin, (2) always monitoring blood glucose and urine ketones at least every 2 to 4 hours, (3) always providing plenty of fluids, (4) using supplemental insulin, if necessary, to break ketosis, and (5) contacting the health care team or seeing a physician if there is a fever, persistent vomiting,

---

BOX 10-1

SICK DAY MANAGEMENT: WHEN TO SEEK MEDICAL ASSISTANCE

Seek immediate medical assistance if any of the following occur:
   Shortness of breath, or respiratory difficulty
   Severe abdominal pain
   Persistent vomiting
   Chest pain
   Severe dehydration
   Acute visual loss
Seek medical attention if any of the following persist:
   Elevated preprandial blood glucose (>250 mg/dl) that is not responding to changes
   Ketonuria
   Persistent diarrhea
   Fever above 100° F
   Other unexplained symptoms

---

persistent presence of large ketones or symptoms of DKA, or the presence of other severe symptoms suggesting a significant underlying medical problem (Box 10-1). The physician should be available to evaluate the patient for underlying illnesses and provide rapid treatment, as indicated by the patient's condition and course. If the person's own physician is not readily available, a visit to an emergency clinic or hospital emergency room is in order.

Monitoring is an essential part of the management of diabetes, and this is even more important during an intercurrent illness. Whenever a person with diabetes is ill, regardless of the symptoms or the blood glucose, urine ketones should be monitored. Likewise, whenever the blood glucose is unexpectedly high (more than 240 mg/dl), urine ketones should be monitored regardless of whether there are any symptoms. Ketones indicate insulin deficiency or stress-related insulin resistance and are nearly always an indication for an additional insulin dose. A large amount of urinary ketones is usually accompanied by hyperglycemia; however, even if the blood glucose is not elevated, large ketonuria warrants the use of sick day guidelines.

Fluids are an essential part of managing diabetes during a sick day (for further discussion see Chapter 4). It is usually recommended that a teenager or young adult attempt to take 6 to 8 ounces of fluid each hour, if possible. If not possible, careful monitoring for the presence or development of dehydration should be implemented. More frequent ingestion of small quantities of fluid (3 to 4 ounces every half hour) is usually better tolerated by persons with gastrointestinal illness than less frequent ingestion of larger quantities. Young children, of course, should take proportionately less (perhaps 3 to 6 ounces every hour). Ingestion of food is not essential during the few-day course of a brief illness, but an inability to take fluids by mouth is a clear indication for intravenous therapy. If meals are not being taken, carbohydrate-containing fluids should be taken to compensate for the carbohydrate intake of the usual meal plan. Additional fluids should be carbohydrate-free as long as hyperglycemia is present. However, once the blood glucose falls to below the 150 to 200 mg/dl range, additional fluids should contain carbohydrates. In some cases, even dehydrated patients can be managed without hospitalization if oral intake is good and close follow-up is ensured. However, when developing a plan to rehydrate a patient at home, it is helpful to obtain the patient's weight and follow weight changes, as well as blood sugar and urinary ketones, throughout treatment. As the patient feels better and vomiting resolves, gradual resumption of the usual meal plan can begin.

In the presence of ketonuria, supplemental doses of insulin are usually required. If intravenous therapy is not indicated, supplemental insulin should be subcutaneous short-acting Regular insulin. A dose equivalent to approximately 10% of the total daily dose is usually recommended; this should be repeated every 2 to 4 hours until ketosis is clearing. If hyperglycemia is absent or minimal in conjunction with significant ketones, supplemental insulin should be given anyway, and additional sugar, in the form of carbohydrate-containing beverages, is used to prevent hypoglycemia. Ketosis accompanied by an inability to take oral fluids, especially if the blood glucose drops to below 150 to 200 mg/dl before successful oral intake can be reestablished, is a clear indication for intravenous fluid therapy. If intravenous fluids and insulin are indicated, it is best to follow the guidelines similar to those reviewed for the treatment of severe DKA (see earlier discussion).

During any sick day, it is imperative that blood glucose, urine ketones, hydration status, and patient symptoms and well-being be monitored at least every few hours. Any deterioration should be promptly reported to the health care team and consideration should be given to having the patient seen by the physician for evaluation. Maintaining a flowsheet of the individual's status is often helpful in following response to therapy. If the individual demonstrates resolution of ketones, improvement of hydration status, and resolution of the symptoms, it is appropriate to continue the sick-day regimen at home and resume the customary insulin dose and meal plan when the individual is ready to resume eating meals. However, if vomiting persists, symptoms worsen, or signs of severe DKA occur, a medical evaluation should be performed without delay.

Diabetes itself, or its complications, can mimic other serious health problems. Any underlying illness must be addressed. Laboratory studies should include electrolytes, BUN, creatinine, and assessment of acidosis, as well as other studies necessary to help rule out underlying causes. However, other serious health problems need to be considered if the history or examination is suggestive. Symptomatic treatment for mild illness, such as with analgesics, decongestants, or antihistamines, is appropriate, unless contraindicated because of diabetes complications or other medical problems. However, antiemetics should be used only with great caution and after evaluation by a physician. Many nonprescription medications can be used by persons with diabetes without major effects on blood glucose. However, patients should be instructed to read the label for warnings. Aspirin and acetaminophen (Tylenol)—the mainstays in treating minor illnesses—are generally well tolerated and safe, except in persons allergic to them. In commonly used doses, they do not interfere with blood or urine sugar or with monitoring of glucose or ketones. Of course, many pediatricians advise parents not to use aspirin in children with flulike or viral illnesses because of the association with Reye's syndrome.

Persons with diabetes should use over-the-counter cold medications—particularly those containing decongestants—with caution. Some contain substances that not only raise blood glucose but also create symptoms mimicking hypoglycemia. Other nonprescription drugs, such as cough syrups, may contain sugar and alcohol, although in limited quantities; the effects on diabetes are usually negligible. In general, the effects of these over-the-counter medications on blood glucose are small and can be easily compensated for by the changes in insulin therapy made during sick day management. Use of decongestant medications may also be inadvisable in persons with hypertension or heart disease.

SURGERY IN THE PATIENT WITH DIABETES MELLITUS

It has been estimated that a patient with diabetes has a 50% chance of undergoing surgery sometime during his or her lifetime.[2] The risk associated with surgery and anesthesia may be increased in diabetic patients as compared with healthy individuals, especially if diabetic control is poor or diabetic complications are present. Poor metabolic control is associated with impaired response to infection, poor wound healing, increased protein breakdown, and electrolyte imbalance. The risk of hypoglycemia in the surgical patient and in the patient recovering from anesthesia is increased, especially since he or she may not be unable to sense or communicate symptoms and needs. Insulin requirements often increase in response to the stress of illness or surgery. In addition, stress can precipitate ketosis or DKA. DKA can mimic other conditions, including abdominal symptoms that suggest a need for surgical intervention.

The metabolic effects of surgery and anesthesia are principally those of the stress response. Catecholamines, cortisol, glucagon, and growth hormone all increase, leading to increased glycogenolysis and gluconeogenesis, protein catabolism, and lipolysis. Insulin resistance also occurs. The net effect of this response is the development of hyperglycemia, protein breakdown, lipolysis, and ketogenesis. Insulin is necessary to overcome this stress hormone response and prevent the intraoperative development of a catabolic and ketotic state. In general, the response to surgery itself is greater than the response to anesthesia, and the magnitude of the metabolic response relates to the severity of the surgery and underlying illness. The response to general anesthesia is greater than the response to local or spinal anesthesia, which has a minimal effect on metabolism.

The primary goal of management for the persons with diabetes undergoing surgery is to avoid hypoglycemia, marked hyperglycemia, ketoacidosis, and fluid and electrolyte imbalance. Normalization of blood glucose during surgery and the immediate postoperative period is not essential and may not even be desirable. Mild hyperglycemia is preferable to unrecognized hypoglycemia. The regimens used to reach the goals should minimize the possibility of error and be widely applicable to the variety of conditions that pertain to surgical wards and operating theaters.

Elective surgery offers the greatest opportunity to anticipate and identify problems. Persons with diabetes requiring elective surgery should be in the best possible metabolic control before admission. If acceptable metabolic control cannot be achieved before elective surgery, hospitalization of the patient for 2 or 3 days may be warranted to establish good control. Elective surgery should be postponed in the presence of ketosis. Screening for diabetic complications should be done before elective surgery; this should include testing for renal, cardiovascular, neuropathic, and retinal disease as directed by the age and duration of disease of the patient. Surgery should be scheduled as early as possible in the day to avoid prolonged fasting. Short-acting (Regular) and intermediate-acting (NPH or Lente) doses of insulin should be altered on the day of surgery. Long-acting (Ultralente) insulin doses should be reduced 1 or 2 days before surgery, if possible, and supplemental regular insulin given as needed to control hyperglycemia. Oral hypoglycemic agents should be held for 1 or 2 days before surgery.

In general, insulin should be used in all patients with diabetes (whether insulin-treated or not) during major surgery or any surgery requiring general anesthesia. In some cases of minor surgery under local or spinal anesthesia, no change in therapy is warranted, except as dictated by change in dietary intake. If surgery is relatively minor and will not involve prolonged periods without oral intake, the use of subcutaneous insulin during the perioperative period seems appropriate. The simplest regimen seems to be using a reduced dose of intermediate-acting insulin alone (one half to two thirds of the usual morning dose of NPH or Lente) before surgery and then dextrose-containing intravenous fluids. Together, these should be adjusted to maintain the blood glucose between 150 and 200 mg/dl. These adjustments can be made based on readings from a reflectance meter. A small amount of Regular insulin can be added if significant hyperglycemia is present. If ketosis is present, it may be best to postpone elective surgical procedures, if this is feasible.

The operative and postoperative health care teams must understand the management objectives during surgery in patients with diabetes (Box 10-2). The clinician should learn specific techniques and plan the preoperative, intraoperative, and postoperative management of these patients before the surgery actually takes place. The management technique should be individualized to meet the specific needs of the patient and his or her situation; one regimen will not be applicable to all situations. The reader is referred to Chapter 12 and to the Reference List for a more detailed description of various regimens.[2,82,148]

If surgery will require prolonged periods of general anesthesia, if hypoperfusion, shock, or electrolyte imbalance are likely during surgery, or if ketosis is present and surgery cannot be postponed, it is best to use intravenous insulin and dextrose. Serum electrolytes, BUN, creatinine, urine ketones, and hydration status should be determined before surgery and monitored during surgery. The usual subcutaneous insulin should be omitted on the day of surgery. Insulin should be administered at 0.05 to 0.1 U/kg/hr and IV fluid begun with a 5% to 10% dextrose solution to give approximately 5 mg/kg/min. Potassium can be added to the IV fluid as necessary to prevent hypokalemia. Blood glucose should be monitored by meter every 4 hours before surgery, hourly during surgery, and at least every 2 to 4 hours after surgery until well into the recovery phase. Blood glucose should be kept in the 150 to 200 mg/dl range. Intravenous infusions should be continued until it is appropriate to resume subcutaneous insulin.

After surgery, meals, or at least carbohydrate-containing oral fluids, should be resumed as quickly as possible. If the patient cannot eat or drink for more than 1 day, intravenous insulin and dextrose should be continued or Regular insulin given every 4 hours throughout that time. Blood glucose monitoring should be performed every 1 to 4 hours. Adults typically require IV dextrose at 150 to 200 g/day and children about 2 to 4 g/kg/day. When meals are

---

BOX 10-2

GUIDELINES FOR THE MANAGEMENT OF PATIENTS WITH DIABETES MELLITUS DURING SURGERY

General goals of perioperative therapy

Prevent hypoglycemia, ketoacidosis, electrolyte and fluid imbalance

Control hyperglycemia: blood glucose 115 to 140 mg/dl is ideal; 150 to 200 mg/dl is acceptable in most settings

Resume oral intake as soon as possible

Use human insulin when insulin required in patient who is not usually treated with insulin

Schedule surgery early in the morning

Specific guidelines

Stabilize glucose before surgery, whenever possible

Use insulin during surgery for:

(1) All insulin-requiring patients

(2) All major surgical procedures

(3) Procedures requiring general anesthesia

(4) Minor surgery, if hyperglycemia or ketosis is present

For type II patients managed on diet and/or oral hypoglycemic agents alone:

(1) Hold oral agent for 1 to 2 days before surgery, if possible

(2) No specific therapy on day of surgery if:

Surgery minor

Local or spinal anesthesia

Fasting blood glucose less than 125 mg/dl

No ketones

Modified from Albert KGMM, Gill GV, Elliot MS: *Diabetes Care* 5(suppl 1):65-77, 1982; and from *Physicians guide to non–insulin-dependent (type II) diabetes: diagnosis and treatment,* Alexandria, Va, 1988, American Diabetes Association, Inc.

---

fully tolerated, the patient's customary insulin regimen should be resumed along with supplemental regular insulin to compensate for elevated blood glucose and ketones.

Emergency surgery may not permit sufficient time to stabilize the patient. In persons who require emergency surgery and are in DKA, treatment of DKA must begin without delay (see the section on treatment of DKA) and should be continued vigorously throughout surgery and into the postoperative period until DKA has resolved. Careful monitoring of electrolytes, blood glucose, rehydration, and urine output is essential throughout surgery. Intravenous Regular insulin should be used in all cases of emergency surgery accompanied by DKA. If possible, surgery should be delayed until the acidosis is beginning to improve. Whenever possible, emergency surgery in a patient in DKA should be performed at a center with appropriate medical and surgical intensive care available.

Individuals with diabetes undergoing local anesthesia (such as dental or spinal anesthesia) should be scheduled as early in the day as possible to avoid prolonged fasting. Oral hypoglycemic agents should be held for 1 to 2 days before surgery and on the morning of surgery. Insulin should be decreased on the morning of surgery. Depending on the length of surgery, Regular insulin can be decreased or omitted. Often one half to two thirds of the usual dose of intermediate insulin dose can be given. Careful monitoring of blood glucose by meter should be performed before, during, and after surgery as just outlined. Blood glucose in excess of 240 mg/dl can be treated with supplemental Regular insulin, and low blood glucose (less than 70 mg/dl) can be treated with intravenous dextrose or oral carbohydrate, as tolerated. Typically, the usual insulin or oral hypoglycemic agent regimen and meal plan can be resumed with the first scheduled postoperative dose of insulin or meal. In cases of extensive dental work, soft foods or liquids containing carbohydrates should be given until oral feeding is reestablished. Careful monitoring of blood glucose and urine ketones should occur as with general anesthesia.

ALTERNATIVES TO STANDARD INSULIN THERAPY FOR THE TREATMENT OF IDDM

Essentially all persons with IDDM receive insulin subcutaneously. Some success has been achieved with rectal or nasal administration of insulin, but neither of these routes has become popular nor has either demonstrated any distinct advantage over subcutaneous insulin. The intraperitoneal route of insulin administration using implantable infusion pumps has been successful on a limited basis over the past few years. However, as of this writing, implantable insulin pumps continue to be available only to a limited number of patients through a limited number of centers. Many, including us, would still consider implantable insulin pumps to be somewhat investigational. Of course, if a reliable continuous glucose sensor could be developed and linked to an implantable pump, thus creating an "artificial endocrine pancreas," the appropriateness of such a device for the treatment of IDDM would be greatly and rapidly expanded.

Subcutaneous insulin is most commonly given in the form of injection. The use of portable infusion pumps to deliver subcutaneous insulin is discussed later. Numerous injection aids are available. These facilitate the insertion of the needle through the skin and may be particularly applicable for young children. Forced-air (or jet) injectors are also available for insulin delivery.[134] These are effective but are relatively expensive and offer little advantage for most young people with IDDM. A recent summary of injection aids and other diabetes care–related devices and supplies is available.[3] The available supplies and devices on the market change rapidly.

Over the past few years, there has been considerable interest in the use of insulin analogs in the treatment of IDDM. These analogs are being developed in hopes of altering the absorption and/or action of insulin to improve glycemic control. The most exciting analog at the time of this writing is the so-called insulin lispro (lysine and proline), which has two amino acid substitutions relative to human insulin. Insulin lispro forms fewer aggregates in solution, is absorbed more rapidly, and has a shorter half-life after subcutaneous injection than regular human insulin itself. This analog is likely to be more effective than regular human insulin at blunting postprandial hyperglycemia without causing subsequent hypoglycemia before the next meal 4 to 5 hours later. Although insulin lispro is available in some countries, as of this writing, it is not yet commercially available in the United States. However, because of the demonstrated improved time course of action, it is likely that insulin lispro and other analogs will be used widely when they do become available.

INTENSIVE DIABETES THERAPY

Insulin is the primary hormonal regulator of carbohydrate metabolism and an important regulator of protein and fat metabolism as well. For the individual without diabetes, insulin is secreted by the β-cells of the islet into the portal vein where it circulates to the liver and subsequently to the rest of the body. The modulation of pancreatic insulin release is under numerous mechanisms of control, including the ambient glucose concentration, autonomic nervous system input, gut hormonal stimulatory factors, and the hormonal milieu. The hormonal factors include circulating endocrine effects, as well as intraislet paracrine effects. As a result of these factors, insulin release by the pancreas and the circulating insulin concentration is modulated to produce the rapid changes necessary to normalize carbohydrate metabolism and maintain blood glucose in the very narrow range of 70 to 140 mg/dl (3.9 to 7.8 mM).

A consistent pattern of insulin release, measured as circulating plasma insulin concentration, is reproduced with each meal. With the ingestion of each meal, the circulating insulin concentration rises tenfold to fifteenfold, from a baseline concentration of 5 to 10 µU/ml to a peak of 50 to 150 µU/ml. This peak insulin concentration is reached about 1 hour after ingestion of the meal, and the insulin concentration then rapidly declines, returning to its baseline level after about 4 to 6 hours. This pattern repeats itself with the ingestion of the next meal. During the postabsorptive and fasting states, the circulating insulin concentration remains low but is not absent. This low level of insulin is required to prevent hyperglycemia from unchecked glycogenolysis and gluconeogenesis.

As discussed elsewhere, the rapid decline in circulating insulin after its postprandial peak is a key component of glucose counterregulation during the postprandial period, that is, the prevention of postprandial hypoglycemia. Likewise, the rapid rise of insulin during the first postprandial hour is a key component in preventing postprandial hyperglycemia. This can be demonstrated by the postprandial hyperglycemia associated with the blunted or delayed first-phase insulin release seen in persons with early IDDM and in some persons with NIDDM. In addition, in insulin-deficient persons, a 15-minute delay in the administration of an intravenous dose of insulin that would otherwise normalize blood glucose results in postprandial hyperglycemia.[33] Therefore the maintenance of blood glucose within the narrow normal range throughout the day is dependent on rapid modulation of insulin release and circulating insulin concentration.

The exogenous administration of insulin as one or two injections per day of fast-acting Regular and/or intermediate-acting NPH or Lente insulin does not result in the rapid modulation of circulated insulin concentrations necessary to normalize carbohydrate metabolism and blood glucose. Instead, conventional insulin therapy results in a slow rise, followed by a gradual decline, of circulating insulin and relatively constant hyperinsulinemia throughout most of the day, with declining insulin overnight. Along with this highly unphysiologic pattern of insulinemia, it is not unexpected that glycemic con-trol is less than perfect. In addition, meal, snack, and exercise timing are relatively inflexible.

Intensive diabetes therapy is the term commonly used to refer to therapy aimed at achieving normal or near-normal blood glucose levels in subjects with diabetes. The benefits and risks of intensive therapy to improve glycemic control have only recently been proven. Since the previous edition of this book, both the Diabetes Control and Complications Trial (DCCT)[48a] and the Stockholm Diabetes Intervention Trial[119a] have shown that lowering blood glucose using intensive diabetes therapy substantially reduces the development and progression of long-term microvascular and neuropathic complications of IDDM in adolescents and younger adults (see later discussion for more details about the results and implications of the DCCT).

A key component of intensive diabetes therapy as implemented in the DCCT is intensive insulin therapy. *Intensive insulin therapy (IIT)* is the term used to describe therapeutic regimens of insulin delivery that are designed to mimic physiologic insulin release and normalize blood glucose. Before launching into a discussion of insulin administration in IIT, it is essential to note that any diabetes care regimen, whether it be conventional or intensive, is more than simply insulin administration. Regardless of the insulin regimen used, meal planning, exercise, monitoring, education, psychosocial support, and close follow-up by a team of highly trained and motivated health care professionals are important components of any diabetes care regimen and no diabetes care plan can succeed without the proper implementation of all these aspects of care. A discussion of these follows, as well as in a recently published guide by the American Diabetes Association.[3b]

Approaches to Insulin Replacement

Four basic approaches to insulin replacement therapy are aimed at mimicking physiologic insulinemia and normalizing blood glucose. These include (1) pancreas or islet cell transplantation, (2) the "closed loop," feedback-controlled artificial pancreas,[124] (3) continuous subcutaneous insulin infusion (CSII),[127] and (4) multiple daily insulin injections (MDII). CSII and MDII are discussed here.

All IIT regimens must combine two components of insulin delivery. The first is rapid rise of insulin followed by a rapid decline back toward baseline following each meal. In CSII and MDII regimens, this is accomplished by what is called the *mealtime bolus,* or simply *bolus,* dose. Because of the desired timing of the postprandial insulin needs, the bolus must be given in the form of rapidly acting insulin or Regular insulin. Even when giving subcutaneous Regular insulin (the use of intravenous insulin as part of an IIT regimen is not discussed here), the peak action does not correspond to the desired time of 1 hour postprandial, but rather occurs 2 to 3 hours later. Optimal benefit can therefore be obtained by administering the dose 30 to 45 minutes before the meal. At least three studies have demonstrated benefit to such a delay.[53,90,164] The use of insulin analogs with more rapid absorption from the subcutaneous injection sites (see discussion above) may eliminate the need for this waiting time between insulin administration and meal ingestion. With any IIT regimen, mealtime bolus doses are given before each meal. The specific dose and timing may vary depending on current blood glucose, time of day, site of injection, planned carbohydrate intake, and anticipated exercise or activity. Patients using IIT require extensive education and assistance with problem-solving, and trial-and-error techniques to learn to consistently administer the correct premeal bolus dose under the varying situations of day-to-day life.

The second component of insulin delivery in an IIT regimen is referred to as the *basal insulin*. The basal insulin is a slow, relatively continuous supply of insulin throughout the day and night that provides the low, but present, insulin concentration necessary to balance glucose consumption (glucose uptake and oxidation) and glucose production (glycogenolysis and gluconeogenesis). Basal insulin needs are usually about 10 to 15 mU/kg/hr and account for 30% to 50% of the total daily insulin needs. However, considerable individual variation is seen. In addition, basal insulin needs may vary from one time of day to another, especially as part of the dawn phenomenon (see earlier discussion).

The implementation of IIT using continuous subcutaneous insulin infusion (CSII) involves the use of an externally worn portable infusion pump.[102,124,127] The reservoir or syringe of the pump is filled with Regular insulin, which is infused continuously through a catheter that is placed subcutaneously. The catheter is not permanent and is replaced every 1 to 3 days. The pump is preprogrammed to infuse insulin continuously at a constant, or variable, basal rate throughout the day and night. The infusion rates are predetermined and adjusted as necessary. The pump is instructed to rapidly (over a few minutes) administer a bolus dose of Regular insulin before each meal. Each of these mealtime bolus doses is under the control of the patient. Over the years, numerous devices for CSII have been available.[3]

IIT using multiple daily insulin injections (MDII) usually involves three or more injections of insulin per day. Regular insulin is injected before each meal. Basal insulin is provided using various combinations of intermediate- or long-acting insulin. The most popular MDII regimens are NPH or Lente at bedtime or Ultralente once or twice a day. When bedtime NPH or Lente is used to provide overnight basal insulin needs, basal insulin (NPH or Lente) is usually not necessary throughout the waking hours if mealtime bolus doses are given at least every 4 to 6 hours. The initial trials of MDII with Ultralente insulin to provide the basal insulin needs were done before the marketing of human Ultralente. Beef/pork Ultralente was usually divided and given twice daily, although once daily was effective in many persons. Beef/pork Ultralente is no longer available, however. Human Ultralente has a shorter duration of action and nearly always needs to be given twice a day (breakfast and supper, or breakfast and bed). It has been observed that some subjects using MDII with Ultralente insulin appear to require much higher basal insulin doses (more than 50% of the total dose) than expected. The reason for this is not clear.

The choice of CSII versus MDII as the method for implementation of IIT is usually an individual one. One regimen has not been consistently shown to be better than the other. Although some subjects might respond better to CSII than MDII or vice versa, most persons respond equally well to either mode.

Regardless of whether CSII or MDII is chosen as the means of implementing IIT, mealtime bolus doses need to be regularly adjusted based on measured blood glucose and anticipated dietary intake and exercise. Breakfast bolus doses are usually higher (for equivalent carbohydrate intake) than are lunchtime or suppertime doses. Occasionally, bolus doses may be required before snacks, especially if the snack is large. However, snacks become a less essential part of the regimen, since they are no longer required to counterbalance the poorly timed hyperinsulinemia associated with prebreakfast NPH insulin administration. Bedtime snacks are still recommended, however, to help prevent nocturnal hypoglycemia. Algorithms for adjustment of insulin doses during IIT have been developed by many investigators.[140] Similar algorithms have been developed for use with conventional insulin regimens.[141]

In the DCCT, initiation of an intensive insulin therapy regimen was done in an inpatient setting in which extensive education and close monitoring can be performed. Inpatient initiation of IIT may still seem optimal, especially when starting CSII therapy. However, in the current wave of health care reform and attempts to reduce cost, IIT is usually initiated on an outpatient basis. However, since major changes in insulin doses are required, extensive education and very close follow-up are essential when implementing IIT. Insulin requirements during IIT may be considerably different from those used during conventional therapy. Basal insulin doses are often calculated as 30% to 50% of the usual daily insulin dose, but this can be done only if the total daily dose the patient is receiving is thought to be appropriate. Alternatively, the basal needs can be estimated using a variable-rate intravenous infusion based on hourly blood glucose measurements, as described by White and associates,[159] but this requires an inpatient stay. Basal insulin requirements are usually 10 to 15 mU/kg/hr. However, for those with a significant dawn phenomenon, lower insulin delivery rates of 8 to 12 mU/kg/hr may be adequate during the early night, whereas higher rates of 15 to 20 mU/kg/hr may be needed during the dawn or prebreakfast period.

Mealtime bolus doses will vary considerably from person to person. Although results calculated from intravenous infusions or taken from artificial pancreas use (Biostator GCIIS, Miles Laboratories, Elkhart, Ind) can be used effectively to determine mealtime bolus doses, this is rarely necessary. In most cases, the breakfast dose is 0.15 to 0.30 U/kg, the lunchtime dose 0.10 to 0.20 U/kg, and the suppertime dose 0.15 to 0.25 U/kg. Snacks are not always covered with a bolus dose but can be covered with about 0.05 U/kg. Of course, the mealtime bolus doses are adjusted based on blood glucose, anticipated activity, and planned carbohydrate intake. Many algorithms, such as those of Skyler and associates,[140,141] have been developed for this purpose. After initiation of IIT, changes in both the basal and bolus insulin doses and insulin adjustment algorithms are made based on self-monitored blood glucose determinations and individually determined goals. Monitoring usually needs to be done four times each day with additional readings taken overnight at least once each week to most safely and effectively make the necessary adjustments. For those with a history of nocturnal hypoglycemia or hypoglycemia unawareness, overnight readings should be recommended a few times each week to detect unrecognized nocturnal hypoglycemia.

Although the goals of intensive diabetes therapy in the Diabetes Control and Complications Trial (DCCT) were for preprandial glucoses between 70 and 120 mg/dl, postprandial glucoses below 180 mg/dl, and a glycated hemoglobin (HbA_{1c}) within two standard deviations of the nondiabetic mean,[51] this target may not be achievable for all persons.[48,48a,48b,48c] Glycemic targets must be individualized. If hypoglycemia unawareness or severe hypoglycemia becomes a problem, glycemic targets may need to be adjusted upward to prevent or reduce the occurrence of all hypoglycemia. In some cases, goals related to flexibility of life-style may be primary and blood sugar targets less rigid. Many subjects find that the use of IIT as part of an intensive diabetes therapy regimen increases their ability to control their diabetes while maintaining an active and flexible life-style, even if their overall glycemic control, as measured by blood glucose and glycated hemoglobin determinations, does not change. However, even if the specific target of near-normalization of blood glucose is not a primary goal, intensive diabetes therapy should not be implemented without the appropriate monitoring, motivation, and support just discussed.

Benefits and Risks of Intensive Diabetes Therapy

At the time of the previous edition of this book, all the benefits and risks of intensive diabetes therapy had not yet been fully defined.[45] The potential benefits included (1) increased flexibility of life-style, (2) better glycemic control resulting in reduced prevalence, delayed onset, slowed progression, or reversal of diabetic complications, (3) better glycemic control during pregnancy with better fetal outcome,[63,65] and (4) an increased feeling of well-being and control. The increased flexibility comes as a result of using premeal bolus doses instead of twice a day "split-mixed" insulin for IIT. Insulin doses are given and timed based on planned meals and activities, whereas in a conventional insulin regimen, meals and activities need to be planned and timed around the insulin doses. Snacks are often an essential part of any conventional therapy regimen because of the peaking insulin action between meals and during periods of activity. With IIT, inappropriately timed peaks of insulin action are not usually present and many of these snacks are no longer essential. Exercise snacks may still be needed, especially for strenuous or prolonged exercise. A bedtime snack is still recommended as protection against nocturnal hypoglycemia.

The potential risks of intensive diabetes therapy include (1) an increased rate of severe hypoglycemia, (2) an increased rate of mild hypoglycemia, (3) excessive weight gain, and (4) the possibility of life-threatening DKA or hypoglycemia as a result of pump malfunction in those using CSII. This latter complication is now unusual using modern pump technology and well-educated, conscientious patients. However, severe hypoglycemia continues to be a major concern, and this could become more of a problem with the development of autonomic neuropathy, hypoglycemia unawareness, defective glucose counterregulation, or hypoglycemia-associated autonomic failure* (see earlier discussion). Mild hypoglycemia is also more common, but this is not usually thought of as a major risk unless hypoglycemia-associated autonomic failure develops or hypoglycemia is frequent enough to interfere with maintenance of a normal life-style. Intensive diabetes therapy had also been associated with excess weight gain.

Preliminary studies reported more than a decade ago demonstrated that intensive diabetes therapy does not reverse diabetes complications at the later stages, and such therapy can result in transient worsening at earlier stages.[57] Studies also showed that intensive diabetes therapy could reverse some of the early subclinical measures associated with complications.†

---

*References 37a, 37b, 40a, 147a, 161a, 161b, 161c.
†References 119, 125, 157, 160, 161.

Table 10-4   Reduction of Diabetes-related Complications in the DCCT

Diabetes-related complication	Risk reduction (95% CI)*
Retinopathy	
First appearance	27% (9-41)
3-Step progression	63% (52-71)
Severe background or proliferative	47% (15-67)
Laser photocoagulation therapy	51% (21-70)
Microalbuminuria (>40 mg/day)	39% (21-52)
Proteinuria (>300 mg/day)	54% (10-74)
Clinical neuropathy	60% (38-74)

Modified from DCCT Research Group: *New Engl J Med* 329:981, 1993.
*Percent risk reduction (95% confidence interval).

However, it has only been over the past couple of years that the benefits of intensive diabetes therapy have been clearly demonstrated.

Both the DCCT[48a] and the Stockholm Diabetes Intervention Trial[119a] have now clearly demonstrated the effectiveness of intensive diabetes therapy aimed at reducing blood glucose in preventing the onset and slowing the progression of diabetic complications. Specifically, the DCCT clearly demonstrated that lowering hemoglobin A_{1c} from a mean of 9.0% (in the conventional group) to 7.1% (in the intensive group) reduced the rate of development and progression of retinopathy, nephropathy, and neuropathy by 23% to 76%.[48a] (See Table 10-4.) There was also a suggestion of reduction in macrovascular disease as a result of intensive diabetes therapy. However, these benefits were not without some risk. Severe hypoglycemia was 3.2 times more likely in the intensively treated patients than in those conventionally treated.[48b] In addition, the intensively treated patients gained an average of 4.6 kg more than the conventionally treated patients during the study. The overall benefit and risk results in the DCCT were similar for the adolescents (younger than 18 years at enrollment) as for the adults.[48c] (See Table 10-5.) This is despite the fact that the glycemic control of the adolescents was worse than that of the adults; hemoglobin A_{1c} and hypoglycemia rates were higher in the adolescents in both groups than those of the adults. The reader is referred to the references 44 to 46 and 48a to 48c for a more detailed description and summary of the DCCT. The major references 48a to 48c and various commentaries 3a and 161a to 161c related to the DCCT should be considered essential reading for all health care professionals who deal with diabetic patients.

Now that the results of the DCCT are known, intensive diabetes therapy should be considered the treatment of choice for many diabetic subjects. It should be noted that the participants in the DCCT were carefully screened and selected for their motivation to complete this important 10-year clinical trial, and the professional staff overseeing their management were specifically trained and highly motivated. Diabetes-related care and supplies were provided at minimal or no cost to reduce barriers to implementation as much as possible. Despite this, intensive diabetes therapy was not perfect. Some patients were unable to achieve and maintain the goals of the intensive group. Therefore the decision to implement intensive diabetes therapy, and particularly intensive insulin therapy, must be individualized.

Table 10-5   Comparison Between DCCT Results in Adolescents and Adults

	Adolescents	Adults	p-value*
HbA$_{1c}$ (%; mean ± SEM)			
Intensive	8.06 ± 0.13	7.12 ± 0.03	<0.001
Conventional	9.76 ± 0.12	9.02 ± 0.05	<0.001
Difference	1.70 ± 0.18	1.90 ± 0.06	0.134
Risk reduction (%) (95% CI)†			
Retinopathy			
Any	30 (−9, 55)	27 (9, 41)	0.819
Progression	61 (30, 78)	63 (51, 71)	0.802
Albumin >40 mg/day	35 (−7, 60)	45 (20, 55)	0.886
Severe hypoglycemia			
Rate‡ (intensive group)	85.7	56.9	0.004
Relative risk§	2.93	3.30	0.753

Modified from DCCT Research Group: *J Pediatr* 125:186, 1994.
*Adolescent versus adult.
†Percent risk reduction (95% confidence interval).
‡Events per 100 patient-years.
§Intensive compared with conventional.

Experience with IIT in young children is still limited, and experience with implementing this therapy in teenagers has been mixed.[11,136] Despite the demonstrated benefits of intensive therapy in adolescents,[48c] many teenagers are not adequately motivated and lack the appropriate support to successfully and safely implement IIT. Caution must also be used in implementing IIT in older adults and those with advanced complications or cardiovascular disease. Although it is likely that patients with NIDDM will benefit from lower blood glucose, the risks and benefits of IIT in NIDDM remain to be determined. (See sections following for additional age-related considerations in infants and young children, adolescents, and older adults.)

The decision to implement intensive diabetes therapy should be made only after careful consideration of the risks and benefits by a team of health care professionals experienced in the care of persons with diabetes. The patient's level of education and motivation, as well as support systems, need to be considered. A health care team familiar with the patient and knowledgeable and experienced in intensive diabetes therapy should be available at all times.

AGE-RELATED CONSIDERATIONS: INFANTS AND CHILDREN

IDDM is by far the most common cause of diabetes in infants and children. Prompt diagnosis and treatment of new-onset IDDM in infants and young children is of critical importance because delay may result in increased morbidity and mortality. A delay in diagnosis can be caused by the nonspecific nature of symptoms in this age-group. Vomiting, dehydration, irritability, fever, and frequent urination can commonly be seen in infants and children with illness other than IDDM. Kussmaul breathing in an infant or young child may be confused with a respiratory disorder such as asthma or pneumonitis. Metabolic acidosis, and even ketoacidosis, can occur in certain inborn errors of metabolism. During infancy, a high degree of suspicion is necessary to lead one to screen for IDDM by measuring urine glucose and ketones. Of course, establishing a definite diagnosis of diabetes requires measurement of blood glucose; diagnosis of diabetes mellitus should never be made using urine glucose alone.

The medical history should focus on the classic signs and symptoms of diabetes mellitus, including increased urination, extreme thirst, and weight loss. Parents may report that the child's urine has become "sticky" as a result of glycosuria. Parents often describe that their child will "drink anything and everything," including water from toilets, pets' bowls, the bath, or watering cans for plants. Diabetes insipidus can also be mistaken for diabetes mellitus in this age group.

Hyperglycemia or diabetes presenting in the first few days of life is quite rare. Although IDDM can be present very early in life, other types of diabetes need to be considered if hyperglycemia presents within the first few weeks of life. Disorders that need to be considered in this setting include agenesis of the pancreas, genetic mutations of the insulin gene (biologically defective insulin or hereditary hyperproinsulinemia[145]) or insulin receptor, or transient neonatal diabetes mellitus (TNDM).[14,109] TNDM is a rare and unusual disorder manifested by neonatal onset of extreme hyperglycemia without ketosis but associated with severe failure to thrive. The condition lasts between 1 and 18 months and subsequently resolves with no residual identifiable abnormality of carbohydrate metabolism. However, during the period of abnormality, treatment with low doses of insulin is essential to establish normal growth[18] and prevent marked hyperglycemia. The etiology of TNDM is unknown but may represent a process of pancreatic islet cell dysmaturity.[109]

Luckily, IDDM is uncommon during infancy. The initial management of IDDM in infants and children is a therapeutic challenge that can be overwhelming for even the most capable of families[74] (see Chapters 17 and 18). After the diagnosis of IDDM has been made in an infant or toddler, the family should be referred to a center with a multidisciplinary diabetes health care team experienced in the management of children with diabetes.[94] The goals of treating an infant or toddler with IDDM should differ from those of treating older patients. The major goals should be (1) avoidance of hypoglycemia, (2) maintenance of normal growth and development, (3) avoidance of DKA, (4) maintenance of emotional well-being, and (5) freedom from persistent symptoms. Euglycemia and normalization of glycated hemoglobin are not primary goals in these patients because the risk of severe hypoglycemia may be too great. In 1961 Ack and associates[1] reported lower IQ scores in children with IDDM diagnosed before the age of 5 years. Both EEG abnormalities and deficits of cognitive function have been reported in children diagnosed before 4 years of age and in children who have had previous bouts of severe hypoglycemia.[77,122,143]

Initiating Therapy

Hospitalization is necessary for most infants and toddlers with new-onset IDDM. In this environment, initiation of insulin hormone replacement therapy, family education, and close monitoring of the patient and progress of the parents in learning diabetes care skills can be carefully followed. Most infants and toddlers will require an initial insulin dose of about 0.5 U/kg/day. Though not universal, some pediatric endocrinologists feel that pork insulin is preferable to human insulin in infants and toddlers because of its longer time course of action. However, most pediatric endocrinologists initiate therapy using human insulin at all ages. Most patients are begun on intermediate-acting insulin (NPH or Lente) alone, or a split-mixed regimen, with doses before breakfast and supper. Changes of insulin doses should be made as indicated by blood glucose monitoring after observing 1 or 2 days of blood glucose values. It can be anticipated that the child's activity and appetite in the hospital environment will not be equivalent to what it will be at home. It is often necessary to decrease insulin dose after discharge from the hospital when the child's activity is greater and as the honeymoon phase begins.[142] Intensive insulin therapy is unproven in this age-group and should not be employed until it has been studied further.

Management Strategies

For children who weigh less than 10 kg and require less than 5 U of insulin per day, it is often necessary to adjust insulin by fractions of a unit.[71,74] Because doses this small are difficult to precisely measure using U-100 insulin, a diluted insulin (usually U-10) can be used. Diluent is available from most insulin manufacturers. Diluted insulin should be clearly labeled, and each vial should usually not be used for longer than 1 month. Despite the recent literature suggesting that some of the variability of insulin absorption and blood sugars can be reduced by using the same anatomic site[9] (i.e., not rotating), rotation of injection sites continues to be important in infants and young children. Because of the relatively small area for injection at each anatomic site, lipodystrophy may develop if injection sites are not rotated. In addition, parents are rarely comfortable using the abdominal injection sites in infants and toddlers, although these sites can be used.

It is normal for children to be frightened of shots and for the parents to harbor much anxiety about giving injections. Many parents feel that they are hurting their child both physically and emotionally when they give injections. Injections should be given quickly and without a need to firmly restrain the child. Discussion and debate with the child about his or her receiving injections usually prolongs the anticipated concern related to the injection for both patient and parents and usually increases the anxiety. Most often the young child forgets the discomfort of the injection shortly after the injection is given. The child (and parent) need to be reassured about their fear of injections from the beginning of therapy. Most young children become quickly acclimated to receiving injections and to monitoring blood glucose when the parents express less anxiety about it. Infants and toddlers are obviously too young to give their own injections, although some school-age children can learn to help with parts of the procedure. Forced-air or jet insulin injectors are not usually recommended for infants and young children with IDDM because they are designed for use in older patients, are not necessarily without pain, and do not obviate the anxiety related to insulin administration. Other injection aids are often useful.

Nutritional planning for the infant or young child with IDDM is also uniquely different from that of older patients.[71] Children under 4 years of age are usually unpredictable in their eating habits. Infants are fed around the clock and on demand. Behaviors typical of the "terrible twos" can certainly last more than just 1 year. A specific, rigid meal plan may not be a reasonable goal at this age. The child should be offered a well-balanced diet usually consisting of four to six feedings a day for infants and three meals and three snacks a day for toddlers. Avoidance of concentrated sweets should be encouraged. A pediatric nutritionist with experience in the treatment of infants and young children with IDDM should be consulted initially and should be available to the family to help answer questions and solve problems. Force feeding of the child who refuses to eat should be discouraged. Rather, a reduction of insulin dose of 10% to 20% and looser blood sugar goals should be used. Variability of blood sugars is to be expected, since variability in dietary intake and activity is unavoidable. Avoidance of hypoglycemia should be a primary goal in this age-group.

Normal growth is also of utmost importance. Growth and development of the child should be determined and plotted on standard growth curves at each visit. Most diabetic children grow within the normal percentiles of the appropriate growth curve when taking into account parental height. However, children with poor diabetic control grow slightly slower[154] and can develop growth failure[95] (see discussion under "Growth Failure in Diabetes and Mauriac's Syndrome"). A decline in growth velocity or poor weight gain may indicate underinsulinization, undernutrition, hypothyroidism, or other chronic medical illness. Excessive weight gain is uncommon in toddlers with IDDM but may reflect overinsulinization and/or overfeeding.

The question remains as to what the optimal degree of metabolic control is for infants and toddlers with IDDM.[36] Parents tend to be anxious about diabetes complications and their relationship with blood glucose control. This relationship is not well established for young children, however, and the risks related to hypoglycemia are well established. Many investigators have recently suggested that the postpubertal duration of IDDM is a more accurate determinant of the development of microvascular complications than total duration, suggesting that the contribution of the prepubertal years of diabetes to the development of long-term complications may be minimal.* To prevent severe hypoglycemia, preprandial blood glucose values of 80 to 150 mg/dl (4.5 to 8.4 mM) are generally recommended, although targets need to be individualized.

Self-monitoring of blood glucose

Parents of all children with IDDM should be instructed in self-monitoring of blood glucose (SMBG). Urine glucose monitoring is unreliable and will not detect low blood glucose. Collection of urine can be difficult to obtain when needed. At least two preprandial blood glucose determinations, as well as a bedtime determination, should be requested each day in this age-group. Parents should check the child's glucose if hypoglycemia is suspected. Urinary ketones should be checked whenever blood glucose is unexpectedly greater than 240 mg/dl (13.4 mM) or if the child is ill. Urine can often be obtained from diapers or bedding. Glycated hemoglobin determinations should be obtained every 3 to 4 months at routine visits. Before 6 to 9 months of life, determinations of glycated hemoglobin need to be performed

---

*References 8, 42, 89, 120, 155.

by a method in which hemoglobin F does not interfere, such as a total glycated hemoglobin by affinity chromatography.

Hypoglycemia

Hypoglycemia in the infant and toddler deserves special consideration because these children are limited in how they can respond to low blood glucose and their response is easily confused with other needs. Early recognition and treatment of hypoglycemia is important, and families should be taught, before the patient's discharge from the hospital, how to recognize and treat both mild and severe insulin reactions. In the infant, hypoglycemia may present as fussiness, irritability, crying, pallor, somnolence, unconsciousness, or convulsion. In the toddler, hypoglycemia may present as night terrors, temper tantrums, voracious appetite, moodiness, sweating, shaking, staring, or seizure. It has been suggested that severe hypoglycemic reactions during the period of neurologic development may be a cause of cognitive deficits later in life.[1,77,122,143] Unrecognized nocturnal hypoglycemia is of great concern to these families. Restlessness during sleep, night terrors, and sweating may be signs of nocturnal hypoglycemia. Blood glucose determinations during the night at the time of peak action of the evening NPH or Lente insulin may help detect unrecognized nocturnal hypoglycemia. These blood glucose determinations are often suggested soon after discharge from the hospital, when increases in the evening insulin dose are recommended, and when symptoms suggestive of hypoglycemia are occurring during sleep.

Treatment of severe hypoglycemia should not await confirmation by blood glucose determination (see Chapters 17 and 18). Mild reactions can be confirmed by the blood glucose meter. Mild insulin reactions in a conscious child can be treated with 2 to 4 ounces of fruit juice or regular soft drink. Glucose paste or cake frosting in a tube is a good alternative that can be easily carried out of the home. Glucose tablets and candy present a risk of aspiration in this age-group and are not recommended. Severe insulin reactions should be treated immediately with glucagon. Administration of glucagon should not be delayed until the child is unconscious or convulsing but may be given when the risk of aspiration or ability to drink is in question.

Glucagon is available in a standard 1-mg vial with 1 ml of diluent. Children weighing less than 30 kg should receive 0.5 mg (0.5 ml) of glucagon, and children heavier than 30 kg should receive 1 mg (1 ml). Nausea and vomiting are not infrequently seen after glucagon administration. When glucagon is administered, the family should be instructed to contact the child's physician without delay. If vomiting should occur, the child should be taken to an emergency room so intravenous dextrose can be administered. After the occurrence of severe hypoglycemia, a precipitating cause should be sought. In infants and toddlers, if no cause is found, the insulin dose should empirically be reduced by 10% to 20%.

Psychosocial Considerations

Emotional growth and well-being present particular difficulties for the preschool-age child with IDDM and for his or her parents. The young child's limited cognitive ability to cope with the stress of diabetes and its management may lead to other coping strategies such as aggression, noncompliance, withdrawal, and psychosomatic complaints. A child's resolution of separation anxiety and development of self-confidence may be impeded by life with IDDM. These concerns may contribute to risk of developing general adjustment difficulties to the behavioral demands of IDDM.[165] It is easy to understand how many parents feel overwhelmed by the responsibility of daily care for their child with IDDM. It is important that both parents learn daily diabetes care together and share the responsibilities of home management for their child. Equally important is the involvement of the diabetes health care team and primary care physician in helping to problem solve and provide psychosocial support to the family. More detailed discussion of care for the infant and young child is addressed in Chapters 17 and 18.

AGE-RELATED CONSIDERATIONS: ADOLESCENCE TO ADULTHOOD

Another very difficult period of life for diabetes management is that of adolescence and the transition to adulthood (see Chapters 19 and 20). Deterioration of glycemic control at the time of adolescence is multifactorial, including psychosocial, physiologic, emotional, and developmental factors. Puberty is associated with a component of insulin resistance. This can be demonstrated in nondiabetic adolescents as higher insulin levels during an oral glucose tolerance test[19] and in teenagers with and without diabetes by using glucose clamp studies.[5] The cause of this insulin resistance is not known but probably relates to the normally occurring hormonal changes of puberty. Because of this relative insulin resistance, many teenagers require as much as 1.0 to 1.5 U/kg/day of insulin. Furthermore, it is becoming increasingly apparent that puberty is a risk factor for the initial development of complications in patients with IDDM.* The period of adolescent development begins with both physical and behavioral changes. It is during this period of development that independence from dependent relationships (family and parents) begins and peer acceptance gains more importance. Body awareness and physical appearance become paramount, and independent cognitive, biophysical, psychologic, social, and sexual identity develops. Diabetes self-care requires balancing many metabolic and life-style factors, and each person must make many diabetes-related choices each day. Problem-solving on these new constructs sets the stage for rebellion and anxiety as self-esteem and confidence fluctuate on a daily basis.

Diabetes Education

The challenge of diabetes education during adolescence is to provide a transition of care from the parents to the child that not only addresses metabolic control of the disease but empowers the developing young adult to gain understanding of diabetes self-care and the consequences based on his or her own goals and choices. Few adolescents will accept complete parental control of their diabetes, but many will do poorly without some continued parental support.[86] This challenges the drive for independence and peer acceptance. Empowerment is a process by which people gain mastery over their own affairs.[117] Empowerment places emphasis on the whole person (biopsychosocial). Components of empowerment include (1) finding personal strengths rather than shortcomings, (2) identifying the learning needs of the patient, (3)

---

*References 8, 42, 89, 120, 155.

negotiating common goals, (4) transferring decision making to the patient, (5) encouraging self-generation of solutions to problems, (6) analyzing failure to achieve goals as a problem to solve rather than as personal failure, (7) encouraging use of support networks, (8) promoting the patient's inherent drive toward health and wellness, and (9) recognizing behavior change as an achievement.[66] The physician and other health care providers should be willing to compromise on almost all aspects of the diabetes care in meeting the personal goals of the patient as he or she learns self-care. Even the slightest acceptance of self-care should be encouraged, and failure of an agreed treatment goal must be evaluated as a problem to solve and not as a personal deficit. Health care providers should act as a resource and objective sounding board for the patient so as to not be viewed as a surrogate parent by the patient.

During office or clinic visits, the adolescent should be seen alone and a summary session held with the parents at the end of the visit. This promotes a relationship between health care provider and patient, yet keeps parents informed and provides them with an opportunity to discuss areas of concern with the clinician and their child. Treatment regimens and goals should be kept as simple as possible. SMBG and record keeping seem to be particularly difficult tasks for adolescents to perform. Patients who refuse to perform self-care should not be abandoned, and any agreement to perform monitoring should be praised. Health care providers should be willing and ready to make major alterations in diabetes self-care expectations. The health care provider needs to remember that the transition from surrogate care to self-care is a long process; patient empowerment should ultimately promote this process.

Risk Behaviors

Important issues to adolescents, such as alcohol, recreational drug use, dating, sex, pregnancy planning, driving, employment, college, sports, and chronic complications from IDDM, must be openly discussed in an objective and nonjudgmental manner. Emphasis should be placed on how drugs and alcohol can affect blood glucose levels. Smoking should be strongly discouraged. Patients should be informed about how to prevent unwanted pregnancy and sexually transmitted diseases. Ready access to birth control counseling should be made available to the patient. Those patients planning a pregnancy should be informed of the importance of achieving excellent metabolic control before conceiving and maintaining it throughout pregnancy[63,65] and should also be referred to expert obstetric care. Often genetic counseling is helpful for these patients to answer questions about probability of their child developing IDDM. Medic alert badges should be worn by all persons with IDDM operating a motor vehicle. Hypoglycemia and unrecognized low blood glucose are important issues to address when discussing driving. Adolescents with IDDM can participate safely in all types of sports and activities as long as they are taught how to adjust food or insulin in relation to their activity. A carbohydrate source to treat insulin reactions should be available during and after exercise. Exercise snacks are often necessary. The potential benefit of regular physical activity should be explained.

As the adolescent makes transition to young adulthood, the option of intensive insulin therapy (IIT) should be discussed. Although, in general, IIT is usually less successful in adolescents than in adults, the benefits and risks associated with IIT are similar for adolescents as for adults.[48c] In addition to the demonstrated long-term benefits, life-style considerations make IIT a preferred mode of treatment for many young adults with IDDM. IIT can be particularly helpful in negotiating new work or school schedules that may not be as predictable as desired. IIT also provides an opportunity to master the schedules of adult life and more independence in self-care without sacrificing any degree of diabetic control.

AGE-RELATED CONSIDERATIONS: THE OLDER ADULT

The older adult with diabetes also faces special considerations and has special needs (see Chapter 21). As a person becomes older, he or she faces physiologic, cognitive, financial, and personal changes over which he or she may have little control. These developmental changes can include changes in cognitive functioning, alterations in sensory systems, decreased visual and auditory acuity, and declining dexterity, mobility, and physical strength. In addition, older persons may be faced with the loss of a spouse or loved one and the loss of financial self-determination.

The diagnosis of diabetes mellitus often brings with it the initiation of a treatment program that is likely to dictate changes in life-style. This may be particularly difficult for an older person, especially if spousal or family support is lacking. Dietary and exercise habits are already well ingrained and difficult to change. Initiation of an exercise program may be complicated by the presence of other medical conditions, disabilities, or diabetic complications. Insulin injections and blood or urine monitoring may be difficult when vision and dexterity are declining. Devices developed to help the visually impaired persons with diabetes (such as auditory additions to blood glucose meters, special syringes and magnifiers, and jet injectors) may help in some cases.

Factors related to economic and social support may become paramount. Loss of income and health benefits often results in an inability of the older patient to obtain appropriate and consistent medical care and the necessary medical supplies. Public assistance (such as Social Security or Medicare) often falls short of meeting all the needs. Loss of the spouse and unavailability of consistent help and support by family and friends also impair ability to manage diabetes and receive continued medical care. Many older persons with diabetes will not have the physical and mental capability and family and financial support to continue with an independent life-style. Adult foster care or nursing home placement may be necessary, but diabetes care may be suboptimal and very expensive in these settings.

Careful assessment of patient ability and available resources is essential. The health care team needs to be prepared to assist the individual in obtaining appropriate help with management of diabetes. This help needs to include diabetes education appropriate for age and cognitive abilities and appropriate financial and social support (e.g., supplies, transportation, in-home assistance). The diabetes care regimen needs to be designed to meet the patient's needs and to be within the patient's capabilities. Development and implementation of such regimens requires the involvement of a multidisciplinary team of experienced health care professionals, including physicians, nurse clinicians and nurse educators, a nutritionist, a social worker, and perhaps a psychologist. The reader is referred to the Reference List[74a] and to Chapter 21 of this text for more specific guidelines related to managing diabetes mellitus in older persons.

REFERENCES

1. Ack M, Miller I, Weil WB: Intelligence of children with diabetes mellitus, *Pediatrics* 28:764-770, 1961.

2. Alberti KGMM, Gill GV, Elliot MJ: Insulin delivery during surgery in the diabetic patient, *Diabetes Care* 5(suppl 1):65-77, 1982.

3. American Diabetes Association, Inc: 1994 Buyer's guide to diabetes supplies, *Diabetes Forecast* 46:48-87, 1993.

3a. American Diabetes Association: Position statement: implications of the diabetes control and complications trial, *Diabetes* 42:1555-8, 1993.

3b. American Diabetes Association: *Intensive diabetes management,* Clinical Education Series, Alexandria, Va, 1995, American Diabetes Association, Inc.

4. Amiel SA and others: Effect of intensive insulin therapy on glycemic thresholds for counterregulatory hormone release, *Diabetes* 37:901-907, 1988.

5. Amiel SA and others: Impaired insulin action in puberty: a contributing factor to poor glycemic control in adolescent diabetics, *N Engl J Med* 315:215-219, 1986.

6. Amiel SA and others: Defective glucose counterregulation after strict glycemic control of insulin-dependent diabetes mellitus, *N Engl J Med* 316:1376-1383, 1987.

7. Atiea JA and others: Early morning hyperglycemia in IDDM: acute effects of cholinergic blockade, *Diabetes Care* 12:443-448, 1989.

8. Bach LA, Jerums G: Effect of puberty on initial kidney growth and rise in kidney IGF1 in diabetic rats, *Diabetes* 39:557-562, 1990.

9. Bantle JP and others: Rotation of the anatomic regions used for insulin injections and day-to-day variability of plasma glucose in type I diabetic subjects, *JAMA* 263:1802-1806, 1990.

10. Beaufrere B and others: Dawn phenomenon in type 1 (insulin-dependent) diabetic adolescents: influence of nocturnal growth hormone secretion, *Diabetologia* 31:607-611, 1988.

11. Becker DJ and others: Current status of pump therapy in childhood, *Acta Paediatrica Japonica* 26:347-358, 1984.

12. Bergada I and others: Severe hypoglycemia in IDDM children, *Diabetes Care* 12:239-244, 1989.

13. Bergenstal RM and others: Lack of glucagon response to hypoglycemia in type I diabetes after long-term optimal therapy with a continuous subcutaneous insulin infusion pump, *Diabetes* 32:398-402, 1983.

14. Bilginturan AN, Jackson RV: Transient hyperglycemia in infancy and childhood, *Clin Pediatr* 17:338-342, 1978.

15. Birk R, Spencer ML: The prevalence of anorexia nervosa, bulimia, and induced glycosuria in IDDM females, *Diabetes Educ* 15:336-341, 1989.

16. Blackard WG and others: Morning insulin requirements: critique of dawn and meal phenomena, *Diabetes* 38:273-277, 1989.

17. Blackman JD and others: Hypoglycemic thresholds for cognitive dysfunction in humans, *Diabetes* 39:828-835, 1990.

18. Blethen SL and others: Plasma somatomedins, endogenous insulin secretion, and growth in transient neonatal diabetes mellitus, *J Clin Endocrinol Metab* 52:144-147, 1981.

19. Bloch C, Clemons P, Sperling MA: Puberty decreases insulin sensitivity, *J Pediatr* 110:481-487, 1987.

20. Bolli GB and others: Abnormal glucose counterregulation in insulin dependent diabetes mellitus: interaction of anti-insulin antibodies and impaired glucagon and epinephrine secretion, *Diabetes* 32:134-141, 1983.

21. Bolli GB and others: Effects of long-term optimization and short-term deterioration of glycemia control on glucose counterregulation in type I diabetes mellitus, *Diabetes* 33:394-400, 1984.

22. Bolli GB and others: Demonstration of a dawn phenomenon in normal human volunteers, *Diabetes* 33:1150-1153, 1984.

23. Bolli GB and others: A reliable and reproducible test for adequate glucose counterregulation in type I (insulin-dependent) diabetes mellitus, *Diabetes* 33:732-737, 1984.

24. Bolli GB and others: Role of hepatic autoregulation in defense against hypoglycemia in humans, *J Clin Invest* 75:1623-1631, 1985.

25. Bolli GB, Gerich JE: The "dawn phenomenon"—a common occurrence in both non-insulin-dependent and insulin-dependent diabetes mellitus, *N Engl J Med* 310:746-750, 1984.

26. Bolli GB and others: Glucose counterregulation and waning of insulin in the Somogyi phenomenon (posthypoglycemic hyperglycemia), *N Engl J Med* 311:1214-1219, 1984.

27. Bolli GB and others: Defective glucose counterregulation after subcutaneous insulin in noninsulin dependent diabetes mellitus, *J Clin Invest* 73:1532-1541, 1984.

28. Boyle PJ and others: Absence of the dawn phenomenon and abnormal lipolysis in growth hormone deficient IDDM's, *Diabetes* 38(suppl 2):3A, 1989.

29. Boyle PJ and others: Plasma glucose concentrations at the onset of hypoglycemic symptoms in patients with poorly controlled diabetes and in nondiabetics, *N Engl J Med* 318:1487-1492, 1988.

30. Campbell P and others: Pathogenesis of the dawn phenomenon in insulin-dependent diabetes mellitus: accelerated glucose production and impaired glucose utilization due to nocturnal surges in growth hormone secretion, *N Engl J Med* 312: 1473-1479, 1985.

31. Campbell PJ, Bolli GB, Gerich JE: Prevention of the dawn phenomenon (early morning hyperglycemia) in insulin-dependent diabetes mellitus by bedtime intranasal administration of a long-acting somatostatin analog, *Metabolism* 37:34-37, 1988.

32. Campbell PJ, Gerich JE: Occurrence of dawn phenomenon without change in insulin clearance in patients with insulin-dependent diabetes mellitus, *Diabetes* 35:749-752, 1986.

33. Chisholm DJ and others: Programming of insulin delivery with meals during subcutaneous insulin infusion, *Diabetes Care* 4:265-268, 1981.

34. Clarke WL, Haymond MW, Santiago JV: Overnight basal insulin requirements in fasting insulin-dependent diabetics, *Diabetes* 29:78-80, 1980.

35. Clutter WE and others: Epinephrine plasma metabolic clearance rates and physiologic thresholds for metabolic and hemodynamic actions in man, *J Clin Invest* 66:94-101, 1980.

36. Copeland KE: Too uptight about tight control? *Diabetes Care* 13:1089-1091, 1990.

36a. Cox DJ, Gonder-Frederick L, Clarke W: Driving decrements in type I diabetes during moderate hypoglycemia. *Diabetes* 42:239-243, 1993.

37. Cryer PE: Glucose counterregulation in man, *Diabetes* 30:261-264, 1981.

37a. Cryer PE: Iatrogenic hypoglycemia as a cause of hypoglycemia-associated autonomic failure in IDDM, *Diabetes* 41:255-260, 1992.

37b. Cryer PE: Hypoglycemia begets hypoglycemia in IDDM, *Diabetes* 42:1691-1693, 1993.

38. Cryer PE and others: Conference summary: hypoglycemia is IDDM, *Diabetes* 38:1193-1199, 1989.

39. Cryer PE, Gerich JE: Glucose counterregulation, hypoglycemia and intensive insulin therapy in diabetes mellitus, *N Engl J Med* 313:232-239, 1985.

40. Cryer PE, White NH, Santiago JV: The relevance of glucose counterregulation systems to patients with insulin dependent diabetes, *Endocrine Rev* 7:131-139, 1986.

40a. Dagogo-Jack S, Craft S, Cryer PE: Hypoglycemia-associated autonomic failure in insulin-dependent diabetes mellitus: recent antecedent hypoglycemia reduces autonomic responses to, symptoms of, and defense against subsequent hypoglycemia, *J Clin Invest* 91:819-828, 1993.

41. Dahl-Jorgenson K and others: Effect of near normoglycemia for two years on progression of early diabetic retinopathy, nephropathy and neuropathy: the Oslo Study, *Br Med J* 293:1185-1189, 1986.

42. Dahlquist G, Rudberg S: The prevalence of microalbuminuria in diabetic children and adolescents and its relation to puberty, *Acta Paediatr Scand* 76:795-800, 1987.

43. Davidson MB and others: Suppression of sleep-induced growth hormone secretion by anticholinergic agent abolishes dawn phenomenon, *Diabetes* 37:166-171, 1988.

44. The DCCT Research Group: The diabetes control and complications trial (DCCT): an update, *Diabetes Care* 13:427-433, 1990.

45. The DCCT Research Group: Are continuing studies of metabolic control and microvascular complications in IDDM justified? The diabetes control and complications trial (DCCT), *N Engl J Med* 318:246-250, 1988.

46. The DCCT Research Group: The diabetes control and complications trial (DCCT): design and methodological considerations for the feasibility phase, *Diabetes* 35:530-545, 1986.

47. The DCCT Research Group: Effects of age, duration and treatment of IDDM on b-cell function: observations during eligibility testing for the diabetes control and complications trial (DCCT), *J Clin Endocrinol Metab* 65:30-36, 1987.

48. The DCCT Research Group: The diabetes control and complications trial: results of the feasibility study (phase II), *Diabetes Care* 10:1-19, 1987.

48a. The Diabetes Control and Complications Trial Research Group: The effect of intensive treatment of diabetes on the development and progression of long-term complications in insulin-dependent diabetes mellitus. *N Engl J Med* 329:977-986, 1993.

48b. Diabetes Control and Complications Trial Research Group: Epidemiology of severe hypoglycemia in the Diabetes Control and Complications Trial, *Am J Med* 90:450-459, 1991.

48c. Diabetes Control and Complications Trial Research Group: Effect of intensive diabetes treatment on the development and progression of long-term complications in adolescents with insulin-dependent diabetes mellitus: Diabetes Control and Complications Trial. *J Pediatr* 125:177-188, 1994.

49. DeFeo P and others: The adrenergic contribution to glucose counterregulation in type I diabetes mellitus: dependency on A cell function and medication through beta$_2$ adrenoreceptors, *Diabetes* 32:887-893, 1983.

50. DeFeo P and others: Modest decrements in plasma glucose concentration cause early impairment in cognitive function and later activation of glucose counterregulation in the absence of hypoglycemic symptoms in normal man, *J Clin Invest* 82:436-444, 1988.

51. *Diabetes Control and Complications Trial* (Full-scale Clinical Trial-Phase III) Protocol, NIH, Pub No 88-2951, Washington, DC, 1987, US Government Printing Office.

52. Deleted in proofs.

53. Dimitriadis GD, Gerich JE: Importance of timing of preprandial subcutaneous insulin administration in the management of diabetes mellitus, *Diabetes Care* 6:374-377, 1983.

53a. Drash AL: The child, the adolescent, and the Diabetes Control and Complications Trial, *Diabetes Care* 16:1515-1516, 1993.

54. Dux S, White NH, Santiago JV: The dawn phenomenon: an increased insulin clearance rate during the prebreakfast period in diabetic and nondiabetic subjects, *J Pediatr Endocrinol* 1:171-176, 1985.

55. Dux S and others: Insulin clearance contributes to the variability of nocturnal insulin requirements in insulin-dependent diabetes, *Diabetes* 34:1260-1265, 1985.

56. Edwards GA and others: Effectiveness of low-dose continuous intravenous insulin infusion is diabetic ketoacidosis, *J Pediatr* 91:701-705, 1977.

57. Ellis D and others: Diabetic nephropathy in adolescence: appearance during improved glycemic control, *Pediatrics* 71:824-829, 1983.

58. Faich GA, Fishbein HA, Ellis SE: The epidemiology of diabetic acidosis: a population-based study, *Am J Epidemiol* 117:551, 1983.

59. Fajans SS: Scope and heterogeneous nature of MODY, *Diabetes Care* 13:49-64, 1990.

59a. Fanelli CG and others: Meticulous prevention of hypoglycemia normalizes the glycemic thresholds and magnitude of most of neuroendocrine responses to symptoms of, and cognitive function during hypoglycemia in intensively treated patients with short-term IDDM, *Diabetes* 42:1683-1689, 1993.

60. Floyd JC and others: An insulin infusion test as a predictor of metabolic events during continuous subcutaneous infusion of insulin in type I diabetes mellitus, *Diabetes Res Clin Pract Suppl* 1:S171, 1985.

61. Floyd JC and others: Prevalences of impaired secretion of pancreatic polypeptide and of cardiovascular neural signs as indicators of autonomic neuropathy in type I diabetes, *Diabetes* 36(supp 1)86A, 1987.

62. Foster DW, McGarry JD: The metabolic derangement and treatment of diabetic ketoacidosis, *N Engl J Med* 309:159-169, 1983.

63. Freinkel N, Dooley SL, Metzger BE: Care of the pregnant woman with insulin-dependent diabetes mellitus, *N Engl J Med* 313:96-101, 1985.

64. Friedenberg GR and others: Diabetes responsive to intravenous but not subcutaneous insulin: effectiveness of aprotinin, *N Engl J Med* 305:363-368, 1981.

65. Fuhrmann K and others: Prevention of congenital malformations in infant of insulin-dependent diabetic mothers, *Diabetes Care* 6:219-223, 1983.

66. Funnell MM and others: Empowerment: an idea who's time has come in diabetes education, *Diabetes Ed* 17:37-41, 1991.

67. Gale E, Kurtz A, Tattersall R: In search of the Somogyi effect, *Lancet* 2:279-282, 1980.

68. Gerich JE and others: Prevention of diabetic ketoacidosis by somatostatin: evidence for an essential role of glucagon, *N Engl J Med* 292:985-989, 1975.

69. Gill GV and others: Clinical features of brittle diabetes. In Pickup JC, editor: *Brittle diabetes,* Oxford, 1985, Blackwell Scientific Publications.

70. Golden M, Herrold A, Orr D: An approach to prevention of recurrent diabetic ketoacidosis in the pediatric population, *J Pediatr* 107:195-200, 1985.

71. Golden MP and others: Management of diabetes mellitus in children younger than five years of age, *Am J Dis* 139:448-452, 1985.

72. Goldgewicht C and others: Hypoglycaemic reactions in 172 type 1 (insulin-dependent) diabetic patients, *Diabetologia* 24:95-99, 1983.

73. Gray DL and others: Chronic poor metabolic control in the pediatric population: a stepwise intervention program, *Diabetes Educ* 14:516-520, 1988.

74. Grunt JA and others: Problems in the care of the infant diabetic patient, *Clin Pediatr* 17:772-774, 1978.

74a. Halter JB, Christensen NJ, editors: Diabetes mellitus in elderly people, *Diabetes Care* 13(suppl 2):1-98, 1990.

75. Hansen I and others: The role of autoregulation of hepatic glucose production in man: response to a physiologic decrement in plasma glucose, *Diabetes* 35:186-191, 1986.

76. Hanson CL, Henggeler SW, Burghen GA: Race and sex differences in metabolic control of adolescents with IDDM: a function of psychosocial variables? *Diabetes Care* 10:313-318, 1987.

77. Haumont D, Dorchy H, Pelc S: EEG abnormalities in diabetic children: influence of hypoglycemia and vascular complications, *Clin Pediatr* 18:750-753, 1979.

78. Havlin CE, Cryer PE: Nocturnal hypoglycemia does not commonly result in major morning hyperglycemia in patients with diabetes mellitus, *Diabetes Care* 10:141-147, 1987.

79. Henderson G: The psychosocial treatment of recurrent diabetic ketoacidosis: an interdisciplinary team approach, *Diabetes Educ* 17:119-123, 1991.

80. Herold KC and others: Variable deterioration in cortical function during insulin-induced hypoglycemia, *Diabetes* 34:677-685, 1985.

81. Hilsted J and others: No response of pancreatic hormones to hypoglycemia in diabetic autonomic neuropathy, *J Clin Endocrinol Metab* 54:815-819, 1982.

82. Hirsch IB and others: Role of insulin in management of surgical patients with diabetes mellitus, *Diabetes Care* 13:980-991, 1990.

83. Hirsch IB and others: Failure of nocturnal hypoglycemia to cause daytime hyperglycemia in patients with IDDM, *Diabetes Care* 13:133-142, 1990.

84. Hoeldtke RD and others: Reduced epinephrine secretion and hypoglycemia unawareness in diabetic autonomic neuropathy, *Ann Intern Med* 96:459-462, 1982.

85. Johnson NB and others: Twice-daily Humulin ultralente insulin decreases morning fasting hyperglycemia, *Diabetes Care* 15:1031-1033, 1992.

86. Johnson PD and others: Nonsupportive maternal behaviors are associated with poorer glycemic control in adolescents with type I diabetes (IDDM), *Diabetes* 39(suppl 1):163A, 1990.

87. Keller U, Berger W: Prevention of hypophosphatemia by phosphate infusion during treatment of diabetic ketoacidosis and hyperosmolar coma, *Diabetes* 29:87-95, 1980.

88. Kleinbaum J, Shamoon H: Effect of propranolol on delayed glucose recovery after insulin-induced hypoglycemia in normal and diabetic subjects, *Diabetes Care* 7:155-162, 1984.

89. Kostraba JN and others: Contribution of diabetes duration before puberty to development of microvascular complications of IDDM, *Diabetes Care* 12:686-693, 1989.

90. Kraegen EW, Chrisholm DJ, McNamara ME: Timing of insulin delivery with meals, *Horm Metab Res* 13:365-367, 1981.

91. Krane EJ and others: Subclinical brain swelling in children during treatment of diabetic ketoacidosis, *N Engl J Med* 312:1147-1151, 1985.

92. Kreisberg RA: Diabetic ketoacidosis: new concepts and trends in pathogenesis and treatment, *Ann Intern Med* 88:681-695, 1978.

93. The Kroc Collaborative Study: Blood glucose control and the evolution of diabetic retinopathy and albuminuria: a preliminary multicenter trial, *N Engl J Med* 311:365-372, 1984.

94. Kushion W and others: Issues in the care of infants and toddlers with insulin-dependent diabetes mellitus, *Diabetes Educ* 17:107-110, 1991.

94a. Lasker RD: The Diabetes Control and Complications Trial: implications for policy and practice, *New Engl J Med* 329:1035-1036, 1993.

95. Lee RGL, Bode HH: Stunted growth and hepatomegaly in diabetes mellitus, *J Pediatr* 91:82-84, 1977.

96. Lerman IG, Wolfsdorf JI: Relationship of nocturnal hypoglycemia to daytime glycemia in IDDM, *Diabetes Care* 11:636-642, 1988.

97. Levandoski LA, White NH, Santiago JV: How to weather the sick-day season, *Diabetes Forecast* 36:30-33, 1983.

98. Levine SN, Loewenstein JE: Treatment of diabetic ketoacidosis, *Arch Intern Med* 141:713-715, 1981.

99. Levitt NS and others: Impaired pancreatic polypeptide responses to insulin induced hypoglycemia in diabetic autonomic neuropathy, *J Clin Endocrinol Metab* 50:445-449, 1980.

100. MacDonald MJ: Postexercise late-onset hypoglycemia in insulin-dependent diabetic patients, *Diabetes Care* 10:584-588, 1987.

101. MacGorman LR, Rizza RA, Gerich JE: Physiological concentrations of growth hormone exert insulin-like and insulin antagonistic effects on both hepatic and exahepatic tissues in man, *J Clin Endocrinol Met* 53:556-559, 1981.

102. Mecklenburg RS and others: Clinical use of the insulin infusion pump in 100 patients with type I diabetes, *N Engl J Med* 307:513-518, 1982.

103. Meyers EF, Alberts D, Gordon MO: Perioperative control of blood glucose in diabetic patients: a two-step protocol, *Diabetes Care* 9:40-45, 1986.

104. Miles JM and others: Effects of acute insulin deficiency of glucose and ketone body turnover in man: evidence for the primacy of overproduction of glucose and ketones bodies in the genesis of diabetic ketoacidosis, *Diabetes* 29:926-930, 1980.

105. Muhlhauser I and others: Incidence and management of severe hypoglycemia in 434 adults with insulin-dependent diabetes mellitus, *Diabetes Care* 8:268-273, 1985.

106. Munro JF and others: Euglycaemic diabetic ketoacidosis, *Br Med J* 2:578-580, 1973.

107. Orr DP and others: Surreptitious insulin administration in adolescents with insulin-dependent diabetes mellitus, *JAMA* 256:3227-3230, 1986.

108. Orr DP and others: Characteristics of adolescents with poorly controlled diabetes referred to a tertiary care center, *Diabetes Care* 6:170-175, 1983.

109. Paglira AS, Karl IE, Kipnis DB: Transient neonatal diabetes: delayed maturation of the pancreatic beta cell, *J Pediatr* 82:97-101, 1973.

110. Paulsen EP, Courtney JW, Duckworth WC: Insulin resistance caused by massive degradation of subcutaneous insulin, *Diabetes* 28:640, 1979.

111. Perriello G and others: The effect of asymptomatic nocturnal hypoglycemia on glycemic control in diabetes mellitus, *N Engl J Med* 319:1233-1239, 1988.

112. Pezzarossa A and others: Perioperative management of diabetic subjects: subcutaneous versus intravenous insulin administration during glucose-potassium infusion, *Diabetes Care* 11:52-58, 1988.

113. Pickup JC: Preface. In Pickup JC, editor: *Brittle diabetes,* Oxford, England, 1985, Blackwell Scientific Publications.

114. Pickup JC: Clinical features of patients unresponsive to continuous subcutaneous insulin infusion. In Pickup JC, editor: *Brittle diabetes,* Oxford, 1985, Blackwell Scientific Publications.

115. Popp DA, Shah SD, Cryer PE: The role of epinephrine mediated β-adrenergic mechanisms in hypoglycemic glucose counterregulation and posthypoglycemic hyperglycemia in insulin dependent diabetes mellitus, *J Clin Invest* 69:315-326, 1982.

116. Pramming S and others: Cognitive function during hypoglycemia in type 1 diabetes mellitus, *Br Med J* 292:647-650, 1986.

117. Rappaport J: Terms of empowerment/exemplars of prevention: toward a theory for community psychology, *Am J Commun Psychol* 15:121-148, 1987.

118. Raskin P: The Somogyi phenomenon: sacred cow or bull, *Arch Intern Med* 144:781-787, 1984.

119. Raskin P and others: The effect of diabetic control on the width of skeletal-muscle capillary basement membrane in patients with type I diabetes mellitus, *N Engl J Med* 309:1546-1550, 1983.

119a. Reichard P, Nilsson B-Y, Rosenqvist U: The effect of long-term intensified insulin treatment on the development of microvascular complications of diabetes mellitus, *New Engl J Med* 329:304-309, 1993.

120. Rogers DG and others: The effect of puberty on the development of early diabetic microvascular disease in insulin-dependent diabetes, *Diabetes Res Clin Pract* 3:39-44, 1987.

121. Rosenbloom AL and others: Cerebral edema complicating diabetic ketoacidosis in childhood, *J Pediatr* 96:357-361, 1980.

122. Ryan C, Vega A, Drash A: Cognitive deficits in adolescents who developed diabetes early in life, *Pediatrics* 75:921-927, 1985.

123. Santiago JV and others: Epinephrine, norepinephrine, glucagon, and growth hormone release in association with physiologic decrements in the plasma glucose concentration in normal and diabetic man, *J Clin Endocrinol Metab* 51:877-883, 1980.

124. Santiago JV and others: Closed-loop and open-loop devices for blood glucose control in normal and diabetic subjects, *Diabetes* 28:71-84, 1979.

125. Santiago JV and others: Ocular fluorophotometry: studies in experimental and human diabetes. In Irsigler K and others, editors: *New approaches to insulin therapy,* Lancaster, England, 1981, MTP Press.

126. Santiago JV, Sargeant DT, White NH: The syndrome of excessive degradation of subcutaneously injected insulin: treatment with aprotinin. In Irsigler K, editor: *New approaches to insulin therapy,* Lancaster, England, 1981, MTP Press.

127. Santiago JV, White NH, Skor DA: Mechanical devices for insulin delivery. In Santiago J, Natrass M, editors: *Recent advances in diabetes,* Edinburgh, 1984, Churchill Livingstone.

128. Santiago JV and others: Defective glucose counterregulation limits intensive therapy of diabetes mellitus, *Am J Physiol* 247:E215-E220, 1984.

129. Schade DS: Surgery and diabetes, *Med Clin North Am* 72:1531-1543, 1988.

130. Schade DS and others: The etiology of incapacitating brittle diabetes, *Diabetes Care* 8:12-20, 1985.

131. Schade DS and others: A clinical algorithm to determine the etiology of brittle diabetes, *Diabetes Care* 8:5-11, 1985.

132. Schmidt MI and others: Fasting early morning rise in peripheral insulin: evidence of the dawn phenomenon in nondiabetics, *Diabetes Care* 7:32-35, 1984.

133. Schwartz NS and others: Glycemic thresholds for activation of glucose counterregulatory systems are higher than the threshold for symptoms, *J Clin Invest* 79:777-781, 1987.

134. Selam J-L, Charles MA: Devices for insulin administration, *Diabetes Care* 13:955-979, 1990.

135. Shalwitz RA and others: Prevalence and consequences of nocturnal hypoglycemia among conventionally treated children with diabetes mellitus, *J Pediat* 116:686-689, 1990.

136. Shiffrin AD and others: Intensified insulin therapy in the type I diabetic adolescent: a controlled trial, *Diabetes Care* 7:107-113, 1984.

137. Skor DA and others: Influence of growth hormone on overnight insulin requirements in insulin-dependent diabetics, *Diabetes* 34:135-139, 1985.

138. Skor DA and others: Relative roles of insulin clearance and insulin sensitivity in the prebreakfast increases in insulin requirements in insulin dependent diabetic patients, *Diabetes* 33:60-63, 1984.

139. Skor DA and others: Examination of the role of the pituitary-adrenocortical axis, counterregulatory hormones, and insulin clearance in variable nocturnal insulin requirements in insulin-dependent diabetes, *Diabetes* 32:403-407, 1983.

140. Skyler JS, Seigler DE, Reeves ML: Optimizing pumped insulin delivery, *Diabetes Care* 5:135-147, 1982.

141. Skyler JS and others: Algorithms for adjustment of insulin dosage by patients who monitor blood glucose, *Diabetes Care* 4:311-318, 1981.

142. Sochett EB and others: Factors affecting and patterns of residual insulin secretion during the first year of type I (insulin-dependent) diabetes mellitus in children, *Diabetologia* 30:453-459, 1987.

143. Soltesz G, Acsadi G: Association between diabetes, severe hypoglycemia and electroencephalographic abnormalities, *Arch Dis Child* 64:992-996, 1989.

144. Somogyi M: Exacerbation of diabetes by excess insulin action, *Am J Med* 26:169-191, 1959.

144a. Steindel B, Kaufman F, Roe T: Continuous subcutaneous insulin infusion (CSII) in poorly controlled patients (PT) with type I diabetes mellitus (DM), *Diabetes* 42 (Suppl 1):184A, 1993.

145. Steiner DF and others: Lessons learned from molecular biology of insulin gene mutations, *Diabetes Care* 13:600-609, 1990.

146. Stephenson JM, Schernthaner G: Dawn phenomenon and Somogyi effect in IDDM, *Diabetes Care* 12:245-251, 1989.

147. Tordjman KM and others: Failure of nocturnal hypoglycemia to cause fasting hyperglycemia in patients with insulin-dependent diabetes mellitus, *N Engl J Med* 317:1552-1559, 1987.

147a. Vaneman T and others: Induction of hypoglycemia unawareness by asymptomatic nocturnal hypoglycemia, *Diabetes* 42:1233-1237, 1993.

148. Watts NB and others: Postoperative management of diabetes mellitus steady-state glucose control with bedside algorithm for insulin adjustment, *Diabetes Care* 10:722-728, 1987.

149. Wayne EA and others: Focal neurologic deficits associated with hypoglycemia in children with diabetes, *J Pediatr* 117:575-577, 1990.

150. Weber ME, Abbassi V: Continuous intravenous insulin therapy in severe diabetic ketoacidosis: variations in dosage requirements, *J Pediatr* 91:755-756, 1977.

151. White N and others: Plasma pancreatic polypeptide measurements as a marker for defective glucose counterregulation in insulin-dependent diabetes, *Diabetes Res Clin Pract Suppl* 1:S601, 1985.

152. White NH and others: Plasma pancreatic polypeptide response to insulin induced hypoglycemia as a marker for defective glucose counterregulation in insulin-dependent diabetes mellitus, *Diabetes* 34:870-875, 1985.

153. White K and others: Unstable diabetes and unstable families: a psychosocial evaluation of diabetic children with recurrent ketoacidosis, *Pediatrics* 73:749-755, 1984.

154. White NH, Robinson GH: Impaired growth in children with poorly controlled type I diabetes (IDDM), *Pediatr Res* 21:349A, 1987.

155. White NH and others: Puberty as a risk factor for complications of diabetes mellitus (IDDM), *Pediatr Res* 25(part 2):204A, 1989.

156. White NH, Santiago JV: Clinical features and natural history of brittle diabetes in childhood. In Pickup JC, editor: *Brittle diabetes,* Oxford, 1985, Blackwell Scientific Publication.

157. White NH, Santiago JV: What can be achieved with and what are the complications of the insulin pump? In Raptis S, Church J, editors: *Diabetes mellitus: achievements and scepticism,* London, 1984, Royal Society of Medicine.

158. White NH and others: Identification of Type I diabetic patients at increased risk for hypoglycemia during intensive therapy, *N Engl J Med* 308:485-491, 1983.

159. White NH, Skor D, Santiago JV: A practical closed loop insulin delivery system for the maintenance of overnight euglycemia and the calculation of basal insulin requirements in insulin-dependent diabetics, *Ann Intern Med* 97:210-213, 1982.

160. White NH and others: Comparison of long-term intensive conventional therapy and pumped subcutaneous insulin on diabetic control, ocular fluorophotometry and nerve conduction velocities. In Brunetti P and others, editors: *Artificial systems for insulin delivery,* New York, 1983, Raven Press.

161. White NH and others: Reversal of abnormalities in ocular fluorophotometry in insulin-dependent diabetes after five to nine months of improved metabolic control, *Diabetes* 31:80-85, 1982.

161a. White NH: The risk of hypoglycemia during intensive therapy of IDDM: from research to practice, *Diabetes Spectrum* 7:231-265, 1994.

161b. White NH: Hypoglycemia: a limiting factor in implementing intensive therapy, *Clin Diabetes* July/August 1994, pp 101-105.

161c. White NH: Controversies in intensive insulin therapy, *Current Opinions in Endocrinology and Diabetes: Diabetes and the Endocrine Pancreas,* 2:45-50, 1995.

162. Wilson HK and others: Phosphate therapy in diabetic ketoacidosis, *Arch Intern Med* 142:517-520, 1982.

163. Winter WE and others: Maturity-onset diabetes of youth in black Americans, *N Engl J Med* 316:285-291, 1987.

164. Witt MF, White NH, Santiago JV: Roles of site and timing of the morning insulin injection in type I diabetes, *J Pediatr* 103:528-533, 1983.

164a. Wolfsdorf JI and others: Split-mixed insulin regimens with human ultralente before supper and NPH (Isophane) before breakfast in children and adolescents with IDDM, *Diabetes Care* 14:1100-1106, 1991.

165. Wysocki T and others: Adjustment to diabetes mellitus in preschoolers and their mothers, *Diabetes Care* 12:524-529, 1989.

11 Diabetes and Pregnancy

Priscilla Hollander

Before the introduction of insulin as a therapy in 1923, pregnant women with insulin-dependent (type I) diabetes mellitus (IDDM) were at high risk for maternal mortality and at even higher risk for perinatal mortality.[45,68] Once insulin was available, maternal mortality over the following decade fell dramatically, from 45% to 2%, for all pregnancies.[67] Perinatal mortality also improved, but more slowly, decreasing from 60% to 20% for all pregnancies by midcentury. This rate was still high when compared with the rate for nondiabetic pregnancies (Fig. 11-1).[67,111]

Not until the role of meticulous blood glucose control during pregnancy was understood and emphasized did the perinatal mortality rate reach its present level of 3% to 5%. The linear relationship between blood glucose level and perinatal mortality was demonstrated in a landmark study published by Karlsson and Kjellmer in 1972.[76] Numerous other studies have

---

CHAPTER OBJECTIVES

- Compare management of pregnancy complicated by pregestational versus gestational diabetes.
- Address issues related to the physiology of pregnancy and diabetes.
- Identify necessary components of care, including the diabetes team approach.
- Discuss complications associated with diabetes treatment during pregnancy.
- Discuss the relationship of vascular disease to diabetes and pregnancy.
- Describe outcome measures as they relate to maternal, prenatal, and neonatal complications.
- Describe management of diabetes complicated by pregestational and gestational diabetes.

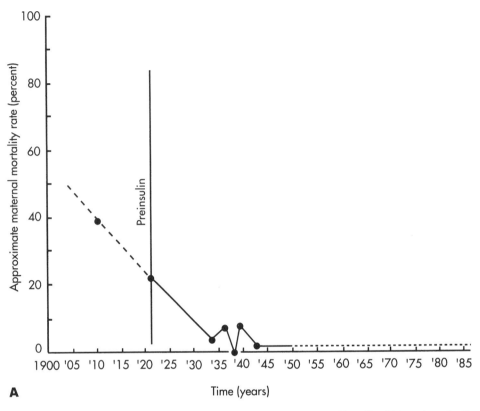

Fig. 11-1   **A,** Maternal mortality before and after the discovery of insulin. Although a decline in perinatal death was observed, this decline was gradual over time. **B,** Maternal mortality before and after the discovery of insulin. A precipitous decline in maternal deaths is depicted shortly after the discovery and use of insulin. (From Reece E: *Diabetes and pregnancy: principles and practices,* ed 2, New York, 1994, Churchill Livingstone.)   *Continued*

supported their findings (Fig. 11-2). Confirmation of the glycemic hypothesis, as shown by the results of the Diabetes Control and Complications Trial (DCCT), has further emphasized the importance of glucose control as a major determinant in achieving and maintaining an optimal metabolic environment in individuals with diabetes.[27] Two hundred and seventy pregnancies were followed in the DCCT with equal occurrence in both the experimental, intensified treatment group and the standard treatment group. Individuals in the standard group who desired pregnancy were identified and their diabetes control intensified before conception. No significant difference in fetal survival rate was found between groups, and perinatal mortality was equivalent to that seen in nondiabetic pregnancies.[74] In addition to the emphasis on blood glucose control, advances in the obstetric care of women with high-risk pregnancies have also contributed to the successful outcome of the pregnancy complicated by diabetes.[21,55]

However, some problems still are associated with the pregnancy complicated by diabetes. One of the major concerns is the high rate of congenital malformations, which ranges from

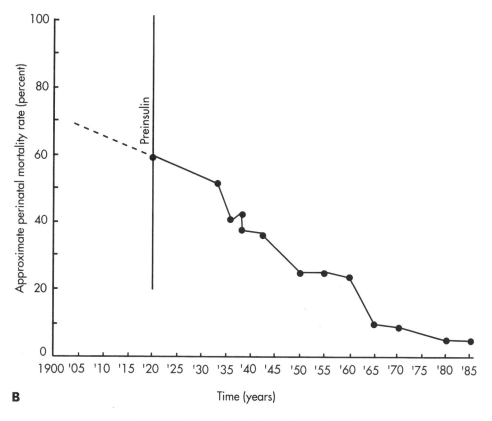

Fig. 11-1, cont'd. For legend see p. 406.

4% to 12% in various studies.[43] This risk has been related to poor glucose control during the first weeks of pregnancy and can be minimized by preconceptual glucose control.[57,79] The risks of pregnancy for the woman with pregestational diabetes also include a higher incidence of maternal complications such as toxemia, premature labor, and delivery by cesarean section and neonatal complications such as respiratory distress syndrome, macrosomia, hyperbilirubinemia, and hypoglycemia. There is also a small but significantly higher incidence of stillbirth.[18]

The concept of pregnancy complicated by gestational diabetes (glucose intolerance occurring during pregnancy that disappears following delivery) was formulated as recently as 1952; however, studies before and many after that time have shown an association between glucose intolerance diagnosed during pregnancy and maternal and neonatal morbidity.[10,64,110] How to define, diagnose, and treat diabetes optimally continues to be controversial, although there is increasing emphasis on tightening blood glucose criteria for both diagnosis and treatment.[58]

Not all the questions about diabetes and pregnancy have been answered. Nevertheless, based on present knowledge and the current approach to treatment of the pregnancy complicated by diabetes, one can assure the pregnant woman with pregestational or gestational

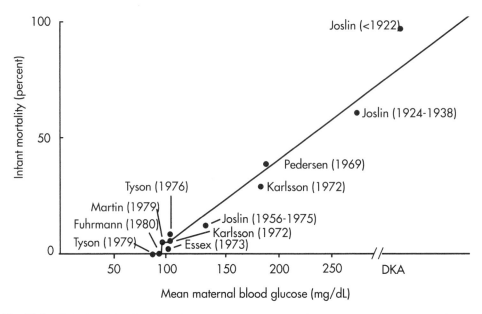

Fig. 11-2   Relationship of perinatal mortality rate to mean plasma glucose levels over the past 60 years, *DKA,* Diabetic ketoacidosis. (From Jovanovic L, Peterson CM: *Diabetes Care* 3:63, 1980.)

diabetes that her chances for a successful pregnancy are very close to those of the woman without diabetes.

Physiology of Pregnancy

The condition of pregnancy is characterized by major physiologic changes in the woman without diabetes. Every aspect of intermediary metabolism is affected. Thus it is not surprising that the combination of pregnancy and diabetes can provide the setting for the development of major metabolic dysfunction, with marked effects on the integrity of the fetus and the health of the mother. Since the goal of the optimal treatment of diabetes during pregnancy is to establish a normal or near-normal metabolic milieu for the fetus, an understanding of fetal and maternal metabolism in both the nondiabetic and the diabetic woman is important for implementing the best approach.

Maternal metabolism

The metabolic state in pregnancy has been characterized as one of "accelerated starvation." What does this phrase mean? To maintain blood glucose within accepted bounds in the fasting and postabsorptive state, the balance depends on the production and utilization of glucose. In the fasting state, glucose availability depends on the liver. The major hormonal signal regulating production of glucose by the liver is the decrease in circulating insulin levels that occurs in a fasting condition. In pregnancy, as early as perhaps the fourteenth week of gestation, fasting blood glucose levels are at 15% to 20% mg/dl lower than in the nonpregnant state.[39] Because of this decrease in blood glucose levels, the fasting insulin concentration may decrease, and this in turn may lead to an exaggeration of what is called *starvation ketosis;* that is, more fat tissue will be metabolized, leading to increased blood levels of ketones, including beta-hydroxybutyric acid and acetoacetic acid. Factors that contribute to the lower fasting blood glucose are thought to be increasing glucose utilization by the fetus and an increase in the volume of glucose distribution.

In the nongravid woman, when nutrients are ingested, they are rapidly assimilated and utilized for fuel, for replacement of tissue, and as storage in the form of glycogen or triglycerides. Ingestion of food is followed rapidly by an increase in insulin, which facilitates the utilization of the nutrients. Because of this system, blood glucose variations are somewhat limited, and blood glucose levels during the day for a nonpregnant, nondiabetic individual are maintained within a very narrow range, from 60 to 160 mg/dl.

During pregnancy, several characteristic metabolic responses occur in response to feeding. Insulin response, blood glucose levels, and triglyceride levels increase when compared with the nonpregnant state.[40,131] A diminished sensitivity to insulin also occurs, leading to increased plasma insulin levels in pregnancy. The hyperinsulinemic effect is most noted in the third trimester. During the pregnancy the amount of insulin produced by the pancreas may increase by two- to threefold.[16] Studies have indicated that tissue sensitivity may be reduced by as much as 80% in pregnancy. This insulin resistance in pregnancy is thought to be related to the increased production of the hormones of pregnancy, including human placental lactogen, progesterone, and estrogen.[65,75,128] Another factor that may be related to increasing insulin resistance during pregnancy is the increase in both maternal weight and fetal and placental weight.

Because of the decreased responsiveness of maternal tissues to insulin during normal pregnancy, an exaggerated rise in plasma glucose concentration may be seen after a meal compared with the nonpregnant state. For individuals who may have an inherited defect in beta-cell function, the secretion of insulin by the mother may fail to keep up with the insulin demands of the pregnancy. If this is the case, an increase in blood glucose levels may occur, resulting in the appearance of overt diabetes, that is, the condition termed *gestational diabetes.*

Fetal metabolism

The fuel requirements of the developing fetus are met mainly by glucose.[6] The level of glucose in fetal blood is generally 10 to 20 mg/dl below that in the maternal circulation.[7] Therefore diffusion favors the movement of glucose from the mother to the fetus. In contrast to the movement of glucose to the fetus, maternal insulin and glucagon do not traverse the placenta.[37] Therefore fetal glucose utilization is not directly dependent on maternal insulin availability.

Fetal insulin is thought to play an important role in the growth of the fetus. Insulin has been shown to be present as early as 9 weeks of gestation.[89] Not only is glucose transferred across the placenta, but amino acids are actively transported from the maternal to the fetal circulation. Transfer of free fatty acids from the maternal to the fetal circulation is limited to the provision of essential fatty acids.[37] Unfortunately, ketones such as

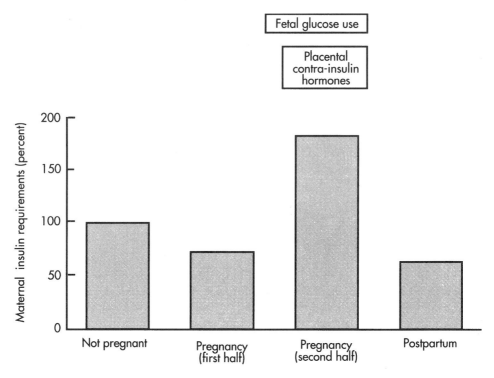

Fig. 11-3   Influence of pregnancy on insulin requirements. The prepregnancy insulin dose is shown as 100%. (Modified from Felig P, Coustan C: In Burrows G, Ferris F: *Medical complications during pregnancy,* Philadelphia, 1987, Saunders.)

beta-hydroxybutyrate and acetoacetate are also readily transferred to the fetus through a diffusion process.[124]

Because the volume of glucose transferred across the placenta is related to the level of maternal blood glucose in a pregnancy complicated by diabetes, the level of glucose available to the fetus could vary enormously. At times adequate substrate might not be available, but, more often, there may be excess glucose delivery. The effects of high concentrations of glucose have been observed in animal experiments.[127] If a continuously high level of glucose is presented to the fetus, fetal insulin production will increase and hyperinsulinemia will result. According to the Pederson hypothesis,[112] increased levels of insulin in the fetus lead to increased fat deposition and macrosomia. Since ketones are also transferred across the placenta, high blood levels of ketones present in the mother could be present in the fetus.

Overview of insulin requirements during pregnancy

Fig. 11-3 illustrates the relationship of maternal insulin requirements to the changes in glucose metabolism. During the early stages of pregnancy, the main factor influencing carbohydrate metabolism is the transfer of glucose and amino acids to the fetus. This transfer may result in symptomatic hypoglycemia in the mother. Some women may actually need a reduction in insulin dosage during the first trimester.[141] The increased risk for hypoglycemia may prevail for up to 12 to 18 weeks, but its occurrence can vary with the individual pregnancy.

During the second half of the pregnancy, the diabetogenic actions of the placental hormones start to become increasingly evident, and their effect will outweigh the use of maternal glucose by the fetus. Insulin needs increase most dramatically between 20 and 29 weeks in most patients, but individual changes may vary greatly. In a recent study by Steel and others,[132] the average increase in insulin need during the pregnancy is 52 U, ranging from 5 to 100 U. Changes may be rapid, so dosage must be adjusted frequently. With the increase in insulin resistance that occurs during this phase, ketogenesis may be more active in some women. During the last 3 to 4 weeks of pregnancy, insulin requirements may level off, or, in some women, decrease. Episodes of moderate or even severe hypoglycemia may occur.

Why insulin requirements may decrease toward the end of the pregnancy is unclear. Placental detachment or decreasing placental activity may underlie this phenomena. In the study by Steel and others,[131] however, a decrease in insulin requirements was seen in 15% of women but was not associated with poor fetal outcome. McManus and Ryan[96] also found no association between a third-trimester decrease in insulin requirements and fetal outcome.

After delivery the concentrations of human placental lactogen, estrogen, and progesterone fall rapidly.[15] In fact, within hours the insulin requirements are rapidly reduced to prepregnancy needs or less. No insulin may be required on the day of delivery and for up to 24 to 48 hours thereafter. Insulin requirements generally return to prepregnancy levels within 4 to 8 weeks. Special dietary needs, such as increased caloric intake for nursing or decreased caloric intake for weight loss, may also play a role in determining postpregnancy insulin requirements.

MANAGEMENT OF PREGNANCY COMPLICATED BY PREGESTATIONAL DIABETES

The primary goal of treatment for the pregnancy complicated by pregestational diabetes is strict metabolic control. This approach starts with preconceptual glucose control to decrease the rate of fetal malformation and continues throughout the pregnancy. Although the importance of blood glucose control has been widely advocated, what blood glucose goals should be sought during pregnancy has led to some discussion. Pregnant women without diabetes have fasting plasma glucose values averaging 74 to 88 mg/dl and 1-hour postprandial mean values of 90 to 100 mg/dl (Fig. 11-4).[69] Such a woman rarely has plasma glucose exceed 130 mg/dl. As early as 1972, in a study of pregnancy complicated by diabetes, Karlsson and Kjellmer[76] reported perinatal mortality rates of 3.68 if the average blood glucose level was kept below 100 mg/dl. Other research studies have also demonstrated that the best outcomes are achieved when blood glucose profiles approximate those of the pregnant woman without diabetes.

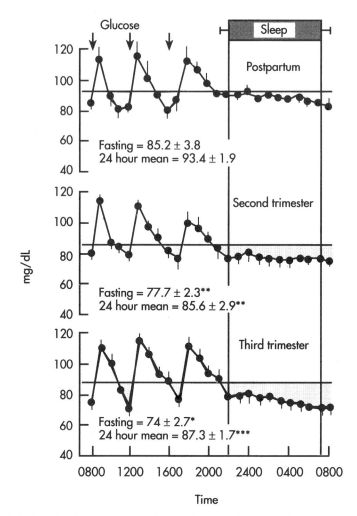

Fig. 11-4 Variations in plasma glucose levels during a 24-hour blood glucose profile in six normal pregnant women during the second and third trimesters of pregnancy and 6 to 11 weeks' postpartum. Meals are indicated by ↓. Data points reflect ± SEM. Horizontal lines represent the 24-hour mean. *$p < 0.05$; **$p < 0.01$; ***$p < 0.005$. (From Cousins L and others: *Am J Obstet Gynecol* 136:483, 1980.)

Recent studies have resulted in a better definition of goals. The importance of postprandial glucose in the development of macrosomia has been more clearly defined, and keeping the 1- to 2-hour postprandial glucose value at less than 120 mg/dl should be emphasized more strongly.[12] At present or until other data are available, target goals for the pregnancy complicated by diabetes should include fasting plasma glucose levels in the range of 60 to 90 mg/dl and 1-hour postprandial blood glucose values of approximately 120 mg/dl. Glycated hemoglobin goals should be well within the normal range of the assay used for monitoring.

Components of Care

Setting the optimal blood glucose goals is important for the treatment of the pregnant woman with diabetes, but the challenge lies in helping the woman achieve these goals. A well-structured treatment program with different care components is needed for success.

Team Approach

Many high-risk pregnancy treatment centers have found that the most effective way to treat the pregnant woman with diabetes is to use a team consisting of an obstetrician who specializes in high-risk pregnancy, a diabetologist, a nurse educator, and a nutritionist. In some centers the perinatologist may also be part of the team. Often a psychologist or social worker is of benefit as well. The team members should know and understand their responsibilities, and communication should be open. In some cases the physical location of the team members may be different, with the diabetes team located in one area and the obstetric team in another. Such physical separations may be overcome by preset guidelines for written and oral communication.

The most important member of the team is the woman with diabetes. She must undertake the major responsibilities of carrying out the day-to-day regimen. If she does not accept and understand the goals of the program, the risk for complications during the pregnancy will increase. Her personal support system is also key. The father and other family members must support and help the woman in performing the rigors of her daily diabetes self-management program.

The responsibilities of the diabetes management team once the woman is pregnant include an initial assessment of the woman's current diabetes regimen and development of a plan for consistent and routine follow-up (Boxes 11-1 and 11-2).

Appointments for the pregnant woman should be frequent. In some centers these appointments are set up every 2 weeks with both the obstetrician and the diabetes management team. Some appointment schedules will need to be individualized, and initially the patient may need to see the diabetes team more often, with more frequent obstetric appointments as the pregnancy proceeds.

Automatic hospitalization of a pregnant woman with IDDM or non-insulin-dependent diabetes mellitus (NIDDM) to achieve metabolic control is not necessary in most cases. If glucose control is poor and factors such as intellect, compliance, and social situations make achieving diabetes control on an outpatient basis difficult, it is best to hospitalize the individual for 5 to 7 days. For women with diabetic complications, such as poorly controlled hypertension, renal disease, neuropathies, or a history of severe hypoglycemia, the goal of treatment, whether through inpatient or outpatient programs, is to bring the blood glucose levels into the target range within 1 to 2 weeks. The hospital may be the proper setting to help them achieve blood glucose control.

Self-monitoring of blood glucose

The development of the technology for self-monitoring of blood glucose (SMBG) has been a major advance in the ability to treat diabetes and has been especially beneficial for the monitoring of blood glucose during pregnancy. By using the technique of SMBG,

---

BOX 11-1

BASELINE ASSESSMENT OF THE PREGNANT WOMAN WITH DIABETES

Endocrinologist

1. Discuss diabetes and pregnancy and risks for mother and child.
2. Discuss importance of blood glucose control during pregnancy and outline blood glucose goals.
3. Assess current insulin regimen and past history of blood glucose control.
4. Medical history
   a. General health
   b. Risk factors
   c. Obstetric/gynecologic history
   d. Current medications
   e. Smoking, alcohol use
5. Physical examination
   a. Height, weight, blood pressure
   b. Head, eyes, ears, nose, throat (HEENT)
      (1) Assess retinopathy.
      (2) Assess thyromegaly.
   c. Heart, lungs, abdomen
   d. Extremities
      (1) Edema
      (2) Pulses
      (3) Neurologic status

Diabetes nurse specialist

1. Explain team concept.
2. Blood glucose monitoring
   a. Discuss rationale for capillary monitoring.
   b. Teach or assess motivation technique.
   c. Assess meter reliability.
   d. Review frequency of monitoring and recording of results.
3. Blood glucose goals
4. Urine ketone testing
   a. Review or teach technique.
   b. Instruct on appropriate times for testing.
5. Hypoglycemia
   a. Assess knowledge of symptoms and treatment.
   b. Review or teach appropriate treatment.
   c. Review or teach use of glucagon follow-ups.

Continued

capillary glucose values can be measured daily and insulin adjustments made in a timely manner.

SMBG can be of great value in pregnancy, but to use it well, its limitations must be understood. Falsification of data, both by pregnant and nonpregnant individuals with diabetes, has been documented.[86,95] Memory reflectance meters can be helpful for detecting this

---

BOX 11-1

BASELINE ASSESSMENT OF THE PREGNANT WOMAN WITH DIABETES—cont'd

Diabetes nutrition specialist

1. Diet recall
2. Assess nutrient adequacy of diet and recommend changes or additions.
3. Describe goals of diet for pregnant women with diabetes and make recommendations for mother's diet.
4. Write a meal plan for appropriate weight gain.
5. Discuss nutrition factors to consider during pregnancy.
6. Address issues concerning caffeine and alcohol ingestion.

Laboratory evaluation

1. Glycated hemoglobin
2. Thyroid studies
3. Hemoglobin
4. Urinalysis
5. Creatinine and potassium levels (history of renal disease or hypertension)
6. Routine follow-up (visits every 2 weeks)

---

problem. Poor technique can also result in either falsely low or falsely high readings. Meter technique and meter reliability should be assessed at the beginning of the pregnancy and reviewed periodically. Most of the commonly used blood glucose reflectance meters are hematocrit dependent, and a low hematocrit may lead to falsely high blood glucose levels.[5] Some women will develop anemia during pregnancy that, if severe enough, could affect the validity of the capillary glucose readings.

During pregnancy, blood glucose testing ideally should be done four to seven times a day. How often it is done may vary depending on the viewpoint of the managing team; however, premeal tests should be done routinely. Many programs would advocate 1-hour or 2-hour postprandial tests as well. If problems exist with fasting blood glucose levels, 2 AM or 3 AM blood tests should be done to help determine why the level is not in the target zone.

For adequate monitoring of blood glucose control during pregnancy, SMBG should not be the exclusive measure of blood glucose. Glycated hemoglobin, although not useful on a day-to-day basis, is very helpful in confirming overall blood glucose control. When using this test, the woman should remember that blood glucose levels may improve within days, but it takes longer for the glycated hemoglobin to reflect this decrease. However, a downward trend should occur, and once blood glucose control has been stable over 6 to 8 weeks, the blood glucose levels should match the glycated hemoglobin values. A discrepancy between the glycated hemoglobin and blood glucose values at this point may indicate problems with falsification of data. Glycated hemoglobin testing is done every 2 weeks in some programs and monthly in others.

BOX 11-2
___

ROUTINE FOLLOW-UP APPOINTMENTS OF THE PREGNANT WOMAN WITH DIABETES

Endocrinologist

1. Discuss blood glucose results.
2. Make recommendations for changes in insulin.
3. Discuss weight and blood pressure.
4. Assess any intercurrent illness or other medical concerns.
5. Perform brief physical examination, including eyes, thyroid, and extremities.

Diabetes nurse specialist

1. Consult by phone once or twice a week for insulin adjustment.
2. Review self-monitoring of blood glucose (SMBG) technique at periodic intervals.
3. See patient every other visit.

Diabetes nutrition specialist

1. See patient every other visit.
2. If concerns with weight or blood glucose problems, see more frequently.
3. Review meal plans and adjust accordingly.

The *fructosamine test* is a blood test that reflects blood glucose control over 2 to 3 weeks. This shorter measurement interval may make it a better test in pregnancy than glycated hemoglobin, as suggested in a study by Roberts and associates.[122] If the test is available to the health care team, it may be a helpful adjunct for monitoring blood glucose during pregnancy.

Diet

Diet plays a major role in the management of diabetes in any individual, as described in Chapter 4, but it may be even more important in managing diabetes in pregnancy. In planning a meal plan for the pregnant woman, three factors should be considered: optimal caloric intake to achieve blood glucose control, appropriate weight gain, and prevention of starvation ketosis. Severe calorie restriction and weight reduction programs during pregnancy are totally inappropriate. Present dietary guides emphasize avoidance of calorie restriction and prevention of excess weight gain.[13,137]

The Recommended Dietary Allowances (RDAs) for pregnancy in 1980 advised an additional food intake of 300 cal/day above basal requirements during the second and third trimesters, 30 g additional protein/day (1.3 g protein/kg body weight), 30 to 60 mg elemental supplemental iron, and a diet or vitamin supplement that would provide additional amounts of all vitamins and minerals, including an additional 400 mg calcium and 400 mg folacin. These guidelines and the 1979 American Dietetic Association recommendations have provided the basis for nutritional counseling of the pregnant woman with diabetes during the past decade.[13] In 1989 the RDAs were revised and estimates of requirements for pregnancy

Table 11-1 Recommended Weight Gain for Pregnant Women Based on Prepregnancy Body Mass Index (BMI)

Weight-for-height category	Recommended weight gain	
	Kilograms	Pounds
Low (BMI* < 19.8)	12.5–18	28–40
Normal (BMI of 19.8 to 26)	11.5–16	25–35
High (BMI > 26 to 29)	7.0–11.5	15–25
Obese (BMI > 29)	~6	~15

Modified from Subcommittee on Nutritional Status and Weight Gain During Pregnancy. Food and Nutrition Board, National Academy of Science: *Nutrition during pregnancy,* Washington, DC, 1990, National Academy Press.
*BMI = weight/(height)^2, weight in kilograms; height in meters.

lowered for several nutrients.[104] The recommended increment in protein was reduced from 30 to 10 g/day and iron from 30 to 60 mg to 15 mg/day. Allowances of nutrients are 50% lower for all adults, with 80 mg/day recommended for nonpregnant women and 400 mg/day during pregnancy. Recommendations for calcium and calorie intake remained the same.

Nutritional and caloric needs during pregnancy continue to be reevaluated. In assessing calorie requirements during pregnancy, the RDA guidelines do not address or acknowledge pregestational weight and optimal weight gain in that regard. In the book, *Nutrition During Pregnancy,* the Subcommittee on Nutritional Status and Weight Gain During Pregnancy[136] recommended new guidelines regarding desired weight gain ranges for pregnancy based on a woman's prepregnancy body mass index (BMI) (Table 11-1). These guidelines were predicated in regard to women delivering term babies weighing 3 to 4 kg. These are general guidelines for pregnancy that can serve as a framework for examining desired weight gain in the pregnancy complicated by diabetes.

In light of new guidelines for weight gain, studies have indicated that 300 cal/day above basal caloric requirements during the second and third trimesters may not be optimal. Recommendations of no extra calories during the first trimester and 150 cal in the second and third trimesters have been made.[31]

Routine and consistency of food intake should be stressed to aid in attaining optimal control. Most individuals should divide calorie intake into six times per day, including breakfast, midmorning snack, lunch, midafternoon snack, evening meal, and bedtime snack. Distribution of food groups may need to be examined carefully to achieve glycemia. Postprandial glucose variations after breakfast are notoriously difficult to control. Limiting carbohydrate intake during that meal, such as eliminating cereal and replacing it with peanut butter toast or eggs, can result in improved postprandial glucose.

Dietary monitoring. The woman should visit the dietitian shortly after diagnosis of the pregnancy. Subsequent visits can be scheduled as needed. The number of visits will vary depending on how well the patient is meeting weight and blood glucose goals. Weight should be monitored at each routine diabetes visit. Food records are an excellent tool for initial evaluation of diet and for ongoing monitoring of food intake. Their correlation with the blood glucose values can be very helpful in determining a possible need for changes in the basic insulin regimen and insulin supplement scales.

An important consideration in planning an adequate diet for the pregnant woman with diabetes is the problem of starvation ketosis. This type of ketosis does not carry the major risk of diabetic ketoacidosis; however, urinary ketones may be a sign of inadequate insulin and/or inadequate calories, especially carbohydrate calories. Most often, starvation ketosis occurs in the morning. This problem can be avoided by increasing the number of calories in the evening snack and, if needed, by increasing overnight insulin.

Certain aspects of the pregnancy complicated by diabetes can make planning an appropriate diet and evaluating weight gain difficult. True weight gain can be difficult to assess, especially during the last trimester, since the diabetic pregnancy is more often complicated by toxemia, hydramnios, and increased fluid retention.

Early in the pregnancy, hyperemesis may cause problems. Often, insulin may need to be adjusted to allow for minimal caloric intake at various times of the day, most often in the morning. Some women may have gastroparesis with symptoms of fullness, nausea, and vomiting, which may persist throughout the pregnancy.

Women with poor blood glucose control before pregnancy may have been eating excess calories but not gaining weight because of glycosuria. Instead of increasing calories, these women may need to decrease their calorie intake, in some cases substantially, to prevent excess weight gain during pregnancy. Another problem is weight gain related to hypoglycemia. If a woman is having frequent hypoglycemic episodes and treats them with extra calories, problems with additional weight gain may ensue.

Exercise

Exercise and physical activity can play an important role in determining the blood glucose level. Physical activity results in the utilization of glucose and often can cause a decrease in the blood glucose level. Exercise, however, can exacerbate problems with blood glucose control, as discussed in Chapter 5.

If exercise is poorly timed, hypoglycemia can occur. Overtreatment of the hypoglycemia can lead to hyperglycemia. Exercise needs to be carefully controlled and timed for an optimal effect on blood glucose level during pregnancy. The best time to exercise may be after meals rather than before meals. Activity during this time may help decrease the rate of hypoglycemia secondary to exercise, but it also can be very helpful in limiting postprandial glucose variations. By testing blood glucose before and after activity, insulin and food can be adjusted to help maintain stable blood glucose levels.

Mild exercise is encouraged during pregnancy; vigorous exercise is not.[2] Walking and swimming are suitable for pregnant women, but high-impact aerobics, running, and contact sports are not recommended. For women with complications of pregnancy such as toxemia and preterm labor, physical activity may need to be extremely limited.

Insulin treatment

Insulin is the treatment of choice as a blood glucose–lowering agent in diabetes and pregnancy. Oral hypoglycemic agents have previously been used in pregnancy, but their effect

Table 11-2   Insulin Regimens in Pregnancy

Breakfast	Lunch	Supper	Bedtime
R/I	—	R/I	—
R/I	—	R	I
R/I	R	R/I	—
R/I	R	R	I
R	R	R	I
R/UL	R	R/UL	—
R/UL	R	R	—
R	R	R/UL	—
R	R	R	UL

R, Regular; *I,* NPH or Lente; *UL,* Ultralente.

on the fetus has not been adequately evaluated.[11,92,142] They may cross the placenta and stimulate fetal insulin secretion. Patients with NIDDM taking oral hypoglycemic agents should be switched to insulin treatment if they are planning pregnancy or if they become pregnant.

The principal goal of insulin replacement in the treatment of the pregnant woman with diabetes is to achieve normal daily blood glucose profiles. The most optimal insulin regimen is one that best mimics the function of the normal pancreas. This regimen generally cannot be accomplished with less than two shots of insulin a day. In most patients, three or four injections of insulin daily are required to maximize blood glucose control. Besides *multiple daily insulin injections* (MDII), another method of insulin delivery that has been used during pregnancy is *continuous subcutaneous insulin infusion* (CSII). This method employs an insulin pump that can be programmed to deliver low basal rates of insulin and also boluses of insulin before meals.[24]

Over the years, different insulin programs for pregnancy have been recommended. Jovanovic and Peterson[68] reported excellent results for blood glucose control and perinatal outcome with a multiinjection regimen of regular and NPH insulin. Insulin intensification programs in general have used a number of different regimens (Table 11-2). In the DCCT, more than 39 different insulin regimens have been used with patients. Whether CSII or MDII is more advantageous in pregnancy was studied by Coustan and associates in a randomized trial.[24] No difference between the two groups of women was found in regard to glycated hemoglobin, fetal outcome, or adverse effects such as hypoglycemia.

Is there one "right" approach to insulin therapy in pregnancy? The most optimal insulin program for any patient may depend on the individual's present regimen and the experience and preference of the diabetes team. For the woman already on an intensified program with either MDII or CSII, no fundamental changes may be needed. If an individual is on a basic program such as an injection of regular and NPH insulin at breakfast and dinner, an initial change would be to split the dinner injection to regular insulin at dinner and NPH insulin at bedtime. A new insulin program can be constructed for any woman, using her initial insulin regimen as a foundation. There are two key points in constructing a new regimen: (1) the guide for changes should be the target preprandial and postprandial blood glucose levels, and (2) changes must be made in a timely and expeditious manner. The level of blood glucose control at the time the woman is seen by the diabetes team will determine the need for a change in insulin regimen.

The details of intensified insulin regimens are beyond the scope of this chapter. However, certain problems in setting up such regimens are common in pregnancy and are addressed here. First, not all insulin regimens are equal. Certain characteristics of insulins make them more or less desirable for use during pregnancy. Human Ultralente may provide a lower background insulin than the intermediate-acting insulins but also may have an unpredictable peaking effect. Control of the morning glucose level can also be more difficult with this insulin. NPH or Lente may be more effective choices for background insulin during pregnancy, since their time course and peak effect are usually more consistent and predictable.

One of the more difficult problems in meeting glucose target goals during pregnancy may be stabilization of the fasting blood glucose level. Nighttime hypoglycemia and an early-morning rise in the glucose level (the *dawn effect*) can create challenges for an insulin regimen. Postmidnight hypoglycemia is often eliminated when NPH/Lente is given at bedtime rather than dinner, but not in all cases. Human Ultralente given at bedtime or at dinner may be more effective in such patients. Bedtime NPH may not always work well if there is a major dawn effect, since to minimize the glucose rise effectively, the dose may have to be so large that hypoglycemia may be induced at 1 or 2 AM. Because of its lower level and delayed peak, human Ultralente may work better in this regard than NPH. In a rare individual a combination of Lente and Ultralente given at bedtime may be a solution. In some cases it is not possible to control the dawn effect with the intermediate-acting or long-acting insulins. In such patients, subcutaneous infusion of regular insulin via ambulatory insulin infusion pump may be effective. The pump can be preprogrammed to increase basal insulin at 3 to 4 AM and stabilize the fasting blood glucose with minimal risk of hypoglycemia. Interestingly, when faced with this problem, some patients, rather than shifting to pump therapy, elect to awaken at 4 AM and take an injection of regular insulin.

Insulin administration

One important aspect of using multiple injections of regular insulin during pregnancy is the timing of injections. In general, injections should be given 30 minutes before a meal; however, the rate of insulin absorption may vary from patient to patient. Establishing the right timing for the injection is essential because of its effect on postprandial blood glucose control and the occurrence of hypoglycemia. Optimal individual absorption rates may vary from 15 minutes to 1 hour. A recent study indicated that absorption is more routine and reliable when injections are given at one site.[4] Certainly, if problems with control arise, the use of one site during pregnancy may be important. Many pregnant women give injections in the abdomen.

Timing the insulin injection and meals based on the level of the premeal blood glucose level is not encouraged. It has been suggested that if blood glucose is high, waiting a longer interval until eating after the injection of regular insulin will help bring down the glucose level. Conversely, if blood glucose is low, injection of insulin after the meal will work to maximize glucose levels. This is not an optimal approach, either during pregnancy or for the nonpregnant patient on an intensified insulin regimen. Delaying the meal can predispose to hypoglycemia, whereas injecting regular insulin during or after the meal will generally result in a marked postprandial glucose rise, occasionally with subsequent hypoglycemia. It is more precise and predictable to increase or decrease the regular insulin bolus based on blood glucose level.

Insulin preparation

Human insulin is recommended for new patients starting an insulin regimen and for patients who may be having problems with insulin antibodies, lipoatrophy, hypertrophy, and allergies. At present there is no general recommendation that all individuals with diabetes taking nonhuman insulins should be changed to human insulin.

Should all women seeking pregnancy and those already pregnant be changed to human insulin? There have been theoretic concerns that maternal insulin antibodies in women treated with nonhuman insulins may pass to the fetus and in some way be harmful. Such antibodies may stimulate insulin production in the fetus and play a role in the development of macrosomia. A recent study demonstrated that insulin antibodies apparently do pass through the placenta; however, a definite link between maternal insulin antibodies and fetal risk has not been established.[97] A study by Jovanoric and others[73] showed no link between human insulins versus animal insulins and fetal antibodies. A slightly higher incidence of macrosomia was seen in the animal insulin–treated group than in the human insulin–treated group, which was related to more postprandial hyperglycemia in the latter group. At this time the choice of insulin species for treatment during pregnancy usually depends on the decision of the health care team and the patient. However, animal insulins are being discontinued, and their continued availability remains uncertain. Thus it may be prudent for women who are treated with animal insulins and interested in pregnancy to be changed to human insulins.

Adjustment of insulin dosage

Self-adjustment of insulin is a key part of an intensified insulin program in pregnancy. Without this component, it is almost impossible to achieve targeted blood glucose goals. Each woman should be provided with an individualized set of algorithms to help her adjust her insulin on a day-to-day basis.

Self-adjustment of insulin usually refers to changing the dose of regular insulin. Insulin changes can be based on several different parameters. The three most common are blood glucose levels, anticipated activity, and changes in diet. The terms *anticipatory supplement* and *compensatory supplement* are used to describe this process. The goal of supplementing is to ensure that the next premeal glucose value is in the goal range. Table 11-3 illustrates fairly simple algorithms set up on the basis of blood glucose levels. For example, a woman is on a basic insulin regimen of 20 U NPH and 5 U regular insulin before breakfast, 4 U regular insulin before lunch, 6 U regular insulin at dinner, and 20 U NPH at bedtime. If her blood glucose is 150 mg/dl before lunch, according to the algorithms she would add 1 U regular insulin to the usual 4 U regular insulin dose, in anticipation of bringing the next premeal blood glucose level into the target range. This is a very simple algorithm; some women have different scales for each meal. More complicated algorithms may be used if the woman wants to vary exercise. Some women are able to master a fairly complicated supplemental scale, whereas others may be able to use only a very simple scale.

Table 11-3 Algorithms for Compensatory Insulin Adjustments*

Premeal blood glucose (mg/dl)	Adjustment
<70	Reduce regular insulin by 1 to 2 U.
71-120	Take prescribed regular insulin.
121-150	Increase regular insulin by 1 U.
151-200	Increase regular insulin by 2 U.
201-250	Increase regular insulin by 3 U.
>250	Increase regular insulin by 4 U.

*Do not use these algorithms at bedtime.

Algorithms are generally based on experience, and as the pregnancy progresses, the algorithm may need to change. Insulin supplements given for extra food also need to be worked out on an individual basis. During pregnancy, however, too much flexibility in diet is discouraged because of the increased difficulty in achieving target blood glucose levels and the concern about weight gain.

Complications of Diabetes Treatment

Ketoacidosis

Ketoacidosis is associated with up to a 50% rate of fetal death and was the major contributor to both fetal and maternal mortality before the introduction of insulin.[30,90] At present, ketoacidosis usually occurs during pregnancy in the setting of an intercurrent illness, such as influenza or urinary tract infection, and is also more likely to occur in women whose diabetes control during pregnancy is poor. The diabetogenic effect of pregnancy and the increased level of ketones produced during pregnancy can set the stage for mild intercurrent illness and cause ketoacidosis in the woman with poor diabetes control.

Routine monitoring for ketones is important to help identify ketosis associated with poor blood glucose control and also to identify starvation ketosis. Many protocols suggest that women check for urinary ketones every morning. Ketoacidosis has also been described in pregnancy with mild elevations of the blood glucose level, so testing for ketones whenever the blood glucose test is greater than 200 mg/dl is important. To help minimize the incidence of ketoacidosis, all women should have protocols that include guidelines for insulin use and diet changes when they are ill. Women should be instructed to call their health care provider early in the course of an illness if blood glucose levels are not in the target range or if moderate to large ketones are present in the urine.

Hypoglycemia

The main concern in seeking strict blood glucose goals during pregnancy is maternal hypoglycemia because of its effect on the mother and its possible effects on the fetus. Studies of nongravid women and men treated with intensified insulin programs have found a higher rate of hypoglycemia than in individuals receiving conventional insulin therapy.[27,82] Coustan and others[24] reported that both MDII and CSII were associated with a high frequency of both symptomatic and biochemical hypoglycemia in pregnancy. In this group, 3 of 11 patients taking CSII and 5 of 11 taking MDII had a total of 31 episodes of severe hypoglycemia. Not all reviews show such a high incidence of severe hypoglycemia, but it is a risk in individuals pursuing normal blood glucose goals.

Few studies have been done and at present there is minimal evidence to suggest that severe hypoglycemia has an adverse effect on perinatal mortality or on subsequent mental and motor function of offspring of mothers with diabetes.[24,123] In a study by Rovergi and associates,[123] insulin doses were increased until the patient manifested symptoms of hypoglycemia. The doses were then decreased slightly, and the patients were maintained through pregnancy on the brink of symptomatic hypoglycemia. Perinatal mortality rate in this study was approximately 2.7% when congenital anomalies incompatible with life were excluded.

Risks to the mother from hypoglycemia are unclear. Maternal deaths from hypoglycemia have been reported but are rare.[46] Neurobehavioral outcomes related to hypoglycemia were monitored in the DCCT, and no difference in results was seen between the group of volunteers treated with standard insulin therapy and the volunteers treated with intensified therapy. Episodes of severe hypoglycemia also did not appear to affect neurobehavioral outcomes.[28]

Evidence indicates that risk from maternal hypoglycemia to the fetus is minimal and that prolonged hyperglycemia is a much greater danger. Maternal risk from hypoglycemia appears to be low and no greater than that seen for individuals on intensified insulin regimens. One group of women, those with a history of severe hypoglycemia or hypoglycemic unawareness, may need to have blood glucose goals set at a higher level than other women with diabetes.

Severe hypoglycemia can be characterized in several ways. Its strictest definition is hypoglycemia requiring hospitalization, an emergency room visit, or a paramedic visit with intravenous administration of glucose or intramuscular administration of glucagon. This definition is often expanded to mean any episode of hypoglycemia that cannot be self-treated.

The best approach to avoiding maternal hypoglycemia is a treatment plan that combines the appropriate insulin regimen with a consistent routine of diet and activity. The patient must also always be alert to the possible occurrence of hypoglycemia. Unusual changes in schedule or activity should be avoided. Deleting food from the meal plan, especially dropping the evening snack, can be a major cause of hypoglycemia.

At the beginning of the pregnancy the patient's and family members' knowledge of the recognition and treatment of hypoglycemia should be evaluated. Such an assessment is important even for women who appear knowledgeable about hypoglycemia. An episode of severe hypoglycemia during pregnancy should not be the stimulus for a belated educational effort.

The optimal treatment of hypoglycemia, including mild, moderate, and severe forms, should be reviewed with the pregnant woman and her family at the beginning of the pregnancy (see Chapter 4 for treatment guidelines). Overtreatment, especially for mild to moderate episodes, should be avoided. The recommended treatment for mild to moderate hypoglycemia for the typical patient with diabetes can be applied in pregnancy. Tablets of glucose are especially useful for treating a reaction with the right amount of carbohydrate. With severe hypoglycemia, the woman's family and possibly co-workers should be trained in the administration of glucagon and the appropriate time to use it.

BOX 11-3

REVISED WHITE CLASSIFICATION (1980)

Gestational diabetes

Abnormal glucose tolerance test (GTT), but euglycemia maintained by diet alone
Diet alone insufficient; insulin required

Diabetes diagnosed before pregnancy

Class A: treatment with diet alone; any duration or onset at any age
Class B: onset at age 20 years or older, duration less than 10 years
Class C: onset at age 10-19 years or duration of 10-19 years
Class D: onset at age under 10 years; duration more than 20 years, background retinopathy, or hypertension (not preeclampsia)
Class R: proliferative retinopathy or vitreous hemorrhage
Class F: nephropathy with greater than 500 mg/day proteinuria
Class RF: criteria for both classes R and F
Class H: arteriosclerotic heart disease clinically evident
Class T: previous renal transplantation

Modified from Hare J, White P: *Diabetes Care* 3:394, 1980.

Vascular Disease

Concern about the effect of diabetic vascular disease on pregnancy outcomes in women with diabetes has long been evident. In the past, perinatal mortality rates were significantly higher among patients with diabetic vascular complications. Because of this relationship, a classification system of perinatal outcome related to the extent and severity of the mother's diabetic complications was set up by Dr. P. White, an early pioneer in the care of the pregnancy complicated by diabetes (Box 11-3).[148] Because of recent advances in assessment and treatment of diabetic complications and improved obstetric care, this classification has not been as helpful or useful as in the past. Women with vascular complications who may have been previously advised against pregnancy may now consider it.

The fear that pregnancy will aggravate existing vascular complications or promote the development of future problems has also been a major concern. Studies on the effect of pregnancy on diabetic vascular complications are still somewhat limited, but available evidence indicates the effect of pregnancy, at least in individuals with mild to moderate complications, is minimal.

Retinopathy

Fears about the effect of pregnancy on the progression of retinopathy initially arose from reports of individual cases. Early formal studies of this question did not examine control groups of nonpregnant women, and their results are inconclusive and contradictory.[130,134]

More recently, it has been shown that the institution of tight blood glucose control may cause progression of diabetic retinopathy.[82] Thus progression of retinopathy in an individual woman during pregnancy may relate to rapid improvement in blood glucose control rather than the pregnancy itself.

In a recent population study on retinopathy, Klein and associates[81] found a small increase in the incidence of advanced retinopathy in women with a history of pregnancy compared with the general population of women with diabetes. These data did not show a relationship between number of pregnancies and worsening retinopathy.[80] Data from the DCCT found no differences in outcomes for retinopathy in patients who became pregnant versus those who did not.[28] Blood glucose control was not materially different during pregnancy in the standard treatment group versus the intensified treatment group.

At present, unless it is unstable and proliferative, the presence of retinopathy should not stop a woman from considering pregnancy. All women who are pregnant should have an eye examination early in the pregnancy and further examinations scheduled as needed. Assessment and treatment of retinopathy during pregnancy do not differ from treatment of the nongravid woman with diabetes.

Nephropathy

Nephropathy can affect the outcome of pregnancy. An increased incidence of intrauterine fetal growth retardation, preterm delivery, stillbirth, and poorer perinatal survival has been seen in pregnant patients with kidney disease, as described by Kitzmiller and associates.[78] They combined the results of several studies on pregnancy and renal disease and showed a 91.2% perinatal survival in diabetic pregnancies complicated by renal disease versus a 97% perinatal survival for diabetic pregnancies not complicated by nephropathy.[124] Pregnancy associated with nephropathy is accompanied by a higher risk of maternal and fetal morbidity. The woman with advanced disease is at higher risk for perinatal mortality. Pregnancy for a woman with advanced renal disease is not recommended.

Can pregnancy affect the course of renal disease? Kitzmiller and others[78] have examined available data and concluded that pregnancy in women with early renal disease does not contribute to progressive loss of function.

Neuropathy

Peripheral diabetic neuropathy does not appear to be aggravated or worsened in a permanent way by pregnancy, although meager data exist in this area. Carpal tunnel syndrome, which is more common in pregnancy and in people with diabetes, certainly may worsen or develop during pregnancy. Symptoms improve or disappear after delivery. Problems with autonomic neuropathy may appear or worsen during pregnancy. Gastroparesis can be the greatest challenge. The hyperemesis of pregnancy can combine with or be aggravated by underlying gastroparesis. The bulk of pregnancy can also increase problems with bloating, nausea, and vomiting. Metoclopramide (Reglan) can be used during pregnancy and may be helpful. Experience with the drug Propulsid in pregnancy is very limited, and its use cannot be recommended at present. Occasionally, lower bowel problems may worsen or develop. Either constipation or diarrhea can cause difficulties for the pregnant woman.

Macrovascular disease

Macrovascular complications of concern in diabetic pregnancy are heart disease and cerebrovascular accident (CVA, stroke). Although it is unusual for a woman of childbearing age to have known coronary artery disease (CAD) or cerebral vascular disease, it does occur and with greater frequency in women with diabetes.[1] Pregnancy is generally not advisable for a woman with a history of known CAD or CVA.

Outcome Measures

Both maternal and fetal outcomes in the pregnancy complicated by diabetes have improved dramatically, but diabetic pregnancy is still characterized by a variety of complications that affect both the mother and the fetus. Fetal mortality, at least in tertiary care centers, has been reduced to the range of 3% to 5%; however, there are still isolated primary care areas where fetal mortality rates are higher.[78]

Maternal Complications

Hypertensive disorders

Hypertensive disorders are more often seen in pregnancies complicated by diabetes than in nondiabetic pregnancies. Their increased incidence is thought to be related to underlying diabetic vasculopathy. Somewhat inconsistent definitions of preeclampsia make it difficult to give exact rates of occurrence, but an incidence of 10% to 15% of all diabetic pregnancies has been frequently reported.[66,94] Some women with pregestational diabetes already have a diagnosis of either essential hypertension or hypertension related to diabetic nephropathy.

Treatment of preeclampsia in the pregnancy complicated by diabetes does not differ from the approach in the nondiabetic pregnancy. Most of the newer medications used in the treatment of essential or diabetes-related hypertension, such as calcium channel blockers, have not been well tested in human pregnancy, and their effect is unknown. Captopril (Capoten), an angiotensin-converting enzyme (ACE) inhibitor, has been shown to have detrimental effects on the fetus in animal experiments, although the calcium channel blocker nifedipine has been used to treat toxemia during labor with no apparent problems.[9,143] Beta-blockers such as atenolol (Tenormin) have been tested in pregnancy and have not been associated with increased neonatal or perinatal morbidity or mortality.[144] Because this class of drug may block the adrenaline-induced symptoms of hypoglycemia in some individuals, their use in the woman with diabetes is generally not recommended. Both methyldopa (Aldomet) and hydralazine (Apresoline) are regarded as safe and effective drugs for treatment of preexisting hypertension in the pregnant woman with diabetes.[118] The use of diuretics is discouraged but may be necessary for blood pressure control and edema control in some women.[49] If a woman is planning pregnancy and is being treated with one of the newer drugs, switching treatment to a drug such as methyldopa may be the best approach.

Hydramnios

Hydramnios historically has been associated with diabetes mellitus in pregnancy, but its true incidence is difficult to document, and a detrimental effect on perinatal mortality has not been shown. Its incidence has been reported at about 15% to 16% in diabetic pregnancy.[77]

Pyelonephritis

Pyelonephritis has been reported in up to 4% of all pregnancies complicated by diabetes and may be more common in individuals with severe diabetes.[77] A urine culture should be done for a baseline and once a trimester. Additional cultures should be done if the woman has symptoms of a urinary tract infection.

Preterm labor

Different studies have found varying incidences of preterm labor in the pregnancy complicated by diabetes. Reports have ranged from 6.1% to 9.2% for women with diabetes compared with 3.9% for nondiabetic pregnant women.[77,90] Various agents are available for treatment of preterm labor such as the beta-agonists. Isoxsuprine (Vasodilan) and terbutaline (Brethine) can be very effective for individual patients but have been associated with deterioration of blood glucose control.[3] If a woman is started on oral medication as an outpatient, she may need major insulin adjustments to control blood glucose. If preterm labor is so severe that hospitalization for treatment with intravenous magnesium sulfate or terbutaline is necessary, intravenous insulin infusions may be needed to maintain blood glucose control.

Cesarean section

One of the more common problems of the pregnancy complicated by diabetes is the increased rate of cesarean section. Early studies indicated a 40% to 60% rate of cesarean section in women with pregestational diabetes, compared with a norm of 20%.[36,77,141] At present, more emphasis is being placed on achieving a vaginal delivery. This is especially true in women with diabetes of shorter duration and in those with minimal problems during the pregnancy. One major contributor to this approach has been the improvement in monitoring and assessment of fetal status.

Maternal mortality

The ultimate obstetric complication is maternal death, which was common before the availability of insulin, when as many as 50% of pregnancies resulted in death. The present maternal mortality rate is approximately 0.5%. However, this rate is still about 10 times that seen in women without diabetes.[14] Leading causes of mortality include sepsis, hemorrhage, ketoacidosis, hypoglycemia, cardiac arrest, and myocardial infarction.[44]

Perinatal and Neonatal Complications

Intrauterine fetal death

The perinatal mortality rate among pregnant women with diabetes has improved remarkably. In 1975 the fetal death rate was about 4% to 12%, which was three to eight times higher than stillbirth rates in the general population.[38] Recently, stillbirth rates of 1% to 4% have been reported.[129] This dramatic decline can be attributed to the emphasis on improved glycemic control, decreased incidence of ketoacidosis, improvement of antepartum monitoring, and the ability to determine the best time to deliver the fetus.

Neonatal mortality

Another success story has been the reduction in neonatal mortality rates, now at about 1% to 5%. Respiratory distress syndrome (RDS) was a major cause of neonatal mortality, as is described later in this section. The incidence of RDS has been reduced from 25% to 35% to rates of about 3% to 10%.[47,129] Deaths from this problem are becoming so rare that the current major cause of neonatal mortality is congenital anomalies.

Congenital anomalies

Major congenital anomalies continue to affect 4% to 12% of all infants of mothers with diabetes.* Congenital heart defects are the most common, and their incidence is increased fivefold over that of the general population. Neural tube defects are also common.[119] Since organogenesis occurs during the first 3 to 8 weeks after conception, attention has focused on hyperglycemia during this period as a major factor in development of anomalies. A number of studies, both retrospective and prospective, have shown a link between hyperglycemia and incidence of congenital malformation.[100,101,133] More recently, several studies have indicated that preconceptual control of blood glucose can lower the incidence of malformation to that of the nondiabetic pregnancy.[57,79,133]

What level of glycemia is necessary to achieve these results? The major link between glycemia and malformation apparently is strongest in mothers who have extremely elevated blood glucose levels during the first weeks of pregnancy. In a recent Swedish study the cutoff point appeared to be at a hemoglobin (Hb) A_{1c} 7 to 10 standard deviations above the mean of the normal level.[57] In a recent study, Kitzmiller and associates[79] established a cutoff point of Hb A_{1c} 1.7 times that of the mean. In terms of actual Hb A_{1c}, this level can be defined. Using a DCCT normal range of 4% to 6%, an Hb A_{1c} less than 7.2% would be associated with normal risk for congenital anomalies.

The Diabetes in Early Pregnancy Study (DIEP) was initiated in 1980 to examine the high rate of congenital anomalies in pregnancies complicated by diabetes.[101] Three groups of patients were enrolled: 347 women were entered early in pregnancy (within 3 weeks of the diagnosis of pregnancy), a second group of 279 women were entered later in pregnancy, and 389 nondiabetic pregnant women made up the control group.[97] Major malformations occurred in the infants of 2.1% of the control group, 4.1% of the early-entry subjects, and 9% of the late-entry diabetic women. This study also supports a link between a greatly elevated Hb A_{1c} and an increased malformation rate. The rate of anomalies for the early-entry group was significantly elevated compared with that for the control group of nondiabetic pregnancies, even though average Hb A_{1c} was low. This discrepancy may relate to a number of the women in the early-entry group already being 3 weeks pregnant when they entered the study, and overall glycemic control may not have approached the level seen in the previously cited studies.

---

*References 43,50,100,101,125.

Substantial evidence indicates that blood glucose control is important in preventing congenital anomalies but that euglycemia is not absolutely necessary to prevent the problem. If initial glycated hemoglobin is within the normal range or 1 to 1.5 units above the top of this range, the risk for congenital malformation appears to be similar to the rate in the pregnancy not complicated by diabetes.

Respiratory distress syndrome

RDS has been a major contributor to neonatal death. The ability to perform in utero tests for pulmonary maturity has helped bring about the dramatic decrease in its incidence.[47,129] These tests include the lecithin/sphingomyelin (L/S) ratio and the phosphatidylinositol test. Recently the reliability of the mature ratio for predicting the absence of RDS in offspring of mothers with diabetes has been questioned.[99] The cause of the increased incidence of RDS in infants of women with diabetes continues to be unclear but is probably multifactorial. Delays in fetal lung maturation may be secondary to fetal hyperglycemia and hyperinsulinemia. The fetus in a diabetic pregnancy is often delivered prematurely, which may also contribute to the increased incidence of RDS.

Macrosomia and microsomia

Excessive fetal size for gestational age, or fetal macrosomia, has long been recognized as a common complication of the pregnancy associated with diabetes.[45] Infants have a characteristic body habitus, including a round, puffy face and an increased length, which may be proportionate to their weight.

The increase in body weight is related to an increase in body fat, mainly of the viscera; non-insulin-sensitive tissues such as the brain are generally not enlarged.[33] Fetal macrosomia can be explained by the Pederson hypothesis that maternal hyperglycemia leads to fetal hyperglycemia.[112] In response to the hyperglycemia, the fetal pancreas produces increased amounts of insulin. This hyperinsulinemia is thought to stimulate growth in utero. This hypothesis has been supported by animal experiments.[137] Large infants result in an increased rate of cesarean section and also can cause complications for vaginal delivery, including shoulder dystocia.

On the opposite end of the spectrum is the fetus who is small for date of delivery. This condition is often seen in women with severe vascular complications and may be related to vascular disease in the uterine vessels that leads to decreased availability of nutrients despite maternal hyperglycemia. Some have speculated that poor blood glucose control also may lead to infants who are small for date of delivery.

Hypoglycemia

Neonatal hypoglycemia is considered to be a common finding in infants of mothers with diabetes, affecting 20% to 60%.[77] The definition of hypoglycemia in the newborn is a blood glucose level less than 30 mg/dl and 20 mg/dl in a premature neonate. Endogenous insulin levels are generally high in the fetus of the mother with diabetes and may remain so after delivery. Since maternal glucose delivery has stopped and the infant's glucagon system may be inhibited, glucose production by the neonate may not increase or may even be reduced immediately after delivery. Hypoglycemia may be prolonged in some infants, lasting up to 48 to 72 hours. Hypoglycemia in the neonate is usually asymptomatic, but if severe and prolonged, it may be accompanied by tremors, apnea, or cyanosis.[59] Long-term consequences have not been established. The best approach to avoiding neonatal hypoglycemia is strict control of maternal blood glucose levels during the pregnancy and labor.

Hypocalcemia

Hypocalcemia has been seen variably in infants of the mother with diabetes. Studies indicate that 8% to 22% of offspring may have hypocalcemia.[77] Its etiology is unclear, but may be related to maternal hyperparathyroidism.

Hyperbilirubinemia

Neonatal jaundice can be seen in any infant. Its incidence has been reported to be as high as 20% in the infants of mothers with diabetes.[77,140] Prematurity is thought to contribute to this incidence.

A higher incidence of neonatal morbidity certainly has been associated with diabetes. Recent reassessment of this incidence has shown that some problems, most notably hyperbilirubinemia, hypoglycemia, hypocalcemia, and RDS, may be associated more with delivery at an early gestational date than with diabetes itself.[63]

Obstetric Treatment

The importance of comprehensive obstetric monitoring of the pregnancy complicated by diabetes cannot be overemphasized. Most obstetricians have their own approach; in general, however, the routine diabetic pregnancy should be followed every 2 weeks initially, once a week at the seventh month, and then biweekly at 34 weeks. The actual timing and frequency of visits will depend on the individual woman's needs.

All usual testing done for the nondiabetic pregnancy should be performed for the pregnancy complicated by diabetes. This includes a baseline evaluation of the mother at the first office visit. Biochemical evaluation of the fetus starts at 16 to 17 weeks of gestation in the form of maternal serum alpha-fetoprotein screening for neural tube defects.

Ultrasound evaluation of the fetus should be done at 16 to 18 weeks for assessment of major congenital anomalies. If concern exists about viability of the pregnancy, such as poor heart tones, an ultrasound examination may be done earlier, at 10 to 12 weeks of gestation. Another ultrasound may not be done until the third trimester at 34 weeks. If there is concern about a large-for-gestational-age infant, an ultrasound may be performed later in the pregnancy to help determine the optimal method of delivery. Some programs suggest ultrasound evaluations at 4-week intervals until delivery. This protocol allows for better and earlier detection of polyhydramnios or oligohydramnios, abnormal fetal growth, or late-onset abnormalities.[121] Maternal estrogen levels once were used to help manage a high-risk pregnancy. Dooley and associates, in a major review,[29] concluded this assay is of little value in the management of the pregnancy and may even contribute to inappropriate deliveries.

The mainstay of antepartum monitoring at present is biophysical assessment. The *nonstress test* (NST), which is based on the presence or absence of fetal heart accelerations associated with fetal movement, is a key component of this assessment. A major collaborative study published in 1970 showed significantly increased morbidity and mortality during pregnancy in the presence of a nonreactive NST.[41] The study also evaluated the *oxytocin challenge test* (OCT), which was found to be a more sensitive test than the NST; however, it is more expensive and on occasion may induce labor.[42] The most common approach is to do either weekly or twice-weekly NSTs and to follow up with an OCT if the NST is suspicious or nonreactive. This testing should begin at 30 to 32 weeks but may be started earlier in some women.

Another aspect of the biophysical assessment is the *biophysical profile* (BPP). Although both the NST and OCT are nonphysiologic, the BPP is physiologic in that it evaluates the status of the fetus in the absence of uterine contractions. The battery is made up of the NST, fetal breathing movements, quantitative amniotic fluid volume, gross body movement, and fetal tone. Each of these parameters is given a score. A score of 8 to 10 generally indicates fetal well-being. A score of 4 or less may indicate that the fetus is seriously compromised and that delivery needs to be imminent.[54] Additional important measures of fetal maturity can be obtained by measuring the L/S ratio in amniotic fluid and performing a variety of other tests of amniotic fluid, which allow accurate evaluation of pulmonary maturity.

Do all patients need close fetal monitoring? A recent study divided pregnant women with IDDM into two groups: those with evidence of vasculopathy, a history of hypertension, or nephropathy and those without such problems. Both groups had early and extensive fetal monitoring. Early delivery based on abnormal fetal profile was seen only in the group of women with vasculopathy.[85] More evidence is needed before monitoring recommendations are changed, but in the future it may be possible to characterize better which woman needs more or less monitoring.

Timing and management of delivery

Historically, the timing of delivery in a pregnancy complicated by diabetes was usually at 36 weeks of gestation. Delivery was a compromise between the increasing incidence of stillbirth after 36 weeks and the fetal risk of developing RDS if delivery was too early. The development of better methods of assessing the maturity of the fetus has allowed many deliveries to be delayed to at least 38 weeks and longer if the cervix is not ripe. Arbitrary early delivery is no longer mandatory in women with diabetes.[19] The longer the delivery can be delayed, the more likely the possibility of a vaginal delivery. Moreover, maternal diabetes does not have to be a primary indication for cesarean section. The decision for such a delivery should be made on the basis of general obstetric indications. Some exceptions to this rule may exist, such as the woman who has or develops active retinopathy during the pregnancy; active labor may aggravate her eye disease.

Diabetes management during delivery

The goal in management of diabetes during labor is to achieve and maintain euglycemia. Administration of excess glucose during labor can lead to maternal hyperglycemia and contribute to neonatal hypoglycemia. Recent data have shown that many women with diabetes may not need exogenous insulin during labor to maintain blood glucose control.[53,70] The current approach for the woman who has been in good metabolic control during the pregnancy is to make sure the day before induction that she follows her usual routine and that the fasting blood glucose level is within the 60 to 100 mg/dl range. On induction morning, insulin and breakfast should be withheld, and an infusion of dextrose and saline initiated at a rate of 75 to 100 ml/hr. Capillary glucose measurements can be done at the bedside every 1 to 2 hours. In most cases the patient can perform her own measurements, but if not, a nurse or technician can obtain the values. If blood glucose does exceed target levels of 60 to 120 mg/dl, an insulin infusion should be started at 1 U/hr. The insulin dosage and intravenous glucose can be adjusted on the basis of the blood glucose values.

If an elective cesarean section is planned, the patient should also follow her usual meal and insulin regimen on the day before the procedure. The cesarean section should be planned for very early in the morning. An intravenous line with normal saline can be started. If the procedure is done quickly and expeditiously, the patient may not need glucose or insulin.

If the woman does not have euglycemia on the morning of induction or cesarean section, insulin and glucose infusions may need to be started immediately. For a woman with a known history of poor blood glucose control, hospitalization before delivery may be necessary to optimize control.

In the postdelivery period, insulin resistance rapidly declines and blood glucose levels often decrease. Hypoglycemia may occur. Frequent monitoring of blood glucose after delivery is necessary to avoid such problems. Until the trend in the blood glucose level is ascertained, insulin should not be given. Women who have injected an intermediate-acting or long-acting insulin shortly before an unexpected delivery (i.e., one related to spontaneous labor with vaginal delivery or an unplanned cesarean section) may have special problems with postdelivery hypoglycemia and should be monitored very closely. Many women may not need insulin for up to 24 to 48 hours after delivery.

When restarting a daily insulin regimen, a cautious approach should be taken. Insulin requirements in most women will have dropped substantially below the predelivery requirement. Often the question will arise as to what type of insulin regimen should be started. Most women will have been on an intensified regimen during the pregnancy, whereas some will have been on a conventional insulin regimen before becoming pregnant. Most women should be encouraged to pursue an intensified regimen to continue optimal glucose control.

Long-Term Outcome of Infants of Mothers With Diabetes

The role of heredity in the determination of IDDM and NIDDM has long been recognized. Epidemiologic studies done in the past allow one to predict the risk for development of IDDM in the offspring of parents with diabetes. For children of a mother with IDDM, the rate of diabetes development is approximately 1.2%. The rate is substantially higher for children of a father with IDDM, up to 6.8%.[14] If both parents have IDDM, the chances of the child developing diabetes increases significantly—20% to 30%.[145] The mother's age may make a difference in the offspring's risk for developing IDDM. A recent study found that the incidence of IDDM in children of mothers over age 25 approached that of the nondiabetic population.[132] The reasons for this difference are unclear.

HLA typing of the offspring can be done to identify the child with a high-risk profile for developing IDDM. If such identification is made, the question becomes how closely the child should be monitored for the development of diabetes. Islet cell antibodies may precede the development of IDDM by a number of years; currently, however, no successful intervention or preventive therapy is available for treating these individuals.[52]

Heredity plays a more important role in determination of NIDDM than IDDM. NIDDM is probably inherited as a dominant trait but with incomplete penetrance. Thus 50% of offspring could inherit the predisposition for this disease. Identical twins may have 100% concordance for NIDDM. The chances of inheriting NIDDM appears to be equal in terms of paternal versus maternal diabetes. If both mother and father have NIDDM, the risk for the offspring could be higher than 50%.[139]

Besides genetic concerns, many questions have arisen about the effect of maternal environment in causing long-term problems for the infant. Children of mothers with diabetes may be at increased risk for obesity, as shown in studies of the Pima Indian population.[115] Studies in other populations, including one from the Joslin Clinic, have supported these findings.[148] Excess obesity seen in offspring of women with diabetes may not be inevitable and can be prevented if the child is of normal birth weight and is placed on a carefully controlled diet.[33]

A study of the Pima Indian population indicated that the maternal blood glucose environment may also affect the development of glucose intolerance in offspring.[115] The rate of diabetes was higher in offspring of women with onset of diabetes before pregnancy than in the offspring of women who did not have diabetes at the time of the pregnancy but developed it later.

Some studies have examined the effect of diabetes in the mother during the pregnancy on subsequent neurologic development and IQ. Most of these studies have found no difference in neurologic outcome between the children of women with and without diabetes.[56,113] Glucose control may have some effect on the subsequent development of offspring of a pregnant mother with IDDM. A follow-up assessment of offspring from the DIEP study (see previous discussion) found that in tests of verbal intelligence at age 3 years, the offspring of women from the late-entry group scored lower than the offspring of the control and early-entry groups.[126]

Prepregnancy Counseling

All women with pregestational diabetes who are capable of childbearing should be well informed about pregnancy and diabetes (Box 11-4). The problems and concerns of the pregnancy must be understood, as well as the excellent chances for a successful pregnancy if the right treatment program is followed. Careful patient teaching regarding prepregnancy planning needs to be carefully followed. Involvement of the entire diabetes team is critical to optimal patient education. The importance of optimal blood glucose control at the time of conception and during the pregnancy must be strongly emphasized.

The question of initial poor blood glucose control on the outcome of a pregnancy can be a difficult one. Some women find themselves unexpectedly pregnant and are not sure they want to continue the pregnancy. They want definite answers about the risk of congenital abnormalities and other problems for themselves and the fetus.

BOX 11-4

EDUCATION PRINCIPLES: PREGESTATIONAL DIABETES

Emphasize the importance of prepregnancy care.

Work with the patient, her partner, her family, and other health care providers to improve the patient's nutrition, exercise program, and blood glucose control.

Recommend that conception be delayed until the patient's blood glucose control is excellent and the glycated hemoglobin level is normal or near normal.

Explain the risks of birth defects and adverse perinatal outcomes and the need for fetal surveillance.

Recommend that the patient's vascular condition be thoroughly evaluated before she becomes pregnant. Explain that pregnancy may exacerbate advanced diabetic retinopathy but generally does not permanently worsen diabetic nephropathy.

Explain that, overall, pregnancy does not shorten the life expectancy of a woman with diabetes but does increase her risk for hypoglycemia and ketoacidosis and associated mortality.

Inform patients with coronary atherosclerosis that their risks for morbidity or mortality may be greater during pregnancy.

Discuss the emotional and financial demands of pregnancy with the patient, her partner, and her family.

Inform patients about life-style elements, such as drinking alcoholic beverages and smoking, that increase the risk for a poor outcome of pregnancy. Emphasize that patients will need to modify such behaviors before becoming pregnant.

Modified from US Department of Health and Human Services, Public Health Service: *Prevention and treatment of complications of diabetes: a guide for primary care practitioners,* Atlanta, 1991, Center for Chronic Disease Prevention and Health Promotion, Division of Diabetes Translation, Centers for Disease Control.

Many women also have concerns about the effects of vascular complications of diabetes on the success of a pregnancy and, conversely, the effect of pregnancy on vascular complications, such as retinopathy and nephropathy. These questions must be covered thoroughly in prepregnancy counseling.

Counseling on birth control should also be part of the routine care for all women who are capable of childbearing. This includes not only women 20 to 40 years of age, but teenagers as well.

Many educational materials about diabetes and pregnancy are now available and can be used either as handouts or for interactive sessions between the prospective mother and the health care provider. Some diabetes centers have participated in programs that actively seek out women with diabetes who are interested in pregnancy to enroll them in an education program that addresses the problems of a pregnancy complicated by diabetes. A recent study showed that such interventions led to a decrease in congenital anomalies and complications of pregnancy.[75]

If a woman is seeking pregnancy, her diabetes control should be assessed. If it is not adequate, a program for achieving optimal blood glucose control can be instituted. How long the patient should be in optimal blood glucose control before conception is unclear. Many programs advise at least 3 to 6 months before attempting to achieve pregnancy.

Pregestational Diabetes and Pregnancy: Conclusion

The present approach to treatment of the pregnancy complicated by diabetes has made successful pregnancy very possible for the vast majority of women with diabetes who desire children. The key to success is a treatment program that utilizes a number of components, including preconceptual counseling, intensive efforts at tight blood glucose control before and during the pregnancy, frequent evaluations by the diabetes team and the high-risk obstetrics team, regular noninvasive measurements of fetal integrity, appropriate timing of delivery, and provision of neonatal care.

MANAGEMENT OF PREGNANCY COMPLICATED BY GESTATIONAL DIABETES

As many as 5% of all pregnant women experience gestational diabetes, making it one of the most common complications of pregnancy.[2] Gestational diabetes is defined by the Second International Workshop-Conference on Gestational Diabetes Mellitus as carbohydrate intolerance of variable severity with onset at first recognition during the present pregnancy.[117] This definition neither depends on the need for or use of insulin nor precludes the possibility that the condition existed before the present pregnancy and that it may be permanent. For the vast majority of women the condition will disappear at the end of the pregnancy. Statistics indicate that in 97% of women with gestational diabetes, glucose tolerance returns to normal after delivery.[105,116]

Gestational diabetes has been associated with increased fetal and maternal morbidity.[1,17,47,147] Therefore careful management of this condition is crucial. Over the past decade, increased awareness of the problems of gestational diabetes has led to a reevaluation of treatment programs and exploration of new approaches. Questions include the following:

- How tightly controlled should blood glucose levels be to ensure optimal outcome for both mother and child?
- How should the diagnosis be made?
- What is the risk to women with gestational diabetes for subsequent diabetes?

Physiology

As discussed earlier, insulin resistance increases and insulin requirements rise steeply during pregnancy. In some women, possibly because of genetic factors, the production of insulin by the beta cells appears to be limited. In these women, at some point in the pregnancy, insulin demand exceeds supply and hyperglycemia occurs. Because insulin requirements start to rise sharply around the twenty-fourth to twenty-eighth week of gestation, gestational diabetes is unlikely to appear at this time. Once delivery occurs, insulin requirements decrease dramatically, generally within hours.

Screening

In the past, most health care providers have screened pregnant women for diabetes on the basis of certain risk factors. Current recommendations of the American College of Obstetricians and Gynecologists (ACOG) are to screen all women over age 29 and screen those under age 29 based on the presence of traditional risk factors. Coustan and others,[25] in a survey of 6000 pregnancies, showed that one-half the cases of gestational diabetes would be missed if these recommendations were followed. This has led the American Diabetes Association (ADA) to recommend that all pregnant women be screened for abnormal glucose metabolism between the twenty-fourth and twenty-eighth week of gestation. Screening before 24 weeks might also be recommended if the presence of risk factors dictates. Risk factors that have been considered important for the development of gestational diabetes include a history of stillbirth or abortion, a family history of diabetes, previous delivery of an infant weighing more than 9 pounds (4 kg), previous gestational diabetes, a history of toxemia, urinary tract infections, hydramnios, advanced maternal age, glycosuria, and obesity. Interestingly, the incidence of gestational diabetes is significantly higher in pregnancies complicated by twins.[32]

The recommended screening method for gestational diabetes is the *glucose challenge test*. A 50 g oral glucose load is given regardless of previous meal or time of day. The venous plasma glucose level is measured 1 hour later. If this level is 140 mg/dl or greater, a full 3-hour, 100 g oral *glucose tolerance test* (GTT) is recommended.[109] In this test, 100 g oral glucose in at least 400 ml liquid is given in the morning after an overnight fast. An unrestricted diet containing at least 150 g carbohydrate should be eaten on the day before the test. The venous plasma glucose level is measured after fasting and at 1, 2, and 3 hours after glucose loading, during which the patient remains seated and does not smoke. The current criterion for a definitive diagnosis is two or more blood glucose values in excess of the following: fasting blood glucose, 105 mg/dl; 1 hour, 190 mg/dl; 2 hour, 165 mg/dl; and 3 hour, 145 mg/dl (Table 11-4). If only one of these values is elevated or the woman has a clinical history indicating possible glucose intolerance, the GTT is repeated at 32 weeks. If an individual has a previous history of gestational diabetes, it is often recommended that they be screened earlier than the 24- to 28-week period. Testing at 18 to 20 weeks has been suggested. If the screen is negative, a retest should be done at 24 to 28 weeks.

Table 11-4 Criteria for 100 g Oral Glucose Tolerance Test (GTT) in Pregnancy

Time	O'Sullivan*	NDDG adaptation†
Preglucose	90 mg/dl	105 mg/dl
1 hour	165 mg/dl	190 mg/dl
2 hours	145 mg/dl	165 mg/dl
3 hours	125 mg/dl	145 mg/dl

*O'Sullivan JB, Mahan CM: *Diabetes* 13:278, 1964.
†National Diabetes Data Group: *Diabetes* 28:1039, 1979.

Because of discrepancies between capillary and whole venous blood glucose levels, the use of capillary blood glucose determinations are not recommended by the ADA for the initial glucose challenge test.[72,83] Also, problems with precision and individual operator error make the use of reflectance meters questionable in screening. However, a recent study that compared the use of a reflectance meter operated by a single individual with laboratory-run venous samples found no difference in sensitivity or specificity between the two methods.[102] In this study the cutoff value for the capillary blood was 155 mg/dl. The glycated hemoglobin also should not be used for the diagnosis of gestational diabetes, since it is not sensitive enough to identify the changing glucose intolerance in gestational diabetes.[18]

Is it always necessary to do an oral GTT for diagnosis of gestational diabetes? This question, as with so many areas in gestational diabetes, is controversial. If the screening test result is greater than 200 mg/dl, some consensus exists that gestational diabetes is present and that further testing is not necessary. A few pregnant women will present with symptomatic hyperglycemia, with random blood glucose values in the 200 to 300 mg/dl range. These women need to be treated as if they have pregestational diabetes and started on insulin immediately. Some of these women will have new-onset type I diabetes; others may have delayed-onset type I diabetes or incipient type II diabetes and will revert to normal glycemia after delivery, but usually only for limited periods.

Currently the 3-hour oral GTT is regarded as the "gold standard" of diagnosis in gestational diabetes. Questions have been raised as to whether the present criteria allow enough specificity not to miss cases of gestational diabetes as defined by perinatal morbidity. Much of this concern has related to the individual with only one abnormal blood glucose level on the test. Langer and others[88] followed women with only one abnormal test and found increased macrosomia. Tallarigo and co-workers studied the relationship of the 2-hour plasma glucose levels on an oral GTT to fetal and maternal morbidity. They found that women with 2-hour levels in the range of 120 to 160 mg/dl, values that would be called normally present and accepted criteria for the oral GTT, had an increased incidence of macrosomia, toxemia, and cesarean section.[138] There should be ongoing evaluation and reassessment of methods of screening and diagnosis in gestational diabetes. The current recommendations from the ADA are to screen all pregnant women for gestational diabetes and to diagnose it on the basis of the O'Sullivan criteria.

Morbidity and Mortality

Studies have shown that the infant of a mother with gestational diabetes is at increased risk for a number of different conditions, including hypoglycemia, polycythemia, hyperbilirubinemia, and RDS. The incidence of intrauterine death, premature delivery, and neonatal mortality is also increased.[17,47,147] Macrosomia is more common in gestational diabetes and can lead to difficulties in delivery that may affect the infant and the mother.[16] In addition to increased problems with neonatal complications, there is increased risk for maternal complications, including pregnancy-induced hypertension, hydramnios, and an increased incidence of cesarean section.[23] Two recent studies have shown that the average cesarean rate for patients with gestational diabetes approximates 30%.[22,61]

A pregnancy complicated by gestational diabetes must be considered a high-risk pregnancy. Once the diagnosis is made, the mother and fetus should be under close scrutiny. Some gestational diabetes programs emphasize the team approach to management, with the involvement of a diabetologist and an obstetrician specializing in high-risk pregnancy. Other professionals important to an effective treatment program are a nurse educator and dietitian. Involvement of a psychologist or a counselor can be helpful in many cases. The diagnosis of gestational diabetes may create severe anxiety and concern in the pregnant woman. Her major fears usually focus on risk to the fetus and future maternal risk for permanent diabetes. Concerns may be especially pronounced in a woman with a family history of diabetes.

Approaches to Therapy

Traditionally, therapy for gestational diabetes has been based on the results of a 3-hour oral GTT. If a woman presents with a fasting blood glucose level greater than 105 mg/dl, she is started on a program of insulin and diet therapy. A woman with a fasting blood glucose level less than 105 mg/dl, but with abnormal post–glucose challenge values, is usually started on diet therapy alone. Metabolic goals for these women are fasting blood glucose levels less than 105 mg/dl, 1-hour postprandial glucose levels less than 140 mg/dl, and 2-hour postprandial levels less than 120 mg/dl.[117] Blood glucose goals in gestational diabetes are currently being reevaluated in light of levels found in the nondiabetic pregnancy. The blood glucose values seen in a nondiabetic pregnancy are lower than traditionally accepted treatment goals for gestational diabetes. In the third trimester of a nondiabetic pregnancy, fasting blood glucose levels generally range from 50 to 90 mg/dl and 1-hour postprandial levels from 80 to 120 mg/dl.[35] Langer and others[87] found that a treatment program based on blood glucose values compatible with those seen in nondiabetic pregnant women resulted in a marked decrease in perinatal complications in a group of women with gestational diabetes. This result was also shown by Hollander and associates.[61] Goals of a fasting glucose of 105 mg/dl and a 2-hour postprandial glucose of 120 mg/dl are still suggested in the report of the Third International Workshop on Gestational Diabetes; however, the evidence for tighter glucose goals continues to mount.[58]

Monitoring

An important aspect of any treatment program for gestational diabetes is ongoing monitoring of blood glucose. In the traditional approach to treatment of gestational diabetes, women may visit their physician's office once or twice a week for preprandial and postprandial blood glucose values. This frequency of monitoring does not give adequate information to make decisions on therapy in a timely manner. Moreover, in many cases the patient will be on her best behavior in regard to diet on the days those values are obtained, and thus they do not provide reliable data. As already noted, glycated hemoglobin is also not helpful in monitoring gestational diabetes, since it is not sensitive enough to detect the degree of maternal hyperglycemia that needs treatment. Daily SMBG can provide the necessary data to implement the current, more intensive treatment programs in gestational diabetes. Most investigators suggest that both premeal and postmeal blood glucose levels be checked. Such a program involves testing at least four to six times a day, including 1- or 2-hour postprandial values.[61,87] For SMBG to be useful, technique and machine reliability must also be consistently evaluated.

Diet Therapy

Diet therapy is a key part of treatment for gestational diabetes, whether used alone or with insulin therapy. The basic goals in regard to calorie planning are the maintenance of euglycemia (i.e., blood glucose levels within the target range) and appropriate weight gain. Goals for weight gain are the same for pregnancies complicated by pregestational diabetes and by gestational diabetes. (See the earlier discussion of caloric intake and weight gain.) Certain aspects of diet therapy for gestational diabetes are challenging. The primary example is that a disproportionate number of obese women develop gestational diabetes, and at diagnosis many women have already gained excess weight.

Diet counseling in a gestational diabetes program should begin with a meeting between the woman and the dietitian. A diet with a specific calorie goal should be set based on prepregnancy weight and desired weight gain during the pregnancy.

Weight and calorie intake must be monitored closely throughout the program. Some women make extreme calorie cuts to control blood glucose levels and avoid insulin therapy and may not achieve proper weight gain. Many women are eating excess carbohydrate in the form of simple sugars such as soda, ice cream, and other desserts. Often the elimination of these simple sugars can make a significant difference in blood glucose control. It is not unusual to see a plateau in weight gain for 1 or 2 weeks in most women after starting their new diet.[61] However, if subsequent weight gain is not appropriate, calorie level may need to be increased. As in pregestational diabetes and pregnancy, the breakfast postprandial glucose is very difficult to control. Shifting away from a high-carbohydrate breakfast can be very helpful. Limited exercise after meals can also help limit postprandial glucose variations.

Insulin Therapy

Insulin therapy should be started if blood glucose goals are not met with diet treatment alone. As in pregestational diabetes, oral hypoglycemic agents are not recommended for treatment of gestational diabetes.[92] Several different insulin regimens have been used for the treatment of gestational diabetes. Although it has been suggested that all women with gestational diabetes should be treated with insulin, most current programs initiate insulin therapy on the basis of maintaining blood glucose goals.[8,22,61,87]

Coustan[20] described a program of insulin treatment in which women are treated initially with a dose of 30 U insulin daily, with 20 U NPH and 10 U regular insulin in the morning. If hyperglycemia persists, adjustments are made in the specific components based on the blood glucose pattern. Board and associates[8] describe a program of insulin therapy for gestational diabetes similar to an intensive program for women with pregestational diabetes, that is, a four-shot regimen that uses both NPH and regular insulin.

Hollander and colleagues[62] describe a mixed injection of regular and NPH insulin given before breakfast and dinner. In this regimen a high ratio of regular insulin to NPH is used to control postprandial blood glucose variation. All these groups have shown good outcomes with insulin treatment.

For most women with gestational diabetes, insulin can be started on an outpatient basis. Arrangements should be made so that insulin can be adjusted quickly and consistently. This goal can be accomplished by frequent contact with the diabetes management team, such as telephone calls twice a week, and by weekly or biweekly appointments. Simple algorithms for self-adjustment of insulin by the patient can also be helpful. If a woman initially has extremely elevated blood glucose levels and ketones, hospitalization is mandated.

Human insulin is the insulin of choice in the treatment of gestational diabetes. Since these women have not been exposed to nonhuman insulins, using human insulin significantly decreases the chance of developing insulin antibodies during the pregnancy. This may be important for the subset of women who will develop diabetes in the future and will require insulin. Although severe hypoglycemia is rare in insulin-treated gestational diabetes, mild episodes may occur. The patients should be taught to recognize the symptoms of hypoglycemia and how to treat it effectively.

Certain problems that may arise close to term, such as premature labor, can result in challenges for glucose control. Terbutaline, a common treatment for this problem, can cause hyperglycemia.[114] Thus control can worsen, and a patient doing well on diet may have to be changed to insulin or, if taking insulin, to a more aggressive program. Some have suggested that any pregnant woman placed on terbutaline therapy should be screened or rescreened for gestational diabetes.

Obstetric Care and Fetal Evaluation

A key aspect of any gestational diabetes treatment program is antepartum monitoring. Once the diagnosis of pregnancy is made, the woman should have close follow-up by her obstetrician. Increased frequency of antenatal monitoring of the fetus is necessary, especially in the insulin-treated mother. In women whose blood glucose control is not optimal or who have a history of maternal complications such as pregnancy-induced hypertension, this monitoring should begin early; 34 weeks has been suggested, and by 36 weeks all fetuses should be monitored closely. This assessment may consist of a weekly NST, followed by an OCT if necessary. BPPs may also be helpful.[84] Generally, it is not advisable to allow delivery to go beyond term.

Postpartum Follow-up

At present, most women are tested with a 75 g oral GTT at 6 weeks postpartum.[103] Whether this test is optimal or necessary is currently being questioned. For instance, if women who have overt diabetes immediately after delivery are eliminated, glucose tolerance will be normal in 99% of the women tested.[105] Other methods of testing for diabetes, such as a fasting blood glucose or glycated hemoglobin, are simpler, more reliable, and less expensive. Besides being inappropriate for diagnosis, the relevance of an oral GTT in a nonpregnant woman as a predictor of future diabetes must be questioned.

Another approach to postpartum evaluation of glucose intolerance is to continue capillary blood testing for individuals whose anticipated risk for the development of diabetes in the postpartum period is high. Women who initially have elevated fasting blood glucose levels or elevated glycated hemoglobin during pregnancy are the best candidates for this approach.

Long-Term Outcomes

What are the long-term outcomes for women with gestational diabetes? Most women are concerned about the chance of recurrent gestational diabetes with future pregnancies and the possibilities of developing clinical diabetes at some point in their life. Because of these fears, discussion of potential future problems with the woman is essential. If gestational diabetes has occurred once, the chances of recurrence in a subsequent pregnancy are about 50%.[91] For most women, recurrent gestational diabetes should not be a major factor in the decision for or against another pregnancy, since repeat episodes of gestational diabetes do not appear to contribute to a greater incidence of future diabetes.[106] Parity itself does not seem to increase the incidence of NIDDM in women.[93]

The development of clinical diabetes later in life should be a major concern. Twenty percent of nonobese and about 60% of obese women with gestational diabetes will develop clinical diabetes within 15 years of pregnancy[107] (Fig. 11-5). Women with a history of gestational diabetes have also been shown to have an increased mortality rate and a higher incidence of cardiovascular disease than the general population of women.[108]

In the past, gestational diabetes was thought to be a predictor of NIDDM. However, recent studies indicate that some women with gestational diabetes will eventually develop IDDM. Studies of islet cell antibody levels and determination of HLA antigens in several populations of women with gestational diabetes have identified a number of women with profiles characteristic of pre-IDDM individuals.[44,135] In some women with gestational diabetes, islet cell antibody positivity may be as high as 30% to 48%.[50]

About 3% of all women with gestational diabetes will remain diabetic after delivery.[105] According to Metzger and associates,[98] if fasting hyperglycemia is identified during pregnancy, diabetes is more likely to persist after delivery. In their series, women with fasting blood glucose levels of 105 to 130 mg/dl had a 43% chance of remaining diabetic. If fasting blood glucose exceeded 130 mg/dl, this probability rose to 83%.

Gestational diabetes is one of the most reliable predictors of future clinical diabetes mellitus. Most women will develop NIDDM, whereas a minority will develop IDDM. A woman with a history of gestational diabetes should be screened periodically for diabetes. Annual testing should be a minimal requirement. Since obesity is a risk factor for NIDDM, some women may be able to delay or even prevent its onset by controlling their weight. Studies have also indicated that routine physical exercise can delay or possibly prevent the onset of NIDDM in the genetically predisposed individual.[60]

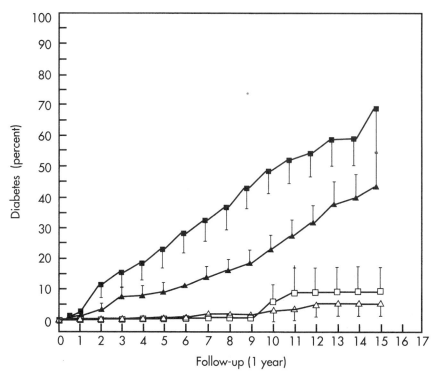

Fig. 11-5 Cumulative incidence of diabetes in overweight women *(black squares)* and normal-weight women *(black triangles)* with gestational diabetes; overweight *(white squares)* and normal-weight *(white triangles)* controls. Percentage +/≥ SE. (From O'Sullivan JB: *JAMA* 248:949, 1982.)

The importance of patient education for all women with gestational diabetes, as well as for those with a positive history of risk for gestational diabetes, is imperative (Box 11-5). The diabetes health care team is crucial to a positive outcome for both the woman with diabetes and her child. As previously addressed, close monitoring before conception, as well as during and after pregnancy, is related to optimal outcomes for mother and child. Patient education principles that guide the health team in caring for the woman with gestational diabetes need to be carefully administered. Precise documentation of care is also necessary, with follow-up and progress comprehensively recorded.

CASE PRESENTATION

A.W. is a 29-year-old white woman with a 16-year history of type I diabetes. She has been referred to the diabetes clinic by her obstetrician at 8 weeks' gestation. This is not a planned pregnancy, and her HbA_{1c} obtained by the obstetrician is 9.2% (normal, 4% to 6%). The patient's diabetes care has been

---

BOX 11-5

EDUCATION PRINCIPLES: GESTATIONAL DIABETES

For women with gestational diabetes

Work with the patient, her partner, her family, and other health care providers to improve the patient's nutrition, exercise program, and blood glucose control.

Explain the risks of adverse perinatal outcomes and the need for fetal surveillance.

Inform patients that they are at increased risk both for developing gestational diabetes during future pregnancies and for developing overt diabetes later in life.

Encourage physical activity and postpartum weight loss to decrease the likelihood of developing diabetes later in life.

Recommend a postpartum evaluation at 6 to 8 weeks and annually thereafter for detecting the development of diabetes.

For women with a history of gestational diabetes

Recommend screening for overt diabetes before subsequent pregnancies.

Recommend early screening for the onset of carbohydrate intolerance during subsequent pregnancies.

Modified from US Department of Health and Human Services, Public Health Service: *Prevention and treatment of complications of diabetes: a guide for primary care practitioners,* Atlanta, 1991, Center for Chronic Disease Prevention and Health Promotion, Division of Diabetes Translation, Centers for Disease Control.

---

intermittent, and she has mainly seen her primary care physician for acute problems. Prepregnancy weight was 121 lb; height is 5 ft, 4 in; and current weight is 124 lb. She does not follow a diet plan and has a high intake of simple carbohydrates and fat. She takes two injections of insulin a day, regular/NPH in the AM and in the PM. Capillary blood glucose testing is not routine. Her most common testing time is in the morning and is usually greater than 150 mg/dl. She supplements regular insulin almost at random, usually for a "high blood glucose" or for extra food. A.W. states that she feels "low" if blood glucose falls below 100 mg/dl.

A.W. has heard that good glucose control is important for pregnancy but had not thought she would become pregnant. Birth control had been sporadic use of condoms and foam. She has decided that she wants to proceed with the pregnancy.

A.W. does have a history of background retinopathy, but her last eye examination was 2 years ago. She denies any symptoms of neuropathy and does not know if she has any evidence of nephropathy.

This is the first pregnancy for A.W. She is married and works as a manager for a food service.

DISCUSSION

Ideally, all women of childbearing age should have preconceptual counseling in regard to the importance of optimal glucose control both before and during the pregnancy. However, cases such as A.W.'s do occur and present a major challenge to the diabetes care team.

The chances of success for such pregnancies may depend on the psychologic and intellectual makeup of the woman and her ability to perform the behaviors necessary to lower the glucose levels and maintain them throughout the pregnancy.

A.W. was seen by the diabetes care team. Initial discussion centered on the importance of glucose control and what would be required of her to meet those goals. Her initial HbA_{1c} placed her in the highest-risk category for major congenital anomalies, and this was also discussed. A.W. had made the decision to go on with the pregnancy, and therefore emphasis was placed on the use of ultrasound and amniocentesis to identify major problems early in the pregnancy.

The next step is to assess the patient's skills in SMBG and knowledge of diet, insulin action, and causes and treatment of hypoglycemia. It is important to bring blood glucose levels down quickly. Can this be done safely and effectively in an outpatient setting, or should a patient such as A.W. be hospitalized? Besides technique and knowledge, the patient's degree of compliance must be estimated. In many cases, hospitalization may be best for a patient, and after initial evaluation, the health care team thought this would be best for A.W. on the basis of her previous history of compliance and deficits in diabetes education. While A.W. was in the hospital, diet, insulin regimens, hypoglycemia, and meter use were reviewed. An attempt to follow the patient's usual routine in terms of meals and exercise should be made in the hospital. A.W. was started on a four-injection insulin regimen: AM, regular/NPH; noon, regular; PM, regular; and bedtime, NPH; also, a simple supplement scale was set up. Appropriate laboratory testing, including tests for nephropathy, was done. She was negative for microalbuminuria and mild background retinopathy when seen by the ophthalmologist. After 4 days, A.W. was discharged.

Not all women with elevated HbA_{1c} need to be hospitalized. Depending on their past record or on a detailed past history from newly referred patients, an outpatient setting may be appropriate. The availability of personnel for daily telephone contact to review blood glucose values with the patient is essential for using an outpatient approach.

A.W. was seen for her first follow-up visit 1 week after leaving the hospital. She had been in telephone contact with the clinic. She had gone back to work, and her base regular insulin dose at lunch was decreased because of activity at work. Her bedtime NPH dose was raised to control fasting blood sugar further. She complained of continuing to "feel low" at blood sugar levels of 70 to 120 mg/dl and complained of blurred vision. These two phenomena may occur in patients whose blood glucose is decreased rapidly from previously high levels. In many patients, their "glucostat" needs to be reset to recognize the normal range of blood glucose. This resetting can take up to several weeks.

The blurred vision usually results from changes in the refractive index of the lens of the eye. These changes occur as the concentration of glucose in the lens changes secondary to improvement of glucose control. It may take several weeks for stabilization. However, for such patients as A.W., other concerns exist in relation to the eyes. In patients who have preproliferative or proliferative retinopathy, rapid intensification may stimulate progression of the eye disease. Thus it is important to establish baseline status of the eye and monitor appropriately through the pregnancy as needed.

A.W. was seen again in 2 weeks, at that point, 12 weeks' gestation. Her weight was 134 lb, and she was concerned that she was becoming too fat. A review of her food records showed that she still was including too much simple carbohydrate in her diet and covering it with supplemental regular insulin. Often, patients such as A.W., if not always consciously, use poor control to maintain weight in the form of glycosuria. This point often needs to be discussed with patients to help them focus on what it means to match appetite to calories to insulin. Review of blood glucose records showed that most of A.W.'s blood glucose levels were in the targeted range. She was complimented on her achievement. Support and reinforcement for the patient's accomplishments are important in promoting ongoing compliance and progress.

A repeat HbA_{1c} test was done, and it had dropped about 0.7%, to 8.5%. This is an appropriate decrease for several weeks of good control. It is essential to obtain periodic HgA_{1c} values during pregnancy to ensure that fabrication of values is not occurring, especially in patients such as A.W.

A.W. is off to good start. She has a major role in promoting the success of the pregnancy, and in many cases such as A.W.'s, the patient will do very well throughout the pregnancy.

REFERENCES

1. American College of Obstetricians and Gynecologists: *Exercise during pregnancy and the postnatal period,* Washington, DC, 1985, ACOG.

2. American Diabetes Association Workshop: Conference on Gestational Diabetes: summary and recommendations, *Diabetes Care* 3:499-501, 1980.

3. Angel J and others: Carbohydrate intolerance in patients receiving oral tocolytics, *Am J Obstet Gynecol* 159:762, 1988.

4. Bantle JP and others: Rotation of the anatomic regions used for insulin injections and day-to-day variability of plasma glucose in type I diabetes, *JAMA* 263:1802, 1990.

5. Barreau P, Buttery J: The effect of the haematocrit value on the determination of glucose levels by reagent strip methods, *Med J Aust* 147:286, 1987.

6. Battaglia FC, Meschia G: Principal substrates of fetal metabolism, *Physiol Rev* 58:499, 1978.

7. Beard A and others: Neonatal hypoglycemia: a discussion, *J Pediatr* 79:314, 1971.

8. Board PJ and others: Gestational diabetes: definition, diagnosis and treatment strategies, *Pract Diabetol* 5:1, 1986.

9. Broughton-Pipkin F, Symonels E, Turner S: The effect of captopril on the mother and fetus in the chronically cannulated ewe and pregnant rabbit, *J Physiol* 323:415, 1982.

10. Carrington ER, Shuman CR, Reardon H: Evaluation of the prediabetic state during pregnancy, *Obstet Gynecol* 9:664, 1957.

11. Coetzee EJ, Jackson WPU: Metformin in management of pregnant insulin-dependent diabetics, *Diabetologia* 16:241, 1979.

12. Combs C and others: Relationship of fetal macrosomia to maternal postprandial glucose control during pregnancy, *Diabetes Care* 15:1251, 1992.

13. Committee on Dietary Allowances, Food and Nutrition Board, National Academy of Sciences: *Recommended dietary allowances,* ed 9, Washington, DC, 1980, US Government Printing Office.

14. Corwin RS: Pregnancy complicated by diabetes mellitus in private practice: a review of ten years, *Am J Obstet Gynecol* 134:156, 1979.

15. Costrini NV, Kalkhoff RK: Relative effects of pregnancy, estradiol, and progesterone on plasma insulin and pancreatic islet insulin secretion, *J Clin Invest* 50:992, 1971.

16. Cousins L: Pregnancy complications among diabetic women: review 1965-1985, *Obstet Gynecol Surv* 42:140, 1987.

17. Cousins L, Jacoby J: Infant and maternal outcomes in gestational diabetes mellitus: a prospective control study, *Diabetes* 36(suppl 1):818A, 1987.

18. Cousins L and others: Glycosylated hemoglobin as a screening test for carbohydrate intolerance in pregnancy, *Am J Obstet Gynecol* 150:455, 1984.

19. Coustan D: Delivery timing, mode, and management. In Reece E, Coustan D, editors: *Diabetes mellitus in pregnancy: principles and practice,* New York, 1988, Churchill Livingstone.

20. Coustan D: Management of gestational diabetes. In Reece E, Coustan D, editors: *Diabetes mellitus in pregnancy: principles and practices,* New York, 1988, Churchill Livingstone.

21. Coustan D: Obstetrical complications. In Reece E, Coustan D, editors: *Diabetes mellitus in pregnancy: practices and principles,* New York, 1988, Churchill Livingstone.

22. Coustan D, Imarah J: Prophylactic insulin treatment of gestational diabetes reduces the incidence of macrosomia, operative delivery, and birth trauma, *Am J Obstet Gynecol* 150:836-842, 1984.

23. Coustan D, Berkowitz RL, Hobbins JC: Tight metabolic control of overt diabetes in pregnancy, *Am J Med* 68:845, 1980.

24. Coustan D and others: A randomized clinical trial of the insulin pump vs. intensive conventional therapy in diabetic pregnancies, *JAMA* 255:631, 1986.

25. Coustan D and others: Maternal age and screening for gestational diabetes: a population-based study, *Obstet Gynecol* 73:557, 1989.

26. Davin JP Jr: Screening of high-risk and general populations for gestational diabetes: clinical application and cost analysis, *Diabetes* 34(suppl 2):24, 1985.

27. The DCCT research: Diabetes Control and Complications Trial: results of the feasibility study, *Diabetes Care* 10:1, 1987.

28. Diabetes Control and Complications Trial Research Group: The effect of intensive treatment of diabetes on the development and progression of long-term complications in insulin dependent diabetes mellitus, *N Engl J Med* 329:977, 1993.

29. Dooley S and others: Urinary estriols in diabetic pregnancy: a reappraisal, *Obstet Gynecol* 64:469, 1984.

30. Drury MI, Greene AT, Strong JM: Pregnancy complicated by clinical diabetes mellitus: a study of 600 pregnancies, *Obstet Gynecol* 49:519, 1977.

31. Durin J: Energy requirements of pregnancy: an integration of the longitudinal data from the five-county study, *Lancet* 2:1131, 1987.

32. Dwyer PL and others: Glucose tolerance in twin pregnancy, *Aust NZ J Obstet Gynecol* 22:131, 1982.

33. Enzi G and others: Development of adipose tissue in newborns of gestational-diabetic and insulin-

dependent diabetic mothers, *Diabetes* 29:100, 1980.

34. Enzi G and others: Postnatal development of adipose tissue in normal children on strictly controlled calorie intake, *Metabolism* 31:1029, 1982.

35. Espinosa de los Monteros AM and others: Periprandial blood glucose and insulin values during the third trimester of normal pregnancies, *Diabetes Care* 7:180, 1984.

36. Fadel H, Hammond S: Diabetes mellitus and pregnancy: management and results, *J Reprod Med* 27:56, 1982.

37. Felig P: Body fuel metabolism and diabetes mellitus in pregnancy, *Med Clin North Am* 66:43, 1977.

38. Felig P, Coustan D: Diabetes mellitus. In Burnow A, Ferris T, editors: *Complications of pregnancy,* ed 2, Philadelphia, 1982, Saunders.

39. Felig P, Lynch V: Starvation in human pregnancy: hypoglycemia, hypoinsulinemia, and hyperketonemia, *Science* 170:990, 1970.

40. Fisher PM, Sutherland HW, Bewsher PD: Insulin response to glucose infusion in normal human pregnancy, *Diabetologia* 19:15, 1980.

41. Freeman RK, Anderson G, Dorchester W: A prospective multi-institutional study of antepartum fetal heart rate monitoring. I. Risk of perinatal mortality and morbidity according to antepartum fetal heart rate test results, *Am J Obstet Gynecol* 143:771, 1982.

42. Freeman RK, Anderson G, Dorchester W: A prospective multi-institutional study of antepartum fetal heart rate monitoring. II. Contraction stress test versus nonstress test for primary surveillance, *Am J Obstet Gynecol* 143:778, 1982.

43. Freinkel N: Of pregnancy and progeny, *Diabetes* 29:1023, 1980.

44. Freinkel N and others: Gestational diabetes mellitus: heterogeneity of maternal age, weight, insulin secretion, HLA antigens and islet cell antibodies and the impact of maternal metabolism on pancreatic beta-cell and somatic development in the offspring, *Diabetes* 34(suppl 2):1, 1985.

45. Gabbe SG: Management of diabetes in pregnancy: six decades of experience. In Pitkin RM, Zlatnik FJ, editors: *Yearbook of obstetrics and gynecology. Part I. Obstetrics,* Chicago, 1980, Yearbook.

46. Gabbe S, Mestman J, Hibbord L: Maternal mortality in diabetes mellitus: an 18-year survey, *Obstet Gynecol* 48:549, 1986.

47. Gabbe SG and others: Management and outcome of class A diabetes mellitus, *Am J Obstet Gynecol* 127:465, 1977.

48. Gabbe SG and others: Management and outcome of pregnancy in diabetes mellitus, classes B to R, *Am J Obstet Gynecol* 129:723, 1977.

49. Gant NF and others: The metabolic clearance rate of dehydroisoandrosterone sulfate. III. The effect of thiazide diuretics in normal and future preeclamptic pregnancies, *Am J Obstet Gynecol* 123:159, 1975.

50. Gillis S, Hisa D: The infant of the diabetic mother, *J Doctor Child* 97:1, 1959.

51. Ginsberg-Fellner F and others: Islet cell antibodies in gestational diabetes, *Lancet* 2:362, 1980.

52. Ginsberg-Fellner F and others: HLA antigens, cytoplasmic islet cell antibodies, and carbohydrate tolerance in families of children with insulin-dependent diabetes mellitus, *Diabetes* 31:292, 1982.

53. Golde SH and others: Insulin requirements during labor: a reappraisal, *Am J Obstet Gynecol* 144:556, 1982.

54. Golde SH and others: The role of nonstress tests, fetal biophysical profile and contraction stress tests in the outpatient management of insulin-requiring diabetic pregnancies, *Am J Obstet Gynecol* 148:269, 1984.

55. Gyves MT and others: A modern approach to management of pregnant diabetics: a 2-year analysis of perinatal outcome, *Am J Obstet Gynecol* 128:606, 1977.

56. Hadden DR and others: Physical and psychological health of children of type I (insulin-dependent) diabetic mothers, *Diabetologia* 26:250, 1984.

57. Hanson U, Persson B, Thowell S: Relationship between haemoglobin A in early type 1 (insulin-dependent) diabetic pregnancy and the occurrence of spontaneous abortion and fetal malformation in Sweden, *Diabetologia* 33:94, 1990.

58. Hare J: Levels of glycemia as management goals, Third International Workshop-Conferences on Gestational Diabetes Mellitus, *Diabetes* 40(suppl 2):92, 1991.

59. Haworth JC, McRae KN, Dilling LA: Prognosis of infants of diabetic mothers in relation to neonatal hypoglycaemia, *Dev Med Child Neurol* 18:471, 1976.

60. Helmrich S and others: Physical activity and reduced occurrence of non-insulin-dependent diabetes mellitus, *N Engl J Med* 325:147, 1991.

61. Hollander P and others: Optimal therapy for improved outcome in gestational diabetes, *Diabetologia* 30(suppl 1):224A, 1987.

62. Hollander P and others: Insulin therapy and improved outcome in gestational diabetes, *Diabetes* 37(suppl 1):261A, 1988.

63. Hunter D and others: Influence of maternal insulin in insulin dependent diabetes on neonatal morbidity, 149:47, 1993.

64. Jackson WV: Studies in prediabetes, *Br Med J* 2:690, 1952.

65. Javier Z, Gershberg H, Hulse M: Ovulatory suppressants, estrogens, and carbohydrate metabolism, *Metabolism* 17:443, 1968.

66. Jervell J and others: Diabetes mellitus and pregnancy: management and results at Rikshopitalet Oslo 1970-1977, *Diabetologia* 16:151, 1979.

67. Joslin EP and others: *The treatment of diabetes mellitus,* ed 8, Philadelphia, 1948, Lea & Febiger.

68. Jovanovic L, Peterson CM: Management of the pregnant insulin-dependent diabetic woman, *Diabetes Care* 3:63, 1980.

69. Jovanovic L, Peterson CM: Optimal insulin delivery for the pregnant diabetic patient, *Diabetes Care* 5:24, 1982.

70. Jovanovic L, Peterson CM: Insulin and glucose requirements during the first stage of labor in insulin-dependent diabetic women, *Am J Med* 75:607, 1983.

71. Jovanovic L, Douzin M, Peterson C: Effect of euglycemia on the outcome of pregnancy in insulin dependent diabetic women as compared to normal control subjects, *Am J Med* 71:921, 1981.

72. Jovanovic-Peterson L, Peterson CM: Screening for gestational diabetes with solid-phase reagent strips, *Diabetes Professional* 20:5, 1988.

73. Jovanovic-Peterson L, Kitzmiller J, Peterson KC: Randomized trial of human versus animal species insulin in diabetic pregnant women: improved glycemic control, not fewer antibodies to insulin, influences birth weight, *Am J Obstet Gynecol* 167:1325, 1992.

74. Kahkonen D and others: Outcomes of pregnancies in the Diabetes Control and Complications Trial (DCCT), *Diabetes* 44:13a (suppl), 1995.

75. Kalkhoff RK, Jacobson M, Lemper D: Progesterone, pregnancy and the augmented plasma insulin response, *J Clin Endocrinol* 31:24, 1970.

76. Karlsson K, Kjellmer I: The outcome of diabetic pregnancies in relation to the mother's blood sugar level, *Am J Obstet Gynecol* 112:213, 1972.

77. Kitzmiller J and others: Diabetic pregnancy and perinatal morbidity, *Am J Obstet Gynecol* 131:560, 1978.

78. Kitzmiller JL and others: Diabetic nephropathy and perinatal outcome, *Am J Obstet Gynecol* 141:741, 1981.

79. Kitzmiller J and others: Preconception care of diabetes: glycemia control prevents congenital anomalies, *JAMA* 265:731-736, 1991.

80. Klein B, Klein R: Gravidity and diabetic retinopathy, *Am J Epidemiol* 119:564, 1984.

81. Klein B, Moss S, Klein R: Effect of pregnancy on progression of diabetic retinopathy, *Diabetes Care* 13:17-22, 1990.

82. The Kroc Collaborative Study: Blood glucose control and the evolution of diabetic retinopathy and albuminuria, *N Engl J Med* 311:372, 1984.

83. Landon MB, Cembrowski GS: Capillary blood glucose screening for gestational diabetes: a preliminary investigation, *Am J Obstet Gynecol* 155:717, 1986.

84. Landon MB, Gabbe SG: Antepartum fetal surveillance in gestational diabetes mellitus, *Diabetes* 34(suppl 2):50, 1985.

85. Landon M and others: Fetal surveillance in pregnancies complicated by insulin dependent diabetes, *Am J Obstet Gynecol* 167:617, 1992.

86. Langer O, Mazze RS: Diabetes in pregnancy: evaluation self-monitoring performance and glycemic control with memory-based reflectance meters, *Am J Obstet Gynecol* 155:635, 1986.

87. Langer O and others: Gestational diabetes: insulin requirements in pregnancy, *Am J Obstet Gynecol* 157:669, 1987.

88. Langer O and others: The significance of one abnormal glucose tolerance test value on adverse outcome in pregnancy, *Am J Obstet* 157:758, 1987.

89. Like A, Orci L: Embryogenesis of the human pancreatic islets: a light and electron microscopic study, *Diabetes* 21:511, 1972.

90. Lufkin G and others: An analysis of diabetic pregnancies at Mayo Clinic 1950-79, *Diabetes Care* 7:539, 1984.

91. Lupo VR, Stys SJ: Recurrence of gestational diabetes in subsequent pregnancies. In Weiss PAM, Coustan DR, editors: *Gestational diabetes,* Vienna, 1988, Springer-Verlag.

92. Malins JM and others: Sulphonylurea drugs in pregnancy, *Br Med J* 3D:187, 1964.

93. Manson J and others: Parity and incidence of NIDDM, *Am J Med* 93:137, 1992.

94. Martin T, Allen A, Stinson D: Overt diabetes in pregnancy, *Am J Obstet Gynecol* 133:275, 1979.

95. Mazze R and others: Reliability of blood glucose monitoring by patients with diabetes mellitus, *Am J Med* 77:212, 1984.

96. McManqus R, Ryan E: Insulin requirements in insulin-dependent diabetes and insulin-requiring GDM women during the final month of pregnancy, *Diabetes Care* 15:1323, 1992.

97. Menon R and others: Transplacental passage of insulin in pregnant women with insulin-dependent diabetes: its role in fetal macrosomia, *N Engl J Med* 321:15, 1990.

98. Metzger B and others: Gestational diabetes mellitus: correlations between the phenotypic and genotypic characteristics of the mother and

abnormal glucose tolerance during the first year postpartum, *Diabetes* 34(suppl 2):111, 1985.

99. Meueller-Beubach E and others: Lecithin/sphingomyelin ratio in amniotic fluid and its value for the prediction of neonatal respiratory distress syndrome in pregnant diabetic women, *Am J Obstet Gynecol* 130:25, 1978.

100. Miller E and others: Elevated maternal hemoglobin A in early pregnancy and major congenital anomalies in infants of diabetic mothers, *N Engl J Med* 304:1331, 1981.

101. Mills J and others: Lack of relation of increased malformation rates in infants of diabetic mothers to glycemic control during organogenesis, National Institute of Child Health and Human Development, Diabetes in Early Pregnancy Study, *N Engl J Med* 318:671, 1988.

102. Murphy J and others: Screening for gestational diabetes with a reflectance photometer, *Obstet Gynecol* 83:1038, 1994.

103. National Diabetes Data Group: Classification and diagnosis of diabetes mellitus and other categories of glucose intolerance, *Diabetes* 28:1039, 1979.

104. National Research Council: *Recommended dietary allowances,* Washington, DC, 1989, National Academy Press.

105. O'Sullivan JB: Long-term follow-up of gestational diabetes. In Camerini-Davolos RA, Cole HS, editors: *Early diabetes in early life,* Orlando, Fla, 1975, Academic Press.

106. O'Sullivan JB: Gestational diabetes: factors influencing rates of subsequent diabetes. In Sutherland HW, Stowers JM, editors: *Carbohydrate metabolism in pregnancy and the newborn,* New York, 1978, Springer-Verlag.

107. O'Sullivan JB: Body weight and subsequent diabetes mellitus, *JAMA* 248:949, 1982.

108. O'Sullivan JB: Subsequent morbidity among gestational diabetic women. In Sutherland HW, Stowers JM, editors: *Carbohydrate metabolism in pregnancy and the newborn,* Edinburgh, 1984, Churchill Livingstone.

109. O'Sullivan JB, Mahan CM: Criteria for the oral glucose tolerance test in pregnancy, *Diabetes* 13:278, 1964.

110. O'Sullivan JB and others: Gestational diabetes and perinatal mortality role, *Am J Obstet Gynecol* 116:901, 1973.

111. Papaspyros NS: *The history of diabetes mellitus,* Stuttgart, 1952, Thieme.

112. Pederson J: *The pregnant diabetic and her newborn,* Baltimore, 1977, Williams & Wilkins.

113. Persson B, Gentz J: Follow-up of children of insulin-dependent and gestational diabetic mothers, *Acta Paediatr Scand* 73:349, 1984.

114. Peterson A and others: Glucose intolerance as a consequence of oral terbutaline treatment for preterm labor, *J Fam Pract* 36:25, 1993.

115. Pettitt D and others: Excessive obesity in offspring of Pima Indian women with diabetes during pregnancy, *N Engl J Med* 308:242, 1983.

116. Pettitt D and others: Congenital susceptibility for development of NIDDM, *Diabetes* 37:622, 1988.

117. Proceedings of the Second International Workshop-Conference on Gestational Diabetes Mellitus, 1984, Chicago, *Diabetes* 34(suppl 2):1-30, 1985.

118. Rednon C: Treatment of hypertension in pregnancy, *Kidney Int* 18:267, 1980.

119. Reece EA, Robbins JC: Diabetic embryopathy: pathogenesis, prenatal diagnosis, and prevention, *Obstet Gynecol Surv* 41:325, 1986.

120. Reece EA and others: Diabetic nephropathy: pregnancy performance and fetomaternal outcome, *Am J Obstet Gynecol* 159:66, 1988.

121. Rigg L, Petrie R: Fetal biochemical and biophysical assessment. In Reece E, Coustan D, editors: *Diabetes mellitus in pregnancy: principles and practices,* New York, 1988, Churchill Livingstone.

122. Roberts AB and others: Fructosamine estimation: a possible screening test for diabetes mellitus, *Br Med J* 287:863, 1983.

123. Rovergi GD and others: A new approach to the treatment of diabetic pregnant women, *Am J Obstet Gynecol* 135:567, 1979.

124. Sabata V, Wolf H, Lausmann S: The role of fatty acids, glycerol, ketone bodies and glucose in the energy metabolism of the mother and fetus during delivery, *Biol Neonate* 13:7, 1968.

125. Sadler TS: Effects of maternal diabetes on early embryogenesis. I. The teratogenic potential of diabetic serum, *Teratology* 21:339, 1980.

126. Sellis R and others: Long-term developmental follow-up of infants of diabetic mothers: Diabetes in Early Pregnancy Study, 125:9, 1994.

127. Silfen SL, Wapner RJ, Gabbe SG: Maternal outcome in class H diabetes mellitus, *Obstet Gynecol* 55:749, 1980.

128. Soler NG, Nicholson HO, Malins JM: Serial determinations of human placental lactogen in the last half of normal and complicated pregnancies, *Am J Obstet Gynecol* 120:214, 1974.

129. Soler N, Soler S, Malins J: Neonatal morbidity among infants of diabetic mothers, *Diabetes Care* 1:340, 1978.

130. Soubrane G, Conivet S, Coscas G: Influence of pregnancy on the evolution of background retinopathy, *Int Ophthalmol Clin* 8:249, 1985.

131. Spellacy WN, Goetz FC: Plasma insulin in normal late pregnancy, *N Engl J Med* 268:988, 1963.

132. Steel J and others: Insulin requirements during pregnancy in women with type I diabetes, *Obstet Gynecol* 83:253, 1994.

133. Steel SM and others: Can pregnancy care of diabetic women reduce the risk of abnormal babies? *Br Med J* 301:1070-1074, 1990.

134. Stephens JW, Page OC, Hare RL: Diabetes and pregnancy: a report of experiences in 119 pregnancies over a period of ten years, *Diabetes* 12:213, 1963.

135. Stowers JM, Sutherland HW, Kerridege DF: Long-range implications for the mother: the Aberdeen experience, *Diabetes* 34(suppl 2):106, 1985.

136. Subcommittee on Nutritional Status and Weight Gain During Pregnancy, Food and Nutrition Board, National Academy of Sciences: *Nutrition during pregnancy,* Washington, DC, 1990, National Academy Press.

137. Susa J and others: Chronic hyperinsulinemia in the fetal rhesus monkey, *Diabetes* 28:1058, 1979.

138. Tallarigo L and others: Relation of glucose tolerance to complications of pregnancy in nondiabetic women, *N Engl J Med* 315:989-992, 1986.

139. Tattersal R, Pyke D: Diabetes in identical twins, *Lancet* 2:1120, 1972.

140. Taylor P and others: Hyperbilirubinemia in infants of diabetic mothers, *Biol Neonate* 5:289, 1963.

141. Troug AI and others: Pregnancy and diabetes: the improving progress, *Ulster Med J* 52:116, 1983.

142. Tyron F: Medical aspects of diabetes in pregnancy and the diabetogenic effects of oral contraceptives, *Med Clin North Am* 55:947, 1971.

143. Ulmsten U: Treatment of normotensive and hypertensive patients with labor using oral nifedipine, a calcium antagonist, *Arch Gynecol* 236:69, 1984.

144. Walker J and others: Antihypertensive therapy in pregnancy, *Lancet* 1:932, 1983.

145. Warram J, Martin B, Krolewski A: Risk of IDDM in children of diabetic mothers decreases with increasing maternal age at pregnancy, *Diabetes* 40:1679, 1991.

146. Warran JH and others: Differences in risk of insulin-dependent diabetes in offspring of diabetic mothers and diabetic fathers, *N Engl J Med* 311:149, 1984.

147. Widness JA and others: Neonatal morbidities in infants of mothers with glucose intolerance in pregnancy, *Diabetes* 34(suppl 2):61, 1985.

148. White P: Childhood diabetes: its course and influence on the second and third generations, *Diabetes* 9:345, 1960.

12 Surgical Management of Diabetes

Irl B. Hirsch

INTRODUCTION

No recent surveys have examined the frequency of surgery during the lifetime of an individual with diabetes. During the 1960s it was estimated that persons with diabetes had a 50% chance of undergoing surgery at some point during their lifetime.[36] Because of the increased risk compared with the general population and the many persons with undiagnosed diabetes, it is not surprising for diabetes to be discovered in the perioperative period. Byyny[13] estimated that one in four previously undiagnosed individuals with diabetes would have his or her diabetes discovered perioperatively.

Because of the long-term complications of diabetes, the risk of surgery is increased. For example, in 1980 11.3% of procedures performed on diabetic patients in the United States involved the cardiovascular system, compared with 4.3% in patients without diabetes. Similarly, ophthalmologic procedures for individuals with diabetes involved 5.5% of all surgery, compared with 3.3% for those without diabetes.[73]

CHAPTER OBJECTIVES

- Describe the metabolic effects of surgery in the patient with diabetes mellitus.
- Discuss preoperative evaluation for elective surgery in the patient with diabetes mellitus.
- Review preoperative evaluation for emergency survey in the patient with diabetes mellitus.
- Summarize intraoperative management of patients with IDDM undergoing general and local anesthesia.
- Summarize intraoperative management of patients with NIDDM undergoing general and local anesthesia.
- Explain the postoperative management of insulin-receiving patients.

During the past decade there has been a documented increase in individuals with diabetes having cardiac surgery, from 4.4% in 1984 to 12.9% in 1990. Furthermore, in one survey those with diabetes were shown to have a mortality risk 1.5 times the nondiabetic population.[56] Other reports show no differences in perioperative mortality for diabetic patients having coronary bypass surgery.[10,49] However, some,[39,77] but not all,[38] studies have shown that diabetes is an independent risk factor for postoperative complications for other procedures requiring general anesthesia. Despite this, overall perioperative morbidity and mortality clearly have improved greatly for persons with diabetes over the last 70 years.[56,60] The ultimate goal should be no differences in surgical complications for those with diabetes compared with their nondiabetic counterparts.

Unfortunately, some disagreements still exist regarding optimal glycemic targets or the most effective protocol to manage individuals with diabetes during the perioperative period. This results in part from the lack of studies examining critical end points such as mortality, infection, wound healing, and length of hospital admission. Still, consensus exists for preoperative evaluation of diabetic complications, especially coronary artery disease, autonomic dysfunction, and diabetic nephropathy, and frequent metabolic (especially blood glucose) monitoring, with the avoidance of hypoglycemia, "excessive" hyperglycemia, ketosis, and electrolyte disturbances.* The greatest unresolved issue pertains to insulin administration perioperatively. This chapter discusses the rationale for the options available for perioperative diabetes management.

METABOLIC EFFECTS OF SURGERY

In simplest terms the regulation of metabolic homeostasis under usual conditions is the result of a balance between insulin (the primary anabolic hormone) and the counterregulatory hormones (those with chiefly catabolic effects), which include epinephrine, glucagon, cortisol, and growth hormone. This concept is too elementary, however, when considering the interrelated metabolism of glucose, protein, and fat. Table 12-1 presents an overview of these relationships, but a detailed discussion of this topic is beyond the scope of this chapter. The interested reader is referred to several recent reviews.[15,36]

Surgery and anesthesia stimulate a neuroendocrine "stress" response with release of adrenocorticotropic hormone (ACTH), growth hormone, catecholamines, and to varying degrees, glucagon.† This pronounced catabolic response occurs simultaneously, with an associated relative decrease in insulin secretion. Therefore, not surprisingly, hyperglycemia may be present even in nondiabetic individuals.[24,36,47,80] In the person with diabetes who is unable to secrete sufficient insulin, unrestrained catabolism may be present with increased hepatic glucose production (glycogenolysis and gluconeogenesis), lipolysis and ketosis, proteolysis, and decreased glucose utilization (Fig. 12-1). The magnitude of the counterregulatory response is related to the severity of surgery and any complications that may develop, such as sepsis.[63]

---

*References 1, 6, 18, 26, 36, 56, 60.
†References 11, 18, 26, 36, 47, 55, 60.

Table 12-1   Hormonal Maintenance of Metabolic Homeostasis

	Insulin	Epinephrine	Glucagon	Cortisol	Growth hormone
Anabolic effects					
Glycogenesis	+	−	−	±	0
Lipogenesis	+	0	0	±	0
Protein synthesis	+	0	0	−	+
Catabolic effects					
Glycogenolysis	−	+	+	−	−
Gluconeogenesis	−	+	+	+	+
Lipolysis	−	+	+*	+	+
Proteolysis	−	−	+	+	+†

+, Stimulatory effect; −, inhibitory effect; 0, no effect; ±, stimulatory in presence of insulin, inhibitory in its absence.
*At nonphysiologic levels.
†In absence of insulin.

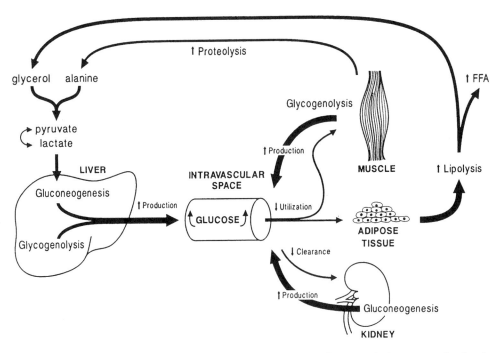

Fig. 12-1   Factors resulting in hyperglycemia during surgery. Increased glucose production is caused by hepatic and muscular glycogenolysis and hepatic and renal gluconeogenesis. Renal clearance of glucose from the circulation may be decreased during volume depletion. Relative insulin deficiency inhibits glucose utilization. (From Hirsch IB, McGill JB: *Diabetes Care* 13:980, 1990.)

In contrast to general anesthesia, epidural anesthesia has minimal effects on glucose metabolism. This results from a lack of change in lactate, alanine, free fatty acids, glycerol, ketones, cortisol, and growth hormone levels.[36] Indeed, splanchnic sympathetic outflow is abolished and epinephrine secretion is reduced, resulting in decreased hepatic glucose production. Thus insulin resistance generally is not changed in this situation, and a greater risk for hypoglycemia may exist,[8,68] especially in the absence of sufficient blood glucose monitoring.

To minimize the adverse effects of these metabolic effects, detailed attention to metabolic control is required. The clinician always needs to recall that (1) major surgery with general anesthesia will cause greater metabolic stress than a minor procedure with local anesthesia[64] and (2) individuals with insulin-dependent diabetes mellitus (IDDM) with absolute insulin deficiency are more prone to a metabolic catastrophe if little attention is given to the diabetes management.

TREATMENT GOALS

Although some controversy still exists regarding exact perioperative glycemic goals, all agree that the principal goal of therapy should be to avoid excess morbidity and mortality compared with the nondiabetic population. As already noted, impressive improvements have occurred in the outcomes for diabetic individuals requiring surgery, but this ultimate goal has not yet been accomplished.

There are a variety of reasons to control glycemia during the perioperative period. For any person with diabetes, acute metabolic complications are the most important concern. Hypoglycemic symptoms may be altered in the sedated patient[8] and are absent in the patient receiving general anesthesia. Signs of hypoglycemia in the anesthetized patient may include electrocardiographic (ECG) (ischemic)[52] or electroencephalographic (EEG)[33] changes, hypothermia,[44] and hyperthermia.[16] The frequency of hypoglycemia during surgery or immediately afterward is unknown but is probably more common than appreciated, especially in individuals with IDDM.[37] Hypoglycemia is the most important metabolic concern of anesthesiologists and is the main reason why many of these providers aim for higher levels of blood glucose.[21]

Other acute perioperative metabolic complications of diabetes include diabetic ketoacidosis (DKA) and hyperosmolar hyperglycemic nonketotic syndrome.[48,59,69] Patients undergoing surgery in a catabolic state are at greater risk for either of these complications. Even individuals with mild glucose intolerance require adequate attention to glucose levels because of other potential complications from perioperative hyperglycemia, including electrolyte abnormalities and volume depletion from osmotic diuresis.

Infection is another reason usually cited to defend glucose control. Unfortunately, no controlled prospective studies directly compare different levels of perioperative glycemia with rates of infection. Although not all the data are in agreement,[70] hyperglycemia appears to interfere with the leukocyte functions of chemotaxis, opsonization, and phagocytosis.[32,53] It appears that both plasma glucose levels greater than 200 mg/dl (11.1 mM) and high serum ketones provide a permissive milieu for the development of infectious complications.[40,81]

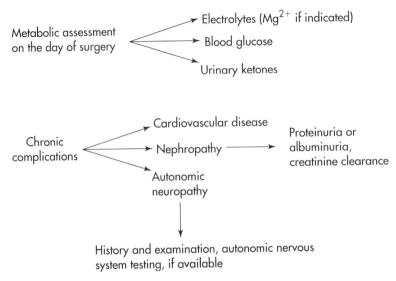

Fig. 12-2 Preoperative evaluation for the individual with diabetes includes metabolic evaluation on the day of surgery and assessment of cardiovascular disease, nephropathy, and autonomic dysfunction.

Studies in animal models of diabetes also implicate plasma glucose levels greater than 200 mg/dl (11.1 mM) and insulin deficiency as factors contributing to impaired wound strength and wound healing.[29,85] Deficient formation of granulation tissue probably is one reason for these findings.[84] Unfortunately, human studies regarding this issue are lacking.

Taken together, it seems that the glycemic goals during the perioperative period for individuals with diabetes should be blood glucose levels that minimize the risk for hypoglycemia but are low enough to prevent any acute complications from diabetes and postoperative morbidity. For this reason, most authors agree a reasonable goal would be to strive for blood glucose levels of approximately 120 to 180 mg/dl (6.7 to 10.0 mM).[6,26,36]

PREOPERATIVE MANAGEMENT
Preoperative Evaluation for Elective Surgery Requiring General Anesthesia
(Fig. 12-2)

Preoperative evaluation may be separated into two categories: assessment of the acute metabolic status and appraisal of the chronic complications of diabetes that may affect surgical outcome. In regard to the former, since metabolic decompensation may occur in a relatively short time, especially in the person with IDDM, preoperative blood glucose, electrolytes, and urinary ketones should be measured *on the day of surgery*. The common practice of "preoperative assessment" and "surgical clearance" before surgery should not be considered complete until the patient's metabolic status is known just prior to surgery. Also, magnesium deficiency is common in patients with IDDM[62] or non-insulin-dependent diabetes mellitus (NIDDM).[67] Although routine measurement for all patients is not recommended, patients with a high risk of hypomagnesemia should be screened before surgery. These include patients using certain drugs (e.g., diuretics or digoxin), patients with congestive heart failure, those with poor glycemic control (especially ketoacidosis), those who abuse ethanol, those with potassium or calcium deficiency of any etiology, and pregnant patients.[3]

In regard to the assessment of the various chronic complications, perhaps the most important is the evaluation of cardiovascular disease, since this is the leading cause of mortality in persons with diabetes. Fifty-five percent of patients with diabetes mellitus will die of cardiovascular complications, while cardiovascular disease accounts for 65% of deaths for those diagnosed with diabetes over age 40.[20] What makes this an even greater problem is that both asymptomatic myocardial ischemia[57] and infarction[58] are more common in patients with diabetes. Not surprisingly, diabetes is an independent risk factor for postoperative myocardial ischemia.[39] Since routine exercise stress testing results in a greater number of false-positive and false-negative studies in patients with diabetes compared with the general population, pharmacologic testing for myocardial perfusion should be considered for high-risk patients before surgery.[22,25,83] Specific details regarding the preoperative workup of cardiovascular disease are beyond the scope of this chapter, but excellent reviews are available.[46,50,83]

Preoperative evaluation should also include assessment for diabetic nephropathy. The surgical setting accounts for 18% to 47% of all inpatient cases of acute renal failure, and for persons with diabetic nephropathy, this risk is higher. Individuals with renal disease are particularly more prone to contrast nephropathy and renal failure from aminoglycosides.[45] Since the hallmark of diabetic nephropathy, proteinuria, develops years before the onset of renal insufficiency,[34,66] measurement of the serum creatinine level alone is not sufficient for this evaluation. The assessment of renal disease at least should include a dipstick for urinary protein. If positive, a more complete evaluation would include a timed (e.g., 24-hour) urine collection for proteinuria and creatinine clearance. This best quantifies the stage of the renal disease. If the urinary dipstick is "negative" or "trace" for proteinuria, ideally an evaluation for microalbuminuria (30 to 300 mg albuminuria/day) should be performed.[4] Although it is not known if patients with microalbuminuria have an increased rate of perioperative renal failure, it seems reasonable to avoid any renal insult in these individuals if at all possible. Furthermore, since microalbuminuria is an independent risk factor for cardiovascular death in patients with NIDDM,[54] this population should be considered a high-risk group for coronary artery disease and should therefore be screened appropriately before surgery.

Controversy has surrounded the best management of these patients when a nephrotoxic agent is unavoidable, such as a radiocontrast agent for angiography. It was recently reported in a group of subjects with renal insufficiency (about half with diabetes) that hydration with 0.45% saline for 12 hours before and 12 hours after the administration of the radiocontrast agent prevented acute decreases in renal function better than hydration with mannitol or furosemide.[74] Therefore hydration should be emphasized in all diabetic persons with albuminuria requiring radiocontrast, and low-osmolality contrast agents are preferred.[9]

Autonomic nervous system function also needs consideration preoperatively. Patients with diabetic autonomic neuropathy have an increased risk of perioperative hypotension.[12] Severe autonomic neuropathy increases the risk of postoperative cardiorespiratory arrest and death.[14] Unfortunately, sensitive testing for cardiovascular autonomic dysfunction is cumbersome and unavailable for most clinicians. Therefore preoperative assessment should include at least specific attention to possible autonomic dysfunction in the history and physical

---

BOX 12-1

DIABETES AND EMERGENCY SURGERY

1. Immediately test glucose, urea nitrogen, creatinine, electrolytes, and pH.
2. Obtain electrocardiogram (ECG).
3. Begin intravenous fluids; if hypotensive, begin normal saline.
4. Examine for signs of DKA (volume depletion, fruity breath).
5. If DKA is present, delay surgery (if possible) until metabolically stable.
6. Begin insulin infusion if blood glucose is greater than 120 mg/dl (6.7 mM) for insulin-requiring patients and greater than 180 mg/dl (10.0 mM) for non-insulin-requiring patients.
7. Begin glucose at 5 g/hr, and administer potassium chloride (KCl) if appropriate.
8. Measure blood glucose level at bedside hourly and potassium (K^+) concentration every 4 hours.

---

examination. Is there a history of early satiety, bloating, and nausea to suggest gastroparesis? Is there a history of constipation and diarrhea? Are symptoms present to suggest a neurogenic bladder, gustatory sweating, or orthostasis? On examination, is tachycardia present, and are there orthostatic changes? Is the anal sphincter tone normal? Although there are now excellent computers to help clinicians quantify autonomic function, they are not in widespread use. Therefore, for most clinicians, attention to the history and physical examination will have to suffice.

Preoperative Evaluation for Emergency Surgery

Past studies have suggested that perhaps as many as 5% of all persons with diabetes will require emergency surgery at some time during their lives.[36] Many of these individuals will be in poor metabolic control; some may even have DKA.

Box 12-1 summarizes the key points for preparing these patients for emergency surgery. The first priority is to assess glycemic, acid-base, and electrolyte status. Physical examination may be misleading, since DKA may present as rebound abdominal tenderness, and this sign may resolve with the treatment of the medical emergency. In all patients with ketoacidosis, it is best to delay the surgery *if possible* until after treatment of the metabolic crisis.

Preoperative Management of the Patient with IDDM

Earlier reviews have recommended that these patients be admitted at least 24 hours before surgery with the goal to maximize glycemic control. That is rarely possible in today's medical climate, even with major procedures such as coronary artery bypass grafting and transplantation. Fortunately, most patients may be admitted in reasonable control, with blood glucose levels less than 200 mg/dl (11.1 mM), partly because of the widespread use of home blood glucose monitoring. For certain patients, however, early admission may be desirable. For example, some with severe visual impairment (especially if recent), who do not yet have a special glucose meter available for visually impaired diabetic patients, may benefit from early admission. Ideally, family members can assist these patients with their care, and early admission will not be required. Patients with poorly controlled diabetes and recurrent DKA are another group who could benefit from early admission.

Traditionally, patients using Ultralente insulin would have their regimen changed to an NPH or Lente program 2 or 3 days before surgery. Since the older animal-species Ultralente insulins are no longer available, the shorter duration of the human Ultralente insulin[35] makes this practice unnecessary. Any insulin regimen used may be continued until the day before surgery. The one situation in which insulin requirements may change is if the diet is changed (e.g., a liquid diet before colon surgery). Home blood glucose monitoring should be performed at least before meals and at bedtime, and adjustments should be made with the advice of a physician or diabetes nurse specialist.

Preoperative Management of the Patient with NIDDM

Similar guidelines for blood glucose control should be followed for NIDDM patients. Even for those with poorly controlled diabetes, every effort should be made to maintain blood glucose levels less than 200 mg/dl (11.1 mM). Previous authors have recommended individuals using sulfonylureas (especially chlorpropamide) discontinue the medication up to 48 to 72 hours before surgery and use insulin to manage glycemia when appropriate. This recommendation has never been tested, is complicated, and is probably unnecessary. In addition, it is rarely followed. Most patients do well by simply omitting the sulfonylurea on the day of surgery (intraoperative management is discussed later), although because of the long action of chlorpropamide, it is reasonable to discontinue this drug 24 hours earlier.

Hypertension is quite common in this population: 70% among blacks with NIDDM and 63% among whites with NIDDM, compared with a prevalence of 41% and 32% in nondiabetic blacks and whites, respectively.[31] Therefore preoperative blood pressure control requires special attention. The primary goal of therapy for adults should be to decrease blood pressure to less than 130/85 mm Hg. For patients with isolated systolic hypertension of 180 mm Hg or higher, the goal is a blood pressure less than 160 mm Hg. For those with a systolic blood pressure of 160 to 179 mm Hg, the goal is a reduction of 20 mm Hg.[5]

INTRAOPERATIVE MANAGEMENT OF THE PATIENT WITH IDDM: GENERAL ANESTHESIA
Insulin

Much of the controversy regarding insulin delivery has been resolved during the past few years. Most authors now recommend either a variable-rate intravenous (IV) insulin infusion or a glucose-insulin-potassium (GIK) infusion for all patients with IDDM requiring general anesthesia.[1,6,26,36] In actual practice, however, subcutaneous insulin is administered most of the time,[37] and some authors reserve IV insulin only for certain situations (shock, DKA, pregnancy, high-dose steroids, sepsis, transplantation, cardiopulmonary bypass [CPB]).[60] Under the best of circumstances, subcutaneous insulin is quite unpredictable.[35] From a purely theoretic point of view, with the blood pressure and fluid shifts that occur during surgery resulting in significant changes in peripheral blood flow, subcutaneous insulin will be more variable than usual. A continuous IV insulin infusion, with a half-life of 4 to 5 minutes and a biologic half-life less than 20 minutes,[78] allows predictable insulin delivery and the opportunity to change insulinemia immediately as the situation dictates. Prospective studies, although few, certainly support the effectiveness and increased safety of the continuous IV insulin infusion.[41,61,79] It must be emphasized that any effective regimen will require frequent bedside blood glucose monitoring (see following discussion).

There has been recent enthusiasm regarding the use of IV bolus insulin for perioperative insulin administration. Raucoules-Aime and colleagues[65] showed that IV bolus administration of insulin every 2 hours was as effective as a fixed-rate IV insulin infusion, with supplemental bolus insulin administered for blood glucose levels greater than 200 mg/dl (11.1 mM). Although there was a biphasic glucose response to the IV bolus insul-in group, compared with constant blood glucose levels in the fixed-rate insulin group, glycemia was only different at one time point. The authors concluded that IV bolus insulin can be used when an insulin infusion pump is not available. Unfortunately, these data are not applicable to individuals with IDDM. Twenty-nine of the study subjects were using oral hypoglycemic agents and classified as having NIDDM. The other 31 subjects were receiving insulin treatment at home and were classified as having IDDM.[65] It seems likely that some, if not many, of these insulin-treated individuals actually had NIDDM, especially since the mean age of the subjects was 52 years. This important point is a common problem with the literature regarding perioperative diabetes management. Patients are misclassified, or a study includes a heterogeneous mix of patients, and conclusions are extrapolated to all patients. No data suggest that IV bolus insulin is efficacious or safe in individuals with IDDM, and the potential for causing dangerous iatrogenic hypokalemia, hypophosphatemia, and hypomagnesemia should limit its use for all persons with diabetes.

An important theme from both the literature and experienced clinicians is that blood glucose concentrations need to be measured frequently with appropriate interpretation by well-trained staff.* The optimal frequency for blood glucose measurement has not been studied. American authors recommend more frequent monitoring than the British.[1,6,26,36] Increased monitoring can only result in greater efficacy and safety no matter how the insulin is delivered.

Box 12-2 provides an example of an insulin algorithm. No optimal concentration exists for the insulin infusion, but if fluids need to be limited, a more concentrated mixture would be desired. The absorption of insulin to the plastic tubing is a theoretic problem, thus the recommendation for the flushing of the insulin solution.[26,36] However, this issue has not been reexamined with human insulin, and therefore the continued need for this practice is not clear. Both the initial starting rates and the algorithm for insulin rate changes may need adjustment

---

*References 1, 6, 26, 30, 36, 56.

BOX 12-2

INTRAVENOUS INSULIN PROTOCOL

1. Standard insulin concentration is 1 U regular insulin/10 ml saline; a convenient solution is 25 U regular insulin mixed with 250 ml saline.
2. The tubing should be flushed with 30 ml solution before use.
3. Capillary glucose is measured hourly for the first 6 to 8 hours while receiving the insulin infusion and hourly during surgery; if blood glucose levels are stable, less frequent monitoring (every 2 hours) is acceptable. Hourly monitoring may be indicated for critically ill patients or those with very unstable glycemia.
4. A conservative initial insulin infusion rate would be 1.0 U/hr for patients with NIDDM and men with IDDM; thin women with IDDM may be started at 0.5 U/hr.
5. Algorithm:

Capillary glucose	Action
<70 mg/dl (3.9 mM)	Discontinue infusion for 30 minutes and administer 15 to 20 ml 50% dextrose; remeasure glucose in 30 minutes and restart insulin infusion at 1 U/hr after blood glucose >100 mg/dl (5.6 mM); continue glucose infusion.
70-120 mg/dl (3.9-6.7 mM)	Decrease rate by 0.3 U/hr.
121-180 mg/dl (6.7-10 mM)	No change
181-240 mg/dl (10.1-13.3 mM)	Increase by 0.3 U/hr.
241-300 mg/dl (13.4-16.7 mM)	Increase by 0.6 U/hr.
>300 mg/dl (16.7 mM)	Increase by 1 U/hr.

6. Most adults require a minimum of 5 g glucose/hr and additional potassium chloride (KCl); 5% glucose in 0.45% sodium chloride (NaCl) with 20 mEq/L KCl at 100 ml/hr may be infused separate to the insulin infusion.

---

because of catastrophic hypoglycemia or hyperglycemia. However, this regimen, which is similar to the algorithm of Watts and associates[79] has proved to be effective and safe for individuals with IDDM or NIDDM (unpublished observations).

Because normal insulin requirements may differ widely, even for a homogeneous group of individuals with IDDM, it is not surprising that perioperative insulin requirements also vary.[79] Higher insulin requirements are required for obese patients, those with severe infection, those receiving steroid therapy, some patients with liver disease, and those undergoing CPB.[6,26,36,60] Reasons for increased insulin requirements for CPB include the use of sympathomimetic drugs, pump priming with glucose-enriched solutions, and hypothermia.* The optimal frequency of blood glucose monitoring during CPB has not been determined, but hourly is probably not sufficient.[18,36] Some authors recommend blood glucose monitoring during CPB every 15 to 30 minutes.[18]

---

*References 26, 36, 47, 75, 80.

The other mechanism for IV insulin delivery is the GIK infusion. This is less flexible than the variable-rate IV infusion but nevertheless preferred by some authors because of its ease of use.[1,42] Since the insulin is mixed directly into the bag of maintenance fluid (usually 0.45% normal saline), the entire bag must be changed each time the plasma glucose is outside of target values. This problem also adds to the cost if the bag must be changed frequently. A recent study of individuals with IDDM comparing the variable-rate and GIK infusions reported no differences in intraoperative and postoperative glycemia but lower blood glucose levels when resuming normal diabetes therapy with the variable-rate infusion compared with the GIK infusion (133 versus 198 mg/dl [7.4 versus 11.0 mM], $p<0.001$). Nursing satisfaction was greater ($p<0.001$) and more insulin rate changes were made with the variable-rate infusion.[72] The GIK infusion is probably best suited for elective procedures in individuals with NIDDM during which insulin requirements are not expected to vary tremendously.[26] Box 12-3 outlines guidelines for a GIK infusion.

Whichever method is used for IV insulin delivery, the insulin and glucose infusions should be started in the morning, preferably at about the same time the morning injection is usually administered. Ideally, surgery for all patients with diabetes should be the first scheduled in the day. In actual practice, this often is not the case. Indeed, unfamiliar health care providers may ask their patients to withhold their insulin. This is disastrous advice for those with IDDM because DKA may result. With the use of the IV insulin infusion, glycemia may be stable before surgery, even if the procedure is not scheduled until later in the day. Using a fraction of the insulin dose in the morning involves a large amount of guesswork, but it also may cause a large release of unexpected depot insulin after the surgery is underway. Since bovine Ultralente insulin is no longer available, any insulin regimen, including continuous subcutaneous insulin infusion (CSII), may be easily converted to the IV insulin infusion early in the morning. However, for those using CSII it is not critical to begin the IV infusion early in the day, since these individuals may continue with their basal insulin via their pump. Finally, the IV insulin infusion makes the problem of unstable glycemia easier to manage after surgery during periods of nausea and vomiting. Often, this is the most difficult time for managing blood glucose levels, especially in persons with IDDM.

Glucose and Fluids

Quantitative kinetic studies of glucose requirements during surgery, in either diabetic or nondiabetic patients, are lacking, and therefore the actual amount of glucose needed to prevent unnecessary fat and protein catabolism is unknown. The traditional rate of 5g glucose/hr[6,26,36] (1.2 mg/kg/min for a 70 kg man) may not be sufficient to suppress glycerol, free fatty acid mobilization, and the development of a negative nitrogen balance.[23,82] For this reason, others suggest the use of 10 g glucose/hr, since in addition to the greater quantity of glucose administered, a more anabolic insulin dose is required.[1] Whichever glucose infusion rate is used, for patients requiring an IV insulin and glucose infusion for more than 24 hours, the measurement of urinary ketones should be considered. Significant ketonuria suggests inadequate glucose and/or insulin administration.

BOX 12-3
<u></u>

GLUCOSE-INSULIN-POTASSIUM (GIK) PROTOCOL

1. The maintenance fluid consists of 5% glucose in 1 L 0.45% normal saline with 20 mEq/L KCl.
2. For patients treated with diet, oral agents, or less than 50 U insulin/day:
   a. Add 10 U regular insulin to the fluid.
   b. The solution should be infused at 100 ml/hr (5 g glucose/hr, 1 U insulin/hr).
   c. For capillary blood glucose <120 mg/dl (6.7 mM): decrease insulin by 5 U.
   d. For capillary blood glucose of 120-180 mg/dl (6.7-10 mM): make no change in insulin.
   e. For capillary blood glucose >180 mg/dl (10.0 mM): increase insulin by 5 U.
   f. For any capillary blood glucose <80 mg/dl (4.4 mM): stop the infusion and administer an IV bolus of 50% dextrose in water (25 ml). Remeasure capillary blood glucose in 15 minutes. If capillary blood glucose is still <80 mg/dl, repeat the IV glucose bolus and remeasure in 15 minutes; if > 4.4 mM, restart the infusion with 5 U regular insulin added to 1 L 0.45% normal saline.
3. For patients treated with more than 50 U insulin/day:
   a. Add 15 U regular insulin to the fluid.
   b. The solution should be infused at 100 ml/hr (5 g glucose/hr, 1.5 U insulin/hr).
   c. For capillary blood glucose <120 mg/dl (6.7 mM): decrease insulin by 5 U.
   d. For capillary blood glucose of 120-180 mg/dl (6.7-10 mM): make no change in insulin.
   e. For capillary blood glucose > 180 mg/dl (10.0 mM): increase insulin by 5 U.
   f. For any capillary blood glucose <80 mg/dl (4.4 mM): stop the infusion and administer an IV bolus of 50% dextrose in water (25 ml). Remeasure capillary blood glucose in 15 minutes. If capillary blood glucose is still <80 mg/dl, repeat the IV glucose bolus and remeasure in 15 minutes; if > 4.4 mM, restart the infusion with 10 U regular insulin added to 1 L of 0.45% normal saline.

Modified from Gavin LA: *Endocrinol Metab Clin North Am* 21:457, 1992.

If adequate insulin, glucose, and potassium are provided, any additional fluids administered during surgery (e.g., to treat intraoperative blood loss) should not contain glucose. As noted earlier, glucose is provided in a solution of 5% or 10% dextrose in 0.45% normal saline. However, if fluids need to be restricted, the glucose may be administered in 20% or 50% solutions at lower rates. These latter solutions are best administered through a central venous catheter because of the increased risks of peripheral venous thrombosis.

The use of lactated Ringer's (LR) solution during surgery for individuals with diabetes is controversial. In a classic investigation of individuals with NIDDM, Thomas and Alberti[76] showed higher plasma glucose levels when LR was administered compared with no fluids. Theoretically, lactate may be acting as a gluconeogenic precursor, resulting in an increase in hepatic glucose output. Further studies regarding optimal fluid administration for patients with diabetes are needed. If LR is used, insulin requirements may be increased.

INTRAOPERATIVE MANAGEMENT OF THE PATIENT WITH IDDM: LOCAL ANESTHESIA

Since less data are available regarding the IDDM patient and local anesthesia, there is also more controversy. The most widely quoted study showed improved glycemia with a GIK infusion compared with subcutaneous insulin,[17] but the clinical significance of this is not clear. Since the hormonal changes appearing with general anesthesia do not occur with local procedures (see previous discussion), it is not surprising that most patients requiring the latter do well with subcutaneous insulin.

If subcutaneous insulin is used, the traditional recommendation of administering a fraction (50% to 60%) of the dose of intermediate-acting (NPH or Lente) insulin and regular insulin usually works well. Regular insulin should be decreased even further (if not withheld) for preoperative hypoglycemia. A higher dose of regular insulin should be considered for significant preoperative hyperglycemia (e.g., greater than 180 mg/dl [10 mM]). Individuals receiving Ultralente insulin would be best served to receive their entire dose (but with a fraction of their regular insulin dose), and those using CSII do well receiving their basal insulin needs, with "bolus" insulin administered for blood glucose levels greater than 180 mg/dl (10 mM). For all persons with IDDM, a minimum of 5 g/hr of glucose should be administered. For marked hyperglycemia (blood glucose levels greater than 300 mg/dl [16.7 mM]) or acidemia, a variable-rate IV insulin infusion or a GIK infusion should be considered. In addition, postoperatively, those with gastroparesis will likely do better with an IV insulin infusion, since the matching of glucose and insulin is better guaranteed after eating is allowed. Since postoperative nausea and vomiting account for 18% of all unanticipated admissions after ambulatory surgery,[28] and, at least theoretically, individuals with gastroparesis should have a greater risk of this complication, an IV insulin infusion should be considered for this population as well.

INTRAOPERATIVE MANAGEMENT OF THE PATIENT WITH NIDDM: GENERAL ANESTHESIA

For persons diagnosed with diabetes after age 20 years, 90% to 95% have NIDDM.[20] However, it is critical not to assume that all patients diagnosed over age 20 have NIDDM, since IDDM may present at any age.[43] A thin or normal-weight individual less than 40 years old without a family history of diabetes but with newly diagnosed diabetes should suggest that the correct diagnosis is IDDM. When the diagnosis is not clear (which does occur during the first few years after diagnosis in this age group), a conservative strategy would be to manage these patients similarly to those with IDDM.

For those requiring general anesthesia, most authors agree that special treatment other than frequent blood glucose monitoring (hourly during surgery) is not required for patients who are *well controlled* (fasting blood glucose less than 120 mg/dl [6.7 mM]) on diet therapy alone.[18,26,36] Because of the hyperglycemic response of surgery, many of these patients will require insulin. As a general rule, if *any* patient with diabetes needs insulin during a procedure requiring general anesthesia, it should be administered as a continuous infusion (either variable-rate or GIK infusion).[1,2,36]

For individuals with NIDDM receiving general anesthesia who are not taking insulin at home, the insulin infusion should be started if the blood glucose exceeds 200 mg/dl (11.1 mM). As noted earlier, wound healing and resistance to infection both appear to be impaired with blood glucose above this level.* In addition, the renal threshold for glucose excretion is 180 to 200 mg/dl (10.0 to 11.1 mM).[19] Blood glucose levels greater than this result in an osmotic diuresis and predisposes patients to volume depletion. Furthermore, high urine volumes suggest adequate volume status, although this may not actually be the case.

Debate surrounds the optimal way to manage those with NIDDM treated with an oral agent (sulfonylurea or biguanide). One author suggests administering sulfonylureas with a small amount of water on the morning of surgery, at least for those with good glycemic control.[60] Another author suggests omitting all oral agents on the morning of surgery.[1] This is perhaps the most reasonable solution, since during general anesthesia it will be difficult to match insulin requirements to the unpredictable absorption of the oral agent from the gut. As already noted, most agree that long-acting sulfonylureas such as chlorpropamide should be discontinued at least 24 hours before surgery.[1,36,60] A shorter-acting agent may be substituted in its place. In regard to metformin, a relatively safe biguanide that generally does not result in lactic acidosis, except with renal or liver disease,[7] it is recommended to stop this drug at least 2 days before surgery because of the higher risk of hyperlactemia during surgery.[1]

For patients with NIDDM who are usually treated with insulin, a continuous IV insulin infusion is recommended.[1,6,26,36] There are no data comparing the variable-rate insulin infusion with the GIK infusion for this population. Recommendations regarding fluid and glucose administration and frequency of blood glucose monitoring are similar to those for IDDM.

INTRAOPERATIVE MANAGEMENT OF THE PATIENT WITH NIDDM: LOCAL ANESTHESIA

Treatment decisions for individuals with NIDDM receiving local anesthesia are similar, except that *well-controlled* patients who are treated with diet alone or diet with oral agents probably will not require additional insulin. It was reported that 93% of patients with NIDDM can achieve acceptable blood glucose control without insulin.[41] Therefore, unless blood glucose levels rise above the targeted values, no further therapy will be required. Since splanchnic sympathetic outflow is abolished and epinephrine secretion is reduced, resulting in decreased hepatic glucose production and potentially an increased risk for hypoglycemia,[8,68] administering the oral agent on the morning of surgery appears to be unnecessary.

For procedures using local anesthesia, individuals with NIDDM who are poorly controlled with oral agents or those who are treated with insulin at home will require insulin

---

*References 29, 32, 40, 53, 70, 81, 84, 85.

to be maintained within the targeted blood glucose levels. No consensus exists regarding the best treatment strategy for this situation. Either an IV insulin infusion or subcutaneous insulin is acceptable, although for more significant hyperglycemia (e.g., 350 mg/dl [19.4 mM] or higher), the IV route is preferred.[36]

Precise recommendations for subcutaneous insulin for poorly controlled persons with NIDDM who do not use insulin at home are difficult. From 4 to 6 U of regular insulin is a reasonable initial dose for a surgical patient not previously treated with insulin.[36] The typical "sliding-scale" regimens used in most American hospitals are irrational and potentially dangerous.[27,71] However, the typical hyperglycemic obese person with NIDDM is also often immune to the dangers of this strategy of retrospective glycemic management. At the very least, those who are receiving subcutaneous regular insulin for the first time should have blood glucose monitoring every 2 or 3 hours. A second dose of insulin then may be administered based on the response of the first dose. For patients who are clearly "oral agent failures,"[51] this is an opportune time to discuss initiating insulin therapy.

The decision to begin an insulin infusion versus using subcutaneous insulin in patients receiving local anesthesia should be based on several factors. First, the patient's current metabolic status needs to be considered; those with severe hyperglycemia (350 mg/dl [19.4 mM] or higher) or acidemia would be best served with an insulin infusion. Next, one asks, how soon will food be allowed after the procedure? If it is known preoperatively that little or no food will be allowed immediately after surgery (e.g., after an oral surgery), the insulin infusion would be the better option. The timing of the procedure during the day should also be considered; since there is less guesswork with the IV insulin infusion, it is reasonable to use this regimen for procedures scheduled later in the day, especially in the afternoon.

Individuals with insulin-requiring NIDDM may be managed similarly to patients with IDDM (see previous discussion). Many of these patients are insulin deficient and thus behave metabolically similar to those with IDDM.

POSTOPERATIVE MANAGEMENT OF THE PATIENT RECEIVING INSULIN

Continuation of either a variable-rate IV insulin infusion or a GIK infusion into the postoperative period is a simple and flexible approach to management. Capillary glucose is monitored for 1 to 2 hours, with continuation of the insulin infusion and appropriate adjustments, as outlined in Box 12-2. Serum electrolytes should be measured immediately after surgery for all diabetic patients and at least daily (for the first few days) at the minimum for those receiving an insulin infusion for a prolonged period.

If food is not tolerated for more than 24 hours, urinary ketones should be measured daily in all patients. This is necessary, since the development of ketonuria in the presence of well-controlled glycemia indicates the need for greater quantities of glucose (starvation ketosis) or, in individuals with IDDM, may identify early DKA, which may be exacerbated by starvation. "Euglycemic DKA" refers the development of diabetic ketoacidosis with plasma glucose levels less than 300 mg/dl (16.7 mM).[36] The frequency of this situation in the postoperative period is unknown, but significant ketonuria (moderate or large) with blood glucose levels below this level should alert the clinician that a metabolic emergency may be developing.

It is easiest to continue the insulin infusion until solid food is tolerated. Thus, if nausea and vomiting are present, glucose and insulin will not be interrupted. If solid food is permitted for the lunch or supper meal on the day of surgery, the regular home dose of insulin may be administered 15 to 20 minutes before the meal and the insulin (and glucose) infusion stopped during or just after the meal. If regular insulin is not usually given before the lunch meal, 4 to 6 U of subcutaneous regular insulin may be administered, but this will need to be individualized. It should be emphasized that the infusion is discontinued only *after* the subcutaneous insulin regimen is initiated, to avoid leaving gaps in insulin coverage that might permit loss of metabolic control.

SUMMARY

The endocrine environment during the perioperative period promotes protein and fat catabolism and glucose production. The metabolic consequences of these processes may have devastating consequences in persons with diabetes, and sufficient insulin and glucose must be administered to prevent tissue breakdown.

Large trials examining optimal medical management and the relationship to surgical outcome of patients with diabetes unfortunately are lacking. Although minor disagreements about certain details of insulin administration do exist, most agree with overall approaches to perioperative management (Table 12-2). Blood glucose levels ideally should remain below 200 mg/dl (11.1 mM) while avoiding hypoglycemia. All insulin-requiring patients who are receiving general anesthesia should be managed by the infusion of IV insulin. Those with IDDM who have procedures with local anesthesia can be managed with either subcutaneous or IV insulin, although the literature supports the latter. For short procedures using local anesthesia or for patients using Ultralente insulin or CSII, subcutaneous insulin usually works well. Unfortunately, the least amount of information exists about the most common situation, the poorly controlled patient with NIDDM receiving local anesthesia. For these patients, there is probably no advantage in using IV insulin compared with subcutaneous insulin.

Perhaps most important, all the providers caring for persons with diabetes must be in agreement with the general strategy for each situation. Differences in practice patterns are common, even within the same institution.[37] Ideally, providers should communicate frequently with each other to provide the best possible perioperative diabetes management.

Table 12-2   Summary of Insulin Strategies for Perioperative Diabetes Management

	General anesthesia	Local anesthesia
IDDM	Insulin infusion	Subcutaneous insulin or insulin infusion*
NIDDM	Insulin infusion	Subcutaneous insulin or insulin infusion†

*Most controversial; many patients do well with subcutaneous insulin, especially for short procedures; patients receiving Ultralente insulin or CSII may continue to receive their basal subcutaneous insulin delivery.
†Well-controlled patients often do not require supplemental insulin.

CASE PRESENTATION

A 55-year-old man with a 15-year history of NIDDM presents to his physician with a chief complaint of dyspnea on exertion. His symptom has been worsening during the past few weeks and is now limiting him from taking his usual walk in that he becomes short of breath after only one block. He denies chest pain, palpitations, orthopnea, or paroxysmal nocturnal dyspnea. He denies symptoms suggesting symmetrical polyneuropathy or autonomic dysfunction, although he recently noted erectile dysfunction. His only medications are insulin (a fixed ratio of 70% NPH and 30% regular), 100 U daily split equally before breakfast and supper, and hydrochlorothiazide, 25 mg daily.

On examination, his blood pressure is 150/100 both supine and standing. Microaneurysms, arteriolar narrowing, and hard exudates are noted bilaterally. There are no signs of congestive heart failure, and his heart rate is 90 beats/min. He has no ankle edema, vibratory perception is diminished, and ankle jerks are absent.

Laboratory testing reveals a glycohemoglobin of 10% (normal, 4% to 6%), normal electrolytes, and a creatinine level of 1.3 mg/dl (normal, 0.3 to 1.2 mg/dl). Twenty-four hour urine studies reveal 1.8 g of proteinuria with a creatinine clearance of 65 ml/min. Captopril therapy is initiated.

Chest x-ray films and ECG are both unremarkable. Dypyridamole thallium testing reveals several perfusion defects. After adequate IV hydration, coronary angiography is performed, and significant stenoses are identified in three vessels. One week after the procedure, the patient's serum creatinine is 1.4 mg/dl.

Before coronary artery bypass, formal autonomic nervous system testing reveals abnormal ''R-R variation'' to deep breathing.

On the morning of surgery, the following laboratory results are noted: fasting blood glucose, 140 mg/dl; potassium, 4.8 mEq/L (normal, 3.5 to 5.1 mEq/L); magnesium, 1.3 mEq/L (normal, 1.5 to 2.0 mEq/L); and creatinine, 1.3 mg/dl. An insulin infusion is initiated at 1.5 U/hr, and over the course of the next 2 hours before surgery, the patient's insulin dose is increased to 2.1 U/hr. IV magnesium is administered. Five percent dextrose in 0.45% saline is administered at 125 ml/hr. Blood glucose levels are measured hourly, except during CPB, when it is measured every 30 minutes. Insulin requirements increase to 4.0 U/hr by the end of surgery (and reached 10.0 U/hr during CPB), and the blood glucose level remains below 200 mg/dl for the entire surgery and is 150 mg/dl on arrival to the recovery room. His electrolytes, including magnesium, are normal, except for a potassium concentration of 3.4 mEq/L.

DISCUSSION

Unfortunately, this scenario occurs too frequently for those with diabetes. A man with longstanding, poorly controlled diabetes has an atypical presentation for coronary artery disease, perhaps because of the development of autonomic dysfunction. During the evaluation, it is also determined he has significant proteinuria consistent with diabetic nephropathy. His hypertension is poorly controlled on a diuretic, and he has developed hypomagnesemia.

Several points regarding his perioperative evaluation and management should be emphasized. Since he is at a high risk for hypomagnesemia (poorly controlled diabetes and diuretic use), it would have been appropriate to measure his magnesium before admission to the hospital. Low magnesium levels in cardiac patients need to be avoided, and his magnesium stores could have been repleted with oral magnesium.

The cardiac catheterization did not cause a significant rise in his serum creatinine. Adequate hydration and low-osmolality contrast agents have made these procedures safer. The history did not suggest any neuropathy, but the examination revealed early symmetrical polyneuropathy. The modest tachycardia was consistent with autonomic (parasympathetic) dysfunction, and the formal testing confirmed this. Fortunately, there were no problems with intraoperative hypotension.

Most anesthesiologists measure electrolytes several times during open-heart surgery. Since the patient was receiving an angiotensin-converting enzyme inhibitor before surgery and he had early renal insufficiency, it was appropriate not to initiate IV potassium with the other fluids at the beginning of surgery. The most likely reason for his mild hypokalemia afterward was a combination of the IV insulin infusion and an IV loop diuretic, which is usually administered during this procedure.

Because severe insulin resistance is common during CPB, blood glucose monitoring should be done more frequently. The short half-life of IV insulin allows any changes in the rate of the infusion to result in rapid changes in insulinemia and blood glucose levels.

Perhaps the most difficult aspect of these cases is changing back to subcutaneous insulin. It is probably easiest to continue with the insulin and glucose infusions until it is clear the patient will be able to tolerate food. For an insulin-resistant individual such as this patient, it would be appropriate to administer only half the usual dose of insulin before the first meal, either breakfast or supper. Since this individual will be hospitalized for at least several days, no advantage exists to initiating subcutaneous insulin before lunch, a time he does not usually administer insulin. The insulin and glucose infusions may be discontinued after the subcutaneous insulin is administered.

Patients such as this man can be managed quite effectively when the basic principles of preoperative evaluation and intraoperative management are followed and all members of the diabetes team agree with their implementation.

REFERENCES

1. Alberti KGMM: Diabetes and surgery, *Anesthesiology* 74:209, 1991 (editorial).
2. Alberti KGMM, Thomas DJB: The management of diabetes during surgery, *Br J Anaesth* 51:693, 1979.
3. American Diabetes Association Consensus Statement: Magnesium supplementation in the treatment of diabetes, *Diabetes Care* 16 (suppl 2):79, 1993.
4. American Diabetes Association Consensus Statement: Consensus development conference on the diagnosis and management of nephropathy in patients with diabetes mellitus, *Diabetes Care* 17: 1357, 1994.
5. American Diabetes Association Position Statement: Standards of medical care for patients with diabetes mellitus, *Diabetes Care* 17:616, 1994.
6. Arauz-Pacheco C, Raskin P: Surgery and anesthesia. In Lebovitz HE, editor: *Therapy for diabetes mellitus and related disorders,* ed 2, Alexandria, Va, 1994, American Diabetes Association.
7. Bailey CJ: Biguanides and NIDDM, *Diabetes Care* 15:755, 1992.
8. Baraka A, Nader A, Samahu S: Hypoglycemia of the diabetic patient during spinal anesthesia, *Middle East J Anesthesiol* 12:177, 1993.
9. Barrett BJ, Parfrey PS: Prevention of nephrotoxicity induced by radiocontrast agents, *N Engl J Med* 331:1449, 1994 (editorial).
10. Barzilay JI and others: Coronary artery disease and coronary artery bypass grafting in diabetic patients aged ≥65 years (report from the Coronary Artery Surgery Study [CASS] registry), *Am J Cardiol* 74:334, 1994.
11. Boyle PJ: Cushing's disease, glucocorticoid excess, glucocorticoid deficiency, and diabetes, *Diabetes Rev* 1:301, 1993.
12. Burgos LG and others: Increased intraoperative cardiovascular morbidity in diabetics with autonomic neuropathy, *Anesthesiology* 70:591, 1989.
13. Byyny RL: Management of diabetes during surgery, *Postgrad Med* 68:191, 1980.
14. Charlson ME, Makenzy CR, Gold JP: Preoperative autonomic function abnormalities in patients with diabetes mellitus and hypertension, *J Am Coll Surg* 179:1, 1994.
15. Chipkin SR, Kelly KL, Ruderman NB: Hormone-fuel interrelationships: fed state, starvation, and diabetes mellitus. In Kahn CR, Weir GC, editors: *Joslin's diabetes mellitus,* ed 13, Malvern, Pa, 1994, Lea & Febiger.
16. Chochinov R, Daughaday WH: Marked hyperthermia as a manifestation of hypoglycemia in long-standing diabetes mellitus, *Diabetes* 24:859, 1975.
17. Christiansen CL and others: Insulin treatment of the insulin dependent diabetic patient undergoing minor surgery, *Anaesthesia* 43:533, 1988.
18. Conill AM, Horowitz DA, Braunstein S: The surgical patient with diabetes mellitus. In Goldman DR, Brown FH, Guarnieri DM, editors: *Perioperative medicine,* New York, 1994, McGraw-Hill.
19. DeFronzo RA, Matsuda M, Barrett EJ: Diabetic ketoacidosis: a combined metabolic-nephrologic approach to therapy, *Diabetes Rev* 2:209, 1994.
20. *Diabetes 1993 vital statistics,* Alexandria, Va, 1993, American Diabetes Association.
21. Dunnet JM and others: Diabetes mellitus and anaesthesia: a survey of the peri-operative management of the patient with diabetes mellitus, *Anaesthesia* 43:538, 1988.
22. Eagle KA and others: Combining clinical and thallium data optimize preoperative assessment of

cardiac risk before major vascular surgery, *Ann Intern Med* 110:859, 1989.

23. Feinstein R, McGill JB, Hirsch IB: Glucose metabolism in nondiabetic subjects during the perioperative period, *Anesthesiology* 75:A622, 1991 (abstract).

24. Fellander G and others: Lipolysis during abdominal surgery, *J Clin Endocrinol Metab* 78:150, 1994.

25. Garber AJ: Noninvasive cardiac testing. In Lebovitz HE, editor: *Therapy for diabetes mellitus and related disorders,* ed 2, Alexandria, Va, 1994, American Diabetes Association.

26. Gavin LA: Perioperative management of the diabetic patient, *Endocrinol Metab Clin North Am* 21:457, 1992.

27. Genuth SM: The automatic (regular insulin) sliding scale or 2, 4, 6, 8—call H.O., *Clin Diabetes* 12:40, 1994.

28. Gold BS and others: Unanticipated admissions to the hospital following ambulatory surgery, *JAMA* 262:3008, 1989.

29. Gottrup F, Andreassen TT: Healing of incisional wounds in stomach and duodenum: the influence of experimental diabetes, *J Surg Res* 31:61, 1981.

30. Hall GM: Insulin administration in diabetic patients: return of the bolus? *Br J Anaesth* 72:1, 1994.

31. Harris MI: Noninsulin-dependent diabetes mellitus in black and white Americans, *Diabetes Metab Rev* 6:71, 1990.

32. Herskowitz IC, Matsutani A, Permutt MA: Leukocyte dysfunction in diabetes is proportional to metabolic control of the diabetic state, *Diabetes* 39 (suppl 1):7A, 1990 (abstract).

33. Himwich HE and others: Cerebral metabolism and electrical activity during insulin hypoglycemia in man, *Am J Physiol* 125:578, 1939.

34. Hirsch IB: Current concepts in diabetic nephropathy, *Clin Diabetes* 12:8, 1994.

35. Hirsch IB, Farkas-Hirsch R, Skyler JS: Intensive insulin therapy for treatment of type I diabetes, *Diabetes Care* 13:1265, 1990.

36. Hirsch IB, McGill JB: Role of insulin in management of surgical patients with diabetes mellitus, *Diabetes Care* 13:980, 1990.

37. Hirsch IB, White PF: Management of surgical patients with insulin-dependent diabetes mellitus, *Anesthesiol Rev* 21:53, 1994.

38. Hjortrup A and others: Influence of diabetes mellitus on operative risk, *Br J Surg* 72:783, 1985.

39. Hollenberg M and others: Predictors of postoperative myocardial ischemia in patients undergoing noncardiac surgery, *JAMA* 268:205, 1992.

40. Hostetter MK: Handicaps to host defense: effects of hyperglycemia on C3 and *Candida albicans, Diabetes* 39:271, 1990.

41. Husband DJ, Thai AC, Alberti KGMM: Management of diabetes during surgery with glucose-insulin-potassium infusion, *Diabetic Med* 3:69, 1986.

42. Jaspers CAJJ, Elte JWF, Olthof G: Perioperative diabetes regulation with the help of a standard protocol, *Neth J Med* 44:122, 1994.

43. Karjalainen A and others: A comparison of childhood and adult type I diabetes mellitus, *N Engl J Med* 320:881, 1989.

44. Kedes LH, Field JB: Hypothermia: a clue to hypoglycemia, *N Engl J Med* 271:785, 1964.

45. Kellerman PS: Perioperative care of the renal patient, *Arch Intern Med* 154:1674, 1994.

46. Kelly KG, Levy WK: The surgical patient with coronary artery disease. In Goldman DR, Brown FH, Guarnieri DM, editors: *Perioperative medicine,* New York, 1994, McGraw-Hill.

47. Kennedy DJ, Butterworth JF: Endocrine function during and after cardiopulmonary bypass: recent observations, *J Clin Endocrinol Metab* 78:997, 1994.

48. Kitabchi AE and others: Diabetic ketoacidosis and the hyperglycemic, hyperosmolar nonketotic state. In Kahn CR, Weir GC, editors: *Joslin's diabetes mellitus,* ed 13, Malvern, Pa, 1994, Lea & Febiger.

49. Laurie GM, Morris GC Jr, Glaeser DH: Influence of diabetes mellitus on the results of bypass surgery, *JAMA* 256:2967, 1986.

50. Lavie CJ and others: Diabetes and cardiovascular disease. In Bergman M, Sicard GA, editors: *Surgical management of the diabetic patient,* New York, 1991, Raven Press.

51. Lebovitz HE: Sulfonylurea drugs. In Lebovitz HE, editor: *Therapy for diabetes mellitus and related disorders,* ed 2, Alexandria, Va, 1994, American Diabetes Association.

52. Lloyd-Mostyn RH, Oram S: Modification by propranolol of cardiovascular effects of induced hypoglycaemia, *Lancet* 1:1213, 1975.

53. Marhoffer W and others: Impairment of polymorphonuclear leukocyte function and metabolic control in diabetes, *Diabetes Care* 15:256, 1992.

54. Mattock MB and others: Prospective study of microalbuminuria as predictor of mortality in NIDDM, *Diabetes* 41:736, 1992.

55. Mickler TA: The physiologic response to surgery and anesthesia. In Goldman DR, Brown FH, Guarnieri DM, editors: *Perioperative medicine,* New York, 1994, McGraw-Hill.

56. Milaskiewicz RM, Hall GM: Diabetes and anaesthesia: the past decade, *Br J Anaesth* 68:198, 1992.

57. Nesto RW and others: Angina and exertional myocardial ischemia in diabetic and nondiabetic

patients: assessment by exercise thallium scintigraphy, *Ann Intern Med* 108:170, 1988.

58. Niakan E and others: Silent myocardial infarction and diabetic cardiovascular autonomic neuropathy, *Arch Intern Med* 146:2229, 1986.

59. Ockert DBM, Hugo JM: Diabetic complications with special anaesthetic risk, *S Afr J Surg* 30:90, 1992.

60. Palmisano JJ: Surgery and diabetes. In Kahn CR, Weir GC, editors: *Joslin's diabetes mellitus,* ed 13, Malvern, Pa, 1994, Lea & Febiger.

61. Pezzarossa A and others: Perioperative management of diabetic subjects: subcutaneous versus intravenous insulin administration during glucose-potassium infusion, *Diabetes Care* 11:52, 1988.

62. Pickup JC and others: Hypomagnesaemia in IDDM patients with microalbuminuria and clinical proteinuria, *Diabetologia* 37:639, 1994 (letter).

63. Porte D Jr, Woods SC: Neural regulation of islet hormone and its role in energy balance and stress hyperglycemia. In Rifkin H, Porte D Jr, editors: *Diabetes mellitus: theory and practice,* ed 4, New York, 1990, Elsevier.

64. Rao MV and others: Role of epidural analgesia on endocrine & metabolic responses to surgery, *Indian J Med Res* [B] 92:13, 1990.

65. Raucoules-Aime M and others: Comparison of two methods of i.v. insulin administration in the diabetic patient during the perioperative period, *Br J Anaesth* 72:5, 1994.

66. Reddi AS, Camerini-Davalos RA: Diabetic nephropathy: an update, *Arch Intern Med* 150:31, 1990.

67. Resnick LM and others: Intracellular and extracellular magnesium depletion in type II (non-insulin-dependent) diabetes mellitus, *Diabetologia* 36:767, 1993.

68. Romano E, Gullo A: Hypoglycemic coma following epidural analgesia, *Anaesthesia* 35:1084, 1980.

69. Seki S: Clinical features of hyperosmolar hyperglycemic nonketotic coma associated with cardiac operations, *J Thorac Cardiovasc Surg* 91:867-873, 1986.

70. Sentochnik DE, Eliopoulos GM: Infection and diabetes. In Kahn CR, Weir GC, editors: *Joslin's diabetes mellitus,* ed 13, Malvern, Pa, 1994, Lea & Febiger.

71. Shagan BP: Does anyone here know how to make insulin work backwards? Why sliding-scale insulin coverage doesn't work, *Pract Diabetol* 9:1, 1990.

72. Simmons D and others: A comparison of two intravenous insulin regimens among surgical patients with insulin-dependent diabetes, *Diabetes Educ* 20:422, 1994.

73. Sinnock P: Hospital utilization for diabetes. In Jarrison MI, Hamman RF, editors: *Diabetes in America* NIH Pub No 85-1468, Washington, DC, 1985, US Department of Health and Human Services.

74. Solomon R and others: Effects of saline, mannitol, and furosemide on acute decreases in renal function induced by radiocontrast agents, *N Engl J Med* 331:1416, 1994.

75. Stephens JW and others: The effect of glucose priming solutions in diabetic patients undergoing coronary artery bypass grafting, *Ann Thorac Surg* 45:544, 1988.

76. Thomas DJB, Alberti KGMM: Hyperglycemic effects of Hartmann's solution during surgery in patients with maturity onset diabetes, *Br J Anaesth* 50:185, 1978.

77. Treiman GS and others: The influence of diabetes mellitus on the risk of abdominal aortic surgery, *Am Surg* 60:436, 1994.

78. Turner RC and others: Measurement of the insulin delivery in man, *J Clin Endocrinol* 33:279, 1971.

79. Watts NB and others: Postoperative management of diabetes mellitus: steady-state glucose control with bedside algorithm for insulin adjustment, *Diabetes Care* 10:722, 1987.

80. Werb MR and others: Hormone and metabolic responses during coronary artery bypass surgery: role of infused glucose, *J Clin Endocrinol Metab* 69:1010, 1989.

81. Wilson R, Reeves W: Neutrophil phagocytosis and killing in insulin-dependent diabetes, *Clin Exp Immunol,* 63:478, 1986.

82. Wolf RR, Peters EJ: Lipolytic response to glucose response in human subjects, *Am J Physiol* 252:E218, 1987.

83. Wong T, Detsky AS: Preoperative cardiac risk assessment for patients having peripheral vascular surgery, *Ann Intern Med* 116:743, 1992.

84. Yue DK and others: Abnormalities of granulation tissue and collagen formation in experimental diabetes, uremia, and malnutrition, *Diabetic Med* 3:221, 1986.

85. Yue DK and others: Effects of experimental diabetes, uremia, and malnutrition on wound healing, *Diabetes* 36:295, 1987.

PART TWO

Psychosocial Contexts of Diabetes Care and Education

13 Sociocultural Concerns of Diabetes Care

Linda K. Sussman

INTRODUCTION

To communicate with and treat diabetes adequately in individuals of ethnically diverse groups, it is important to understand the nature of medical systems cross-culturally, the process of health maintenance and health seeking by individuals, and sociocultural factors that influence health care decisions and behavior. In this chapter, common attributes of medical systems across cultures are described, emphasizing especially the process of managing illness. This is followed by a discussion of three sociocultural factors and their impact on illness management: medical beliefs, social structure and organization, and cultural values and history. The chapter concludes with a description of a culturally sensitive approach to diabetes care and patient education, including specific pointers and pitfalls concerning selected components of diabetes care.

With advances in biomedicine in the twentieth century, the number of individuals living with chronic disease has increased considerably. Diseases such as diabetes, which in the recent past were not treatable, may now be "managed," allowing individuals to lead full, productive lives. Illness exists among all peoples, and each culture has devised its own ways of dealing with it. Throughout human history and across cultures, medical systems have focused

---

CHAPTER OBJECTIVES

- Discuss medical systems from a crosscultural perspective.
- Describe the common components of culturally diversed medical systems.
- Describe the health-seeking process.
- Summarize sociocultural factors, including belief systems, social structure, and cultural values, that affect health-seeking and illness management.
- Review approaches to culturally sensitive diabetes care and education.

predominantly on curing illness and reducing pain. Chronic illness represents a special and, to many lay people across cultures, a rather peculiar case of illness in that the goal of biomedical treatment is not a cure but rather lifelong management. Biomedical treatment for diabetes requires both routine medical care and ongoing daily management and monitoring in the home by patients and their families.

The prevalence of diabetes in the United States is higher among many ethnic minorities, notably African Americans and Hispanic-American and Native-American groups, than among the white majority.[2] (See Chapters 2 and 3.) Compared with non-Hispanic whites, with a 6.2% prevalence rate, age-standardized prevalence rates of non-insulin-dependent diabetes mellitus (NIDDM) are 50% to 60% higher among Cubans (9.3%) and African Americans (10.2%) and 110% to 120% higher among Mexican Americans (13%) and Puerto Ricans (13.4%).[29] Similar patterns are reported for the prevalence of both NIDDM and insulin-dependent diabetes mellitus (IDDM) combined.[24] Native-American groups exhibit very high prevalence rates, with the Pima of Arizona experiencing the highest rates (50% among adults over age 35)[77] and the Hopi experiencing a doubled rate in the past 20 years.[9] High prevalence rates among ethnic minorities are often also accompanied by a higher incidence of complications[70] and by higher morbidity and mortality rates.[18,33] For example, death rates from diabetes are four times higher for Mexican Americans in South Texas than for other whites,[61] and the rate of lower extremity amputations resulting from peripheral vascular disease is 1.5 to 2.5 times higher for African Americans than white Americans with diabetes.[18]

More than 29 million African Americans reside in the United States, making up about 12% of the population.[4] Hispanics, numbering more than 15 million, represent over 7% of the population.[24] Of this group, Mexican Americans are the most numerous (more than 12 million) and the most rapidly growing minority.[99] Given current rates of population increase, it has been predicted that in the next century Hispanics will be the largest U.S. minority group.[15] It is therefore important to understand the medical beliefs and practices that may influence diabetes management among ethnic minorities. Moreover, levels of adherence to treatment regimens by all groups and subgroups have been found in numerous studies to be far from ideal.[21,75,76,91] It cannot be assumed that the lay system of medical beliefs and behavior of even most Americans necessarily corresponds to the biomedical model.

MEDICAL SYSTEMS IN CROSS-CULTURAL PERSPECTIVE

Culture is a set of guidelines (both explicit and implicit) which individuals inherit as members of a particular society, and which tells them how to *view* the world, how to experience it *emotionally,* and how to *behave* in it in relation to other people, to supernatural forces or gods, and to the natural environment. . . . To some extent, culture can be seen as an inherited "lens," through which individuals perceive and understand the world that they inhabit, and learn how to live within it. Growing up within any society is a form of *en*culturation, whereby the individual slowly acquires the cultural "lens" of that society.

One aspect of this "cultural lens" is the division of the world, and the people within it, into different *categories.* . . . For example, kinsfolk or strangers, normal or abnormal, . . . , healthy or ill. And all cultures have elaborate ways of moving people from one social category into another (pp. 2-3).[32]

Shared Elements of Medical Systems

All human societies possess beliefs and practices related to illness. These reflect the "cultural lens"[32] through which members of the society view the world; they do not exist as isolated "folk beliefs" or "folk remedies" removed from the wider culture.

Within a society, the "medical system" is a cultural system just as are the religious, political, and economic systems. It is composed of all the health knowledge, beliefs, skills, and practices of members of the group. It "includes the ways that people become recognized as ill,' the ways that they present this illness to other people, the attributes of those they present their illness to, and the ways that the illness is dealt with" (p. 7),[32] as well as "patterns of belief about the causes of illness; norms governing choice and evaluation of treatment; socially-legitimated statuses, roles, power relations, interaction settings, and institutions" (p. 24).[46]

Most complex societies are composed of members of ethnic and religious minorities, including recent immigrants from other cultures. Each group may possess its own cultural beliefs, norms, and practices, while individual members of the group may become acculturated to varying extents to the culture of the larger society.

Despite the great diversity of "medical systems" throughout the world, a number of components have been found to be common to all, including biomedicine. These include the following:

1. **Conceptual components**
   a. An *illness classification system,* composed of labels for various symptoms and illnesses (nosology)
   b. A system of *beliefs concerning the possible causes* of illness (etiology)
   c. A means of *attributing causes and applying labels* (diagnosis) to specific episodes
   d. A set of *appropriate treatments* for specific illnesses
   e. *Expectations* regarding course of the illness and treatment outcome (prognosis)
2. **Personnel.** *Healing specialists* who possess specialized knowledge or power are usually respected members of the community and have a set of paraphernalia for diagnosis and treatment that sets them apart from other members of the community. Healing specialists may belong to the *professional sector,*[46] as members of organized healing professions such as biomedicine, Ayurveda, Chinese medicine, or chiropractics, in which some group control exists over training, licensing, and so on, or to the *folk sector,*[46] as nonprofessional, nonbureaucratic specialists.
3. **Behavioral components**
   a. *Norms regarding treatment seeking and illness management:* criteria for defining oneself as ill and labeling others as "sick," culturally appropriate sick role behavior, and expectations regarding the identities of those responsible for making health care decisions and caring for sick persons.
   b. *Norms regarding consultations with healing specialists:* appropriate content (e.g., brief description of physical symptoms; discussion of feelings, social relations, or moral dilemmas; context in which symptoms developed), modes of interaction (e.g., formal questions/answers, patient narratives, physical examinations, ritual ceremony), location of consultation and identification of individuals who may or should attend consultations

(e.g., client/patient, kin group, friends), role of healing specialist (e.g., expert, authority, counselor, advisor), nature of specialist's advice (e.g., suggests explanations, orders course of treatment), method and amount of payment (e.g., cash, livestock, food; mandatory or voluntary; payment given for each consultation or after cure has been effected).

Medical systems worldwide consist of the *lay* ("popular"[46]) sector and the *specialist* ("folk" and "professional"[46]) sectors. Each sector has its theories of causation, explanatory models, methods of treating illness, and criteria for guiding treatment seeking and treatment evaluation. In most societies today a number of different therapeutic systems (specialist subsectors) coexist within the specialist sector, although one system may dominate. This is called *medical pluralism.* * The belief systems and treatment practices of the different specialist subsectors may differ significantly from each other. The United States is an example of a society with a plural medical system in which biomedicine dominates but coexists with other formalized systems, such as chiropractics and osteopathy, along with faith healers, herbalists, homeopaths, and healers of ethnic minorities.

In societies with plural medical systems and a multicultural population, the situation may be fairly complex. The theories and practices of each of the specialist subsectors (e.g., biomedicine, chiropractics, homeopathy) differ to varying extents from each other, as do the medical beliefs and practices of ethnic groups (lay subsectors) in the lay sector. Of particular importance to health care practitioners is that different therapeutic systems may be used by an individual either for different illnesses or for a single illness with little or no perceived ideologic conflict.† For example, it has been estimated that 65% to 70% of Mexican Americans in San Jose, California, who eventually consult a physician have first tried some other form of treatment. Treatment may include home herbal remedies, herbalists, curanderas, chiropractors, and homeopaths.[13]

The degree to which the medical system of a *lay* subsector matches that of a specialist subsector varies from ethnic group to ethnic group (Fig. 13-1). Thus, although patterns of health care and treatment seeking of individuals in a particular group (E_1 to E_8 in Fig. 13-1) *may reflect norms and values of that group, they may not concur with patterns advocated in some specialist subsectors, such as biomedicine (B in Fig. 13-1).* Even for the white majority in the United States and Europe, the biomedical and lay sectors are not necessarily synonymous.[32,46] One consequence of this is that self-care actions of patients may go unrecognized by medical personnel because they do not fit the medical model of appropriate self-care.[37] It is therefore important to recognize the existence of the lay sector, to respect it, and to take it into account when treating and communicating with patients.

Patterns of health seeking and health maintenance are products and integral parts of the sociocultural systems in which they occur, and decisions about the seeking of care, the choice of care, and chronic illness management vary across cultural groups.‡ Leininger,[54] therefore, suggests the need to study health care from an anthropologic

---

*References 17, 28, 32, 43, 65, 93, 103.
†References 4, 13, 16, 17, 67, 80, 83, 84, 92, 93, 96, 104.
‡References 4, 13, 32, 46, 63, 74, 80, 97.

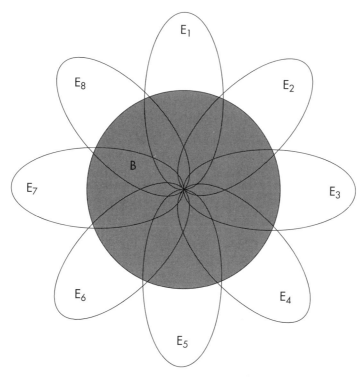

Fig. 13-1   Schematic representation of biomedical subsector *(B)* and lay subsectors (ethnic groups E_1 to E_8).

perspective, which approaches people in their natural and familiar life environments to learn their language, customs, problems, and aspirations. Illnesses are "lived experiences."[78] As such, Gibbs,[26] in a discussion of older African Americans, identifies the need to study the present circumstances of individuals, emphasizing the interplay between social and institutional factors and personal experience. Rimer and colleagues[72] conclude that an ecologic model that takes into account the influence of intrapersonal, interpersonal, community, and health policy factors is the most appropriate perspective for research on minority health behavior.

Health-Seeking Process: The Lay Perspective

The customary view is that professionals organize health care for lay people. But typically lay people activate their health care by deciding when and whom to consult, whether or not to comply, when to switch between treatment alternatives, whether care is effective, and whether they are satisfied with its quality. In this sense, the popular sector functions as the chief source and most immediate determinant of care (p. 51).[32]

In the lay sector, most illness beliefs and health-seeking behavior patterns are not formally learned in school but, starting in childhood, are "picked up" piecemeal from

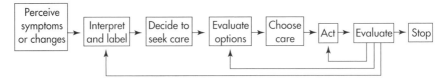

Fig. 13-2   The health-seeking process

experience, observation, and teaching within the household and social group. They continue to be learned and modified over one's lifetime as experiences with illness accumulate.

Illness is first experienced by individuals, their households, and families, and it is usually within this context that illnesses are managed, with or without the advice or help of a healing specialist. Most illness episodes in Western and non-Western societies are treated within the lay sector with no recourse to specialists.[47,108] Kleinman,[46] for example, found that in two districts of Taipei, 93% of all illness episodes in a 1-month period were first treated in the family and 73% of all episodes were treated exclusively in the family. Cross-culturally, most illnesses and conditions requiring special care are recognized, interpreted, and managed by a lay "therapy management group,"[39,42] the composition of which varies from culture to culture (e.g., the individual patient, nuclear family, mother and grandmother, paternal kin, extended family). This group may obtain advice and suggestions from others in their "therapeutic network," composed of culturally appropriate informal and formal sources of advice and care.

The *health-seeking process* is a decision-making process engaged in by individuals in the lay sector.* It includes (1) decisions about the need for care and associated role changes, (2) choices concerning source of care, and (3) ongoing health maintenance decisions. It is a dynamic process and may be conceptualized as involving the following steps (Fig. 13-2):

1. Identify presence of symptoms or physical or other changes.
2. Perceive and attend to those symptoms or changes.
3. Interpret and label them.
4. Decide to treat (or not).
5. Delineate and evaluate the options, including self-treatment and no treatment.
6. Choose treatment or source of care.
7. Act on choice and treat or seek care.
8. Evaluate the outcome.
9. *Then either:*

    a. Continue the same treatment or source of care, with ongoing evaluation (8 and 9).

    or

    b. Cease current treatment/care and (1) cease treatment seeking, or (2) delineate/evaluate other care options, choose care, and so on, (5 to 9); or (3) reinterpret and relabel symptoms or changes and so forth (3 to 9).

---

*References 4, 12, 26, 46, 55, 59, 60, 92, 97.

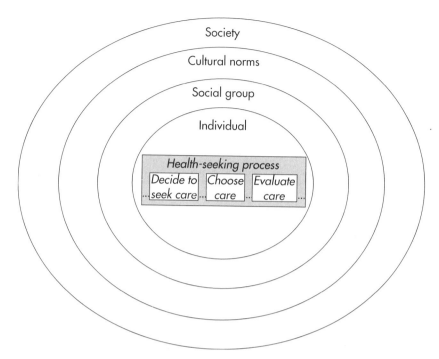

Fig. 13-3   Context of the health-seeking process.

For acute or self-limiting illnesses, this process may be relatively short and uncomplicated. For chronic illness and symptoms, it may be quite complex and represent a lifetime of trying different sources of care, modifying treatment regimens, and evaluating outcomes.

Context of the Health-Seeking Process

The health-seeking and health maintenance process is shaped by the interaction of individual, social group, subcultural norms, and societal characteristics.[94] These are represented by four concentric circles in Fig. 13-3. The inner circle represents the *individual,* who is imbedded in a *social group,* which is imbedded in the *culture* of the (minority) group, which in turn is imbedded in the *society,* which represents the sociocultural and institutional components of the majority culture. It is important to realize that although these levels are separated conceptually, they are inextricably linked, and constant interaction and feedback occur among all levels.

Humans are social beings who develop primarily through learning and experience. Individual thought and behavior are viewed as developing through interaction among the individual, social group, subculture, and society at large. A major emphasis of this model is that individuals reflect the layers of influence that surround them in the form of social group, subcultural norms, and the social, political, and economic realities of the society at large.

Learning and development are ongoing, and changes in one level of the model may result in changes in other levels. For example, changes in a nation's health care policy may lead to changes in patient behavior; alternatively, changes in patient choices and expectations may lead to changes in physician behavior or health care policy. This dynamic, multilevel model is particularly appropriate for both research and medical treatment, with the goals of identifying, understanding, and addressing the multiple factors influencing the health-seeking process and illness management among minority groups.

Some components of the four levels follow.

Individual characteristics may include (1) individual health status; (2) personal resources such as economic resources, insurance coverage, and housing; and (3) cognitive factors such as knowledge, beliefs, attitudes, and expectations about illness and health care.

Characteristics of the social group refer to (1) characteristics of groups of kin and friends such as composition, proximity, and frequency of contact; (2) characteristics of interactions between the individual and social groups such as the type of support received from and obligations and responsibilities to the various groups; and (3) beliefs, attitudes, and values of group members regarding illness and health. Since the immediate social group of family and friends is cross-culturally the primary source of care and support as well as the locus of many health care decisions, examination of the characteristics of this group can provide important information concerning the relation between the structure and nature of family social life and decisions concerning chronic illness management.

Cultural characteristics include *shared group norms* of thought and behavior, values, and preferences, as well as shared history. Some cultural components relevant to the health-seeking process include (1) medical belief systems; (2) social structure and organization (e.g., the locus of responsibility for health care decisions and care of the sick, roles and statuses of individuals of various age-groups and gender groups); (3) values regarding individual attributes and behavior, characteristics of social interaction, and spiritual or religious obligations; and (4) history of the cultural group, especially its relevance to contemporary perceptions of the relationship of the minority group to the majority culture and its institutions. These four components are discussed in detail later.

Societal characteristics include the health care, economic, social, and political systems of the society within which the individual lives. Some specific components relevant to health care and chronic illness management include (1) the health care system, such as the distribution, cost, quality, and policies of the health care resources; (2) the economic system, such as the distribution and abundance of economic resources in the minority group in relation to the majority, and social welfare policies; and (3) demographics, including educational attainment and occupational status, geographic distribution of the group, neighborhood resources, and availability of transportation or particular food items.

SOCIOCULTURAL FACTORS AFFECTING HEALTH SEEKING AND ILLNESS MANAGEMENT

The following sections focus specifically on selected sociocultural factors affecting the health-seeking and health maintenance process:

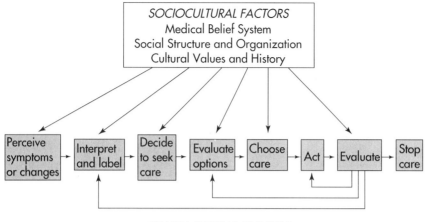

HEALTH-SEEKING PROCESS

Fig. 13-4   Sociocultural factors influencing the health-seeking process.

1. Medical belief systems
2. Social structure and organization
3. Cultural values and history

These provide the lens through which patients and families of different ethnic groups perceive and interpret symptoms and illness and the context in which they decide whether or not to seek care, choose sources of care, develop treatment goals and expectations, evaluate treatment, and decide whether to continue, cease, change, or supplement care (Fig. 13-4).

Medical Belief Systems

To communicate effectively with a patient about his illness or treatment regimen, a physician must know something about how the patient conceives of disease, its etiology, and therapeutics in general. When the patient comes from a different sociocultural milieu than the physician, the likelihood is great that the two will face each other with quite different views on these matters (p. 1153).[30]

It [lay belief system of African Americans] is a coherent medical system and not a ragtag collection of isolated superstitions. If the underlying premises are accepted, it makes just as much sense to the believer as the principles of orthodox medicine do to the graduate of an accredited medical school (p. 83).[83]

Medical belief systems provide individuals with an explanatory framework with which to view illness. This framework guides the interpretation of symptoms, decisions to seek care, decisions about where to seek care, the ways in which symptoms are presented to physicians and other healing specialists, and the evaluation of treatment outcomes. It also provides the lens through which patients view physicians, physician behavior and interaction, and physician statements concerning the diagnosis, nature of the disease, and logic of treatment.

In all medical classification systems, symptoms are generally attributed to particular causes on which treatment is based. The problem facing biomedical physicians is that the lay classification system may not correspond to the biomedical system. The medical consultation may then be viewed as a transaction between the lay and professional "explanatory models,"[46] in which the clinician must strive to make the explanation of the illness and its treatment "make sense" to patients while respecting patients' experiences and interpretations of their illness. Consensus must be reached regarding a shared model of the illness.[32]

Although medical belief systems may differ considerably from culture to culture, they share some themes or characteristics. Two themes that exist in many systems are (1) the belief in multiple causes of illness and (2) the belief that illness reflects and is caused by some type of imbalance or disharmony. Since these themes are so prevalent worldwide and among U.S. ethnic groups, they are described in some detail next. This is followed by a discussion of specific ways that belief systems may shape health seeking and illness maintenance.

Multicausal belief systems

Owing to his lack of knowledge, the ordinary man cannot attempt to resolve conflicting theories or conflicting advice into a single organized structure. He is likely to assume that the information available to him is on the order of what we might think of as a few pieces of an enormous jigsaw puzzle.

From this perspective, the presence of plural medical philosophies is a reflection of a generally pluralized conception of the Universe. There are many gods, many roads to Heaven, many scriptures, many intellectual traditions, and many kinds of people. That unity arises out of this plurality is an article of faith. It is not for the ordinary man to attempt to reconcile diversity or to find it surprising when his neighbor holds different views of the nature of things (pp. 185-186).[6]

The concept that illness may be caused by multiple factors is found in many medical belief systems throughout the world. This does not mean that illness may be caused by germs or exposure or heredity, but that different categories of factors may cause illness and that different types of treatment or healers are effective in treating different causes.

Among the most widespread is the belief that illness (and other forms of misfortune) may be caused by either *natural* or *unnatural* (or *supernatural*) factors and agents. This has been reported in Africa* and Asia,[6,11,46,98] as well as in the New World among African Americans, Bahamians, Cubans, Haitians, Puerto Ricans, Trinidadians, the Garifuna of Belize, Mexicans, Mexican Americans, and Native Americans, as well as among white ethnic groups.†

Natural illnesses may result either immediately or later in life from constitutional weaknesses or exposure to forces of nature such as cold air; impurities in air, food, and water; or germs. In many cultures they are viewed as part of the world as God, the creator, intended it to be. God is thus viewed as part of the natural world or as the creator, and source, of the natural world. In several cultures, "natural" illnesses are referred to as "illnesses of God."‡ In some cultures, such illnesses may be interpreted in a more "personalistic" framework. They may be believed to result from the will of God, being sent by God as punishment to victims or their kin or sent for other reasons unknown to the victims. For example, they may be sent to teach lessons to individuals or to improve their character.

---

*References 39, 43, 64, 92, 96.
†References 4, 13, 34-36, 80, 82-86, 89, 107.
‡References 39, 92, 93, 96, 105.

Unnatural or *supernatural illnesses* often represent some sort of upset in the natural world and often result from impaired social relations. Although sinners, who lack God's protection, may fall prey to demons and evil spirits, the most common causes of these illnesses are witchcraft and sorcery, usually based on sympathetic, imitative, and contagious magic frequently implemented through adulterated food. These illnesses are thus frequently caused by some malign human intervention calling on supernatural resources. Among some groups, divine retribution (e.g., punishment by the ancestors or saints) for improper behavior toward other people, deceased ancestors, or other spiritual beings may be included in this category or in a category of supernatural illnesses. Possession by various types of spirits, often not the fault of the victim, would also fall under this category.

Although specific symptoms are not always related to particular causes of illness (in which case the context in which the illness occurred is diagnostically more important than symptoms themselves), some types of symptoms do seem cross-culturally to be related to "unnatural" causes. They tend to be those that occur suddenly and unexpectedly in healthy individuals, such as fainting and dizziness. They may involve otherwise unexplainable behavior changes or physical changes, such as sudden bouts of violence or aggressiveness, sudden changes in mood, extreme lethargy, or weight loss with no significant changes in diet. The similarity between these and some symptoms that may be experienced by individuals with diabetes is noteworthy.

It is important to keep in mind that medical beliefs and associated forms of treatment are part of an internally logical system and closely intertwined with a host of other cultural norms, values, and world views. For example, in research on low-income African Americans residing in Arizona but who were socialized in the rural south or maintained kin ties to the South, Snow[83] finds a coherent system of medical beliefs and practices that is a composite of many sources, including earlier classic medicine, European folklore, African elements, and selected beliefs from biomedicine. "The whole is inextricably blended with the tenets of fundamentalist Christianity, elements from the Voodoo religion of the West Indies, and the added spice of sympathetic magic" (p. 83). Snow[83] states quite emphatically that it is most important for the physician to remember that although a composite of many elements, this is a coherent system of belief and practice.

Working with Puerto Ricans with NIDDM in Boston, Quatromoni and others[68] remark how strongly religious beliefs impact health beliefs. They find that the religious belief system seems "to override all other belief systems related to preventive health and nutritional behaviors" (p. 872). It is believed that personal health is controlled by God. He brings health, He brings illness, and He is the only one who knows why. He can also give people the strength to deal with illness. From this perspective, diabetes is viewed as a disease that makes one's health worse but also as a disease that has to be endured because it is the result of God's will. This belief system, which involves an "external locus of control" of health, can pose significant barriers to achieving adherence to a medical regimen for diabetes and long-term, sometimes extensive, changes in life-style and behavior.

Fatalism has also been reported among other Hispanic groups, in which preventive health measures are viewed as ineffective in preserving health or preventing illness.[68] Likewise, Hopper and Schechtman,[38] focusing on low-income, predominantly African-American women with NIDDM, find that a considerable proportion are fatalistic about their diabetes and express a lack of belief in the possibility of having control over one's health.

An important implication is that some believe those whom God has made ill cannot be healed by physicians. On the other hand, individuals afflicted with illness, for whatever cause, may be healed through God's intervention,[75] and individuals may be protected by God from all types of illness, even those caused by microorganisms. For example, Snow[83] states, "One woman, a Pentecostal evangelist, spends much time at a local hospital praying for the sick. She understands that there are illnesses caused by micro-organisms but believes that while she is making her hospital rounds, God puts an invisible barrier around her that germs cannot penetrate" (p. 84). Clark,[13] however, notes that among some Mexican Americans, although illness is believed to result from God's will, physicians may also be viewed as instruments of God in healing individuals.

Belief systems based on the concept of balance

Another prevalent theme in medical belief systems is the concept of balance, in which health is viewed as a manifestation of proper balance or harmony and ill health as a result of imbalance or disharmony. This is widespread and found in such diverse regions as Latin America, North America, Asia, and Africa.* In some belief systems the balance required for health involves mainly physical and behavioral factors, whereas in others, optimal health is maintained only when balance, order, or harmony exists in the physical, social, and spiritual (or moral) spheres of life.

In traditional Chinese medicine, health is conceived of as a balance between the principles of *yin* (dark, moist, watery, and female) and *yang* (hot, dry, fiery, and male).[32] In the Indian Ayurvedic medical system the five elements *(bhutas)* of ether, wind, water, earth, and fire are the basic constituents of all life and make up the three bodily humors *(dosas)* of wind, bile, and phlegm. Illness results from a lack of balance among the three humours, and hot and cold foods and remedies are used to restore appropriate balance.[32]

A number of belief systems emphasizing the role of balance in health classify illnesses, conditions, foods, and medicines into categories of "hot" and "cold." Although also found in Asia and North Africa, they are especially prevalent among Latin-American groups and are thus particularly relevant to medical care in the United States.

Hot/cold theories. The hot/cold systems of disease etiology and classification found in Latin America are largely derived from the humoral theory of disease, developed in the fifth century BC by Hippocrates and elaborated by Galen in the second century AD. According to this theory, health was viewed as a state of balance among four humors: blood, phlegm, black bile, and yellow bile. Health was manifest in a warm, moist body. Illness, on the other hand, was manifest in an excessively dry, wet, hot, or cold body, which was caused by humoral imbalance.[30]

In the centuries that ensued, Galen's theories spread throughout the Roman world as well as into the Islamic world, translated into Arabic. Spanish and Portuguese adopted humoral theory and later carried it to the New World in the sixteenth and seventeenth centuries.[32] There

---

*References 7, 28, 30, 32, 46, 52, 53, 56, 64, 82, 98, 107.

it was taught in medical schools and also taught by medical practitioners to indigenous and mestizo populations. Variations of it were incorporated into Latin-American folk medical practice and continue to persist today. Although variations exist between groups, the wet/dry dichotomy was largely dropped, and the hot/cold distinction predominates in most current systems.[13,30] In this classification, illnesses are categorized as either "hot" or "cold," as are foods, herbs, and modern medications.

Puerto Ricans in New York City group illnesses into "hot" and "cold" but categorize foods and medicines into three groups of "hot," "cold," and "cool."[30] They treat cold illnesses with hot medicines and foods and hot illnesses with cool medicines and foods. Harwood[30] notes that this system is firmly rooted among New York City Puerto Ricans and exhibits considerable vitality, since new medicines and foods are being incorporated into the system according to their effects on the body. Penicillin, for example, is classified as "hot" because it can cause symptoms such as rash or diarrhea, which are "hot." Drugs that may cause effects such as muscular spasms, however, would be classified as "cold." However, variations exist between cultural groups and between individuals within groups in the actual content of the classifications. They may be related to the degree of acculturation of individuals to mainstream American society or to idiosyncratic ways in which particular foods or medicines affect their bodies.

Medical beliefs and illness management: some examples

Respect for the patient's tradition and an ability to work with the therapeutic choices inherent in it allow for development of a treatment regimen with the patient which does not contravene his deeply held ideas about illness and will stand a much better chance of success (p. 1158).[30]

Clearly, medical belief systems are of utmost importance in decision making regarding health and illness management and influence all the steps in the health-seeking and health maintenance process. Symptoms are categorized, labeled, and interpreted according to the cultural lens of patients and their families. This in turn affects decisions about whether or not to seek care and from whom to seek care. The diagnosis, treatment, and explanation of the health care provider are then evaluated in terms of the medical belief system to determine whether it makes sense. For short-term acute illnesses that may be rapidly cured, this may not pose a great problem for biomedical physicians as long as the patient decides to follow the treatment prescribed for a short time. However, for chronic illnesses that require constant ongoing maintenance at home and regular checkups with the physician, the nonconcurrence of the medical belief systems of patient and physician can create a great barrier to maintaining adequate medical management from a biomedical perspective. According to Helman,[32] describing results of research in Pakistan by Mull and Mull[62]:

. . . Some [rural Pakistani mothers] . . . saw the diarrhoea—which was very common in the area—as a "natural" and expected part of teething and growing up, and not as an illness. Some believed it was dangerous to try to stop the diarrhoea, lest the trapped "heat" within it spread to the brain and cause a fever. Others explained infant diarrhoea as due to certain folk illnesses, . . . which should be treated with traditional remedies or traditional folk healers without recourse to ORT. . . . Many mothers in the group saw diarrhoea as a "hot" illness, . . . which required a "cold" form of treatment—such as a change in maternal diet, or giving certain foods and herbs to the infant—to restore the sick infant to a normal temperature. They classified most Western medicines, such as antibiotics and even vitamins, as also "hot," and therefore inappropriate for a diarrhoeal child. . . . Health care programmes should always be designed not only to address medical concerns, but also to take into account what the people in the community actually believe about their own ill-health and how it should be treated (p. 10).

Symptom perception and interpretation. Perceptions and interpretations of symptoms are shaped by beliefs about their etiology, treatability, and curability. First to consider is *whether the patient views the symptoms as abnormal* and as requiring any treatment at all. For example, in many regions of the world, diarrhea is quite common in infants and children. Oral rehydration therapy (ORT) is inexpensive and widely available, but many reject its use for diverse reasons. In the previous example, some mothers viewed diarrhea in their infants as normal, and some even believed that it would be dangerous to try to stop it.

It is important to understand concepts of human development and ideas about what is viewed as "normal" for different age-groups or gender groups. For example, Reid[71] has found that among aged African Americans with diabetes, age is seen as a period of general decline, and a symptom such as fatigue is viewed as a normal part of old age, as is a loss of control over one's body. There is also a sense that if one is too old, treatment for certain problems such as eye or vision problems and incontinence is useless. Such beliefs may greatly impact symptom perception and interpretation as well as subsequent health-seeking and health maintenance decisions.

What about instances in which an asymptomatic individual has been medically diagnosed as having a disease? The question to consider under these circumstances is, *can the patient conceptually be "sick" in the absence of symptoms?* Such distinctions between patient and clinical views have been addressed in social science through the concepts of "disease," "illness,"[20] and "sickness."[106] Although "disease" is a biologically defined, pathologic bodily state, "illness" refers to an individual's experience of a disvalued change of state that may include symptoms or disease. "Sick" is a socially bestowed label and culturally defined role assigned to individuals. Given these definitions, an individual can have a disease but not have an illness and not be sick. Conversely, an individual can have an illness and be "sick" but not have a "disease."

Clark,[13] for example, notes that a thin Mexican-American male "whose lack of abdominal fat permits the palpation of the abdominal aorta may promptly seek treatment for latido, a dread folk disease" (p. 228). He is "sick," although biomedicine does not recognize his "pounding stomach" as a sign of disease. Clark further remarks:

In Sal si Puedes illness is generally defined as a state of bodily discomfort. A person who has no debilitating symptoms is usually held to be well and healthy even though the diagnostic tests of scientific practitioners may reveal such serious pathological processes as carcinoma, tuberculosis, or heart disease. It is difficult for the people to understand how a sick person can feel well and go about his normal tasks without discomfort. To say to a patient without symptoms, 'You are sick,' is to invite confusion and disbelief (p. 228).

Staiano[89] comments that for the Garifuna of Belize, although the biomedical terms for common chronic diseases such as diabetes and hypertension are accepted and incorporated into the lay system, the concepts of these as chronic diseases do not completely concur with those of biomedicine. For example, if an individual with a chronic disease experiences relief from symptoms, this is often thought of as a "cure." If symptoms return, the individual is then thought of as "catching" the illness again.

Regarding preventive care, or early care of those diagnosed with a disease, the idea of preventive measures to avoid illness or stop the further progression of illness exists in many medical belief systems. Among Mexican Americans, for example, "susto" is an illness resulting from a frightening event. However, an individual may not develop symptoms until some time after the event and, if preventive measures are taken, may avoid the illness altogether.[13] Other examples are widespread and may include such diverse practices as wearing talismans to protect former victims of sorcery against subsequent attacks or drinking herbal decoctions during pregnancy or the postpartum period to prevent the development of specific illnesses.[95] Clark[13] notes that perhaps the value of preventive care or of care during the "preclinical" stage of disease has not been accepted by many lay people because it "has not been presented to the people in familiar terms" (p. 228).

Treatment options and choices. Next to consider is *whether the illness is believed to be treatable by biomedicine.* In the earlier example from Pakistan, some respondents believed the diarrhea was caused by factors (e.g., spirits, other supernatural causes) requiring traditional rather than biomedical treatment.[62] Beliefs about the role of God in causing, preventing, or curing illnesses may lead one to believe that biomedical care is unnecessary for health maintenance or will be ineffective in curing particular illnesses.

On the other hand, biomedical care might be sought based on beliefs that are not completely concurrent with biomedical theory. Such care may be sought because it is believed that the illness is "natural" and caused, for example, by a weak constitution or by past exposure to particular stimuli, or that it is a new illness that has been brought by outsiders. Biomedical disease terms, such as *diabetes, cancer, tuberculosis,* and *measles,* are frequently incorporated into different medical systems and languages and used by patients when interacting with biomedical physicians. However, associated concepts about the disease, its etiology, and its treatment may differ significantly from biomedical concepts. Clark,[13] for example, asked Mexican-American patients at a county tuberculosis sanitarium how they thought they contracted the disease. One patient explained that he got sick after going to a dance at which he danced a lot, got very hot, and then drank a bottle of very cold soda. He felt that he was never well after that, exemplifying an explanation derived from "hot/cold" theories of balance. Another patient believed she got sick because she had given blood at the blood bank for her mother's surgery, illustrating the possible deleterious effects of blood loss in this medical belief system. A third patient thought his tuberculosis was brought on by his diabetes, which was viewed as a dangerous disease that can "cause a lot of other things" (p. 181).[13] Only 1 of 10 patients questioned believed they had acquired tuberculosis from contact with an infected person.

Health care among U.S. ethnic minorities frequently includes nonbiomedical practitioners and nonbiomedical treatments.* (Indeed, the use of nonbiomedical care occurs even among members of the majority culture in North America and Europe.†) For example, in a study of

---

*References 4, 5, 13, 22, 34, 52, 53, 68, 73, 80, 82-86.
†References 5, 19, 32, 36, 58.

Bahamians, Cubans, Haitians, Puerto Ricans, and African-Americans in Miami, Scott[80] found that each group has their own system of medical beliefs, set of health care resources, and patterns of using these resources. The type of healing practitioner chosen for a particular illness or condition depends largely on the presumed cause of the illness.

Cubans rely almost exclusively on Cuban sources of care. For illnesses with presumed "natural" causes, they resort to their own clinics and pharmacies with medicines, plants, and botanicas; for those of "unnatural" or "supernatural" origin, they consult faith healers, espiritistas, and santeros. The other ethnic groups Scott studied in Miami do not have access to such an extensive array of healing resources within their own group. They tend to rely as much as possible on their own knowledge and on whatever healers are available from their group, using biomedicine sparingly. Bahamians seek biomedical care only in crises and, even then, in conjunction with folk medicine. Haitians largely treat illness at home with herbs and other remedies. When deemed necessary, they use hospital emergency rooms and a few selected physicians and clinics. They also consult Vodun cult priests and priestesses or pray to God because He is believed to have the power to heal. Puerto Ricans in Florida use biomedicine the least. They believe they are not treated with respect by Cuban and other biomedical doctors and rely heavily on the use of herbs and folk remedies. African Americans, although using biomedical clinics frequently, also exhibit high rates of self-treatment and typically use home herbal remedies, faith healers, spiritualists, and root doctors, many of whom have legendary reputations in the South.[4,80,83,85]

Diabetic individuals of diverse Hispanic groups have been reported to use traditional healers, home herbal remedies, and praying in conjunction with biomedical care for their diabetes.[22,68,73] Quatromoni and co-workers[68] found that every participant in their focus groups of Puerto-Rican patients with diabetes in Boston used some traditional remedy consisting of either herbs, liquid mixtures, extracts, or foods. These same focus group participants also exhibited preferences for Spanish-speaking health care providers, who were believed to be more willing to combine biomedical and traditional forms of treatment. The patients thus thought that Hispanic physicians would exhibit greater tolerance for traditional treatment methods, implying that other physicians would have a greater tendency to reject traditional beliefs and treatments. It has been noted that, in general, patients tend not to inform physicians about other treatments or remedies.[5,68,83] Even among Anglos, Bauwens[5] found frequent use of home remedies, especially those containing honey, which is not thought to be bad for diabetes. She noted that the "individuals studied are aware that orthodox medicine often minimizes or discredits the value of folk medicines, and therefore, they note that they generally do not tell the physician about the home remedies they've used" (p. 268).

Different types of health care practitioners and treatments may be used in a variety of ways, depending on the culture and situation.[46] To a great extent, although not exclusively, decisions regarding the type of care to seek are guided by medical beliefs. One pattern of utilization reported in several societies involves the use of different types of care for illnesses with different causes. This has been termed *compartmentalization*. A simple case would be one in which biomedical physicians are consulted for illnesses diagnosed within the lay sector to be "natural," and priests are consulted for those diagnosed as "unnatural."

A second pattern is one in which health care options are positioned in a *hierarchy of resort*,[79] with options being sought in a particular order, according to culturally based criteria. Different types of care are thus sought consecutively until, it is hoped, the desired outcome is achieved. This pattern of utilization is consistent with medical systems in which it is believed that illness may have many causes and that a cure exists for every illness if the right practitioner can be found.[6,83,89,92] In addition, responses of an illness to particular treatments in some societies are used to make further diagnostic judgments. For example, in many societies, treatment appropriate for "natural" illnesses are usually sought first.* If an illness originally believed to be "natural" is not cured by biomedicine and other appropriate treatments, this may provide good grounds for suspecting it to be an "unnatural" illness.[84,89,92] This may lead to a tendency to reject notions concerning the chronicity or incurability of particular diseases.

A third pattern of health care utilization involves the *concurrent* or *complementary use* of two or more systems of care. For example, an individual may consult both a physician and an espiritista, or a patient may consult a physician and follow the biomedical regimen while also taking herbal remedies prepared at home. One reason for this might be to counteract presumed ill effects of one of the treatments; if a physician prescribes a "hot" medication, a patient also may take a "cool" herbal tea to counteract the heat. A common variation of this pattern, especially among those with chronic diseases, is to alternate care between two systems. On Mauritius, for example, individuals with chronic illnesses requiring ongoing medication, such as diabetes and hypertension, often alternate between taking physician-prescribed medication and herbalist-prescribed remedies to rest the body from strong medicines and their side effects.[93]

Complementary treatment from two distinct therapeutic systems may also be sought to address multiple causes of an illness, such as an underlying supernatural cause and a resultant physical cause. On Mauritius, individuals may consult sorcerers to remove magical objects from their bodies resulting from sorcery against them and simultaneously may consult biomedical physicians to heal the physical injury caused by the magical objects. A typical case involved a woman diagnosed by a physician as having severe bleeding ulcers that were not responding well to treatment. A sorcerer was consulted, who diagnosed the underlying cause as a magical thorn inserted into her stomach through sorcery. He was employed to remove the thorn and conduct a ritual to prevent further magical insertions, thereby enabling biomedical treatment to be effective. Likewise, among African Americans, physicians may be consulted to treat physical symptoms while faith healers are consulted simultaneously to address the underlying cause.[85]

Treatment expectations, goals, evaluation, and adherence. Last to consider is *whether the prescribed biomedical treatment conflicts with the patient's concept of the illness and its appropriate care.* Lay concepts of a particular disease (as denoted by a specific label, such as "diabetes") may differ significantly from biomedical concepts. Nevertheless, the lay concepts shape patient treatment expectations, goals, and evaluation and largely determine whether particular treatment recommendations "make sense" to patients. Unless the underlying assumptions of patients concerning the disease are elicited by health care

---

*References 64, 89, 92, 93, 96, 105.

professionals, patients and medical personnel may be operating within different conceptual systems. In many ways they may be using the same words but speaking different languages.

Once again, the example of diarrhea in Pakistan serves to exemplify this issue. Many mothers viewed diarrhea as a "hot" illness that requires treatment by "cold" foods, herbs, and remedies. Most Western medicines, however, were classified as "hot," and therefore biomedical recommendations to use ORT were rejected as inappropriate.[62]

Treatment expectations. If it is believed that an illness is the result of divine retribution or witchcraft, expectations from biomedical treatment may be quite low, since it logically follows that medical treatment will have little effect. Some beliefs also contribute to a fatalistic attitude about health in general and a belief that one has little control over one's health, again leading to low expectations from biomedical treatment and preventive care. Such fatalistic beliefs have been found to be related both to adherence to prescribed regimens for diabetes and to diabetes control. For example, Hopper and Schechtman[38] found that among low-income, predominantly African-American women who were clinic patients with diabetes (95% with NIDDM), beliefs in the controllability of one's health and in the likelihood that treatment will help were associated with lower mean annual fasting blood glucose levels. Cohen and colleagues[14] reported a positive correlation between effective diabetes management and concurrence between the "explanatory models" of diabetes of the physician and patient.

A strong sense of fatalism concerning the inevitability of diabetes[84] and of its complications[68] has been reported for African Americans and Hispanic groups. For example, in Boston, members of focus groups of Puerto Ricans with NIDDM tended to believe that diabetes was inevitable if it was in the family, and they saw preventive health measures as generally ineffective in preserving health.[68] Although expressing fear about the complications of blindness and amputations, they exhibited little appreciation for the role of diet, exercise, or the monitoring of glucose levels in the development, treatment, or prognosis of the disease. They were unclear about the role of diet in diabetes management or in its long-term prognosis, believed that exercise was good for diabetes but did not sense that it would help their prognosis, and did not view self-monitoring of blood glucose levels as important for avoiding complications. With such low expectations from medical care, there would be little reason for making the sometimes extensive changes in life-style recommended by physicians for diabetes care.

Treatment goals. Closely linked to expectations, goals may also differ between patients of different ethnic groups and between physician and patient.[75] When the patient and the physician are from different sociocultural backgrounds, distinctions between physician and patient goals may be considerable.[70]

Hopper and Schechtman[38] found that among low-income, predominantly African-American individuals under medical care for diabetes, the phrase "treatment will help" meant to the overwhelming majority that treatment would make them feel better or decrease the frequency or severity of symptoms; only 4% to 5% viewed "helping" as lowering or controlling blood sugar levels. The authors note, "Such data may suggest the saliency of immediate body states in determining an individual's perception of treatment helpfulness" (p. 282) and thus the need for physician-patient communication regarding the goals of treatment.

In general, individuals frequently tend to place more emphasis and importance on how they feel and on their ability to maintain their way of life rather than on a physiologic state measured by a laboratory test.[37,75] In rural Puerto Rico, older adults with diabetes were most concerned about the impact of the disease on their lives and bodies, whereas their physicians were primarily concerned with its impact on their bodies only.[73] In Boston, Puerto-Rican patients stated that feeling well was more important to them than knowing their glucose levels and keeping them low. In fact, it was generally expressed that high but stable glucose levels were better than lower but more varied levels.[68]

Diabetes may be especially problematic in this regard because of the significance attributed to blood in many medical systems.[32,84] This is reflected in the many different ways in which blood is described in medical systems throughout the world: high versus low blood, thick versus thin blood, hot versus cold blood, living versus sleeping blood, impure versus pure blood, dirty versus clean blood, new versus used blood, and good versus bad blood. Moreover, in many regions, including parts of Latin America, blood is not believed to be regenerative, which could certainly lead to a reluctance by patients to part with their blood for testing.

Snow[83] describes an example of how differing concepts of "stroke" held by a physician and an African-American woman were related to conflicting treatment goals and led to the rejection of medical treatment. The woman had had a mild cerebrovascular accident (CVA) and was recuperating at home, sitting up in bed. Stroke, she believed, was caused by "high blood," or too much blood that boiled up and gave her "blood on the brains." Sitting up, she thought, would make the blood go back down more quickly. She had thrown away the medication prescribed by a physician because he had told her that she would have to take it all her life. Since she believed "high blood" to be a temporary condition, her reaction was, "Now that don't make no sense" (p. 92), and she was considering a home remedy to bring the high blood down. New blood is believed to be constantly generated, and when the volume becomes too high ("high blood"), substances such as lemon juice and vinegar may be used to open the pores so the excess blood can be sweated out.[84]

"Low blood," on the other hand, although terminologically similar to low blood pressure, is conceptually related to anemia.[84] Low blood, or not enough blood, is believed to result in symptoms of weakness and fatigue and is equated with the medical diagnosis of anemia. If individuals are informed by a physician that they have both hypertension (high blood) and anemia (low blood), they may change physicians because logically it makes no sense to have both high and low blood at the same time.[83]

According to some concepts, "high sugar" in the blood or body is a temporary state. A frequently reported remedy is the ingestion of bitter or sour substances such as eggplant, grapefruit juice, lemon juice, or other bitter medicinal plants to counteract the sugar.[68,73,83,84] The belief that sugar is *produced* or *overproduced* by the body has been reported among Puerto Ricans in Puerto Rico,[73] along with a belief among aged African Americans that individuals with diabetes should drink a large amount of water to flush the sugar out of the body.[71] The perceived goal of treatment for those holding such notions is to relieve a temporary condition. As such, it makes sense to take some medication or remedy to lower the sugar, but the continual use of medication or insulin and the implementation of lifelong dietary changes do not make sense.

The notion that chronic diseases such as hypertension and diabetes are "cured" but may come back has been reported among some groups. Among rural African Americans with hypertension and diabetes, Roberson[75] found that treatment regimens effective in stopping symptoms, especially when patients were able to discontinue their medication, were believed to have cured the illness. "Such a person was typically described as no longer having high blood pressure or diabetes. Rather than describing themselves as having high blood pressure which was controlled, some informants stated that they 'used to have high blood pressure' but did not have it anymore" (p. 15).

Among African Americans, Snow,[84] for example, found little understanding of chronic disease. Individuals generally believed that every illness should be cured relatively quickly:

Many informants reported that they expect alleviation of symptoms within two or three days after the inception of treatment. This is true both for home remedies and those of professional practitioners. Illnesses considered chronic by physicians, e.g., diabetes or hypertension, are considered curable if the proper means is found. Lack of a cure may: reflect failure to try the right medicine, find the right doctor, a lack of faith, or something more ominous. If an illness has gone on for some time, therefore, and the sufferer has tried everything, then witchcraft may be the final diagnosis (p. 71).

Staiano[89] reports a similar finding among the Garifuna of Belize. Although she notes that the concept of chronic illness is not generally understood and that chronic illnesses are most likely to be classified as "unnatural," illnesses such as diabetes and hypertension that are common in the community and can be labeled by a physician are likely to be classified as "natural." However, symptom relief in such illnesses is often conceptualized as a cure, and the return of symptoms is thought of as catching the illness again.

Treatment evaluation and adherence to prescribed regimens. Evaluation and adherence are closely linked to each other. Treatment evaluation may at first appear to be a straightforward appraisal of "Does it work?" but is also a culturally based process.[23] Treatment is evaluated according to its effectiveness in meeting treatment goals, its perceived necessity and importance vis-à-vis treatment expectations, and its logic vis-à-vis the patient's medical belief system. According to Sbarbaro and Steiner[76]:

Much of compliance research assumes that noncompliance is a remediable disease, much like a urinary tract infection, and can be "cured" if we educate, communicate, and initiate appropriate strategies of behavior modification. In short, we have assumed that compliance is ultimately under our control as physicians.

Such an assumption may not tell the whole story. Researchers in the social sciences who have studied chronic diseases from the patient's perspective have proposed an alternative explanation of the causes of variation in compliance. For patients with chronic illness, . . . seeing doctors is only one of a wide range of tactics. . . . The goal of this process is not to subvert their doctors, but to regulate their own lives and to reconcile their treatment with their understanding of the disease. Failing to recognize the motive for this behavior, we stigmatize it by calling it "noncompliance" (p. 274).

Patients who are active in managing illness but may have treatment goals different from those of the physician often will alter the treatment regimen to fit their needs, life-styles, and goals without informing the physician. Roberson[75] found this to be the case among rural African Americans with chronic illnesses. She notes that although many individuals she studied would be seen by their physicians as noncompliant, they "saw themselves as managing their chronic illnesses and treatment regimens effectively" (p. 24).

Prescribed regimens may be totally rejected as senseless, ineffective, or objectionable or may be altered according to the expectations, goals, and beliefs of patients and their therapy management groups. These sociocultural factors do not include the many other social, psychologic, economic, and other practical factors that may influence evaluation, adherence, and subsequent management practices. Not surprisingly, therefore, adherence, as biomedically defined, is low among not only members of ethnic minorities, but also among individuals of all ethnic groups and backgrounds.*

Puerto Ricans and other Hispanic groups have been reported to be skeptical about biomedical treatment for diabetes. In fact, Quatromoni and others[68] found that most Puerto-Rican focus group members had a negative view of the effect of insulin on the health of individuals with diabetes. They believed that insulin actually increases the severity of the disease and that the more one takes, the more likely one is to develop complications and to experience side effects such as weight gain, dizziness, nausea, and memory loss. The majority thought that medical therapy leads to undesirable side effects, whereas traditional remedies are acceptable and useful. Puerto-Rican elders in Puerto Rico report low levels of adherence to both insulin and dietary regimens.[73] It should not be surprising that biomedical care for diabetes receives such a poor evaluation and such low levels of adherence by members of some ethnic groups given prevalent lay concepts of diabetes and resultant treatment goals and expectations.

The initial medical encounter is particularly important in developing an atmosphere of respect and in gaining the trust and confidence of patients and their families. If this is not attended to, one runs the risk of immediate rejection of explanations and recommendations. For example, Clark[13] points out that Mexican Americans "rarely blame the patient for getting sick" (p. 230). Whereas Anglos accept the role of negligence or elements of life-style in the development of particular diseases, "[a] medical worker who implies that a sick person is at fault and is somehow responsible for his condition may find his statements received with indignation or hostility. To the patient and his family, such a view is unjust or even malicious" (p. 230).

In addition to evaluating explanations of illness and the actual effectiveness of a specific treatment, patients and their families also evaluate treatment and medical encounters according to whether they meet prevailing cultural norms of interaction and expectations regarding the role of healing specialists. For example, Clark[13] states:

[Mexican Americans], who expect a curer to be warm, friendly, and interested in all aspects of the patient's life, find it difficult to trust a doctor who is impersonal and "clinical" in his manner. Nor do they accept his authority to "give orders." He may suggest or counsel, but an authoritarian or dictatorial approach on his part is resented and rejected. His behavior, culturally sanctioned in his own society, is often interpreted by Spanish-speaking patients as discourtesy if not outright boorishness (pp. 230-231).

---

*References 4, 5, 31, 32, 75, 76, 91.

Although some medical belief systems may lead to overall rejection of or low levels of adherence to treatment regimens, others may be compatible with overall adherence but at times require temporary suspension of the regimen. For example, according to some belief systems emphasizing hot/cold distinctions, certain conditions require special care, which may include restrictions on what may be ingested, including both particular types of food and medicines. Common conditions of this type include pregnancy, the postpartum period, menses, and menopause.* For example, Mexican-American women may avoid "cold" foods such as fresh citrus fruit, tomatoes, and green vegetables during menstruation, fearing that they will cool the womb and interrupt menstrual flow.[87] These are also usually avoided during lactation.[13] The treatment of some common illnesses, such as colds, influenza, or diarrhea, may also contraindicate specific categories of food or medicine, such as "hot" medicines. Religious rituals, ceremonies, or holidays may impose certain restrictions or demands on individuals, such as fasting, refraining from eating particular foods, and observing particular time schedules that may conflict with the diabetes management plan.

Most lay medical belief systems reflect an eclectic approach to health and healing. A wide array of causes is recognized, and diverse types of healing specialists are accepted as legitimate. Individuals working within the system are pragmatic and eclectic, base their judgments and evaluation on empiric observations (made through their cultural "lens"), and may simultaneously or sequentially use a diversity of healing specialists and remedies representing different theories and ideologies.[6,13,92,93] This may pose a problem for biomedical practitioners intent on convincing patients that the biomedical system is *the only valid system for the treatment of all illnesses,* but it provides an opportunity for those content with convincing patients that biomedical treatment is *a valid and effective one for the particular illnesses they are currently experiencing.* Medical belief systems, while internally coherent, are not closed and static; rather, they are open and changing. New elements— theories of causation, illness categories, illness labels, and forms of treatment—may be and are incorporated into them, but they are incorporated in forms congruent with the underlying values and principles of the system as a whole.

Social Structure and Organization

People in Sal si Puedes do not act as isolated individuals in medical situations. In illness as well as in other aspects of life, they are members of a group of relatives and compadres. Individuals are responsible to their group for their behavior and dependent on them for support and social sanction. Medical care involves expenditure of time and energy by the patient's relatives and friends. Money for doctors and medicines comes from the common family purse; many of a sick person's duties are performed during the period of illness by other members of his social group. Illness is not merely a biological disorder of the individual organism—it is a social crisis and period of readjustment for an entire group of people (p. 203).[13]

The pattern of reserving for the group the right to control the medical treatment of its members is sometimes in conflict with the expectations of Anglo health personnel. In the society to which most

---

*References 13, 57, 81, 84, 86, 87.

American doctors and nurses belong, the concept of individual responsibility and self-determination is a well-developed pattern; in Sal si Puedes, it is almost nonexistent.

... The authority of the family group also supersedes that of the professional medical workers. Opinions of doctors and nurses certainly influence family decisions, but they are not accepted as absolute fact. The unwillingness of barrio people to look upon members of the medical profession as the final authority in medical matters sometimes leads to conflict and antagonism (p. 205).[13]

It is overwhelmingly within the context of the family and household that illness is recognized and managed throughout the world. The conditions of individuals are assessed and labeled by the social group as "sick," thereby assigning individuals to the "sick role" and granting them culturally defined rights, privileges, and obligations of that role. The lay "therapy management group"[39,42] makes decisions in regard to seeking care and following particular treatment regimens, and specific individuals are delegated the task of caring for sick members of the group. Social structure and organization provide the means for implementing cultural beliefs, norms, and values through the delineation of those individuals responsible for the various aspects of illness management.

Decision makers

Across cultures, great diversity exists in how people organize themselves into groups and what roles and statuses individuals assume within those groups. When treating patients, it is especially important for health care providers to understand the patient's role and status and to identify those individuals responsible for making health care and illness management decisions.

American health care professionals may assume that individual patients, as long as they are physically and mentally able, are in charge of their illness management. With children the assumption is likely to be that the parents are responsible for management decisions. Worldwide, however, this is not necessarily the case, and family groups and responsibilities extend well beyond the household and nuclear family. In some cultures the male head of household is ultimately responsible for such decisions, not only about his children but about his wife (or wives) and his daughters-in-law as well. Within extended kin groups, as in some parts of Africa, the male head of a kin group may be responsible for a number of individuals related to him in a variety of ways. In cases of serious or prolonged illness or extensive treatment or expense, the authority of yet other family members, who may not even reside in the same village or city, may be called into play. Individuals of highest authority may be consulted only for the most serious or problematic illnesses, allowing those at the lower levels of the hierarchy to make most decisions.

The potential complexity of the decision-making process can be seen from the following example from southwest Madagascar. In this culture, nuclear families are grouped into extended kin groups based on biologic relationship through males. An adult male typically lives in a household with his wife (wives) and unmarried children. This same adult male, if his father is deceased and if he is the eldest male child, may head a kin group composed of his wife (wives), his children, his unmarried sisters and their resident children, his mother, his widowed paternal aunts, his younger brothers and their wives and children, and so forth. Furthermore, this male is a member of a larger, patrilineal lineage, whose head is the eldest male in the most senior generation, traced back through males. The head of the lineage is the ritual leader for the lineage and ultimately is responsible for making important decisions about lineage members. Minor daily health care decisions are usually left to individual male heads of household, but those regarding more serious illness or expensive treatment options may be made by the head of the extended kin group or even by the head of the lineage. To make matters more complicated, although males and the heads of their extended kin groups are usually responsible for their wives' well-being, in cases of serious illness the woman's father and possibly the head of her patrilineal lineage must be notified and brought into the decision-making process, since they ultimately are responsible for her even though they may live in distant villages.

This example may appear "exotic" and not applicable to ethnic groups residing in the United States today, but most minority U.S. ethnic groups exhibit social structures and norms that differ from those of the white majority. The importance of family and kin group in medical decisions and care has been noted, for example, among African Americans regarding decisions to seek prenatal care.[90] Clark[13] clearly documents the powerful impact of the social group among Mexican Americans, as described in the excerpt at the beginning of this section. In 2 full days of observation at a county clinic, *not a single Mexican-American patient* [was] *unaccompanied by friends or relatives"* (p. 231). Clark reports that individuals do not have the authority to decide whether or not they are ill; members of the social group must also be convinced. Furthermore, decisions regarding care are made by the social group rather than the individual who is ill; during clinical encounters, patients are not free to make immediate decisions or enter into agreements about their care. "When a Spanish-speaking person is asked to make an on-the-spot medical decision on his own initiative, he is placed in an embarrassing, impossible situation" (p. 205). Although decisions cannot be made until other family members have been consulted, at the time the patient may agree with whatever the physician or nurse has presented so as to be courteous and avoid conflict. Subsequent family decisions may result in the breaking of appointments, cancellation of tests or treatments, and lack of adherence to the plan, "much to the confusion and exasperation of medical workers" (p. 205).[13]

One recurring theme among minority groups is respect for elders. This may be found among various Hispanic and Asian groups, African Americans, and Native Americans, each of whom possess different social structures and organizations and "therapy management groups." Individuals in the therapy management groups may be members of senior generations who have experienced different levels of exposure to and acceptance of American culture and biomedicine than younger family members who may be ill.

Social structure and organization therefore determine to a great extent the identity of those individuals who have the authority to make health care decisions, including decisions regarding the need to seek care, the source of care, the evaluation of treatment, and the adherence to and continuation of care. In general, it is important not to underestimate the complexity of the decision-making process and the sources of advice (if not authority) used by patients and their families in making health care decisions. It is better to overestimate the complexity of the process and discover that it was less complex than expected than to care for a patient assuming that the patient is the sole decision maker, only to discover later that this was not the case.

Furthermore, health care decision makers frequently turn to various individuals for advice in times of illness. The identities of formal and informal sources of health care advice ("therapeutic networks") are also influenced by cultural norms and may consist of parents and other relatives, friends, other health care professionals such as pharmacists and nurses, priests and ministers, other knowledgeable community members, as well as popular literature. The extensive reliance on lay referral networks and informal sources of advice regarding illness has been noted, for example, among African Americans.[4,26,63] These may be used before, instead of, or in combination with formal sources of care. Biomedical practitioners must recognize that even for patients of the majority culture, they may be only one of several sources of advice concerning health and illness management.

Individuals responsible for caregiving

After a decision has been made to seek care and follow a particular treatment regimen, the identity of those who will assume the responsibility for care is largely determined by cultural norms and the roles and statuses of individuals within the group. For instance, whereas fathers in a particular culture may be responsible for making decisions about the health care of their children, the mothers may be responsible for implementing the tasks of caring for sick children. Elderly spouses, daughters, and daughters-in-law may be delegated the responsibility of caring for elderly males.[22] In reaching a decision about a treatment regimen, not only the patient but also those responsible for the patient's care need to be identified and consulted.

In many cases, especially concerning NIDDM among adults, the patients themselves will be responsible for the management of their illness. Although this may appear to be a case in which all that needs to be done is to "educate" patients and determine whether they are willing to follow the prescribed regimens, this view may be deceptively simple and misleading. Once again, it is important to understand the role, status, rights, and obligations of individual patients within their sociocultural context. Individuals in particular categories (e.g., women, daughters-in-law, sons) may be of lower status, possess fewer rights, or be expected to fulfill obligations, which may make some of the rather drastic life-style changes required in diabetes management difficult to realize despite patients' desire and willingness. Those of lower status frequently are responsible for such tasks as cooking and caring for others, which may make it difficult for them to follow their own diets and medication and eating schedules.

Even among groups without strict prescriptive rules regarding status, roles, rights, and obligations, there are cultural norms regarding these. For example, among African Americans, grandmothers frequently assume the responsibility of caring for their grandchildren. Given this sometimes great responsibility, such older women, if diagnosed with NIDDM, may have difficulty both caring for the children and making recommended changes in diet, exercise, and scheduling of meals and medication. Some evidence suggests that individuals who live alone may have better-than-average adherence to dietary regimes,[48] suggesting that family interactions, although positive and important in some respects, may inhibit adherence in large or multigenerational households.[49] Once again, it must be determined whether obligations to other individuals and household needs to meet the food requirements and preferences of young children, adolescents, and older adults will interfere with following the suggested regimen. If so, adjustments must be made in the regimen, which should be discussed with the other individuals concerned.

Cultural and social isolation

The previous sections have shown how social and cultural group membership may affect the management of illness and how important it is to understand the social context in which patients live. Isolation from one's cultural and social group may also influence individuals' capabilities to manage illness, especially a chronic illness such as diabetes. Scheder,[77] for example, discusses the need to take this issue into account when treating Mexican-American migrant workers with diabetes. It is important both in determining appropriate treatment regimens and in evaluating individuals' abilities to adhere to them.

The migrant workers with diabetes in Scheder's study experienced frequent life changes and stressful events related to loss. These probably play a significant role in the ability of individuals to maintain adequate glucose levels. The migrant workers were culturally isolated, making up a very small percentage of the population in some states. In Wisconsin, although 90% of the migrant workers were U.S. citizens, more than 40% did not speak English, and 29% of the adults had less than 5 years of formal education (functionally illiterate according to the government definition). They were linguistically and educationally isolated from the host communities, separated from family networks, and experienced frequent moves to different work sites.[77] In short, health care workers must take into account the social context in which their patients live, which may include cultural isolation, lack of family support networks, little control over diet and schedule, and frequent changes inherent in the life-style, resulting in high levels of stress.

Cultural Values and History

Medical beliefs and social orders reflect a larger system of cultural values. Moreover, the history of a cultural group, as well as of a minority group in relation to the majority, may play a significant role in the development of cultural values and health care norms and beliefs.

Gender-related values

Some cultures show a preference for the offspring of one gender. This may be related to a variety of other factors, such as marriage rules and practices (e.g., presence of "bridewealth" or "brideprice," sons residing in father's village, daughters marrying outside the village), rules regulating group membership (e.g., patrilineality versus matrilineality), economic or other social support benefits derived from sons versus daughters, or rights and status earned by having a son as opposed to a daughter. Among some peoples this may be exhibited as a mild preference; among others it may be quite marked because substantial benefits may hinge on the child's gender. Moreover, in some cultures, rights and status of the mother may depend on both bearing a son and having that son survive into adulthood.

Such preferences may influence treatment-seeking, illness management, and even nurturing decisions. In parts of India, for example, male offspring are more highly valued than female offspring for various reasons. This has been found to be related to sons being given priority of access to food, which is particularly significant under conditions of scarcity;

differential feeding practices of infant boys and girls;[101] and tendencies to seek medical care more frequently and more quickly for males. Williams and colleagues[101] present a striking example of the potential impact of such differential care through a photograph of a mother and her twin infants: one, a healthy, well-developed breast-fed baby boy; the other, a severely stunted, malnourished baby girl. Such practices may clearly lead to poor health and at times the death of young females. In some cultures these practices may not be normative, but cultural values may nevertheless lead to differential care of sons and daughters, especially when resources are scarce. Similarly, these values, linked to differential status of men and women, may play a part in decisions regarding the care given to and resources expended on adult members of various subgroups.[101]

Values related to generation and birth order

The status and roles of members of different generations or of siblings occupying particular positions in the birth order may also have an impact on decisions regarding illness management. Where elders are highly respected and hold positions of high status, many economic and human resources may be expended to maintain their health. Likewise, children holding a specific place in the birth order, often first sons, may be given preferential treatment.

Combinations of medical beliefs and cultural values may affect health care decisions. If it is believed that individual health slowly degenerates in old age and that nothing can be done to prevent this, acceptance of ill health and fatalism regarding death may prevail. Likewise, if productivity and full functioning of older adults in the society are valued, health conditions obviating the ability to play a productive role in society may lead to the acceptance of death as superior to life maintenance efforts.

Affirmation or rejection of ethnic identity

Medical beliefs and practices may be used by individuals to declare something about themselves.* Individuals may affirm and assert pride in their ethnic identity or religious affiliation through the endorsement of traditional medical beliefs, the use of healers from one's own ethnic group (either traditional or biomedical practitioners), the use of traditional home remedies, and the consumption of particular foods. On the other hand, rejection of traditional beliefs and practices and acceptance and use of those of the majority culture or of Western culture may reflect a desire to demonstrate one's level of acculturation, one's education, one's status, or one's acceptance into mainstream society.

Therefore many reasons may exist for using both nonbiomedical care and biomedical care. Choice of care may reflect (1) adherence to a particular system of medical beliefs; (2) acceptance (or rejection) of the experience, judgment, and status of others in one's social group; and (3) a desire to declare one's values and pride in (or rejection of) one's heritage.

Another issue faced by members of minority groups is "double consciousness and double self-identity," described as the desire or attempt to be American while retaining one's ethnic identity and not being viewed as "white."[50] This may result in ambivalence toward treatment regimens and programs and alternation between adherence and nonadherence.

---

*References 4, 7, 10, 17, 82.

Health professionals must take care when addressing cultural medical beliefs and practices because they are integral parts of patients' cultural heritage. They frequently reflect deep-seated moral and social values, world views, and religious beliefs that transcend specific beliefs about human anatomy, physiology, and pathology. Likewise, health care professionals must refrain from stereotyping individuals; this could be quite detrimental, especially with patients who are, for example, attempting to assert their dissimilarity from others in their ethnic group.

Cultural meanings and values associated with food and body weight

Food is more than just a source of nutrition. In all human societies it plays many roles, and is deeply embedded in the social, religious and economic aspects of everyday life. For people in these societies it also carries with it a range of symbolic meanings, both expressing and creating the relationships between man and man, man and his dieties, and man and the natural environment. Food, therefore, is an essential part of the way that any society organizes itself—and of the way that it views the world it inhabits (p. 31).[32]

Their clinical significance is that they [food categories] may severely restrict the types of foodstuffs available to people—and that diet may be based on cultural, rather than nutritional, criteria (p. 32).[32]

When there are perceived contradictions between clinical values assigned to food and social cultural values, clinical advice regarding diet may be ignored (p. 819).[37]

Food may be associated with or may symbolize cultural values, such as cooperation, sharing, and generosity. In times of scarcity, households in many societies are expected to share their food supply with other kin who are in need, emphasizing the cultural value of sharing and cooperation. The value placed on generosity is exemplified in many societies by the prescribed conduct toward visitors, who are given special treatment by being served particularly large portions or foods that are highly valued. In households with limited resources, this may restrict the quality or quantity of food available to household members. The roles and status of individual members are also frequently reflected in their priority of access to food, either in portion size, variety of food, or order in which individuals serve themselves.

Foods, often classified as "sacred" or "profane," may possess religious or ritual significance. For example, individuals may be required to consume particular foods or beverages, including alcoholic beverages, during ceremonies and to eat or fast at particular times of day. Within the "profane" category, certain foods may be highly valued because of relative scarcity or expense. The diet of a household not only may reflect taste preferences and decisions based on nutritional criteria, but also may represent a declaration of status or wealth, serve to affirm ethnic identity and pride, or symbolize acculturation to another culture.

Health and well-being may be conceived of differently in different cultures and in turn may reflect different values, experiences, and histories. Biomedically defined "normal" weight may not be viewed as normal, or even desirable, in other cultures, where being thin may reflect poor health, inadequate diet, and deprivation, while being heavy may reflect good health, abundance of food, and wealth. Historically seen as a sign of health, obesity may be seen by older African Americans as a sign of beauty.[49] Moreover, role changes, such as the assumption of grandmotherhood, occur early among African Americans, and the value of low weight may decrease as individuals age and assume different roles.[50] It has also been reported that among African Americans, weight gain is seen as a normal part of the aging process, and it is viewed as inappropriate to try to lose weight to improve one's appearance. Losing weight specifically to improve one's health, however, is acceptable.[71] Moreover, some may believe that adequate rest is more important for health than exercise and being thin.[50] Therefore one cannot assume that individuals are motivated to be thin or that those who are biomedically defined as overweight consider themselves to have a weight problem or to be unattractive.[50] The fact that 36% of African Americans aged 20 to 79 (44% of African-American women) and that 34% of Mexican Americans, 31% of Puerto-Rican Americans, and 31% of Cuban Americans aged 20 to 74 are overweight[70] will certainly influence the motivation of and social support for individuals to lose weight and remain thin. Mexican Americans have been reported to be skeptical about the desirability of weight loss and tend to view non-Hispanic whites as too occupied with being thin.

Norms, ideals, and preferences regarding weight therefore may differ significantly across cultures and must be respected and taken into account by health care professionals.[50] As pointed out by Hopper,[37] since food and diet are so tied to cultural norms and values, medical advice or counseling may become "politicized," with white middle-class professionals appearing to demean or disvalue traditional diets, traditions, and values.

Cultural history

The history of a group may be particularly relevant to current medical beliefs, patterns of health seeking, and attitudes toward particular types of healing specialists. For example, historic group tensions in California and the Southwest between Anglos and Mexican Americans may lead to feelings of hostility by Mexican Americans toward Anglo health care personnel or to feelings of discomfort, fear of discriminatory treatment, and sensitivity to Anglo criticism.[13]

The ancestors of present-day African Americans, forcefully removed from their homelands, social groups, and cultural resources and until recently denied access to medical care of whites, had to develop their own unique system of medical beliefs and treatment methods based on diverse medical systems from Africa and available knowledge and resources in their new environment.* These developed over time and, although resulting in responses to conditions not of their own making, came to be part of African-American culture.

Likewise, slaves received the least desired foods and found ways to survive on them, preserve them, and make them palatable. Particular food items and dishes then became part of African-American cultural traditions. They may serve as markers of membership in the group and could also be viewed as symbolizing the history and strife of the group. Culturally insensitive attempts by white middle-class health care professionals to alter diet and patterns of use of biomedical care may understandably be viewed by African Americans as debasing their cultural traditions and blaming these traditions, originally developed as adaptive responses to white oppression, for their current health states.

---

*References 4, 44, 83, 84, 88.

African-American culture has been associated with values of affiliation, collectivity, sharing, obedience of authority, respect for the older adults, spirituality, acceptance of fate, and respect for the past. These values, derived from African roots and developed over hundreds of years in the New World, differ from or are in conflict with the majority value system.[66] Treatment regimens and programs such as weight loss programs need to be designed with these in mind. For example, Kumanyika and co-workers[50] contend that weight control programs do not "operate in a culture-free context. . . . Weight control programs may be inherently biased toward the needs and values of the dominant culture and, therefore, may be less attractive to or less successful with those who are not members of the majority" (p. 166). For instance, African Americans place high value on kin networks and are highly oriented toward family. This may be described as "family centeredness" as opposed to the "self-centeredness" more common among the white majority. Kumanyika and others[50] observe that in weight loss programs, "African-American women appeared to have a limited inclination or ability to assume the self-centered posture that is encouraged in behavioral counseling programs, whereas this approach appeared acceptable to the white women" (p. 172). The question is then raised as to "whether what is theoretically sound for white Americans, raised on an ethic of survival through self-reliance, is also theoretically sound for African Americans, who have been raised on an ethic of survival through mutual aid and interdependence. . . . The family or social network may be more appropriate than the individual as a unit of treatment" (pp. 173-174).

Similarly, Native-American groups experienced extensive oppression at the hands of whites settling their homelands. In speaking of the causes and development of diabetes among tribe members, the Dakota, for example, tend to view the disease not only as the result of specific dietary practices and physical conditions (e.g., obesity) of individuals, but also within the social and historic perspective of the tribe, of Native Americans in general, and of their interactions with whites.[52,53] Diabetes is seen as a new illness that has been brought to them by whites; it did not exist in former times, when their cultural traditions and ability to hunt for and produce their own fresh food were intact. Whites forced them to eat unhealthy canned foods, which have now been incorporated into a traditional food system. Dakota patterns of eating large quantities of food are frequently explained and described within the context of periods in their history of grave deprivation and hardship. As described by Lang,[52] "Food preferences and styles of cooking mark family (and individual) orientations, community solidarity vis-à-vis other Dakota communities of the region, Dakota identity vis-à-vis other Native American groups, . . . and Indian identity vis-à-vis white society. Foods likewise provide a means by which Dakota make connections with an idealized past" (pp. 319-320). As with African-Americans, attempts by biomedical practitioners, representatives of white society, both to implicate diet in the development of diabetes and to change the diet, originally imposed on them by whites but now an integral part of current traditions, may not be well accepted by Native Americans. Dietary changes are rarely followed by Dakota individuals with diabetes; in fact, they are viewed as yet "another 'imposition' on Indian people by a non-Indian world" (p. 320).[52]

Diet is so intimately intertwined with religion, politics, social structure, and centuries of history that medical advice that appears to place blame on the victims for their illness because of poor diet and obesity is unlikely to succeed. However, if presented differently, dietary recommendations may be made more acceptable among Native Americans and other minority groups. Brenton[9] suggests encouraging inclusion of former traditional Native-American (Hopi) food items and placement of high value on the traditional diet.

CULTURALLY SENSITIVE DIABETES CARE AND EDUCATION

Diabetes educators and health care providers need to take into account specific ethnic beliefs, customs, food patterns, and health care practices, with the goal of incorporating these cultural factors into a practical and beneficial treatment regimen (p. 313).[70]

A treatment regimen suggesting changes which are not only difficult but also culturally unacceptable or incomprehensible will likely be rejected by the patient. Compliance, therefore, largely depends on developing management programs which incorporate, rather than pre-empt, the patient's culture (p. 279).[99]

Patient education cannot be successful when an individual's pride is threatened (p. 820).[37]

Approach

The following eight components of diabetes care and education are important in (1) creating a culturally sensitive atmosphere of interaction and care, (2) obtaining adequate information concerning sociocultural factors affecting illness management, and (3) developing mutually agreeable and implementable treatment goals and regimens.

I. *Maintain respect for cultural differences in medical beliefs, social organization, religious beliefs, world views, and values.* Although these may differ from your own and from those of biomedical science, you must remember that they, as with yours, are part of a cultural heritage of which individuals may (and should) be proud. Direct negation of the validity of beliefs usually leads only to the rejection of one's own beliefs and alienation of patients.[4] Folk illnesses, such as the "evil eye" or fright, are very real to individuals; they have seen them. Some examples of how medical practitioners may avoid questioning the validity of patient beliefs were supplied by Clark[13] many years ago and are still applicable today:

> With those who are convinced of the validity of their beliefs it might be possible to work within the context of folk medicine. For example, if a mother suggests that her child is suffering from "fallen fontanelle," a doctor or nurse might point out that Anglos call this disorder by another name—dehydration. Differences in ideas of etiology might simply be ignored. Conflict might also be avoided by saying, "Yes, I know about that disease, but it seems to me that this is something else" (p. 226).

Keep in mind that you are a cultural outsider and, depending on the ethnic group of the patient, that you may also be viewed as a representative of a group historically associated with oppression and intolerance.

II. *Obtain information on sociocultural factors related to diabetes management.* Inquire about beliefs, management practices, and concerns in a nonjudgmental way. Listen carefully. Be attentive to all factors mentioned by patients and their families, since although some may not at first seem particularly important within the biomedical model, they are important to your patients. Pay attention to references to beliefs, the causes and nature of diabetes and its complications, the use of home remedies and other healing specialists, the observance of food restrictions, social influences and barriers, values, specific treatment goals, expectations, and concerns. Helman[32] provides some short "clinical questionnaires" that may be useful to practitioners in structuring questions concerning sociocultural factors relevant to illness management.

III. *Strive to reach a negotiated understanding of the illness and mutual agreement regarding management.* If you begin with the assumptions that patients are active in illness management, that views of patients and health care practitioners may represent different ways of understanding disease in general and diabetes in particular, and that cultural distinctions may amplify such differences, it follows that a primary goal of the therapeutic encounter should be to reach a negotiated understanding of the disease and its management. This may require some change and compromise by both patients and health care practitioners. To reach this goal, seek to gain in a nonjudgmental manner an understanding of patients' views, communicate to patients the views of biomedicine, engage in a dialogue with rather than a lecture to patients, participate in joint problem solving regarding perceived barriers to treatment, and engage in cooperative planning of a treatment regimen with specified goals and expected results.[28a]

IV. *Work within cultural systems as much as possible.* Individuals seek advice and information from many sources in their attempts to make sense of illness. The biomedical practitioner is but one of many sources consulted concerning diabetes. If what the practitioner says does not make sense to patients or questions their values and beliefs, they most likely will reject the advice. Therefore treatment recommendations and "health education programs may be more effective if their health messages are consistent with the values and norms of the target population" (p. 183).[3]

Attempt to make as few changes as possible in current ways of life. Reinforce cultural traditions that support biomedical beliefs and treatment. Some traditional food items and dishes may be particularly appropriate for diabetes,[1,13,69,99] and traditional herbal remedies may actually possess hypoglycemic properties[102] that could be beneficial if the physician is informed about their use and takes them into account in the treatment regimen. Do not suggest the rejection of those practices or beliefs that, while not conforming to the biomedical model, do not conflict or interfere with biomedically based treatment regimens.[13,25] Positive and neutral elements may be incorporated "into the treatment as a complementary component that enhances the confidence of the patient" (p. 315)[70] and may serve to establish you as someone who is respectful and tolerant of cultural differences. Do not underestimate the strength of religious convictions or feel the need to "secularize everything" (p. 227).[13] Patients who believe in faith healing, for example, may believe that physicians may be able to heal because God works through them. Although this may not concur with physicians' views of themselves, there may be no need to dispute this view among patients.

If you find that specific components of the cultural system oppose biomedical views and present barriers to following appropriate treatment regimens, present the biomedical view as an *alternate* view of the *disease* or *symptoms* rather than as the *right* view of the *world*. Give supporting evidence that a particular type of treatment or change in life-style has been observed to produce specific results. For example, you might begin by saying, "Doctors have found that if individuals with diabetes do *x,* then *y* usually occurs," or "Doctors find that too much fat and sugar lead to health problems and that it is best for people with diabetes to eat *z.*" In this way, individuals are presented with an observation and may then make their own informed decisions about their own lives.[9] If an individual expresses the belief that a specific illness episode or set of symptoms is of "unnatural" origin (e.g., evil eye), you may offer an alternative explanation without calling into question the entire belief system.[25] You might begin by saying, "These symptoms may be caused by many things. From my exam and your description of the symptoms, I'm convinced that it's *x* and that we should treat it by *y.*"

Most medical systems are open, dynamic, and able to incorporate new theories of illness causation, new illness labels, and new forms of treatment, as long as they do not directly require rejection of beliefs and values underlying the system. New elements tend to be integrated into medical systems in forms congruent with the existing system; they rarely completely replace existing elements.*

V. *Be sensitive to culturally based interaction styles, rules, and preferences.* Different individuals and members of different ethnic groups may respond best to different types of interaction. Some may respond well to direct, rather formal questioning on specific topics (if not too intrusive and not judgmental), whereas others may respond best to more informal, indirect questioning, such as open-ended requests to describe particular aspects of current diabetes management. Keep in mind that you are likely to be responded to as an authority figure, which is not particularly conducive to open, frank discussion.

Furthermore, roles of healing specialists differ from culture to culture. In some cultures an authoritative mode of interaction may be expected; in many, healers are expected to assume the role of interested counselor or advisor to patients and their kin. Be sensitive to norms of modesty and discomfort of individuals in discussing particular topics they may view as inappropriate to speak about with health care workers or in the presence of particular family members. Although all patients may experience some discomfort or embarrassment discussing, for example, genitourinary problems or sexual dysfunction and their diabetes, members of some ethnic groups may experience heightened levels based on cultural norms and values.

VI. *Involve relevant family members in discussions on diabetes management.* This is done to ensure that they play a role in, understand, and support management decisions. Family members important to include might be those involved in medical decisions; those in charge of care, cooking, and food shopping; those dependent on the patient for care and cooking; or those identified by the patient as posing a barrier to or as providing strong support for diabetes management. Keep in mind the statuses of individuals in the social group so as not to undermine those in authority and not to place unrealistic demands on lower-ranking members.[28a]

VII. *Use appropriate language and culturally relevant educational materials.* Attempt to present explanations of illness and treatment and other educational materials in the primary language of patients. Ensure that materials and explanations are appropriate for the formal educational levels of patients.[99]

---

*References 8, 11, 27, 40, 41, 45, 51, 100, 103.

In education programs, materials and presentations should address issues that are relevant to the particular group and meaningful to them in terms of their experiences and values.[3] Some materials may be designed to address, for example, culturally specific issues of diabetes care, such as traditional food items and dishes, alternate ingredients or cooking methods, quantity of food consumed, mealtimes, and discrepancies or confusion in the specific terms used in different languages or cultural groups related to food attributes, symptoms, and diseases. The inclusion of individuals belonging to the target group in photographs, drawings, and videos is helpful.

VIII. *Use an interdisciplinary team approach to diabetes care and education.* Diabetes management can be influenced by such a wide array of factors that it is unlikely that a single individual trained in a single field could have the time, inclination, or expertise to address them all. An interdisciplinary team of, for example, physicians, nurses, social workers, nutritionists, and educators could address physiologic, social, economic, educational, and cultural issues affecting diabetes management.

Furthermore, attempts should be made to staff health care facilities with some individuals from relevant ethnic minorities in regions with culturally diverse patient populations. Interactions among multicultural staff will contribute to increased understanding of and sensitivity to different cultural systems. Patients belonging to minority groups may also experience higher levels of comfort and familiarity with the health care setting if members of their own ethnic groups are employed as staff.

Some Pointers and Pitfalls

General issues

- Take care not to offend individuals by questioning the validity of firmly rooted cultural belief and value systems. Offer alternative labels, explanations, or treatment for the specific symptoms or illness in question while avoiding direct negation of culturally based beliefs and values.
- Be sensitive about topics that patients may view as inappropriate for medical encounters.
- Be aware of the culturally accepted roles of health practitioners and valued attributes (e.g., authority versus advisor, impersonal versus warm and interested).
- Avoid statements that appear to blame patients (or their kin) for their conditions.
- Beware of differences between both long-term and short-term treatment goals and expectations of health care provider and patient. How might these be related to different concepts of the disease (e.g., temporary state versus chronic disease)?
- Gain an understanding of the status and role (rights and obligations) of the patient in relation to other household/kin group members and associated implications for diabetes management.
- Identify individuals other than the patient involved in illness management decisions and implementation and include them in management planning sessions.
- Beware of nonequivalent uses of the same terms in different languages and between different cultural groups (e.g., "high and low blood").
- Identify concurrent alternate sources of care and home remedies.

Food-related issues: diet, mealtimes, and weight

- Become familiar with food items, dishes, and cooking methods used and preferred as well as customs regarding service of and order of access to food.
- Gain an understanding of the cultural, religious, and social significance of food and mealtimes and how these may affect diabetes management and responses to biomedical recommendations to avoid particular items or preparation modes.
- Become familiar with food classification systems; of particular relevance are categories based on hot/cold distinctions. Identify symptoms (e.g., diarrhea, flu, coughs), conditions (e.g., pregnancy, lactation, menses), and events (e.g., religious rituals) associated with food and medicine prohibitions.
- Identify individuals responsible for food-related activities, such as meal planning, shopping, and cooking, along with their statuses and roles vis-à-vis the patient.
- Identify positive aspects of traditional diets and home remedies.
- Attempt to change current diet and life-style as little as possible. Encourage the use of traditional food items, cooking methods, and home remedies that are congruent with diabetes management regimens. Whenever possible, instead of substituting new items into the diet, encourage greater use of beneficial foods already in the diet.
- Become familiar with cultural norms and preferences regarding ideal body weight and attitudes about weight gain, weight loss, dieting, and exercise by members of different age-groups and gender groups.
- Beware of cultural differences in the use and understanding of food/nutritional terms (e.g., "rich," "starch," "fat").

Insulin and medications

- Identify attitudes about medication along with other patient concerns (e.g., insulin makes diabetes worse; side effects; prefer traditional herbal hypoglycemic agents).
- If any prescribed medications are derived from plants, it may be helpful to point this out, given the confidence that members of many groups have in herbal preparations.[13]
- Clarify patient understanding of the role of sugar, insulin, and other medications in diabetes management, along with expected results of treatment.
- Reach a joint agreement on a medication schedule that is implementable by the patient and household.

Regular checkups and monitoring

- Identify and address any beliefs or attitudes reflecting fatalism about health and the prevention of illness or complications related to diabetes. How are these related to treatment expectations, specific goals, and adherence to prescribed regimens?
- Identify patient concerns regarding daily blood glucose monitoring based on cultural conceptions of blood and its attributes.
- Explicitly address relationships among specific aspects of the regimen, symptom control, metabolic control, and ongoing care and the prevention of complications.

SUMMARY

Four major themes are emphasized throughout this chapter.

1. What are frequently called "folk beliefs" are not isolated beliefs and practices or "holdovers" from different times and places. Rather, medical belief systems are coherent, logical systems of beliefs, practices, norms, and values that are intimately tied to social structure and organization and cultural norms, values, world views, and history.

2. Individuals who are ill, along with individuals in their social group, are active: they use their own knowledge and experience and seek that of others in attempts to make sense of illness and to find relief and cure. Although they may not consistently or completely follow treatment regimens advised by biomedical practitioners and thus may be labeled as "nonadherent," they are most likely doing something (other things) and may consider themselves to be effectively managing their illness. For an illness such as diabetes, which requires extensive self-management or home management, the tendency to be active in illness management should be encouraged, and practices may be thoughtfully and sensitively guided to conform with biomedical guidelines.

3. Lay medical belief systems are open and dynamic, constantly changing, adapting to new conditions, incorporating new elements, and even modifying past elements. Moreover, most permit and many encourage individuals to be pragmatic and eclectic in their quests for cure. Beliefs in multiple causes of illness and acceptance of the legitimacy of a variety of distinct therapeutic systems actually provide a framework conducive to the acceptance of biomedical management of diabetes.

Therefore the task of biomedical health workers is to work within the lay belief system to convince patients and kin that biomedical treatment is an appropriate and effective way to control and manage diabetes. Recognition of the illness by biomedical practitioners, their ability to label it, and their knowledge of a treatment for it provide some evidence to patients that the illness is within the scope of expertise of biomedicine.

4. The concepts of chronic illness, illness management or control without cure, and being "sick" while feeling "well" may be difficult to incorporate into lay belief systems without resultant misunderstanding. If health care workers understand these difficulties, however, they can strive to reach negotiated understandings of the disease and its management that are congruent with biomedicine, make sense to patients and their kin, do not threaten and devalue the basic lay belief and value systems, and are implementable within patients' social systems.

In conclusion, no attempt has been made in this chapter to present a list of "to do's" and "not to do's" for each of the many ethnic groups represented in the United States. Not only are there too many groups to attempt this, but more importantly, so much variation exists between individuals within groups and so many factors (individual, social, economic, and political as well as cultural) may shape illness management that oversimplified characterization of cultural groups, or stereotyping, is misleading and counterproductive as well as potentially offensive. Rather, this chapter has strived to convey an appreciation for the many "lenses" through which illness may be viewed and an understanding of the multiple sociocultural issues and processes that may shape and underlie health decisions and illness management practices. Armed with this understanding, health care providers will possess a conceptual framework they can use systematically to explore, identify, and discuss specific factors influencing diabetes management in the daily lives of their individual patients.

RECOMMENDED READING

The two volumes listed here may be of particular interest to health care practitioners. Both are written by physician-anthropologists, are addressed to health care personnel, and present medical anthropologic theory within the context of clinical experience. Helman also includes a useful set of "clinical questionnaires" addressing selected relevant sociocultural issues.

- Helman CG: *Culture, health and illness: an introduction for health professionals,* ed 3, Oxford, 1995, Butterworth Heinemann.
- Kleinman A: *Patients and healers in the context of culture: an exploration of the borderland between anthropology, medicine, and psychiatry,* Berkeley, University of California Press.

REFERENCES

1. American Diabetes Association: Clinical practice recommendations: nutritional recommendations and principles for individuals with diabetes mellitus, *Diabetes Care* 15(suppl 2):21-28, 1992.
2. American Diabetes Association: *Direct and indirect cost of diabetes in the United States in 1992,* Alexandria, Va, 1993, American Diabetes Association.
3. Auslander WF and others: Community organization to reduce the risk of non-insulin-dependent diabetes among low-income African-American women, *Ethnicity Dis* 2(2):176-184, 1992.
4. Bailey E: *Urban African American health care,* Lanham, Md, 1991, University Press of America.
5. Bauwens E: Medical beliefs and practices among lower-income Anglos. In Spicer EH, editor: *Ethnic medicine in the Southwest,* Tucson, 1977, University of Arizona Press.
6. Beals AR: Strategies of resort to curers in South India. In Leslie C, editor: *Asian medical systems: a comparative study,* Berkeley, 1976, University of California Press.
7. Beckerleg S: Medical pluralism and Islam in Swahili communities in Kenya, *Med Anthropol Q* (NS) 8(3):299-313, 1994.
8. Bledsoe CH, Goubaud MF: The reinterpretation and distribution of Western pharmaceuticals: an example from the Mende of Sierra Leone. In van der Geest S, Whyte R, editors: *The context of medicines in developing countries,* Dordrecht, Netherlands, 1988, Kluwer Academic.
9. Brenton BP: Don't worry, be Hopi: biocultural perspectives on diet and health. Paper presented at the Annual Meeting of the American Anthropological Association, San Francisco, 1992.
10. Carrier AH: The place of Western medicine in Ponam theories of health and illness. In Frankel S,

Lewis G, editors: *A continuing trial of treatment: medical pluralism in Papua New Guinea,* Dordrecht, Netherlands, 1989, Kluwer Academic.
11. Carstairs GM: Medicine and faith in rural Rajasthan. In Paul BD, editor: *Health, culture, and community: case studies of public reactions to health programs,* New York, 1955, Russell Sage Foundation.
12. Chrisman NJ: The health seeking process: an approach to the natural history of illness, *Culture Med Psychiatry* 1:351-377, 1977.
13. Clark M: *Health in the Mexican-American culture: a community study,* ed 2, Berkeley, 1970, University of California Press.
14. Cohen MZ and others: Explanatory models of diabetes: patient practitioner variation, *Soc Sci Med* 38(1):59-66, 1994.
15. Council on Scientific Affairs: Hispanic health in the United States, *JAMA* 265:248-252, 1991.
16. Counts DR, Counts DA: Complementarity in medical treatment in a West New Britain Society. In Frankel S, Lewis G, editors: *A continuing trial of treatment: medical pluralism in Papua New Guinea,* Dordrecht, Netherlands, 1989, Kluwer Academic.
17. Crandon-Malamud L: *From the fat of our souls: social change, political process, and medical pluralism in Bolivia,* Berkeley, 1991, University of California Press.
18. *Diabetes: 1991 vital statistics,* Alexandria, Va, 1991, American Diabetes Association.
19. Eisenberg DM and others: Unconventional medicine in the United States: prevalence, costs, and patterns of use, *N Engl J Med* 328(4):246-252, 1993.
20. Eisenberg L: Disease and illness: distinctions between professional and popular ideas of sickness, *Culture Med Psychiatry* 1:9-23, 1977.

21. Eraker SA, Kirscht JP, Becker MH: Understanding and improving patient compliance, *Ann Intern Med* 100:258-268, 1984.

22. Espino DV, Moreno CA, Talamantes M: Hispanic elders in Texas: implications for health care, *J Texas Med* 89(10):58-61, 1993.

23. Etkin NL: Cultural constructions of efficacy. In van der Geest S, Whyte R, editors: *The context of medicines in developing countries,* Dordrecht, Netherlands, 1988, Kluwer Academic.

24. Flegal KM and others: Prevalence of diabetes in Mexican Americans, Cubans, and Puerto Ricans from the Hispanic Health and Nutrition Examination Survey, 1982-1984, *Diabetes Care* 14(7)(suppl 3):628-638, 1991.

25. Foster GM: Relationships between theoretical and applied anthropology: a public health program analysis, *Hum Org* 11:5-16, 1952.

26. Gibbs T: Health-seeking behavior of elderly Blacks. In Jackson JS, editor: *The Black American elderly,* New York, 1988, Springer.

27. Gould HA: Modern medicine and folk cognition in rural India, *Hum Org* 24:201-208, 1965.

28. Greenwood B: Cold or spirits? Choice and ambiguity in Morocco's pluralistic medical system, *Soc Sci Med* 15B:219-235, 1981.

28a. Haire-Joshu D: Cultural sensitivity in diabetes education. In Dittko VP, Godley K, Meyer J: *A core curriculum for diabetes educators, ed 2,* Chicago, 1993, American Association Diabetes Educators and AADE Research Foundation.

29. Harris MI: Epidemiological correlates of NIDDM in Hispanics, whites, and blacks in the US population, *Diabetes Care* 14(7)(suppl 3):639-648, 1991.

30. Harwood A: Hot-cold theory of disease: implications for treatment of Puerto Rican patients, *JAMA* 216:1153-1158, 1971.

31. Haynes RB, Taylor DW, Sackett DL, editors: *Compliance in health care,* Baltimore, 1979, Johns Hopkins University Press.

32. Helman CG: *Culture, health and illness: an introduction for health professionals,* ed 2, Oxford, England, 1990, Butterworth Heinemann.

33. Herman WH, Tentsch SM: Kidney diseases associated with diabetes. In Harris MI, Hamman RF, editors: *Diabetes in America,* NIH Pub No 85-1468, Washington, DC, 1985, US Government Printing Office.

34. Heyer KW: *Rootwork: psychosocial aspects of malign magical and illness beliefs in a South Carolina Sea Island community,* Doctoral dissertation, Farmington, 1981, University of Connecticut.

35. Hill CE: Black healing practices in the rural South, *J Popular Culture* 6:849-853, 1973.

36. Hill CE: A folk medical belief system in the rural South: some practical considerations, *South Med* 16:11-17, 1976.

37. Hopper SV: Meeting the needs of the economically deprived diabetic, *Nurs Clin North Am* 18:813-825, 1983.

38. Hopper SV, Schechtman KB: Factors associated with diabetic control and utilization patterns in a low-income, older adult population, *Patient Educ Counsel* 7:275-288, 1985.

39. Janzen JM: *The quest for therapy in Lower Zaire,* Berkeley, 1978, University of California Press.

40. Janzen JM: The comparative study of medical systems as changing social systems, *Soc Sci Med* 12(2):121-129, 1978.

41. Janzen JM: The need for a taxonomy of health in the study of African therapeutics, *Soc Sci Med* 15B:185-194, 1981.

42. Janzen JM: Therapy management: concept, reality, process, *Med Anthropol Q* (NS) 1(1):68-84, 1987.

43. Janzen J, Prins G, editors: Causality and classification in African medicine and health, *Soc Sci Med* 15B(3), 1981 (special issue).

44. Jordon JW: The roots and practice of voodoo medicine in America, *Urban Health* 8:38-41, 1979.

45. Katz SS, Katz SH, Kimani VN: The making of an urban *Mganga:* new trends in traditional medicine in urban Kenya, *Med Anthropol* 6(2):91-112, 1982.

46. Kleinman A: *Patients and healers in the context of culture,* Berkeley, 1980, University of California Press.

47. Kleinman A, Eisenberg L, Good B: Culture, illness, and care: clinical lessons from anthropologic and cross-cultural research, *Ann Intern Med* 88:251-258, 1978.

48. Kouris A, Wahlquist ML, Worsley A: Characteristics that enhance adherence to high-carbohydrate/high-fiber diets by persons with diabetes, *J Am Diet Assoc* 88(11):1422-1425, 1988.

49. Kumanyika SK, Ewart CK: Theoretical and baseline considerations for diet and weight control of diabetes among blacks, *Diabetes Care* 13(11)(suppl 4):1154-1162, 1990.

50. Kumanyika SK, Morssink C, Agurs T: Models for dietary and weight change in African-American women: identifying cultural components, *Ethnicity Dis* 2(2):166-175, 1992.

51. Kunstadter P: Do cultural differences make any difference? Choice points in medical systems available in Northwestern Thailand. In Kleinman A and others, editors: *Medicine in Chinese cultures: comparative studies of health care in Chinese and other societies,* DHEW Pub No (NIH) 75-653, Washington, DC, 1975, John E Fogarty International Center for Advanced Study in the Health

Sciences, US Department of Health, Education, and Welfare.

52. Lang GC: "Making sense" about diabetes: Dakota narratives of illness, *Med Anthropol* 11:305-327, 1989.

53. Lang GC: Talking about a new illness with the Dakota: reflections on diabetes, food and culture. In Winthrop RH, editor: *Culture and the anthropological tradition: essays in honor of Robert F. Spencer,* Lanham, Md, 1990, University Press of America.

54. Leininger M: Futuristic approaches to nursing care of the elderly with a transcultural focus. In Leininger M, editor: *Transcultural nursing care of the elderly: concepts, theories and models in use,* Salt Lake City, Utah, 1978, Wiley Medical.

55. Leventhal H, Nerenz DR, Straus A: Self-regulation and the mechanisms for symptom appraisal. In Mechanic D, editor: *Symptoms, illness behavior and help-seeking,* New York, 1982, Prodist.

56. Luecke R, editor: *A new dawn in Guatemala: toward a worldwide health vision,* Prospect Heights, Ill, 1993, Waveland.

57. MacCormack CP, editor: *Ethnography of fertility and birth,* London, 1982, Academic.

58. McGuire MB: *Ritual healing in suburban America,* New Brunswick, NJ, 1988, Rutgers University Press.

59. Mechanic D: The concept of illness behavior, *J Chron Dis* 15:189-194, 1962.

60. Mechanic D: *Medical sociology: a selective view,* New York, 1968, Free Press.

61. Mexican-American Policy Research Project: *The health of Mexican-Americans in South Texas,* Austin, 1979, Lyndon Baines Johnson School of Public Affairs.

62. Mull JD, Mull DS: Mothers' concept of childhood diarrhoea in rural Pakistan: what ORT program planners should know, *Soc Sci Med* 27:53-67, 1988.

63. Neighbors HW, Jackson JS: The use of formal and informal help: four patterns of illness behavior in the Black community, *Am J Community Psychol* 12:629-644, 1984.

64. Ngubane H: *Body and mind in Zulu medicine: an ethnography of health and disease in Nyuswa-Zulu thought and practice,* London, 1977, Academic.

65. Pearce TO: Lay medical knowledge in an African context. In Lindenbaum S, Lock M, editors: *Knowledge, power, and practice: the anthropology of medicine and everyday life,* Berkeley, 1993, University of California Press.

66. Pinderhughes E: Afro-American families and the victim system. In McGoldrich M, Pearce J, editors: *Ethnicity and family therapy,* New York, 1982, Guilford.

67. Press I: Urban illness: physicians, curers and dual use in Bogota, *J Health Soc Behav* 10(3):209-218, 1969.

68. Quatromoni PA and others: Use of focus groups to explore nutrition practices and health beliefs of urban Caribbean Latinos with diabetes, *Diabetes Care* 17(8):869-873, 1994.

69. Raheja BS: Diabetes-associated complications and traditional Indian diet, *Diabetes Care* 10(3):382-383, 1987.

70. Raymond NR, D'Eramo-Melkus G: Non-insulin-dependent diabetes and obesity in the black and Hispanic population: culturally sensitive management, *Diabetes Educ* 19(4):313-317, 1993.

71. Reid BV: "It's like you're down on a bed of affliction": aging and diabetes among Black Americans, *Soc Sci Med* 34(12):1317-1323, 1992.

72. Rimer BK and others: Task Group V: the role of theory in health behavior research in minority populations. In Becker DM and others, editors: *Health behavior research in minority populations: access, design, and implementation,* NIH Pub No 92-2965, Washington, DC, 1992, US Department of Health and Human Services.

73. Rios Iturrino H: *Hispanic diabetic elders: self-care behaviors and explanatory models,* Doctoral dissertation, Iowa City, 1992, University of Iowa.

74. Rivers WHR: *Medicine, magic, and religion,* New York, 1924, Harcourt Brace.

75. Roberson MHB: The meaning of compliance: patient perspectives, *Qualitat Health Res* 2:7-26, 1992.

76. Sbarbaro JA, Steiner JF: Noncompliance with medications: vintage wine in new (pill) bottles, *Ann Allergy* 66:273-275, 1991 (guest editorial).

77. Scheder JC: A sickly-sweet harvest: farmworker diabetes and social equality, *Med Anthropol Q* (NS) 2(3):251-277, 1988.

78. Scheper-Hughes N, Lock M: 'Speaking truth' to illness: metaphors, reification, and a pedagogy for patients, *Med Anthropol Q* 17:137-140, 1986.

79. Schwartz LR: The hierarchy of resort in curative practices: the Admiralty Islands, Melanesia, *J Health Soc Behav* 10:201-209, 1969.

80. Scott CS: Health and healing practices among five ethnic groups in Miami, Florida, *Public Health Rep* 89:524-532, 1974.

81. Scott CS: The relationship between beliefs about the menstrual cycle and choice of fertility regulating methods within five ethnic groups, *Int J Gynecol Obstet* 13:105-109, 1975.

82. Shutler ME: Disease and curing in a Yaqui community. In Spicer EH, editor: *Ethnic medicine in the Southwest,* Tucson, 1977, University of Arizona Press.

83. Snow LF: Folk medical beliefs and their implications for care of patients, *Ann Intern Med* 81:82-96, 1974.

84. Snow LF: Popular medicine in a Black neighborhood. In Spicer EH, editor: *Ethnic medicine in the Southwest,* Tucson, 1977, University of Arizona Press.

85. Snow LF: Sorcerers, saints and charlatans: black folk healers in urban America, *Culture Med Psychiatry* 2:60-106, 1978.

86. Snow LF: *Walkin' over medicine,* Boulder, Colo, 1993, Westview.

87. Snow LF, Johnson SM: Folklore, food, female reproductive cycle, *Ecol Food Nutr* 7:41-49, 1978.

88. Spector R: *Cultural diversity in health and illness,* New York, 1979, Appleton-Century-Crofts.

89. Staiano KV: Alternative therapeutic systems in Belize: a semiotic framework, *Soc Sci Med* 15B(3): 317-332, 1981.

90. St. Clair PA and others: Social network structure and prenatal care utilization, *Med Care* 27:823-832, 1989.

91. Stimson GV: Obeying doctor's orders: a view from the other side, *Soc Sci Med* 8:97-104, 1974.

92. Sussman LK: Unity in diversity in a polyethnic society: the maintenance of medical pluralismon Mauritius, *Soc Sci Med* 15B:247-260, 1981.

93. Sussman LK: The use of herbal and biomedical pharmaceuticals on Mauritius. In van der Geest S, Whyte R, editors: *The context of medicines in developing countries,* Dordrecht, Netherlands, 1988, Kluwer Academic.

94. Sussman LK: Discussion: critical assessment of models. In Becker DM and others, editors: *Health behavior research in minority populations: access, design, and implementation,* NIH Pub No 92-2965, Washington, DC, 1992, US Department of Health and Human Services.

95. Sussman LK: Routine herbal treatment for pregnant women, neonates, and postpartum care among the Mahafaly of Southwest Madagascar, Working Paper #251, *Women and international development,* East Lansing, 1995, Michigan State University.

96. Sussman LK: Medical beliefs and practices among the Mahafaly of Southwest Madagascar. In *Proceedings of the Sixth International Congress on Traditional and Folk Medicine,* Austin, Texas, 1995, American Botanical Council (in press).

97. Sussman LK, Robins LN, Earls F: Treatment-seeking for depression by black and white Americans, *Soc Sci Med* 24(3):187-196, 1987.

98. Topley M: Chinese traditional etiology and methods of cure in Hong Kong. In Leslie C, editor: *Asian medical systems: a comparative study,* Berkeley, 1976, University of California Press.

99. Urdaneta ML, Krehbiel R: Cultural heterogeneity of Mexican-Americans and its implications for the treatment of diabetes mellitus type II, *Med Anthropol* 11(3):269-282, 1989.

100. Welsch RL: Traditional medicine and Western medical options among the Ningerum of Papua New Guinea. In Romanucci-Ross L, Moerman DE, Tancredi LR, editors: *The anthropology of medicine: from culture to method,* South Hadley, Mass, 1983, Bergin.

101. Williams CD, Baumslag N, Jelliffe DB: *Mother and child health: delivering the services,* ed 3, New York, 1994, Oxford University Press.

102. Winkelman M: Ethnobotanical treatments of diabetes in Baja California Norte, *Med Anthropol* 11:255-268, 1989.

103. Wolff RJ: Modern medicine and traditional culture: confrontation on the Malay Peninsula. In Lynch LR, editor: *The cross-cultural approach to health behavior,* Rutherford, NJ, 1969, Fairleigh Dickinson University Press.

104. Woods CM: Alternative curing strategies in a changing medical situation, *Med Anthropol* 1(3): 25-54, 1977.

105. Yoder S: Knowledge of illness and medicine among Cokwe of Zaire, *Soc Sci Med* 15B:237-246, 1981.

106. Young A: The anthropologies of illness and sickness, *Ann Rev Anthropol* 11:257-285, 1982.

107. Young JC: *Medical choice in a Mexican village,* New Brunswick, NJ, 1981, Rutgers University Press.

108. Zola IK: Studying the decision to see a doctor, *Adv Psychosom Med* 8:216-236, 1972.

14 Environmental Influences on Diabetes Management: Family, Health Care System, and Community Contexts

Wendy Auslander and Daniele Corn

INTRODUCTION

The environment of individuals with diabetes has a great influence on management and disease control. Part 3 of this text describes the impact of diabetes as it interacts with the unique developmental and psychosocial milestones of each stage of the life cycle. However, it is important to view these developmental influences within a *social-environmental context.*

Diabetes management and regimen-related behaviors are influenced not only by intraindividual factors but also by the system that surrounds the individual. The *ecologic* or *biopsychosocial model* has emerged as a paradigm that has replaced the traditional biomedical model and maintains that disease and behavior are functions of the interaction among biologic, psychosocial, developmental, sociocultural, and ecologic factors.[22] The model is broadly based on the general systems approach, which proposes that bidirectional influences exist between a person and the environment and that multiple factors interact to influence health and disease. This broad framework can be used to conceptualize the influence and interaction of family, health care system, and community environments on individuals with diabetes (Fig. 14-1). Theories that are consistent with the ecologic or biopsychosocial perspective are critical to further understanding the complex nature of how health behaviors are influenced by social and environmental factors. Thus far, most of

---

CHAPTER OBJECTIVES

- Provide an overview of several theoretic frameworks that have been used to examine the environmental influences on diabetes management, specifically the family, health care system, and community contexts.
- Provide examples of empiric studies that have addressed the role of family, health care system, and community factors in diabetes management and prevention.
- Provide intervention strategies relating to each of the environmental contexts that may be adapted by health professionals.

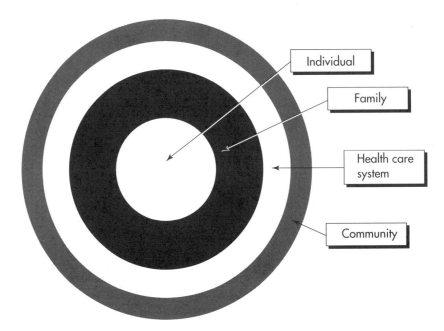

Fig. 14-1   Theoretic framework of influences on diabetes management.

the research has focused on the family environment, with relatively little attention on the health care system and community contexts.

THE FAMILY CONTEXT

The family is the most frequently mentioned social context in the psychosocial literature on diabetes. Although many studies have examined the associations between family and disease factors, it is generally accepted that bidirectional influences exist among family, disease, and regimen-related factors.[1] Because the family is so important in child development, most of the literature on the family's influence on diabetes management focuses on children and adolescents with diabetes. Relatively few studies examine family influences on adults with diabetes.

Family Interactions

One of the earliest theoretic perspectives to link family interactional patterns with the health status of diabetic children was Minuchin's structural family systems perspective in his work with psychosomatic families. Specifically, Minuchin and colleagues[51] formulated the view that four family characteristics—enmeshment, overprotectiveness, extreme rigidity, and lack of conflict resolution—are necessary for the development of "psychosomatic diabetes" in children. Although it is important to note that less than 5% of diabetic children are considered "psychosomatic" (i.e., containing all four characteristics accompanied by metabolic instability),[50] the work of Minuchin and colleagues triggered a wealth of research that examined the associations between family system variables and metabolic control.

Several consistent findings across studies have emerged relating to family interactions and metabolic control in children and adolescents with insulin-dependent diabetes mellitus (IDDM). Anderson and associates[2] found that high levels of cohesion or expression of support among family members and low levels of conflict were significantly associated with better metabolic control. Evidence of the association between family cohesion and children's metabolic control was provided by other studies as well.[5,32,41] Family conflict has also been shown to relate to the children's metabolic control, with higher levels of conflict associated with poorer control of diabetes.[5,41,61] Other studies have focused on family behaviors or factors that support adherence to the treatment regimen. For example, nonsupportive family behaviors were associated with poorer adherence to glucose testing, diet, and insulin injections among diabetic adults.[59] Among children with diabetes, patterns of sharing diabetes-related responsibilities between mothers and children were related to metabolic control. Disagreements between mothers and children about who is assuming responsibility for regimen tasks were significantly associated with poorer metabolic control.[3] These findings provide evidence for the strong linkage among family interaction patterns, adherence behaviors, and metabolic control.

Family Protective Factors

A second framework for understanding family influences to diabetes management draws from the child development literature, specifically from work of the last two decades on *protective factors* or *resiliency* among children who are exposed to adverse or stressful conditions.[25,26,46] This framework emphasizes the strengths or protective factors of families rather than focusing on individual vulnerability or risk factors of persons from disadvantaged environments. According to Garmezy,[26] evidence indicates that broad groups of variables may be considered protective in that they have the potential to reduce the risks associated with stressful life conditions or impoverished environments. These variables include (1) *personality features* of the individual with diabetes, such as self-esteem, cognitive skills, and skills to cope with new situations; (2) *family cohesion,* the presence of a caring adult, and the absence of marital discord; and (3) the presence of *external support systems,* such as a strong maternal substitute, a teacher, or an institutional structure (e.g., church, caring agency).[25,26]

Few studies have explicitly utilized the resiliency framework to investigate the role that family protective factors play in the development of resiliency among children who are forced to manage a chronic illness such as diabetes. One such study suggests that resiliency in diabetic adolescents is likely to be influenced by family protective factors on two levels: (1) the *macro level,* which includes family composition, family roles, and family environment, and (2) the *micro level,* which includes family interaction and communication patterns.[34] Studies that examine the macro level, specifically those that focus on family environmental characteristics, indicated that family orientations toward independence, participation in social-recreational activities, and organization were strongly associated with the diabetic adolescent's perception of competence and adjustment to diabetes.[33]

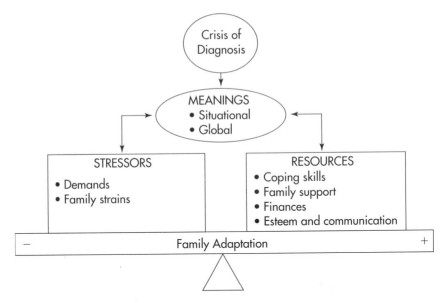

Fig. 14-2 The family adjustment and adaptation response (FAAR) model. (Modified from Chilman CS, Nunnally EW, Cox FM, editors: *Chronic illness and disability,* Newbury Park, Calif, 1988, Sage.)

The resiliency framework of Garmezy[26] and Rutter[57] has application to minority families. For example, much has been written recently about the cultural "protective" factors of African-American families in discussions of their strengths. Extended intergenerational family networks, religion and spirituality, and flexible roles of family members[47] are considered protective factors that can buffer the effects of chronic stressors such as the stress of managing diabetes. More attention should be given to enhancing the resiliency of families by focusing on family strengths. This is in contrast to deficit models of human and family development that emphasize reducing the psychosocial risks associated with diabetes.

Family Stress and Resources

A third theoretic perspective that has guided research on family factors and diabetes is the *family adaptation and adjustment response,*(FAAR) or *double ABCX model* formulated by McCubbin and Patterson.[49] Briefly, this is a resource-demand model that examines the interaction of family stressors (demands) and resources (coping skills, extended family support, finances, esteem, communication) to determine the degree to which a family adapts to the crisis of diagnosis (Fig. 14-2). According to this model, families with greater resources and fewer stressors are likely to adapt and cope more effectively with the crisis of diagnosis and subsequent treatment.

Recent research has used this perspective to study families coping with the diagnosis of diabetes. Assessments were performed 1 year after diagnosis. Family stressors were found to be the strongest predictor of the children's metabolic control when controlling for C peptide levels and family resources.[8] These data indicate that family variables such as stress are more strongly associated with metabolic control than the child's level of endogenous insulin after the first year following diagnosis. This is an important finding, given other research (e.g., Kovacs and colleagues[45]) that challenges the notion that family variables significantly impact the health status of diabetic children. Results from other investigations that include measures of family stress, coping, and levels of metabolic control have been contradictory. Several studies of diabetic children have found stressful family life events to be significantly associated with poor metabolic control.[10,14,31] In contrast, others have found no significant relationship between frequency or severity of stress and metabolic control.[13,18] Inconsistent findings across studies are probably a result of differences in the patient populations, in instruments used to measure stress and coping, and whether a family or individual perspective is examined. In addition, as McCubbin's model indicates, the impact of chronic stress on individuals and families with diabetes varies according to the resources available to buffer the impact and the definition or perception that the individual or family attributes to the stressor.[48] Several resources have been identified as potential buffers to the stress of managing a chronic illness in the family: family esteem and communication, sense of mastery, financial well-being, and extended family social support. Certainly, these resources represent potential areas of intervention with diabetic individuals and their families.

Intervention Strategies with Families

Most family interventions reported in the literature are descriptive in nature and do not systematically evaluate the impact of the intervention on medical and behavioral outcomes. However, a few family-based interventions have been minimally evaluated and merit adaptation by health professionals, given the wealth of evidence that the family context strongly impacts psychosocial and medical outcomes in diabetes.

In an innovative approach to strengthening the supportive aspects of the family, Satin and colleagues[58] delivered and evaluated the impact of a 6-week, multifamily group intervention with diabetic adolescents and their parents. The investigators chose to treat the families in a group format, with approximately three families per group. There are several advantages of a multifamily group approach versus family therapy with single families: (1) it is a ready-made source of social support for youth and parents, (2) it includes role modeling of solutions or strategies to cope with diabetes management problems, (3) it is cost-effective for health professionals to offer, and (4) less stigma is associated with it when compared to traditional family therapy.[15] Results of the evaluation of the intervention indicated that multifamily groups have a positive impact on metabolic control when groups are limited to three or four families per group. However, because the sample was small (32 families), replication of this intervention is necessary before firm conclusions can be made regarding its effectiveness with diabetic adolescents and parents.

Another family-based intervention[4] was piloted with six adolescents with poorly controlled diabetes and their parents. Specifically, the goals of the intervention were to improve diabetes-related communication between parents and children and to increase supportive interactions related to diabetes treatment. The brief family intervention was based on a problem-solving approach that has been used extensively in short-term family therapy in health care settings. (See Ell and Northen[21] for a discussion of this approach). This approach was adapted to address problems related to family communication and sharing of diabetes-related responsibilities among family members. The outcomes of the intervention were twofold: (1) to help family members identify their roles and responsibilities in disease management and (2) to identify positive ways in which family members can communicate with one another about diabetes.[4] It was suggested that these two intermediate outcomes would lead to improved adherence and metabolic control in the long term. Results of this pilot study indicated that families receiving the intervention showed improvement by increasing their level of cooperation and reducing parenting strains and family conflict. Conversely, the families in the control condition showed evidence of deterioration in that family stress increased and cooperation among family members decreased.[4]

Phases of Chronic Illness and Family Impact

Although the importance of the developmental stage of the individual with diabetes is acknowledged as an important variable in the education and medical management of the disease, less attention has been given to the different phases of an illness (i.e., crisis phase, chronic phase, and terminal phase[52]) and how each phase affects the educational and psychosocial needs of diabetic patients and their families. This is related in part to the difficulty that researchers experience in conducting longitudinal studies, in addition to the fact that health professionals rarely follow a chronically ill patient throughout the illness life cycle. More attention is warranted in diagnosing the educational and psychosocial needs of the patient with diabetes and the family at each illness phase.

Several family-based studies of children with IDDM have acknowledged that the phase after diagnosis may be unique in terms of the needs of diabetic families, and thus these studies have focused on recently or newly diagnosed children and adolescents with diabetes and their families. One study examined the predictors of the acquisition of diabetes knowledge within the year following diagnosis in children and adolescents with diabetes and their parents.[6] Problem-solving knowledge relating to disease management was poorer than general knowledge in both parents and children. Both demographic (age, family, socioeconomic status [SES]) and family variables (family communication skills, financial resources) were predictive of general information and problem-solving knowledge, suggesting that family factors should be considered as well as demographics in the education of newly diagnosed children and families.

Another investigation of newly or recently diagnosed children and families found that coping with the diagnosis and early impact of diabetes lasts up to 9 months for most children and that psychiatrically diagnosable reactions were more likely among children of lower-SES families and from families with marital distress.[44] Other studies of recently diagnosed children and families examined predictors of compliance[39] and family environmental characteristics of diabetic versus acutely ill adolescents.[33]

Research that has taken into account the illness phase has primarily focused on newly or recently diagnosed individuals and their families. The interest in newly diagnosed families is based on the assumption that if health care professionals intervene immediately after diagnosis, new patterns of cooperation and interaction can be learned that would facilitate the successful integration of the treatment regimen into daily routines. In doing so, the prevention of psychosocial and management problems could be attained. One such study trained newly diagnosed children with diabetes and their families in self-monitoring of blood glucose (SMBG) and its application in the home.[19] Results showed that compared with supportive counseling, SMBG training was more effective in preventing the deterioration of metabolic control at the end of the "honeymoon" period. The study emphasized the importance of teaching patients to *use* systematically the results of SMBG to alter their behavior (e.g., increase insulin dosages, delay mealtimes, eat more or less), depending on their blood glucose values.

Because most health professionals rarely work with only newly diagnosed patients and their families, more information is needed regarding the family reactions, needs, and types of coping with diabetes at other phases of the illness. Diabetes is a disease characterized by predictable crises or predictable complications in its course. Health professionals, with their expertise and knowledge of the disease course, can prepare families to anticipate, prepare, and cope with diabetes-related complications at each phase of the disease. Family members and persons with diabetes would benefit from *anticipatory coping*.[29] Specifically, anticipatory coping would include gaining knowledge about what may happen in the near future regarding the disease, preparing themselves attitudinally and emotionally, gaining the necessary problem-solving and disease management skills, gaining confidence that the family can successfully cope with the disease and treatment changes, and eliciting social support from others outside of the family.

THE HEALTH CARE SYSTEM CONTEXT

The health care system is another critical context that influences individuals and families in their management of diabetes. The quality of the patient-provider relationship and patient-practitioner communication have emerged as critical determinants to health outcomes such as patient adherence,[24] patient satisfaction with treatment,[43] and the amount of information delivered and retained during the medical encounter.[16,56] Diabetes is a chronic disease managed primarily by the patient, with frequent consultations with health care professionals for ongoing education, support, and modification of treatment. During times of medical crises and hospitalizations, the individual with diabetes and the family experience intensive interactions with health care professionals. Because of this unique relationship, there has been considerable interest in the impact of the patient-practitioner relationship on disease management and related medical outcomes.

Patient satisfaction with health care has been identified as an important determinant of compliance.[43] In particular, satisfaction with verbal and nonverbal communication between patient and practitioner has been examined. In general, practitioners who use a more affiliative communicative style, characterized by warmth, empathy, genuineness, and a nonjudgmental attitude, rather than a controlling, authoritative style, receive more favorable evaluations by patients. One study found that satisfaction of mothers in a pediatric setting was associated with a physician who addressed the mothers' concerns by answering questions and who expressed warmth and empathy.[42,43] In addition to the personal qualities of the health professional, patient perceptions of the professional's competence and accessibility and convenience of medical care (time and effort needed to make an appointment and receive treatment) have been identified as important determinants of patient satisfaction.[60]

The practitioner's ability to deliver medical information to patients is one aspect of professional competence that has received much attention. One study found that noncompliance to medication among patients with diabetes was largely attributed to miscommunication from the practitioner to the patient and not to intentional behaviors of the patient.[38] More recent studies have examined patient-practitioner communication as a two-way interaction, not simply from provider to patient, but as a dyadic interaction during which patients are active participants. Increasing patient participation in medical care and in encounters with physicians has been the focus of several investigations. This emphasis has partly been in response to the recognition that diabetes and other chronic illnesses are self-management diseases and rely on the patient's active participation in treatment. As a result, several interventions have been described in the literature.

Intervention Strategies in the Health Care System

Several intervention strategies are described in the literature that can be adapted for use by health professionals. One of the earlier intervention studies to increase patient satisfaction and patient compliance was implemented by Roter[55] with chronically ill patients who were predominantly low-income, African-American, and female. The intervention involved "patient activation," or increasing patient participation in the negotiation of care with providers. It was hypothesized that patient activation through increased question asking during the medical visit would increase patient compliance with appointment keeping and satisfaction with the medical encounter. Patient activation involved meeting for 10 minutes with a health educator in the waiting room of the clinic before the medical visit to help the patient identify questions he or she might have regarding treatment. Results indicated that the intervention was effective in increasing questions asked by the patients and increasing the number of appointments kept, but patient satisfaction decreased. It was suggested that the decrease in patient satisfaction may have resulted from patients not receiving adequate responses to their questions. Thus it was concluded that because communication is a two-way process, providers need to be prepared for an "activated" patient.[55]

In an intervention that builds on Roter's study, the effects of increasing patient participation in medical care decisions among adults with diabetes mellitus were examined.[27] The rationale for the study was that patients who actively negotiate treatment plans with their physicians are more likely to have that treatment plan fit into their life-styles and thus are more likely to be compliant. The intervention consisted of a 20-minute session before the visit to the provider, during which an assistant reviewed the medical record with the patient and helped the patient identify medical decisions likely to arise during the visit, particularly issues likely to be affected by life-style changes. Then the patient was encouraged to use the information gained to negotiate medical decisions with the provider. The study's findings indicated that when compared to a standard educational session of equal time, the patient participation group had improved metabolic control and patient functioning in everyday life. However, the precise mechanism by which metabolic control improved was not clear, since the intervention did not make changes in the treatment regimens of the patient groups who participated more in medical decision making. It was suggested that feelings of being in more control over one's life may have contributed to improvements in metabolic control. In a replication of this study, similar findings resulted with respect to increases in functional status among individuals with diabetes who participated in a patient activation intervention.[54]

In summary, interventions with individuals with diabetes that increase their participation in medical decision making and that increase their sense of control over their lives appear to be promising in improving health status outcomes and compliance with appointment keeping. Improvements in the overall relationship between patients and the health care system are necessary for subsequent improvements in patient satisfaction, adherence to treatment, and communication between patient and provider. The self-help and consumer health movements, coupled with home SMBG technology, have contributed to patients taking more responsibility for diabetes management than patients have done previously. However, recognizing that communication is a two-way interaction, changes in the health care system are necessary to maximize the benefits associated with positive patient-provider relationships.

THE COMMUNITY CONTEXT

Health education and promotion has primarily focused on facilitating behavior change through interventions that target the individual rather than the environment. Within the biopsychosocial framework, however, health behaviors are a function of the reciprocal effects of individual, family, health care system, and community factors. The community is the environmental context of individuals who may share similar values, culture, social groups, economics, and institutions. Community components or subsystems that can enhance the health status of individuals are churches, volunteer associations, schools, neighborhood groups, and extended family networks.[36] Community features that can have adverse effects on health include poverty, crime, unemployment, gang violence, and drug and alcohol abuse. These characteristics are often conceptualized as risk factors or strengths that influence an individual's health status. One often thinks of the impact of risk factors such as poverty and unemployment independently. In reality, however, risk factors related to the community context cluster together and, when combined, may influence health status exponentially rather than additively. For example, a study of the health needs of Hispanic children suggested that the combined effects of economic disadvantage and the discrimination and powerlessness associated with minority status increased their risk of health problems.[28] Thus evidence indicates that the impact of multiple risks on physical health is much greater than the summation of each individual risk factor.

Recently the community context of individuals with diabetes has received much attention, partly because of the disparity in health status between ethnic and Caucasian groups in the United States and the subsequent attempts to identify features of the community context that contribute to poor health. The following disparities related to diabetes between certain ethnic groups and Caucasians have been noted. According to the National Diabetes Data Group (NDDG), the rate of non-insulin-dependent diabetes mellitus (NIDDM) in African Americans is 50% to 60% higher than that in Caucasians. The rate of diabetes among African-American women is alarming: 1 in 4 black women over age 55 has diabetes.[53] Among Native Americans the diabetes-related mortality rates are 2.3 times higher than those in the general population. The prevalence rate of NIDDM for the Pima Indians is the highest in the world: 10 to 15 times the rate for the general U.S. population. African Americans and Native Americans incur higher rates of three complications of diabetes: end-stage renal disease, blindness, and amputation.[35] The disparity in the health status between ethnic and Caucasian groups has been noted also in pediatric populations with IDDM. In one study of recently diagnosed children and adolescents,[5] youths from African-American families had significantly poorer metabolic control than children from Caucasian families, when controlling for family factors and SES levels. Moreover, this pattern persisted 2 and 3 years after diagnosis. Likewise, a study comparing African-American and Caucasian children with IDDM revealed that African-American children were in poorer metabolic control, were hospitalized more frequently for diabetic ketoacidosis, and missed more clinic visits than did their Caucasian counterparts.[20] A third study found that adolescent African-American females had poorer metabolic control than their white, male, adolescent counterparts.[30]

What are some of the community factors that contribute to the poorer health status within some minority communities? Lower SES levels among minority individuals explain part of the effects of race on the diabetic individual's metabolic control, since fewer financial and educational resources are associated with lower quality of medical services and less emphasis on preventive care.[28] However, in many of the studies such as those just mentioned, the difference in health status between African Americans and Caucasians was not explained entirely by SES levels. Other social and environmental factors that cluster together with poverty or low SES may partly explain the poorer health status of some ethnic groups. Evidence suggests that characteristics of the environments of those who live in poverty may have a negative impact on health status.[40] For example, environmental factors such as overcrowding, noise, pollution, neighborhood crime, and inadequate housing are associated with lower-SES communities and may negatively influence health. Characteristics associated with lower-income families, such as inadequate money for food, medical care, or medicine, directly affect health. Also, minimum-wage or low-wage jobs characterized by activities that are repetitive, difficult, and fast paced can create non-health-promoting work environments.[40]

Other factors that contribute to poor health among certain ethnic groups *may* be unique to their minority status. For example, evidence indicates that minority populations experience more stress than nonminorities through interactions with a racist climate that denies personal values, identity, and economic opportunities.[47] Chronic stress can influence health in two ways: (1) *directly,* through physiologic and biochemical pathways (e.g., increases in blood pressure and lipid levels, changes in immune function), and (2) *indirectly,* through behavioral mechanisms (e.g., decreases in compliance with regimens and in protective behaviors such as eating healthy, getting adequate sleep, and exercising).[11] Moreover, cultural barriers to effective communication and treatment planning between minority patients and health care providers may also contribute to the disparity in health status between minority and nonminority populations. For example, in a study of low-income, predominantly African-American older adults with NIDDM, diet was reported as the most problematic aspect of the regimen.[37] The authors suggest that this may partly be related to the lack of sensitivity to sociocultural factors in the assessment and prescription of the dietary component of the treatment regimen.

Intervention Strategies in Communities

Many of the intervention strategies implemented at the community level are designed to build on community strengths to enhance both community competence and individual health-promoting behaviors. One strategy, *community organization,* has been used to promote health through citizen participation in the defining, planning, and implementing of a smoking cessation program in low-income, African-American neighborhoods.[23] This program used key community organization strategies, as described by Bracht and Kingsbury,[12] such as integrating the intervention activities into already existing informal and formal neighborhood networks. Implicit in this approach is the strategy of *empowerment*—to provide the neighbors with ownership and control over the program and simultaneously to provide opportunities for gaining skills, knowledge, and control over their lives and circumstances. Community organization as a strategy to prevent diabetes and its complications is an approach that may prove to be an effective strategy in minority and low-income communities where more traditional methods have failed.

A second community-based study combined community organizational strategies with *peer models* ("nutrition neighbors") to promote knowledge and skills related to reduced-fat dietary habits among African-American women at risk for diabetes caused by obesity.[7] The results of the pilot program indicated that compared with a dietitian-led intervention, peer educators were more effective in increasing dietary skills such as label reading and knowledge about fat in the diet among participants.[9] Other community-based health promotion programs have targeted churches and clergy to promote positive health behaviors; others have enlisted schools, work settings, and social service organizations; and still others have used peer leaders in local bars and taverns to promote "safer sex" messages within the gay community.

The overall objective for many community-based programs is to focus on changing community norms, which in turn will lead to mobilization of neighborhood resources and informal networks to support long-term health-promoting behaviors. It has become increasingly clear that without the support, ownership, and active participation of educational organizations, coalitions, and informal social and religious groups within communities, health-promoting programs will not result in long-term positive changes.

SUMMARY

The biopsychosocial approach to diabetes management involves the interaction of persons with their environment. Health professionals are traditionally trained in the biomedical model that emphasizes individual influences on diabetes management: physiologic, physical, and developmental factors. Of equal importance, however, are the environmental contexts in which individuals with diabetes live, primarily because of the environment's influence on human behavior, particularly health preventive and management behaviors. Three social contexts—the family, the health care system, and the community—have considerable impact on individuals with diabetes throughout their lives. Consideration of the social context is critical in the design and implementation of interventions with these individuals. The interventions presented in this chapter represent potential strategies that can be adapted by health professionals, particularly social workers and health psychologists, to prevent or manage diabetes better by addressing the family, health care system, and community contexts of the individual. Adherence to treatment and improved metabolic control are important outcomes of interventions. These outcomes have been highlighted by the recent findings from the Diabetes Control and Complications Trial (DCCT),[17] which indicated that glycemic control can reduce the risk of long-term complications. To reach the goals outlined by the DCCT, health care professionals are faced with the challenge of understanding the complex interactions among social-environmental factors, health behaviors, and health outcomes. In doing so, health care providers can then develop strategies that target the family, the health care system, and the community contexts and not solely individuals with diabetes, isolated from their environments.

REFERENCES

1. Anderson BJ, Auslander WF: Research on diabetes management and the family: a critique, *Diabetes Care* 3:696-702, 1980.
2. Anderson BJ and others: Family characteristics of diabetic adolescents: relationship to metabolic control, *Diabetes Care* 4:586-594, 1981.
3. Anderson BJ and others: Assessing family sharing of diabetes responsibilities, *Pediatr Psychol* 15:477-492, 1990.
4. Auslander WF: A brief family intervention to improve family sharing of diabetes responsibilities and communication, *Spectrum* 6:330-333, 1993.
5. Auslander WF and others: Risk factors to health in diabetic children: a prospective study from diagnosis, *Health Soc Work* 15:133-142, 1990.
6. Auslander WF and others: Predictors of diabetes knowledge in newly diagnosed children and parents, *J Pediatr Psychol* 16:213-228, 1991.
7. Auslander WF and others: Community organization to reduce the risk of non-insulin-dependent diabetes among low-income African-American women, *Ethnicity Dis* 2:176-184, 1992.
8. Auslander WF and others: Family stress and resources: potential areas of intervention in recently diagnosed children with diabetes, *Health Soc Work* 18:101-113, 1993.
9. Auslander WF and others: Increasing diet-related skills and knowledge among low-income African American women at risk for NIDDM. Paper presented at the Society For Behavioral Medicine, Boston, 1994.
10. Barglow P and others: Diabetic control in children and adolescents: psychosocial factors and therapeutic efficacy, *J Youth Adolesc* 12:77-94, 1983.
11. Baum A: Behavioral, biological, and environmental interaction in disease processes. In *New Research Frontiers in Behavioral Medicine, Proceedings of the National Conference,* National Institutes of Health, Washington, DC, 1994, US Government Printing Office, 61-69.
12. Bracht N, Kingsbury L: Community organization principles in health promotion. In Bracht N, editor: *Health promotion at the community level,* Newbury Park, Calif, 1990, Sage.
13. Brand AH, Johnson JH, Johnson SB: Life stress and diabetic control in children and adolescents with insulin-dependent diabetes, *J Pediatr Psychol* 11:481-495, 1986.

14. Chase HP, Jackson GG: Stress and sugar control in children with insulin dependent diabetes mellitus, *J Pediatr* 98:1011-1013, 1981.

15. Citrin W, La Greca AM, Skyler JS: Group intervention in type I diabetes mellitus. In Ahmed PI, Ahmed N, editors: *Coping with juvenile diabetes,* Springfield, Ill, 1985, Charles C. Thomas.

16. Cline RJ: Interpersonal communication skills for enhancing physician-patient relationships, *Md State Med J* 32:272-278, 1983.

17. The DCCT Research Group: The effect of the intensive treatment of diabetes on the development and progression of long-term complications in insulin-dependent diabetes mellitus, *N Engl J Med* 329:977-986, 1993.

18. Delamater AM and others: Stress and coping in relation to metabolic control of adolescents with type I diabetes, *Dev Behav Pediatr* 8:136-140, 1987.

19. Delamater AM and others: Randomized prospective study of self-management training with newly diagnosed diabetic children, *Diabetes Care* 13:492-498, 1990.

20. Delamater AM and others: Racial differences in metabolic control of children and adolescents with type I diabetes mellitus, *Diabetes Care* 14:20-25, 1991.

21. Ell K, Northen H: *Families and health care: psychosocial practice,* New York, 1990, Aldine de Gruyter.

22. Engel GH: The need for a new medical model: a challenge for biomedicine, *Science* 196:129-136, 1977.

23. Fisher EB and others: Community organization and health promotion in minority neighborhoods, *Ethnicity Dis* 2:252-271, 1992.

24. Friedman HS, DiMatteo MR: Patient-physician interactions. In Shumaker SA, Schron EB, Ockene JK, editors: *The handbook of health behavior change,* New York, 1990, Springer.

25. Garmezy N: Stress resistant children: the search for protective factors. In Stevenson J, editor: *Recent research in developmental psychopathology,* Oxford, 1985, Pergamon.

26. Garmezy N: Resiliency and vulnerability to adverse developmental outcomes associated with poverty, *Am Behav Scientist* 34:416-430, 1991.

27. Greenfield S and others: Patients' participation in medical care: effects on blood sugar control and quality of life in diabetes, *J Gen Intern Med* 3:448-457, 1988.

28. Guendelman S: At risk: health needs of Hispanic children, *Health Soc Work* 10:183-190, 1985.

29. Hamburg BA, Inoff GE: Coping with predictable crises of diabetes, *Diabetes Care* 6:409-416, 1979.

30. Hanson CL, Henggeler SW, Burghen GA: Race and sex differences in metabolic control of adolescents with IDDM: a function of psychosocial variables, *Diabetes Care* 10:313-318, 1987.

31. Hanson CL, Henggeler SW, Burghen GA: Social competence and parental support as mediators of the link between stress and metabolic control in adolescents with insulin dependent diabetes mellitus, *J Consult Clin Psychol* 55:529-533, 1987.

32. Hanson CL and others: Family system variables and the health status of adolescents with insulin-dependent diabetes mellitus, *Health Psychol* 8:239-254, 1989.

33. Hauser ST and others: The contribution of family environment to perceived competence and illness adjustment in diabetic and acutely ill adolescents, *Fam Relations* 34:99-108, 1985.

34. Hauser ST and others: Vulnerability and resilience in adolescence: views from the family, *J Early Adolesc* 5:81-100, 1985.

35. Heckler MM: *Report of the Secretary's Task Force on Black and Minority Health, 1985, executive summary,* Washington, DC, 1985, US Government Printing Office.

36. Hill RB: Research on the African-American family: a holistic perspective, Westport, Conn, 1993, Auburn House.

37. Hopper SV, Schechtman KB: Factors associated with diabetic control and utilization patterns in a low-income, older adult population, *Patient Educ Counsel* 7:275-288, 1985.

38. Hulka BS and others: Doctor-patient communication and outcomes among diabetic patients, *J Community Health* 1:15-27, 1975.

39. Jacobson AM and others: Psychologic predictors of compliance in children with recent onset of diabetes mellitus, *J Pediatr* 110:805-811, 1987.

40. Kaplan G: Reflections on present and future research on bio-behavioral risk factors. In *New Research Frontiers in Behavioral Medicine, Proceedings of the National Conference,* National Institutes of Health, Washington DC, 1994, US Government Printing Office.

41. Klemp SB: Adolescents with IDDM: the role of family cohesion and conflict, *Diabetes* 36(suppl 1):18A, 1987.

42. Korsch BM, Negrete VF: Doctor-patient communication, *Sci Am* 227:66-74, August 1972.

43. Korsch BM, Gozzi EK, Francis V: Gaps in doctor-patient communication, *Pediatrics* 42:855-871, 1968.

44. Kovacs M and others: Initial coping responses and psychosocial characteristics of children with insulin-dependent diabetes mellitus, *J Pediatr* 106:827-834, 1985.

45. Kovacs M and others: Family functioning and metabolic control of school-aged children with insulin-dependent diabetes mellitus, *Diabetes Care* 12:409-414, 1989.

46. Masten A, Garmezy N: Risk, vulnerability, and protective factors in developmental psychopathology. In Lahey BB, Kazdin AE, editors: *Advances in clinical child psychology,* vol 8, New York, 1985, Plenum.

47. McAdoo HP: Societal stress: the black family. In McCubbin HI, Figley CR, editors: *Coping with normative transitions,* New York, 1983, Brunner/Mazel.

48. McCubbin HI, Patterson JM: Family adaptation to crisis. In McCubbin HI, Cauble E, Patterson JM, editors: *Family stress, coping, and social support,* Springfield, Ill, 1982, Thomas.

49. McCubbin HI, Patterson JM: The family stress process: the double ABCX model of adjustment and adaption, *Marr Fam Rev* 6:7-37, 1982.

50. Minuchin S, Rosman BL, Baker L: *Psychosomatic families,* Cambridge, Mass, 1978, Harvard University Press.

51. Minuchin S and others: A conceptual model of psychosomatic illness in children, *Arch Gen Psychiatry* 32:1031-1038, 1975.

52. Rolland JS: Toward a psychosocial typology of chronic and life threatening illness, *Fam Sys Med* 2:245-263, 1984.

53. Roseman JM: Diabetes in Black Americans. In *Diabetes in America,* NIH Pub No 85-1468, Washington, DC, 1985, US Government Printing Office.

54. Rost KM and others: Change in metabolic control and functional status after hospitalization: impact of patient activation intervention in diabetic patients, *Diabetes Care* 14:881-889, 1991.

55. Roter DL: Patient participation in the patient-provider interaction: the effects of patient question asking on the quality of interaction, satisfaction and compliance, *Health Ed Mong* 5:281-315, 1977.

56. Roter DL: Physician/patient communication: transmission of information and patient effects, *Md State Med J* 32:260-265, 1983.

57. Rutter M: Protective factors in children's responses to stress and disadvantage. In Kent MW, Rolf JE, editors: *Primary prevention of psychopathology.* Vol 3. *Social competence in children,* Hanover, NH, 1979, University Press of New England.

58. Satin W and others: Diabetes in adolescence: effects of multifamily group intervention and parent simulation of diabetes, *J Pediatr Psychol* 14:259-275, 1989.

59. Schaefer LC, McCaul KD, Glasgow RE: Supportive and nonsupportive family behaviors: relationships to adherence and metabolic control in persons with type I diabetes, *Diabetes Care* 9:179-185, 1986.

60. Ware JE, Davies-Avery A, Stewart AI: The measurement and meaning of patient satisfaction, *Health Med Care Serv Rev* 1:1-15, 1978.

61. White K and others: Unstable diabetes and unstable families: a psychosocial evaluation of diabetic children with recurrent ketoacidosis, *Pediatrics* 73:749-755, 1984.

15 Application of Health Behavior Models to Promote Behavior Change

Cheryl A. Houston and Debra Haire-Joshu

Diabetes mellitus has biologic, psychologic, and social impacts. Consequently, the individual with diabetes must understand and act on a variety of complicated clinical information to attain adequate self-management.[2,36,38] To do this effectively, persons with diabetes must interact with various members of the health care team to solicit the knowledge and skills needed to care for themselves successfully. Effective diabetes education therefore involves all disciplines of the health care team (e.g., physicians, dietitians, nurses, physical therapists, social workers, psychologists).[36,38,42,47] In addition, these team members must apply skills associated with the teaching/learning process in a systematic manner. The patient and members of the health care team must also consider diabetes within the context of multiple levels of influence. These levels of influence include intrapersonal, interpersonal, organizational, community, and policy factors, which, when considered together, create an ecologic perspective toward health promotion in general[30] and diabetes self-management in particular. Thus the ultimate goal of our teaching is to interact with the individual with diabetes and the family so that the skills needed to modify behavior effectively can be obtained within a larger environmental context.

CHAPTER OBJECTIVES

- Consider diabetes from an ecologic perspective.
- Discuss several health behavior models and theories to help guide the diabetes educator in the selection of intervention strategies.
- Discuss teaching methods and skills applied to diabetes self-management.
- Present an example of how to apply teaching models to diabetes education. The transtheoretical, or stages of change, model is used as an illustrative example of how skills can be applied to diabetes teaching.[40,41]
- Address the diabetes care relationship and its association with self-management.

ECOLOGIC MODEL APPROACH TO DIABETES SELF-MANAGEMENT

Health behavior theories provide an organizing framework to increase our understanding of the determinants of health-related problems and behaviors. As such, theories offer insight into the design of effective intervention strategies and methods to be employed in the field.[22,52]

In the past, diabetes patient education programs focused on changing the behavior of individuals. Other models stressed the need to change the systems and environments in which the individual with diabetes lives. A recent trend attempts to integrate both approaches into what is known as an *ecologic model of health promotion*.[30] The ecologic model addresses factors associated with five levels of influence, which are targets for diabetes education interventions. These five levels of influence include intrapersonal, interpersonal, organizational, community, and public policy factors. The ecologic model stresses the importance of directing change strategies and techniques at all five levels of influence. It assumes a type of reciprocal causation in that the individual, his or her behavior, and the environment influence each other simultaneously. For example, a person with diabetes might delay having his or her eyes screened for retinopathy. The reason for this inaction may be prematurely labeled as "nonadherence." However, one or more levels of influence may have an impact on the situation. The individual may lack understanding about the relationship between having diabetes and the need for an eye examination or may fear finding that he or she is going blind *(intrapersonal factors)*. The physician may fail to recommend the examination *(interpersonal factors)*. The individual may lack physical access to skilled medical personnel to conduct the screening *(community factors)* and/or inability to pay because of inadequate insurance coverage *(organizational and public policy factors)*.

Each of these factors is addressed by particular theories of health behavior change, as noted in Table 15-1. A discussion of a select number of these theories in relation to the ecologic model is detailed next.[17,30] Although varied in perspective, all recognize the critical need for a theoretic base as a guide for organizing teaching activities.

Intrapersonal Factors

Intrapersonal factors are characteristics of the individual. These "within individual" characteristics include knowledge, attitudes, self-concept, and personality traits. Several models, or theories, have been used to explain health-related behavior or program development at this level.[40,41,44] One such model, the *health belief model* (HBM), was originally developed to explain participation in screening programs, but its application has been broadened to understanding patient adherence to therapeutic regimens (e.g., following a low-fat diet). The HBM addresses a person's perception of a threat of a health problem (e.g., for the person with diabetes, this might be susceptibility to developing neuropathy and the perceived potential severity that may result) and a personal assessment of the perceived benefits and barriers that would remove this threat (e.g., tight control as a means of limiting the symptoms of neuropathy). The desire to take action can be triggered by an individual's cognitions *(internal factors)* or via *external factors* such as print or mass media messages about health issues. The concept of self-efficacy was added to the HBM in 1977 to improve

Table 15-1   The Ecologic Perspective: a Multilevel Approach to Diabetes Management

Level of influence	Definition	Applied model
Intrapersonal factors	Characteristics of the individual that influence behavior, such as knowledge, attitudes, self-concept, and personality traits	Health belief model Transtheoretical (stages of change) model
Interpersonal factors	Formal and informal social networks and social support systems, such as family, friends, work group, and health professionals	Social learning theory Social support Interpersonal communication Social networks
Organizational factors	Rules, regulations, and policies in formal structures that may have an impact on an individual's health-related behavior	Organizational development Organizational stage theory

Community factors	Social networks and norms, or standards, that exist formally or informally among organizations and individuals within organizations	Community organization:
		  Locality development
		  Social planning
		  Social action
		Diffusion of innovation
		Social marketing

Public policy factors	Local, state, and federal policies and laws that influence disease prevention and treatment practices	Social learning theory Organizational development Community organization (emphasizing media advocacy for social action) Diffusion of innovation

Modified from Glanz K, Rimer BK: *Theory at a glance: a guide for health promotion practice,* Bethesda, Md, 1995, Office of Cancer Communication, National Cancer Institute.

its explanatory power and is defined as "the conviction that one can successfully execute the behavior required to produce the outcomes."[44] Demographic, social, structural, and personality factors are included in some versions of the model as modifying factors, since they may indirectly influence behavior.[34]

Another model often applied at the intrapersonal level is the *transtheoretical,* or *stages of change, model.*[40,41] This model focuses on an individual's motivation or readiness to change a given behavior. The model identifies five distinct stages: precontemplation, contemplation, preparation, action, and maintenance. The definition of each stage and the application of this model to identify intervention strategies for the person with diabetes are covered in detail later in this chapter. It is important to note at this point that these stages represent a *circular,* not linear, *relationship.* Individuals can move forward and backward among the stages. *Relapse* and *relapse prevention skills* are important components of the model. The transtheoretical model may help the educator understand why a person is not making a particular change at a given point in time and offers intervention strategies based on each stage that might be useful in moving a person forward in making positive health-related behavior changes.

Interpersonal Factors

Interpersonal factors involve formal and informal social networks and social support systems, including the family, work group, health professionals, and friendship networks. At this level the individual is seen as influencing and being influenced by the social environment. Appropriate interventions that focus on interpersonal factors change the nature of existing social relationships. Models of interpersonal influence include social support, interpersonal communication, social networks, and *social learning theory* (SLT).[15] SLT, also referred to as *social cognitive theory* (SCT), is a complex theory with a basic premise of *reciprocal determinism* (i.e., human behavior is determined by the interaction among the personal factors of the individual, the environment, and the behavior itself).[37]

On an interpersonal level, the patient and educator can identify barriers to the patient's ability to complete the diabetes regimen. A synthesis of the data from a detailed learning assessment, together with the information about the environmental context of the person with diabetes, can identify self-management problems on which the diabetes team and the individual can focus their efforts.[24] Emphasis is placed on providing skills training to improve behavioral capability, encourage improved self-efficacy, identify appropriate role models (observational learning), and provide reinforcements such as incentives, rewards, and praise.[15,17] For example, nonadherence may be touted as the educational diagnosis when poor metabolic control is present in a young person with insulin-dependent diabetes mellitus (IDDM); in fact, further assessment may reveal an interaction effect among intrapersonal factors (insufficient knowledge of complex information about diabetes) and interpersonal factors (lack of family support) that are interfering with successfully following the diabetes regimen recommendations.

Organizational Factors

The next level of influence concerns organizations. From childhood to adulthood, most individuals spend a great amount of their time each day in organizational environments such as formal day care, schools, colleges and universities, and work sites. As such, these environments affect individual health and health-related behavior.[30] For example, work conditions can have a profound impact on the diabetic person's ability to carry out regimen recommendations. Simple scheduling (e.g., shift work, overtime, irregular hours, timing of meals) can make diabetes management difficult. Job demands (e.g., set routine, consistency in activity levels) can promote self-management in the work environment (e.g., having time and a private area at work to monitor blood glucose and inject insulin).[21]

Accommodations to support employees with chronic diseases such as diabetes are possible, but change is not always easy to accomplish. Organizational change is best promoted at multiple levels within the organization. The most successful interventions focus on changing (1) organizational norms (e.g., employee health is a priority), (2) rules and regulations (e.g., smoking restrictions), and (3) structure of work (e.g., flexible lunch hour so that employees with diabetes may consume a meal when blood sugar levels, not the clock, dictate).[17]

Community Factors

Community factors describe relationships among organizations (e.g., local voluntary agencies, health departments, schools), informal networks (also called mediating structures, including families, friendship networks, neighborhoods), and geographic and political boundaries.[30]

Community organization theory includes locality development, social planning, and social action. *Locality development* focuses on gaining broad community participation and citizen ownership. *Social planning* emphasizes identifying community needs and goals and designing intervention strategies to achieve these goals. *Social action* involves social policy, legislation, and advocacy to create change.[46] These theories are rarely used in isolation. Intervention strategies at the community level often adopt strategies from each model. Useful techniques at this level include focus groups, coalition development, and media advocacy.[15]

Comprehensive diabetes control strategies at the community level are essential for the well-being of community members. However, program development and integration of existing efforts are often time-consuming. To assist individuals interested in diabetes programming at the community level, a course called *Diabetes Today!* has been developed by the Centers for Disease Control and Prevention (CDC).[9] Based on the *PATCH* (*p*lanned *a*pproach *t*o *c*ommunity *h*ealth) approach, this program provides health professionals and community volunteers with the skills and information necessary to plan, implement, and evaluate community-based diabetes programs.[8] The program consists of six training sessions:

1. An overview of diabetes
2. Strategies for identifying and involving community members and techniques for conducting a community needs assessment
3. Methods for selecting target groups
4. Prioritizing of diabetes-related community needs and goal setting
5. Planning of intervention strategies
6. Evaluation of the diabetes program developed

Such a program provides an effective means of positively impacting the individual via intervention at a community level.[9]

Public Policy Factors

Public policy encompasses local, state, and national laws, including those that restrict behavior (e.g., no smoking policies in public buildings), those that contain behavioral incentives (e.g., reduction in insurance premiums for positive health behaviors), and those that affect access to certain health programs (e.g., coverage for diabetes education). Diabetes educators, persons with diabetes, and community members can influence interventions at this level by lobbying and voting for health-promoting legislation (e.g., clean indoor air legislation, tax on cigarettes), increasing public awareness about health and policy issues, and organizing coalitions.[30]

Process of Promoting Behavior Change

The ecologic model provides a comprehensive framework from which to promote behaviors associated with optimal diabetes self-management. This perspective guides the planning of self-management strategies that address or are sensitive to each level of the model. Comprehensive diabetes education needs to be organized in a systematic manner that reflects the designated model to ensure that important components are not omitted.

This section describes steps associated with a systematic teaching/learning process designed to promote self-care behaviors. These steps are applicable to interventions planned for each level of the ecologic model.

Step 1: Assessing Learning Needs

The best way to identify important factors at each level of influence that may impact the educational process is by conducting a thorough learner assessment. Assessment represents the first step of gathering a variety of physical and psychosocial data necessary to determine an appropriate educational plan for diabetes self-management training. The term *learning assessment* should not imply a review of diabetes knowledge or skills alone. Rather, a learning assessment results from the compilation of an accurate and thorough health and life-style history.[3,4] Such a history identifies strengths and weaknesses or past and present susceptibility or resistance to psychologic as well as physical stresses. Just as a clinical determination is necessary before adjustment of insulin, an educational assessment is necessary to determine the best strategies for incorporating diabetes management into the individual's life.

One issue that arises when conducting assessment is the lack of time. Assessment may prove to be very time-consuming, with studies reporting that up to 55% of an interaction reflects the assessment phase.[39] However, the collection of comprehensive data lends itself to more effective translation of information to the individual with diabetes. As such, it should be carefully conducted, with as much time devoted to careful completion as is needed.

Information sources

The collection of data for the assessment of learning needs may come from a variety of sources, including the individual, medical records, family members, and other health care team members. For example, the physical aspects of the assessment generally come from the medical and nursing history, while a more detailed psychosocial/developmental history may be obtained from a social worker's or psychologist's assessment. The ability to coordinate such findings makes for a very comprehensive picture of the individual and enables one to identify an appropriate learning diagnosis.[20]

Assessment variables

As discussed earlier, a variety of factors may influence the learning assessment of the individual with diabetes. A brief discussion of each of these factors follows.

Demographic factors. Gender, age, and years of formal education are important variables in any assessment. Documentation of diabetes knowledge, such as might be reflected on a knowledge test, is also important.[13,16]

Cultural factors. Information regarding members of household, role and position in household, and position in the extended family are important cultural variables.[2,48] The *role* in the household refers to the tasks and responsibilities assumed by the patient, and the *position* refers to placement in the structure of the household. For example, many women have the role of the breadwinner, mother, and homemaker. Position in the extended family refers to the individual with diabetes as grandparent, aunt, cousin, or sibling. In some situations the grandparent, not the parent, assumes the role of primary caregiver for the child. For a working parent without family support, the day-care worker assumes the status of major caregiver. These assessment data describe the "actual" life situation of the individual and suggest other persons who may play a significant role in the person's diabetes education.

Environmental factors. A description of the neighborhood in which the individual lives, pattern of moving, and description of home are helpful. A description of the neighborhood highlights the relationships with neighbors, location in reference to established health care facilities, and environmental risks, such as violence.[13] Persons who move frequently, such as may be found in lower socioeconomic groups, also tend to have less opportunity for establishing support systems and using community resources. They are therefore at higher risk for less than optimal care, which further necessitates careful planning of educational interventions.

Finally, consideration should be given to a description of the community at large. What diabetes-related resources (e.g., local chapter of the American Diabetes Association, diabetes support groups, educational programs at local hospitals) are available? Is transportation available if these resources exist?

Economic profile. Is the individual with diabetes employed? If so, an understanding of the type of occupation, work setting, and job requirements is essential for planning how the diabetes regimen can best be incorporated into his or her life-style. What is the nature of the work? How are work and breaks structured? Does the person have a flexible work environment so that he or she can leave his or her desk as needed to take care of diabetes-related tasks, such as checking blood sugar levels and taking medication? Does this person have health insurance, and to what extent are the current health care costs impacting personal finances? How much does the individual spend on diabetes care in an average month? What percentage of this is monthly income? What other major economic expenditures does the individual and his or her significant others face?

Activities of daily living. What are the usual activities of a given day? What are the normal sleep and activity patterns? Such information enables the health care provider to determine the amount of time devoted to leisure versus work and gives some sense of the extent to which diabetes is a focus of the person's life.[13] In the case of the child with diabetes, such information provides insight into parental fatigue and stress, which often are associated with a "nonsleeping" child.

Current health beliefs and practices. What is the patient's philosophy of health care? For example, does he or she exhibit a particular interest in preventive health care by seeking regular health care for diabetes management? In contrast, does he or she rely on the emergency room as a primary health care source? What is this individual's view on maintaining metabolic control? What is his or her attitude toward risky health behaviors, such as obesity and alcohol or drug abuse? Does he or she smoke, and if so, how many cigarettes per day?[20]

Psychosocial assessment. Diabetes causes a variety of emotional responses in the per-son with diabetes as well as in significant others. These responses need to be clearly identified so that they can be carefully assessed with regard to the behavior change process. On diagnosis of diabetes, patients move through various stages of acceptance in response to this diagnosis, such as shock and disbelief, anger, guilt, depression, and acceptance.[20] In what stage is the person with diabetes? To what extent is the individual accepting the diagnosis of diabetes? Is there a perception that parents, family, and friends assist with diabetes management? How would the patient describe the current level of emotional family support or support from other social networks? How many close friends does he or she identify? How does developmental status, as discussed in other chapters of this text, influence adjustment to diabetes?

Physical status. This information is secured from laboratory or physical findings, typically found with the medical history. How long has the individual been diagnosed with diabetes? What is the type of diabetes, physical and nutritional assessment, complication status, history, and current level of metabolic control?

Prescribed regimen. What is the current method of prescribed management of the diabetes? To what extent is the individual following *each component* of the regimen (medication, diet, exercise, etc.)? Is the patient satisfied with the regimen? What is the most difficult part of the regimen for this person, or the most important problem?

Learner priorities. Documentation of what the individual sees as a priority of care is essential to a thorough educational assessment. What is the greatest overall concern for the patient at this time in life? What is the major concern regarding diabetes management? What type of benefits, if any, does the person perceive he or she will receive from following the regimen? How confident is the person that he or she will be able to follow each component of the regimen? Discussion with the individual as to how identified priorities compare with those noted by the diabetes health care team is important. Ultimately, it is the person with diabetes who will be asked to make any behavior changes or carry out any regimen.[20,45] As such, it is necessary to determine the extent to which the changes are seen as important and to determine whether the individual possesses adequate skills and resources to complete the regimen.

Step 2: Setting Behavioral Goals

Goals are broad statements describing what will be accomplished by the person with diabetes.[18] For example, one goal might be that the patient will maintain desirable body weight by following a low-fat diet. The goal is generally a result of the behavioral diagnosis, which identifies a specific problem area that has been recognized and that needs modification.

Goal setting focuses efforts on progression toward an ultimate accomplishment. The goal should be established with the input of the person with diabetes. As previously noted, individuals must be involved in a collaborative effort to set goals if long-term changes are to be realized. The health care provider works with this person in setting concrete, understandable goals that serve as positive reinforcers for self-management.

Specific guidelines for establishing treatment goals include negotiating individualized treatment goals to meet the patient's needs. If the necessary skills are not within the individual's repertoire, easier goals should be employed until those skills are accomplished. Ultimately, the goals must lead to meaningful rewards for the individual.

Step 3: Developing Behavioral Objectives

Before one can teach or evaluate progress, the health care team must know what learning outcomes are expected. What behavior does the individual exhibit at the beginning of the educational intervention? How does this contrast with the expected behavior at the conclusion of the educational experience? What knowledge and understanding should the individual possess? What skills should be displayed?

This section defines and describes various types of behavioral objectives. *Behavioral objectives* are learning outcomes that establish direction by stating expected changes in the individual's behavior. According to Mager, measurable objectives "are useful in pointing to the content and procedures that lead to successful instruction, help to manage the instructional process itself, and help to provide the means of finding out whether the instruction has been successful."[28] Without measurable behavioral objectives, learning cannot be successfully planned or evaluated. Behavioral objectives are as follows[18,28,40]:

- Measure the individual's behavior rather than health care educator's duties and techniques.
- Establish the direction for learning.
- State the "ends" of the desired performance rather than the "means" of the individual's performance.
- Indicate a specific behavior rather than general behavior for the individual to fulfill.
- Communicate to the individual his or her expected performance by identifying the performance itself, the standard or criterion by which the performance is to be judged, and the condition under which performance takes place.
- Contain only one specific action verb.
- Assist the diabetes educator in developing evaluation instruments.

Taxonomies of learning

There are various "types" of objectives. Objectives typically are written using various action verbs. These action verbs imply a level of learning; some verbs imply a higher level of learning than others. These levels have been characterized as taxonomies of learning. This is a detailed classification system of objectives. It divides objectives into three major areas: the cognitive, affective, and psychomotor domains (Fig. 15-1).[18]

Each of these domains can be further divided into categories that "break down" each step of the learning process within the areas described next. In other words, each domain

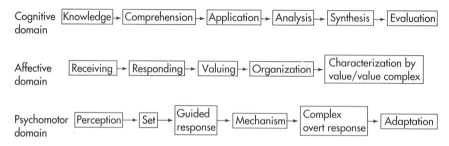

Fig. 15-1 Examples of verbs for taxonomies of learning.

has steps of difficulty (or performance levels) that help the health care provider plan for well-rounded and comprehensive learning experiences. The taxonomy may be of value to the provider, since one can plan for the individual's growth in learning by presenting the individual with measurable performance objectives that range from "low" to "high" in level of difficulty. This is especially important when dealing with patients of varying ages. Box 15-1 depicts the taxonomy and an example of how verbs reflect the more advanced understanding associated with each domain. This list is not all inclusive and is meant to serve as an example.

Cognitive domain. This domain is concerned with knowledge outcomes and intellectual abilities and skills (e.g., understanding the difference between hypoglycemia and hyperglycemia) (see Fig. 15-1).[5] The cognitive domain classified intellectual responses in a hierarchic order, ranging from simple rote memory to complex problem-solving thought processes. The cognitive processes are those processes whereby " . . . we organize, interrelate, and respond to the data of the experience and the range of intellectual activities one is capable of performing in order to sort, interpret, and respond to stimuli in the environment."[5] The cognitive domain comprises six levels that reflect simple to complex knowledge:

1. *Knowledge.* This is the lowest level of performance in the cognitive domain, a measure of the person's ability to recall or recognize information in the same format it was presented. Before an individual can reach higher learning, he or she must have a basic knowledge of the material. For example, an individual with diabetes should be able to list the symptoms of hypoglycemia.

2. *Comprehension.* This is defined as a measure of understanding at the most rudimentary level. This level takes the learner one step beyond knowledge or memorization. For example, the patient can explain why treatment of hypoglycemia is important to diabetes care.

3. *Application.* This is a measure of the person's ability to select and apply previously acquired information and requires a higher understanding of material than in the previous levels. The individual is expected to apply previously learned material to new situations or settings. For example, the patient recognizes the symptoms of hypoglycemia that dictate the use of glucagon versus less substantial treatment.

4. *Analysis.* This level is a measure of the person's ability to separate complex communication into its component parts and to recognize relationships among common parts of a particular communication. For example, the individual is able to discuss the components

---

BOX 15-1

MEASURABLE VERBS IN TAXONOMIES OF LEARNING FOR USE IN WRITING BEHAVIORAL OBJECTIVES

Cognitive (knowledge) domain

Analyzes	Describes	Illustrates
Applies	Differentiates	Interprets
Compares	Discusses	Lists
Debates	Explains	Names
Defines	Identifies	Recalls
Demonstrates		

Psychomotor (skill) domain

Adjusts	Imitates	Practices
Administers	Incorporates	Produces
Carries out	Manipulates	Return demonstrates
Computes	Operates	Skillfully demonstrates
Constructs	Performs	Utilizes
Follows instructions		

Affective (attitude) domain

Accepts	Cooperates	Seeks opportunities
Acknowledges	Defends	Shares
Agrees	Judges	Shows interest
Approves	Listens	Values
Argues	Responds	Volunteers
Assumes responsibility		

Modified from Istre SM: *Diabetes Educ* 15:67-75, 1989.

---

that interact to produce good control (e.g., diet, exercise, medication) and also is able to recognize that insulin is potentiated by exercise.

5. *Synthesis.* The individual should be able to "reorganize" the material that has been learned. For example, the patient with diabetes realizes that hypoglycemia may occur during exercise and that exercise potentiates the impact of insulin. Thus the person arranges for additional snacks to cover activity during this period.

6. *Evaluation.* The individual is able to form judgments based on agreed criteria concerning the value of ideas, plans, and so forth. For example, the patient recognizes the need to modify dietary activities further based on the occurrence of rebound hyperglycemia caused by excessive treatment of low blood sugar levels during exercise.

Affective domain. Affective objectives attempt to provide feedback to the health care educator concerning an individual's feelings or attitudes regarding a particular topic or situation. Affective objectives can be distinguished from cognitive objectives, since affective objectives reflect a voluntary attitude or feeling, whereas cognitive objectives reflect a competency necessary for effective performance.[26] The five levels of the affective domain, progressing from simple to more complex, are as follows:

1. *Receiving.* This means the learner is aware of and interested in the material being presented. For example, the individual with diabetes is interested in learning about multiple injections as a means of maintaining metabolic control.

2. *Responding.* The individual displays interest in the teaching/learning interaction by discussing pertinent information with the health care educator.

3. *Valuing.* The individual displays behaviors that suggest he or she has a degree of commitment or conviction to the accepted value. For example, great care is taken to follow a daily multiple-injection routine in the belief that metabolic control will improve his or her quality of life.

4. *Organization.* The individual analyzes a concept and compares it with others with which he or she is familiar. For example, physical exercise is incorporated into weekly activities in the belief that such activities assist diabetes management.

5. *Characterization by a value or value complex.* This means that the individual responds in a consistent manner, based on his or her values. For example, the patient who values metabolic control as an outcome of personal behavior may exhibit a life-style that consistently promotes this as a goal.

Psychomotor domain. This domain deals with skill development, such as skills associated with diabetes management. There are six performance levels associated with this domain.[28] The components of the domain include the following:

1. *Perception.* This is a process of becoming aware of objects or qualities by way of auditory, visual, or other sensory organs. An example is when the individual recognizes the visual differences indicating blood glucose level on the strips.

2. *Set.* This implies the individual is prepared for the learning experience (e.g., the individual has all the materials needed to perform blood glucose monitoring).

3. *Guided response.* The person performs the activity (e.g., blood glucose monitoring) under the guidance of the diabetes educator.

4. *Mechanism.* At this point the learned response becomes more habitual. Various aspects of trial and error may also take place, with the individual finding a means of performing the task most appropriate to him or her.

5. *Complex overt response.* The person now effectively and routinely performs the skill. For example, the individual accurately performs blood glucose monitoring, as validated by laboratory measures.

6. *Adaptation.* This implies an ability to alter motor activities pending the demands of new and problematic situations.

Writing objectives

Objectives should reflect the taxonomies of learning (cognitive/knowledge, psycho-motor/skill, affective/attitude), encouraging learner progression. The structure for writing objectives always addresses the learner (e.g., parent of child with diabetes), the performance (e.g., plans a daily menu for a school-age child using the exchange list), the standards for the performance (e.g., correct 90% of the time), and the conditions under which the performance takes place (e.g., diabetes clinic).[28,51]

Objectives might also be written using the "who," "what," "when," "where," and "how" terms. The who is the learner or individual with diabetes. The what is the content or information the individual should acquire. The how is the measurable behavior the individual will exhibit, such as "will describe." The when or where describes the circumstances under which the learner will achieve the objective. For example, at the conclusion of the clinic or office visit (when/where), the individual with diabetes (who) will be able to demonstrate (how) the proper way to examine his or her feet (what).[2,28,51]

Step 4: Identifying Behavioral Change Strategies

Once the behavioral objectives are readily defined, one can identify various teaching strategies that are available for use by diabetes educators to enhance the individual's understanding and attainment of objectives. In general, learning is facilitated through reinforcement in an atmosphere in which persons with diabetes are given adequate time to assimilate information and skills at appropriate intervals. It is also important that patients are made aware of their progress at intervals through feedback.[27,32]

Although not intended to be all inclusive, the following section identifies several strategies that are very effective in promoting behavior change.

Self-monitoring

This is a behavior modification technique based on the assumption that awareness of actions is a first step toward changing actions. The use of self-monitoring procedures in diabetes care is already an integral part of the regimen. The establishment of behavioral objectives and the self-monitoring of these objectives have a substantial impact, since it is easier to monitor a behavior than a goal. Thus it is easier for the individual with diabetes to realize what the behavioral objective is and to evaluate his or her effectiveness in achieving this objective.[1,27] To facilitate this process, it is helpful to have the individual identify positive behavioral changes, for example, how many times per week the person *did* exercise as opposed to *did not* exercise.

Behavioral Contracting

Once behavioral objectives are developed, they can be included in a useful technique called *behavioral contracting*. This contracting process involves concrete discussion of specific behaviors that might be beneficial and how they might be carried out to fulfill the contract.[1,6,12] The critical ingredient in using behavioral contracting is the negotiation of the contract by the individual and the provider.

Box 15-2 outlines specific guidelines for formulating a contract, which include the following[23,38]:

- A clear and detailed description of the required instrumental behavior should be set (e.g., *the individual with diabetes will walk 30 minutes a day, three times per week*).

BOX 15-2

GUIDELINES TO FOLLOW IN FORMULATING A BEHAVIORAL CONTRACT

1. State a clear, detailed description of the required instrumental behavior.
2. Set some criterion for the time or frequency limitations constituting the goal of the contract.
3. Have the contract specify positive reinforcements contingent on fulfillment of the criterion.
4. Make provisions for some aversive consequences contingent on nonfulfillment of the contract within a specified time or with a specified frequency.
5. Ensure a bonus clause indicates the additional positive reinforcements obtainable if the person exceeds the contract's minimal demands.
6. Have the contract specify the means by which the contract response is observed, measured, and recorded; a procedure is stated for informing the patient of his or her achievements over the duration of the contact.
7. Arrange for the timing for delivery of reinforcement contingencies to follow the response as quickly as possible.

Example of behavioral contract
Health care contract

Contract goal: (specific outcome to be attained)

I, (patient's name), agree to (detailed description of required behaviors, time and frequency limitations) in return for (positive reinforcements contingent on completion of required behaviors; timing and mode of delivery of reinforcements).

I, (provider's name), agree to (detailed description of required behaviors, time and frequency limitations).

(Optional) I, (significant other's name), agree to (detailed description of required behaviors, time and frequency limitations).

(Optional) Aversive consequences: (negative reinforcements for failure to meet minimal behavioral requirements)

(Optional) Bonuses: (additional positive reinforcements for exceeding minimal contract requirements)

We will review the terms of this agreement and will make any desired modification on (date). We hereby agree to abide by the terms of the contract described above.

Signed: (patient)

Signed: (significant other, if relevant)

Signed: (provider)

Contract effective from (date) to (date)

Modified from Kanfer FH, Gaelick L: In Kanfer FH, Goldstein AP, editors: *Helping people change,* ed 2, New York, 1986, Pergamon.

- Some criterion should be set for the time or frequency limitation constituting the goal of the contract (e.g., *for 2 weeks*).
- Specific positive reinforcements are contingent on fulfillment of the criterion (e.g., *after which she will buy a new dress*).
- Bonus clauses should indicate the additional positive reinforcements obtainable if the person exceeds the minimal demands of the contract (e.g., *and see a movie if he walks 5 days a week*).
- Means are specified by which contract response is observed, measured, and recorded (e.g., *to be documented by her spouse*).
- Timing for delivery of reinforcement contingencies (e.g., *with the rewards to be received within 2 weeks of completion of the contract*).

Behavioral skills training

In order for an individual to manage diabetes, he or she must have component skills, such as planning, stress management, and assertiveness. Enhancement of problem-solving skills may also benefit the individual with diabetes. *Problem solving* is a form of skills training. Problem solving forces the focus on one specific aspect associated with diabetes care and also identifies any solutions. Such strategies are especially effective when one considers that patients need less information on pathophysiology and more on ways of integrating information into their regimen. Knowledge about one's regimen, not about one's disease, is predictive of clinical outcome. Problem solving encourages a critical look at specific problems and suggests the need for collaborative efforts toward solutions. It further demands the involvement of the patient in the process. Problem solving relies on oral questioning to generate strategies for resolving the problem. Through oral questioning, the diabetes educator helps the patient do the following[23]:

- Recall what has been learned.
- Think critically.
- Apply concepts.
- Become more actively involved in diabetes care.
- Learn more on his or her own.
- Become more interested in diabetes care.
- Develop a positive self-concept.
- Become motivated to take greater responsibility for care.

Evaluation of the adequate use of problem-solving techniques and development of skills demand an assessment of the process. Box 15-3 lists some steps one might evaluate to ensure proper use of this technique.

Providing appropriate educational materials

Carefully selected educational materials can contribute substantially to the individual's learning. Various materials are available that are pertinent to different groups; availability of materials is usually not a problem. However, two major concerns before using any diabetes material is whether the material is appropriate to the ethnic background and reading level of the individual or group who is to receive it.[13,33,35] Critical characteristics that need to be

---

BOX 15-3

PROBLEM-SOLVING SKILLS

Assist the patient to do the following:

1. Define the problem clearly in behavioral terms (give examples).
2. Analyze what one cannot do and why.
3. Generate possible solutions to each problem.
4. Evaluate the pros and cons of each proposed solution.
5. Rank the solutions from least to most practical and desirable.
6. Try out the most acceptable and feasible solution.
7. Reconsider the original problem in light of this attempt at problem solving.

Table 15-2 Contrasting Values by Culture

Anglo-American values	Alternative culture values
Personal control over the environment	Fate
Change	Tradition
Time dominates	Human interaction dominates
Human equality	Hierarchy/status
Individualism/privacy	Group welfare
Competition	Cooperation
Future orientation	Past orientation
Informality	Formality

From Haire-Joshu D: In Peragallo-Dittko V, Godley K, Meyer J, editors: *A core curriculum for diabetes education,* ed 2, Chicago, 1993, American Association of Diabetes Educators and the AADE Education and Research Foundation.

considered with educational materials include cultural sensitivity and literacy level of materials.

Delivery of diabetes education for cultural groups requires the application of comprehensive educational principles that respect the cultural differences of the specific ethnic group, as discussed in Chapter 13 and depicted in Table 15-2. This requires a level of cultural competence. *Cultural competence* is a multidimensional concept involving knowledge and skills that allow the educator to increase his or her understanding and appreciation of cultural differences and similarities within, among, and between groups. The educator also needs to display cultural sensitivity to other groups in practice by selecting strategies and materials that are sensitive to differences and effective in using cultural symbols to communicate messages. Table 15-3 provides a schematic representation of a framework depicting cultural competence. Informed awareness of the role of culture in health care choices by the individual with diabetes and incorporation of sociocultural components into the program are critical to being able to address minority health concerns.[2]

Table 15-3   A Framework of Cultural Competence

	Culturally incompetent	Culturally sensitive	Culturally competent
Cognitive domain	Oblivious	Aware	Knowledgeable
Affective domain	Apathetic	Sympathetic	Committed to change
Skills	Unskilled	Lacking some skills	Highly skilled
Overall impact	Destructive	Neutral	Constructive

From Haire-Joshu D: In Peragallo-Dittko V, Godley K, Meyer J, editors: *A core curriculum for diabetes education,* ed 2, Chicago, 1993, American Association of Diabetes Educators and the AADE Education and Research Foundation.

Table 15-4   Variables Used in Selected Readability Formulas

Formula name	Variables used in each formula
SMOG	Average number of words of three syllables or more per 30 sentences
Flesch-Kincaid	Average number of words per sentence Average number of syllables per word
Gunning's FOG	Average number of words per sentence Average number of words of three syllables or more per 100 words
Flesch Reading Ease	Average number of words per sentence Average number of syllables per 100 words
Fry Graph	Average number of syllables per 100 words Average number of sentences per 100 words

Modified from Hosey GM and others: *Diabetes Educ* 16(5):407-414, 1990.

Literacy level of materials is critical in planning behavior change interventions. There are various methods for assessing readability of materials (Table 15-4). In general, successful methods attempt to grade an individual in terms of reading skills based on sentence length, number of syllables or word length, number of words per page, and number of illustrations per number of words.* These formulas are typically easy to use and ensure the appropriateness of materials to the individual or group.

Step 5: Follow-up/Evaluating Individual Outcomes

Evaluation results provide the answer to the question, How effectively has the individual progressed toward meeting the behavioral goals and objectives? Careful documentation of teaching/learning activities and of progress during the teaching session is necessary if communication among diabetes team members is to be clear. Substantial evidence indicates that persons with diabetes forget or do not recall the specifics of what they have been told by the physician or health care educator once they have left the office. Consistent follow-up is an important mechanism to include in any educational experience as a means to promote

---

*References 14,19,25,29,50.

learning.[31] Follow-up in the form of mailings or telephone contacts, as well as additional appointments or memory aids (refrigerator stickers), may be important to those who are learning new information and who may be anxious regarding the new expectations.[27,38] Documentation of successes and problem areas should occur at the time of the teaching and should not be postponed until a later date. After documentation, team discussion of modifications of the behavioral diagnosis is not only appropriate but also critical to good education as well as to the instructional plan.

"PULLING IT ALL TOGETHER": APPLICATION OF THE TRANSTHEORETICAL MODEL TO IMPROVE TEACHER/LEARNER EFFECTIVENESS

This section provides an example of how the process of promoting behavior change is related to theoretic models of health promotion. An example of linking strategy to patient need is illustrated by the transtheoretical, or stages of change, model.[40,41] This model consists of five stages: precontemplation, contemplation, preparation, action, and maintenance. Intervention strategies are matched to the person's readiness for change. Originally designed to understand readiness to change single behaviors, such as smoking or drinking alcohol, this model has now been suggested for application to more complex models of behavior, such as those required for diabetes self-management. The model provides the educator with a means of targeting interventions based on the individual's readiness to change specific behaviors associated with each component of the diabetes regimen. For example, the patient may be in precontemplation for exercise, contemplation for dietary change, preparation for self-monitoring of blood glucose (SMBG), and action for medication taking. Intervention strategies differ for each behavior at each stage of readiness.

Staging of Individuals for Readiness to Change

In order to target interventions, the patient must be staged as to readiness to change specific self-care behaviors. The educator frequently asks the question, "How do I identify what stage of change an individual is in so that I can apply the appropriate educational interventions?" Box 15-4 lists sample questions used to assess readiness to change behaviors related to diabetes along with answers. It is important to remember that these questions should be asked *for each* component of the diabetes regimen. The example provided only describes the process for SMBG and diet. Questions should be posed for additional components of the diabetes regimen, such as exercise, stress management, eye examination, foot care, and dental examination.

Once the individual is staged, the educator can apply interventions appropriate to the readiness of the patient to learn with regard to each self-management behavior. Examples of each stage and the role of the diabetes educator within each stage are described in more detail next.

Precontemplation stage

Individuals in this first stage are not yet ready to commit to making a change in their behavior in the near future. A 6-month period is generally used as a reference.

BOX 15-4
_____

SAMPLE STAGING QUESTIONS FOR DIABETIC PATIENTS

Self-monitoring of blood glucose (SMBG)

Do you always check your blood sugar (glucose) in the way you were instructed?
  Yes, I have been for more than 6 months (maintenance).
  Yes, I have been for less than 6 months (action).
  No, but I plan to in the next month (preparation).
  No, but I plan to in the next 6 months (contemplation).
  No, and I do not intend to in the next 6 months (precontemplation).

Diet

Do you always follow your diet in the way you were instructed?
  Yes, I have been for more than 6 months (maintenance).
  Yes, I have been for less than 6 months (action).
  No, but I plan to in the next month (preparation).
  No, but I plan to in the next 6 months (contemplation).
  No, and I do not intend to in the next 6 months (precontemplation).

_____

Modified from Ruggiero L, Prochaska JO: _Diabetes Spectrum_ 6(1):23, 1993.

Individuals with diabetes may be in this stage for several reasons, including lack of knowledge or emotional barriers such as anger and denial. They may not even be aware that a problem exists.[40,41] The educator should conduct a thorough learner assessment, as described earlier in this chapter, to assist in the identification of benefits and barriers to making change at this point in time.

In terms of decisional balance (i.e., pros versus cons in a given situation), precontemplators tend to overestimate barriers or negative thoughts associated with change and underestimate the positive outcomes, in terms of both improved physical and improved psychosocial end points of behavioral change. For the person with diabetes, the cons associated with SMBG (e.g., inconvenience, extra expense, physical discomfort) outweigh the pros of making this change (e.g., feeling in control of one's life, reducing risk for complications associated with hypoglycemia and hyperglycemia). The role of the diabetes educator at this point is to inform the patient about the need to alter his or her behavior. Providing behavioral skills training would not be an appropriate or effective strategy for an individual in this stage because the innovation (change idea) does not meet the patient's current needs. Instead, providing personalized information that attempts to alter knowledge and attitudes would be more appropriate. The diabetes educator might also call on several constructs from the HBM described earlier, such as perceived threat (perceived susceptibility and severity) to make the change more salient to the patient.

Although educational strategies appropriate at this stage (i.e., one-to-one counseling, providing printed or audiovisual materials) seem to indicate reliance on one-way communication from the diabetes educator to the patient, this is not the case. For the linkage to be effective, feedback from the patient must be received by the educator so that modifications in strategies can be made.[43]

Contemplation stage

Individuals in this stage are thinking about changing their behavior within the next 6 months. Contemplators consider the pros and cons of their behavior as equivalent or the cons only slightly outweighing the pros. For example, an individual with diabetes in the contemplation stage may believe that there are as many disadvantages as advantages to beginning an exercise program. With contemplators, the role of the diabetes educator is to establish an information-exchange relationship. The educator should emphasize the benefits of making a change to help the individual tip the decisional balance scale to favor the pros of making the behavioral change(s). Once a need for change has been created, the educator must strive to build rapport with the patient so that the patient feels comfortable with and has confidence in the educator. The educator should try to increase patient feelings of self-efficacy, thereby increasing confidence in one's ability to adopt recommended behaviors. At this stage, it is important to recognize the impact of interpersonal factors (family members, other social networks) on the patient's ability to comply.[40,41] Once again, information gathered during the assessment of learner needs can provide insight into existing interpersonal factors influencing the patient's behavior.

Preparation stage

Individuals are characterized as being in the preparation stage if the intent to change behaviors is expected to occur within the next month. Often, individuals in this stage have made some small step toward change. For example, the person with diabetes may be making some change in the diet, such as switching from whole to 2% milk, although more changes are required to meet dietary recommendations.

At this point the pros outweigh the cons of making behavior change. However, individuals often need assistance in making specific plans. The role of the diabetes educator is to translate the intent to change into an action plan for change. The educator should be sure to reinforce any small positive changes made to date. It is important at this stage *not* to make general recommendations (e.g., follow a low-fat diet). The educator should help the patient to set specific, achievable goals and behavioral objectives. Measurable, behavioral objectives that consider the three taxonomies of learning (cognitive, affective, and psychomotor domains) should be written, as described earlier. Effective goal setting and the development of appropriate behavioral objectives are critical to the success of the educational intervention targeted to the patient in the preparation stage.

Action stage

In the action stage, individuals are immersed in the change process. For example, the patient with diabetes may be performing SMBG, following a diet, exercising, and taking medication as recommended. In this stage, diabetes educators should offer additional behavioral skills training, rather than simple information generation, and should reinforce

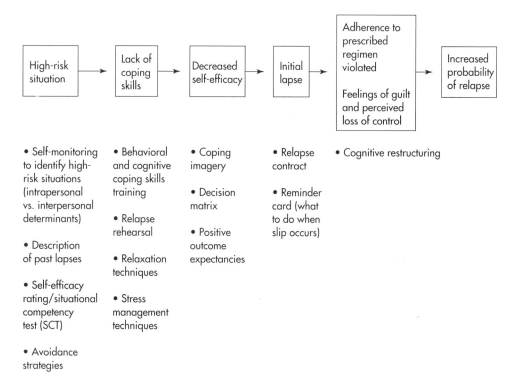

Fig. 15-2   Stages of the relapse process and specific strategies applied at each point. (Modified from Marlatt GA: In Marlatt GA, Gordon JR, editors: *Relapse prevention,* New York, 1985, Guilford.)

the importance of social support networks for continued success. Self-monitoring techniques and behavioral contracting are both useful strategies in this stage. The goal is to help the individual to stabilize the adoption of new behaviors. Although this is a very dynamic stage, it is also the point in time when the patient is at greatest risk for relapsing back into previous patterns of behavior. Relapse prevention techniques are useful strategies at this point (Fig. 15-2).

Once the behavioral objectives are defined in the preparation stage, the diabetes educator can identify various teaching strategies that encourage the individual's progression toward the action stage.[27,32,53]

Maintenance stage

Patients are considered to be in the maintenance stage when behavior change is consistently maintained for at least 6 months. Individuals at this stage should continue to work to avoid lapsing into previous patterns of behavior. The role of the diabetes educator in this stage is to promote self-reliance. Continued praise and support for the positive changes made, regardless of how large or small the change, should be provided. Individuals should continue to receive assistance with strategies for planning ahead to avoid lapse or relapse (Fig. 15-2).

Attention should also be given to enhancing the individual's self-efficacy for maintenance of all new health behaviors.[41]

Limitations to Applying the Transtheoretical Model to Complex Behaviors

One of the disadvantages in using the transtheoretical model is that it is not useful for assessing an individual's stage of readiness to change for *overall* diabetes management. Originally designed to understand readiness to change single behaviors, such as smoking or drinking alcohol, this model has limitations when applied to more complex models of behavior, such as those required for diabetes self-management. An individual can be in a different stage of readiness for each component of the diabetes regimen.

Another disadvantage is that this model is best applied to ongoing and in-depth education rather than initial education. *Initial education* can best be defined as the critical information necessary for the individual to live on his or her own outside the acute care environment. Typically, initial education refers to the content targeted to meet the needs of the newly diagnosed person with diabetes (or to educate those who are undergoing substantial stress and are unable to learn more in-depth information). Initial information varies in content depending on the person's age but tends to focus on such skills and knowledge as appropriate understanding of insulin management and treatment of hypoglycemia.

Staging for readiness to change is best applied to *ongoing* or *in-depth education* when the individual is comfortable with basic skills and is ready to learn more advanced skills related to diabetes management. Information associated with ongoing care focuses on skills associated with sick-day management, intensive exercise therapy, or insulin adjustment based on the need to alternate working days and nights. Information associated with an in-depth level of teaching falls into several categories. First, it might include those who are seeking alternative means of insulin delivery, such as intensive therapy or pump therapy. The correction of errors in learning, such as improper technique in SMBG, might also be addressed. Much of this information is directed to what the individual perceives as the most critical needs, as well as to a continuing assessment of the level of self-care.[20]

THE DIABETES CARE RELATIONSHIP

The purpose of diabetes self-management training is to improve the patient's health through education. The role of the diabetes educator in effecting change within this context is to communicate new health-related ideas or innovations to the patient in an attempt to improve the patient's health-related behavior. Several theoretic models have been described to assist the educator in tailoring his or her message to the needs of the person with diabetes. Regardless of which health behavior model is selected, the educator should develop several major interpersonal skills, which are cited as being imperative for a good diabetes care relationship to be successfully established.[49] Good interaction skills are present when the diabetes educator does the following[7,32,42]:

- Addresses concerns raised by the individual and ensures that the objectives of the visit, even if different from those of the clinician, are consistently being met. Finds out what the patient wants to know. The educator asks the individual directly, "What are your concerns?" and responds directly to the patient regarding the identified concerns.

- Encourages questions. The individual probably has numerous questions related to health care or diabetes concerns. An effective relationship enables and encourages the individual to ask questions. The diabetes educator frequently reinforces asking questions by responding with statements such as, "That's a good question," to support question asking further.
- Presents treatment instructions in a clear, simple manner. The medical language is often complex and technical, and the educator may not realize that individuals may have little understanding of terms such as insulin and hypoglycemia. When a patient uses such terms, the diabetes educator checks to make sure the patient understands the meaning and is not simply repeating jargon.
- Uses concrete advice. The diabetes educator gives detailed, specific advice. For example, the individual should walk for 25 minutes after dinner, as opposed to the individual should take a daily walk. Sensitivity to the timing of the information is noted, with care taken not to overload the learner with information.
- Repeats and stresses the importance of critical components of the advice. The educator reinforces the advice whenever possible with written materials.
- Provides advanced organizers or a brief summary of what is to be said. Explicit categorization is demonstrated when the provider divides the instructions into content categories and announces these before giving the individual diabetes information pertaining to each area. The educator might say, for example, "First I will talk and describe the procedure for foot care, then I will demonstrate, with your assistance."
- Checks the individual's understanding. Persons with diabetes can be asked to demonstrate what they have been shown or asked to restate treatment recommendations.
- Uses a variety of communication channels. Whenever possible, diagrams and models are used. Oral and written materials are also provided (perhaps with simple written instructions that can be taken home).
- Reduces the complexity of the regimen. A substantive amount of evidence indicates that learning and adherence are more likely when the complexity of the regimen is reduced.[32] The diabetes educator asks the individual to make relatively small changes in the beginning. The regimen is then graduated so the treatment is divided into a series of behaviors of increasing difficulty. As the individual achieves behavioral change, components are gradually added, building toward the final regimen. The treatment is tailored to the person's life-style. For example, specific events are anchored around existing routines (e.g., SMBG before brushing teeth).
- Provides feedback. Critical to the feedback process is *how* feedback is provided to the individual. Deci and Ryan[11] suggest two ways in which feedback is most likely given: informational and controlling. *Informational feedback* is perceived by the individual as promoting choice and self-determination while providing information that is useful for a person attempting to interact effectively with the environment. Informational feedback is critical to the goal-setting process in that it implies a mutual agreement for the goal being set and employs the aspect of choice throughout the communication process. *Controlling feedback,* in contrast, implies pressure to achieve a behavioral outcome, often set by the

health care team, as opposed to a mutually agreed-on goal. Controlling feedback also implies a deadline (e.g., you should lose 10 pounds by the next clinic visit, or your glycosylated hemoglobin should be less than 9%). The perception from such communication is that one will feel guilty or incompetent if the goal is not met within the time frame. Such feedback encourages extrinsic motivation, which is less likely to maintain a behavior change.

- Involves significant others whenever possible. Social support is a helpful prerequisite to optimal diabetes care. The involvement of family and significant others in the learning process facilitates environmental adaptations that must frequently be made to accommodate the diabetic regimen.

Self-Assessment

To improve effectiveness in dealing with persons with diabetes, the diabetes educator should periodically evaluate personal teaching skills. One approach that can be implemented on a regular basis is self-assessment. Self-assessment enables the educator to "self-monitor" teaching skills. A format for self-assessment includes the following[10]:

1. *Planning.* Before conducting the educational intervention, ask several questions. What impact will the session have on the individual with diabetes? What should the patient be able to do as a result of the session? What teaching strategies will be used? How will success be measured? What behaviors will the learner exhibit that demonstrate that the teaching experience was successful?
2. *Conduct the session.* Audiotape or videotape the session.
3. *Assessment.* Before reviewing the tape, and as soon after the session as possible, answer the following questions:
   - What is your overall impression of the experience?
   - How do you think the patient felt? Write down some examples that support your interpretation.
   - What went easily? What gave you more difficulty?
   - What, if anything, had you planned or hoped to have happen that did not?
   - If your session did not go as you planned, and if the behavioral objective was not achieved to your satisfaction, try to account for the difference between what you planned and what happened. Focus only on those components that are within your control.
4. *Review the tape.* How similar is what you believed happened to what actually happened? What is different from what you might have expected? Perhaps the individual is being directed by the use of closed instead of open-ended questions, or perhaps some verbal or nonverbal communication is being used that interferes with the establishment of rapport. Maybe the patient is not allowed to express his or her own goals for the session. Finally, what are the problems that are most important to address in improving current teaching skills? Focus on those items first.
5. *Have a colleague review the tape.* To what extent does the colleague validate your assessment?
6. *Identify a strategy for improving your teaching.* Work on one behavior/skill at a time. Schedule additional periods of self-assessment.

SUMMARY

Good diabetes education does not occur by accident. It is the result of time, practice, innovation, and energy on the part of the diabetes team and the individual with diabetes. Models of health behavior provide a foundation on which to organize, apply, and evaluate teaching methodologies. The teaching skills of each of the disciplines, the systematic instruction of the individual, and regular follow-up and evaluation of educational progress are critical to good diabetes education.

REFERENCES

1. American Association of Diabetes Educators and the AADE Education and Research Foundation: Behavioral change. In Peragallo-Dittko V, Godley K, Meyer J, editors: *A core curriculum for diabetes education,* ed 2, Chicago, 1993, AADE.
2. American Association of Diabetes Educators and the AADE Education and Research Foundation: Cultural sensitivity in diabetes education. In Peragallo-Dittko V, Godley K, Meyer J, editors: *A core curriculum for diabetes education,* ed 2, Chicago, 1993, AADE.
3. American Association of Diabetes Educators and the AADE Education and Research Foundation: Educational principles and strategies. In Peragallo-Dittko V, Godley K, Meyer J, editors: *A core curriculum for diabetes education,* ed 2, Chicago, 1993, AADE.
4. American Association of Diabetes Educators and the AADE Education and Research Foundation: Psychosocial assessment and support. In Peragallo-Dittko V, Godley K, Meyer J, editors: *A core curriculum for diabetes education,* ed 2, Chicago, 1993, AADE.
5. Bloom BS, editor: *Taxonomy of educational objectives. Handbook I. Cognitive domain,* New York, 1956, McKay.
6. Boehm-Steckel S: *Patient contracting,* East Norwalk, Conn, 1982, Appleton-CenturyCrofts.
7. Brookfield SD: *Understanding and facilitating adult learning,* San Francisco, 1986, Jossey-Bass.
8. Buckner WP and others, editors: Planned approach to community health (special issue), *J Health Educ* 23(3):131-192, 1992.
9. Centers for Disease Control: *Diabetes today,* National Center for Chronic Disease Prevention and Health Promotion, Atlanta, 1991, US Department of Health and Human Services.
10. Connell K: *Problem solving assessment tool,* Chicago, 1984, Institute for Inquiry in Education (unpublished handout).
11. Deci EL, Ryan RM: *Intrinsic motivation and self-determination in human behavior,* Rochester, NY, 1985, Plenum.
12. Dobson T, Nord W, Haire-Joshu D: The use of goal setting by physicians in the treatment of diabetes, *Diabetes Educ* 15:62-65, 1989.
13. Drury T, Danchik K, Haris M: Sociodemographic characteristics of adult diabetics. In National Diabetes Data Group: *Diabetes in America: diabetes data compiled 1984,* DHHS Pub No (NIH)85-1468, Bethesda, Md, 1985, Public Health Service, National Institutes of Health.
14. Fry EB: Fry's readability graph: clarifications, validity and extension to level 17, *J Read* 21:242-252, 1977.
15. Glanz K, Rimer B: *Theory at a glance: A guide for health promotion practice,* Office of Cancer Communication, Bethesda, Md, 1995, National Cancer Institute.
16. Glasgow RE, Osteen VL: Evaluating diabetes education: are we measuring the most important outcomes? *Diabetes Care* 15(10):1423-1432, 1992, (review).
17. Gottlieb NH, McLeroy KR: Social health. In O'Donnell MP, Harris JS, editors: *Health promotion in the workplace,* ed 2, New York, 1994, Delmar.
18. Gronlund NE: *Measurement and evaluation in teaching,* ed 6, New York, 1990, MacMillan.
19. Hafner L: Cloze procedure, *J Read* 9:415-421, 1966.
20. Haire-Joshu D: Nursing care of adults with disorders of the pancreas. In Beare PG, Meyer JL: *Principles and practice of adult health nursing,* ed 2, St Louis, 1995, Mosby.
21. Heins JM and others: The Americans with Disabilities Act and diabetes, *Diabetes Care* 17(5):453, 1994.
22. Hochbaum GM, Sorenson JR, Lorig K: Theory in health education practice, *Health Educ Q* 19(3):295-313, 1992.
23. Janz NK, Becker MN, Hartman PA: Contingency contracting to enhance patient compliance: a review, *Patient Educ Counsel* 5:165-178, 1984.
24. Jenny J: Knowledge deficit: instructional or behavioral diagnosis? *Patient Educ Counsel* 11:91-93, 1988.
25. Klare GR: Assessing readability, *Read Res Q* 10:62-102, 1974.
26. Krathwohl DR, Bloom BS, Masia BB: *Taxonomy of*

educational objectives. Handbook II. Affective domain, New York, 1964, McKay.

27. Kurtz SMS: Adherence to diabetes regimens, empirical status and clinical applications, *Diabetes Educ* 16:50-56, 1990.

28. Mager RF: *Preparing instructional objectives,* Belmont Calif, 1975, Fearon.

29. McLaughlin GH: SMOG grading: a new readability formula, *J Read* 12:639-646, 1969.

30. McLeroy KR and others: An ecological perspective on health promotion programs, *Health Educ Q* 15(4):351-377, 1988.

31. Mehrens WA, Lehmann IJ: *Measurement and evaluation in education and psychology,* ed 3, New York, 1984, Holt, Rinehart and Winston.

32. Meichenbaum D, Turk DC: Enhancing the relationship between the patient and health care provider. In Meichenbaum D, Turk DC, editors: *Facilitating treatment adherence: a practitioner's guidebook,* New York, 1987, Plenum.

33. Muhlhauser I, Berger M: Diabetes education and insulin therapy: when will they ever learn? *J Intern Med* 233(4):321-326, 1993.

34. Mullen PD, Hersey JC, Iverson DC: Health behavior models compared, *Soc Sci Med* 24(11):973-981, 1987.

35. Overland JE and others: Low literacy: a problem in diabetes education, *Diabetic Med* 10(9):847-850, 1993.

36. Padgett D and others: Meta-analysis of the effects of educational and psychosocial interventions on management of diabetes mellitus, *J Clin Epidemiol* 41:1007-1030, 1988.

37. Perry CL, Baranowski T, Parcel GS: How individuals, environments, and health behaviors interact: social learning theory. In Glanz K, Lewis FM, Rimer BK, editors: *Health behavior and health education:* theory, research, and practice, San Francisco, 1990, Jossey-Bass.

38. Peyrot M, McMurry JF: Psychosocial factors in diabetes control: adjustment of insulin-dependent adults, *Psychosom Med* 47:542-557, 1985.

39. Pichert JW: Teaching strategies for effective nutrition. In Powers MA, editor: *Handbook of diabetes nutritional management,* Rockville, Md, 1987, Aspen.

40. Prochaska JO, DiClemente CC: Stages and pro-

cesses of self-change of smoking: toward an integrative model of change, *J Consult Clin Psychol* 51:390-395, 1983.

41. Prochaska JO, DiClemente CC, Norcross JC: In search of how people change: applications to addictive behaviors, *Am Psychol* 47:1102-1014, 1992.

42. Redhead J and others: The effectiveness of a primary-care-based diabetes education service, *Diabetic Med* 10(7):672-675, 1993.

43. Rogers EM: *Diffusion of innovation,* ed 3, New York, 1983, Free Press.

44. Rosenstock IM: The Health Belief Model: explaining health behavior through expectancies. In Glanz K, Lewis FM, Rimer BK, editors: *Health behavior and health education: theory, research, and practice,* San Francisco, 1990, Jossey-Bass.

45. Roter DL, Hall JA, Katz NR: Patient-physician communication: a descriptive summary of the literature, *Patient Educ Counsel* 12:99-119, 1988.

46. Rothman J: Three models of community organization practice. In Cox FM and others, editors: *Strategies of community organization,* ed 2, Itasca, Ill, 1970, Peacock.

47. Ruby KL and others: The knowledge and practices of registered nurse, certified diabetes educators: teaching elderly clients about exercise, *Diabetes Educ* 19(4):299-306, 1993.

48. Stracqualursi F and others: Assessing and implementing diabetes patient education programs for American Indian communities, *Diabetes Educ* 19(1):31-34, 1993.

49. Street RL Jr and others: Provider-patient communication and metabolic control, *Diabetes Care* 16(5): 714-721, 1993.

50. Taylor WS: Cloze procedure: a new test for measuring readability, *Journalism Q* 30:415-433, 1953.

51. Thompson A, Gibbon C: Setting standards in diabetes education, *Nurs Standard* 7(43):25-28, 1993.

52. Van Ryn M, Heaney CA: What's the use of theory? *Health Educ Q* 19(3):315-330, 1992.

53. Wing RL and others: Behavioral self-regulation in the treatment of patients with diabetes mellitus, *Psychol Bull* 99:78-89, 1986.

16 Systematic Evaluation of Diabetes Self-Management Programs

Debra Haire-Joshu

Evaluation is a critical component of diabetes practice that can be defined as a continuous and systematic process underlying all teaching and learning. Evaluation delineates, obtains, and provides useful information for defining decision alternatives and determines congruence between performance and objectives.[11,18] Evaluation is a means of determining the degree of success in achieving a predetermined objective and comparing an objective of interest against a level of acceptability.[23]

One measures or evaluates characteristics of people, such as their knowledge of diabetes and their willingness to perform certain aspects of the regimen. Alternately, one might measure properties of programs, such as content, materials, and effectiveness. Research methods are a crucial component of evaluation, as depicted in carefully selected data-gathering designs.

CHAPTER OBJECTIVES

- Define evaluation.
- Discuss the general principles of evaluation.
- Compare formative and summative evaluations.
- Discuss evaluation of process, outcome, and efficiency.
- Describe the steps of a systematic program evaluation.
- Explain the various components of program evaluation.
- Analyze various data collection techniques.
- Compare the concepts of reliability and validity.
- Discuss the role of data-gathering design as a component of evaluation.
- Contrast experimental and nonexperimental data-gathering designs.
- Summarize the characteristics of programs with high-quality evaluations.

These designs yield data that assist the evaluation by the health care provider in understanding the learner, planning the learning experiences, and determining the extent to which the instruction and objectives are being achieved in the program. The need for such data is critical to the quality assurance of diabetes self-management, as dictated by the National Standards for Diabetes Patient Education and the American Diabetes Association Review Criteria (see Appendix G).[20] Evaluation provides a dependable basis for making judgments about the teaching/learning process and the effectiveness of the educational program.[17] It also produces a diabetes self-management program that is flexible enough to meet the needs of the individual with diabetes.

The purpose of this chapter is to describe components of a *systematic program evaluation* and its relationship to diabetes self-management. Evaluation of the individual and professional is addressed as *components* of overall programmatic evaluation. However, these components are critical to the comprehensive programmatic evaluation.

DEFINITION OF EVALUATION

Evaluation is the systematic application of procedures for assessing the conceptualization, design, implementation, and use of interventions and intervention programs. Evaluations answer such questions as, What is the nature and scope of the problem? Whom does it affect? What interventions are likely to ameliorate the problem? Is the intervention reaching its target population? Is the intervention implemented in the way planned? and Is it effective in terms of the cost/benefit ratio?[23]

GENERAL PRINCIPLES OF EVALUATION

Several critical principles are associated with evaluation and have been identified by numerous sources. In general, Gronlund[11] summarizes these principles as follows:

1. Evaluation is the process of delineating, obtaining, and providing useful information for judging decision alternatives that underlie all teaching and learning.[8,14] Without evaluation, it is difficult to empirically establish the level at which diabetes programs work. Data from program evaluations are thus necessary if one is to validate programmatic impacts.

2. Comprehensive evaluation requires a variety of evaluation measures. The use of multiple measures in evaluating all aspects of a diabetes self-management program (e.g., teaching skills, educational materials, program effectiveness) ensures that the first principle of evaluation, the delineation of useful information, is met. No single evaluation measure is adequate for appraising the impact of program components on an individual's progress toward all the important outcomes of instruction.[12,23] Most evaluation measures are rather limited in scope, providing unique but focused evidence on some aspect of the behavior of the individual with diabetes. For example, an objective test of factual knowledge regarding diabetes provides important evidence concerning an individual's knowledge but little evidence concerning how attitudes are changing, how he or she will perform in an actual situation requiring application of knowledge, or what influence knowledge might have on personal adjustment. Another example might be the use of glycohemoglobin as a means of documenting metabolic control.

This is an accurate laboratory measure of metabolic control but provides little direct information about subjects such as the individual's knowledge, self-management techniques, or attitudes toward diabetes.

3. Even the best evaluation measures fall short of the precision one would like them to have. The care with which the health care provider ensures the reliability of laboratory measures and the accuracy of results is justified, as in any use of educational/behavioral measures.

4. Evaluation is a means to an end, not an end in itself. Too frequently the purpose of the evaluation is lost while extensive amounts of data are gathered. Ultimately, these data are probably filed away with the hope that someday this information will prove worthwhile. Such data-gathering activities are wasteful of both the professional's and the individual's time and effort. One means of avoiding the trap of collecting "everything" and using "nothing" is to view program evaluation as a systematic process of obtaining information on which to base *decisions*. This implies that the types of decisions to be made will be identified before the evaluation procedures are selected and that no evaluation procedure will be used unless it contributes to improved decisions of an instructional nature.[11]

Overview of Program Evaluation

Program evaluations are done for a variety of reasons and occur at various times. *When* the evaluation takes place often characterizes the general philosophy as to *why* the evaluation is being conducted. Common categories include formative and summative evaluations. The categories clarify purpose and lend further guidance to the selection of materials, techniques, and tasks for conducting the evaluation.[11,18]

Formative evaluations

Formative evaluations are designed to help develop the programs themselves. These evaluations focus on tasks associated with program planning, development, and pretesting as a means of guiding the design process. Formative evaluations are a systematic collection of data used to construct a profile of the learning program and to obtain feedback that allows ongoing modification of the program. Many programs fail because insufficient time and resources were invested in formative efforts either in the design phase or during early periods of operations. Formative evaluations may include pilot testing and assessing a diabetes program at one or a few sites before full implementation.[11,18,23]

Health care providers may use the formative approach as part of the decision-making process during routine education. An individual's progress is assessed so that a determination can be made as to the immediate learning and clinical needs. Feedback to the individual provides reinforcement for successful learning and identifies the specific learning errors that need correction (e.g., accurate injection procedures). Feedback to the team provides information for modifying diabetes information and providing additional assistance in the form of referrals to community programs. Formative evaluation depends heavily on specifically prepared evaluative procedures for each segment of instruction. Decisions made as a result of formative evaluation are likely to address staffing, activities, organization, and

Table 16-1 Categories of Evaluation

Formative evaluation	Summative evaluation
General purpose	
How can the diabetes program be improved?	Is the diabetes program worth continuing or expanding?
How can it become more efficient or effective?	What conclusions can be made about the effects of the diabetes program or its various components?
Types of questions answered	
What are the goals and objectives of the diabetes program?	What are the goals and objectives of the diabetes program?
What are the program's most important characteristics: materials, staffing, activities, administrative arrangements?	What are the program's most important characteristics: activities, services, staffing, administrative arrangements?
How are the program's activities supposed to lead to attainment of the objectives?	Does the program lead to goal achievement?
Are the program's important characteristics being implemented?	How effective is the diabetes program compared with alternative programs?
Are the program's components contributing to achievement of the objectives?	
Which activities or combinations best accomplish each objective?	
What adjustments in the program's management and support might lead to better attainment of the objectives?	
Is the program, or some aspect of it, better suited to certain types of participants?	Is the program differentially effective with particular types of participants and in particular locales?
What problems exist and how can they be solved?	How costly is the program?
What measures and designs could be recommended for use during summative evaluation of the diabetes program?	

Modified from Herman J, Morris L, Fitz-Gibbon C: *Evaluator's handbook,* Newbury Park, Calif, 1987, Sage.

other materials of the program.[12] Table 16-1 lists sample questions that might be asked as a component of formative evaluation.

Summative evaluations

Summative evaluations help to determine whether a program should be started, continued, or chosen from among alternatives. Summative evaluations have a sense of finality; a program might end depending on the outcome of the evaluation. Examples of summative evaluations include a postprogram evaluation that generally occurs immediately after a formal program, or at 6- and 12-month intervals, to assess impact. Decisions associated with summative evaluation are more likely to reflect whether a program should continue or be discontinued, or whether to expand or reduce it.[11,18] Table 16-1 lists questions answered by a summative evaluation.

Types of Evaluations

The type of evaluation is characterized by its focus or scope. Several types of evaluation are pertinent to diabetes self-management programs. These include an evaluation of need, or needs assessment; process evaluation or program monitoring; outcome or impact evaluation; and efficiency.[23]

An *evaluation of need* is frequently the first step in program development or design and typically is a component of formative evaluation. Needs assessment is a component not only of evaluation but also of planning. Such an assessment provides information as to the need *for* the program and the needs *of* the program.

Process evaluation is also referred to in terms of *program monitoring.* To manage and administer a program properly, a means must exist for identifying, quantifying, and qualifying what was done. Program monitoring is a means of providing systematic assessment of whether or not a program is operating in conformity to its design and is reaching its specific target population. To what extent is the diabetes program implemented as designed and serving the target group?[23]

A third type of evaluation is *outcome evaluation,* or *program impact.* This type of evaluation provides information about the extent to which a program produces the desired outcome. For example, an impact assessment might compare a new diabetes program with a standard program to determine the extent to which the new program improves diabetes knowledge and control. In this instance, evaluation focuses on the immediate impact of the program or some aspect of it, particularly as it affects the individual. Have short-term goals been met? Is a health risk to the person with diabetes reduced? Has detection or treatment changed as a result of this program?[23]

Program efficiency assesses the benefit of the program in relation to costs (cost-benefit versus cost-effectiveness analyses). Such an evaluation provides a systematic means of addressing both costs and benefits of any program, identifying and comparing the actual or anticipated costs with the known or expected beneficial outcomes. Since many programs operate under financial constraints, such evaluations are invaluable. Frequently, efficiency analyses can be considered an extension of, rather than an alternative to, impact or outcome evaluations.[6,25]

Examples of each of the types of evaluation follow. Staff members of an outpatient diabetes clinic are concerned about a recent increase in diabetic foot ulcers. They perceive that adequate information regarding foot care is not being appropriately delivered to patients and want to institute a foot care and education program. To verify the problem, an evaluation of need would first be conducted. Patients might be surveyed about current knowledge of foot care procedures, where this information was obtained, and interest in additional types of information. If a need is determined, an intervention that draws from the current literature (e.g., foot care video shown in waiting room) would be developed and conducted. A process evaluation would determine whether the film was shown, how frequently, how many patients should have seen the film, and how many actually were present when the film was shown. Such an evaluation would also validate reasons the film was not shown. The impact evaluation would be a measure of how many individuals with diabetes who were sitting in the waiting room can recall the specifics of the film demonstration and can demonstrate foot care. This evaluation would focus on increased self-reporting of foot examinations. Finally, the program efficiency would be evaluated in terms of cost of staff time and equipment needed to show the film versus its impact on improved foot care. Was the benefit of decreased clinic visits for foot problems among individuals who viewed the film equal to or greater than the financial costs of such an intervention?

Tailoring Evaluations

Evaluations need to be tailored to meet the needs of the diabetes program. Evaluations will vary depending on whether the program is new or innovative, an established program being evaluated, or a program that is in place but being modified or "fine-tuned."[23] Evaluations of new programs generally are undertaken to determine the program's impact and efficiency. Such evaluations frequently require program staff and sponsors to rethink some of the program aspects. Existing programs almost always are difficult to evaluate in terms of their impact and efficiency. The evaluation is limited to assessing the extent that the program objectives are relevant to the interests of program sponsors, staff, and others and to assessing whether or not the program is conforming to plans and reaching the target audience.

Modification or fine-tuning of diabetes programs is a common practice. These evaluations frequently result in redefining the target population, changing the delivery system, or otherwise modifying the program to increase its effectiveness, efficiency, or both. Evaluations of efforts to modify programs often resemble those of new programs in that impact assessment is emphasized.[23] Table 16-2 summarizes tailoring aspects of evaluations.

A MODEL OF SYSTEMATIC PROGRAM EVALUATION

Any program evaluation will generally include the formulation of the objective(s), identification of the criteria to be used in measuring success, and determination and explanation of the degree of success.[10,26] More detailed steps, as depicted in Fig. 16-1, are guided by these general characteristics.

Step 1: Who Is Involved

Relevant persons who are involved with and impacted by the diabetes self-management program should participate in the evaluation.[9] In particular, members of the multidisciplinary diabetes team are critical to involve in the evaluation. Various persons who might participate or become interested in the evaluation process and its results include the following[23]:

1. *Policymakers and decision makers:* persons responsible for deciding whether a diabetes program is to be continued, discontinued, expanded, or curtailed

Table 16-2   Tailoring Program Evaluations for Diabetes Care

Evaluating new and innovative programs	Evaluating established programs	Modifying or fine-tuning programs
Conceptualizing		
1. Defining and describing diabetes program	1. Determining evaluability	1. Identifying needed diabetes program changes
2. Operationalizing objectives	2. Developing evaluation model	2. Redefining objectives
3. Developing intervention model	3. Identifying potential for modification	3. Designing program modifications
4. Defining extent and distribution of target population	4. Determining accountability or evaluation criteria	
5. Specifying delivery system		
Implementing		
1. Performing formative research and development	1. Implementing process evaluation or program monitoring	1. Doing research and developing refinements
2. Monitoring	2. Performing accountability studies	2. Monitoring program changes
Assessing		
1. Doing impact studies	1. Doing impact studies	1. Doing impact studies
2. Performing efficiency studies	2. Performing efficiency studies	2. Performing efficiency studies

Modified from Rossi P, Freeman H: *Evaluation: a systematic approach,* Newbury Park, Calif, 1993, Sage.

2. *Program sponsors:* organizations that initiate and fund the diabetes program to be evaluated
3. *Evaluation sponsors:* organizations that initiate and fund the evaluation of the diabetes program
4. *Target participants:* individuals with diabetes, families, or others who participate in the program or receive the services being evaluated
5. *Program management:* the group responsible for overseeing and coordinating the program
6. *Program staff:* health care providers responsible for actual delivery of the program
7. *Evaluators:* groups or individuals who are responsible for the design and who conduct the evaluation
8. *Community:* persons from the community who can pass judgment on program value

When conducting a program evaluation, one would include members of the diabetes self-management team and members of the organizational staff not directly associated with the program. In addition, it is often appropriate to involve statistical and administrative personnel in the evaluation process. Finally, individuals with diabetes who are affected by the

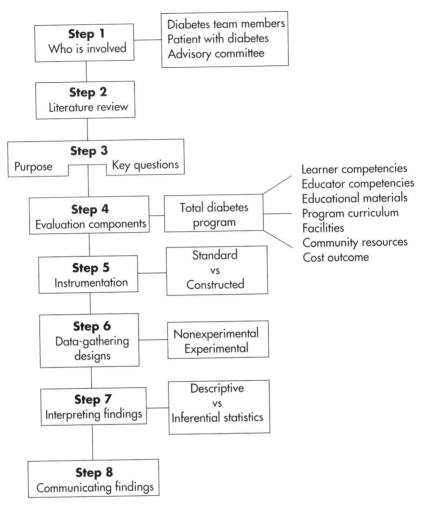

Fig. 16-1 A model of systematic evaluation.

program should be represented in any evaluative procedure, since they are the ones most affected by changes. The formation of an advisory committee is an effective strategy for incorporating multiple views.

Step 2: Literature Review

An examination of previous evaluations that have been conducted assists in determining the most effective means for conducting the current evaluation, as well as familiarizing the evaluation team with the state of the literature in their area.[9] The literature review identifies the measures developed or used, how reliable those measures are, the findings, the issues that were or were not addressed, and potential resources for consulting assistance with the current planned evaluation. Just as importantly, the literature review should provide the theoretic background for conducting the evaluation. An understanding of the theory that guides any interventions is critical to all aspects of evaluation, including selection of measures and interpretation of findings.

Step 3: Purpose and Key Questions

A major initial task of any evaluation is to identify the purpose and key evaluation questions that are to be answered. The evaluation's purpose can most succinctly be defined as "who wants to know what and why." The answer to this question clarifies for the provider and any other members of the evaluation team what is being undertaken.[31]

The purpose statement gives direction to the evaluation process.[12,14,23] Examples of an evaluation's purpose might be the following:
- To determine the effectiveness of the outpatient diabetes self-management curriculum
- To determine the availability of community resources
- To determine the cost-effectiveness of a diabetes program

The key evaluation questions are drawn from the evaluation's purpose. The key questions serve to focus specifically the evaluation from the purpose statement down to the individual parts or segment of the component being evaluated.[12,23] Some examples of key questions follow:
- Is the learning module of a dietary education component more efficient than the traditional, didactic approach?
- Is a comprehensive listing of community resources used by the diabetes program?
- What is the average cost spent on educational materials for the diabetes program?

Step 4: Evaluation Components

Program evaluation is a comprehensive assessment of effectiveness in obtaining program objectives.[12,14,23] The following list, not intended to be all inclusive, identifies some of the core components critical to any program evaluation.[4]

1. *Learner competencies.* Does systematic diabetes self-management demonstrate significant improvements in learner knowledge, skills, and self-care behaviors across the life span?[3] Evaluation of diabetes education includes information specific to what one wants the learner to know by program conclusion:
- What can the learner and the learner's family expect to receive from the diabetes self-management program?
- Does a list of behavioral objectives guide the learning experience for the individual with diabetes?
- Are educational assessment techniques thorough and conducted with regularity?
- How are basic and more complex skills assessed?
- What are the strengths and weaknesses of the individual with diabetes with regard to learning, and how can the diabetes health care team meet these needs?
- Is there a documented learning plan to assist in meeting the needs of the individual with diabetes?

2. *Educator competencies.* Extensive work has been done in identifying the key skills associated with good teaching (see Chapter 15).[2,5,22] Evaluation of these skills is critical to program effectiveness. The diabetes educator needs to be carefully and regularly evaluated as to teaching skills and competency. As addressed in Chapter 15, self-assessment is one means of evaluating teaching. Other methods include peer or learner evaluation of the educator. Such information needs to focus on skills related to comprehensive teaching ability, including ability to develop or plan programs, command of subject, and effectiveness of teaching techniques.[30] Other questions related to the evaluation process include the following:

- How frequently has the health care provider been evaluated by a peer or person with diabetes regarding teaching skills?
- Does the diabetes educator effectively implement the teaching/learning process?
- How thoroughly does the diabetes educator assess the learner?
- How recently has the diabetes educator attended continuing education courses or sought additional formal instruction?
- What evidence shows that the professional alters practice based on new information?

3. *Educational materials.* Instructional materials are tools or aids that facilitate the learning process and are products of the diabetes self-management program. These include both print and nonprint products, such as films, transparencies, brochures, or pamphlets. These materials should meet standards for use that are appropriate to the individual with diabetes. To determine appropriateness, one must assess the means of identifying seldom-used media, outdated or inadequate media, or new materials.[7,13,15,19] To secure consistent and objective data, information as to effectiveness of the materials should be carefully documented on evaluation forms, an example of which appears in Box 16-1. Such a form can be modified to reflect the particular specifics of other educational materials.

Other questions that should be considered when evaluating materials include:

- Is the learner involved in the evaluation of the instructional aids?
- What measures are used to evaluate the materials?
- How is this information analyzed and summarized?
- How is the diabetes team made aware of current materials?
- Is there an ongoing procedure for discarding inappropriate materials and piloting new materials?
- How are decisions made to purchase materials?

4. *Program curriculum.* The program curriculum reflects the overall organization and implementation of all components of diabetes self-management. Questions include:

- How is the curriculum sequenced?
- How is it determined that the goals of the individual with diabetes were or were not achieved?
- What is the impact of the program on persons other than the individual with diabetes (e.g., family members)?
- Is there accurate compilation of formative and summative evaluation data?

5. *Evaluation of facilities.* Location and adequacy of space for teaching/learning are

---

BOX 16-1

PROGRAMMED INSTRUCTIONAL MATERIALS EVALUATION FORM

Reviewer's name _____

Review date _____

Title _____

Source _____

Date of publication _____

Type of material (e.g., book, video, self-study module) _____

_____

_____

General criteria	Yes	No
Is this material congruent with course or program objectives?	___	___
Is the material technologically accurate?	___	___
Is the material up to date?	___	___
Is the material free from racial and sexual bias?	___	___
Is the reading level appropriate to grade level of users?	___	___
What is the cost of the materials? _____		

Appraisal of content and organization	Poor		Average		Excellent
Clarity of instructions to learner	0	1	2	3	4
Sequence of information	0	1	2	3	4
Continuous involvement of learner	0	1	2	3	4
Allows response from learner	0	1	2	3	4
Material can be easily pretested	0	1	2	3	4
Material is relevant to subject	0	1	2	3	4
Program sets desired goal for learner	0	1	2	3	4
Repetition of material	0	1	2	3	4
Availability of cues	0	1	2	3	4

Technical quality

Printing	0	1	2	3	4
Photography	0	1	2	3	4
Sound	0	1	2	3	4

Composite rating _____

Evaluation comments:

General course information		Cost information						
1	2	3	4	5	6	7	8	9
Diabetes self-management program components	Number of patients	Equip-ment	Supplies	Books	Media	Travel	Other	Total

Fig. 16-2   Educator/cost data instrument.

important program components. Questions to be addressed in any program evaluation include:

- What data are available regarding adequacy of existing facilities?
- Is there a need for renovation of facilities or modernization?
- What are the priorities for space?
- More specifically, is there available space to conduct diabetes self-management classes adequately?

6. *Referral and use of community resources.*

- Are there adequate and available community resources to facilitate additional diabetes education?
- Is there a comprehensive listing of available resources for use by individuals with diabetes?
- How are the resources evaluated, and is this evaluation ongoing?
- How much communication occurs between the community resources and the diabetes program?

7. *Cost outcome evaluation.* The cost outcome analysis is crucial to making resource allocation decisions, providing accountability indices, and determining the advisability of financing the development of new programs.[1,6,25,28] Information is provided related to the efficacy of a program or intervention in achieving a given outcome in relation to the program costs.[23] It also provides information as to ways of decreasing the costs of the program and provides assistance in choosing among instructional alternatives. A major area of concern includes how frequently the provider collects cost data on all aspects of the program (e.g., salary, instructional materials expenditure, equipment, travel, administrative costs, community service costs, capital outlay, including fixed building costs). Fig. 16-2 provides a sample of a cost summary data sheet that might be used to record pertinent information.

BOX 16-2

SAMPLE DATA COLLECTION TECHNIQUES

Interviews

Interviews can be structured with a form or interview schedule that specifies the questions to be asked of each respondent. Interviews can also be open ended, with the use of a topical outline that guides the interviewer in knowing what areas should be probed. The interview can be conducted face to face or by telephone.

Questionnaires

Questionnaires are printed forms designed to collect information and judgments from respondents. They can include many different types of items, including checklists, graphic rating scales, multiple-choice items, numeric rating scales, and matching items. Questionnaires can be administered by mail or distributed personally. In either case a strong follow-up effort is essential to ensure an adequate, representative response.

Chart review

Chart review/audit involves the analysis of already-existing information that may be of secondary use. It can be done formally using checklists or other structured instruments.

Testing

The administration of patient tests can provide valuable information. Testing can focus on cognitive, affective, and psychomotor behaviors. Instruments used in testing can include paper-and-pencil tests, inventories, simulation tests, and performance tests.

Observation

Observations can provide descriptive information regarding the way something is constructed or behaves. Observations can be unstructured or structured through a special recording form. Observations can be open, secret, or visually recorded.

Modified from Shea ML, Boyum PG, Spanke MM: In *Clinical evaluation: theory and practice in health occupations,* Springfield, Ill, 1985, Illinois State Board of Education.

Step 5: Instrumentation

Instrumentation is the process of selecting or developing methods appropriate for measuring specific objectives.[12] One of the most challenging but vulnerable aspects of the evaluation process is the measurement of the variables. Multiple types of measurement provide more assurances that the measures are accurately quantifying the variable in question. For example, the health care team might use a variety of techniques to determine the type of information the learner should receive, including pretests on diabetes information, self-report inventories, and observational techniques. Box 16-2 lists other techniques of data collection.

What is measured?

What is measured is determined by the evaluation question. However, just as objectives can be classified according to a taxonomy of behavioral outcomes (as described in Chapter 15), so can measurement devices.[11,18] Cognitive instruments are tests of a participant's knowledge of or achievement in a specific content area. They can be used to assess the accomplishment of objectives before and after an educational program. Cognitive measures are the most frequently used types of instruments and often are written tests (e.g., diabetes patient knowledge tests).[27]

Affective measures seek to determine interests, values, and attitudes. Such measures are important if the evaluation question focuses on programmatic impact on the participant's attitude toward diabetes. The most direct approach to determining the patient's attitude is to ask the individual with diabetes directly about his or her attitudes or interests. Self-report inventories are designed to yield measures of adjustment, appreciation, attitudes, interest, temperament, and so forth and may provide an indicator of change in affective behavior. Another means of determining affective change is to conduct interviews or engage in role-playing activities.[27]

Psychomotor measures are generally focused toward performance of a skill and typically reflect task analysis procedures.[27] The particular task is broken down into individual steps, with an observer evaluating the individual's performance at each step. An example of this would be evaluation of the individual with diabetes performing an insulin injection.

Who constructs the measurement instrument?

Standardized measures are typically developed for wide use in the measurement of specific constructs. For example, norms regarding general knowledge tests are established and generally available. However, standardized measures for the evaluation of components of diabetes self-management programs are not typically available, and the diabetes team must construct or supplement instruments in an effort to measure the program outcome in question.[11,18]

Various sources are available that detail the methods for constructing measures.[12,23] In general, however, the process includes developing items that adequately assess the attainment of the given behavioral or programmatic objectives. The objectives and their proposed measurement techniques should be reviewed carefully by other educators and members of the health care team to ensure comprehensive inclusion of all data needed for accurate measurement. The instrument is then revised based on suggestions by the reviewers. After revision, the educator should pilot the instrument on a small group of individuals closely related to the ones who will be using the measure on a regular basis. Feedback from these groups is very helpful in further refining the measure. Determination of reliability and validity of the measure, as described next, is also necessary.

How reliable is the measure?

Reliability refers to consistency in measurement.[18] Factors that affect this consistency include the manner in which the measure is coded, characteristics of the measure itself, the physical state of the learner at measurement time, and properties of the situation in which the measure is administered, such as the room. For example, one would expect that glycohemoglobin reflects an accurate reading of metabolic control from one time of measurement to another. A paper-and-pencil measure of diabetes knowledge should also reflect an accurate measure of knowledge from one time to another.

Reliability refers to *results* obtained with an instrument and not to the instrument itself. Reliability is primarily statistica! in nature, with analysis of test results providing information as to how reliable the measure is. All measures should undergo testing for reliability. Table 16-3 describes some of the more common tests.

The degree of reliability required depends on the planned use of the measure. How confident does the group need to be with their results? If they are measuring blood glucose level, they would want a reliability of *at least* 95%, since they need to be very confident in how the individual with diabetes is progressing physically in terms of his or her diabetes. If evaluators are measuring attitudes toward diabetes care, they may be willing to accept a reliability of 80%. The most important consideration is that, *if reliability is low, one must not treat the scores as highly accurate.*[18] Factors that may also influence decisions regarding reliability include the ease of administration, the time required for administration, and the ease of scoring and interpretation.

How valid is the measure?

Validity refers to the extent to which the results of an evaluation serve the uses for which they are intended. If the results are to determine the individual's attitude toward diabetes, evaluators need to be sure they are not measuring knowledge instead. As previously noted, reliability refers to the consistency of evaluation results. If evaluators obtain similar scores over time, they are somewhat confident that the measure is reliable. However, validity indicates that they *do* measure what they say is being measured. In short, they can have a very reliable measure, but it may have low validity.[18,23]

Several characteristics are associated with validity. First, validity pertains to the results of a test and not to the instrument itself. Second, validity is a matter of *degree;* it is *not* present

Table 16-3   Methods of Estimating Reliability

Type	Reliability measure	Procedure
Test-retest method	Measure of stability	Give the same test twice to the same group with any time interval between tests, from several minutes to several years.
Alternate-forms method	Measure of equivalence	Give two forms of the test to the same group in close succession.
Test-retest with equivalent forms	Measure of stability and equivalence	Give two forms of the test to the same group with increased time interval between forms.

Modified from Gronlund NE: *Measurement and evaluation in teaching,* ed 3, New York, 1976, MacMillan.

on an all-or-none basis. Finally, validity is always specific to some particular use and is not a general quality. For example, a test may be a valid measure of cognitive knowledge of diabetes but not of psychomotor knowledge.

There are three basic types of validity: content, criterion related, and construct[11,18] (Table 16-4).

Step 6: Data-Gathering Designs

Data-gathering designs are the methods used to test the effectiveness of the intervention or the program. These designs are used for *all* components of program evaluation. For example, at its simplest level, evaluating a specific program component, a data-gathering design may be used to assess the effectiveness of an educator's teaching protocol before and after completion of a self-assessment protocol. At a more complex programmatic level, a specific data-gathering design may be used as a means of testing the effectiveness of a hospital-based diabetes self-management program versus a peer-based program. In either case the design selected will depend primarily on the evaluation's purpose.

This selection of design is influenced by a number of support factors, including the following:

- Who is available to conduct or coordinate the evaluation.
- Amount of money available for consultation time, computer time, and instrument development.
- Effort of the individual required to obtain the needed data.
- Size of the program to be studied.

Table 16-4   Types of Validity

Type	Meaning	Procedure
Content	How well the test measures the subject matter content and behaviors under consideration	Compare test content to the content and behaviors to be measured.
Criterion related: Another validity obtained	How well test performance predicts future performance or estimates current performance on some valued measure other than the test itself	Compare test scores: With measure of performance at a later date (for prediction)
or Concurrently		With another measure of performance obtained (for estimating present status)
Construct	How test performance can be described psychologically	Experimentally determine factors that influence scores on the test.

Modified from Gronlund NE: *Measurement and evaluation in teaching,* ed 3, New York, 1976, MacMillan.

Two of the major differences among data-gathering designs are whether they are experimental or nonexperimental.[14] *Nonexperimental designs* provide an accurate description of what exists in the particular program or how one factor corresponds with another in the program (e.g., counseling is related positively to lower glycohemoglobin). These are frequently used when external financial support for program evaluation is not available. *Experimental designs* are generally conducted as a part of evaluation research and are usually reserved for those situations in which it is possible to randomize subjects to treatment, a control group is desired or necessary, or cause-and-effect relationships are of interest. Such designs are frequently supported with funds specific to program evaluation activities. For the purposes of this chapter, nonexperimental and experimental designs are generally discussed and characterized as to major differences and feasibility with regard to program evaluation. More detailed information can be attained by reviewing various resources cited in the References.

Nonexperimental designs

The simplest and often most practical evaluation designs are nonexperimental designs, which are frequently used by diabetes educators.

Single-group posttest design. The single-group posttest design (Fig. 16-3) identifies a single point during which program participants complete the selected measure. For example,

Single-Group Posttest Design

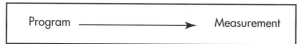

Single-Group Pretest-Posttest Design

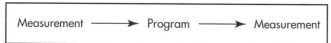

Nonequivalent Control Group Design

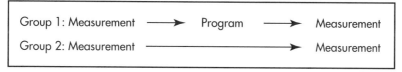

Nonequivalent Comparison Group Design

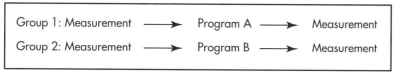

Fig. 16-3   Nonexperimental designs.

if this design were used at the conclusion of a diabetes self-management program, one could characterize the knowledge, attitudes, or beliefs of the participants regarding diabetes care. However, it would be impossible to state how much change there had been in these variables as a result of the program, since only a one-time postmeasure was used.[9]

Single-group pretest-posttest design. The addition of a pretest before the initiation of a program lends strength to findings by providing data as to what changes have occurred. Although this design is stronger than the single-group posttest design, however, it does not enable the diabetes educator to attribute any change to the program.[14] Such a design provides evidence of some type of relationship between the program and behavior change, but one cannot say this relationship is causal, only that it is present. The best example of this is the maturation that occurs in children during a given period. With a diabetes program, such maturation may be the factor that most impacts attitudes toward diabetes.[26]

Nonequivalent control group design. One way of accounting for rival explanations that may limit the strength of findings in the single-group pretest-posttest design is to add a control group.[14] The control group comprises persons who have not received the program that is being offered. In other words, the control group is untreated. An example of this would be if the provider measured knowledge of individuals who have received diabetes education with those who have not yet received the education. The advantage to such a design is that it enables the diabetes educator to say, with more confidence, what the impact this component of the program had on a specific group of subjects.

Nonequivalent comparison group design. This design allows the diabetes educator to compare one program to another[14] (see Fig. 16-3). Such a comparison may assist in determining which program components are more effective. For example, if a diabetes educator is comparing the impact of group versus individual education, one might use this design.

Controlled experimental designs

Data-gathering designs that require *randomization* of subjects to either a control/usual care or intervention/experimental condition promote equivalence between groups. This facilitates the likelihood that any significant differences between groups will be related to the program being offered. Such designs include randomization as a component and are most frequently used in evaluation research.[14]

Randomization procedures allow the generalization of findings to other programs or to a larger population and are therefore an important aspect of evaluation research. In simple random sampling, each and every unit of the study (e.g., all persons with diabetes) has an equal and independent chance of being selected for study. Thus, by chance, one can assume persons with diabetes selected to be evaluated are representative of the entire group of persons with diabetes. Two examples of these designs follow.

Pretest-posttest control group design. Randomization occurs in this design, ensuring that each individual could have been assigned to either the experimental or the control group[14] (Fig. 16-4). Final assignment to a group depends on chance alone. For example, 100 individuals with diabetes attending a program have an equal chance of being assigned to a control group, receiving the usual brochure information on diet and diabetes, or to an experimental group, in which they receive information from a dietitian. Any differences

Pretest-Posttest Control Group Design

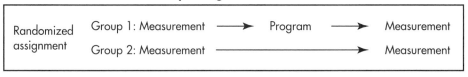

Pretest-Posttest Comparison Group Design

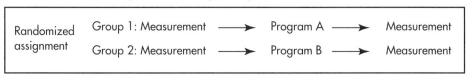

Fig. 16-4   Experimental designs.

between groups, as established by comparing the pretest and posttest scores, have a significant chance of being caused by the intervention.

Pretest-posttest comparison group design. Instead of a control group, individuals are randomized to a comparison group program in this design (Fig. 16-4).[14] For example, in this case the diabetes team is interested in whether a group-oriented diabetes program is more effective than a modular self-study program given over the same length of time. Since individuals are randomized to one of the two conditions, any changes would most likely be a result of the intervention. Such a design is frequently used as a component of a research study.

Step 7: Interpreting Findings

Interpretation of findings can range from a simple task, when only a few measures and subjects are involved, to a very complicated task requiring extensive data analysis.[9] Any statistical analysis that might be conducted is concerned with the collection, organization, and interpretation of data according to well-defined procedures. The objective of statistical analysis is then to draw conclusions and understand more about the sources of the data.[16,21,29]

There are two general types of statistics: descriptive and inferential. *Descriptive statistics* are procedures for summarizing, organizing, graphing, or describing quantitative information.[14,29] Percentages, means, and correlations are examples of descriptive statistics. These statistics may suggest whether or not a relationship exists, but not that one factor causes another. For example, an individual has a perfect score on a diabetes knowledge test and excellent metabolic control, as determined by glycated hemoglobin levels. One cannot say that a high level of knowledge causes excellent metabolic control, only that a positive relationship exists between knowledge and control.

Inferential statistics allow one to examine relationships in terms of causality and are typically used when experimental data-gathering designs have been implemented.[14,29] For example, using inferential statistics, one may infer, from a random sample of persons with diabetes who attend a diabetes self-management class, the average level of knowledge for the entire population of persons attending diabetes self-management classes. This can be done *without* sampling every person. This contrasts with descriptive or correlational relationships, which are simply observed as they occur in the natural environment.

The program's design often determines the type of analysis to be used. Nonexperimental data-gathering designs tend to reflect descriptive statistics. Experimental designs use both descriptive and inferential statistics.

Step 8: Communicating Findings

Effective writing and presentation of evaluation results are critical if the findings are to result in improvements or necessary changes. A clear, concise report of evaluation results is the first step to using findings effectively.

The report of evaluation results should contain five sections[23,27]: (1) purpose and key questions, (2) description of the program or program component being evaluated, (3) description of the evaluation methodology used, (4) evaluative findings, and (5) conclusion and recommendations.

Purpose and key questions should open with a discussion that asks, "Who wants to know what and why?" The key questions of the evaluation are presented. An introductory paragraph is also helpful, such as providing a description of the program, including demographic information such as who is in charge, how long has the program been operational, and the major characteristics of the setting.[12,26]

The *program/program component description* provides an overview of what is being evaluated. For example, in a program evaluation the reader should be able to determine program context, resources, and problems. This section might also include program goals, educational objectives, available program staff, and other characteristics.[12,26]

A detailed description of the *data-gathering methods and measures* (e.g., chart audit, questionnaire) should be included. The procedures section should address the actual method of data collection in sufficient detail, including a discussion of subject protection, with guarantees of confidentiality and anonymity. A copy of the questionnaire might also be included for the reader.[12,26]

Findings or outcomes of the evaluation activities, including a display of information collected, should be presented. Data should be presented as clearly as possible, with tables being an effective way to accomplish this. The findings section can range from very brief, if only one question was examined during the evaluation, to very lengthy. Typically the results are presented without interpretation of their findings.[12,26]

The most important section of the report contains the *interpretations, conclusions, and recommendations* based on the evaluation results.[12,26] There are general areas in which information might be used, including changing the diabetes curricula to better meet the needs of the learners, informing administrators of activities and needs, promoting staff development, supporting equipment requests, recruiting persons with diabetes to the program, and discontinuing programs or program components. However, the evaluation is not complete until a plan is in place to act on any results. What if some action is needed based on the evaluation process? How will the results be used?

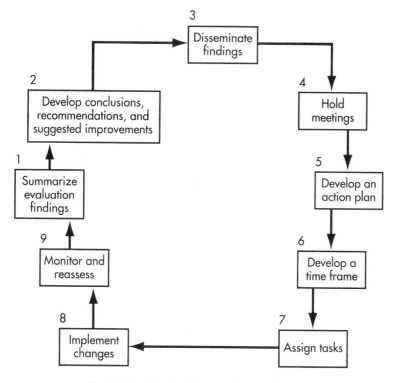

Fig. 16-5   Model of evaluation results.

   To facilitate constructive change based on the findings, a plan for how the results are to be used should be included. A model for such a plan appears in Fig. 16-5. The inclusion of a plan ensures that change and improvement become an acceptable, common process that is a logical extension of any evaluation activity associated with diabetes care and education.

SUMMARY

Systematic evaluation should be incorporated into every activity associated with diabetes self-management. It is a critical ingredient whereby the diabetes educator has objective and concrete feedback on which to base future educational decisions as they may impact the individual patient and the comprehensive program. Without systematic evaluation, diabetes care and management will not achieve the quality standards necessary to promote optimal care. Systematic feedback leads to characteristics associated with high-quality evaluation. The number of characteristics present frequently defines the quality of the evaluation. These characteristics, summarized by Rubenstein and colleagues,[24] can be applied to diabetes self-management as follows:

1. Diabetes interventions or programs should have a sound theoretic basis that allows for further testing and dissemination of interventions.
2. Diabetes self-management program goals and objectives should be explicit and closely related to measurable changes in process, outcome, and/or efficiency. Failure to define

clearly the goals and objectives of the self-management program is the most common reason for an unsuccessful evaluation. Theoretic perspectives regarding measurable changes in structure, process, and outcomes may be one of the most important contributions of evaluation.

3. Measures of process, outcome, and/or efficiency used in the evaluation are relevant to educational or program goals and are evaluated for their performance characteristics (e.g., reliability and validity). Measures must reflect the goals and objectives of the diabetes self-management program being evaluated. If the goals are not clearly defined, the measures will not provide effective data for evaluating the intervention or program.

4. Data-gathering methods should be documented and justified in relationship to defined purpose, goals, and objectives. The data used in diabetes program evaluations can come from a variety of sources. Each method should be described, including the reasons for its selection and its properties in terms of reliability and validity of the instruments used to gather the data.

5. Analysis methods should be documented, updated, and available for review. Findings are explained in relation to key study questions, the baseline characteristics of the sample, educational or program theory, program goals, strengths and limitations of the evaluation, and significance.

6. Results of the evaluation should be summarized, reported, and disseminated.

In conclusion, systematic evaluation is critical to the quality of interventions designed to promote diabetes self-management. This process promotes ongoing planning and implementation of interventions for the individual patient. These interventions have characteristics associated with successful outcomes and quality diabetes care at the level of the self-management program.

REFERENCES

1. American Diabetes Association: Third-party reimbursement for outpatient education and nutritional counseling, *Diabetes Care* 16(5):42-43, 1993.
2. Anderson R and others: The diabetes care and education provided by nurses working in physicians' offices, *Diabetes Educ* 14:532-536, 1988.
3. Bloomfield S and others: A project in diabetes education for children (Department of Child Life and Health, University of Edinburgh, UK), *Diabetic Med* 7:137-142, 1990.
4. Brown SA: Effects of educational interventions in diabetes care: a meta-analysis of findings, *Patient Educ Counsel,* 16(3):189-215, 1990.
5. Davis E: Role of the diabetes nurse educator in improving patient education, *Diabetes Educ* 16:36-38, 1990.
6. Elixhauser A: Cost-effectiveness of preventive care of diabetes, *Diabetes Spectrum* 2(6):349-353, 1989.
7. Farrell-Miller P, Gentry P: How effective are your patient education materials? Guideline for developing and evaluating written educational materials (professional development), *Diabetes Educ* 15:418-422, 1989.

8. French D, Wittman J, Gallagher P: Evaluation of diabetes education programs: getting the answers you need, *Diabetes Educ* 15:176-180, 1989.
9. Garrard J and others: Clinical evaluation of the impact of a patient education program, *Diabetes Educ* 16:394-400, 1990.
10. Green L, Lew F: *Measurement and evaluation in health education and health promotion,* Palo Alto, Calif, 1986, Mayfield.
11. Gronlund N: *Measurement and evaluation in teaching,* ed 3, New York, 1976, MacMillan.
12. Herman J, Morris L, Fitz-Gibbon C: *Evaluator's handbook,* Newbury Park, Calif, 1987, Sage.
13. Hosey G and others: Designing and evaluating diabetes education material for American Indians, *Diabetes Educ* 16:407-414, 1990.
14. IOX Assessment Associates: *Diabetes education: program evaluation handbook,* Los Angeles, 1988, IOX.
15. Joint Committee on Standards for Educational Evaluation: *The standards for evaluations of educational programs, projects, and materials,* New York, 1981, McGraw-Hill.
16. Kachigan SK: Statistical analysis: an interdiscipli-

nary introduction to univariate and multivariate methods, New York, 1986, Radius.

17. Lorenz R, Pichert J: Evaluation of education program developments: illustration of the research and development cycle, *Diabetes Educ* 25:253-257, 1989.

18. Mehrens W, Lehmann I: *Measurement and evaluation in education and psychology,* New York, 1973, Holt, Rinehart and Winston.

19. Mulrow C and others: Evaluation of an audiovisual diabetes education program: negative results of a randomized trial of patients with non-insulin-dependent diabetes mellitus, *J Gen Intern Med* 2:215-219, 1987.

20. National Standards for Diabetes Patient Education and American Diabetes Association Review Criteria, *Diabetes Care* 16(suppl 2):113-118, 1993.

21. Norusis MJ: *The SPSS guide to data analysis for release 4,* Chicago, 1990, SPSS.

22. Peragallo-Dittko V, Godley K, Meyer J, editors: *A core curriculum for diabetes education,* ed 2, Chicago, 1993, American Association of Diabetes Educators and the AADE Education and Research Foundation.

23. Rossi P, Freeman H: *Evaluation: a systematic approach,* Newbury Park, Calif, 1993, Sage.

24. Rubenstein L and others: Evaluating generalist education programs: a conceptual framework, *J Gen Intern Med* 9(suppl 1):S64-S72, 1994.

25. Rubin RJ and others: Health care expenditures for people with diabetes mellitus, 1992, *J Clin Endocrinol Metab* 78(4):809A-809F, 1994.

26. Shadish W, Cook T, Leviton L: *Foundations of program evaluation: theories of practice,* Newbury Park, Calif, 1991, Sage.

27. Shea ML, Boyum PG, Spanke MM: Health occupations: clinical teacher education series for secondary and post-secondary educators. In *Clinical evaluation: theory and practice in health occupations,* Springfield, Ill, 1985, Illinois State Board of Education.

28. Skaburskis A: Cost-benefit analysis: ethics and problem boundaries, *Evaluation Rev* 11(5):591-611, 1987.

29. Tabachnick B, Fidell L: *Using multivariate statistics,* ed 2, New York, 1989, Harper-Collins.

30. Wentling T and others: *Student evaluation of instruction,* Springfield, Ill, 1978, Illinois Office of Education.

31. Wheeler ML and others: Diabetes patient education programs: quality and reimbursement, *Diabetes Care* 15(suppl 1):36-40, 1992.

PART THREE

Individualizing Diabetes Care Across the Life Span

17 Diabetes Mellitus and the Preschool Child

Sharon L. Pontious

INTRODUCTION

The diagnosis of insulin-dependent diabetes mellitus (IDDM) during childhood can be devastating to the child and parent(s). When that child is less than 6 years old, the impact is even more pronounced. The daily life of the child and family is affected by the additional constraints imposed by the treatment regimen, which includes changes in content and timing

---

CHAPTER OBJECTIVES

- Describe how the specific aspects of normal growth and development are affected by IDDM and its required care.
- Summarize common concerns of parents and siblings living with a young child with diabetes.
- Address practical applications of the diabetes meal plan for infants, toddlers, and preschoolers.
- Discuss typical health concerns in terms of diabetes management.
- Describe the role of BGM as a tool in making daily decisions about diabetes management.
- Review considerations in selecting and preparing a day-care provider or babysitter to care safely for the infant and young child with diabetes.
- Address approaches to BGM and giving injections to young children.
- Address techniques helpful in approaching and communicating with a young child.
- Discuss guidelines for managing hypoglycemia and sick days in the infant, toddler, and preschool child.

The author acknowledges the contribution of Barbara Schreiner to Chapter 11 of the first edition of this book, from which this chapter is revised.

of meals, frequent blood glucose monitoring (BGM), insulin injections and dose adjustments, and exercise. Parents of children newly diagnosed with IDDM must deal with the loss of health of their previously healthy child; the potential of shortened life expectancy for that child; the subsequent episodes of hypoglycemia, hyperglycemia, diabetic ketoacidosis (DKA), and rehospitalizations; and the daily stresses caused by adherence to the treatment regimen's constraints on the family's life-style.[49] In addition, each family member may experience one or more of the following feelings in reaction to these added constraints: anger, guilt, sadness, rejection, and frustration. Promoting healthy growth and development of each of the children and of the family becomes more difficult. However, diabetes in very young persons can be managed effectively, both metabolically/physiologically and psychosocially/emotionally. The guiding principle is to help the family to develop a balance between "ideal" care and metabolic control and what is "realistic" or practical for the child of this particularly vulnerable age-group.

An interdisciplinary diabetes health care team must work closely with the child and family to develop optimal therapeutic management strategies. A necessary overall goal is to promote "normal" growth and development of the child less than 6 years old while maintaining good metabolic control (hemoglobin A_{1c} [Hg A_{1c}] values of 7% to 11%). Other goals of long-term therapy include (1) avoidance of severe ketosis and hypoglycemia, (2) maintenance of physical and psychologic health, (3) reduction of symptomatic hyperglycemia or hypoglycemia, and (4) institution of preventive measures for long-term complications.[79] A knowledge of normal physical, cognitive, and psychosocial development is essential to assess and plan for the care of the infant, toddler, or preschooler with IDDM. In this chapter, *infants* are children up to 1 year of age, *toddlers* are 1 to 3 years old, and *preschool children* are 3 to 5 years old.

DIAGNOSIS OF IDDM

Diagnosis of IDDM in infants is rare. However, the incidence of IDDM in young children appears to be increasing. The diagnosis of IDDM may not be identified quickly in infants because most parents and physicians rarely think about diabetes as a diagnosis for infants. The added stress of being ill may increase the infants' insulin deficiency.[54] Thus, by the time they are diagnosed, they frequently have very high values for blood glucose and ketones and are seriously ill.

Early clues leading to a diagnosis of IDDM include enuresis and nocturia in a previously "dry" child combined with drinking large amounts of water. Weight loss despite an excellent, often increased appetite is frequently present at the initial diagnosis. If these early signs persist for several months, growth failure may result.[79] Hyperglycemia with dehydration is common. If DKA is present, marked hyperglycemia, severe dehydration (weight loss, sunken anterior fontanel, dry mucous membranes), stomach ache, vomiting, a fruity odor on the breath, and Kussmaul respirations are seen. Infants and young toddlers may also be lethargic, irritable, tired, and weak. One young toddler was so weak that he began to crawl everywhere instead of standing up to walk.

The diagnosis of diabetes mellitus is made when one of the following occurs:

1. A repeat random plasma glucose level is 200 mg/dl or higher 2 hours after a meal (after an initial randomly taken plasma glucose level greater than 200 mg/dl).
2. Nocturia, polydipsia, polyuria, glycosuria, ketonuria, and plasma glucose values are greater than 200 mg/dl with or without weight loss or fatigue.
3. Fasting plasma glucose values are between 115 and 140 mg/dl and a 2-hour postprandial value is less than 200 mg/dl, but an oral glucose tolerance test (OGTT) yields two of the measured values above 200 mg/dl fasting plasma glucose level.[24,79]

It is common for parents to blame themselves for their child having IDDM, especially when parents have a family history of diabetes and know IDDM has a genetic component. They blame themselves for not seeing the problem sooner and for initially discounting the signs of the illness. They blame themselves for disciplining the child for enuresis or trying to restrict the child's liquid intake before the diagnosis. They also blame themselves for not being able to protect their child from both the physical pain of treatments and tests and the emotional pain of "being different." Often, parents add guilt by giving extra time to the child with IDDM, and then feel they are neglecting their other children. In general, the guilt parents feel has little to do with the reality of the child's condition or their own actions. Some believe they are being punished through their child's illness, or they may see their child's illness as their own personal failure. Unfortunately, once parents accept guilt, it leads to more negative consequences, such as feeling incompetent and unworthy of being parents.

The interdisciplinary diabetes health team must help parents of children with newly diagnosed IDDM to manage their sense of guilt. Some healthy ways to deal with guilt include accepting the guilt and moving past it, acknowledging that many events are beyond their control, and learning about IDDM and how to treat hyperglycemia and hypoglycemia to gain a sense of control. Parents must be helped to see what they are doing right and to celebrate their children's successes.

Siblings of children with IDDM may also have problems with and possibly negative reactions to their brother or sister being diagnosed with IDDM. They may feel guilty because they were angry with their sibling and think they magically caused him or her to become ill, may be fearful that they will "catch" IDDM too, may feel left out because of the increased attention focused on the child with IDDM, and may have difficulty understanding the disease.

The diabetes team needs to help family members express their feelings and concerns. Dealing openly with them at the time of diagnosis is believed to facilitate their long-term adjustment.[80]

An assessment of family functioning using the Diabetes Family Behavior Scale; the Family Concept Inventory, which results in a Family Effectiveness Score that reflects the degree to which the family is characterized by open communication, ability to resolve conflict, family loyalty, and satisfaction and close familial relations; or the Moos Family Environment Scale helps the team to identify strengths and resources that can be used to cope with the disease.* Evidence of family dysfunction requires referral to a mental health professional for

---

*References 5, 27, 76, 88, 96.

evaluation and therapy. It is now known that families who are highly cohesive and organized, have open communication, use appropriate consistent guidance and control with effective problem-solving skills, and are warm and nurturing are more likely to have children with IDDM in good metabolic control.[5,40,76,88] Dysfunctional families, families in conflict, and families with less organization or less cohesion and with parental incongruence are predictive of children with poor adherence to the therapeutic regimen and thus in poor metabolic control.*

PHYSICAL DEVELOPMENT

Maintaining a normal growth rate is a major and attainable goal in the treatment of IDDM for infants, toddlers, and preschoolers. In general, growth is predictable and orderly but progresses at varying rates for each individual. In addition, growth "spurts" and growth "slow downs" normally occur. For example, during the first year of life, infants typically triple their birth weight and grow 10 to 12 inches (25 to 30 cm). Infants have large appetites and require approximately 1000 calories per day. Thereafter, toddlers and preschoolers typically gain 3 to 5 pounds and grow 2 to 3 inches (5 to 7.5 cm) per year.

Growth rate in children is characterized by periods of acceleration, or "spurts," occurring at different times but in similar sequences for healthy children.[53] By age 2 the child has achieved 50% of his or her adult height.[94] By age 3 years the child is expected to be 3 feet (90 cm) tall. Linear growth is rapid in the first year of life, then slowly decelerates until puberty.[53] From 1 to 6 years, there is an average annual increase in height of 3 inches (7.5 cm).[77]

Despite growth delays caused by disease or nutritional deprivation, catch-up growth is possible if the initial problem is corrected or managed. Once an adequate diet or recovery from illness occurs, the child may experience a rapid acceleration in growth.[45] How much of lost linear growth can be recovered is determined by the timing, severity, and duration of the interruption. Children who are newly diagnosed with IDDM have typically lost some weight during the days or weeks before the diagnosis. This is especially true for toddlers and preschoolers who have smaller and "picky" appetites. Once these children have been taking insulin for a few days, their appetite increases dramatically. The diabetes health care team typically increases the insulin dosages to allow these children to eat enough to gain back the weight lost. Children of this age have daily requirements of 1000 plus 100 calories for each year of age over 1 year for normal growth and development;[89] they need even more during this catch-up period. After this catch-up time of a few weeks, children's appetites usually return to normal, at which time the insulin dosage and food requirements are often stabilized.

During the first few weeks after diagnosis, many children begin to produce some insulin again, the time called the "honeymoon period." Very little insulin may be needed to achieve excellent glycemic control during the honeymoon period, which may last months but is more likely to be of shorter duration in prepubertal children. Current evidence suggests that endogenous insulin secretion can be sustained for longer periods with efforts that maintain

*References 40, 56, 72, 76, 80, 88.

lower mean blood glucose levels. The insulin requirements gradually increase over several weeks as the honeymoon period comes to an end. Before puberty, most children require about 0.6 to 0.9 U of insulin/kg of weight/day.[79] More insulin is required during growth spurts, periods of high stress, and when infections are present.

Sequential measurements of growth plotted on standardized growth charts are used to evaluate the rate and pattern of normal growth and to detect changes in linear growth.[38] Children with IDDM should have their height and weight measured and recorded every 4 to 6 months. An in-depth evaluation of growth should be conducted for those children with IDDM whose (1) height and weight patterns deviate from their usual pattern; (2) height and weight patterns deviate more than usual from standardized norms; (3) height at diagnosis falls under the fifth percentile or over the ninety-fifth percentile without concomitant percentiles for weight for age; or (4) height or weight demonstrates a loss or gain of several standardized percentiles. Such an evaluation should include physical assessment, previous history of illness, history of nutrition, and family patterns of growth. Specialized growth charts allow for the parents' heights to be considered in assessing the child's growth potential.[90]

Children up to 2 years of age should have head circumference monitored. At birth the neonate's head circumference measures 14 inches (34 to 35 cm). The infant's head may increase by 4 inches (10 cm) in the first year. By the end of infancy, growth in head circumference slows to ⅘ to 2 inches (2 to 5 cm)/year. By age 5 years the child's head circumference is expected to increase less than ½ inch (1.25 cm)/year. Head circumference typically equals chest circumference by ages 1 to 2 years.

Neuromuscular Development

Neuromuscular growth occurs rapidly and in a predictable sequence. At birth the human brain is 25% of its adult size. By the end of the first year of life, the brain has grown to two-thirds its final size, and by the end of age 5, 90% of brain mass is present. Although brain growth is nearly complete by school age, the following are critical times of especially rapid brain cell replication: at 15 to 20 weeks' gestation and from 30 weeks' gestation to the end of the first year of life. A growth spurt occurs first and fastest in the cerebellum, the site of coordination and balance. Later, growth predominates in the forebrain and brainstem. Nerve cell myelination sheathes and protects neurons and allows impulses to travel more rapidly and accurately. Myelination follows a cephalocaudal direction, with the pathways for sensory nerves myelinating before motor pathways. Myelination in the spinal cord allows for the gross motor development in the toddler. This nervous system development depends on a constant, unfailing supply of glucose as nerve cell replication and myelination progresses.[82,94] Central nervous system (CNS) damage from recurrent or severe hypoglycemia is a concern for young children whose brain is still developing and is more susceptible to permanent injury.[54,79]

Development of Other Systems

The child's gastrointestinal (GI) system is also in a state of rapid growth and change from infancy through young childhood. At birth the infant's stomach is very small and empties relatively quickly (2 to 6 hours). In infancy, regurgitation is common because of an immature cardiac sphincter. Because of these anatomic characteristics, young children with IDDM require small, frequent meals and three snacks daily.

Voluntary control of elimination occurs at about ages 18 to 24 months, following CNS maturation. Children at these ages not only can detect a full bladder but also can often control its emptying. Bowel control precedes bladder control, and daytime toilet training precedes nighttime control. It is helpful for parents of children with IDDM to know that hyperglycemia with concomitant enuresis is likely during infections and periods of stress such as holidays. Children should not be punished for lack of bladder control during these times and should be told it is not their fault but rather is caused by having too much sugar in their system.[51]

Sleep and Rest Patterns

Sleep and rest in the young child progressively change in both quantity and quality. Infants sleep as much as 15 hours a day. By age 3 months, newborns demonstrate diurnal patterns of waking and sleeping. By 4 to 6 months, the child is often sleeping through the night. The 1- to 2-year-old child may be taking one to two naps daily, decreasing to one nap by age 3 and no naps by 5 years.[2]

Parents should be alerted that *nocturnal* (1 AM to 4 AM) *hypoglycemia* is relatively frequent. "Night terrors" or "nightmares" may be symptoms of hypoglycemia. Other symptoms include apnea, pallor, and unexpected lethargy or hypotonia. Causes of nocturnal hypoglycemia include peak activity from the suppertime NPH insulin dose, failure to eat a bedtime snack, and unusually intense physical activity the previous day. Children's blood glucose should be checked at 2 to 3 AM, especially when the suppertime or bedtime dose of intermediate insulin is being adjusted to lower morning glucose levels or when any of the previously listed symptoms occur. Every attempt should be made to keep the 2 to 3 AM blood glucose value greater than 65 mg/dl without causing morning hyperglycemia (above 180 mg/dl). One way to prevent nocturnal hypoglycemia is to add supplements (extra milk, cheese, peanut butter, or a complex carbohydrate) to bedtime snacks when bedtime glucose is low.[79] Young children with nocturnal hypoglycemia frequently want a 2- to 4-ounce bottle or glass of milk to fall back asleep; in my experience, however, substituting water is less likely to cause hyperglycemia later.

HEALTH CONCERNS FOR THE YOUNG CHILD
Physical Injuries and Accidents

Injuries and accidents are the leading cause of death in young children whether or not they have IDDM. Falls, aspiration of small objects, poisoning, burns, and drowning contribute to infant mortality and morbidity. Many accidents in this age-group result from the parent's lack of knowledge of normal child development. Knowing the general age when a child will roll over, reach for objects, and begin crawling are important to making his or her environment safe. For the infant a safe environment includes an infant car seat, medications and household chemicals locked away, small objects and toys out of reach, and pacifiers, toys, and clothing that are well made, fire resistant, and appropriate for age.

Injury prevention for the toddler includes use of approved car seats; close supervision at playgrounds, ponds, swimming pools, and lakes; and locking away medicines, firearms, and house and garden chemicals. Toddlers and preschool children can begin to understand safety precautions, and therefore teaching them about general safety precautions is essential.

Immunizations

Immunization against childhood diseases is an essential component of children's health care for this age-group (Table 17-1).

The neonate has received passive immunity to many viral and bacterial organisms through the transplacental transfer of maternal immunoglobulin G (IgG).[94] This maternal IgG is virtually the neonate's only protection against infection. By 3 months of age, maternal IgG is waning and the infant is actively producing his or her own immunoglobulin. By age 1 year the child is producing about 40% of the adult levels of IgG.[97] Other immunoglobulins (A, D, and E) are produced more gradually, with maximum levels reached in early childhood, leaving infants and young children prone to upper respiratory illnesses and common childhood diseases. It is especially important for children with IDDM to be up to date on their immunizations, since they tend to develop ketosis and DKA with stress hormone release during illnesses.[54]

Infants and toddlers require a series of immunizations against measles, mumps, and rubella (MMR), polio, diphtheria, and tetanus. The recommended age to begin immunizations is 2 months, with repeat inoculations at scheduled intervals throughout childhood. MMR and hepatitis B virus (HBV) inoculations are given at 12 to 15 months; they may be given at 12 months in high-risk areas. Normal consequences from immunizations include fever, malaise, and pain or swelling at the injection site. Some children have malaise or feeding irregularities after their immunizations. Children with elevated temperature (greater than 39.5° C) for more than 48 hours should be evaluated further.[82,94] Blood glucose levels of children with IDDM should be monitored more closely after immunizations for both hypoglycemia and hyperglycemia with or without ketones. Adjustment of insulin doses may be necessary.[81,82,92]

Dental Care

Once teeth begin to erupt, oral hygiene should be implemented. Removing plaque and food particles is the parent's responsibility for several years, until children's dexterity allows for self-care. Visits to the dentist should begin no later than 2 to 2½ years old. An initial appointment simply to meet the dentist and his or her staff is recommended to decrease children's anxiety. Routine checkups allow the dentist to establish a relationship and begin preventive measures for healthy dentition.[82,94]

The child with IDDM is prone to gum infections and dental problems because the oral mucosa and gums are bathed in glucose during periods of hyperglycemia. Strict oral hygiene and controlling glucose levels are necessary. Children with diabetes are generally not exposed

Table 17-1 Recommended Ages for Administration of Currently Licensed Childhood Vaccines—August 1995

Vaccines are listed under the routinely recommended ages. Solid bars indicate range of acceptable ages for vaccination. Shaded bars indicate new recommendations or vaccines licensed since publication of the Recommended Childhood Immunization Schedule in January 1995. Hepatitis B vaccine is recommended at 11-12 years of age for children not previously vaccinated. Varicella Zoster Virus vaccine is recommended at 11-12 years of age for children not previously vaccinated, and who lack a reliable history of chickenpox.

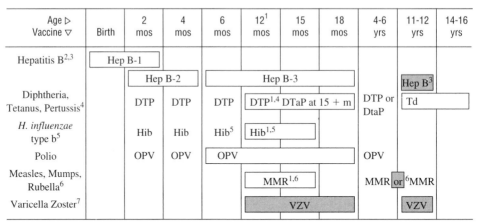

Age ▷ Vaccine ▽	Birth	2 mos	4 mos	6 mos	12[1] mos	15 mos	18 mos	4-6 yrs	11-12 yrs	14-16 yrs
Hepatitis B[2,3]	Hep B-1									
		Hep B-2			Hep B-3				Hep B[3]	
Diphtheria, Tetanus, Pertussis[4]		DTP	DTP	DTP	DTP[1,4] DTaP at 15 + m			DTP or DtaP	Td	
H. influenzae type b[5]		Hib	Hib	Hib[5]	Hib[1,5]					
Polio		OPV	OPV	OPV				OPV		
Measles, Mumps, Rubella[6]					MMR[1,6]			MMR or [6]MMR		
Varicella Zoster[7]					VZV				VZV	

From American Academy of Pediatrics.

1 Vaccines recommended in the second year of life (12-15 months of age) may be given at either one or two visits.

2 Infants born to HBsAg-negative mothers should receive 2.5 μg of Merck Sharp & Dohme (MSD) vaccine (Recombivax HB) or 10 μg of SmithKline Beecham (SKB) vaccine (Engerix-B). The second dose should be given between 1 and 4 months of age, if at least one month has elapsed since receipt of the first dose. The third dose is recommended between 6 and 18 months of age.

Infants born to HBsAg-positive mothers should receive immunoprophylaxis for hepatitis B with 0.5 ml Hepatitis B Immune Globulin (HBIG) within 12 hours of birth, and either 5 μg of MSD vaccine (Recombivax HB) or 10 μg of SKB vaccine (Engerix-B) at a separate site. In these infants, the second dose of vaccine is recommended at 1 month of age and the third dose at 6 months of age. All pregnant women should be screened for HBsAg in an early prenatal visit.

3 Hepatitis B vaccine is recommended for adolescents who have not previously received 3 doses of vaccine. The 3-dose series should be initiated or completed at the 11-12 year-old visit for persons not previously fully vaccinated. The 2nd dose should be administered at least 1 month after the first dose, and the 3rd dose should be administered at least 4 months after the first dose.

4 The fourth dose of DTP may be administered as early as 12 months of age, provided at least 6 months have elapsed since DTP3. Combined DTP-Hib products may be used when these two vaccines are to be administered simultaneously. DTaP (diphtheria and tetanus toxoids and acellular pertussis vaccine) is licensed for use for the 4th and/or 5th dose of DTP vaccine in children 15 months of age or older and may be preferred for these doses in children in this age group. Td (tetanus and diphtheria toxoids, absorbed, for adult use) is recommended at 11–12 years of age if at least 5 years have elapsed since the last dose of DTP, DTP-Hib, or DT.

5 Three H. influenzae type b conjugate vaccines are available for use in infants: HbOC [HibTITER](Lederle Praxis); PRP-T (ActHIB; OmniHIB)(Pateur Mérieux, distributed by SmithKline Beecham; Connaught); and PRP-OMP (PedvaxHIB) (Merck Sharp & Dohme). Children who have received PRP-OMP at 2 and 4 months of age do not require a dose at 6 months of age. After the primary infant Hib conjugate vaccine series is completed, any licensed Hib conjugate vaccine may be used as a booster dose at 12–15 months.

6 The second dose of MMR vaccine should be administered EITHER at 4–6 years of age OR at 11–12 years of age, consistent with state school immunization requirements.

7 Varicella zoster virus vaccine (VZV) is routinely recommended at 12–18 months of age. Children who have not been vaccinated previously and who lack a reliable history of chickenpox should be vaccinated by 13 years of age. VZV can be administered to susceptible children any time after 12 months of age. Children under 13 years of age should receive a single 0.5 mL dose; persons 13 years of age and older should receive two 0.5 doses 4–8 weeks apart.

BECAUSE THE AAP, ACIP AND AAFP HAVE AGREED TO FORMALLY REEVALUATE THE IMMUNIZATION SCHEDULE ANNUALLY, ANY SUBSEQUENT REVISIONS WILL BE PUBLISHED IN THE "RECOMMENDED CHILDHOOD IMMUNIZATION SCHEDULE/ UNITED STATES—JANUARY 1996" IN THE JANUARY 1996 ISSUE OF PEDIATRICS.

©1995 American Academy of Pediatrics

to as many cariogenic snacks as other children. However, selecting snack foods that limit plaque formation is recommended. Popcorn and raw fruits and vegetables provide a mechanical cleaning of the teeth while the child is enjoying the snack. Sweet foods are less damaging to the teeth when eaten immediately after a meal than when eaten alone. This practice is better in blunting the postprandial glucose rise as well.[55,82]

Nutrition

The demand for adequate nutrition and calories is greatest during infancy and childhood. Infants require 110 to 120 kcal/kg/day, and toddlers require about 100 kcal/kg/day. Providing a suitable diet for growing young children demands a combination of parental creativity, patience, and perseverance. Eating behaviors are closely linked to other aspects of cognitive and social development. Consequently, young children's "food jags," mealtime rituals, and dawdling at mealtimes provide challenging situations for busy parents.[4,52]

Between 3 and 4 months of age, infants must transition from sucking and swallowing to eating solid foods. During the first year, infants are introduced to new flavors and new textures. Foods should be offered in small amounts, simply prepared but with variety.[52] Typically, infants and toddlers prefer individual foods rather than mixtures of foods. As infants gain dexterity and fine motor skills, self-feeding should be encouraged.

Infants with IDDM should be fed frequently because of the risk of hypoglycemia and possible brain damage. Some diabetologists order an unmeasured diet consisting of three meals and one to three snacks per day that excludes concentrated sweets (any foods containing sugar, honey, or frosting) for infants and young toddlers. Other diabetologists refer nutritionists to teach the parents how to use the diabetes exchange diet. There are proponents of both approaches.

Parents must understand whatever diet is recommended and that the bedtime snack should be emphasized. Whenever the infant refuses to eat solids or finger foods, parents can feed 2 to 4 ounces of infant formula (if less than 12 months of age) or whole milk (not 2% or skim) if over 12 months of age. The American Academy of Pediatrics (AAP) recommends whole milk be used for children older than 12 months of age to decrease the tendency for GI bleeding and iron deficiency anemia in younger infants fed milk. Skim or 2% milk is not recommended because it does not provide sufficient calories or essential fatty acids for growth and development.[54] Similarly, restrictions in dietary fat are not necessary in preschool children.[79] Older infants generally eat some baby foods and some table food. Parents must learn to check the label of each baby food jar to avoid added sugar.

When infants become "picky" and "finicky" and refuse to eat certain foods, parents should not become too worried. If infants refuse to eat most of the meal, parents can increase the size of the subsequent snack or can feed 2 to 4 ounces of infant formula along with one or two crackers. Parents must maintain a positive attitude toward eating and make appropriate diet substitutions instead of battling with children at mealtime to avoid feeding problems later.[54] Parents should maintain a low-key attitude when children do not eat well instead of becoming excited or anxious to prevent reinforcing children for this behavior.

Table 17-2 lists a typical food plan.

Table 17-2   Suggested Serving Portions for Toddlers and Preschoolers

Type of food	Suggested portion					Number per day
	1 year	2 years	3 years	4 years	5 years	
Milk	4 oz	5 oz	6 oz	6 oz	6 oz	Total intake of 16-24 oz
Meats and alternatives	1 tbsp	2 tbsp	3 tbsp	4 tbsp	4 tbsp	3-4 servings
Egg	1	1	1	1	1	0-1
Cooked legumes	1 tbsp	2 tbsp	3 tbsp	4 tbsp	4 tbsp	0-2 servings
Fruits and vegetables						At least 4
Citrus juice or other vitamin C source	¼ cup	¼ cup	⅓ cup	½ cup	½ cup	1 serving
Dark-green, leafy, or yellow vegetables	1 tbsp	2 tbsp	3 tbsp	4 tbsp	5 tbsp	1 serving on alternate days
Other fruits and vegetables	1 tbsp	2 tbsp	3 tbsp	4 tbsp	5 tbsp	
Breads (enriched or whole grain)	¼ slice	⅓ slice	⅓ slice	½ slice	½ slice	4 or more servings
Cooked cereal	1 tbsp	2 tbsp	3 tbsp	4 tbsp	4 tbsp	0-2 servings
Ready-to-eat dry cereal	2 tbsp	¼ cup	⅓ cup	½ cup	½ cup	0-2 servings

From McWilliams M: *Nutrition for the growing years,* ed 4, New York, 1986, Wiley.

Children require a combination of foods from all the food groups. Variety is important not just in the type of food but also in its texture. A balance of dry and moist foods should be offered to the toddler. One recommendation is to serve one soft food, one chewy food, and one crisp food at each meal. Children may prefer meals served at room temperature, since very hot foods are sometimes frightening.

Factors that help to shape food patterns in young children include parents' food preferences, the sweetness and familiarity of foods, food preparation, parents' nutrition knowledge, and other influences such as television.[52] Overcooking, for example, has been cited as the most common offender in children's dislike for vegetables and other foods.[34] A relaxed mealtime, with simply prepared foods of balanced nutrients, encourages an appropriate food intake (Box 17-1).

Parents worry about their children's food intake, especially between 2 and 4 years of age. During this time, children's appetite may be erratic and unpredictable. Play and other distractions make them "picky eaters." Toddlers should be offered small, frequent meals rather than large amounts of food at mealtimes. Parents should remove the plate at the end of the meal (15 to 25 minutes) regardless of the amount eaten.[23] No foods should be offered until the next planned eating/snack time. Some parents worry that children's nutrient intake will suffer with this approach. Keeping a food diary for several days and consulting the pediatrician or dietitian should assure parents that nutritional needs are being met. Some nutritionists are now recommending the addition of vitamins for all

---

BOX 17-1

MEALS AND SNACKS

1. Stress the terminology "meal plan," not "diet." Diet denotes restriction; meal plan allows for flexibility.
2. Give child no more than 25 minutes to eat a meal and no longer than 15 minutes for snacks. (Set a timer, and throw away all supper or snacks from the child's plate when the time is up. Save no foods for later.)
   a. Make meal time pleasant and enjoyable; food can be fun! Be creative (e.g., place smile faces on top of the pancakes with the fruit exchange). Let children choose between two vegetables they help prepare (this also gives them a sense of control).
   b. For "picky" eaters, use a large plate (e.g., food platter) to make the quantity of food appear smaller. You can present one item at a time, but let the child know quantity of items to follow.
   c. Substitute: 1 bread = 1 fruit exchange and 1 milk = 1 fruit + 1 meat exchange. Most important things to eat are protein and carbohydrate; do not worry as much about vegetables and fats.
   d. Use nutrient-dense foods if the child is a "problem eater" (e.g., raisins, dry fruit) because the amounts are smaller.
   e. Preferred foods can be used as reinforcers.
   f. Give only free foods in between meals. Try sugar-free Jellos and flavored frozen drinks. Be careful: do not give so many as to fill the child up before meals and snacks.
3. The parents should eat what the child eats. For example, if the child is expected to eat chicken, rice, broccoli, and peaches, the parents eat this dinner as well.
4. If the child is more active, let him or her have an extra bread, fruit, *or* meat and record it. If this happens 2 or 3 days in a row, call for a diet adjustment.
5. Do not allow frequent snacking.
6. Ensure meals are structured—same place, same time, with no television or radio.
7. If the child "cheats," do not focus on it; do not nag. Ask, "Are you eating because you are "hungry," or because you just want a treat?"
8. Say nothing (no nagging) about food not eaten.
9. If the child is still hungry, the nutritionist will help you increase food and insulin proportionately.
10. Your child will have "food jags." Call immediately for help to decrease the insulin to compensate for his or her lack of food. Food jags are normal, not harmful. It does not really matter if the child eats the same foods repeatedly; however, keep reintroducing new foods.
11. Parties are difficult because food is never put away. It helps to talk to the child about all the extra food and "temptations" before going to parties. Plan so the child is not so "different" (e.g., ½ rice cereal bar and ½ cupcake instead of 1 cupcake). Discuss this before going.
12. Encourage toddlers to do "finger sticks" on dolls by themselves. (This helps them work through many emotions.) Preschoolers may want to do their own finger sticks. It may hurt less when they do it themselves and gives them a sense of control and mastery over the situation.

who have IDDM—specifically, vitamins C and E and magnesium supplements.[7] The diabetes team may recommend reducing the following day's insulin dose whenever a child with IDDM becomes hypoglycemic because of being in a particularly finicky stage or on specific food jags.

"Food jags" and rituals are normal developmental stages for young children; they may persist for several days or even weeks. Sometimes, food jags are related to children's physical development. For example, many youngsters prefer carbohydrate-rich foods over protein foods because they are easier to masticate. Chewing is a challenging activity for the 1- to 4-year-old child. Allowing toddlers their preferred food is appropriate if the food wanted is reasonably nutritious. Finger foods, such as carrot sticks, green beans, small sandwiches, or hard-boiled eggs cut in quarters, are ideal snack and meal items. Serving small portions of food on large plates encourages eating because children of this age perceive there is less food.[32,65]

Food rituals are normal for the toddler and preschooler. Children may prefer a certain food preparation or utensil. For example, some always want the crust cut from the sandwich or drink milk only from a special cup. Allowing toddlers to have food jags and rituals is appropriate as long as they are within reason. Unrealistic expectations of toddlers make meals a battleground, and the child may become manipulative (e.g., agreeing to eat only at fast-food restaurants).[51]

Regular mealtimes and snack times are important for the picky eater. Snacks should be offered more than 1 hour before the next meal. Snacks are important adjuncts to the typical American plan of three large meals daily and hold particular importance for the child with IDDM. In the young child, glycogen stores in the liver are limited and easily depleted between meals. Snacks provide a more constant source of glucose for energy and storage.

Role of Play Activities

Play has been termed the "work of childhood,"[6,19] since during play children learn about self and others. Play is "extraordinary and supremely serious."[19]

There are several primary types of play. *Practice* or *sensorimotor play* is the infant's and toddler's mechanism for investigating self and the world by using his or her body, motion, and senses to explore and manipulate objects. Young infants (0 to 6 months) enjoy *exercise play*—repetition of actions and sounds for pleasure (e.g., putting their feet into their mouths, kicking at toys hung above their crib, rolling over, babbling).[61] Older infants (6 to 12 months) enjoy *exploratory play*—attainment of pleasure by causing effects and reconfirming skills (e.g., playing "pat-a-cake," throwing mashed potatoes on the floor to see what will happen).

Toddlers (12 to 24 months) are developmentally driven to explore and manipulate their environment. Play is used to practice their newly developed physical skills of walking, running, and climbing. They also test and reexamine objects from all angles for shape, size, weight, texture, color, function, spatial relationship, and interaction with themselves.

Toddlers (18 to 36 months) enjoy *deferred imitation*—imitating previously observed actions (not the reasons for or purposes of actions) from memory.[61] For example, they pretend to be "daddy" and "shave," walk outside to "go to work," then come back inside and snore to "take a nap." At this age, play is parallel and personal rather than reciprocal or interactive. Conflicts are common as the youngster claims his or her "property rights."

By the preschool years, play is more interactive and cooperative. Preschoolers engage in *symbolic play*—play in which they represent or reenact experiences and reflect on people, things, and events they have experienced.[6,61] Symbolic play enables children to turn reality into what they wish reality was (e.g., imaginary friends are common).

Research suggests that parental expectations and resources for play vary across cultures and socioeconomic backgrounds. Parents in lower socioeconomic brackets, for example, play less often with their children and speak less often to them during play.[94]

The interdisciplinary diabetes team members can use play to teach toddlers about their diabetes, help them express their feelings, and facilitate their attainment of a sense of control over their environment. Using a doll with organs inside a zip-open body can help younger children understand the location and appearance of the pancreas. Having them prick a doll's fingers to check for blood sugar and giving the doll insulin with syringes helps older toddlers and preschoolers feel in control of events occurring to them. Children often demand to check their dolls' blood sugar and give dolls their insulin just before or immediately after receiving their own.

Impact of Television

Children between 2 and 11 years of age average 4 hours daily in front of the "electronic babysitter."[23] As a solitary activity, television viewing promotes increased passivity and decreased physical activity and social interaction.[17,97] Frequent viewing is not conducive to the development of imaginative capacities[86] and competes with the child's sports and exercise.

On average, children are exposed to 20,000 television commercials each year. Typically, sugary treats or fast foods are advertised, influences of special concern for the parents of children with IDDM. In addition, frequent television viewing is associated with an increased consumption of snack foods and indirectly may promote obesity in some children. Parents need to help children with IDDM find alternative snacks to those advertised on television.

Physical Examination

The young child with diabetes needs a physical examination at least quarterly, with special attention paid to the following aspects[50,82]:

- Height and weight (plus head and chest circumferences until age 2 years) measurements and comparison with standardized norms
- Cardiac (including pulse and blood pressure), neurologic, dental, and ophthalmoscopic examinations
- Thyroid palpation
- Skin examination, including inspection of injection sites for lipodystrophies and infection or redness of fingertips to determine frequency of blood glucose testing and to identify errors in technique
- Laboratory tests for glycohemoglobin, urine ketones, and protein.

If findings indicate, a fasting lipid profile, urine culture, and thyroid function tests are added. The child who has ketones, is not gaining weight or growing, or appears wasted or dehydrated may have had hyperglycemia for days or weeks and may need hospitalization for determination of causes and for a major adjustment in insulin dose.

Growth Retardation

On a more long-term basis, IDDM can affect the young child's linear growth.[91] The complex interactions among insulin, growth hormone, and somatostatin result in a normal growth pattern. When this balance is altered, as in IDDM, growth may be affected. Golden and associates[34] found that intensified management with frequent BGM and multiple injections resulted in a more normal growth pattern when compared with a group of children managed less optimally. Jackson[45] reported that catch-up growth is possible in children formerly in poor metabolic control. Once glycemic balance was achieved, these children reestablished and maintained normal growth. Other authors have noted that growth velocity greatly improves with intensification of insulin treatment.[60]

Central Nervous System Growth and Hypoglycemia

Without an available source of glucose, the CNS will not develop normally. Animal studies suggest that prolonged hypoglycemia results in diminished brain weight, cellularity, and protein content. Myelinization is also decreased. Complex motor functions require an intact CNS. Thus probably the most serious impact of IDDM for the infant, toddler, and preschooler is the potential for severe, prolonged, or frequent hypoglycemia.[46] Because of these children's inability to communicate hypoglycemic symptoms accurately, most diabetes specialists recommend maintaining blood glucose levels between 100 and 200 mg/dl as a precaution against undetected hypoglycemia. Intensive insulin therapy, as carried out in the Diabetes Control and Complications Trial (DCCT) study, is not recommended for children under age 5.[25]

Schedules

Ideally the management of IDDM requires a fairly rigid schedule of meals, snacks, BGM, insulin injections and dose adjustment, and exercise. Young children are often inconsistent in their activity levels or appetite, although they do well with a structured routine. Balancing the management of IDDM with young children's routine is demanding and often difficult. The diabetes team needs to prepare parents for negative behaviors such as regression to clinging, bedwetting or soiling, temper tantrums, and nightmares. Parents should be cautioned to avoid power struggles, overprotection, outbursts of temper, and feeling pity or guilt for the child.[51] Consistent discipline must be maintained. Providing parents with distraction methods to help with painful BGM and children's dislike of being restrained for insulin injections is helpful. For example, one parent can shake a favorite toy in front of the infant while talking to him or her as the other parent administers the insulin.[54] Parents should also take turns in doing BGM and giving the insulin injections so one does not always feel like the "bad guy." Using new syringes each time will decrease the pain of injections from duller needles and will prevent infections. Having toddlers choose and then hold the bandaid during these procedures gives them a sense of control. Treating the IDDM management activities in a businesslike, matter-of-fact manner without bribing or cajoling children helps to minimize their manipulation of parents later.

Parents often worry about how children with IDDM will fare during the night or during nap time. What will happen to blood glucose levels? Will children awaken if hypoglycemic? Before nap time and sleep time, parents should check children's blood glucose values. Naps should follow either a meal or a snack, particularly if insulin will peak during the sleep period. **Parents should not allow the child to nap through a meal or snack.** Parents may be reassured that most children will awaken when hypoglycemic and that their normal counterregulatory hormones will provide some safety in buffering low blood glucose.[13] However, diabetes team professionals must emphasize the importance of the bedtime snack.

Bedtime BGM and snacks are especially important for young children with IDDM because they can prevent the relatively common occurrences (approximately once a week) of silent nocturnal hypoglycemia. This is a problem partly because nocturnal insulin requirements are lower between 1 and 2 AM.[22,84] Nocturnal hypoglycemia is manifested by nightmares, sleep walking or sleep talking, and restlessness, as well as the common daytime symptoms such as pallor, sweating, increased lethargy, and feeling starved. The best predictor of 1 to 3 AM hypoglycemia is the blood glucose level at bedtime.[84,98] Children with a bedtime glucose level lower than 120 mg/dl who have skipped the bedtime snack or who have had an unusual amount or intensity of exercise the previous day frequently have a subsequent episode of hypoglycemia at 1 to 4 AM. The bedtime snack can be used to reduce the risks of nocturnal hypoglycemia by doubling its protein content if any of the previous events has occurred or if the blood glucose level is less than 120 mg/dl at bedtime. If the bedtime blood glucose value is greater than 300 mg/dl, parents should eliminate the carbohydrate portion of the usual bedtime snack but still give the protein component. **The bedtime blood glucose check and snack should never be skipped.**

Illnesses and Diabetes

Young children with IDDM who are in relatively good metabolic control are *not* more likely to be ill than children without IDDM. However, infections in children with IDDM stimulate wide fluctuations in blood glucose levels; some infections cause hypoglycemia, whereas others, especially chronic infections, tend to cause hyperglycemia and insulin resistance. Infections frequently stimulate the development of the stress response and DKA. Thus insulin requirements vary during illness episodes. In general during illness, children with IDDM need frequent BGM and urine ketone testing, along with increased variable amounts of insulin based on the glucose and ketone levels during illness. Young children often exhibit *low* blood glucose because of smaller glycogen reserves and loss of appetite during illness. Many clinicians recommend sugar-containing liquids during this time. When blood glucose values are greater than 250 mg/dl, ingested clear liquids should not contain carbohydrates; diet soda or unsweetened tea should be given. After glucose levels drop below 250 mg/dl, carbohydrate-containing liquids such as regular soda, clear juices, flavored gelatin dessert, or

---

BOX 17-2

SICK-DAY MANAGEMENT

Check for ketones in urine if blood glucose value is greater than 250 mg/dl.
Use full-liquid and/or clear-liquid diet if child cannot or will not eat.
Have child drink 4 to 8 ounces fluid every 2 hours and retest if ketones present.
Call diabetes team at _(tel. no.)_ if:
    Ketones persist after child drinks 4 to 8 ounces fluid every 2 hours.
    Child has stomach or abdominal pain and vomiting.
    Child has moderate or severe ketone levels.
    Child vomits 2 or more times.
Give supplemental regular insulin per diabetes team's recommendation.

---

other glucose drinks should be used.[79] Children who have high blood glucose or ketones should be given large amounts of fluids to drink (4 to 8 ounces fluid each hour for 2 to 3 hours). Giving children something very salty will stimulate their thirst and promote their drinking of the fluids. If the blood glucose and ketones do not decrease after 2 to 3 hours of drinking increased fluids, parents should call the diabetes team for a supplemental insulin dose to bring them down.

Children with IDDM are especially susceptible to dehydration. During illness, especially when diarrhea occurs, these children should be taken off solid foods for 4 to 8 hours and encouraged to drink 4 to 8 ounces of fluid every hour. If they are unable or unwilling to ingest fluids, they need to be taken to the physician's office or emergency room for intravenous (IV) fluid therapy. Whenever children with IDDM are sick for any reason, "sick-day" management rules should be followed (Box 17-2).

Insulin requirements can vary considerably during illness episodes. Generally the parent should continue to administer the routine insulin doses even if the child is unable to eat, with additional amounts based on blood glucose fluctuations. Since infection may cause insulin resistance, the insulin dose may need to be increased. It is best to give the supplemental insulin needed during illness in the form of regular insulin. A supplemental dose equivalent to about 10% to 20% of the total daily dose every 4 to 6 hours or more frequently may be needed to control severe hyperglycemia and ketosis.[79] If, however, the ill child's blood glucose falls below normal, a reduction in the usual insulin dose will be necessary. Parents should be in close contact with the diabetes team or pediatrician during their child's illness.

COGNITIVE AND LANGUAGE DEVELOPMENT
Cognitive Development

Just as physical development follows predictable patterns, cognitive development has established milestones. Infants learn about the world through their developing senses. Sucking and grasping are early means for experiencing the environment. Young infants have relatively no sense of time. Gradually they begin to appreciate object permanence. Play becomes more goal directed. By the first birthday, infants understand some cause and effect and can remember events. Cuddling and comforting an infant after a painful procedure will assist the infant in feeling loved. Once the infant remembers events, however, just the site of the BGM device or the syringe may stimulate crying.

Toddlers begin to use symbols and can recall past events. By the fourth year, children begin to understand the perspective of others and use classification, although nonsystematically. Children ages 3 to 5 years have an active imagination and explain much of their world in terms of fantasy. These children are particularly vulnerable to medically invasive procedures.

Piaget[32,62-64] described two developmental stages for children from birth to 7 years of age: (1) sensorimotor (0 to 2 years) and (2) preoperational (2 to 7 years). Each of these stages has characteristic attributes that affect how children perceive, comprehend, problem-solve, and reason about themselves and their environment.

Sensorimotor stage

Infants and young toddlers (birth to 2 years) are in Piaget's sensorimotor stage of cognitive development. Their senses and motor skills are actively used to define and interpret objects and events.[65] Infants learn about their environment through reflex activity, simple repetitive behaviors, imitation, and ultimately trial-and-error problem solving. Infants in this stage love to shake a rattle, but, if they drop it, the rattle no longer exists. Infants ages 4 to 6 months have a growing interest in the results or consequences of their actions. These infants can recognize the bottle from seeing only a portion of it hidden under a blanket. They are able to use combinations of reflexes and senses purposely. From 6 to 12 months of age, infants demonstrate purposeful actions and an understanding of object permanence. For example, an infant will begin crying as soon as an alcohol pad is wiped on the skin, anticipating the stick to follow.[65]

Around 12 months of age, toddlers begin to problem solve by using familiar actions to achieve results. However, they perceive only the whole, not parts, which results in connecting a series of separate actions or ideas into one confused whole.[62] For example, if a toddler wants the squeaky toy to make noise, he or she "reasons" that the toy squeaks when dad touches it, so the toy is taken to dad and the child cries if dad fails to make it squeak. Toddlers begin to experiment with new means of achieving familiar results. For example, the child will slowly pour out supper on the floor to watch the effects on the food and on the behavior of those present.

Toddlers ages 18 to 24 months use combinations of mental processes to solve problems. "Out of sight, out of mind" no longer works with this age-group. If daddy goes into another room and closes the door, the toddler knows that he still exists behind that door.

Preoperational stage

Children 2 to 4 years old are in Piaget's preoperational phase and have an increasingly sophisticated use of language, but they interpret the world in egocentric ways. Objects and events occur only in relationship to themselves, and this age-group does not see another person's point of view.

By ages 4 to 7 years, children enter a time of more concrete, tangible thinking. Thought is dominated by what is seen, heard, and experienced. These children can make simple seriations and begin to understand weight, length, size, and time. They love to classify objects, separate them into groups, and sort them into categories. Conservation occurs when children understand that changing the outward appearance of an object does not change its permanent characteristics (e.g., a popsicle is a frozen flavored drink and is the same as a liquid drink melted from a popsicle).

Fantasy and play predominate preschool children's lives, and inanimate objects take on rich and sometimes frightening lives of their own. For example, the syringe likes to hurt them. Preschool and school-age children differ in how they think.[23] As previously noted, toddlers and young preschoolers exhibit *egocentrism* and *absolutism,* which means they perceive situations only in terms of immediate personal outcomes (things they enjoy are good, things that hurt or frustrate them are bad, and anything bad is always bad). For example, a finger stick or injection either hurts or does not hurt; it can not hurt just a little. *Artificialism,* the belief that natural events are created by humans, influences 2- to 5-year-old children to believe someone made them become sick. *Animism* is the belief that inanimate things have intentions, feelings, and thoughts. Children of this age often ask, "When do the stars go to bed?" "Where does the sun play when it rains?" and "Why does my body make me sick with so much sugar?" *Irreversibility,* the belief that actions or thoughts *cannot* be reversed or compensated for, causes children of this age who receive finger sticks or injections to think that all their blood will leak out of this hole and that they will die if a bandaid is not placed on it.[65]

Preoperational-stage children exhibit *magical thinking,* the belief that their own thoughts or actions influence events outside their control. For example, an angry child who wishes a sibling would no longer be there to pester him or her feels guilty when the sibling becomes ill, believing his or her wish came true. The cognitive development from infancy through preschool has implications for diabetes management, as discussed later in this chapter.

Speech and Language

Infants are particularly responsive to high-pitched voices and react to the cadence and melody of voice. By 3 months old they are cooing and reciprocating certain sounds with the caregiver. By 4 months infants laugh, and by 6 months they babble in monosyllables. By the end of the first year, children are attentive to their own name and knowingly use "ma-ma" or "da-da."

Toddlers begin using short sentences and have a vocabulary of 50 to 200 words. Clearly, they understand more than they can verbalize. However, misunderstanding of words often occurs.

Children ages 3 to 5 years have a much larger vocabulary, ranging from 850 to 2000 words. By 3 years, children put two or three sentences together.[42] As their social world expands to include peers, repetitive phrases and songs become tools for language development.

It must be emphasized that preschoolers do not necessarily understand the meaning of the words used unless they have had direct contact in learning to apply them.[11,65] Words used in relation to time, causality, and left and right frequently are incorrectly employed because children of this age do not understand these concepts. Homonyms, words spelled differently but sounding the same, are confusing to them.

It is imperative that health care professionals know the cognitive development of the specific child they are working with to understand what the child is thinking and the best way to communicate information. Parents and professionals must explain any special medical treatments or tests before their occurrence, using words and phrases that children understand. When no explanation is given, toddlers and preschoolers will conjure up their own reasons that contain elements of self-reproach and punishment.[6,11,65] For example, telling children you will "take their temperature" connotes taking something from them; it is better to say you are "checking" it. "Testing" often implies determining if they are good or bad, whereas, "checking" is less challenging.

Developing Concepts of Health and Illness

Preschoolers' understanding of health and illness is very much linked to their cognitive development and is key to understanding children of this age with IDDM. Health is viewed as a positive state, associated with the ability to play, whereas being sick or having a disease such as IDDM is associated with feeling bad and staying in bed.[31] Young children newly diagnosed with IDDM frequently think they no longer have IDDM when they go home from the hospital and can go outside to play. They then think their parents continue to give them "shots" and prick them for BGM because they are bad or their parents want to hurt them. The diabetes team needs to help parents understand IDDM and its therapeutic regimen from their child's point of view.

Robinson[67] studied preschool children in an effort to determine how children explain illness causality. In general, they understood illness better than health. They thought a person could be sick and healthy at the same time and that the relative degree of health or illness was determined by the kind of activity permitted. For example, one with a cold could still play inside and was healthier than one who had to stay in bed. Often, children interpreted ill health as the result of some misdeed or as punishment. They thought the transfer of illness was accomplished magically.[12,31,65]

Verbal explanations contribute minimally to children's understanding of illness or health care procedures and treatments; describing sensory experiences is more helpful. Preparing children for health care encounters should therefore include the expected sights, sounds, and sensations.

PSYCHOSOCIAL DEVELOPMENT
Erikson's Theory of Personality Development

According to Erikson,[28] infants are characterized by the stage of *trust versus mistrust*. Successful development of trust results in being able to maintain hope, optimism, and faith in their environment and abilities. Caring, consistent parenting is necessary to this development of trust. Lack of such care or inconsistency results in children's inability to trust the caregiver and presumably later to lack a sense of faith and confidence. The development of "fear of strangers" is positive in that infants demonstrate bonding to their primary caregivers and learn to be wary of those they do not yet know.

Toddlers are in Erikson's stage of *autonomy versus shame and doubt.* They must establish autonomy by gaining control of their body, its functions, and its mobility. If repeatedly thwarted in attempts at self-control or overprotected, toddlers begin to question their abilities with a sense of shame and self-doubt. Central to this stage is children's desire to imitate their parents' actions.

Preschoolers are in Erikson's *initiative versus guilt* stage. Imagination guides these children into new adventures, and their inner voice warns of limits in the environment. Successfully starting (but not necessarily completing) tasks results in a long-term sense of direction, purpose, and competence. Conflicts, with frequent severe criticisms of efforts, leave children of this age feeling guilty and worthless.

Family Systems

The social domain for infants, toddlers, and preschoolers is the family. For infants, parents (especially the mother) are the borders of the social world. As children mature and are exposed to other social systems (day care, babysitters), siblings, peers, and extended family members become increasingly important to social development.

Families as units have developmental tasks and responsibilities. From providing physical needs to allocating resources to socializing its members, the family system is responsible for ultimately incorporating its members into the society at large. The family provides developing children with the "rules" for society. Each family has its own system of communication and interaction, with unwritten rules for expressing affection and aggression. The family must interface with society, through interaction with work, church, school, day care, or extended family members, and must maintain motivation and morale in its members by rewarding achievements, confronting personal and family crises, setting goals, and developing family values.[18] Interactions within and outside the family in a variety of contexts, a sense of coping and mastery of the members, and a flexible internal organization characterize the "energized" family.[66]

Families who are highly organized and cohesive with less conflict have more successful initial adaptation to their child's diagnosis of IDDM.[5,40,76,88] Hauser and others[40] found the strongest predictor of adherence to the IDDM treatment regimen, improvement in adherence, and overall higher levels of patient adherence was the parents' and children's perceptions of family cohesion. Standen and associates[88] found the degree of metabolic control was related to parental involvement with the nondiabetic children and to many aspects of the Family Environment Scale, including parental incongruence.

Parenting Styles

Children seem to cycle in their behavioral patterns of equilibrium and disequilibrium. The smooth, consolidated behaviors of the 2-year-old child become the disturbed, erratic behaviors of the 2½-year-old child, which become the rounded, balanced, and happy patterns of the

3-year-old child, and so on.[44] Such flux in behavior typically marks surges of growth toward new developmental challenges. Parents, however, often find that although one approach to parenting was effective for the toddler, that same technique no longer works with the preschooler.

Parenting styles seem to fit one of three patterns: authoritarian, permissive, or authoritative.[94] The *authoritarian style* sets absolute standards for behavior and is highly structured. The *permissive style* is tolerant, allowing for considerable self-regulation by the child. Few demands are made for mature behavior. The *authoritative style* sets standards, expects developmentally appropriate behavior, encourages independence, and allows for open communication between parents and children in decision making.

Setting limits and maintaining consistency in reinforcing those limits are concerns for most parents. Structuring children's interpersonal and physical environment to minimize misbehavior and applying behavior management techniques when misbehavior has occurred are skills parents often learn by doing them. Minimizing the opportunity for misconduct includes setting clear and simple rules, modeling appropriate actions, frequently reminding children about the established rules, and rewarding children when they are demonstrating good behavior.

Despite a parent's best efforts, misbehavior will occur. Common strategies for discipline include "time-out," reasoning or scolding, ignoring, or using natural and logical consequences.[58,59]

Regardless of the approach, parents should initiate discipline immediately. Young children have short attention spans, and immediate feedback is necessary for them to attach the discipline to the precise action. In selecting a discipline style, parents must consider the temperament of their child and the severity of the misbehavior. Furthermore, after the behavior is disciplined, the parents should express concern for the child's feelings and should consider the issue closed.

Temperament

Temperament has been defined as the way in which an individual typically behaves, the stylistic aspects of behavior, or the manner of thinking, behaving, or reacting that characterizes an individual. Temperament is an important component to consider in terms of planning the diabetic regimen because it reflects constitutional or dispositional characteristics of a child's behavior.[68,97] Chess and Thomas[21] identified nine qualities contributing to differentiations in temperament: (1) motor activity or activity level, (2) rhythmicity (biologic regularity), (3) approach-withdrawal, (4) adaptability, (5) threshold of responsiveness, (6) intensity of reaction, (7) quality of mood, (8) distractibility, and (9) attention span and persistence. The child's response to new stimuli is assessed in terms of the amount of mobility the child displays, how quickly the child approaches a new stimulus, the energy level of the response, and how easily the child is distracted from the stimulus.

Vaughan[94] has warned that labeling infants and children in this way may promote a self-fulfilling prophecy. Rather, the classifications should be considered in terms of how well the child's temperament fits with the environment and specifically with the parent's personality and styles. Behavior problems are more likely to occur when the child's approach to the world differs greatly from the parent's expectations or childrearing practices.

A study by Rovet and Ehrlich[88] validated that children with IDDM did not differ in overall temperament from sibling controls and did not display a unique temperamental profile. In addition, they found that five of the nine temperament categories (in order of importance: activity level, biologic regularity, intensity of response, distractibility, and mood) consistently accounted for more than 40% of the variance in metabolic control, as measured by HbA_{1c}. Children who were in better metabolic control had normal activity levels, were more predictable and liked regularity, reacted moderately, were easily distracted, and were prone to negative moods. Children in poor metabolic control were less active and predictable, displayed stronger reactions, were less distractible, and had better moods.[68] Unfortunately, this study was completed on school-age children, so these findings cannot be generalized to toddlers or preschoolers. Another study found children with IDDM who reported more extensive disease-related coping repertoires and more frequent use of particular coping strategies to regulate negative emotions had higher HbA_{1c} values.[47] It is important that parents and health care professionals assess the type of coping styles used, since certain styles may be associated with poorer outcomes. This will enable parents and providers to assist children with IDDM by encouraging behavioral coping styles that are more adaptive and predictive of good glycemic control, such as being more active and exercising regularly, both of which help one cope with stress. One study found better glycemic control was associated with children's negative and unpleasant emotions, and thus parents and providers must remember the psychosocial well-being of the child with IDDM is as important as metabolic control.[47]

Fears and Stresses of Young Childhood

Psychologic or physiologic stress negatively affects glucose control. Specific metabolic responses to stress that influence serum glucose levels include the body's production of counterregulatory hormones such as glucagon, catecholamines, growth hormone, cortisol, and thyroid hormone. These hormones increase the release of glucose from the liver through gluconeogenesis and glycogenolysis. Glucagon and catecholamines are rapid acting. Cortisol, growth hormone, and thyroid hormone are longer acting and involved in long-term control of glucose release. Peripheral resistance to insulin may also be increased by the release of these insulin antagonists. In addition, anxiety and stress may indirectly affect glycemic control by negatively affecting adherence behaviors. Parents and children under high stress are less likely to follow the IDDM meal plans and to monitor blood glucose or insulin dosages appropriately. Both need to learn positive coping behaviors.

The nature and impact of childhood fears and stressors are related to children's level of cognitive development, temperament, and overall vulnerability to stress (Table 17-3). Children who are active, energetic, resourceful, and willing to take risks are more resilient to the effects of stress than children who are more withdrawn, timid, stubborn, impulsive, or dependent.[97]

Infants are frightened by loud noises or by loss of physical support. Older infants (6 months to 1 year) fear strangers, heights, things looming over them, and separation from the

Table 17-3   Children's Fears by Age and Behaviors Indicative of Fears

Age	Major fears	Behaviors
Infants (0-3 months)	Sudden movements Loud noises Loss of physical support	Generalized total body reaction, crying Clinging to adult

Infants (4-12 months)	Strange objects and people
	Heights
	Anticipation of previous uncomfortable situations
	Change in routines
	Separation from loved ones
		Crying
		Clinging to adult
		Pulling away, crying
		
		Difficulty eating and sleeping
		Separation anxiety
		  Protest
		  Despair
		  Denial, detachment

Toddlers (1-3 years)	The unknown, the dark Being alone and separation Large or scary animals Loss of control Body injury/pain	Delaying bedtime Separation anxiety Crying, clinging to adult Regression, negativism, temper tantrums, resistance Physical aggression, verbal uncooperativeness
Preschool (3-5 years)	The unknown, the supernatural Monsters and ghosts Separation and abandonment Loss of control Change in routine Body injury and pain Fear of body mutilation	Refusing to sleep Aggressive behavior Separation anxiety, aggression Regression, withdrawal, guilt, anxiety Aggression, withdrawal anxiety

caregiver. By ages 2 to 4 years, toddlers are particularly frightened by certain animals, scary masks, and the darkness. Bedtime, visits to the physician, loss of routines, and loss of a security toy also may be sources of stress. Because the sense of personal boundaries is poorly defined, toddlers fear the loss of body parts.

For preschoolers, fears include fantasies about ghosts and concerns about bodily harm and castration. Invasive procedures, such as needle sticks, are a real threat to body integrity. Stressors for these children center around changes in their routines. Nightmares are common.

According to the primary-secondary control model, a model of cognitively based coping, children use two broad coping approaches: a more *immature* type of coping aimed at modifying the objective sources (objects or events) of stress *(primary control)* and a more subtle, *mature* type of coping aimed at modifying one's own subjective experience or psychologic state (mood, expectations, wishes, interpretations) *(secondary control)*. For example, children might seek to reduce their perception of pain from BGM by directing their parents to be very careful and gentle when doing the finger stick (primary control) or by telling jokes during the finger stick (secondary control).[8] Other examples of primary control include taking insulin to keep from becoming sick, telling oneself that it is bad to eat sweets in order to eat less candy, or talking to friends about diabetes so they know what to do to help if something happens. Additional examples of secondary control include sticking to the meal plan so one feels good about oneself, telling oneself it is good to have the BGM test done so one does not have to worry until the next time, or talking to parents about having diabetes so one can feel good about oneself even if one has IDDM. One study of school-age children found that coping styles at preoperational levels of cognitive development were characterized by the use of primary control, such as seeking emotional support from others who may help children influence objective circumstances. The authors purported that this coping strategy may enhance children's sense of control over IDDM and its treatment requirements.[8] Future studies need to validate these findings with toddlers and preschoolers.

Helping children to master a problem may also encourage cognitive and psychosocial development.[87,97] Ways to help children cope with fears might include giving the child who is fearful of the dark a flashlight and giving a child who is afraid of finger sticks or injections a doll and syringes so he or she can give the doll injections. (NOTE: children will not do painful or fear-provoking procedures on their favorite dolls because they do not want to hurt them.) Also, children use drawings to master their fears, such as drawing a picture of the scary creature and then tearing it up in a ritualized banishing. One 5-year-old child drew a picture of a green monster coming to get her in the lower bunk bed. On questioning about the picture, the author found out this child had been having nightmares because of frequent nocturnal hypoglycemia. With an increase in protein in the bedtime snack, these nightmares stopped.

IMPACT OF DIABETES ON COGNITIVE DEVELOPMENT
Perceptions and Feelings

The onset of diabetes is harrowing to the parent and necessitates an abrupt life-style change for the family. The sensitive child quickly perceives mother's and father's reactions to testing, injections, and meal plans. The best single predictor of adherence to IDDM treatment and good metabolic control and the best preventive measure of recurrent DKA is a reliable, stable family who has undergone extensive education.[79] A number of studies have demonstrated that families who are highly organized and cohesive with open communication, demonstrate consistent expectations and guidance, and are supportively involved in the IDDM management regimen are more likely to have children with IDDM in good metabolic control.*

According to Brewster,[15] children at this age believe illness is the outcome of wrongdoing. Frequent finger sticks (testing blood glucose levels) and insulin injections validate their beliefs. Parents and children need to be frequently reassured there was nothing they thought or did to cause the diabetes and nothing they could have done to prevent it. Preschoolers whose needs for security, affection, praise, and discipline are met often have the confidence to learn specific parts of their IDDM management regimen. These children may be more likely to develop positive self-esteem and social competence, both of which are helpful in developing continued adherence to their IDDM regimen.

---

*References 5, 40, 56, 76, 88.

Effect of Early Onset of Diabetes

Infants, toddlers, and preschoolers with IDDM are subject to the same cognitive development as children without IDDM. Some studies have demonstrated no difference in the mental and cognitive development of children with IDDM.[5,8] However, a few studies have found that preschool children with chronic illnesses (e.g., IDDM) develop delays in cognition compared with those without chronic illness.[30]

Researchers have shown that even mild hypoglycemia (45 to 60 mg/dl blood glucose) may cause visuospatial, visuomotor, cognitive speed, and global cognitive skills to deteriorate in adults.[74,83,95] Ryan and associates[75] found that after 21 minutes of induced mild hypoglycemia on adolescents, mental efficiency was significantly compromised, especially regarding measures of attention and sustained concentration. Another study found children with early onset of IDDM had lower scores on the Wechsler Intelligence Scale for Children–Revised (WISC-R).[42] Rovet and others[68-71] found that children with earlier onset and longer duration of IDDM and more frequent hypoglycemic seizures scored lower on visuospatial tests. Thus even mild hypoglycemia may impair mental functioning to some degree.[42] At this time it is not known if or how many hypoglycemic events or what magnitude or duration will cause permanent impaired mental functioning. Therefore parents must quickly learn the signs and symptoms of hypoglycemia in their child and its treatment. To help young children be able to tell others they are "low" as soon as possible, parents should always label the signs and symptoms of hypoglycemia for their child as "feeling low" (Box 17-3). Having the child eat sugar cubes or frosting instead of candy to treat the "lows" will minimize the number of times children say they are "low" when in reality they just want the candy. Siblings, day-care and preschool teachers, and other parents must also know what to look for and how to treat hypoglycemia.

IMPACT OF DIABETES ON PSYCHOSOCIAL DEVELOPMENT
Parental Coping

The reactions of parents and family members to IDDM indirectly affect young children's psychosocial development. Family characteristics can directly predict the level of the child's metabolic control.* Therefore early assessment of family functioning is essential.

The key components of healthy family functioning include good organization abilities, coherence, warm nurturance, open communication, and consistent guidance and discipline with effective problem-solving abilities. The perception that the family is highly organized and cohesive by the parents and children predicts compliance with the IDDM therapeutic regimen and lower glycohemoglobin levels.[5,40,76] The use of the *Diabetes Regimen Responsibility Scale* (DRRS), the *Diabetes Family Behavior Scale* (DFBS), and the *Family Environment Scale* (FES) is useful to assess thoroughly responsibility with specific regimen tasks and other important family characteristics.[56,73] The DFRS is a 17-item questionnaire designed to measure an individual's perception of who takes responsibility for tasks categorized as general health maintenance, regimen tasks, and social presentation of diabetes.[5] Some researchers have found the following two measures helpful in assessing diabetes-specific family behaviors

---

*References 5, 8, 47, 49, 56, 73, 76, 88.

BOX 17-3

TREATMENT FOR LOW BLOOD SUGAR LEVELS IN THE DIABETIC CHILD

- Check blood glucose if child is crabby, whiney, or stubborn; is suddenly sleepy; or has clinging behaviors (they may be caused by low blood glucose). Look for other physical/behavioral clues of low blood glucose (e.g., pale, change in activity level, rubbing head, looking for food, shaky, sweaty but cool to touch, "spacey" look in eyes).
- When possible, use the same food item to treat "lows" (e.g., juice, regular soda, sugar cubes, frosting).
- Always have foods to treat the "lows" with you. Even short trips to the grocery store can be extended by unforeseeable complications (e.g., traffic).
- Routine is crucial to blood glucose management with toddlers. Even on weekends, do not vary the schedule more than an hour to maintain good blood glucose control, prevent low blood glucose, and add to toddler's comfort.
- Encourage children to tell you how they felt after a "low" so they learn to recognize their own body's sensations. This will help you to know specific low blood glucose symptoms.
- Praise children when they tell you they feel "low" or "funny" or report symptoms.
- If you are having difficulty getting children to drink when "low," try giving something salty first to increase their desire to drink.
- Always use same word when referring to a decreased blood glucose level (e.g., "low").
- Do not allow child to take extended naps, especially if it will cause the child to miss a meal or snack. Be sure to do a blood glucose check if your child is napping or sleeping longer than usual.

(hypothesized to be important in helping or hindering children to follow the IDDM medical regimen) and in evaluating the coping strategies (in relation to their children's illness) of mothers: the DFBS and the *Coping Health Inventory for Parents* (CHIP).[47,56] The DFBS may be helpful in assessing the family's diabetes-specific functional ability and in identifying diabetes-specific family problem areas that relate to a child's metabolic control level in that particular family system.[56]

Parents and other caregivers experience the full range of emotional reactions when a young child is diagnosed with diabetes, including anger, mild depression, guilt, resentment, blaming, and overall emotional distress.[27,49] As the demands of daily care become more clear, parents can become apprehensive, overprotective, and more depressed and experience more emotional strain.[27,39,49] Researchers found that mothers initially reacted to the diagnosis of IDDM in their children with mild depression and overall emotional distress and that these reactions subsided in about 6 to 9 months. They further found that after the initial adjustment phase, there were slight increments in maternal depressive symptoms over the duration of the illness, especially for mothers from higher socioeconomic levels. Their overall psychologic distress (e.g., anxiety, anger, suspiciousness, dysphoria) also increased with the duration of the illness. The mothers' degree of emotional distress immediately after the medical diagnosis strongly predicted their later symptomatology.[49] However, most parents are able to cope with these feelings in a healthy way after the initial diagnosis with extensive education and continuing support by a diabetes team.[79]

How parents, particularly mothers, adjust to IDDM in their preschool children was studied by Wysocki and associates,[99] who surveyed 20 mothers of preschoolers using various behavioral scales and stress indices. In this sample, mothers of children with IDDM reported more sleep problems, social withdrawal, and somatic complaints in their children, although *overall* the mothers did not score their children as abnormal. The mothers also identified more overall family stress, with the diabetic child seen as the source of that stress.

Parental stress and negative feelings are communicated and responded to by young children.[50] The more attention parents place on diabetes activities, the more children are reminded of being different and the more they resist. Parents of chronically ill children often view them as vulnerable or endangered.[55] For example, the child with IDDM may have activities restricted because of parental fear of hypoglycemia. Choices in foods may be severely limited because of parents' uncertainty about their glycemic effect. At a time when the child is beginning to learn independence, the parent may feel obligated to maintain a rigid schedule of meals and activities.

The cost and stress of managing diabetes can certainly stretch a parent's coping abilities. Horan and associates[43] have speculated that children with IDDM may be at risk for child abuse and neglect. Abuse incidence data are higher in chronically ill children, although no data are available about cases involving children with IDDM specifically. Family conflict, parental hopelessness, unrealistic or exaggerated parental expectations, overprotectiveness, and inconsistent parenting are all indicators of poor adaptation to the child's diagnosis and care needs.[51,56,72] Studies found that preexisting problems in family communication and relationships, conflict over who is expected to do what, less family organization and cohesiveness, less warmth and nurturance, and inappropriate problem solving were directly related to poorer metabolic control of children with IDDM.*

Well-meaning friends may offer a variety of how-to approaches or share stories of what can happen when the management plan is not compulsively followed. Thus, underlying the day-to-day anxieties associated with diabetes self-management, are the parents' worst fears of long-term complications and poor health. The DCCT's findings may validate these fears.[25] Such fears may manifest as overprotective limitations on the child's life.

Parents may benefit from contact with other families with young children with IDDM within the parameters of a diabetes education program.[72,85] Diabetes education programs can provide the opportunity for parents of young children to share other concerns, fears, and anxieties as well as ideas on how to handle problem times such as finger sticks, injections, and meals or snacks. Parents can learn their "worst fears" may be positively handled when others describe their crises, what they did, and the outcome for the child[50] (see Boxes 17-4 to 17-7 and Table 17-4). Parents, especially mothers, have considerable responsibilities for

---

*References 5, 8, 40, 49, 56, 76, 88.

Table 17-4   Effect of Diabetes on the Child and Parents

Developmental tasks	Effect of diabetes on child's development	Effect of diabetes on parents	Suggested approaches
Infancy (0-1 year)			
Trust versus mistrust Sensorimotor stage	Infant is confused by parents inflicting pain. Frequent feedings are required to maintain blood glucose levels. Frequent, severe or prolonged hypoglycemia may be dangerous to developing CNS. Immunizations may elevate blood glucose levels.	Grief over loss of perfect child Selection of day care and babysitters more difficult Anxiety over fear of hypoglycemia	Reassure, cuddle, and hold child after injections and finger sticks. Use finger stick blood glucose tests to monitor and alter care. Use external clues with bedtime and midnight blood glucose levels to detect hypoglycemia during night.
Toddler (1-3 years)			
Autonomy versus shame and doubt Sensorimotor and preoperational stages	Toddler depends on parents for BGM, diet, and insulin. Food jags lead to diet inconsistencies. Childhood illnesses and growth spurts affect blood glucose levels. Older toddler begins to know if "low." Older toddler can begin assisting with finger sticks.	Difficulty distinguishing misbehavior from blood glucose levels Difficulty in allowing child some autonomy	Offer child choices in food selection, injection, and BGM sites. Use matter-of-fact, quick approach with procedures. Use BGM to help identify symptoms. Provide consistency in discipline, setting limits, and routines. Use a flexible insulin program. Prevent mealtime battles. Have a plan for managing sick days. Child needs to be told that he or she did not cause IDDM, and that finger sticks and injections are not punishments.

Preschool (3-6 years)

Initiative versus guilt
Preoperational stage

Child begins to feel different from peers.

Child views any aspects of diabetes management as punishment.

Child fantasizes that finger sticks and injections may result in bleeding to death.

Child needs to control own environment and wants to cooperate

Child fears body mutilation.

Overprotective behaviors as child becomes increasingly independent

Working with preschool teachers

Avoid giving candy or extra attention when hypoglycemia occurs.

Note that 2- to 3-year-old child can identify "low" and tell adult.

Use play and drawings to express feelings.

Encourage child's participation in simple diabetes tasks.

Basic diabetes education includes choosing proper foods, identifying symptoms, and knowing what to do for "lows."

Knowing if blood glucose high; child needs to wait to eat.

If child can do own fingerstick, may try to give own injection.

Plan for parties and holidays to minimize child's feelings of "differentness."

Encourage child's participation in sports, swimming, dancing, and gymnastics.

BOX 17-4

PARENTAL CONCERNS AND THE YOUNG CHILD WITH DIABETES

Fear of hypoglycemia, especially undetected hypoglycemia
Fear of hyperglycemia and long-term complications
Accepting their child has diabetes
Dealing with the opinions of relatives and friends
Lack of support or help from spouse
Adapting to a rigid schedule
Feeling alone
Dealing with siblings' reactions and behaviors
Fear of making a mistake in the management
Finding and trusting other caregivers
Developing a working relationship with the medical community
Guilty feelings about all the invasive procedures

---

their children's treatment-related tasks. The diabetes team members must provide them with liberal emotional and informational support (Box 17-4).[27]

Behavior Management

Knowing when and how to discipline the very young child with diabetes can be quite a dilemma for parents (Box 17-5). The diabetes team must help parents learn to differentiate misbehavior from symptoms of hypoglycemia and hyperglycemia.

The child who is irritable or combative may be having a low blood glucose level (hypoglycemia, insulin shock) or may be having normal difficulty with impulse control. The physical sensations of blood glucose fluctuations are often not recognized by the child and can be misdiagnosed by the parent. Parents need to be taught how to differentiate the symptoms of hypoglycemia and hyperglycemia from behaviors caused by poor impulse control. They should automatically test the child's blood glucose when the child misbehaves.

Hypoglycemic symptoms in young children include the six S's: feeling shaky, sweaty (but cool to touch), sleepy, starving (will happily eat their least favorite foods), stubborn, and "spacey." Young children also may have an abrupt change in activity level and become pale and irritable, whiney, or clinging without provocation.[13,16] Infants may manifest hypoglycemia by appearing unexpectedly sleepy, lethargic, hungry, irritable, pale, or glassy eyed or have a unique specific facial expression or particular behavior. They also might have apnea, hypothermia, cyanosis, hypotonia, or poor feeding.[87] Toddlers and preschoolers may have unique feelings they can identify as they are becoming "low" (e.g., legs feel heavy, feel like they are walking on a cloud or just above the ground, tingling or tightness in their head). Nocturnal hypoglycemia is evidenced by any of these, as well as nightmares, restlessness, or noisy sleep, sleep walking, or sleep talking.

BOX 17-5

BEHAVIORAL MANAGEMENT TECHNIQUES FOR THE DIABETIC CHILD

To encourage and maintain positive diabetes care behaviors, "catch the child being good" and give praise or do a special activity.

Be sure to be specific about what behavior you want from the child. For example, it is better to say, "Hold your arm still when I give you your insulin," than "Be good when you get your insulin."

1. Positively reinforce behaviors that are helpful in diabetes management and care.
2. Avoid only giving attention for behaviors that undermine diabetes management and care.
3. Find out the best rewards for the child and what he or she likes to do (e.g., read a book, color, use molding putty, have a bubble bath).
4. Keep a stash of items the child likes available as rewards for good behavior (e.g., for girls, bracelets, gum, markers; for boys, fantasy and combat toys).
5. Identify the time of day it is most difficult for the child to comply or the one thing the child does not like to do. Reward child for doing well with this particular problem each time child does well. Ignore behavior if not done well.

Hypoglycemia often occurs when children are late for meals, eat only part of their meal, are more active than usual (excess exercise can cause hypoglycemia up to 18 hours afterward), take long naps (especially when they are then late for a meal or snack), when schedules are altered (e.g., holidays, start or end of school), or if their appetite is decreased during illness. Parents should test the blood glucose or, if not possible, treat a possible "low" by giving the child one-half glass of juice or 1 to 2 teaspoons of sugar or pancake syrup. Parents might treat infants by rubbing maple syrup, cake gel, or frosting inside their cheek, especially if they appear too sleepy or weak to drink. Honey should be avoided in children under 1 year of age because of the risk of infant botulism.[87] If the behavior improves and the parent thinks the misbehavior was caused by hypoglycemia, they should be sure to tell the child he or she was "low" and ask how he or she felt at the beginning of becoming "low." Describing this episode and reminding the child how he or she felt will help the child recognize and report a similar incident the next time. If the misbehavior does not decrease within 5 minutes, discipline should be instituted if the hypoglycemic symptoms do not worsen. Candy and extra attention should *not* be given for hypoglycemia because children will use these symptoms for secondary gain.

Children whose symptoms of hypoglycemia worsen and who become unresponsive or go into a coma should be treated immediately with glucagon. For infants under 40 pounds (18 kg), 0.5 ml (half the vial) is given intramuscularly.[87] Children who weigh more are usually given 0.66 (two-thirds vial) to 1.0 ml intramuscularly. The child should regain consciousness within 20 minutes. If nausea and vomiting do not occur, the child should be fed and the physician notified immediately. If nausea and vomiting occur the physician most likely will want to see the child.

It is extremely important that the child wear an identification tag with his or her name and the diagnosis of IDDM. It is helpful if the parents have a card listing the diabetes team members' phone numbers and common symptoms accompanying a hypoglycemic reaction. This prevents parents from being unable to take action the first few times they witness their child having a hypoglycemic reaction.

Hyperglycemia causes children to become thirsty, urinate frequently, feel "lazy" and tired, and become irritable, frustrated, and less able to follow direction. Many infants and toddlers become flushed, cry, or fuss and rub their eyes for no apparent reason. Hyperglycemia occurs when children are not as active as usual, eat more than planned, have an infection, or develop relative insulin deficiency as a result of a growth spurt or inadequate insulin adjustment, especially during growth spurts.

Children with hyperglycemia should be given extra sugar-free fluids and should be encouraged to remain active unless they have ketones, blood glucose level greater than 350 mg/dl, or fever. They should not exercise if these are present. Ketones are checked on infants or toddlers wearing diapers by placing a cotton ball in the diaper to absorb enough urine to yield accurate results.[87] Children with ketones may require additional insulin, according to the recommendation of the physician or diabetes nurse practitioner. In addition, 4 to 8 ounces of fluid per hour for 2 to 3 hours and frequent BGM testing are recommended. If the ketones and blood glucose are not diminishing, if the child cannot drink and retain fluids 1 hour without vomiting, or if the child vomits twice regardless of the cause, the parents should call the diabetes nurse clinician or physician regardless of the time of day (see Box 17-6 for treatment for high blood sugar and ketones).

Siblings

Siblings are children's first peer group. Siblings are important participants in preschooler's social development. As much as one third of the interactions between a toddler and an older sibling consist of imitation.[23] Often older siblings share in parenting responsibilities and provide security and language enhancement.[9] Sibling relationships may have increasing relevance today because of shrinking family size, loss of the expanded family because of geographic mobility, maternal employment, and day care.[9]

The impact of diabetes in the family on well sibling(s) can be profound. Older siblings may feel guilty that their brother or sister developed diabetes or worry that they also will get it. They may assume the management anxieties and worries of their parents. In a study of 30 well siblings, Ferrari[29] found lower self-concept scores when compared with control subjects. Siblings of diabetic children were more concerned about their school status, their personal happiness, and their popularity.

Older siblings should be taught what diabetes is, the signs and symptoms of hypoglycemia, and how to manage it, as well as the basic concepts of the meal plan. If they are responsible for the younger child with IDDM while the parents work, they should be taught how to give glucagon. However, they should never be asked to help restrain or give insulin injections because of the psychologic stress this imposes on the sibling and the resentment it may engender against that sibling by the child with IDDM.[54]

BOX 17-6

TREATMENT FOR HIGH BLOOD SUGAR AND KETONE LEVELS IN THE DIABETIC CHILD

- Do not get in a power struggle over food.
- Always use the same sugar-free drink for high blood glucose.
- Use a sticker on the bottom of the glass to get your child to drink. (Have drinking races between mom, dad, and your child, and have a special prize for the one who finishes first to ensure someone does.)
- Pour a little fluid in a larger glass so that it appears to the child that he or she has to drink less.
- Always use the same word for high blood glucose (e.g., "high").
- Have the child help check for ketones.
- To help the child drink, give him or her something salty (e.g., two or three chips, salty crackers).
- Prepare favorite programs or commercials on videotapes, or use already developed videotapes 60 minutes long to distract child until time to eat (e.g., Disney's *The Little Mermaid* is 82 minutes long, or use *Sesame Street* or Saturday morning cartoons).

Day Care and Babysitters

As increasingly more mothers work outside the home, issues of child care surface. About 50% of infants and approximately two thirds of preschool children have mothers in the workplace.[94] Most mothers feel some guilt over leaving their infants or toddlers in another's care; these feelings may be intensified in mothers of children with diabetes. The American Academy of Pediatrics (AAP) has a reference manual to assist parents in selecting appropriate child care.[1]

Finding adequate and knowledgeable child care is an additional, difficult demand for parents of the child with diabetes. Day-care workers and babysitters must know how to handle hypoglycemia. Emergency protocols include ready access to juice or glucose gels and the administration of glucagon. Mealtimes, snack foods, and what to do if the child will not eat must be clear to and implemented by the day-care workers and babysitter. Access to the parent or a capable family friend by phone, as well as the diabetes team's phone number, should be available.

The diabetes team should provide education for siblings and regular day-care workers and babysitters, preferably at the same time the parents are learning.[33] The AAP or Juvenile Diabetes Foundations have additional resources and classes.

TEACHING AND LEARNING IMPLICATIONS

An underlying philosophy for teaching young children and their parents includes an appreciation that knowledge and skill acquisition can be gradual and that children will eventually attain self-management behaviors.[82] Young children require a gradual introduction of concepts and skills. This introduction should not necessarily be in the same order that adults learn. For instance, it may seem more reasonable to teach drawing up the insulin dose first, followed by injection procedures. Toddlers only have the fine motor and cognitive skills to be able to push the button on the BGM device, hold a bandaid during BGM, or insulin injections, and begin to recognize and report hypoglycemia. Preschoolers (5 to 6 years old) can recognize, report, and treat hypoglycemia; state reasons for wearing diabetic identification; state the insulin schedule; develop the fine motor skills to inject insulin; remember to rotate sites; use a lancet to obtain an adequate blood sample; perform BGM sometimes with supervision; begin to categorize food into groups; remember favorite foods they can and cannot have; and state appropriate actions in response to hyperglycemia.[100] Not until perhaps 8 to 12 years old will the child have the fine motor and the cognitive skills required to draw up and mix insulin doses accurately. Children should have parental supervision while completing IDDM activities through adolescence.[81] Together, parents and professionals should plan for the gradual introduction of self-care skills consistent with the child's developmental level according to the interest and abilities of the individual child and guided by the findings of Wysocki and others' study[100] (see Table 17-4). In addition, diabetes team members should provide ongoing guidance about ways to enhance children's independence, promote adaptive parent-child sharing of responsibilities, and address significant parent-child conflicts concerning IDDM management regimens.[5,27]

Strategies

Teaching and learning strategies for young children with diabetes and their families are dictated by several aspects of learner readiness. Clearly, most of the education will be directed toward the parents and significant caregivers. These individuals must be assessed for their desire and ability to learn the information necessary for safe management of the child. Strategies that enhance learning include early introduction and direct application of necessary diabetes skills, such as injections, finger stick procedures, and record keeping. By becoming actively involved from the beginning, the parent is better able to regain a sense of control. Having a parent perform the necessary IDDM-related procedures seems to be much less threatening for children of this age. Consequently, if hospitalization is necessary at diagnosis, parents should be encouraged to stay with their child and participate actively in his or her care. Often, parents are so overwhelmed at the time of diagnosis that they are unable to attend fully to all the new information. Modeling diabetes skills for these parents assists them to assume the care more quickly in a less threatening manner.

Much anxiety of parental learning about caring for children with IDDM centers around learning to give the insulin injection. The diabetes team needs to insist that parents learn to give insulin injections early during the hospitalization because they need to become accurate and feel competent and comfortable with their skill and knowledge before they go home. It often helps if the diabetes educator gives the parents an injection of saline with the insulin syringe the second day of the hospitalization or as soon as the child's condition is stabilized. This helps parents know the injections are not painful. They are then able to concentrate on learning this skill.

Infants and toddlers will necessarily have very small doses of insulin ordered. Even preschoolers may have less than 2 U of insulin given during the "honeymoon period." A few research studies found that neither parents nor health care providers are accurate with insulin doses less than 2 U.[20] However, parents who give 1 or 2 U of insulin frequently can become more accurate. It is recommended that for those receiving very small doses of insulin, a diluted insulin solution be used because it allows for more accurate regulation of blood sugar.[54] U-10 and U-25 insulin is often used for infants and young toddlers (U-50 concentration may also be used).

Educational techniques directed at adult learning are used for the parents (see Chapters 15 and 20). Understanding how a parent approaches new information is important. Some parents learn best through self-study, some are more visual or auditory learners, and others need more direction from the educator.

In any teaching plan for the very young child, a component of behavior management and parenting skills must be included. How to assess the need for discipline and when to begin helping the child learn some self-care skills must be addressed. Parents need to be given information about what to expect as the child grows, both in terms of predictable changes in IDDM management and in normal child development. Parents should be introduced to the use of positive reinforcement and praise for acceptable behavior and "timeout" for unacceptable behavior.[58,59] Parents often find that the principles of logical and natural consequences of misbehavior are extremely helpful. For example, a natural consequence of not allowing the finger to be washed with warm water before BGM is the necessity to "milk" the finger or reprick it to obtain enough blood for an accurate check. The natural consequence of not eating at mealtime is having the uncomfortable feelings associated with "low" blood sugar.

Teaching toddlers and preschoolers about diabetes is difficult because their cognitive abilities and language skills are limited. Although educational materials are available for young children, diabetes educators and parents need to be extremely creative and use play, videotapes, cartoons, storytelling, and children's drawings to teach them about diabetes.[35,36,51,65] Novo-Nordisk provides *Sam's Day: A Coloring Book,* which can be used to stimulate discussions with preschoolers.[78] Telling a story about another child who has the same symptoms, fears, and behaviors as the toddler or preschooler is very helpful. It becomes even more helpful if the educator uses a doll to demonstrate the BGM and insulin injections and then encourages the toddler or preschooler to "help the doll feel better by" giving the insulin injection or "see if the doll is feeling very sleepy, thirsty, and starving because she has low blood sugar." Emphasizing the child did nothing to cause the diabetes and restating that finger sticks and injections *are not punishment* are essential. The stories can be repeated often, adding new behaviors and feelings of the child.

The young child must be approached slowly with a caring attitude. Young children are fearful of strangers, particularly those dressed in white laboratory coats. The child should be allowed time to observe and inspect the professional from a safe distance, often while securely in the parent's arms. Toddlers and preschoolers are also frightened by prolonged eye contact or staring. It is helpful if the professional averts his or her gaze, talks with the child's toy animal first, and approaches the child slowly, unhurriedly, and quietly. Preschool children need to handle equipment to assure themselves that the stethoscope or reflex hammer is not alive. Analogies escape these children. "Taking your blood pressure" or "giving a little stick on your arm" are taken quite literally.

Asking preschool children to tell the health care professional a story either about another doll or about their drawings helps reveal their thoughts, feelings, and misperceptions. Some preschoolers will tell stories more readily into tape recorders.

Some preschoolers find learning to do their own finger sticks is fun, especially if they first saw a similar peer do one on a videotape and then they were videotaped doing one on themselves.[35] Giving the videotape to the preschooler to show to their parents and day-care classes reinforces their increased self-esteem while demonstrating to adults how capable they are.

Leaving the educator's doll with syringes without needles and practice insulin bottles plus the BGM device without lancets in the open in the toddler's or preschooler's hospital room frequently encourages the child to do these procedures on the doll when he or she is alone or just before the parents actually do it to the child. Children express their anger of having to have these painful and fear-provoking procedures done, release hostility and anger while gaining a feeling of being more in control of the situation, and reveal misperceptions and socially unacceptable thoughts through this type of play. They also become quite proficient at correctly doing the procedures because of this practice. One 2¾-year-old surprised both myself and her parents by announcing she would "prick her own finger today" and quickly did so correctly and competently. This toddler continued to dictate who could "prick her finger" as a healthy means of controlling the situation.

Children should be encouraged to give their doll or stuffed animal "who has diabetes" injections and finger sticks just before and just after they receive their own. This helps them attain mastery and a feeling of control over these situations. It also helps them express their thoughts, feelings, unrealistic fears, and misperceptions so that adults can then help them cope with their feelings and correct their misunderstandings.

Assessment and Planning

Diabetes in the child less than 2 years old is reported to be increasing in most diabetes centers in the United States and Great Britain.[79] The infant and toddler typically are very ill when the diagnosis of IDDM is made. Management of DKA in the very young child focuses primarily on correcting fluid, electrolyte, and acid-base balance along with insulin replacement. (Management of DKA is addressed in detail in Chapter 10.)

Once past the crisis of DKA, the health team's plans are directed at long-term management centered on the goals of adequate blood glucose control with promotion of normal growth and development. To this end, blood glucose and urine ketone testing, a meal plan, insulin therapy, and an activity plan are established with the parents (Table 17-5).

Monitoring Blood Glucose Levels

Self-monitoring of blood glucose (SMBG) has afforded the parents of infants and very young children a practical and expedient means of evaluating effects of the management plan.[16]

Table 17-5   Summary of Approaches to Diabetes Management According to Developmental Stage

Need	Approach
Infants and toddlers	
Parent education	Obtain complete diabetes management information.
Blood tests	Do not delay learning procedure.
	Incorporate into daily routine.
	Reassure child this is not a punishment.
Injections	Swaddle child with sheet or blanket.
	Do procedure slowly.
	Reassure child of love and acceptance after injection.
	Give injection to toddler's doll.
	Rotate sites (e.g., arms one week, thighs next week; use abdomen if enough fatty tissue present when blood glucose high).
Changing eating patterns	Allow child to follow own pattern.
	Do not force-feed.
	Do not get into power struggle over food.
	Remember that finger foods are most loved.
Recognizing and treating hypoglycemia	Note that a sudden change in behavior may be the only symptom.
	Treat calmly with sugar cubes or juice, not candy, and do not give extra attention at this time.
Parental anxiety	Identify health care professional you feel comfortable with and maintain ongoing follow-up.
	Maintain contact with other parents.
Preschoolers	
Parent education	Obtain complete diabetes management information.
Blood tests	Provide child with own record book in which he or she receives stickers or stars for each blood test completed.
	Allow child to test doll's blood.
	Allow child to help by holding cotton or bandaid.
	Always cover hole with bandaid.
	Treat as routine care item.
	Emphasize this is not punishment.
Injections	Note that child may physically resist and be angry.
	Allow child to give injections to doll.
	Give child tasks to do during procedure.
	Reassure child injections are not a punishment.
	Allow child to make choices between acceptable things (left or right arm).
Changing eating patterns	Allow child to follow own eating pattern.
	Determine likes and dislikes.
	Give child reasonable choices.
Recognizing and treating hypoglycemia	Note that a sudden change in behavior, especially dreams, tiredness, and irritability, may be only symptoms.

Continued.

Table 17-5 Summary of Approaches to Diabetes Management According to Developmental Stage—cont'd

Need	Approach
Behavior problems related to diabetes	Treat calmly with sugar cubes or juice, not candy.
	Do not overreact or give unnecessary attention at this time.
	Child must have some control over self; give choices within limits.
	Allow child to feel in control by giving blood tests and injections to dolls and by "helping" with own.
	Give attention when good, not when acting out or refusing care.
Parental anxiety	Maintain frequent contact with health care person of choice.
	Meet with other parents of children with diabetes.

BGM should be completed three or four times each day. Morning and bedtime values are essential. Typical sites include fingertips (outer aspects), ear lobes, and the outer aspect of the heel (for infants). With such small surface areas available, parents need to observe carefully the areas for any skin breakdown or infection. Parents should be cautioned about using the central portion of the finger and heel because repeated punctures in those sites may be associated with loss of touch sensation in fingers and osteomyelitis in the heel.

During the initial education sessions, parents should test their own blood glucose so they know these are painful and can be prepared for their child's reaction. Parents can be taught to use only two or three fingers so they become callused more quickly and then are not as painful for the child. To facilitate obtaining a good drop of blood with one stick, parents may be taught to wash the area with soap and warm water and keep the area below the level of the heart. This avoids the additional pain caused by "milking" the area and makes it easier to obtain the hanging drop with wiggly fingers or toes. Bandaids should be applied after every finger stick and insulin injection to prevent the young children from being afraid all their blood will run out.

As with injections, parents must be quick, matter of fact, and calm to gain the child's confidence. As the child becomes old enough to participate actively, the parent can begin to offer choices (e.g., Which finger? Which bandaid? Do you want to push the button? Do you want to help hold the strip?). Finger sticks can be completed at the kitchen table or in the living room while the child is distracted (e.g., sitting on the couch watching cartoons). Even 2-year-old toddlers like to wash their hands, unwrap and hold the bandaid, and select the finger to be used this time. Most 3- and 4-year-old children like to do the finger stick by themselves (with the parent present). It seems to hurt less and provides them with a sense of accomplishment and control (Box 17-7).

Blood glucose monitors selected for use with young children should operate with accuracy and require small amounts of blood. Most parents prefer those with automatic memories. However, parents should record the blood glucose values by date and time to be able to spot decreasing or increasing trends quickly at specific times of the day to facilitate appropriate changes in the insulin doses.

BOX 17-7

HELPING PARENTS AND TODDLERS/PRESCHOOLERS COPE WITH INJECTIONS AND FINGER STICKS

1. Treat the finger sticks and insulin injections in a calm, matter-of-fact, no-nonsense manner. Do not give in to stalling, and avoid debates with the child. Use a firm but pleasant manner.
2. Ways that the child can help with finger sticks include the following:
   a. Choose finger (can play "eenie-meinee-minie-mo").
   b. Wash finger.
   c. Hold cotton balls on to stop bleeding.
   d. Hold bandaid and help wrap finger.
3. Keep the child's room a safe place by not giving finger sticks or insulin injections there.
4. Children are creatures of habit and are often more comfortable doing procedures in the same place (a comfortable couch).
5. Never do procedures during or immediately after a reprimand or punishment. The child might associate these procedures with being punished. It is best to do them after a story or a favorite TV show, when the child is relaxed.
6. During finger sticks or injections, help the time go faster by singing with your child, saying the ABCs, or talking about the child's interests. If the child screams, remind the child that he or she can scream as loud as he or she wants but must hold the finger, leg, or arm still to complete the procedures quickly and to avoid injury.
7. If child runs from you before the procedure, get him or her immediately. Do not play or become angry; just do what you need to do to complete the procedures.
8. Many children enjoy having their own medical box of equipment, including the following:
   a. Alcohol pads
   b. Washcloth
   c. 3 ml syringes without needles
   d. Finger-sticking device
   e. Bandaids
   f. At 3 years of age, bottle of normal saline
9. Children often need to give their stuffed animal or doll finger sticks or insulin injections immediately after their own. This promotes feelings of mastery and control over these threatening situations.
10. Drawing a body outline of your child and placing stickers where insulin was received help the child identify (and control to some degree) where insulin would be or was given.
11. Be prepared for increased demonstration of emotions when with significant others (e.g., grandparents, aunts, uncles). The child may retest each new person that becomes involved in or watches the diabetes management, (including mom or dad).
12. Expect some dawdling; when your child exhibits desired behavior, praise him or her.

Nutrition

The chief aim of dietary management in this age-group is providing sufficient calories and nutrients for normal growth while limiting the amount of simple sugars. Unlike the adult with diabetes, these children *need* extra calories for impending growth demands.[92,93]

With an infant, demand feeding is allowed, with adjustments made to the insulin program. Mothers who are breastfeeding can be assured that, with BGM and use of a short-acting insulin, their babies' blood glucose can be adequately controlled. Once the switch is made to baby foods, a more standard exchange system is often used.[10]

Toddlers are notoriously picky about their foods. Food jags and faddisms are common. At times they are ravenous and other times refuse food altogether. Such behaviors play havoc on diabetes control but can be managed with insulin adjustments. In general, however, allowing toddlers to eat their "food of the week" (e.g., peanut butter with sugar-free jelly at lunch and at supper) will satisfy both the meal plan and the child's developmental needs. Parents must not allow mealtimes to become battlegrounds or allow children to manipulate them by eating or not eating specific foods. In some cases a parent may be told to give the insulin *after* the child's meal in amounts based on food intake. This is not the ideal approach to good control, but such adaptations sometimes are necessary to prevent future battles and manipulation by certain children at mealtimes. Perhaps when the insulin analog lispro is available, this difficult problem will be minimized because it is purported to be absorbed immediately.

It is important that any child less than 6 years old has small, frequent meals throughout the day (i.e., three meals and three snacks).[48,79] Because of limited storage of glycogen, the child cannot safely delay meals or snacks. Snacks such as finger foods (crackers, fruits, breadsticks, cheese) provide not only the needed nutrition but also the opportunity for fine motor development and independence. Parents need to use creativity in appealing to the young child's appetite. Mixing fruit juice with seltzer and freezing the combination makes a nice alternative to soda pop. Raw vegetables with yogurt dip are an ideal choice for the extra-hungry child.

Mealtime battles may be avoided or managed with a reward system of stars or "smiley faces."[37] Children should be given no more than 25 minutes to eat a meal and 15 minutes to eat snacks, after which time leftover food is removed. No additional food is given until the next meal, or hypoglycemic symptoms begin. If hypoglycemic symptoms begin, blood glucose is tested and treatment initiated. Five minutes after treatment, the child should be reminded that hypoglycemia occurs when he or she does not eat most of the food planned for meals or snacks. Since children do not like to feel hungry or "low," these experiences serve as natural consequences; they are the best teachers (see Box 17-1). In contrast, children who become hypoglycemic after excessive activity should be given an extra bread, fruit, or meat. If hypoglycemia occurs 2 to 3 days in a row, parents should call the diabetes professional for a meal plan and insulin adjustment.

Exercise

Although there is no question that exercise is an important component of the diabetes care plan, it is probably the most inconsistent parameter in the young child. Exercise in the young child is not easy to schedule, and the child does not participate in the same degree each day. For example, once the child begins walking, parents may notice more hypoglycemia and a subsequent need to adjust insulin doses. BGM and diet adjustment are essential to assist in adjusting insulin doses. If prolonged or excess activity is anticipated, a decrease in the insulin dose or additional complex carbohydrates (e.g., peanut butter, cheese and crackers) may be required.

Insulin Management

Infants and young children require correspondingly lower doses of insulin than older children or adolescents. This presents unique management challenges. Insulin syringe manufacturers market syringes measured by 0.5-unit increments, with a total of 25 units (Terumo), and Becton-Dickinson produces a 30-unit U-100 syringe. Both are ideal for small doses.

Infants may require very small portions of an insulin unit. In such cases, diluting the insulin to either U-10 or U-25 concentrations may be required.[82] Diluting insulin is not ideal because of the extra manipulation in preparing the dose, potential error in drawing up insulin in a U-100 syringe, and decreased storage time. If dilution is required, the parent must clearly understand how the conversions are made.

U-10 insulin is prepared by a pharmacist and made up of 1 part insulin with 9 parts diluent (yielding 10 U of insulin in every 1 ml). Likewise, U-25 yields 25 U of insulin in every 1 ml. Parents can be taught to use the phrases "lines of insulin" to denote the volume and "actual units of insulin" to denote the strength. The following is an example of using U-10 concentration, preferably with a 0.5 or 0.3 ml syringe[54]:

Actual units of insulin		Lines of insulin on 0.5 or 0.3 ml syringe
0.1 U	=	1 line on syringe
0.3 U	=	3 lines on syringe
0.5 U	=	5 lines on syringe
0.8 U	=	8 lines on syringe
1.0 U	=	10 lines on syringe
1.3 U	=	13 lines on syringe
2.4 U	=	24 lines on syringe

An example of using U-25 concentration with a 0.5 or 0.3 ml syringe follows:

Actual units of insulin		Lines of insulin on 1 ml syringe
0.25 U	=	1 line on syringe
0.75 U	=	3 lines on syringe
1.25 U	=	5 lines on syringe
2.0 U	=	8 lines on syringe
2.5 U	=	10 lines on syringe
3.25 U	=	13 lines on syringe
6.0 U	=	24 lines on syringe

Current insulin therapy suggests that frequent doses provide a smoother pattern of glycemic control across the day. Often, two mixed doses a day provide adequate glucose control in the young child. More intensive insulin therapy regimens are available, but this increases the risks of frequent and more severe hypoglycemic episodes. Intensive insulin therapy provides doses of regular insulin before meals and an intermediate insulin at bedtime or with the evening meal and allows the parent or physician to make rapid adjustments as appetite and activity levels change. At this time, however, intensive insulin therapy is not recommended for young children because of the potential harm to the developing brain and nervous system.[25] In addition, prepubertal children with IDDM are relatively protected against the development of microvascular complications.[79] The parent and diabetes team members must weigh ideal management against the most practical and reasonable protocol for the young child. Good metabolic control for young children with IDDM is now defined as children who are well adjusted, do not have frequent severe hypoglycemia, and have HbA_{1c} values of 7% to 9%. Values greater than 11% are considered to represent poor metabolic control.[79] It may be necessary to compromise on having HbA_{1c} values between 9% and 11% for infants and toddlers to minimize the number of severe hypoglycemic events.

Because the child is smaller, insulin injection sites are limited. Thighs, arms, and upper buttocks are generally acceptable. The abdomen is acceptable when sufficient subcutaneous tissue is present. Parents must be taught ways to hold the child comfortably while giving the injection.

The child's attitude about injections closely approximates the parents' responses. Parents should be encouraged to approach the procedure in a calm, matter-of-fact manner, quickly preparing and giving the injection, with plenty of hugs and reassurances afterward. Parents often find it helps to give toddlers and preschoolers stickers for holding still and then when five stickers are earned, going to the park or playing a favorite game (see Box 17-5). Pleading and negotiating with the struggling toddler or preschooler are futile and accelerate both the child's and the parent's stress levels and encourage the child to use more manipulative behaviors (e.g., temper tantrums) in an attempt to avoid this procedure.

Unless the parent has personally experienced an injection, he or she may believe that the child feels pain. Simulated injections (with saline in an insulin syringe) are potent teaching aids for frightened and anxious parents, who then find the injection does not hurt as much as they thought. Most parents appreciate the opportunity to practice on the health care professional, themselves, and each other, gaining confidence and skill before giving their child an injection.

For the child who continues to be anxious about injections, therapeutic play with syringes and dolls is beneficial. Extreme behavioral responses may require the expertise of a behavioral specialist such as a child psychologist or psychiatrist.

Several "jet" injector devices are on the market. These needleless injectors operate under high-pressure air blasts that propel the insulin under the skin. Although seemingly a wonderful idea for small children, pressure settings that are not properly adjusted and holding the device at the wrong angle result in bruising or painful "injections." In addition, the cost of these devices (more than $400) is prohibitive for many.

Daily Schedules

Despite careful planning, parents often find that children do not always eat or sleep on schedule and do not always cooperate with testing and injections. Parents need guidance in knowing which aspects of care cannot be changed and which areas of care can be more flexible. For example, there is no question that the child must have insulin two or more times each day. It may be possible, however, to establish a standard routine for weekdays with a more flexible time schedule for weekends. Any alterations in the treatment plan must be carefully monitored with BGM to determine the effect.

Naps should be preceded by a snack. Parents will feel more confident and safe if they observe the sleeping child once or twice during the sleep hours, checking for external symptoms of hypoglycemia, such as pallor, sweating, or restless sleep. Silent nocturnal hypoglycemia occurs between 1 and 4 AM rather frequently, especially if the blood glucose level is less than 120 mg/dl at bedtime.[79,84] If the bedtime blood glucose value is less than 120 mg/dl or if the child has had excess vigorous exercise during the late afternoon or early evening, parents should double the amount of protein in the bedtime snack and check the blood glucose again at 2 AM.[84] The evening intermediate insulin may need to be decreased if blood glucose is consistently low over three nights.

Nighttime hyperglycemia is often detected because of extra wet diapers, enuresis, or frequent trips to the bathroom. If nighttime hyperglycemia occurs more than three of five nights, the evening intermediate insulin (NPH or Lente) may need to be increased.

Children who awake with ketones in the morning either may be "running out of insulin" overnight and may require dosage adjustments or may be experiencing rebound hyperglycemia in response to nighttime hypoglycemia and its treatment. This most frequently occurs in children after the honeymoon period, in those with frequent nocturnal hyperglycemia, and during rapid growth spurts. Parents should be instructed to take their child's 2 AM blood glucose levels for two nights after ketones occur in the morning and then adjust the evening insulin and bedtime snack accordingly. They need to be reminded not to give too much food in response to a nighttime hypoglycemic event. For example, one parent consistently gave the child a half glass of orange juice with 3 tbsp sugar plus a half sandwich and glass of milk each time the child had nighttime hypoglycemia. The child subsequently awoke with hyperglycemia and small to moderate ketone levels that morning.

Management of Acute Problems

Hypoglycemia

As noted earlier, hypoglycemia is often difficult to detect in the preverbal child. Subtle symptoms such as sleepiness, change in personality, fussiness, sweating, pallor, and dilated pupils are typically what alert a parent to problems. Young children also may have an abrupt change in activity level and become pale and irritable, whiny, or clinging without provocation.[13,16] As noted earlier, infants may manifest hypoglycemia by appearing unexpectedly sleepy, lethargic, hungry, irritable, pale, or glassy eyed or may have a unique specific facial expression or particular behavior. They also might have apnea, hypothermia, cyanosis, hypotonia, or poor feeding.[87]

Hypoglycemia is most likely to occur around the peak action of insulin, just before mealtime or snack time or after excessive activity and a poorly eaten meal. For example, with infants who receive a morning dose of intermediate insulin, peak action may occur during the afternoon nap. Parents should be made aware of the subtle changes that indicate hypoglycemia in a sleeping child and taught to establish a pattern of BGM that will help to avoid such problems.

Managing hypoglycemia in an infant or small child is no different in concept than handling hypoglycemia in an older child or adult. The object is to provide an adequate glucose source to raise the blood glucose level. Two teaspoons of most table syrups, molasses, corn syrup, or jelly is an effective treatment. Infants can be fed regular cola or sugar water from the bottle. Honey should generally be avoided in infants because of recent reports of associated infant botulism.

Parents may carry a tube of cake-decorating frosting (in the child's favorite color or flavor) and a can of apple juice in the glove compartment of the car at all times in case of traffic delays. Parents should use the same word ("low," "funny," "need sugar") each time hypoglycemia occurs so the child learns to associate the feelings with the term.

All parents should be taught how and when to administer glucagon. Glucagon is used whenever the child passes out or has a seizure or in situations when oral treatment would be dangerous. For preschool children, one-third to one-half a vial (0.3 mg to 0.5 mg) is recommended, with dilution required immediately before intramuscular administration. If the child does not become conscious and the blood glucose does not improve in 15 to 20 minutes, more aggressive treatment is required by emergency medical personnel. All such episodes should also be reported immediately to the diabetes team (see Box 17-3).

Illnesses and infection

The effect of illness on diabetes control in infants, toddlers, or preschoolers can vary. Some children experience a drop in blood glucose level, especially during the initial illness onset. Others exhibit a rise in blood glucose associated with the release of counterregulatory hormones during illness. As previously noted, routine immunizations may also result in blood glucose variations.

Guidelines for sick-day management are addressed in Chapter 4. For children these guidelines include the following:

1. Monitor blood glucose and urine ketones every 2 to 3 hours. Placing cotton balls in the infant's diaper to absorb urine is one method of more accurately monitoring ketones. Using urine collection bags may be discouraged because of possible damage to the child's skin with repeated use.

2. Ill children with IDDM often need more insulin and usually require more than the usual dose. Parents should call the diabetes team for adjustment of insulin doses whenever the child is ill.

3. If hyperglycemia or ketones are present, give the child 4 to 8 oz of sugar-free fluid hourly (depending on the child's age and size) for 2 to 3 hours and retest. If blood glucose and ketones remain the same or increase, call the diabetes team for insulin dose adjustments.

4. If the child has diarrhea or vomits, omit solid foods and give only clear liquids for the next 4 to 8 hours.

5. Call the diabetes physician immediately if the child vomits more than once in a 4- to 6-hour period or if the child refuses fluids (see Box 17-2).[10,37,82]

IMPLEMENTATION AND EVALUATION
Self-Management

Choices are important for the developing child's growing independence and sense of self. Parents can foster this developmental need even with diabetes care. As previously discussed, the toddler can gather the supplies for testing, select a finger for sticking, press the button on the meter, or compare the color on the strip with the chart. Even before recognizing numbers, preschool children can color in a block on a record sheet to match the color of the glucose strip, help or do BGM under supervision, and recognize, report, and even treat mild-moderate hypoglycemia. Some can even inject the insulin.

Offering choices at mealtime is equally important. Allowing the child to choose between two starch groups or to select which sugar-free drink he or she would like contribute to the child's need to master his or her environment.

Although there may not seem to be many choices in the area of injections, some options can be offered. The preschool child can select which of two sites to use, can wipe the site with alcohol, and can even push the plunger in after the parent injects. Each small step the child participates in moves the child closer to self-care.

Many older preschoolers enjoy going to diabetes camp. Being with other children who have IDDM helps them feel less different. Being encouraged to do as much for themselves as possible further encourages their participation in self-care activities and facilitates their development of positive self-esteem and social competence.

The very young child cannot formulate words to describe symptoms. Parents can foster this language development by identifying symptoms and using simple words to describe the sensations. For example, "You look shaky—shaky means you need sugar." Explaining other aspects of care is also useful. For instance, "It's time for your insulin. Insulin keeps you healthy." Such explanations remind the child that this is a part of daily life.

Role of the Diabetes Health Care Team

The health care team serves the family in various ways. From initial diagnosis and training to long-term follow-up and support, the physician, nurse, dietitian, psychologist, and social worker provide a core group of professionals. Reaching a team member quickly at any time of the day provides immense support and reassurance. Parents need diabetes professionals who are versed in well-child needs and are willing to collaborate with the pediatrician or family physician and the day-care and school staff. Some parents benefit most from a single, continuously available team member who can provide ongoing support and expertise.[3]

Table 17-6   Suggested Diabetes Care and Follow-up for Children

	First year of diabetes						Routine diabetes care after first year				
	Diagnosis	6 weeks	3 months	6 months	9 months	1 year	3 months	6 months	9 months	12 months	Comments
Primary physician	X					X				X	More often as needed
Core diabetes team											
Diabetes physician	X	X	X	X		X	X	X		X	
Diabetes nurse	X	X	X	X	X	X	X	X	X	X	
Diabetes dietitian	X	X		X		X		X		X	
Diabetes consultant team											
Ophthalmologist						X				X	Every 5 years until puberty, then yearly
Dentist						X				X	
Podiatrist			As needed or referred								
Diabetes counselor			As needed or referred								
Laboratory studies											
Glycated hemoglobin (HbA1c)	X		X	X	X	X	X	X	X	X	Every 3 months
Urine for microalbumin	X					X				X	Yearly
Urine for culture (females)	X					X				X	Yearly
Thyroid studies	X									X	Optional: yearly
Lipid studies	X					X				X	Yearly (cholesterol, triglycerides)
Serum creatinine										X	Yearly starting at 5 years' duration at puberty

Developed by Children's Diabetes Management Center, Galveston, 1991, University of Texas Medical Branch.
Home test: blood glucose testing—2 to 8 times/day, minimum—14 tests/week; urine ketone testing—whenever blood glucose is 240 mg/dl or more and during illness.

The diabetes professional working with children must keep current with resources available to families for a variety of problems and must provide case management and appropriate referral services.

The diabetes team is also responsible for offering follow-up assessments. Infants, toddlers, and preschoolers should be evaluated every 3 months (Table 17-6). A typical visit should include height and weight assessments, blood glucose and glycohemoglobin levels, review of current management and knowledge of hypoglycemic and hyperglycemic symptoms and blood glucose levels, and reassessment of IDDM management information and skills. Also, adjustments to the meal plans and insulin doses are required during periods of rapid growth and changes in schedules (e.g., vacations, holidays, summer).

Many families are unable to access an interdisciplinary team and must rely on diabetes care and supervision from their pediatrician or family practice physician. Because of the complexity of the disorder, involvement with a diabetes team is preferred and often necessary. However, the pediatrician can establish a "quasi-team" within his or her community. Working with community health nurses, dietitians, and social workers is one approach.[26] In addition, many communities now provide diabetes classes and diabetes educators in the local hospitals and clinics. Networking with these individuals who know about IDDM in children provides a valuable source of information and support to families followed by a primary care physician.

Role of the Family

Because diabetes is a disease requiring daily and sometimes hourly adjustment and management, the family, especially the parent, becomes the ongoing provider of care. Parents are expected to assume this task and participate in this decision making.

Outcome Evaluation

If the diabetes team and the parents have accomplished their goals, several factors will be apparent. First, the child and parents will have established a relatively comfortable, routine system of managing diabetes. This is not to say that all anxieties and misbehavior will abate. Rather, the family will find a schedule and a routine that are no longer disruptive to the family's overall needs and that do not cause frequent conflicts among family members.

Second, the child will be developing normally—physically, cognitively, and emotionally. Growth will occur as expected, and typical infant, toddler, or preschool behaviors will be apparent. Levels of misbehavior, including temper tantrums, will be no more than expected. The child will achieve normal developmental milestones.

Another outcome is related to metabolic control. Blood glucose and glycohemoglobin levels should reach acceptable ranges (ideally HbA_{1c} between 7% and 10%), with no extremes of severe hypoglycemia or ketosis and few moderate to severe hypoglycemic events.

It is hoped that all members of the family and extended family and others who care for the child will be able to discuss the fact the one child has IDDM, basic concepts of IDDM management, and what to do in emergencies. The child will have a neutral or positive attitude toward having IDDM and will be proud of what part he or she has in the treatment regimen.

Finally, parents will have developed a realistic plan for encouraging the child's growing involvement in self-care. Parental expectations for the child participating in care should be consistent with normal maturation patterns and unique levels of cognitive and musculoskeletal development of that child.

SUMMARY

Infants, toddlers, and preschool children with diabetes present several management challenges. The ideal approach to diabetes management of the young child must be a balance of the ideal with the practical and realistic. Managed with sensitivity by knowledgeable caregivers, young children with diabetes attain realistic levels of metabolic control while having every opportunity to grow and develop physically, cognitively, psychosocially, and emotionally in healthy and positive ways.

CASE PRESENTATION

Jenifer, 31 months old, was admitted to the emergency room (ER) with a blood glucose level of 760 mg/dl, large amounts of urine ketones, serum pH of 6.9 with Kussmaul respirations, and a distinct fruity odor to her breath. She had a temperature of 101° F, heart rate of 143, tenting of the skin, dry oral mucous membranes, and no urine output for 2 hours while in the ER. She was not verbally responsive to the medical personnel but would stare at her parents and whimper continuously. Her weight was 3 pounds less than that recorded in the pediatrician's office 3 weeks ago.

The parents stated that 3 weeks earlier, Jenifer began to be extremely thirsty and lethargic and wanted something to eat every 2 hours but would only take a few bites and then say she was full, even eating her favorite fast-food hamburger. Her mother took Jenifer to her pediatrician, who stated she probably had the flu affecting many children in her day-care center. She continued to be lethargic and refused to go to day care the next week. Her mother took her back to the pediatrician, who prescribed an antibiotic for her runny nose and cough. She was also given a cough suppressant. She had not improved over the last 5 days and had become extremely irritable, had a flushed face, would drink anything her mother gave her but refused to eat more than a few bites, and refused to play. This is extremely unusual, since Jenifer is a very active, verbal toddler who is constantly "on the go." The last couple of days, Jenifer could not seem to walk but instead crawled a few yards to get something she wanted. She began wetting her bed at night and even had some enuretic episodes the last 2 days. Yesterday she cried, saying her "tummy hurt." Her mother noticed she was losing weight (more than 4 pounds on their home scale). The parents brought her to this children's hospital ER because their family pediatrician was out of town, the mother was concerned about how sick Jenifer looked the past 2 days, and Jenifer refused to drink or eat that day. Jenifer was diagnosed with insulin-dependent diabetes mellitus (IDDM), diabetic ketoacidosis (DKA), and moderate dehydration.

Jenifer was admitted to the ninth floor of the hospital, where an intravenous line (IV) was inserted. She was rehydrated by replacing fluids and electrolytes (including added potassium) relatively slowly to prevent cerebral edema and was given IV regular insulin. When her blood glucose dropped to 300 mg/dl, some glucose was added to the IV line. She was not given IV bicarbonate because of the potential risk of cerebral edema. She was monitored via the electrocardiogram (ECG) and watched closely for signs and symptoms of hyponatremia and hypokalemia. Blood glucose was monitored every 1 to 2 hours, and urine ketones were checked at each voiding. Serum electrolytes, pH, and bicarbonate were monitored every 2 hours for the first 8 hours, then every 4 hours until the results were normal. By the following day, Jenifer's blood sugar was less than 250 mg/dl, urine ketones were negative, and serum pH was 7.35. Her glycohemoglobin level returned to 13%.

Jenifer received her first liquids-only meal the evening of the second day. Because she tolerated the regular diet for lunch the third day, she received her first subcutaneous insulin injection that evening. Jenifer started playing actively the evening of the third day. When she saw her nurse come to her room with the blood glucose monitoring (BGM) equipment, she started crying and quickly slid under the hospital bed to hide. Both the nurse and the mother first tried to talk her out from under the bed and then began to bribe her to come out. The nurse clinician was called by the nursing staff to help with this problem.

DISCUSSION

It seems that an increased number of children under age 3 years currently are not diagnosed with IDDM until they are very ill with high blood glucose, DKA, and moderate to severe dehydration. Early symptoms of IDDM are similar to the "flu" (thirst, frequent urination, eruresis, lethargy, irritability, possible flushed face, hunger that is quickly satisfied, some weight loss). Often the early symptoms mimic a cold or flu and precede the diagnosis of IDDM by days or months. For this reason, many infants and toddlers are not diagnosed with IDDM until their blood glucose level is greater than 500 mg/dl and they have moderate to severe DKA, as did Jenifer.

Parents initially react with increased guilt. They blame themselves for not taking the child back to their pediatrician when the child did not improve right away. They begin to mistrust the medical profession, frequently asking, "Are you sure my child has diabetes?" "Why didn't the other doctor diagnose it?" or "If the other doctor had diagnosed high blood sugar 3 weeks ago, could my child have been prevented from having diabetes now?"

On admission to the hospital, the parents should be introduced to the interdisciplinary diabetes team, which consists of a diabetologist, a clinical nurse specialist for diabetes who is a certified diabetes educator (CDE), nutritionist, social worker, and psychologist or child psychiatrist. The physician and nurse CDE met with the parents initially to give them basic information about their child's diagnosis and care and to begin establishing rapport. The physician discussed the diagnoses with the parents and assured them that they did nothing to cause the diabetes and that nothing could have been done to prevent it. The nurse initially obtained a history of the events leading up to this hospitalization and a family assessment to identify potential problems and strengths. She informed the parents that diabetes is not contagious, so other family members will not "catch" it. She described in simple, direct language that IDDM has three triggers that may stimulate onset: genetic, environmental, and viral. She explained that IDDM has a relatively long onset, during which the child's body is triggered to make antibodies that kill off their own insulin-producing cells. This process probably occurred for many months before the actual diagnosis. At this point, Jenifer still has a few insulin-producing cells, but the added infection (flu and/or cold) overwhelmed her ability to make enough insulin to keep her symptom free. The nurse again emphasized there was nothing they could have done to prevent her from developing IDDM. The nurse then set up 1- to 2-hour appointments with the parents for each subsequent day of hospitalization. She helped them determine the best time to meet with her. She encouraged them to include any other regular caregivers, such as grandparents, day-care workers, or babysitters. She offered to give all those involved notes to give to their employers describing the necessity for their presence at the education sessions.

On the second day of Jenifer's admission, the nurse met with the parents at the agreed-on time in the morning. She restated information about the development and onset of IDDM. She then presented the signs and symptoms of hyperglycemia (increased urination, excessive thirst, irritability, muscle weakness, headache, weight loss, possible flushed face) and explained the physiologic reasons for each. In addition, she presented them with the signs and symptoms of DKA (Kussmaul respirations, fruity odor to the breath, nausea, stomach ache, and presence of urine ketones) and again listed the physiologic reasons for them. The parents told the nurse when they noticed each of these symptoms over the last weeks and months. The nurse then discussed their feelings of grief and guilt (anxiety, sadness, depression, hostility, disbelief, numbness, shock) and reemphasized nothing they could have done would have prevented IDDM from occurring and neither one of them was to blame. She gave them time to identify how they were feeling and corrected any misperceptions they currently had. She presented them with flash cards on which were written the signs and symptoms of hyperglycemia and DKA. Other cards included how to treat each of these problems. Since the parents said they were not overwhelmed, she simply stated how to treat these symptoms in the future. Reading materials were given, and a reading assignment was made on BGM, insulin, and the injection procedure.

The afternoon of the second day the nurse met with Jenifer's parents just before BGM was to be done. She described what BGM is and demonstrated how to do it on herself. She then asked each parent to test their own blood glucose, which they did. At this time both parents expressed pity for Jenifer having to be hurt so often. The nurse suggested only two or three fingers be used for BGM to facilitate the development of calluses to minimize the pain. She also told them that Jenifer would pick up their feelings of pity, sorrow, and guilt and use them to make both herself and them feel worse. The nurse strongly suggested they treat BGM as a matter-of-fact event that must be done three or four times each day, just like brushing teeth or washing hands. The nurse stated that, if needed, the parents should take turns restraining Jenifer during the BGM and then immediately afterward cuddle and hug her to show their love. The nurse suggested several distraction techniques, such as having Jenifer watch her favorite show, singing a song with her, or telling a story while BGM was being done. The nurse also suggested ways Jenifer could participate: selecting the finger to be used, selecting and holding the bandaid, and pushing the button on the BGM machine. The nurse also discussed therapeutic play activities that would be started that afternoon with Jenifer (allowing Jenifer to do BGM and give insulin injections to the nurse's doll).

The nurse educator met with Jenifer that afternoon. Jenifer readily went to the playroom with the nurse. After Jenifer played a short time with a stove and a doll, the nurse educator asked her to sit on her lap while she told her a story about her (the nurse's) doll Annie. The nurse told Jenifer that Annie has diabetes just like Jenifer and that sometimes Annie's body makes too much sugar and then Annie feels tired, thirsty, and crabby. Sometimes Annie even wets her bed at night because her body is making too much sugar; Annie's parents don't get mad because they know it's not Annie's fault. To be sure Annie feels good, Annie's mother (the nurse) has to check her blood sugar during the day. The nurse then showed Jenifer how she does this. The nurse also has to give Annie insulin every day to keep her feeling good. Again, the nurse showed Jenifer how she does this. The nurse then told Jenifer that Annie told the nurse she would like Jenifer to take care of her while Jenifer is in the hospital. She asked Jenifer if she would do this. Jenifer smiled and said, "I make her OK." The nurse left Jenifer with Annie in the playroom and watched from the nurse's station. Jenifer immediately "talked with" Annie and slowly started touching the BGM device and different-sized syringes (without needles attached). After 10 minutes, Jenifer put Annie on the floor and methodically used an alcohol swab all over Annie. She then took a 30 ml syringe and began jabbing Annie in her buttocks, on her legs, and on her arms. The jabs became more aggressive and rapid for about 5 minutes. Then Jenifer threw the syringes across the playroom and grabbed Annie and rocked her while saying, "No more hurts." When the nurse reentered the playroom, Jenifer grabbed some syringes and the BGM device, put them in a bag, and carried the bag and Annie back to her room.

That evening the nurse educator walked into Jenifer's room and saw the mother and the staff nurse laying on the floor trying to coax Jenifer out from under the bed. She asked them to stand up, moved the bed, and quickly pulled Jenifer out from under the bed. In a calm and matter-of-fact tone, she told Jenifer it was time for her blood sugar to be checked. She then asked Jenifer if she would like to hold the bandaid and Annie. Jenifer looked at her with a stubborn, angry look on her face and said "NO!" The nurse put Annie next to where Jenifer would sit and helped Jenifer wash her hands in warm soapy water, saying her hands were dirty from the floor. She then sat Jenifer on her lap and quickly activated the finger-sticking device while talking to Jenifer about Annie. She asked Jenifer to help her put the drop of blood on the BGM machine and to push the button, which Jenifer did. Then the nurse gave the finger-sticking device (without the lancet) to Jenifer and sat Jenifer on the window bench next to Annie.

(There were bandaids and two syringes in Annie's pocket.) The nurse educator then talked with the mother and the staff nurse describing what she had done and why. Quietly, she asked them to sneak a peak at Jenifer, who was aggressively sticking Annie's hands, feet, and eyes with the BGM device. She described how toddlers and preschoolers gain a sense of control over painful or fear-provoking events by doing what frightened them to a doll, but not their own special doll. The nurse then described additional techniques of distraction and suggested appropriate ways of rewarding Jenifer's appropriate behavior (e.g., setting up a sticker chart). Each time Jenifer allows her mom or the staff nurse to do BGM or give insulin, she picks a sticker and puts it on the chart. After she has earned three stickers, she gets to go to for a walk or to the big hospital playroom as a treat. After she understands this system, the number of stickers needed for a special activity may be increased gradually.

The morning of the third day, the nurse educator met with Jenifer's parents, both sets of grandparents, and a day-care worker. She summarized the information presented the day before and answered all questions. The grandparents focused on their belief that Jenifer developed diabetes because they gave her too much candy and cookies whenever she visited them and that the parents were too lenient with Jenifer. They vigorously denied that anyone in their families ever had diabetes. The nurse educator discussed a number of myths about diabetes, including that it is "catching," eating sugar causes it, it will go away if the child no longer eats foods with sugar or loses weight, it is God's punishment for something the parents or grandparents did, and Jenifer will outgrow it when she becomes a teenager.

The nurse educator then told them about insulin, demonstrated how it is given, and asked everyone present to allow her to give them a simulated insulin injection (3 U saline). All were surprised that the injection truly did not hurt. The mother said that the nurse's holding of her skin in a bunched position hurt more than the injection. The dad said he didn't even feel the needle go into his skin and just slightly felt the fluid. From then on, everyone was able to pay closer attention to how to draw up insulin and actually give the injection. The nurse educator suggested insulin be kept in the refrigerator during the summer if they were in a non-air-conditioned place or traveling in the car or to keep it in a cooler if they took it with them to the park or on camping trips. A new bottle should be dated with the time and day it is first opened and thrown out after 30 days because it loses its effectiveness after that. Everyone was sent home with an orange, two syringes, a bottle each of "practice regular insulin" and "practice intermediate insulin" plus a list of 15 doses to draw up and give. The mother was to give Jenifer her evening dose that day, and the father was to give Jenifer her morning dose on day 4. The grandparents and day-care worker were to give each other injections of "practice insulin" the next morning under the supervision of the nurse educator.

The nurse educator met with the mother and father late that afternoon to evaluate their skills in accurately drawing up insulin and to supervise their giving it to each other. Both parents were very nervous but accurately drew up five different doses and successfully gave each other injections of "practice insulin." At this time the mother asked her husband to give that evening's injection, which he agreed to do.

The nurse educator supervised the father drawing up the evening insulin dose for Jenifer in the nurse's station before going into Jenifer's room. She suggested the mother check Jenifer's blood glucose first. The mother was surprised by being asked this but successfully completed the BGM in a matter-of-fact manner and encouraged Jenifer to check Annie's. Having the mother do the BGM gave the father some extra time to prepare himself emotionally to give Jenifer the insulin injection, since he appeared very nervous. The father then told Jenifer he was going to give her the insulin tonight and needed her help in holding the bandaid. Jenifer selected one with a large red heart on it, opened it, and held it tightly while Dad gave her the injection. The mother "helped Jenifer hold her leg still for Dad" by restraining it above the knee while Jenifer sat on her lap. The father successfully and quickly gave the insulin and helped Jenifer apply the bandaid. Both he and Jenifer received a "badge of courage" from the nurse educator, which they wore proudly that evening.

The reverse occurred *the following morning.* Unfortunately, Jenifer's blood glucose was 235 mg/dl that morning, and she was irritable and cranky. Dad assertively but matter-of-factly restrained Jenifer with the nurse educator's assistance while Mom gave the insulin injection. Jenifer gave many injections to Annie afterward in a very aggressive manner. Jenifer then asked for her "badge," which the nurse educator had forgotten to give her. Jenifer and Mom proudly showed the physician and the nutritionist their badges later that morning.

The nutritionist met with the parents, grandparents, and the day-care worker the morning of day 4. All were feeling somewhat overwhelmed after this session, so the nutritionist scheduled three additional outpatient educational sessions over the next week.

The nurse educator continued to reinforce the information provided to this point with the parents and continued to have therapeutic play sessions with Jenifer. She scheduled the last in-hospital education session for the *morning of day 5,* since the insurance required they be discharged by 11 AM that day. (Insurance companies are continuing to shorten the amount of time they will pay for children with newly diagnosed IDDM to remain in the hospital. Nurse educators and other diabetes team members need to plan outpatient educational settings to be sure the family receives comprehensive education.)

During this last session the nurse educator discussed the signs and symptoms of hypoglycemia (six S's: shaky, sweaty but cool to the touch, sleepy but not tired, stubborn, "spacey," and starving). Other behaviors Jenifer might exhibit were reviewed and included pallor, abrupt change in activity level, rubbing her head, looking for food, and hypotonia. The nurse then suggested that whenever Jenifer appeared uncooperative or misbehaved, the parents should check her blood glucose level, since they had not yet been able to identify specific ways Jenifer would act when she had hypoglycemia. To treat hypoglycemia, the nurse suggested they give Jenifer two sugar cubes, ½ oz of frosting in a tube, or 3 or 4 oz of fruit juice or regular soda. If hypoglycemia occurs more than an hour from the next meal or snack, they might also want to give two or three crackers and/or 2 to 4 oz of milk, depending on how low the blood glucose is and how long until the next snack or meal. The nurse educator reminded them of the flash cards with the signs and symptoms of hypoglycemia and how to treat it. She then taught them how to give glucagon intramuscularly (0.5 ml or one-half vial) if Jenifer did not respond to oral treatment or if she refused to drink or eat or was unconscious. The nurse emphasized that they should call the diabetes team to report any time they had to use glucagon and to report for an insulin dose adjustment any time Jenifer had two or three hypoglycemic episodes in 2 or 3 days. The nurse explained when hypoglycemia was likely to occur: when Jenifer did not eat most of her meal, when she exercised more than usual, when the schedule varied greatly, during holidays, or if she slept through a snack or into a mealtime.

The nurse educator emphasized that the parents should always check Jenifer's blood glucose and give her a snack at bedtime, even if her blood glucose level was relatively high. In addition, the nurse requested that the parents monitor 2 AM blood glucose at least three times per week for the first 6 weeks or if Jenifer has a nightmare, talks or walks in her sleep, or has restless sleep. Discussion of appropriate treatment for hypoglycemia at 2 AM was discussed, with emphasis placed on not overfeeding Jenifer, since she would be hyperglycemic and possibly have ketones in the morning. The nurse also told the parents that Jenifer must always have her bedtime snack. However, if the bedtime blood glucose is above 300 mg/dl, they can omit the bread exchange and have her eat only the protein exchanges. If the blood glucose is less than 120 mg/dl at bedtime, Jenifer should eat an extra protein exchange in addition to her usual bedtime snack.

Additional education sessions were set up for *four evenings* to include the parents, grandparents, and day-care worker over the next 2 weeks. During these additional sessions the nurse educator discussed additional behavior management strategies; discussed difficulties in eating and suggested additional foods to use; reinforced the symptoms and treatment of hyperglycemia, ketoacidosis, and hypoglycemia; had all demonstrate BGM and insulin and glucagon injections to recheck techniques; and discussed additional myths or advice given by well-meaning friends or family members to correct misperceptions and misinformation.

This family did not need referrals to the psychologist or social worker at this time. On discharge the use of their newly purchased BGM machine was reviewed, they received their Humulin insulin regular and intermediate bottles, extra 0.3 ml syringes, extra lancets for BGM, the booklet in which to record the blood glucose values that they had started in the hospital, an initial Medic-Alert bracelet, and additional resource material from the American Diabetes and Juvenile Diabetes Associations. Jenifer was also given a coloring book developed by one of the drug companies, which she and her parents could use to discuss diabetes.

Parents were instructed to call the nurse educator twice a day for insulin doses for the first 3 weeks, then once a day for the next 2 weeks, then every other day until their first clinic appointment in 6 weeks. During these telephone calls, additional education regarding the interaction of food, activity, and blood glucose levels with insulin dosage was discussed. In addition, any questions that arose about the therapeutic regimen were answered immediately. Additional behavioral strategies were also discussed. These phone calls decreased the parents' anxiety about being "on their own" after only a few days of education, provided the additional support necessary, and reinforced educational concepts presented. New problems developed daily for the parents (ones not anticipated and that can become immense problems if not addressed immediately).

At the *6-week clinic visit,* parents were taught about the "honeymoon period," a phase of residual beta-cell function that results in increased numbers of hypoglycemic events and a need for decreased insulin for weeks to months in young children. The nurse educator emphasized that this does not mean the child does not have IDDM and does not mean that the child will "grow out of " IDDM. Instead the remaining insulin-producing cells erratically produce insulin for a variable and unpredictable period. Therefore Jenifer could have a hypoglycemic event not obviously connected to increased activity, decreased food, or irregular schedule. It also means that the insulin doses need to be adjusted more often throughout this period. Parents were instructed to watch the pattern of blood glucose readings and to call for insulin adjustments whenever the pattern in the morning, at noon, in the evening, or at bedtime reveals a trend of decreasing blood glucose readings or whenever Jenifer has two or three hypoglycemic events in a week at the same time or within 2 or 3 days.

Approximately 10 months after diagnosis, Jenifer became difficult to manage. She began to cry frequently and say she was going to die. She refused to go to day care, refused to allow her mother to give her insulin or do BGM, and started throwing temper tantrums two or three times a day. The family was referred to the team's child psychologist, who, through play therapy and family counseling, was able to identify Jenifer's increasing fear of death as being caused by her perception that her parents let her do things she was not supposed to because she was really sick. After extensive work, Jenifer lost her fear of death, and the family began to use natural and logical consequences successfully in their behavioral management. The psychologist stated that Jenifer reacted so strongly because she was so intelligent and that her advanced verbal abilities helped in the resolution of this problem. At the early age of 4½ years, Jenifer took over her own BGM, under the parents' supervision, for approximately 6 months, after which she turned it back to her parents for more than a year.

Jenifer is now 6 years old and developing cognitively, psychosocially, and physically in an extremely healthy manner. She is the star in her first-grade class, Brownies, and gymnastics and very active in the Juvenile Diabetes Association's activities for young children. This outcome might not have been so positive without the resources and support of the whole interdisciplinary diabetes team.

REFERENCES

1. American Academy of Pediatrics, Committee on Early Childhood, Adoption and Dependent Care: *Health in day care: a manual for health professionals,* Elk Grove Village, Ill, 1987, American Academy of Pediatrics.
2. Anders TF, Carskadon MA, Dement WC: Sleep and sleepiness in children and adolescents, *Pediatr Clin North Am* 27:29-43, 1980.
3. Anderson B: The impact of diabetes on the developmental tasks of childhood and adolescence:
a research perspective. In Natrass M, Santiago J, editors: *Recent advances in diabetes,* London, 1984, Churchill Livingstone.
4. Arky R: Nutrition therapy for the child and adolescent with type I diabetes mellitus, *Pediatr Clin North Am* 31:711-719, 1984.
5. Auslander W and others: Risk factors to health in diabetic children: a prospective study from diagnosis, *Health Soc Work* 15:133-142, 1990.
6. Axline V: *Play therapy,* Boston, 1947, Houghton-Mifflin.

7. Baker D, Campbell R: Vitamin and mineral supplementation in patients with diabetes mellitus, *Diabetes Educ* 18:420-427, 1992.

8. Band E: Children's coping with diabetes: understanding the role of cognitive development, *J Pediatr Psychol* 15:27-41, 1990.

9. Bank S, Kahn M: *The sibling bond,* New York, 1982, Basic Books.

10. Benz M, Kohler E: Baby food exchanges and feeding the diabetic infant, *Diabetes Care* 3:554, 1982.

11. Betz C, Poster E: Communicating with children: more than just words, *Paedovita* 1:11-16, 1984.

12. Bibace R, Walsh M: Development of children's concepts of their illness, *Pediatrics* 69:355-362, 1980.

13. Brambilla P and others: Glucose counterregulation in pre–school-age diabetic children with recurrent hypoglycemia during conventional treatment, *Diabetes* 36:300-304, 1987.

14. Brazelton T: Stress for families today, *Infant Ment Health J* 9:65-71, 1988.

15. Brewster A: Chronically ill hospitalized children's concepts of their illness, *Pediatrics* 69:355-362, 1982.

16. Brouhard B: Management of the very young diabetic, *Am J Dis Child* 139:446-447, 1985.

17. Bryant J, Anderson D: *Children's understanding of television,* New York, 1983, Academic.

18. Burr C: Impact on the family of a chronically ill child. In Hobbs N, Perrin J, editors: *Issues in the care of children with chronic illness,* San Francisco, 1985, Jossey-Bass.

19. Caplan F, Caplan T: *The power of play,* Garden City, NY, 1974, Anchor.

20. Casella S and others: Accuracy and precision of low-dose insulin administration, *Pediatrics* 91:1155-1157, 1993.

21. Chess S, Thomas A: Temperamental differences: a critical concept in child health care, *Pediatr Nurs* 11:167-171, 1985.

22. Clarke W, Haymond M, Santiago J: Overnight basal insulin requirements in fasting insulin-dependent diabetics, *Diabetes* 29:78-80, 1980.

23. Clarke-Stewart A, Friedman S: *Child development: infancy through adolescence,* New York, 1987, Wiley.

24. Davidson J, Krosnick A, Palumbo P: When to screen for diabetes, *Patient Care* 25:39-44, 1991.

25. Diabetes Control and Complications Trial Research Group: The effect of intensive treatment of diabetes on the development and progression of long-term complications in insulin-dependent diabetes mellitus, *N Engl J Med* 329:977-986, 1035-1036, 1993.

26. Drash A, Berlin N: Juvenile diabetes. In Hobbs N, Perrin J, editors: *Issues in the care of children with chronic illness,* San Francisco, 1985, Jossey-Bass.

27. Drotar D, Levers C: Age differences in parent and child responsibilities for management of cystic fibrosis and insulin-dependent diabetes mellitus, *Dev Behav Pediatr* 15:265-272, 1994.

28. Erikson E: *Childhood and society,* ed 2, New York, 1959, Norton.

29. Ferrari M: The diabetic child and well sibling: risks to the well child's self-concept, *J Child Health Care* 15:141-148, 1987.

30. Garrison M, McQueston A: *Chronic illness during childhood and adolescence,* Newbury Park, Calif, 1989, Sage.

31. Garrison W, Biggs D: Young children's subjective reports about their diabetes mellitus: a validation of the Diabetes Pictorial Scale, *Diabetes Educ* 16:304-308, 1990.

32. Ginsberg H, Opper S: *Piaget's theory of intellectual development: an introduction,* Englewood Cliffs, NJ, 1969, Prentice-Hall.

33. Giordano B, Edwards L: Meeting the needs of parents of children with diabetes: a babysitter's course, *Diabetes Educ* 6:26, 1980.

34. Golden M and others: Management of diabetes mellitus in children younger than 5 years of age, *Am J Dis Child* 139:448-452, 1985.

35. Gross A and others: Video teacher: peer instruction, *Diabetes Educ* 10:30-31, 1985.

36. Hahn K: Therapeutic storytelling: helping children learn and cope, *Pediatr Nurs* 13:175-178, 1987.

37. Hall J, Keltz J: What to do when your child won't eat, *Diabetes Forecast,* May-June, 1980, pp 27-29.

38. Hamill PV and others: Physical growth: National Center for Health Statistics percentiles, *Am J Clin Nutr* 32:607-629, 1979.

39. Hauenstein E and others: Stress in parents of children with diabetes mellitus, *Diabetes Care* 12:18-23, 1989.

40. Hauser S and others: Adherence among children and adolescents with insulin-dependent diabetes mellitus over a four-year longitudinal follow-up. II. Immediate and long-term linkages with the family milieu. In Special issue: Adherence with pediatric regimens, *J Pediatr Psychology* 15:527-542, 1990.

41. Holmes C, Richman L: Cognitive profiles of children with insulin-dependent diabetes, *Dev Behav Pediatr* 6:323-326, 1985.

42. Holmes C and others: Verbal fluency and naming performance in type I diabetes at different blood glucose concentrations, *Diabetes Care* 7:454-459, 1984.

43. Horan P, Gwynn C, Renzi D: Insulin-dependent diabetes mellitus and child abuse: is there a relationship? *Diabetes Care* 9:302-207, 1986.

44. Ilg F, Ames L: *Child behavior,* New York, 1955, Harper & Row.

45. Jackson R: Growth and maturation of children with insulin-dependent diabetes mellitus, *Pediatr Clin North Am* 31:545-567, 1984.

46. Jefferson I and others: Insulin-dependent diabetes in under 5 years old, *Arch Dis Child* 60:1144-1148, 1985.

47. Kager V, Holden E: Preliminary investigation of the direct and moderating effects of family and individual variables on the adjustment of children and adolescents with diabetes, *J Pediatr Psychol* 17:491-502, 1992.

48. Kinmonth A, Magrath G, Reckless J: National Subcommittee of the Professional Advisory Committee of the British Diabetic Association: Dietary recommendations for children and adolescents with diabetes, *Diabetic Med* 6:537-547, 1989.

49. Kovacs M and others: Psychological functioning among mothers of children with insulin-dependent diabetes mellitus: a longitudinal study, *J Consult Clin Psychol* 58:189-192, 1990.

50. Kushion W and others: Issues in the care of infants and toddlers with insulin-dependent diabetes mellitus, *Diabetes Educ* 17:107-110, 1991.

51. Lipman T and others: A developmental approach to diabetes in children: birth through preschool. Part 1, *Matern Child Nurs J* 14:255-259, 1989.

52. Lowenberg M: The development of food patterns in young children. In Pipes PL, editor: *Nutrition in infancy and childhood,* ed 4, St Louis, 1989, Mosby.

53. Lowrey G: *Growth and development of children,* Chicago, 1986, Year Book.

54. Martin R and others: The infant with diabetes mellitus: a case study, *Pediatr Nurs* 20:27-31, 1994.

55. McCollum A: *The chronically ill child: a guide for parents and professionals,* New Haven, Conn, 1975, Yale University Press.

56. McKelvey J and others: Reliability and validity of the Diabetes Family Behavior Scale (DFBS), *Diabetes Educ* 19:125-132, 1993.

57. McWilliams M: *Nutrition for the growing years,* ed 4, New York, 1986, Wiley.

58. Patterson GR: *Families,* Champaign, Ill, 1979, Research Press.

59. Patterson GR: *Living with children,* Champaign, Ill, 1980, Research Press.

60. Petersen H and others: Growth, body weight and insulin requirement in diabetic children, *Acta Pediatr Scand* 67:453-457, 1978.

61. Piaget J: *Play, dreams and imitation in childhood,* New York, 1962, Norton.

62. Piaget J: *The construction of reality in the child,* New York, 1971, Ballantine.

63. Piaget J: *The child's conception of the world,* Totowa, NJ, 1976, Littlefield, Adams.

64. Piaget J, Inhelder B: *Memory and intelligence,* New York, 1973, Basic.

65. Pontious S: Communicating with children. In Servowsky J, Opus S, editors: *Nursing management of children,* Boston, 1987, Jones & Bartlett.

66. Pratt L: *Family structure and effective health behavior: the energized family,* Boston, 1976, Houghton-Mifflin.

67. Robinson CA: Preschool children's conceptualizations of health and illness, *J Child Health Care* 16:89-96, 1987.

68. Rovet J, Ehrlich R: Effect of temperament on metabolic control in children with diabetes mellitus, *Diabetes Care* 11:77-82, 1988.

69. Rovet J, Ehrlich R, Hoppe M: Behaviour problems in children with diabetes as a function of sex and age of onset of disease, *J Child Psychol Psychiatry* 28:477-491, 1987.

70. Rovet J, Ehrlich R, Hoppe M: Intellectual deficits associated with early onset of insulin-dependent diabetes mellitus in children, *Diabetes Care* 10:510-515, 1987.

71. Rovet J, Ehrlich R, Hoppe M: Specific intellectual deficits in children with early onset diabetes mellitus, *Child Dev* 59:226-234, 1988.

72. Rubin R, Peyrot M: Psychosocial problems and interventions in diabetes, *Diabetes Care* 15:1640-1657, 1992.

73. Ruggiero L, Mindell J, Kairys S: A new measure for assessing diabetes self-management responsibility in pediatric populations: the Diabetes Regimen Responsibility Scale, *Behav Ther* 14:233-234, 1991.

74. Ryan C, Vega A, Drash A: Cognitive deficits in adolescents who developed diabetes early in life, *Pediatrics* 75:921-927, 1985.

75. Ryan C and others: Deterioration of mental efficiency associated with experimentally induced mild hypoglycemia in children with IDDM, *Diabetes* 38(suppl 2):8A, 1989.

76. Safyer A and others: The impact of the family on diabetes adjustment: a developmental perspective, *Child Adolesc Soc Work J* 10:123-140, 1993.

77. Sahler O, McAnarnwy E: *The child from three to eighteen,* St Louis, 1981, Mosby.

78. *Sam's day: a coloring book,* 1991, Novo-Nordisk Pharmaceuticals.

79. Santiago J, White N, Pontious S: Diabetes in childhood and adolescence. In Alberti K and others: *International textbook of diabetes mellitus,* London, 1992, Wiley.

80. Savinetti-Rose B: Developmental issues in managing children with diabetes, *Pediatr Nurs* 20:11-15, 1994.

81. Schreiner B, Travis L: When your child has diabetes: the preteen years, *Diabetes Forecast* 40:37-41, 1987.

82. Schreiner B, Travis L: The child less than 3 years old. In Travis L, Brouhard B, Schreiner B, editors: *Diabetes mellitus in children and adolescents,* Philadelphia, 1987, Saunders.

83. Schroeder DB and others: Cognitive and motor effects during hypoglycemia and recovery, *J Am Diabetes Assoc* 38(suppl 2):108a, 1989.

84. Shalwitz R and others: Prevalence and consequences of nocturnal hypoglycemia among conventionally treated children with diabetes mellitus, *J Pediatr* 116:685-689, 1990.

85. Simpson O, Smith M: Lightening the load for parents of children with diabetes, *Matern Child Nurs J* 4:293-296, 1979.

86. Singer J, Singer D: *Television, imagination and aggression,* Hillsdale, NJ, 1981, Erlbaum.

87. Smart M, Smart R: *Children: development and relationships,* ed 3, New York, 1977, Macmillan.

88. Standen P and others: Family involvement and metabolic control of childhood diabetes, *Diabetic Med* 2:137-140, 1985.

89. Steranchak L: How big, how tall, *Diabetes Forecast* 45:50-53, 1992.

90. Tanner J, Goldstein H, Whitehouse R: Standards for children's height at 2-9 years allowing for height of parents, *Arch Dis Child* 45:755-762, 1970.

91. Tattersall R, Pyke D: Growth in diabetic children, *Lancet* 2:1105, 1973.

92. Thorp F: Infants and children. In Powers M: *Handbook of diabetes nutritional management,* Rockville, Md, 1987, Aspen.

93. Travis L, Brouhard B, Schreiner B, editors: *Diabetes mellitus in children and adolescents,* Philadelphia, 1987, Saunders.

94. Vaughan VC, Litt IF: *Child and adolescent development: clinical implications,* Philadelphia, 1990, Saunders.

95. Wedin B, Topliffe L, Simonson D: The effect of glycemic control on hypoglycemia-induced neuropsychological dysfunction in IDDM, *Diabetes* 38(suppl 2):4A, 1989.

96. Wertlieb D and others: Adaptation to diabetes: behavior symptoms and family context, *J Pediatr Psychol* 11:463-479, 1986.

97. Whaley L, Wong D: *Nursing care of infants and children,* ed 4, St Louis, 1991, Mosby.

98. White N and others: Identification of type 1 diabetic patients at increased risk for hypoglycemia during intensive therapy, *N Engl J Med* 308:485-491, 1983.

99. Wysocki T and others: Adjustment to diabetes mellitus in preschoolers and their mothers, *Diabetes Care* 12:524-529, 1989.

100. Wysocki T and others: Parental and professional estimates of self-care independence of children and adolescents with IDDM, *Diabetes Care* 15:43-52, 1992.

18 Diabetes Mellitus and the School-Age Child

Sharon L. Pontious

More than 1 million, or 1 in every 500 children, have type I or insulin-dependent diabetes mellitus (IDDM); it is the most common endocrine disease of school-age children.[121] For children with IDDM between ages 6 and 11 years, this means they must master the diabetes care regimen of learning to inject insulin, monitor their blood glucose, and modify their diet

---

CHAPTER OBJECTIVES

- Describe how diabetes mellitus influences the normal physical development of the school-age child.
- Describe the impact of diabetes mellitus on the cognitive and language capacity of the school-age child.
- Summarize cognitive problems associated with school-age children.
- Identify factors associated with diabetes mellitus that impact psychosocial development.
- Describe the family's and child's adaptation process associated with a diagnosis of diabetes mellitus.
- Discuss the importance of individualizing treatment goals for the school-age child with diabetes.
- Summarize the content associated with an individualized, developmentally based program.
- Assess issues related to regimen adherence.
- Address the role of the interdisciplinary diabetes health care team.

The author acknowledges the contribution of Barbara Tesno to Chapter 12 of the first edition of this book, from which this chapter is revised.

and exercise while they also master the common developmental tasks of latency, industry, and concrete cognitive operations.

IMPACT OF DIABETES ON PHYSICAL DEVELOPMENT

IDDM has the highest incidence of all life-threatening diseases of children in the United States.[84,121] Approximately 120,000 young people in the United States,[84] or 1 in every 500 children, will develop IDDM by the end of high school. The non-age-adjusted mortality rate associated with IDDM is at least four times greater than that for non-insulin-dependent diabetes mellitus (NIDDM). Patients with IDDM also develop retinopathy, neuropathy, and renal disease earlier and in more severe forms than those with NIDDM. Thus IDDM is likely the most important and costly chronic illness affecting children in the United States.[104]

IDDM can affect the normal physical development of school-age children in three ways: (1) stunted growth in those very poorly controlled, (2) delayed puberty, and (3) enhanced risk for development of early retinopathy, nephropathy, or neuropathy, particularly during adolescence.[1,8,92,128]

Growth

Healthy children enter the school-age period with a body type and a linear rate of growth of 2 to 3 inches (5 to 7 cm) each year that they maintain until the changes of puberty begin: 10 to 12 years for girls and 12 to 14 years for boys. Children grow approximately 2½ to 3 inches (6 to 7 cm) in height and gain 5 to 7 pounds (2 to 3.5 kg) in weight each year until puberty. It is important for parents, teachers, and physicians to accept that, in general, short children remain short and thin ones thin. Over the past three decades, it has become apparent that the secular trend of constantly increasing size of successive generations of American children has ended. Black and white children have been found to be of essentially the same height.[92] Thus the parents' height and weight are major predictors of their children's ultimate height and weight.

Disproportionate growth of the lower extremities during early and middle childhood gives them a taller and thinner appearance. However, bony epiphyses are largely cartilaginous and soft in early childhood. Thus physical activities for the school-age child should be supervised to avoid bone or joint injuries. Rapidly growing children often complain of knee pains that can be increased by overexertion or injury.[2] These pains are usually not significant if they occur late in the day or night and disappear in the morning, but children with persistent leg pains should be referred to a physician.[144] Facial bones grow faster than the skull because more than 90% of brain growth occurs by age 6.[11]

Overall, school-age children look slimmer and are more graceful and better coordinated than preschool children. Their posture improves and their legs are longer. Movements are more skilled and precise.

Eighty percent of the height and weight measurements of children at a given age are expected to fall between the tenth and ninetieth percentiles of the National Center for Health Statistics' anthropometric charts. Children with height and weight measurements that fall in greatly different percentile groups, as well as those who shift by more than 25 percentiles or fall near to or outside the fifth and ninety-fifth percentiles, need to be referred for potential growth abnormalities. The child who is newly diagnosed with IDDM will usually have lost some weight during the days or weeks before diagnosis; the drop in their percentile for weight compared with their previous measurement or compared with their percentile for weight should alert health care personnel to look for other signs and symptoms of IDDM.

Growth Rate and Height at Diagnosis

Drayer,[41] in a study of 62 children with diabetes, surprisingly found that 4- to 9-year-old boys with IDDM, but not girls, were significantly taller than control subjects. The average height or the age of parents of children with IDDM was not significantly different from that of the control subjects. A more recent study of a population of 200 newly diagnosed children, 187 nondiabetic siblings, and 169 parents at the University of Pittsburgh confirmed and extended these findings. The researchers found that 5- to 9-year-old children with IDDM were consistently taller than the national average, as were their nondiabetic siblings. Children positive for islet cell antibodies were taller than those without these antibodies.[92] The cause of this relatively increased height is not known and is difficult to reconcile with other studies indicating that monozygotic twins with diabetes are shorter at diagnosis than their unaffected twins at diagnosis.

Growth Failure

Previous studies showed that diabetic dwarfism was a common finding when insulin treatment of IDDM was first begun. The growth failure was clearly related to an inadequate amount of insulin and a negative nitrogen and carbohydrate balance. It was frequently associated with Mauriac syndrome, which also includes truncal obesity, round facies, delayed puberty, and an enlarged fatty liver. Growth failure, alone or with other associated physical findings of Mauriac syndrome, is still seen sporadically today, primarily in those children who consistently fail to administer all their prescribed insulin or who falsify their blood glucose records for various reasons and are in poor metabolic control.[2,89]

More recently, several studies have found that children with IDDM are statistically likely to be shorter than their initial genetic makeup would have suggested.[92,135] To date, no evidence suggests that children with IDDM are more likely to be obese or, if they are, that obesity leads to the development of IDDM.[1] It is currently unclear whether or not children in good metabolic control, as measured by glycohemoglobin, attain their full growth potential.[92,109] Conflicting data also exist regarding whether delayed puberty or an abnormal growth spurt exists today for children who are in moderate or good-to-average metabolic control.[26,30,125,133] It does seem that girls with average or good metabolic control no longer have pubertal or menarcheal delay. It is clear that children with IDDM who are in poor metabolic control with glycohemoglobin values indicating average blood glucose values greater than 240 mg/dl have inadequate weight gain, poor growth, delayed pubertal onset and menarche, and decreased peak pubertal height velocity.[92,102]

Children with IDDM who are in poor metabolic control most often have insulin deficiency. This prevents the appropriate maintenance of a positive nitrogen balance, which may be responsible for some of the growth failure observed. In addition, glycosuria leads to urinary loss of minerals and loss of normal vitamin homeostasis. Specifically, a zinc deficiency has been associated with poor growth and delayed puberty.[22] Hypercalcuria and hyperphosphaturia were noted in children with IDDM and correlated closely with reduced height.[98] Two other autoimmune disorders that are found more frequently in children with IDDM, chronic lymphocytic thyroiditis and Addison disease, may also be associated with growth failure or poor weight gain, respectively. Hashimoto thyroiditis may occur in as many as 20% of the white and 5% of the black children with IDDM.[102] The most common findings are an elevated thyroid-stimulating hormone (TSH) value in serum and a modest goiter.

Physiologic growth hormone (GH) peaks have been found to be more pronounced in children with IDDM. Normal stimuli of GH release (i.e., exercise, glucagon, arginine, falling blood glucose levels) also lead to an exaggerated release of GH. However, all these abnormal responses of GH release can be normalized by good control of the blood glucose. On the other hand, somatomedin C (also known as insulin-like growth factor, or IGF-1) levels tend to be lower than normal and negatively correlate with glycohemoglobin.[92] The lower somatomedin C levels may be responsible for poor growth in poorly controlled IDDM.

Diabetes-Related Health Complications

Consistently higher levels of plasma glucose place affected children at a higher risk for the development of specific diabetes-related health complications, such as retinopathy, nephropathy, and neuropathy.[25,65,79,128] The presence of limited joint mobility in the metacarpophalangeal and interphalangeal joints is common, is associated with children's level of glycemic control, and is indicative of an increased risk of microvascular complications.[102] The Diabetes Control and Complications Trial (DCCT) Research Group[38] found that intensive insulin therapy reduced the adjusted mean risk for the development of retinopathy by 76% and reduced the occurrence of microalbuminuria by 39%, that of albuminuria by 54%, and that of clinical neuropathy by 60%. Intensive insulin therapy was attained either by using an external insulin pump (which is controversial for children) or by administering three or more daily insulin injections. Therapy was guided by frequent blood glucose monitoring (BGM) and insulin dose adjustments so that subjects maintained their blood glucose concentrations within 155 ± 30 mg/dl and their glycohemoglobin levels at about 7%. However, the risk of having severe hypoglycemia was three times higher than with conventional therapy, and thus the risk-benefit ratio of intensive therapy is less favorable in children under 13 years of age.[38] The prepubertal child with IDDM is relatively protected against the development of microvascular complications. Furthermore, younger children, especially preschoolers, may be at risk for developing unwanted neurologic sequelae following repeated bouts of severe hypoglycemia. As a result, many recommend that prepubertal children be treated somewhat less aggressively than young adults in terms of target glucose levels. Good control for school-age children with IDDM is defined by the American Diabetes Association (ADA) guidelines and others as children who are well adjusted, do not have frequent severe hypoglycemia, and have hemoglobin (Hb) A_{1c} values of 7% to 9%. Those with HbA_{1c} values greater than 11% are considered to be in poor control and at higher risk for complications of the eyes and kidneys.[121] Thus health care providers should emphasize the importance of maintaining a glycohemoglobin value of 9% or less and a mean blood glucose level below 180 mg/dl to lessen children's risk of developing these dangerous health problems.

Maintaining good glycemic levels is an extremely difficult task for most school-age children and their families. It requires frequent insulin dose adjustment. Insulin replacement regimens rarely duplicate normal patterns because of erratic patterns of absorption of injected insulin. Some degree of individual differences in insulin sensitivity/resistance and the degree to which catecholamines (epinephrine and norepinephrine), glucagon, cortisol, and GH are secreted in response to growth and stress contribute to problems with glycemic control among young persons.[17,29,108,150] Thus frequent and substantial adjustment in the insulin requirements of prepubertal, and especially of pubertal, children are essential to maintain acceptable levels of glycemia.[16,98]

School-age children typically receive 0.5 to 1 U of insulin/kg of body weight/day, with two thirds of their total insulin dose given before breakfast and one third before supper.[121] However, during illness and growth spurts, especially pubertal growth spurts, these same children often require as much as 1.5 U or more of insulin/kg.[2] It is essential that children and their parents learn when and how to change the insulin doses and that insulin requirements change with amount of food, growth, activity, illness, and stress as well as other factors such as erratic absorption. Insulin doses are generally adjusted by 0.5 to 2 U per type of insulin or by no more than 10% of the total insulin per day.

Physical Examination

The physical examination of children with IDDM must include an evaluation of growth and screening for early development of microvascular and macrovascular complications. Evaluation of growth includes recording accurate measurements of the height and weight of children every 3 to 4 months and plotting on the standardized weight and height charts. Discovering a deviation from the child's usual growth pattern enables the practitioner to pick up potential problems quickly, such as poor growth, possibly as a result of too little insulin or decreasing adherence to the diabetes regimen; failure to gain weight, possibly because the child is not eating enough or the child's body is not using the food well; or excessive weight gain, possibly from the child eating too much food or having too much insulin.[132] Blood pressure should be plotted on age- and gender-standardized curves. Determining the specific Tanner stage is important because the pubertal growth spurt routinely requires an increase of 20% to 50% in insulin doses, as well as an increase in food.[17,133] Children with poor growth or abnormal weight should be evaluated for meal plan adherence, insulin deficiency, or autoimmune diseases such as celiac syndrome and Addison disease. If children have a goiter, they should be evaluated for hypothyroidism.

The health care practitioner should routinely assess children to ensure that gross and fine motor coordination improves greatly throughout the school-age period. Exercise is required for developing muscle and muscle tone, refining balance and coordination, gaining strength and endurance, and maintaining normal weight.[141] Exercise is especially important for children with IDDM. It increases insulin sensitivity and decreases insulin requirements and has beneficial effects on blood pressure, blood lipids, and emotional status.[52] During the school-age period, children's muscular strength doubles, so they can play increasingly strenuous games for longer periods. However, it is essential that all school-age children adhere to the following guidelines for sports: proper physical conditioning; proper grouping according to body size, skill, and maturation; use of good protective equipment; periodic health appraisals; and availability of an experienced health professional (knowledgeable in sports and diabetes mellitus) during games and practice sessions. Noncontact sports such as swimming, gymnastics, track and field, martial arts, tennis, and skating are recommended for 6- to 7-year-old children. Later, they can add basketball, volleyball, soccer, and wrestling. Some authorities recommend that collision sports such as football, rugby, and hockey be delayed until age 11.[100]

Finally, children should be screened for the presence of limited joint mobility by having them place their hands in the prayer position. If limited joint mobility is present, children should be carefully examined for the presence of retinopathy, nephropathy, and neuropathy.[92,109]

Nutrition

Caloric, protein, vitamin A, carbohydrate, and calcium needs increase slowly and steadily during the school-age years. A rule of thumb is that children need 1000 calories plus 100 calories for each year of age up to puberty; thus the 6-year-old child generally requires 1600 calories, whereas the 12-year-old child not in the prepubertal growth spurt requires 1000 plus 1200, or 2200, calories. These are only estimates, however, and the actual caloric requirements vary greatly depending on the child's activity level and presence or absence of growth spurts. Girls' pubertal growth spurt usually begins between ages 10 and 12 and ends approximately 2 years after menarche. Maintenance of the basal metabolism of the school-age child uses approximately 50% of the caloric intake.[144]

The school-age child usually eats well and has fewer food fads. Children 9 years of age or younger need to eat every 2½ to 3 hours; children between 9 and 12 years need to eat every 3 to 3½ hours.[131] Midmorning snacks are thus often discontinued in children after age 9. Meals and snacks should be spaced appropriately to counterbalance peaks of insulin actions.

Breakfast is an especially important meal for 6- to 11-year-old children. Those who eat a well-balanced breakfast may perform better academically than those who do not.[137] Because of their desire not to be viewed as different from peers, lunch preferences are often based on whether friends take lunch to school or eat in the school cafeteria. In addition, children often eat as fast as possible to be able to go outside and be with their friends. Thus variable amounts of well-planned lunches are often not eaten, posing potential problems for children with IDDM.

School-age children want and need snacks. The 6- to 8-year-old child benefits from a midmorning snack of milk or juice. Most children want after-school snacks. These snacks can help make up for the lack of food consumed at lunch. Snacks eaten more than an hour before meals do not usually decrease the child's food intake at mealtimes. Acceptable nutritious snacks include milk, cheese, fresh fruits and vegetables, raisins, peanut butter, unsugared nuts, yogurt, and fruit juices.

Dietary adherence is the most difficult part of the diabetes regimen.* The overall nutritional requirements for a child with well-controlled IDDM are essentially the same as those for the same-age child without diabetes. The main difference is that meals should be consumed at similar times and should have similar protein, carbohydrate, and fat distributions from one day to another so that the insulin needs are more predictable. The goals for nutritional management of IDDM in childhood include promoting normal growth, enabling and encouraging normal physical activity for age, and maintaining acceptable blood glucose levels.[80]

Children weighing 20 to 70 kg need 1500 calories plus 20 calories/kg of body weight; the distribution of these calories varies slightly. The ADA recommends between 50% and 65% of the calories be from carbohydrates (of which 70% are from complex carbohydrates), 12% to 20% from protein, and less than 30% from fat.[20] The recommended daily intake of protein is 0.8 g/kg and of fiber is 35 to 40 g/day. Intake of highly refined sugars or simple carbohydrates should be minimized because they tend to exaggerate glucose increments after meals. In general, 25% to 30% of the total caloric intake is at breakfast, 25% to 30% at lunch, and 25% to 30% at supper, leaving 5% to 10% each for midafternoon and bedtime snacks. In older school-age children (9 years and older) the midmorning snack is omitted unless the child is prone to prelunch hypoglycemia as a result of a long delay (more than 4 to 5 hours) between breakfast and lunch.[121]

Currently the ADA does not recommend routine vitamin and mineral supplementation for those with diabetes. However, Baker and Campbell[8] found recent results of studies published in the medical literature suggest that supplementation with vitamins C and E and magnesium may be beneficial in helping prevent some long-term complications and, unless the child with IDDM has severe renal dysfunction, probably will not be harmful. Vitamin C concentration was found to be decreased in animals and humans with diabetes, and a supplementation of 1000 mg twice daily was found by one study of adults with diabetes to inhibit the glycosylation of proteins, which may help prevent or reduce the development of cataracts and nerve disorders. Vitamin E supplementation of 600 to 1200 mg daily was found to reduce protein glycosylation in adults with diabetes, independent of changes in plasma glucose, and possibly to decrease the hypercoagulability and increase the adhesivity of red blood cells (RBCs) because of vitamin E's ability to prevent oxidative damage and thus reduce the incidence of cataracts and vascular disease. Magnesium deficiency has recently been estimated to be present in 25% of those with diabetes. Since magnesium is high in bran cereal, cashews, peanuts, soybeans, whole wheat, chocolate, rice, dried fruits, and shrimp, the use of a magnesium supplement of 20 to 130 mg daily is more practical, since many of these food sources are not recommended for those with diabetes because of their high-calorie, high-sugar, or high-cholesterol content. Children with maturity onset of diabetes in youth (MODY) who take magnesium supplements may have decreased blood glucose levels and require a concomitant decrease in their insulin dose, since magnesium has been found to increase the

---

*References 3, 4, 20, 33, 47, 97, 136.

release of insulin.[8] Although none of these studies used children as subjects, the ADA is presently reviewing the scientific data associated with the use of these vitamin and mineral supplements to determine the need for patients with diabetes.

Meal plans are designed to take into account the consistency, timing, composition, and caloric content of foods ingested and physical activity, age, gender, and pubertal status.[20] The keys to successful adherence to meal plans are allowing flexibility and requiring as few major changes from the family's usual nutrition and meal times as reasonable. However, meal plans must take into consideration the pharmacokinetics of previously injected insulin and the need to consume adequate food to prevent hypoglycemia with exercise.[47] The experienced dietitian typically evaluates the current eating patterns, preferences, and nutritional needs of children before negotiating an acceptable meal plan with them and their families. All members of the multidisciplinary diabetes team must know and consistently reinforce the specific meal plan agreed on by the child and the family.

Maintaining a consistent eating pattern is the most difficult behavioral task for families of children with IDDM.[20] Children who lack predictable daily eating and activity patterns have the greatest difficulty maintaining adequate blood glucose control. Younger children do not possess the cognitive knowledge and skills required for good dietary adherence.[35,97,111]

Both children and their parents have common and substantial dietary knowledge and skills deficits. Research found that on the average, only 54% of the meal plan was accurately recalled, with particularly poor recall of afternoon (40%) and bedtime (42%) snacks.[33,80,81] Even more disturbing was the poor performance (50% or less) of both children and mothers when asked to estimate amounts and identify their exchange groups for 20 food models of common foods. Younger children and mothers of older children were the worst at estimating amounts of foods. Underestimation errors were found for meats and fruits, whereas overestimation errors were found for fats.

More than one third of the children in one study reported problems with adhering to their meal plan.[35] These problems occurred most often for the afternoon snack, while at school or in restaurant, and when with their friends. Children with poor adherence at school and while with their friends were more likely to have worse metabolic control. Thus health care providers' expectation that children and their parents adhere strictly to any prescribed meal plan is not only incorrect but also unrealistic.

Dietary knowledge and skills can be enhanced through the use of behavioral rehearsal, problem solving, role playing, and supervised practice. Demonstrating how to substitute some of the popular "teenage," "snack," or "junk" foods for appropriate bread and fruit exchanges is extremely helpful. Giving and showing the child and the family how to use one or more of the various meal-planning tools is extremely helpful: the basic food pyramid; a list of healthy food choices that provides foods that are low fat, low sugar, low sodium, and high fiber; carbohydrate or fat or calorie counting tools; and the Dietary Guidelines for Americans, a tool produced by the U.S. Department of Agriculture (USDA) that provides various tips and suggestions for lowering the fat content of the diet.[68] Encouraging the whole family no longer to have candy, ice cream, donuts, or high-fat snacks in the house but instead to have more fruits and vegetables available and to use sugar-free sodas and drinks, sugar- and fat-free yogurt, candy, and snacks helps the child with IDDM feel less different and less deprived.

Teaching children self-management strategies for coping with urges while alone at home, especially for the afternoon and bedtime snacks, and for coping with temptation and peer pressure while with friends at school or in restaurants is also very helpful. Ventilating feelings, seeking diversions such as after-school clubs or athletic activities, using humor, and talking with close friends are helpful coping strategies for school-age children. Self-monitoring of blood glucose (SMBG) can be used to demonstrate the effects of various foods on blood glucose values after eating.[136] This is a superb way of demonstrating to children the effects foods have on blood glucose. This also may assist children to feel that controlling what they eat really does affect their blood glucose control.[20]

Parents should avoid getting into power struggles with their child over food. Maintaining an open attitude in which "dietary indiscretions" are openly acknowledged and unconditionally accepted by all parties concerned is crucial. Children who can discuss situations in an honest dialogue with family and health care team members can be helped to problem-solve preplanned eating deviations by increasing activity or insulin.[146] The family that allows some members to consume forbidden foods in front of children probably contributes to the child's dietary indiscretions.[20] It is not surprising that children with IDDM who feel different from, or not adequately supported by, their family and peers "act out" through dietary or insulin administration noncompliance.[117]

Exercise

Regular strenuous exercise by children with IDDM increases insulin sensitivity and lowers insulin requirements. However, hypoglycemia may occur immediately after strenuous activity (up to 24 hours after) if moderately severe exercise is prolonged for several hours.[52] Snacks eaten just before, during, or just after strenuous activity are helpful in preventing hypoglycemia. Foods such as fruit, crackers with cheese or peanut butter, and milk are often recommended for prevention or treatment of hypoglycemic episodes. In addition, some foods such as ice cream or frozen yogurt may be more acceptable at these times because, despite the high carbohydrate content, they contain sufficient protein, fat, and guar gum (used in processing) that blunt the rapid absorption of the carbohydrate. Therefore ice cream or frozen yogurt is a good choice to counterbalance the immediate carbohydrate need after exercise.

Bedtime snacks

Bedtime snacks are an essential part of the meal plan of children with IDDM because they can help prevent the relatively common occurrences (approximately once a week) of often silent early-morning hypoglycemia. Nocturnal hypoglycemia is sometimes manifested by nightmares, sleepwalking, or sleep talking and restlessness as well as the common daytime symptoms such as sweating and feeling shaky, sleepy, or starving.

During the early-morning hours (1 to 4 AM), insulin requirements are lower than at any other time of the day except when the child is in a growth spurt.[121] Common causes of nocturnal hypoglycemia include attempting to achieve optimal glycemic control with a twice-daily insulin injection regimen, peak activity period from the suppertime NPH dose, failure to take a bedtime snack, and unusually excessive physical activity the previous day.[121]

Since most episodes of hypoglycemia during sleep go undetected, it is not surprising some studies found that more than 50% of all episodes of severe hypoglycemia occur during sleep. The best predictor of 1 to 4 AM hypoglycemia is the blood glucose level at bedtime.[126,142] A child who has a bedtime glucose less than 120 mg/dl has an increased chance of a subsequent episode of hypoglycemia at 2 AM. Thus the bedtime snack can be used to reduce the risks of 1 to 4 AM hypoglycemia by increasing calorie and protein content.

Children whose bedtime glucose value is less than 120 mg/dl should eat double the usual amount of protein for their bedtime snack to avoid silent nocturnal hypoglycemia between 1 and 4 AM.[121] In addition, if the blood glucose is greater than 300 mg/dl at bedtime, the carbohydrate portion may be omitted for that bedtime snack, but the protein portion should still be consumed.

Sweeteners

A common concern of most parents is the safety of available nonsugar sweeteners. Recent evidence suggests that the use of alternative sweeteners such as aspartame and saccharin is safe. The Diabetes Task Force Report for the Committee on Nutrition of the American Academy of Pediatrics in 1985 suggested combining alternative sweeteners as a means of limiting their potential toxicity. Aspartame has been found to cause headaches, stomach upsets, and dizziness in a few susceptible people. Its use should be limited in those with phenylketonuria (PKU) because aspartame is a derivative of phenylalanine. The total consumption of nutritive sweeteners should be limited to 10% of the total calories.[20,51]

In summary, the nonnutritive alternative sweeteners aspartame and saccharin can be safely used; fructose and sugar alcohols may also be used in limited amounts. However, more expensive foods sweetened with fructose or sorbitol have no proven ability to help promote weight loss or improve overall blood glucose control in children with diabetes.[51,52]

OTHER HEALTH CONSIDERATIONS

Physical Injury

School-age children are at high risk for physical injuries. Developmental characteristics that place them at risk include independence, growth in height exceeding muscular growth and coordination, daring and adventurous activities, frequently playing in hazardous places, attempting dangerous feats, confidence often exceeding physical capacity, overdoing, and having a strong need for activity.[141] Children who have an attention deficit disorder and immature children are at higher risk for injuries. They often attempt dangerous acts to prove themselves worthy of acceptance and improve their status in their peer group.[91,93] Children with IDDM are at greater risk for hypoglycemic episodes during and after exceptionally aggressive exercise periods.

Motor vehicle accidents are the most common cause of accidental injury and death among 6- to 12-year-old children. Ninety percent of fatal bicycle injuries are the result of collisions with motor vehicles. Their rate of bicycle injuries not involving motor vehicles is twice that of teenagers and four times that of preschool children.[48,59] Bicycle injuries are often related to violations of traffic laws or the result of "dashing out." In addition, the peak incidence of child pedestrian fatalities is between ages 5 and 9 years.[115] Children with IDDM may be at a slightly greater risk for motor vehicle accidents if they experience hypoglycemia when riding bicycles.

Teaching and modeling accident prevention activities such as correct pedestrian behavior, use of restraint systems, door lock mechanisms, appropriate passenger seating and behavior, and use of protective equipment for the more dangerous sports are essential. Children with IDDM should also be taught to be alert to hypoglycemia when participating in sports or riding bicycles.

Children with IDDM must be taught that episodes of hypoglycemia may be increased with strenuous exercise. Most experienced pediatric diabetologists encourage, rather than discourage, normal sports and physical activity. This requires extensive training regarding the causes, recognition, and prompt treatment of exercise-related hypoglycemia. SMBG and diet and insulin adjustments before, during, and after sports or strenuous exercise greatly reduce the risks of hypoglycemia. Children who participate in after-school strenuous athletic practices need help in modifying the composition of the afternoon snack and supper. To avoid postexercise hypoglycemia and assist the child to deal with postexercise anorexia, it may be necessary for the child to eat a very large snack (composed of the exchanges usually included in the afternoon snack plus one half of those usually included in supper) immediately after school and a concomitant small supper (one half of the usual amount of supper). Some children will need to increase their overall caloric intake during supper and at bedtime on the days of extensive exercise to help replace muscle glycogen.

Infections

School-age children with IDDM who have good to excellent metabolic control are not more likely to become ill than children of this age without IDDM. Chronic hyperglycemia, however, may increase risks of common bacterial and viral infections for children with IDDM because of impaired granulocytic and immune function in debilitated children.

Parents of children with IDDM must check their children's urine for ketones whenever a viral or bacterial infection is suspected or they complain of nausea or stomachache, have acetone-smelling breath, have trouble breathing, or develop vomiting or abdominal pain. Regardless of the blood glucose level, the presence of large amounts of ketones in the blood or urine indicates the need for increased insulin.

Children with IDDM who have gastrointestinal upsets or diarrhea are prone to become dehydrated much more quickly. When they are vomiting or have abdominal pain, they should be taken off solid foods and given ample fluids to avoid dehydration—8 to 12 ounces every hour until the ketones are negative and the vomiting or diarrhea is resolved. Those who cannot keep liquids down need to be taken to the emergency room or clinic for rehydration until the vomiting resolves. Although hydration with sugar-free fluids is sometimes done for short periods (4 to 8 hours), carbohydrate-containing fluids and insulin are often required to clear the ketones. A common error that sometimes has disastrous consequences is to attempt to correct hyperglycemia with sugar-free fluids and simultaneously withhold insulin from children who cannot eat or who are vomiting.

Dental Health

Dental health is of particular importance to school-age children because all the permanent teeth, except wisdom teeth, erupt during this period. Prolonged undernutrition, such as might occur with undiagnosed or poorly controlled IDDM, may delay the eruption of permanent teeth. All children should receive regular preventive dental care and supervision in daily hygienic care. Inadequate dental care results in the most prevalent childhood health problems, dental caries, malocclusion, and periodontal disease.[141]

Children with IDDM have been shown to develop early, severe periodontal disease more often than those without IDDM. Poor removal of food debris allows for the development of caries and periodontal disease from proliferation of acid-forming bacteria and dental plaque. Frequent oral hygiene and dental checkups every 6 months are highly recommended for all school-age children. Children with IDDM with extensive dental and periodontal disease often have a worsening of glycemic control as a result of these chronic infections.

Obesity

Obesity typically begins during middle childhood. A combination of factors contribute to obesity: inactive life-styles with too much time spent watching television, frequent snacking to treat hypoglycemia, physical or emotional stress, lower socioeconomic status, and having obese parents. Children receiving intensive insulin therapy to keep their glycohemoglobin between 6% and 8% may also experience weight gain. Overweight children are often teased, ridiculed, and left out of activities, which result in feelings of inferiority, rejection, and isolation. Children then tend to withdraw or act out, which may continue a cycle of rejection and overeating. Overeating then becomes the main source of emotional gratification, exacerbating obesity.

The goal for obese children is to allow them to "grow into their weight" by stabilizing their weight rather than encouraging them to lose large amounts of weight over a short time. Parents can help by removing junk foods from the home and having low-calorie snacks and foods instead. Actively participating in at least 30 to 60 minutes of strenuous activity every day is essential. Overweight children should be encouraged to take part in group activities such as the Boy or Girl Scouts, YMCA or YWCA, and after-school athletic programs.[106] Children with IDDM are taught these same dietary goals as a component of their regimen. Adherence to these goals and scheduled physical activity prove to be of benefit in maintaining appropriate body weight.

Enuresis

Enuresis (bedwetting) is usually nocturnal and occurs in 17% of the children over 5 years of age. *Primary enuresis* occurs in a child who has never attained a dry period and is usually caused by delayed or incomplete neuromuscular maturation of the bladder. *Secondary enuresis,* which occurs after a child has been dry for over a year, may be caused by bladder infections, urinary tract infections or structural disorders, major neurologic deficits, nocturnal epilepsy, chronic renal failure, sickle cell disease, diabetes insipidus, or diabetes mellitus. These organic causes must first be ruled out.[124] Parents need reassurance that bedwetting is not willful misbehavior.[39,40] They should know that punishing, shaming, and scolding are useless and harmful.

Children with IDDM can be taught to avoid IDDM-triggered nocturnal enuresis by keeping blood glucose values less than 200 mg/dl during the night. Children's self-esteem and self-confidence must also be enhanced. They must believe they can help themselves and achieve independent self-control. One way to facilitate this is to teach the children that if their blood glucose level before the bedtime snack is 200 to 300 mg/dl, they should eat one-half their usual carbohydrate but all their protein exchange(s) for that night's snack and that if their blood glucose is greater than 300 mg/dl, they should eat only the protein exchange(s).

YOUNGER SCHOOL-AGE CHILDREN'S NORMAL COGNITIVE AND LANGUAGE DEVELOPMENT

Cognitive Development

During the early school-years, intense intellectual and conceptual growth occurs and reasoning becomes more logical. Cognitively, younger school-age children (6 to 8 years) are in transition between Piaget's *preoperational* and *concrete* stages (Table 18-1). These children have learned to (1) seriate, (2) classify by one primary characteristic, (3) realize that numbers and words stand for objects, events, and feelings, (4) perceive common objects and events from others' perspectives, (5) use systematic trial-and-error problem solving, (6) make judgments based on outcomes to themselves but verbalize the intent behind the actions, and (7) play alone or socially with others.[110,111,113]

Perception

Younger school-age children view the world primarily in terms of how they perceive it or how it appears on the outside; thus they are extremely susceptible to perceptual illusion. For example, 10 raisins spread out are "more" than 20 raisins bunched together. Because of the perceptual illusions, they can easily be tricked into eating or drinking even when they do not want to. Bunching foods together on a large plate or giving an ounce of fluid in a round, fat glass looks like a lot less, so the child may eat or drink it.[114]

Thought

Since children are more sociocentric, they can begin to compare their own thoughts and feelings with those of another person. However, if the person's viewpoints conflict with their own, they still do not comprehend the other's thoughts or feelings. Their thinking is based on their own experiences: literal interpretations of words or parts of things on which they have focused. Thinking is still colored by their beliefs in animism, absolutism, irreversibility, and magical thinking.[111,114]

Table 18-1 Characteristics of School-age Children's Thinking: Transitional and Concrete Stages

Transitional stage (6 to 8 years)	Concrete stage (9 to 11 years)
Major task *Conquest of symbol*	*Mastery of classes, quantities, and relations*
Thought is influenced almost completely by child's own perceptions, personal actions, and experiences. Thinking moves from perceptual illusion and egocentricity (from the child's own viewpoint and in the child's own way) toward the beginning of sociocentricity (socially validated ideas from others' perspectives) and manipulating symbols.	Thought processes are not internalized so that overt actions on objects or experiences are not essential; thought is limited by dependence on reality and past experiences, therefore it is of limited complexity; observation is now accurate (not perceptually bound) and objective.
Perception	
Child is less egocentric and begins to appreciate other persons' points of view and feelings although does not comprehend others' viewpoints when there is conflict with own perspective.	View of world is concrete but objective and can encompass a variety of perspectives of others.
Thought	
Child views world in terms of a combination of own and beginning awareness of others' perspectives. World exists independent of self, but all events still have a purpose. Decentering begins: child can focus on two or more aspects of an event at the same time; begins to seriate and classify by dominant feature. Animism: child believes only things that move have consciousness. Words and numbers: child begins understanding concepts of number and spatial relations. The concepts of length, number, amount, and distance are attained at approximately age 6 to 7 years.	Animism is now confined to natural phenomena, but loss of animism causes need to cope with concept of death. The following concepts are mastered: Reversibility: can perform opposite or compensating act to undo first one Measurement: and use of various measuring devices Association, combination, negation Causality: as different from association or combination Classificaton and seriation Conservation: mass of an object remains the same even if the form and shape change. The following concepts are attained at the approximate ages indicated: 7 to 8 years: substance, area space, mass 9 to 10 years: weight, time 11+ years: volume, speed (time plus distance), velocity, density

Table 18-1   Characteristics of School-age Children's Thinking: Transitional and Concrete Stages—cont'd

Transitional stage (6 to 8 years)	Concrete stage (9 to 11 years)
Reasoning	
Systematic trial-and-error problem solving and reasoning begin. Judgments still are made based on outcomes for self but now verbalizes intent behind actions.	Reasoning is concrete: child does mental experiments on things that were actually sensed previously or currently by directly organizing immediately given or remembered data. Child lacks ability to transfer learnings immediately because the learning is still tied to particular objects and situations. Child progresses from inductive reasoning (8 to 11 years) to deductive reasoning (11 years and older) and uses elementary logic. Child judges actions by logical effect and separates cause and intent from outcome.
Language	
Words: represent one or more common names or uses of things; child still understands words more generally and less completely than adults; has learned the power of words (words as effective in creating reactions than are actions). Questions: child asks now to learn about the "how" of things and to express frustration.	Symbols now truly represent real objects and events as well as those concepts attained so far; structure of language now more important; child progresses toward increasingly more sociocentric verbal exchanges and sharing ideas among people.
Play	
Symbolic: child satisfies self needs and means of coping with conscious or unconscious conflicts by transforming what is real into what is wished was real (e.g., via painting, drawing, puppets, plays). Social: child plays games where rules are collectively made up so everyone wins and has fun (e.g., hopscotch, jump rope, tag).	Symbolic play continues. Collaborative play in groups (detailed rules to maintain equality and mutual respect) progresses toward competition (object is to win after "fair" play).

Animism

Children of this age think animistically and believe nonliving, moving things have their own consciousness and intention. Cars, computers, machines, and even bicycles are believed to have childlike characteristics. They make statements such as, "The candy machine ate my quarters; it didn't want me to have any."[114] Many children have drawn insulin bottles, syringes, and finger-sticking devices with smiles, sad faces, or even "mean-looking" faces with teeth when I have asked them to draw a picture of what it is like to have diabetes.

Absolutism

Absolutism, the belief that things are good or bad, work or do not work, hurt or do not hurt, is still present but now modified. These children say, "The shot hurt but not that long" or "The nurse hurt me when doing my finger stick but she didn't mean to." However, they cannot see the gray areas between right and wrong or good and bad and do not perceive pain or punishment in degrees. Children at this age still believe that if an adult is wrong or has lied about one thing, he or she is wrong or lies about everything.[44] Thus it is essential that all health care providers are honest with children.

Irreversibility

Irreversibility, the belief that actions or thoughts cannot be undone or compensated for, is present only for those things children have not actually seen changing. For example, they know that an intravenous (IV) line is not going to be a permanent part of their arm. However, many believe that a finger stick or cut not covered by a bandage may kill a person because losing blood equals death.[114]

Magical thinking

Children believe their own thoughts or actions influence events outside of their control. For example, a brother, when angry at his sister, wished she would become ill. When he was told she had IDDM, he was certain he had caused it. Many 6- to 8-year-old children newly diagnosed with IDDM have told me that they are sure they caused it by going outside without their hats or coats or by eating too many sweets. In addition, thinking about their internal body parts or functions, which they cannot touch or see, is primitive and fear provoking, and is influenced by fantasy, magical thinking, and absolutism.[113] It is not surprising, therefore, that children under age 9 become panicky when the well-meaning physician says their "islet" (perceived as "eyelid") "cells do not make insulin and they now need insulin injections," since the children reason they will be getting "shots in their eyelids."

Reasoning

Younger school-age children reason inductively, from a particular action or event to a whole group of similar actions or events. For example, children may state, "A nurse sticks me with a needle to help my diabetes," so poking them with any needle (e.g., straight or safety pin) "will help me feel better." Health care providers must show 6- to 8-year-old children how water comes out of the syringe needle so they can reason: "When I push on the syringe, water comes out of the needle, so when I get an injection, medicine called insulin goes into my body."[114]

Language

The 6-year-old child understands 2500 to 3000 words, carries out commands involving three to four actions, and to a large extent, comprehends "if," "because," and "why."

They receive and give information, take turns in conversation, but still make grammatic errors.[54] From the time children enter school, the extent and precision of their speaking vocabulary and reading skills attained will be the predominant factors that determine their success or failure.[14]

It is essential to remember that younger children (6 to 8 years old) still use many words without understanding their meaning because they are simply imitating what they have heard others say.[44,113] Elkind[44] showed that children's imitation and use of words conceal many limitations of their understanding and thinking. One reason is that they assume words convey the particular meaning that they have to others because of their egocentrism. Thus, if they make a word up, they think others know its meaning. They have no concept of relativeness; words are taken extremely literally.

Many terms often used to help children understand diabetes and illness are actually very fear provoking. For example, using *bug* for germ when discussing infections conveys the idea of insects crawling around inside their bodies. *Shot* implies a violent, punishing, or aggressive act and instills fears of being severely hurt or killed. *Take* or *test* implies removal of something from the children.[114] The term *diabetes* implies "die-of-betes"; they become very afraid they are going to die of something called "betes" or "beets." Even *glucagon*, the hormone used for low blood glucose emergencies, stimulates the fear that they will be "shot with gluc from a gun."

Moral Development

Younger school-age children are extremely egocentric and behave to avoid punishment and parental disapproval. They are just beginning to use self-control to resist temptation. Children begin to incorporate the same-sex parent's moral values into their behavior by thinking of these values as precepts, "I must" or "I must not." Thus they apply the rules of right and wrong in a rigid, strict, and absolute manner with no allowances made for extenuating circumstances.[75] This unyielding standard of right and wrong causes children to be very critical of others' behavior and the "unfairness" of uncontrollable events.[144]

Younger school-age children decide whether or not to break a rule based on the type of physical punishment they anticipate. Parents are viewed as all powerful and rules as being rigid and unbreakable.[46] In essence, they feel no guilt for doing things forbidden; they only wish to avoid punishment. Discipline for children of this age needs to include clear limits, with consistent rewards for good behavior and punishment for bad behavior.

OLDER SCHOOL-AGE CHILDREN'S COGNITIVE AND LANGUAGE DEVELOPMENT

Cognitive Development

Older school-age children, 9 to 11 years old, are in Piaget's *concrete* stage of cognitive development. Thought processes of these children are now internalized (concrete objects or experiences are not absolutely necessary), but their thinking is still limited because of their dependence on reality and the limited number and quality of their past experiences.[110,111]

Thought

Older school-age children can use symbols to organize their ideas and manipulate the world around them. They can experience an event without touching or seeing it.[144] The 9- to 11-year-old child now can think about the present, the past, and to some extent the future. Because they can perceive objects and events more objectively, they can correct some perceptual distortions and illusions. However, their thought is still less complex and flexible than that of adults (Table 18-1). The most important concepts needed to understand children of this age are described next.

Animism

The 9- to 11-year-old child believes in animism only for natural events such as tornadoes, hurricanes, and earthquakes. When they lose their animistic belief that objects have intention, these children now must deal with what death is. They begin asking many questions about death, such as: "What happens to your body when you die?" and "Will I die of diabetes?"[114]

Reversibility

Older children now comprehend the concept of reversibility—that an act can be undone by performing an opposite act or be compensated for by other behaviors. They understand a person who feels ill today can feel good tomorrow. In addition, they perceive thoughts, actions, and events from another's point of view.[114]

Conservation

Older school-age children understand conservation; for example, popsicles and fruit drinks are the same even when their form and shape change from frozen to liquid. They now know that the amount of water in a tall, thin glass is the same when poured into a short, fat glass. They are less easily fooled into thinking they are eating less food if it is bunched up on their plates.

Relationships

Older children seriate and classify things by many characteristics simultaneously (e.g., color, size, weight, number). This, along with reversibility, measurement, and conservation, allows them to comprehend relations and degrees of things such as "hurting a little bit." They now can understand the rationale for insulin therapy, the importance of restricting sugar and fat, and the danger of widely fluctuating blood glucose levels. They can recognize times in their schedules when they are to perform BGM or eat their snacks, plan exercise according to short-term blood glucose fluctuations, alter food intake in response to blood glucose levels, and state indications for insulin dose changes.[149] They can recognize signs and symptoms of hyperglycemia or hypoglycemia. In fact, some develop a fear of exercise and sports after experiencing an activity-induced hypoglycemic episode.[122]

Reasoning

Older school-age children can do experiments in their minds instead of requiring the concrete manipulation of objects. However, they cannot always transfer what they learned from one situation to another because they still need actual data to organize and manipulate. They begin to reason deductively, from groups of experiences to a particular experience.[110] For example, "The nurse says injections hurt less if muscles are relaxed, so if I relax the muscles in my leg, this insulin shot will not hurt as much." They can also separate consequences to them from the causes and intentions, "Mom hurt me when she gave my insulin shot, but I need the insulin and she didn't want to hurt me."

Health care providers should determine whether school-age children are in the early or later concrete cognitive developmental stages to know what words and terms are appropriate to use in teaching them.[114] For learning to occur, those in the earlier phase need multisensory teaching techniques and careful use of words, avoiding homonyms and synonyms that may cause misinterpretation of information.[138] Those in the later concrete stage develop fearful misperceptions less often when only pictures or concrete teaching materials are used. School-age children can be motivated to learn procedures, especially those that they fear (e.g., insulin injections, finger pricking for SBGM), by having the opportunity both to view peer children on television and by performing and seeing themselves on a videotape. Watching other children their age with IDDM successfully complete these skills facilitates their learning, since the more similar the model is to the observer, the higher the likelihood that observational learning will occur.[58]

Coping Mechanisms

School-age children use a variety of defense mechanisms and types of coping strategies to cope with feelings of anxiety or inadequacy. Extreme independence is usually expressed in relation to denial of fears. They display the greatest amount of bravado when they are feeling the most helpless. They use compulsive rituals or "magic incantations" to defend themselves from anxiety related to aggression. They believe expressions of their new awareness of death prevents something happening to them.[114] Younger school-age children were found to use mainly primary coping strategies and behaviors such as engaging in direct self-care activities (e.g., finger sticks to check blood sugar levels) or changing their physiologic condition by using insulin to lower their blood sugar level. Older school-age children were beginning to use secondary coping strategies and behaviors to modify or influence their own subjective psychologic state (e.g., moods, expectations, wishes, interpretations). Examples of secondary coping include sticking to the meal plan so they feel good about themselves, telling jokes while giving themselves their own insulin, or telling others not being able to have sugar keeps them from having cavities. Thus secondary control coping often involves reinterpreting events to find meaning or purpose in them and requires more complex cognitive processes.[9] Regardless of the type of coping behaviors used, children who reported using more extensive coping repertoires or particular coping strategies more often also felt better about themselves and their disease and more secure in their relationships with peers.[32,34,61,73]

Language

Language is now used to share ideas, communicate thoughts, and learn others' perspectives.[53] Jokes that play on words are especially appreciated. Because the structure of language is becoming important, children enjoy arguing and trying to stump adults with jokes that have multiple meanings, depending on the way one structures the sentence.[114] For example, "What child can jump as high as a tree?" Answer: "All children because trees can't jump." Using this type of humor during teaching sessions encourages children to pay closer attention to the diabetes educator.

Moral Development

Most children ages 10 to 12 years believe rules should be followed and will try to bargain with others to have those rules and laws to meet their own needs. However, they have no true understanding of abstract concepts such as fairness, loyalty, or laws.[143,144]

Discipline

Adults must establish consistent rules and discuss the issues involved in setting each of the rules. Punishment must be consistent, immediate, appropriate to the nature of the misdeed, and given in a businesslike tone. Experiencing the natural or logical consequences for actions is helpful. Reminding children they felt shaky, sweaty, "spacey," sleepy, stubborn, and starving after strenuous exercise because they forgot to eat their after-school snack helps them understand the importance of the preexercise snack. Children must understand they are punished for the lying about eating candy because it is harmful to them, not because they are not loved or liked as a person.

Lying and Cheating

Kohlberg[75] found that all school-age children cheat and that the amount of cheating varies with the amount of pressure they feel to succeed. Children will cheat to blame others for their misdeeds, to appear more knowledgeable or skilled in activities, to appear more like their peers, and to avoid punishment or a "lecture" from significant adults. Children ages 9 to 12 have a strong need for peer group membership and for approval from authority figures, which may intensify or lessen the frequency and degree of lying and cheating behaviors associated with the diabetes regimen.

Play

Play is the most significant way in which children learn and the chief medium of communicating their ideational and fantasy preoccupations. Because it is self-revealing, it should be used to better understand children's concerns and feelings about IDDM. One must remember that children communicate their unconscious conflicts or wishes through play and create new situations or put real and imagined experiences together in new combinations. Play gives them renewed energy to tackle their problems at a later time.[51] Incorporating therapeutic medical play into diabetes education enables the educator to determine the child's misconceptions and fears so that knowledge can be corrected and fears minimized in later educational sessions.

Cognitive Problems: Learning Problems With and Without Hyperactivity

Approximately 4 million, or 12% of, school-age children have some form of learning problem. Three-fourths are actually diagnosed with a learning disability. Of these, two-thirds are boys. The number of children with learning problems is currently growing at an alarming rate; this means more children with diabetes are likely to have this problem as well. Learning disability is now diagnosed as either an *undifferentiated attention deficit disorder* (ADD: DSM-III-R, 3.400) or as *attention deficit hyperactivity disorder* (ADHD: DSM-III-R, 314.014). The primary difference between these two is that children with ADHD are also hyperactive. Although the etiology is unknown, a strong familial tendency exists. In 1987 the Interagency Committee on Learning Disability defined these disorders as follows[54]:

> Learning disability is a generic term that refers to a heterogeneous group of disorders manifested by significant difficulties in the acquisition and use of listening, speaking, reading, writing, reasoning, or mathematical abilities, or of social skills.

Some educators classify learning disabilities into four types: receptive, integrative, expressive, and *diffuse,* which is a combination of the three previous categories. Children with a *receptive* type of learning disability have trouble getting information into their brains. Those with the *expressive* type have difficulty getting the information out, in speaking, spelling, writing, calculating, or drawing. Those with the *integrative* type can get the information in but have difficulty in organizing their thoughts, as is noted in having difficulty sequencing, understanding clichés, and in analyzing or synthesizing information.[54,90] Although each child is unique, children with ADD or ADHD exhibit most of the specific behaviors identified in Box 18-1.

Parents and educators must know that learning-disabled children function best when they have clear guidelines, structure, routine, and consistency. They should be given directions one or two at a time and not be overwhelmed with having to make a number of decisions at any one time, especially pertinent considerations in teaching with child with IDDM.

Learning occurs best when 5- to 10-minute teaching sessions are given in a quiet room away from any extraneous stimuli. Careful structuring of diabetes content is essential. These children need to feel successful at understanding the previous content before moving onto new ideas. For example, the educator should present *only* six ways they will feel if they have low blood glucose and use a chart with each symptom written and pictures illustrating each one. They should have the children look at the chart, read it aloud, act out each symptom, and then write each one down. When they can state these symptoms, educators should teach them to take five or six sugar cubes or 4 ounces of juice whenever they feel this way. Then eductors should help them transfer this information to various situations they will confront. For example, one should ask, "What should you do if you feel shaky and starving in math class?"

BOX 18-1

BEHAVIORS COMMON TO CHILDREN WHO HAVE ADD AND ADHD

Behaviors common for children with ADD

Hear only the beginning or end of set of directions.
Start work before receiving the directions.
Often lose things necessary for tasks or activities.
Ignore and are impatient with details because they think they have the general idea.
Do not recognize relationships of parts to whole task.
Resist going back over new material.
Resist correcting work.
Want black-and-white, simple, uncomplicated answers.
Do not consider all variations of problems; arrive at quick, simple answers and decisions.

Behaviors common for children with ADHD

All behaviors listed for children with ADD plus:
Have difficulty sustaining attention in tasks or play.
Talk excessively.
Interrupt or intrude on others.
Blurt out answers before question is completed.
Rush into potentially dangerous situations.
Are quick to anger in unpredictable and explosive ways.
Have very short attention spans.
Are easily distracted by extraneous stimuli.
Are constantly moving; have great difficulty in sitting or staying still.
Have difficulty in waiting turns.
Show a lack of concern for rules and the rights of others.

One should suggest they have sugar cubes in the pockets of their athletic shorts or slacks and ask them, "What should you do if you start feeling shaky and spacey at soccer practice?" What should you do if you feel shakey and real sweaty (but your skin is cool) during a basketball game?"

IMPACT OF DIABETES ON NORMAL COGNITIVE AND LANGUAGE DEVELOPMENT

School-age children with IDDM are subject to the same cognitive development as children who do not have IDDM. However, children who experience multiple, severe episodes of low blood glucose may develop learning difficulties or delayed or impaired cognition. It is now believed that a high number of school-age children with chronic illnesses (e.g., IDDM) may have either regressed or delayed cognitive development when compared with those without illnesses.[43,53] In one study 25% of 7- to 10-year-old children with IDDM were still preoperational, whereas none of those without chronic illnesses was preoperational at these ages. This may be especially true for children who have frequent nocturnal or daytime hypoglycemia.

Perceptions of Diabetes

Children's understanding of illness may be determined by their level of cognitive maturation and by the amount of relevant information they have about their body and its functions.[149] Younger school-age children often have numerous misperceptions about what diabetes is. For example, a 7-year-old child said IDDM is "something where you have to take blood out. Getting holes in you." Children in the later stage of cognitive development also have misperceptions about IDDM. For example, "The insulin in your body isn't traveling right. I'm eating too much sugar and it goes into my blood system and blocks the insulin passage." Parents also may have many misconceptions and erroneous beliefs about diabetes; one of the most common is that children develop diabetes because "they ate too much sugar and sweets."

Younger school-age children often think the cause of any disease results from human action or the outcome of wrongdoing (e.g., God gave it to them, they caught it, or they ate too much sugar). Later in this stage they perceive that illness can have multiple causes.[15,19,43,53]

Studies found that school-age children who had diabetes for 1 year perceived their diabetes as caused by several reasons: (1) a mechanical breakdown (e.g., "Insulin-producing cells are sick"), (2) simplified cause and effect, (e.g., "I ate too much candy"), (3) being punished, (e.g., "I got diabetes because I fought with my brother), (4) it just happened, or (5) for a *specific* reason to *help* that child in some way[35,81,134] (e.g., Jeff thought he developed IDDM as a message to give up alcohol, smoking, and hanging around a bad group of kids[19,26,115]).

Feelings About Having Diabetes

Children clearly remember how they felt and what they thought when they first heard they had diabetes. Most children say they were confused, sad, mad, and frightened of needles.[81] In response to a request to "Draw what it's like to have diabetes," newly diagnosed children frequently draw broken hearts or large faces with tears. Other feelings about having diabetes include fear of death and feelings of acceptance or rejection of having IDDM.[21] Feelings of acceptance include statements about the perceived good aspects of having IDDM, such as not getting many cavities, getting to eat snacks at school when others do not, never getting fat, feeling special, and being spoiled. Major negative feelings about having IDDM focus on being "different," feeling alone even with friends or family (primarily because of feeling different), the inconvenience and extra time the diabetes regimen takes every day, having to eat when you are not hungry, and not being able to eat sweet treats whenever friends do.[37,88] It is important to note that having to take "shots" is not usually verbalized as the worst thing about having IDDM, although many younger school-age children draw pictures of oversized, black or red syringes and finger-sticking devices in response to the question, "What is the worst thing about having diabetes?"

Many children are unable to verbalize their feelings. Drawing and painting are extremely useful communication techniques to help children express their thoughts, feelings, and misperceptions in a very nonthreatening and revealing manner.[71] Art is less subject to control by defense mechanisms and allows children to reveal unconscious tensions, feelings, and perceptions of deeper reactions to events.[14,44,114] Children draw what is important to them and what they think and feel, not necessarily reality. This enables them to express taboos and release hostility and other socially nonacceptable feelings through artwork.[114] In addition, drawings provide children with the opportunity to master their feelings and alert health care providers to the misperceptions and fantasies they have about IDDM to facilitate later development of more positive feelings and correct knowledge.[13,52]

Analysis of drawings completed by children with IDDM and their parents indicate common emotions. In one study, Italian children with IDDM drew healthy and ill children smaller than did their nondiabetic peers, indicating these children may not be as well adjusted to their environment. In addition, they seemed to have less clear-cut images or stereotypes of sick and healthy persons.[107] In another as yet unpublished study, drawings completed in response to my question, "What is it like to have diabetes?" yielded the following emotional themes in order of frequency: insecurity, anxiety, ambivalence, rigidity, isolation, anger, sadness, and fear. Parental drawings had similar themes but more frequently included anxiety, insecurity, and powerlessness.

School-age children have varied feelings about each component of the required daily diabetes care regimen, including the diet, insulin, insulin reactions, exercise, and testing. In general, they feel a sense of achievement and pride when they can test their own blood glucose and give themselves insulin injections,[21,37,88] but some complain blood testing takes too much time and that it hurts. Others have misperceptions of these skills. For example, a 9-year-old child used only one finger for blood tests because she thought it was "the only one with blood in it."[88]

IMPACT OF DIABETES ON PSYCHOSOCIAL DEVELOPMENT

The management of diabetes in children requires a complicated treatment regimen that includes one to four daily insulin injections, two to four daily blood glucose tests, dietary regulation, consistent timing of meals and snacks, and careful monitoring of physical activities.[49,82] In addition, both children and their parents must know which behaviors can cause or correct high blood glucose, ketones, and low blood glucose. They must know what to do when any of these occur. These management tasks must be carried out on a daily basis, with no "vacations."[25] Thus diabetes care is time-consuming, difficult, and complex and requires a high degree of self-discipline and regulation and often a change in life-style for children with IDDM and their families.[3,49,69,117]

Children's Reactions to Diabetes

In general, most school-age children with normal psychosocial development adequately cope with diabetes, although some do have considerable difficulty.[82,117] Children more likely to cope with diabetes successfully are those who become immersed in learning about diabetes and are interested in developing a variety of new skills, including diabetes management skills, to master the environment, affirm their sexual identity, and find their place in a peer group. A sense of industry and self-esteem is acquired from frequent successes and from significant others' encouragement and recognition of their achievements. Children gain self-esteem and appreciation of their own worth by being accepted by parents and peers and by having clear, consistent limits flexible enough to permit individual actions.[127] Those with high self-esteem can accept criticism, state their beliefs even if they challenge authority, and confidently enter new situations.

Rubin and Peyrot[117] found in a review of the recent literature on psychosocial problems and interventions in diabetes that children's emotional disturbances (e.g., sadness; feelings of anger, friendlessness, and rejection; social withdrawal) are fairly common after the initial diagnosis of diabetes. It is clear that most children adapt well and quickly to the new illness.[57] They and other authors found that mothers initially felt depressed, angry, sad, and overwhelmed emotionally. Mothers who were most distressed immediately after diagnosis were most likely to remain emotionally upset over a long period and more likely to increase their distress as the duration of the disease lengthened.[6,57,61,77] Several authors have found that successful initial adaptation to diabetes depends on a family environment that is highly cohesive and organized and where expectations of parents were consistent and clear.* Thus efforts by the multidisciplinary diabetes team should include assessment of family environment using the Diabetes Family Environment Scale, the Diabetes Adjustment Scale, or the revised Diabetes Family Behavior Scale or Diabetes Family Responsibility Questionnaire with the Diabetes Regimen Responsibility Scale as well as assessment of the child's ability to cope.† If a family is found to have less organization, cohesion, open communication, warmth and nurturance, or inconsistent expectations, psychosocial and crisis interventions may be needed, including psychologic and biomedical interventions (and even psychotherapy in certain cases) to reduce whatever distress may be present. Referrals and treatment should begin during the initial diabetes education. This may prevent further psychologic distress and the development of other psychopathology such as depression, eating disorders, and self-destructive behavior later. However, if any of these psychopathologic disorders appear, if family dysfunction occurs later, or if disagreements develop between mothers and children in perceptions of who is assuming responsibility for specific diabetes management tasks, the family members involved should be treated as soon as possible to avoid frequent severe hypoglycemic and hyperglycemic episodes along with severe noncompliance with the diabetes treatment regimen.‡ Interventions may include relaxation training, coping-skills training, day or overnight retreats with other families of children with IDDM, individual and family participation in self-help groups, and individual or family therapy.[74,117,129,151] Children with IDDM might attend diabetes camp and find it helps them.

To care adequately for their diabetes, school-age children must comprehend the disease, have positive attitudes toward themselves and their diabetes, and have help and guidance from their peers, significant adults, and their family.[72,73,151] Kager and Holden[74] found research

---

*References 6, 65, 121, 130, 140.
†References 6, 55, 61, 65, 118, 120, 130, 140.
‡References 76, 77, 101, 103, 118.

supported that school-age children have minimal emotional difficulties when they have confidence that they can follow the diabetes regimen, an extensive repertoire of particular coping strategies to regulate negative emotions, and a feeling of being secure in their relationships with peers. Because 6- to 11-year-old children have a very rigid behavior style; they tend to follow rules of the diabetes regimen more closely than children of other age-groups. They complete these tasks in a specific order and continuously practice their newly learned skills. Rules and specific guidelines about what to do in various situations reduce their anxiety and provide an external standard against which to measure themselves.[114,122,144]

Although most families receive extensive instruction regarding the diabetes care regimen, many studies suggest that school-age children have much lower levels of essential skills and knowledge about their regimen than health care professionals expect.[49,149] In fact, a number of studies have demonstrated that children made numerous errors in insulin injections and urine and blood testing.* Most had some understanding of the need for insulin, but many did not comprehend the route insulin takes in the body or the reason for rotating injection sites. Most children know that eating candy is forbidden and eating too much contributes to high blood glucose but do not really understand how choices or the timing of food affects them. Many admitted to sneaking a candy bar[37] and then feeling guilty but did not know *why* they should not eat it. Although some children understand that exercise brings their blood glucose down, many use diabetes as a reason for not participating in activities.[88] Thus children must be provided with individualized, extensive, cognitively appropriate information and hands-on practice sessions to learn how food, exercise, and insulin influence blood glucose levels.[49] They must be frequently helped to apply this information to their daily activities.[7,66,88,95]

Children's cognitive developmental level and an assessment of what they know and what they misunderstand should be the determinant of what they are taught and how they are taught.[70,95,151] One recent study found diabetes educators tended to have too low expectations while parents may have had inordinately high estimates of their school-age children's self-care competence. They found school-age children often could do skills that consisted of rote, motoric action (e.g., perform complete blood glucose test with a meter, use lancet to obtain adequate blood sample), or the consequences of an error tended to be immediate, salient, and aversive (e.g., treat hypoglycemia, anticipate and prevent hypoglycemia).[149] Diabetes educators can use the numbers, water, and clay Piaget-type tasks to identify children's current cognitive level. It may be necessary to reteach some self-care management content each time children reach a new cognitive level because they understand information in new ways. It is essential to reevaluate their skills and knowledge at least twice a year to correct any bad habits or misconceptions they may have developed.

Personality Development

No specific pattern of healthy or unhealthy personality traits have been found to characterize children with diabetes. In addition, the levels of emotional disturbance are no higher among these children than for children with any other chronic illness or even in the general

---

*References 26, 31, 45, 73, 145.

population.[36,105,122] Several studies have found no difference between the levels of behavioral problems or self-esteem of school-age children with and without diabetes.*

Children who do exhibit emotional problems need to be referred for psychologic or psychiatric assistance. Since stress may negatively influence metabolic control of diabetes by increasing the release of glycogen from the liver or by increasing the peripheral resistance to insulin, children with IDDM need to be taught stress reduction techniques and coping skills to modulate their stress reactions and be encouraged to participate in activities and exercise that will help to disperse their anxious feelings.[9,18,78]

Children's Adaptation to Diabetes

School-age children often adapt quite well to the diagnosis of diabetes, at least initially.[50,57,104] Studies of children newly diagnosed with IDDM have illustrated this phenomenon and demonstrated two general modes of coping with the initial strain of living with IDDM. Most school-age children were found to be emotionally resilient and adapted psychologically with comparative ease to the new life demands. In fact, 64% had a rather subdued reaction to the diagnosis throughout the first year. Their reactions consisted of mild sadness, anxiety, feelings of friendlessness, and social withdrawal. The rest of the children exhibited a depressive syndrome that included an anxious, apprehensive, and depressed mood; anger; irritability; suicidal ideation; and excessive somatic complaints. However, recovery from these symptoms occurred over the 9-month period after diagnosis.[117] Another study found children with IDDM coped by ventilating feelings (yelling, blaming others, complaining), ran away from family problems, or relied on close friends to help them cope.[57]

Healthy attitudes toward having diabetes are best developed by a relatively stress-free environment and by parents, teachers, and other significant adults who acknowledge the presence of diabetes but who treat it in a matter-of-fact and supportive manner. Disturbed family environments are often associated with poor diabetic control.† Children from low socioeconomic, single-parent homes are at higher risk for poor diabetes management.‡ Children are also at risk for poor diabetes control if they are from homes in which the family patterns are overprotective and overanxious, overindulgent, and overpermissive; perfectionistic and controlling; or indifferent and rejecting.§ In the school setting, teachers who treat the child with IDDM the same as others and who assist other children in the classroom to understand diabetes promote positive adaptation.

Family's Reaction to Diabetes

Three major factors have an impact on the family's ability to achieve each developmental task and meet the needs of all members: the family's perception of the task, the availability or

---

*References 21, 74, 86, 87, 119.
†References 4, 6, 7, 9, 99, 117, 140.
‡References 6, 65, 121, 140, 149.
§References 65, 78, 120, 130, 140.

resources to achieve each task, and the family's ability to cope with problems. Incorporating the management of children's diabetes into the family can dramatically affect the family's healthy development. It is important to remember to include the siblings to be sure they become positively involved and continue to feel valuable in the family. It is also important to help the family attain organization, cohesion, open communication, and warm, supportive involvement with children with IDDM in the management regimen; have clear expectations of who is responsible for what diabetes management regimen component; and prevent conflict, especially over who is responsible for what.*

The initial goal in the treatment of children with diabetes is to empower the child and family with the knowledge required to participate in and gain independence with self-care management. Formal educational programs are designed to assist the family in learning and integrating two levels of knowledge regarding diabetes. Basic knowledge includes an understanding of the physiologic processes of IDDM and the ability to perform the psychomotor skills, which include insulin administration, blood glucose monitoring, urine ketone testing, and diet management. A higher level of knowledge requires applying the basic information to everyday problems.[49] This level of understanding allows the family to problem-solve actively and negotiate independent decisions about the child's everyday management, such as handling hyperglycemia with or without the presence of ketones before a sporting event and when and how to permit sweets in children's diets.

Diabetes education is best viewed as an ongoing process that must be continually reevaluated and reinstituted as the developmental needs of the children and family change. Parents of younger school-age children have been found to have higher levels of knowledge, especially in the problem-solving area, than parents of older school-age children.[7] Recent research found that mothers are more knowledgeable about children's diabetic management than either fathers or children. In the preadolescent population the mother's knowledge level, not the children's, is closely associated with treatment adherence and metabolic control.[73] The mother feels the greatest burden for maintenance of the diabetes regimen. The diabetes team members need to be sure to provide adequate, ongoing education for all family members and provide continuous, ongoing emotional support for the child with IDDM and the mother.

Family's Adaptation to Diabetes

Healthy family adaptation and rearing children with a chronic illness such as IDDM require collaboration and sharing of responsibilities among all family members; the single largest threat to effective diabetes management is family dysfunction.[117,122] However, the primary responsibility for diabetes care tasks often falls on mothers. Hauenstein and colleagues[63] studied 52 mothers who had children with IDDM and found that more than 50% reported excessive maternal stress caused by negative characteristics of their children. These negative characteristics included poor adaptability, demanding behaviors, and distractibility resulting in mothers' stress. Other subsequent studies have validated these findings.[77,78,101] In another study, school-age males with IDDM were found to have more behaviors associated with

---

*References 6, 65, 76, 77, 130, 149.

neurotic tendencies and personality disturbances than females with IDDM of the same age. Such behaviors included withdrawal, anxiety, hyperactivity, and aggression.[27,70,72,87]

The complex array of daily tasks that must be followed to manage children with IDDM requires families to adjust and rearrange their established routines. Family organization and control are necessary for successful management of children with IDDM.[65,117,139,140] A significant association between parental stress, age of the child, and glycemic control has been found.[77] Low levels of parental stress in mothers of younger school-age children were associated with good glycemic control, but the same levels in mothers of older children were associated with poor metabolic control.[63] Rubin and Peyrot[117] cite several studies that found family functioning is related significantly to regimen adherence or glycemic control. Family support was associated positively with the child's diabetes regimen adherence and good metabolic control; family conflict was associated negatively with adherence and good metabolic control.[6,121] Thus the multidisciplinary team should use diabetes-specific measures of family functioning and support (e.g., Diabetes Family Environment Scale, Diabetes Adjustment Scale, revised Diabetes Family Behavior Scale, or Diabetes Family Responsibility Questionnaire with Diabetes Regimen Responsibility Scale) to assess whether or not the family needs psychologic interventions.[6,101,118,121] Future research needs to describe more definitively the relationships among children's personality, parental stress, family adaptation, and adherence and glycemic control.

Adaptation and coping behaviors of parents of children with IDDM have not been extensively investigated. One study found parental coping methods included expressions of anger, trying again, talking with friends and hospital staff, and learning more.[13] Such coping behaviors may assist parents in becoming more aware of their added responsibilities associated with the care of their children's diabetes.[112]

Participation of *all* family members in the diabetes care regimen is essential for healthy adaptation and good glycemic control.* Research on sharing of diabetes responsibilities among family members found that 72% of the sample families reported areas of disagreement between the child and mother about who took ultimate responsibility for 22 diabetes-related tasks. The mother-child dyads that reported multiple areas of disagreement and whose mothers admitted low levels of adherence to the care regimen had children at risk for poor glycemic control.[4,76,101] These results emphasize the need for clearly defined expectations within the family and the need for each family member to have agreed-on responsibilities for specific diabetes-related tasks.[149]

Adaptation to School

School entry brings about a new set of hurdles for parents and children with IDDM. Normal childhood activities, such as swapping of food between friends and spontaneous exercise sessions, place these children at risk for diabetes problems.[78] Parents worry most about their children's diabetes management while they are at school. They often lack confidence in teachers' abilities to recognize insulin reactions and to understand their children's special

---

*References 24, 56, 118, 120, 140.

dietary needs.[66,134] These concerns are legitimized by recent research that found school-teachers often have an inadequate understanding of IDDM and its management. In one study of more than 400 teachers, 55% could not identify symptoms of hypoglycemia and only 26% could identify when a hypoglycemic reaction is most likely to occur.[94] Tatman and Lessing[134] recommend that an educated diabetes nurse talk with teachers, the principal, and school staff about a newly diagnosed child's diabetic regimen and the parents' main concerns before the child goes back to school and leave information packs and telephone numbers of the multidisciplinary diabetes team members. This nurse should visit each school at least once a year to upgrade their information.

Throughout the elementary-school years, peer relationships become increasingly important and are essential for the child's healthy socialization. Perceived restrictions imposed by the diabetes regimen may hinder some children's active participation in normal childhood activities. Parents agonize over whether or not to allow their child to attend slumber parties, go on outings with friends, and attend birthday parties without parental supervision. It is the uncertainty over whether their children may stray from the diabetes regimen or will become ill and not be properly treated that causes much of this parental anxiety and fear.

Information and support from national organizations, current publications, and community resources are of assistance to families with children who have IDDM. Such organizations and publications offer ideas on living with diabetes and current information regarding new trends in diabetes management.

Assessment of the Family

The success of the health care team in caring for school-age children with IDDM begins with a complete and thorough family assessment, including the use of family assessment tools (e.g., Diabetes Family Environment Scale, Diabetes Adjustment Scale, revised Diabetes Family Behavior Scale or Diabetes Family Responsibility Questionnaire with Diabetes Regimen Responsibility Scale).[6,55,65,120,140] The initial assessment is critical in planning children's education and care, and the ongoing assessment of the family's development reveals current and new information (Fig. 18-1).

The family's socioeconomic status (SES) affects children's compliance with the diabetes regimen and with their glycemic control. Children with IDDM living in a family with a relatively high SES tend to have parents who possess higher education levels, more financial resources, and greater problem-solving skills. These children are able to achieve better metabolic control than those from families with relatively low SES[4,6,7] who continually struggle to meet their basic needs.

Over the past 30 years, changes in the structure of the American family have resulted in a dramatic increase in single-parent homes. According to the U.S. 1984 Bureau of the Census, more than 25% of all children in the United States were living with only one parent, and the percentage has increased greatly since that time. The majority of these families are headed by women and are more likely to live in poverty than are two-parent households.[5] Children with IDDM who live in such families are at risk for poor compliance and poor metabolic control. Auslander and colleagues[7] found the glycohemoglobin levels were 30% higher in

Child's name _____ Age _____ School grade _____
Race _____ Nationality _____ Religion _____

Household members

Name	Relationship to patient	Age	Pertinent information

Family/healthcare/community support

Name	Address	Phone	Comments

Socioeconomic status

Variable	Adequate	Inadequate	Excellent
Income			
Housing			
Neighborhood			
Telephone			
Transportation			
Resources for dietary needs			
Resources for medical equipment			
Resources for health care needs			

Communication patterns/family functioning

Family stability _____
Family flexability _____
Support from extended family _____
Decision-making process _____
Communication patterns _____
Family's feeling of closeness _____
Satisfaction with relationships _____
Sharing of IDDM responsibilities _____
Understanding child development _____
Impact of IDDM on family members _____

Fig. 18-1   An example of a family assessment tool.   *Continued.*

```
┌────────────────────────────────────────────────────────────────────┐
│  Functioning in community                                            │
│  Variable                            Adequate  Inadequate  Excellent │
│  Knowledge of community resources _____  │
│  Utilization of community resources _____  │
│  Social activities of family _____  │
│  Social activities of child _____  │
│  Adequate babysitting resources _____  │
│  Support from school system _____  │
│                                                                      │
│  Treatment knowledge/management skills                               │
│  Ability to learn psychomotor skills _____  │
│  Ability to problem-solve _____  │
│  Knowledge of health care management _____  │
└────────────────────────────────────────────────────────────────────┘
```

Fig. 18-1, cont'd.

children from African-American families and single-parent homes than levels in children from white or two-parent families. This may be true in part because cohesion and emotional expressiveness between members within the African-American and single-parent families are significantly lower than those for the white and two-parent households.[6] Another study found that children with IDDM living with their mothers and a stepfather or with adoptive parents have even worse glycemic control than those living in single-parent homes, regardless of SES.[101]

Families who are organized and cohesive, have open communication patterns, use supportive problem solving, and frequently share ideas create a nurturing atmosphere that encourages learning about diabetes.[65,101,140] Marteau and associates[99] concluded that "... happy families may produce happy children who carry out a diabetic regimen compatible with good control and consequently have good diabetic control."

TEACHING AND LEARNING IMPLICATIONS

It is clear from many studies that school-age children need an individualized, developmentally based education program that not only presents knowledge at an understandable cognitive level but also emphasizes the application of that knowledge in their daily activities.[6,7,122] Since studies also identified variability in the levels of knowledge about diabetes within specific age-groups,[21] educators need to be conscious not only of individual differences but also of the cognitive development level at which children are currently operating.

Frequent reassessment of children's skills and knowledge is essential. Educators can employ children's drawings to assist them to communicate their fears, misperceptions, and current understanding of the various components of the diabetes care regimen.[21,28,114] When fears and anxieties are revealed, parents and health care providers need to let the children know they are recognized and assist them in coping with these feelings.

Individualizing Treatment Goals for the School-Age Child

A common assumption among health care providers is that children with diabetes should assume as much responsibility for self-care as possible. A recent summary of more than 200 diabetes professionals found that the average expectation of mastery for 14 to 20 selected skills was below the age ranges recommended by the ADA in 1983.[148] An even more recent study found that diabetes professionals underestimated the age but that parents may have overestimated the age at which school-age children can and should assume primary and shared responsibility for specific self-care management skills.[149] Therefore numerous diabetes providers and parents have inappropriate age-related expectations for school-age children. In fact, recent research demonstrated that children given more primary responsibility for their diabetes care make more errors, are less adherent, and are in poorer metabolic control than children whose parents are more involved.[49,50,82] Therefore the determination of the amount of self-management responsibility for diabetes care must not be based on age alone. Instead, it should be based on a detailed assessment of the child's cognitive level, current correct information about diabetes, their readiness to learn, and their fine motor skills.

The responsibility for diabetes management must be shared between parents and children, with a gradual increase of more responsibility being assumed by children, as determined by their demonstrating correct skills and wanting more independence. It must be based on the child's social and emotional maturity and family characteristics in addition to the child's cognitive development.[42,149] A recent study found that of 400 children, 50% of those 10 to 11 years old wanted more help with recording their blood glucose values and thought they should be at least 9½ years old before giving their own insulin injections, and 150 wanted their families to keep sweets out of the house.[54] Another study found that children who were more prone to worry and apprehensive had better blood glucose control than those without emotional or adjustment problems.[9,116] Did the children with good glycohemoglobin values experience rigid control and structure that directly affected their personality characteristics, or did they become more negative toward diabetes in reaction to the high structure? It is likely that well-adjusted children are more diligent in monitoring the subjective signs of poor blood glucose control and thus counteract them more effectively. These children also may not take responsibility for their diabetes care, and their dependence on their parents may protect them from the adverse effects of precocious self-care.[50]

Currently, empirical information is needed to define appropriate developmental expectations for acquisition of self-care independence by children with IDDM.[49] Clearly, any guidelines about age-related expectations of children's learning knowledge or assumptions of diabetes care skills must be individualized for that specific child.[122]

Goals of an Individualized, Developmentally Based Education Program

There are four major goals of a developmentally based diabetes education program: (1) to facilitate parents' and children's positive knowledge of and adjustment to diabetes, (2) to help the parents and children attain and maintain shared interdependence and responsibility for assuming diabetes management skills that enhance good metabolic control without frequent severe hypoglycemic events, (3) to enhance parents' and children's self-esteem and independence as part of their normal development, and (4) to encourage the development of normally developing and well-adjusted children with IDDM. To attain these goals, the diabetes health care providers must provide the family with cognitively appropriate knowledge, guidelines for age-related expectations, and information on how to apply the diabetes care knowledge and skills in a flexible way to meet everyday activities and must encourage the learning of appropriate behavioral management strategies.

Several research studies found that to assume responsibility for IDDM self-care, children must be provided with the knowledge base needed via multiple senses, active participation, and behavioral demonstration, not just through verbal information.[35,138,151] Second, it is important to assess the current knowledge and perceptions of both parents and children before beginning an education program. In addition, positive family functioning and parental involvement are critical for school-age children, since parental knowledge, especially the mother's knowledge, has been found to be significantly related to both adherence and control for 7- to 11-year-old children. Knowledge of diabetes care is a necessary, but not sufficient, prerequisite to good self-management, adherence, and metabolic control. Behavioral strategies aimed at improving various skills children need in diabetes-related situations (e.g., social skills) should be included. As previously noted, many studies have shown that even children with good information about diabetes skills make numerous and serious errors in estimating amounts of foods, drawing up insulin doses, and testing and recording urine ketone and blood glucose values.[33,45] These errors are serious enough to have a negative impact on metabolic control. It is also clear that skill or adherence in one area of care does not predict adherence in others.[123]

School-age children are at an ideal age to *begin* taking some responsibility for their own insulin injections, glucose testing, and diet control.[42,149] However, it is important to implement changes gradually, frequently assessing both specific areas of knowledge and specific skills to determine children's readiness and motivation to perform self-care tasks.[42,49,122,149]

Assessing children's current cognitive level via Piaget-type tasks and their ability to manage complex information in areas other than diabetes provides important clues about their ability to manage the multiple and complex aspects of their diabetes.[49] Children who have a positive self-image and demonstrate self-discipline and deductive reasoning abilities in school or in the types of questions they ask educators are most likely to understand more advanced principles of diabetes care and to assume an increased role in diabetes care skills.[122] In these cases the educator should encourage implementation of a *gradual* transfer of appropriate responsibilities from parents to children. The educator must remember that parents should maintain shared responsibility or should oversee all components of their school-age children's diabetes regimen.

Optimal metabolic control (HbA$_{1c}$ values between 7% and 9%) is encouraged in families who value and affirm structure and organization and who also maintain good communication with their children.[121] Parents who provide consistent expectations and guidance to the child with diabetes in a cooperative, shared way without nagging or being perfectionistic promote behaviors that contribute to better metabolic control.[4,7,117] In contrast, overprotectiveness, competitiveness, overachievement, overcontrol, and indifference are associated with poor metabolic control and should be discouraged.[42,149]

The overall goal for diabetes education of school-age children and their parents is to provide both with complete diabetes education and to facilitate the children's ability to become active and knowledgeable participants in diabetes care. Diabetes instruction needs to be geared toward children's conceptual and developmental level, with very strong messages for both parents and children to work as a team. Education programs must teach by using multiple senses, behavioral demonstrations, and unannounced, frequent "spot checks" of parents' and children's performances.

Content of Educational Program

The content for an individualized, developmentally based diabetes education program is similar for both newly and previously diagnosed children with IDDM and their families. (See Appendix F for a list of content provided to children with IDDM and their families by an multidisciplinary team at St. Louis Children's Hospital.) After extensive initial in-hospital education, all families and children with IDDM need frequent reeducation and retraining. Box 18-2 presents topics frequently reevaluated.

Self-monitoring of blood glucose

Children should be taught to select three fingers that are to be used for SMBG so that in 3 to 4 weeks, calluses will develop and the finger sticks will not be so painful. One should ensure that children stick the sides of their fingers to minimize pain and to prevent pads from losing their sense of touch over the next few years.

As these SMBG skills are mastered, the educator should teach the child to try to keep most blood glucose levels between 80 and 180 mg/dl.[121] This is a more realistic target for school-age children than the normal range of 60 to 120 mg/dl. Keeping most glucose values in this target range usually results in adequate glycemia without greatly increasing the number of severe hypoglycemic episodes. However, having many blood glucose levels above 200 mg/dl does constitute poor control and places the child at risk for many renal and eye complications.[121]

Parents and children must be told that maintaining most blood glucose values between 80 and 180 mg/dl is often easier during the first few months when a child's ability to produce insulin temporarily increases. This period, called the "honeymoon," usually lasts for several months during the first year after diagnosis and may result in excellent glucose control even when the diabetes regimen is not followed closely. Subsequently, as maintaining good control becomes more difficult, higher and more erratic blood glucose readings become more common, and children and parents must work harder to keep them down in the target range. Conflicts over who is at fault and who should be responsible for various components of the diabetes regimen are likely to occur at this time. The diabetes team needs to provide educational and emotional support to prevent these conflicts from resulting in family problems or poor glycemic control.

Hypoglycemia and hyperglycemia

As early as possible, children must be taught to recognize when a "low" blood glucose occurs and immediately either to tell someone or treat it. A "low" is defined as having less

---

BOX 18-2

DIABETES EDUCATION FOR SCHOOL-AGE CHILDREN

For younger school-age children

   I. What is diabetes?

      Explain by using an analogy such as blood sugar is like gasoline. Gasoline must get into the car's engine to make it run, and blood sugar must get in so you can run and play.

      Diabetes is not caused by thoughts or misdeed.

      Diabetes is not a punishment.

      Diabetes will not go away.

   II. How to check blood for amount of sugar.

 III. How to check urine for ketones.

 IV. What it feels like to have low blood sugar (shaky, sweaty, sleepy, and starving).

   V. What to do if you have low blood sugar. Tell your mom, dad, teacher, coach, or friend. Always carry cubes of sugar or packs of honey in pocket and keep these in desk at school. Treat low blood sugar by eating 1 tsp sugar, honey, jelly, or syrup or drinking 3 oz unsweetened juice.

 VI. When low blood sugar levels are likely to occur.

      When not all food at a meal is eaten.

      When a snack is skipped.

      When playing sports longer and harder than on other days.

      When too much insulin is accidentally given.

 VII. What it feels like to have high blood sugar levels (thirsty, have to "pee" [or other word] a lot, pee is sticky; feel very tired and crabby).

VIII. What to do if you have high blood sugar. Tell your mom, dad, teacher, coach, or friend. Drink a large glass of water, ice tea, sugar-free fruit drink, or diet soda.

 IX. When likely to have high blood sugar levels.

      When snacks and food are eaten that mom does not know about.

      When an apple is traded for a candy bar with a friend.

      When forget to take insulin injection.

   X. What it feels like to have ketones (sick to stomach, throw up, stomach hurts, breathe funny, and bad breath that does not brush away).

---

than 60 mg/dl blood glucose. The child often can be taught to remember the *six S's of low blood glucose: shaky, sweaty (but cool to touch), sleepy (not tired), starving, stubborn, and "spacey."* Parents should also watch for children to have a quick change in their activity level or become pale, quiet, whiny, or irritable. One should emphasize to parents that candy is not to be used to treat a "low" because some kinds of candy may not have enough sugar, it must be eaten too quickly to enjoy, and many children cannot resist eating the candy even when they know they are not "low." Whenever a "low" occurs more than 1 hour before the next scheduled snack or meal, the child should also drink at least one-half glass of milk or eat three to six saltine crackers with cheese, meat, or peanut butter. This avoids hypoglycemia every 20 to 30 minutes.

BOX 18-2

DIABETES EDUCATION FOR SCHOOL-AGE CHILDREN—cont'd

For older school-age children

I. What is diabetes?

Explain using three-dimensional doll.

Explain location of pancreas and define insulin.

Explain "cells" to child and how insulin is their best friend because it gets sugar into the cells so the body can grow and work well.

Diabetes was not caused by them. It is not a punishment for being bad or lying.

They did not catch diabetes from someone.

II. How to check blood sugars.

III. How to check urine for ketones.

IV. How to give self insulin injections (not until age 10 to 11 years to draw dose up).

Wash hands.

Clean top on insulin bottles.

Place air into NPH insulin bottle.

Place air into regular insulin bottle.

Draw up regular insulin.

Draw up NPH insulin.

Clean off injection site.

Bunch up skin with free hand.

Break skin with needle using a 90-degree angle.

Inject insulin.

Rotate needle before removing.

Remember to rotate site (arms and abdomen 1 week and legs and abdomen the next).

Use abdomen when blood sugar levels are high (insulin is absorbed more quickly).

V. Symptoms of high and low blood sugar levels.

VI. Treatment of high and low blood sugar levels.

VII. Causes of high and low blood sugar levels.

VIII. Problem-solving skills.

What would you do if:

You were locked out of your house and your blood sugar was low?

It was a schoolmate's birthday and the class was having cake?

You are in the middle of a science test and you suddenly realize you forgot to eat lunch?

Children with extremely elevated glucose levels over 240 mg/dl for several hours or more have to urinate often, feel thirsty or exhausted, are crabby, and may develop refractive errors. When blood glucose values are over 240 mg/dl or whenever children with IDDM become ill, someone should check the urine for ketones. Children should avoid strenuous exercise when large amounts of ketones are present in the urine.[60]

If hyperglycemia occurs before a scheduled insulin injection, children and their parents should learn when and how to adjust the insulin dose. When ketones are present, children should drink at least 8 oz of sugar-free liquid per hour for 2 to 3 hours and then retest. If the blood glucose or ketones have not gone down after taking appropriate fluids and/or extra insulin, they should call the diabetes health professional, who may then order a supplemental amount of regular insulin.

Sick-day management

Parents must know that children with IDDM who are ill are very susceptible to dehydration, which can increase the concentration of both glucose and ketones. Children can develop diabetic ketoacidosis (DKA) within a few hours when dehydrated or febrile. Thus sick-day management requires that children drink large amounts of fluids. A rule of thumb is to take children off solid food and have them alternate 6 to 8 oz of sugared fluids with sugar-free fluids every hour. Children should be seen by their physician or brought to an emergency room for IV therapy if they cannot keep liquids down or vomit more than once within 4 to 6 hours.

Giving injections

Giving insulin injections can be frightening for parents and children alike. Diabetes educators can reduce this anxiety by demonstrating and then expecting the parents to give each other saline injections. School-age children who want to and who have the manual dexterity necessary should be encouraged to give the educator saline injections early in the education program. Parents are usually surprised at how little the injections hurt, and children are very proud of themselves afterward. Both must be taught to insert the needle quickly through the skin to minimize pain. Using insulin syringes calibrated to the smallest amount of units possible makes it easier for all to see the unit markings accurately. For example, Terumo makes a 25-unit syringe that is marked in ½ units, and Becton-Dickinson makes a 30-unit syringe for U-100 insulin. However, neither should be used unless the total number of insulin units per dose is 5 U less than the amount held by the syringe. Younger children, during the "honeymoon period," may require ½-unit insulin doses, such as ½ regular and 3½ NPH. Often, parents can be fairly accurate in measuring ½ units on either of the new small insulin syringes just described. However, one study found neither professional staff nor parents were accurate when giving 2 U or less of insulin using currently available syringes.[23] They recommend using diluted U-10, U-25, or U-50 insulin if this small dose of insulin is required.

Parents and children must know that both glucagon and insulin need to be kept between 32° and 86° Fahrenheit; keeping them in the refrigerator is best during warm months. Once opened, insulin should be used within 30 days. Otherwise, unexplained high blood glucose levels are sometimes caused by insulin that has "gone bad." This can be noted when older NPH or Lente insulin appears thready or crystallized or if the bottle appears frosted.

Rotation of injections is extremely important.[10] Injections should be given 1 inch (2.5 cm) apart. Some studies found that insulin is absorbed faster and more completely from the abdomen than from arms, buttocks, and legs.[7] This suggests rotation should not be taught clockwise around the body as previously thought. Instead, all sites on the arms should be used 1 week, then all leg sites should be used on alternate weeks (buttocks used only in children who do not mind). The abdominal sites should probably be used whenever hyperglycemia is present before injections. In addition, injections should be avoided in the legs or arms if the child is about to participate in strenuous activities, using these limbs within the next 2 hours.

Behavioral strategies

Parents help children become active participants in their care by not expecting perfection, making it easy for children to remember care activities by leaving written reminders in visible places, or using simple, matter-of-fact verbal reminders.[124] Parents who encourage their children to be progressively more involved in their self-care, while providing structure and working together with them, send their children the message that they trust them and see them as competent and worthwhile persons who can do increasingly complex skills. Successful parents clearly list each family member's responsibilities. In addition, they set up natural or logical consequences; having a "low" reaction, for example, may be the consequence of being late for a meal, and wetting the bed may be the consequence of eating too many snacks at bedtime at a friend's house. A logical consequence for choosing not to measure blood glucose is the need for a parent to come to a friend's house where the child is sleeping overnight to test blood at bedtime and before breakfast.

Diabetes health care providers need to help parents set up natural or logical consequences for children's actions. This is a much more instructive way for children to learn the consequences of their various actions and may reduce parental guilt or anger.

Health care providers should emphasize to school-age children, in front of their parents, that adults will not become angry with them, like them less, or punish them if their blood glucose values are not within the target range or if they honestly say they ate a candy bar or other food that raised their blood glucose. Encouraging children to be honest and to eat sweet foods, within clearly established limits, prevents the need to sneak foods or lie about blood glucose values.

On the other hand, parents should know the various ways and reasons children "cheat" on their diet and should be encouraged to supervise their children closely. For example, some children place ketchup on their glucose test strips to make the blood test come out within range, whereas others may spit on the blood test strips or run diluted fruit drink or milk over them to obtain low readings and subsequent sweets as treatment of hypoglycemia.

Parents need to be reminded that younger school-age children think differently from adults and cannot comprehend the wisdom of doing something difficult today to prevent something bad from occurring in 5, 10, or more years. Furthermore, causing fear of some dreadful consequence such as loss of a leg or vision is likely to cause them to feel depressed or hopeless instead of encouraging their compliance.

Parents must also be cautioned not to think that children need to eat all their food or have blood glucose values between 80 to 180 all the time; these are unreal expectations for every single blood glucose value. (However, these goals may become more readily accepted since the DCCT study's findings were released in 1993.) Behavioral management strategies, such as the use of sticker charts, earning tokens to be traded in for activities they like to do, and the use of practical positive and negative reinforcers to make diabetes activities easier is helpful. For example, completing three or four "good" behaviors earns a reward. The parent should allow the child to negotiate the reward, such as extra TV time or a walk in the park with parents. It is necessary to change the tasks and rewards biweekly to keep the child interested and motivated.

Parents must also be taught to avoid power struggles with their children over food. It is better to let children experience the "low" as a consequence of not eating all their food or exercising too much without eating extra food than for parents and children to argue about it. Experiencing low blood glucose under parental supervision provides a safe and effective learning experience.

Parents must remember the primary goal is to encourage children to become independent, develop normally, and feel as similar as possible to their peers. Parents must openly be in agreement, as a couple, on the goals they want to establish for their children.[70] Then they must *consistently* encourage their children to attain these goals or discipline them for misbehavior or misdeeds.

DIABETES REGIMEN ADHERENCE ISSUES

The overall level of metabolic control is related to the following categories of variables: regimen adequacy; knowledge and management skills; psychosocial adjustment or dysfunction of children, family, and peers; stress; and adherence or self-care management of the diabetic regimen.[83] Regimen adequacy, self-care or adherence to the diabetes regimen, and stress are directly related to metabolic control. Psychologic adjustment or dysfunction and knowledge and correct management skills are directly related to each other and to self-care or adherence and thus indirectly to metabolic control.

Regimen Adequacy

Encouraging children with IDDM to maintain good metabolic control may reduce the risks of future development of diabetes-related health problems such as retinopathy.[38,128] School age is a time of rapid physical, cognitive, and social change. Thus children undergo difficult development changes while having to follow a complex diabetes regimen. Studies report that 10- to 15-year old children are at very high risk for poor metabolic control because of rapid growth, less parental supervision, inadequate problem-solving ability, and difficulty in adhering to the diabetic regimen.[16,29,84]

Knowledge and Management Skills

Recent research studies have found the following to be associated with good metabolic control:

1. *General and problem-solving levels of knowledge.* Higher levels are related to better control for older adolescents and for parents of younger children.[84] In contrast, the levels of knowledge attained by children are not related to their knowledge of diabetes management.
2. *Age of the child.* Children between 6 and 11 have better control, whereas midadolescents have the worst.[4,6] These data suggest it is not the information per se that is important, but

the child's and family's ability to understand and use the information to solve daily problems and correctly adjust the diabetes regimen.[7,121]

3. *Number of parents in the home, race, SES, and the following characteristics of families*—high cohesion and organization, clear and consistent expectations and routines, less conflict, warm and supportive involvement with child in diabetes management tasks, and use of effective problem-solving techniques—are associated with good glycemic control.*

4. *Gradually increasing the percentage of primary and shared diabetes-related management tasks* that are completed by the child based on the child's motivation, temperament, cognitive level, fine motor coordination, and family characteristics is associated with better glycemic control and continued adherence to the diabetes regimen. Having children perform these tasks too early, without supervision and without their motivation and continued reeducation, is associated with poorer glycemic control.[42,121,149]

Psychosocial Adjustment, Dysfunction, and Stress

Research findings regarding the effects of children's stress on metabolic control are conflicting. Some studies have found stressful life events of children were associated with poor glycemic control,[18,62] whereas others found the frequency and intensity of daily stressors or of laboratory-induced stress did not differentiate between levels of glycemic control.[32,34,77] Anxiety, depression, and interpersonal conflict among children with IDDM have been found to impact glycemic control.[83] These findings indicate that children who are depressed or whose families are in stress (e.g., family conflict, decreased cohesion and organization, financial problems) are more likely to have worse glycemic control.[65,101,117,122]

Adherence and Self-Care

Treatment adherence refers to how closely children or their parents follow the prescribed diabetes management regimen. In general, SMBG alone is not sufficient to achieve good metabolic control.[11,31,147] Knowledge about diabetes management is higher in youths who are responsible for their own self-care and is related to better control.[4] In contrast, children who report more depression and anxiety display less problem-solving knowledge and worse control. Children with the following five temperament characteristics were found to be in poorer glycemic control: (1) lower levels of activity, (2) less regularity in routines, (3) strong reactions to external stimuli, (4) less distractibility, and (5) positive moods.[116] Those who identify barriers to adherence also exhibit poorer control[84] (e.g., meal plan barriers included social interference, planning and problem-solving difficulties, and appetite problems).

Overall, these and other data suggest that adherence-control relationships must take into account the individual child's cognitive and psychosocial development levels, knowledge and management skills, the adequacy of the treatment regimen, effective family functioning, and

---

*References 6, 65, 101, 119, 121, 130, 140.

the presence of stress factors that together contribute to disruptions in metabolic functioning, since even children who adhere to the diabetes regimen may not have improved metabolic control.

ROLE OF THE DIABETES HEALTH CARE TEAM

The interdisciplinary diabetes health care team needs to consist of a physician, nurse, dietitian, social worker, and/or psychologist. Team members need to reassess frequently parents' and children's levels of knowledge, care, and coping skills; reinforce information given by other members; and confer with each other to devise effective management plans. Team members should be available to both parents and children by phone to answer the many questions that arise on a day-to-day basis. However, the team's goal must be to assist parents and children to become independent in diabetes management, not to continue dependence on team members.

RESEARCH IMPLICATIONS

Research is needed to determine the factors that influence the development of positive and negative emotional and psychosocial behaviors in children who have chronic illnesses such as diabetes.[105] In addition, research is needed to define the interrelationships of these behaviors with children's adherence to illness management and ultimately to a good or poor metabolic control outcome.

The critical periods when children are most receptive to basic and advanced knowledge and implementation of diabetes management skills have not been clearly identified.

Future research needs to determine when children with IDDM are best able to assume responsibility for specific components of diabetes management. Guidelines for self-care management skills need to be identified for specific developmental stages, especially for cognitive levels of children.

CASE PRESENTATION

Tony, 9 years old, was accompanied by his grandmother to the endocrine clinic for his quarterly checkup. The clinic's routine health assessment revealed he was in the seventy-fifth percentile for height and the forty-sixth percentile for weight; he had lost 6 pounds (2.7 kg) in the last 3 months and had not grown over the last 6 months. He had a blood glucose level of 325 mg/dl, moderate to large amounts of ketones, and a fruity odor to his breath. His diabetes record documented he had received all insulin injections over the last 3 months and that his blood glucose levels varied between 115 and 175 mg/dl. The nurse educator questioned the veracity of these values because all ended in 5. Grandmother stated proudly that Tony did all his own diabetes care, including SMBG and giving insulin twice daily. However, she was concerned that Tony had been missing too much school recently because of throwing up and having a bad stomachache in the mornings. When she told Tony's mother she thought he should be seen by a physician, mother said Tony just did not like school and she could not take off work to take him. When asked, Tony emphatically stated he loved school. He said he refused to go to school on the days he threw up in the morning because he knew he would throw up again in class and be embarrassed and teased by his friends. He said he wanted to try out for the basketball team but was afraid he was too skinny to make it.

His past medical history revealed Tony had been admitted to the children's hospital with severe DKA 8 and 6 months previously. Tony, his mother, and a little brother live with his 79-year-old grandmother. Tony's mother is a social worker in one of the nearby counties and works from 9 AM to 6 PM. He is essentially cared for by his 79-year-old grandmother, who has type II diabetes mellitus. The family has a history of running out of diabetes supplies, including insulin, and calling the diabetes nurse educator for free BGM strips, syringes, and insulin. The diabetes team decided to admit Tony to the children's hospital for DKA because of his current medical status and recent history of recurrent DKA.

DISCUSSION

The interdisciplinary diabetes team knows that Tony is at risk for nonadherence to the diabetes regimen because he is a child in a single-parent home, cared for by a grandmother, who has type II diabetes but who does not adhere to her own diabetes regimen, and because Tony has essentially been given sole responsibility for adherence to the diabetes regimen. This, plus having been admitted twice within 2 months for moderate to severe DKA, having missed his previous clinic checkup, and currently having moderate DKA, were indications he needed to be readmitted at this time.

The diabetes nurse clinician, who is a certified diabetes educator (CDE), immediately alerted the team's social worker, diabetologist, and child psychologist to Tony's admission. She asked both Tony and his grandmother to complete a diabetes knowledge and application of knowledge test of 49 items. While they were completing this, she arranged for serum electrolytes and pH to be drawn. Blood for glycohemoglobin had already been drawn and sent to the clinic. She retested his blood glucose (335 mg/dl) and urine ketones (large) and obtained an order for 6 U regular insulin to be given. She asked Tony to draw up the dose and give this insulin under her supervision. Tony drew up the appropriate amount of insulin and was about to inject himself in his right thigh. The nurse educator checked the thigh and found his preferred site was hard. When questioned, Tony admitted he always injected himself in his thighs, preferably his right one because it did not hurt there (because of the lipodystrophy). The CDE requested he give the injection in his abdomen because it would be more quickly absorbed there. After a few moments of hesitation, Tony asked her where to give it, saying he had never given an injection in his abdomen. The CDE showed him the appropriate areas, and Tony successfully injected the insulin in his abdomen. While Tony was completing the knowledge and application test, the CDE took his BGM machine to retrieve the values from its memory. She found the values in the BGM machine's memory did not agree with the values written in his BGM record book. In fact, the values in the memory revealed his blood glucose was actually between 173 and 328 mg/dl over the last 4 weeks and that Tony only completed one BGM each day, usually in the morning.

Evaluation of the knowledge and application tests identified that grandmother was able to answer only 28% of the questions correctly and that Tony was able to answer 60% of the knowledge but 25% of the application questions. Looking back at the hospital records, she found that grandmother had refused to take a form of this test before the previous two discharges and that Tony had attained a 75% on the knowledge questions but only 50% on the application questions the previous hospitalization. However, his mother had attained an 80% on the knowledge and 70% on the application portions both previous hospitalizations. It was also recorded that mother said she provided all the diabetes care for Tony.

The CDE held a phone conference with the mother, who was very angry Tony had been admitted to the hospital and who said she would not take off work to attend any more education sessions. She blamed her mother and Tony for not doing what they were supposed to do. She blamed the CDE for "sticking her nose in where it doesn't belong."

The CDE held a case conference with the interdisciplinary diabetes team members. The team decided that in light of the mother's hostility and refusal to participate in the care of her child with diabetes, the grandmother's inability to take responsibility for his care, and his current and recent past health, the social worker should put in a hot-line call and start an investigation of the child's welfare.

Meanwhile, the CDE, nutritionist, and child psychologist were to work with Tony and his grandmother to determine how much each could learn and how much responsibility each was capable of and willing to take.

The next morning, a very angry mother came to the hospital. She stated she had been the one to do all of Tony's BGMs and give his injections, each twice daily. When confronted with the evidence that the blood glucose values in the memory were fewer and much higher than those recorded in Tony's record book, she admitted Tony did SMBG and gave his own injections. She admitted she told him not to check his blood glucose more than once a day because the strips were so expensive, even though she had received 2 months' supply free from the CDE at the last hospital admission. (NOTE: This family's income was adequate to purchase diabetes supplies needed, although the required increase in blood glucose test strips did strain the budget.) The mother still did not want to attend the education sessions. The CDE restated that the social worker would continue the investigation into Tony's home situation if the mother did not attend the education sessions and cooperate with the diabetes team members.

The mother reluctantly agreed to attend further education sessions with the grandmother and Tony. The CDE covered the following topics:
- Causes, signs, and symptoms and treatment of hyperglycemia and DKA
- Causes, signs, and symptoms and treatment of hypoglycemia
- Demonstration and return demonstration of correct SBGM and drawing up and giving insulin, including an individualized rotation of sites (using the arms in the morning, since Tony could not give injections there; the thighs in the afternoon; and the abdomen whenever the blood glucose was above 275 mg/dl)
- Checking blood glucose before bedtime; eating the prescribed bedtime snack of 1 protein, 1 bread, and 1 milk, decreasing the bedtime snack to just 1 protein and ½ milk if the bedtime blood glucose level was greater than 300 mg/dl, and increasing the bedtime snack to 2 proteins, 1 bread, and one milk if the bedtime blood glucose was less than 120; removing donuts, cookies, cake, ice cream, candy, and potato chips from the house and following the prescribed meal plan agreed on by the grandmother, Tony, and the nutritionist (after the initial 4 weeks of compliance, the nutritionist taught Tony and his grandmother how to include sugar-free yogurt or angel food cake into his diet no more than three times a week); and knowing the effects of exercise on blood glucose levels, including the amount and types of snacks Tony should eat just before basketball or soccer practice after school

The overall goal for Tony at this time was that he maintain blood glucose values between 80 and 180 mg/dl; check his blood glucose before breakfast, before supper, and at bedtime; and take the correct amount of insulin before breakfast and before supper each day. In addition, he was to eat three meals per day, a snack before after school exercise, and a bedtime snack each day. He was not to eat at any other time. He was not to eat any candy, cake, cookies, or donuts. He was to follow the new meal plan closely.

Tony drew four pictures for the CDE. One showed him in a wheelchair, with no legs, very thick glasses, and an IV line in each arm, and another showed him on a stretcher going to the operating room to "have his kidneys and liver taken out." He told the CDE that he knew his diabetes would make him go blind and make them cut his legs off and that he would die of kidney failure, so why shouldn't he eat and do what he wanted to do? Tony did not understand that if he followed the diabetes treatment regimen more closely, the likelihood of these things happening decreased.[38] Once he understood this concept, he was much more receptive to SMBG, taking his insulin, and following his diet so he could play soccer and basketball.

The other two pictures Tony drew were all in black and purple with heavy, thick lines. One showed Tony standing alone in front of a single grave in the dark. The grave had his name on it. The other was drawn during daylight with heavy dark clouds in the sky, with Tony standing alone being rained on while other boys were playing basketball together on the other side of the page. The CDE recognized Tony was very fearful of death, depressed, and feeling very much alone. She referred Tony, his mother, and his grandmother to the child psychologist for family therapy and Tony for additional individual therapy.

The CDE contacted the school nurse at Tony's school, who requested the CDE come and talk with herself, Tony's teachers, and the principal, all of whom wanted to understand more about Tony's diabetes. The CDE met for 1 hour three times with the school personnel. Primary topics included the signs and symptoms of hyperglycemia and DKA and how to treat them and the signs and symptoms of hypoglycemia and how to treat it, including the use of glucagon. Additional materials were left for their review. The school nurse offered to supervise Tony's after-school blood glucose checks and his prebasketball or presoccer snacks.

The CDE also called the community health nurse for Tony's area. She informed her of the hot-line call and the education received by the family so far and agreed to send a copy of the diabetes care plan and education outcomes on Tony's discharge. The community health nurse agreed to visit Tony and his grandmother twice each week for the next 12 weeks just before dinner to supervise BGM and insulin injections. At the end of that period, she would reassess Tony's need for her visits.

On the evening of the fourth day, Tony, his grandmother, and his mother were given another form of the diabetes knowledge and application test. This time Tony and his mother attained a 75% on the knowledge portions and 65% and 70%, respectively, on the application section. Grandmother scored 60% on the knowledge and 50% on the application sections. Tony and grandmother were very proud of their new knowledge. The mother was still sullen but cooperative.

At the weekly interdisciplinary team meeting, all members of the team reported on the progress they thought these family members had made. All agreed to discharge Tony home this one last time if the family would agree to follow a written contract that would be supervised by the CDE, the school health nurse, and the community health nurse.

The diabetes team met with Tony, his mother, and his grandmother for 90 minutes early the morning of the fifth day. The seriousness of Tony's condition was emphasized in simple, concrete terms. The object was to ensure all understood the life-threatening consequences of DKA or hypoglycemia but not to scare Tony about possible future consequences. A written contract was signed by each member of the family and of the diabetes team. This contract clearly stated the responsibilities of each family member. For example, Tony's mother was to check his blood glucose and give his insulin each morning before he went to school. Tony was to check his blood glucose before supper and at bedtime each day. Tony was to give his own insulin injection before supper under grandmother's supervision. Grandmother was to watch him do the SMBG and ensure that he gave his insulin in different sites each evening according to a chart the CDE provided. Tony was to call the CDE with his blood glucose values every Wednesday and Friday after school and to record any necessary insulin dose changes made. Each Monday, the mother and Tony were to bring the BGM machine to the clinic, where the CDE would review the memory and match those values to the ones recorded by Tony in his record book.

The contract also indicated the responsibilities of each diabetes team member. For example, the CDE and the diabetologist agreed to answer all Tony's calls within 30 minutes and to make appropriate insulin changes as indicated by the blood glucose values. All agreed that if this contract was followed for 4 consecutive weeks, the intervals between coming to the clinic and Tony's calls would be lengthened. If this contract was not followed, the social worker would pursue relocating Tony in a foster home because his health was in serious danger.

Tony did concretely follow the guidelines of the contract as specifically written out for him. He was rewarded every week by some type of small surprise from the CDE. Ten months later, the grandmother reported the mother no longer was present in the morning for Tony's blood glucose and insulin injections. The diabetes team's social worker called child protective services, and Tony was placed in a foster home for 2 years. The same diabetes team educated the foster parents during the first month Tony lived with them.

At age 12, Tony and his little brother were adopted by this foster family, since Tony's grandmother had recently died and the mother had released them for adoption. Today, Tony is highly recruited as a guard for several college basketball teams. Had Tony not had the interest, support, and follow-through by the interdisciplinary team members and had they not recognized and admitted him because of his moderate DKA in the clinic, the outcome might have been very different.

REFERENCES

1. Abusrewil S, Savage D: Obesity and diabetic control, *Arch Dis Child* 64:1313-1315, 1989.
2. Ainslie M, Spencer M: New approaches to diabetes in the young, *Compr Ther* 14:65-70, 1988.
3. Anderson B: The impact of diabetes on the developmental tasks of childhood and adolescence: a research perspective. In Nattrass M, Santiago J, editors: *Recent advances in diabetes,* London, 1984, Churchill Livingstone.
4. Anderson B and others: Assessing family sharing of diabetes responsibilities, *J Pediatr Psychol* 15:477-492, 1991.
5. Angel R, Worobey J: Single motherhood and children's health, *J Health Soc Behav* 29:38-52, 1988.
6. Auslander W and others: Risk factors to health in diabetic children: a prospective study from diagnosis, *Health Soc Work* 15:133-142, 1990.
7. Auslander W and others: Predictors of diabetes knowledge in newly diagnosed children and parents, *J Pediatr Psychol* 16:213-228, 1991.
8. Baker D, Campbell R: Vitamin and mineral supplementation in patients with diabetes mellitus, *Diabetes Educ* 18:420-427, 1992.
9. Band E: Children's coping with diabetes: understanding the role of cognitive development, *J Pediatr Psychol* 15:27-41, 1990.
10. Bantle JT: Injection site rotation: the downside, *Pract Diabetol* 9:1-3, 1990.
11. Behrman R, Vaughn V, editors: *Nelson's textbook of pediatrics,* ed 12, Philadelphia, 1983, Saunders.
12. Belmonte M and others: Impact of SMBG on control of diabetes as measured by HGBA1: a three year survey, *Diabetes Care* 11:484-488, 1988.
13. Betschart J: Parents' understanding of and guilt over children's blood glucose control, *Diabetes Educ* 13:393-401, 1987.
14. Betz G, Poster E: Communicating with children: more than just words, *Paedovita* 1:11-16, 1984.
15. Bibace R, Walsh M: Development of children's concepts of illness, *Pediatrics* 66:912-916, 1980.
16. Blethen S and others: Effect of pubertal stage and recent blood glucose control on plasma somatomedin C in children with insulin-dependent diabetes mellitus, *Diabetes* 30:868-872, 1981.
17. Bloch C and others: Puberty decreases insulin sensitivity, *J Pediatr* 110:481-487, 1987.
18. Brand A, Johnson J, Johnson S: Life stress and diabetic control in children and adolescents with insulin-dependent diabetes, *J Pediatr Psychol* 11:481-495, 1986.
19. Brewster A: Chronically ill hospitalized children's concepts of their illness, *Pediatrics* 69:355-362, 1982.
20. Brink S: Pediatric, adolescent, and young-adult nutrition issues in IDDM, *Diabetes Care* 11:192-200, 1988.
21. Brown A: School-age children with diabetes: knowledge and management of the disease, and adequacy of self-concept, *Matern Child Nurs J* 14:47-61, 1985.
22. Canfield W, Hambridge K, Johnson L: Zinc nutriture in type I diabetes mellitus: relationship to growth measures and metabolic control, *J Pediatr Gastroenterol Nutr* 3:577-584, 1984.
23. Casella S and others: Accuracy and precision of low-dose insulin administration, *Pediatrics* 91:1155-1157, 1993.
24. Cerreto M, Travis L: Implications of psychological and family factors in the treatment of diabetes, *Pediatr Clin North Am* 31:689-707, 1984.
25. Cerutti F and others: Course of retinopathy in children and adolescents with insulin-dependent diabetes mellitus: a ten-year study, *Ophthalmologica* 198:116-123, 1989.
26. Clarson C and others: Residual beta-cell function in children with IDDM: reproducibility of testing and factors influencing insulin secretory reserve, *Diabetes Care* 10:33-38, 1987.
27. Court S and others: Children with diabetes mellitus: perception of their behavioral problems by parents and teachers, *Early Hum Dev* 16:245-252, 1988.
28. Cross B and others: Metabolic and endocrine function and alterations. In Servonsky J, Opas S, editors: *Nursing management of children,* Boston, 1987, Jones and Bartlett.
29. Cryer P, Gerich J: Relevance of counter regulatory system to patients with diabetes: critical roles of glucagon and epinephrine, *Diabetes Care* 6:95-99, 1983.
30. Daneman D, Ehrlich R: Management of insulin-dependent diabetes mellitus in childhood, *Med Clin North Am* 15:1852-1859, 1984.
31. Daneman D and others: The role of self-monitoring of blood glucose in the routine management of children with insulin-dependent diabetes mellitus, *Diabetes Care* 8:1-4, 1985.
32. Delamater A and others: Stress and coping in relation to metabolic control of adolescents with type I diabetes, *Dev Behav Pediatr* 8:136-140, 1987.
33. Delamater A and others: Dietary skills and adherence in children with type I diabetes mellitus, *Diabetes Educ* 14:33-36, 1988.
34. Delamater A and others: Physiologic responses to acute psychological stress in adolescents with type I diabetes, *J Pediatr Psychol* 13:69-86, 1988.

35. Delamater A and others: Randomized prospective study of self-management training with newly diagnosed diabetic children, *Diabetes Care* 13:492-498, 1990.

36. Delamater A and others: Diabetes management in the school setting: the role of the school psychologist, *School Psychol Rev* 13:192-203, 1984.

37. Delp R: Kids speak up: a special article for the young set, *Diabetes Forecast* 36:38-40, 1983.

38. Diabetes Control and Complications Trial Research Group: The effect of intensive treatment of diabetes on the development and progression of long-term complications in insulin-dependent diabetes mellitus, *N Engl J Med* 329:977-986, 1993.

39. Dische S and others: Childhood nocturnal enuresis: factors associated with outcome of treatment with an enuresis alarm, *Dev Med Child Neurol* 25:67-80, 1983.

40. Doleys D: Behavioral treatments for nocturnal enuresis in children: a review of the recent literature, *Psychol Bull* 84:30-54, 1977.

41. Drayer N: Height of diabetic children at onset of symptoms, *Arch Dis Child* 49:616-620, 1974.

42. Drotar D, Levers C: Age differences in parent and child responsibilities for management of cystic fibrosis and insulin-dependent diabetes mellitus, *Dev Behav Pediatr* 15:265-272, 1994.

43. Eisner C: *The psychology of childhood illness,* New York, 1985, Springer-Verlag.

44. Elkind D: *Children and adolescents: interpretive essays on Jean Piaget,* ed 3, New York, 1981, Oxford University Press.

45. Epstein I and others: Measurement and modification of the accuracy of determinations of urine glucose concentration, *Diabetes Care* 3:535-536, 1980.

46. Esslinger P: The preschooler. In Smith M, Goodman J, Ramsey N, editors: *Child and family: concepts of nursing practice,* New York, 1987, McGraw-Hill.

47. Faro B: Maintaining good control in children with diabetes, *Pediatr Nurs* 9:368-373, 1983.

48. Feldman K: Prevention of childhood accidents: recent progress, *Pediatr Rev* 2:75-82, 1980.

49. Follansbee D: Assuming responsibility for diabetes management: What age? What price? *Diabetes Educ* 15:347-352, 1989.

50. Fonagy P and others: Psychological adjustment and diabetic control, *Arch Dis Child* 62:1009-1013, 1987.

51. Franz M: Use of nonnutritive and nutritive sweeteners, *Diabetes Educ* 14:357-359, 1988.

52. Franz M, Norstrom J: Diabetes—actively staying healthy: your game plan for diabetes and exercise, Wayzata, Minn, 1990, DCI.

53. Garrison M, McQueston A: *Chronic illness during childhood and adolescence,* Newbury Park, Calif, 1989, Sage.

54. Gearheart BR: *Learning disabilities: educational strategies,* ed 4, St Louis, 1989, Mosby.

55. Giordano B, Neuenkirchen G, Banion C: Diabetes management responsibilities: assessment for readiness, Paper presented at American Association of Diabetes Educators Meeting, Cincinnati, 1990.

56. Gray D and others: Chronic poor metabolic control in the pediatric population: a stepwise intervention program, *Diabetes Educ* 14:516-520, 1988.

57. Grey M and others: Initial adaptation in children with newly diagnosed diabetes and healthy children, *Pediatr Nurs* 20:17-22, 1994.

58. Gross A and others: Video teacher: peer instruction, *Diabetes Educ* 10:30, 40, 1985.

59. Guyer B, Gallagher S: An approach to the epidemiology of childhood injuries, *Pediatr Clin North Am* 32:5-15, 1985.

60. Hamburg B, Inoff G: Coping with predictable crises of diabetes, *Diabetes Care* 6:409-415, 1983.

61. Hanson C: Social competence and parental support as mediators of the link between stress and metabolic control in adolescents with insulin-dependent diabetes mellitus, *Consult Clin Psychol* 58:529-533, 1987.

62. Hanson S, Pichert J: Perceived stress and diabetes control in adolescents, *Health Psychol* 5:439-452, 1986.

63. Hauenstein E and others: Stress in parents of children with diabetes mellitus, *Diabetes Care* 12:18-23, 1989.

64. Hausdorf G, Rieger U, Koepp P: Cardiomyopathy in childhood diabetes mellitus: incidence, time of onset, and relation to metabolic control, *Intern J Cardiol* 19:225-236, 1988.

65. Hauser S and others: Adherence among children and adolescents with insulin-dependent diabetes mellitus over a four-year longitudinal follow-up. II. Immediate and long-term linkages with the family milieu. In Special issue: adherence with pediatric regimens, *J Pediatr Psychol* 15:527-542, 1990.

66. Hodges L, Parker J: Concerns of parents with diabetic children, *Pediatr Nurs* 13:22-24, 1987.

67. Holler H: Meal planning approaches: practical application, *Diabetes Educ* 18:388-391, 1992.

68. Hymovich D, Chamberlin R: *Child and family development,* New York, 1980, McGraw-Hill.

69. Ingersoll G and others: Cognitive maturity and self-management among adolescents with insulin-dependent diabetes mellitus, *J Pediatr* 108:620-623, 1986.

70. Jacobson A and others: Psychologic predictors of compliance in children with recent onset of diabetes mellitus, *J Pediatr* 110:805-811, 1987.

71. Johnson BH: Children's drawings as a projective technique, *Pediatr Nurs* 16:11-17, 1990.

72. Johnson S, Rosenbloom A: Behavioral aspects of diabetes mellitus in childhood and adolescence, *Psychiatr Clin North Am* 5:357-369, 1982.

73. Johnson S and others: Cognitive and behavioral knowledge about insulin-dependent diabetes among children and parents, *Pediatrics* 69:708-713, 1982.

74. Kager V, Holden E: Preliminary investigation of the direct and moderating effects of family and individual variables on the adjustment of children and adolescents with diabetes, *J Pediatr Psychol* 17:491-502, 1992.

75. Kohlberg L: The child as a moral philosopher, *Psychol Today* 2:25-30, 1968.

76. Kovacs M and others: Psychological functioning among mothers of children with insulin-dependent diabetes mellitus: a longitudinal study, *J Consult Clin Psychol* 58:189-192, 1990.

77. Kovacs M and others: Prevalence and predictors of pervasive noncompliance with medical treatment among youths with insulin-dependent diabetes mellitus, *J Am Acad Child Adolesc Psychiatry* 31:1112-1119, 1992.

78. Krauser K, Madden P: The child with diabetes mellitus, *Nurs Clin North Am* 18:749-762, 1983.

79. Krolewski A and others: Risk of proliferative diabetic retinopathy in juvenile-onset type 1 diabetes: a 40-year follow-up study, *Diabetes Care* 9:443-452, 1986.

80. Kupper N, Foster M, MacMillan D: Treating children with type 1 mellitus: choosing an appropriate nutritional treatment strategy, *Diabetes Educ* 14:238-242, 1988.

81. Kurtz S: Adherence to diabetes regimens: empirical status and clinical applications, *Diabetes Educ* 16:50-56, 1990.

82. La Greca A: Children with diabetes and their families: coping and disease management. In Field T, McCabe P, Schneiderman N, editors: *Stress and coping across development,* Newark, NJ, 1988, Erlbaum.

83. La Greca A, Skyler J: Psychosocial issues in IDDM: a multivariate framework. In McCabe P and others, editors: *Stress, coping and disease,* Hillsdale, NJ, 1991, Erlbaum.

84. La Greca A, Follansbee D, Skyler J: Developmental and behavioral aspects of diabetes management in youngsters, *Children's Health Care* 19:132-139, 1990.

85. LaPorte R, Cruickshanks K: Incidence and risk factors for insulin-dependent diabetes. In *Diabetes in America,* National Diabetes Data Group, NIH Pub No 85-1468, US Department of Health and Human Services, Washington, DC, 1985, US Government Printing Office.

86. Lask B: Psychosocial factors in childhood diabetes and seizure disorders: the family approach, *Pediatrician* 15:95-101, 1988.

87. Lavigne J and others: Parental perceptions of the psychological adjustment of children with diabetes and their siblings, *Diabetes Care* 5:420-426, 1982.

88. Leach D, Erickson G: Children's perspectives on diabetes, *J School Health* 58:159-161, 1977.

89. Lee R, Bode H: Stunted growth and hepatomegaly in diabetes mellitus, *J Pediatr* 91:82-84, 1977.

90. Lerner J: *Learning disabilities: theories, diagnosis, and teaching strategies,* Boston, 1981, Houghton Mifflin.

91. Levine M: Middle childhood. In Levine M and others, editors: *Developmental-behavioral pediatrics,* Philadelphia, 1983, Saunders.

92. Levitsky L: Growth and pubertal pattern in insulin dependent diabetes mellitus, *Semin Adolesc Med* 3:233-239, 1987.

93. Lewis C, Lewis M: Peer pressure and risk-taking behaviors in children, *Am J Public Health* 74:580-584, 1984.

94. Lindsay R, Jarrett L, Hillman K: Elementary schoolteachers' understanding of diabetes, *Diabetes Care* 13:312-314, 1987.

95. Lipman T and others: A developmental approach to diabetes in children: schoolage-adolescence, *Matern Child Nurs J* 14:330-332, 1989.

96. Lockwood D and others: The biggest problem in diabetes, *Diabetes Educ* 12:30-33, 1986.

97. Lorenz R, Christensen N, Pichert J: Diet-related knowledge, skill, and adherence among children with insulin-dependent diabetes mellitus, *Pediatrics* 75:872-876, 1985.

98. Mann N, Johnson D: Improvement in metabolic control in diabetic adolescents by the use of increased insulin dose, *Diabetes Care* 7:460-464, 1984.

99. Marteau T, Bloch S, Baum J: Family life and diabetic control, *Child Psychol Psychiatry* 28:823-833, 1987.

100. Martens R, Seefeldt V: *Guidelines for children's sports,* 1979, The American Alliance for Health, Physical Education, Recreation, and Dance.

101. McKelvey J, Schreiner B, Murphy J: Reliability and validity of the Diabetes Family Behavior Scale, *Diabetes Educ* 19:125-132, 1993.

102. Menon R, Spearling M: Childhood diabetes, *Med Clin North Am* 72:1565-1576, 1988.

103. Minuchin S and others: A conceptual model of psychosomatic illness in children, *Arch Gen Psychiatry* 32:1031-1039, 1975.

104. Moy CS, LaPorte RE: Why do so many children in U.S. develop diabetes? *Pract Diabetol* 8:1-8, 1989.

105. Nelms B: Emotional behaviors in chronically ill children, *J Abnorm Child Psychol* 17:657-668, 1989.

106. Neumann C: Obesity in pediatric practice: obesity in the preschool and school-age child, *Pediatr Clin North Am* 21:117-122, 1977.

107. Nuvoli G and others: Diabetes and illness image: an analysis of diabetic early-adolescents' self-perception through the draw-a-person test, *Psychol Rep* 65:83-93, 1989.

108. Pedersen O, Beck-Nielsen H: Insulin resistance and insulin-dependent diabetes mellitus, *Diabetes Care* 10:516-523, 1987.

109. Peterson H and others: Growth, body weight and insulin requirement in diabetic children, *Acta Pediatr Scand* 67:453-457, 1978.

110. Piaget J: *The construction of reality in the child,* New York, 1971, Ballantine.

111. Piaget J, Inhelder B: *Memory and intelligence,* New York, 1973, Basic.

112. Pond H: Parental attitudes towards children with a chronic medical disorder: special reference to diabetes mellitus, *Diabetes Care* 2:425-431, 1979.

113. Pontious S: Practical Piaget: helping children understand, *Am J Nurs* 82:112-114, 1982.

114. Pontious S: Communication with children. In Servonsky J, Opas S, editors: *Nursing management of children,* Boston, 1987, Jones and Bartlett.

115. Rivara F, Barber M: Demographic analysis of childhood pedestrian injuries, *Pediatrics* 76:375-381, 1985.

116. Rovet J, Ehrlich R: Effect of temperament on metabolic control in children with diabetes mellitus, *Diabetes Care* 11:77-82, 1988.

117. Rubin R, Peyrot M: Psychosocial problems and interventions in diabetes, *Diabetes Care* 15:1640-1657, 1992.

118. Ruggiero L, Mindell J, Kairys S: A new measure for assessing diabetes self-management responsibility in pediatric populations: the Diabetes Regimen Responsibility Scale, *Behav Ther* 14:233-234, 1991.

119. Saddler A, Hillman S, Benjamins D: The influence of disabling visibility on family functioning, *J Pediatr Psychol* 18:425-439, 1993.

120. Safyer A and others: The impact of the family on diabetes adjustment: a developmental perspective, *Child Adolesc Soc Work J* 10:123-140, 1993.

121. Santiago J, White N, Pontious S: Diabetes in childhood and adolescence. In Alberti K and others: *International textbook of diabetes mellitus,* London, 1992, Wiley.

122. Savinetti-Rose B: Developmental issues in managing children with diabetes, *Pediatr Nurs* 20:11-15, 1994.

123. Schafer L and others: Adherence to IDDM regimens: relationship to psychosocial variables and metabolic control, *Diabetes Care* 6:493-498, 1983.

124. Schreiner B, Travis L: When your child has diabetes: the preteen years, *Diabetes Forecast* 40:37-41, 1987.

125. Schriock E, Winter R, Traisman H: Diabetes mellitus and its effects on menarche, *J Adolesc Health Care* 5:101-104, 1984.

126. Shalwitz R and others: Prevalence and consequences of nocturnal hypoglycemia among conventionally treated children with diabetes mellitus, *J Pediatr* 116:685-689, May 1990.

127. Sieman M: Mental health in school-age children, *Am J Matern Child Nurs* 3:215, 1978.

128. Skyler JS: Why control diabetes? Influence on chronic complications of diabetes, *Pediatr Annu* 16:713-724, 1987.

129. Smith K and others: Issues of managing diabetes in children and adolescents: a multifamily group approach, *Child Health Care* 18:49-52, 1989.

130. Standen P and others: Family involvement and metabolic control of childhood diabetes, *Diabetic Med* 2:137-140, 1985.

131. Steranchak I: When the lunch bell rings, *Diabetes Forecast* 39:32-37, 1986.

132. Steranchak I: How big, how tall, *Diabetes Forecast* 45:50-53, 1992.

133. Stewart-Brown S, Lee T, Savage D: Pubertal growth of diabetes, *Arch Dis Child* 60:768-769, 1985.

134. Tatman M, Lessing D: Can we improve diabetes care in schools? *Arch Dis Child* 4:450-451, 1993.

135. Tattersal R, Pyke D: Growth in diabetic children, studies in identical twins, *Lancet* 2:1105-1109, 1973.

136. Templeton C and others: A group approach to nutritional problem solving using self-monitoring of blood glucose with diabetic adolescents, *Diabetes Educ* 14:189-191, 1988.

137. Tuttle WW and others: Effect on school boys of omitting breakfast, *J Am Diet Assoc* 30:674-678, 1974.

138. Vessey J, Braithwaite K, Wiedmann M: Teaching children about their internal bodies, *Pediatr Nurs* 16:29-33, 1990.

139. Wertlieb D, Hauser S, Jacobson A: Adaptation of diabetes: behavior symptoms and family context, *J Pediatr Psychol* 11:463-479, 1986.

140. Wertlieb D and others: Adaptation to diabetes: behavior symptoms and family context, *J Pediatr Psychol* 11:463-479, 1986.

141. Whaley L, Wong D: *Nursing care of infants and children,* ed 4, St Louis, 1991, Mosby.

142. White N and others: Identification of type I diabetic patients at increased risk for hypoglycemia during intensive therapy, *N Engl J Med* 308:485-491, 1983.

143. Wilcox M: *Developmental journey—a guide to the development of logical and moral reasoning and social perspective,* Nashville, 1980, Abingdon.

144. Wilde J: The school-age child. In Smith M, Goodman J, Ramsey N: *Child and family: concepts of nursing practice,* New York, 1987, McGraw-Hill.

145. Wing R and others: Behavioral skills in self-monitoring of blood glucose: relationship to accuracy, *Diabetes Care* 9:330-333, 1986.

146. Winter R: Special problems of the child with diabetes, *Comp Ther* 8:7-13, 1982.

147. Wysoki T, Green L, Huxtable K: Blood glucose monitoring by diabetic adolescents: compliance and metabolic control, *Health Psychol* 8:267-284, 1989.

148. Wysocki T and others: Survey of diabetes professionals regarding developmental changes in diabetes self-care, *Diabetes Care* 13:65-68, 1990.

149. Wysocki T and others: Parental and professional estimates of self-care independence of children and adolescents with IDDM, *Diabetes Care* 15:43-52, 1992.

150. Yki-Jarvinen H, Kovisto V: Natural course of insulin resistance in Type I diabetes, *N Engl J Med* 315:224-227, 1986.

151. Yoos H: Children's illness concepts: old and new paradigms, *Pediatric Nursing* 20:134-140, 145, 1994.

19 The Adolescent With Diabetes Mellitus

Denis Daneman and Marcia Frank

Anna Freud[43] characterized the period between childhood and young adulthood as follows[42]:

> Adolescence is by its nature an interruption of peaceful growth, and . . . the upholding of a steady equilibrium during the adolescent period is in itself abnormal . . . Adolescence resembles in appearance a variety of other emotional upsets and structural upheavals. The adolescent manifestations come close to symptom formation of the neurotic, psychotic, or dissocial order and merge almost imperceptibly into . . . almost all the mental illnesses.

This view of adolescence, however, which has been supported by many of the earlier commentators, has been based more on "confident assertion than by the presence of well-based knowledge."[108] Even today debate rages as to whether the view of adolescence as a time of turmoil and significant emotional upheaval is fact or fiction. More recent studies

---

CHAPTER OBJECTIVES

- Develop an understanding of teens with diabetes as normal adolescents in an abnormal situation.
- Describe the normal biology and psychology of adolescence.
- Discuss the impact of diabetes on the normal processes of adolescence.
- Summarize the goals of diabetes management in this age-group.
- Explore those factors contributing to poor health outcomes (poor metabolic control).
- Describe the epidemiology of diabetes-related complications in teenagers.
- Explain the effects of exercise, alcohol, drugs, and smoking on diabetes.
- Evaluate the impact of diabetes on career planning.
- Offer strategies to improve metabolic control and general well-being.

have concluded that although adolescent turmoil may be a fairly frequent finding, its psychiatric importance has been greatly overestimated.[64,108]

Similarly, early research on the relationship between both the cause and the course of diabetes on the one hand and psychosocial factors on the other was most influenced by psychoanalytic theory and sought to find a "diabetic personality" that predisposed the individual to this disease. Research and clinical experience have failed to support this concept; nevertheless, interest in the interaction between diabetes and behavioral, social, and emotional factors has flourished.[63,64,78] Thus, although early research on psychosocial aspects of diabetes in adolescence focused primarily on personality issues, current models are much more complex and presume psychosocial adjustment and health status to be the result of multiple patient and environmental variables.

Adolescence is clearly a time of rapid biologic change accompanied by increasing physical, cognitive, and emotional maturity. It is a time of increasing independence from family and the start of peer conformity, experimentation, and limit testing. The presence of a chronic disease such as insulin-dependent diabetes mellitus (IDDM) may have an impact on both biologic and psychologic aspects of adolescent development.

In this chapter we focus on normal adolescent development, both physical and emotional, and the impact of IDDM on this development. We highlight how these interactions may have an impact on both the short-term and long-term outcomes of diabetes. Since the adolescent with diabetes is often characterized as being in poor metabolic control, we also explore the reasons for such metabolic deterioration. We outline a treatment approach to adolescents with IDDM, stress the importance of anticipatory guidance with respect to the long-term microvascular and macrovascular complications, and suggest directions for future research in this population.

PHYSICAL DEVELOPMENT
Growth and Development

The onset of adolescence is heralded biochemically by activation of the "gonadostat," the hypothalamic-pituitary-gonadal axis, through mechanisms that remain largely unknown.[116] This change from tonic suppression of gonadotropin secretion to its pulsatile release begins a period of the most rapid hormonal and physical changes since early infancy. The pulsatile nature of secretion of a number of hormones, including gonadotropins, sex steroids, and growth hormone (GH), are important in both the initiation and the maintenance of sexual maturation. The period ends with the achievement of full sexual and physical development. Very good correlations during adolescence exist between sex hormone concentrations found in the plasma (either in the basal state or in response to dynamic testing) and the stage of physical development achieved.

The onset of puberty in the female (noted by the onset of breast development between 9 and 13 years of age) occurs slightly earlier than that in the male (testicular enlargement starting between 10 and 14 years).[123] Furthermore, pubertal progression in the female is much more rapid, with achievement of peak height velocity soon after the onset of puberty (Tanner stages 2 to 4) and virtual completion of maturation with the onset of menstruation (menarche occurs on average 2 years after the onset of puberty, i.e., 11 to 15 years). In males, peak height velocity is reached later in puberty (Tanner stages 3 to 5). The later onset of puberty and the later achievement of peak height velocity in the male account for the final adult height differential between the genders, with adult men being on average 5 inches (12.5 cm) taller than women. Females appear more sensitive to small changes in gonadotropin-releasing hormone (GnRH) concentrations than males. This explains why puberty begins slightly earlier in girls. The reason for the difference in timing of peak height velocity is uncertain but may relate to differences in sex steroid–growth hormone relationships between the sexes. In females, low levels of estradiol may stimulate GH secretion, whereas high levels block insulin-like growth factor 1 (IGF-1) production. In males, relatively higher levels of testosterone are required to accentuate the effects of GH.[116]

Impact of Diabetes on Physical Development

The relationship between diabetes and adolescence may be viewed from the following three different directions:

1. Do factors during adolescence trigger the onset of the disease and its complications?
2. What is the impact of diabetes on normal adolescent development?
3. What are the effects of the hormonal changes of adolescence on metabolic control?

IDDM affects both genders equally; it can occur at any age but it has its peak incidence in late childhood/early adolescence, with this peak being somewhat earlier in females than males.[36] It remains largely speculative as to the reasons why the peak incidence of IDDM occurs at this age. Whether the changing hormonal milieu is responsible in any way remains unknown. In those with declining B cell mass, a rapid increase in counterregulatory hormones and the metabolic needs for growth may tip the balance, leading to exhaustion of the remaining functional B cells and presentation of the disease. By the end of adolescence the prevalence of IDDM will be 1 in 500 to 600, making it one of the most common chronic disorders of childhood.[36]

The severity of the presenting metabolic derangement tends to be greater in younger children, particularly infants and toddlers, and less so in adolescents. Clinical remission (the "honeymoon period") occurs shortly after diagnosis and is associated with metabolic stability, declining insulin dose requirement, and usually partial recovery of B cell function.[113] This remission period tends to last longer and be of greater magnitude clinically in the adolescent than in the younger child.

The impact of IDDM on adolescent physical and sexual development has been studied ever since the availability of insulin therapy in the 1920s.[8,60,81] At onset of diabetes, children have been reported to be of average to slightly above average height, suggesting that the "preclinical phase of IDDM" (marked by the presence of immunologic abnormalities and also by abnormalities in insulin secretion, but with normal glucose homeostasis) does not impact physical development. After initiation of insulin therapy, normal growth and sexual development depend more on the presence of adequate insulinization than on the achievement of near-normal glycemia.[19]

Early reports suggested that children with IDDM grew more poorly than their nondiabetic peers, entered puberty at a later stage, and achieved a significantly decreased final adult height.[8,60,83] The most striking illustration of the impact of underinsulinization on adolescent growth and development was described in 1934 by Mauriac[86] and others.[88] The Mauriac syndrome, fortunately now quite rare, comprises hepatomegaly, growth failure, and pubertal delay, all resulting from prolonged and profound underinsulinization. Several authors in the 1950s and 1960s reported a significant decrease in height caused by a reduced growth velocity in children studied from 6 months to 3 years after diagnosis.[8,60,81] Some also found a decrease in final adult height in those with IDDM, particularly boys.[8,74] More recent studies have reported that children with diabetes display normal growth patterns and normal onset and progression of pubertal development.[19,61]

We evaluated growth and pubertal development and their relationship to metabolic control in a representative subgroup of 122 children in our diabetes clinic.[19] These children were found to have growth characteristics similar to those of children without diabetes, not only in terms of distribution of height and weight percentiles, but also in terms of height and weight velocity percentiles. Specifically, we were unable to find any relationship between metabolic control, as reflected by glycated hemoglobin (GHb) levels, and growth parameters. We concluded that conventional management of IDDM children should be associated with normal growth and puberty and that normal development did not necessarily indicate optimal, but rather only "average," control.

Among factors that influence growth in children, some, such as genetic background and nutrition, are major determinants of growth velocity, onset of puberty, and final adult height achieved. The contribution of diabetic control to growth may be very small and only apparent at the very extreme of poor metabolic control. Thus the presence of normal growth and physical development in IDDM children should not lull health care providers into a false sense of security that this reflects good metabolic control. Conversely, although extremely poor metabolic control may contribute to poor growth and delayed adolescence, the latter finding in an adolescent with IDDM warrants thorough investigation.

Early data also suggested a delay in the onset of menstruation in IDDM girls compared with their nondiabetic counterparts.[61,117,124] In 1948 Beal[8] reported that diabetic girls continued to increase in height until age 17½ years, indicating a delay in either the onset or progression of puberty. Sterky[117] found menarche to occur 4 months later than normal in 27 girls with IDDM onset before 12 years of age, and Jackson and others[61] reported that delayed menarche occurred in girls with poor metabolic control. The most striking evidence for delayed menarche occurring in association with diabetes was found in the report by Tattersall and Pyke[124]: menarche occurred 4 and 5 years later in the diabetic than in the nondiabetic identical twins. Unlike the earlier reports, more recent research has revealed a normal distribution of the onset of menarche.[19]

Taken together, the earlier data revealed poorer growth in adolescents with IDDM, whereas more recent evidence has suggested that in adolescents with adequately treated IDDM, growth is normal. This change is likely a result of more comprehensive treatment strategies, which include appropriate insulinization and provision of calories.[24] This allows for normal growth and development within a wide spectrum of metabolic control. An extension of this is the finding of excessive weight gain in those IDDM individuals treated more intensively with either continuous subcutaneous insulin infusion systems or with multiple daily injections (three or more) of insulin and in whom normoglycemia has been targeted.[30-34] In the first 5 years of the Diabetes Control and Complications Trial (DCCT), intensively treated adolescent males gained 4.04 kg and adolescent females 3.25 kg more than their conventionally treated peers.[34]

Finally, what is the impact of the changing hormonal milieu during adolescence on the ability to achieve and maintain adequate metabolic control in these children? There is convincing evidence that metabolic control, as noted by increasing GHb levels, deteriorates during adolescence despite significantly higher insulin doses.[11,25] Research has demonstrated that GHb levels increase with age, with the highest levels found in the age-group 12 to 16 years[25] (Fig. 19-1).

This deterioration in GHb levels was more marked in females than males with IDDM. Furthermore, this increase with age was independent of disease duration. Blethen and others[11] reported a similar finding in relation to pubertal staging. This deterioration in control is even more striking when the relative increased insulin dose requirements during adolescence are noted.[11,36] In Blethen's study, for example, GHb levels increased in pubertal boys from 11.6% to 14.1% despite an increase in insulin dose (expressed as U/kg/day) of 36% to 44%.

The report of the DCCT highlights differences between adolescents and adults with IDDM both at onset and throughout the entire duration of the study. First, at randomization into the trial, GHb levels and insulin dosages were significantly higher in the adolescents than in adults.[30,33] For example, in those randomized to conventional insulin treatment, adult volunteers had a mean GHb and insulin dose of 9.0% and 0.65 U/kg, respectively; in the

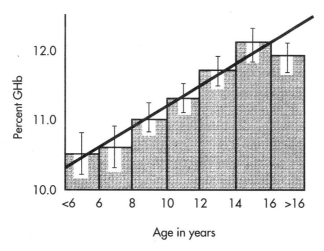

Fig. 19-1   Relationship of age of the patient to glycosylated hemoglobin (*GHb*) (*r* = 0.24, *p* < 0.001). (Modified from Daneman D and others: *J Pediatr* 99:847-853, 1981.)

adolescents these were both significantly higher, 9.8% and 0.94 U/kg. In those randomized to the intensive treatment group, adult GHb of 9.2% and insulin dose of 0.62 U/kg were similarly less than those of the adolescent, 10.1% and 0.95 U/kg, respectively. Second, throughout the study, GHb levels in adolescents remained about 1% higher whether they were assigned to the standard or experimental group. Nevertheless, the reduction in mean GHb and blood glucose levels in the intensively treated adolescents was of the same order of magnitude as that seen in the intensively treated adults when compared with their respective conventionally treated groups.

These data suggest that substantial impediments exist to the achievement of good metabolic control in adolescents with IDDM. The deterioration in metabolic control during adolescence has long been attributed to problems with compliance in these young-sters.[18,58,63,66] However, recent data have emerged that suggest that biologic factors may also be operative, namely, declining peripheral insulin action and changing counterregulatory hormonal responses.[4,12,99,122]

Although IDDM is a disease of B cell destruction, what is also becoming increasingly clear is that peripheral insulin action ("sensitivity") is impaired in all hyperglycemic states and more particularly at certain times, specifically during adolescence and times of poorer metabolic control.[4,12,17] Using the euglycemic, hyperinsulinemic clamp technique, several groups have been able to demonstrate convincingly that peripheral insulin sensitivity is decreased during adolescence in nondiabetic persons when compared with that in younger children and adults.[4] At each stage (Fig. 19-2) of development, insulin action is more impaired in those individuals with IDDM, such that the most impaired insulin action is seen in

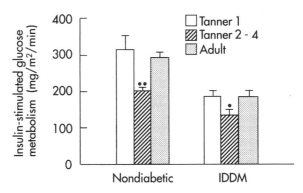

Fig. 19-2 Effect of puberty on insulin-stimulated glucose metabolism in nondiabetic and diabetic subjects. Values (means ± standard error) in prepubertal children (Tanner stage 1) are shown by open bars, those in pubertal (Tanner stages 2 to 4) by hatched bars, and those in adults by the shaded bars. The double asterisk denotes $p < 0.01$ for nondiabetic children in Tanner stages 2 to 4 versus nondiabetic children in Tanner stage 1 and adults; the single asterisk denotes $p < 0.05$ for children with IDDM in Tanner stages 2 to 4 versus children with IDDM in Tanner stage 1. Insulin-stimulated glucose metabolism was also significantly lower in patients with IDDM than in nondiabetic persons at each stage of development ($p < 0.01$). (From Amiel D and others: *N Engl J Med* 315:215-219, 1986.)

adolescents with IDDM.[2] The data also suggest that this "resistance" may be most marked in the female adolescent. The reasons for declining insulin action remain speculative but are likely related to at least some of the attendant hormonal changes. Since sex hormones in adolescents are lower than those in adults, it seems unlikely that these would be the prime suspects. More probably, changes in growth factors, specifically changes in the GH–IGF-1 axis, are involved.[4,12,99] In fact, in the study of Bloch and others,[12] a correlation was noted between insulin resistance and IGF-1 concentrations.

Furthermore, it appears that counterregulatory hormone responses, particularly those of epinephrine, may be more brisk in children with diabetes than in those without, and also more so than in diabetic or nondiabetic adults. In at least one study, epinephrine responses were shown to occur at higher blood glucose concentrations and to reach a greater magnitude in children with diabetes than in adults.[122] These rapid changes in epinephrine may contribute, at least in part, to the metabolic instability that characterizes some adolescents with IDDM.

PSYCHOLOGIC DEVELOPMENT
Normal Development

In attempting to understand the psychosocial impact of diabetes on adolescents and their families, it may be helpful for the health care provider to view these young people as normal teens in an abnormal situation. Such an approach casts adolescents with diabetes in a normalizing framework and permits the use of developmental theories to conceptualize and predict the difficulties that they and their families may encounter.[17,97] This section begins with a review of normal psychosocial and cognitive growth during adolescence and then focuses on the interrelationship between normal development and diabetes.

Adolescence is a term quite distinct from both childhood and adulthood in terms of emotional focus and psychologic needs. Furthermore, within adolescence, three distinct stages of development are recognized: early, middle, and late adolescence.[28,95] Briefly, early adolescence is characterized by rapid physical growth and maturation. These changes are accompanied by intense self-examination; body image is of paramount importance. Young teens need to know that they are normal; reassurance is sought by comparison with peers.[95] Emotional normalcy is tested by acceptance into the peer group. To be excluded is the worst possible scenario.[28] As teens move into midadolescence, the struggle for autonomy and control of personal destiny become more prominent. This period is often associated with varying degrees of parental conflict as the peer group replaces parental influence and sets behavior standards.[17,28,95] With late adolescence comes increasing stability. Successful conclusion of adolescent development is accompanied by the establishment of clear vocational goals and a global sense of personal identity.[38]

In a comprehensive review of normal adolescence, Orr and Ingersoll[95] emphasize the wide variability in adolescent development. They stress that differences occur not only across age-groups but also within age-groups and within individuals. Taken as a whole, however, the teen's central developmental task is to establish a new sense of personal identity that involves adjusting to a new physical self, a new cognitive self, and a new social self. For many persons, this level of maturation is not reached until their mid-20s.

Cognitive development

Included in the many transitions that occur during adolescence are a number of important changes in cognitive abilities. Cognitive development is more than an accumulation of new knowledge; it also involves a new way of thinking and speculating about oneself and the environment.[51,95] Inhelder and Piaget[59] have provided the most useful model for the understanding of development. During preadolescence, children operate on a cognitive level that has been termed *concrete operational thought.* During this early stage, young people require concrete references to solve problems. Clearly, this way of thinking is limiting, and one's ability to adapt to the environment depends on moving beyond this stage. As teens progress through adolescence, it is expected that they will become more capable of abstract thinking and shift into what has been termed *formal operational thought.* Along with increasing cognitive maturity comes more latitude in the adolescent's ability to consider hypothetic situations and to speculate about various possibilities for future consequences based on current actions. Furthermore, as young people progress toward social cognitive maturity, egocentrism diminishes, permitting the adolescent to understand the perspectives of others, to better tolerate ambiguity and differences, and to recognize the interdependence of oneself with others. Orr and Ingersoll[95] point out that all of these attributes can be related to positive health care.

Included in the adolescents' cognitive structure and of particular relevance to the health practitioner are the teen's concepts of health and illness. Theoretically, these views will have an impact on his or her willingness and ability to deal with health-related behaviors. In general, researchers have found that such concepts develop parallel with other aspects of cognitive maturation.[10,88,93] In their study of normal adolescents, Millstein and associates[88] found a shift from magical and mystical thinking in identifying causes of illness in younger children to a more conceptually sophisticated understanding of the disease process in older adolescents. However, they also reported a persistence of concrete explanations for illness in some older adolescents. This variation, which is also described by others who study cognitive development, underlines that qualitative shifts in concepts are age related rather than age dependent.[17,51,97] Consequently, health professionals are wise to avoid assumptions regarding a teen's level of maturity simply on the basis of age and physical maturity.

Social development

Critical to adolescent psychosocial development is the emergence of a new sense of self.[38] Adolescents who successfully complete this task will enter the adult years with a feeling of competence. Preparation for adulthood, however, is a gradual and somewhat painful process. In the context of self-exploration and uncertainty, teens must make some sense out of the world, set realistic goals and limits, learn that rules are not the same for everyone everywhere, and learn to balance their own individual rights with the rights of others. It is not surprising, therefore, that many young people experience a considerable degree of inner turmoil at this time. Epidemiologic studies of normal adolescents summarized by Rutter and co-workers[108] indicate that 14- and 15-year-old children typically experience feelings of misery and self-deprecation. Many reported ideas of reference, that is, feeling that people were looking at them or talking and laughing about them. Only a small percentage had suicidal ideation. The results of these same studies also suggested that adults do not seem to appreciate how miserable these teens may feel.[108]

As teens progress through normal adolescence, their questions about who they are become multifaceted and their self-concept more complex. Self-concept is an accumulation of personal perceptions of one's own physical, social, educational, intellectual, and psychologic characteristics. In their review, Orr and Ingersoll[95] found evidence to support the smooth continuous development of self-concept over the teen years. They also suggest that significant social and psychologic crises, such as a move or a change in schools, may temporarily or permanently alter one's self-concept. The occurrence of major life events and the teen's ability to manage them contributes to adolescents' feelings of self-worth.

Within the context of the social milieu, other important transitions are occurring for the adolescent. Relationships with family members, especially parents, are changing; the peer group is increasingly influential. Teens beg and bargain for more freedom and responsibility; rules and limitations are frequently challenged. Conflict develops when the new values of the adolescent clash with the existing family values. How common and how serious are these conflicts? The epidemiologic studies summarized by Rutter and associates[108] showed parent/adolescent conflict to be very common. Conflict issues, however, were generally trivial, that is, related to clothes, hair, and going out. Major parent/adolescent alienation appeared to be unusual; physical and emotional withdrawal occurred infrequently; most teens were not especially critical of their parents, and very few rejected them. This and other studies indicate that parents continue to have substantial influence on their children through adolescence and into early adulthood. As expected, peer influence increased during the teen years, sometimes to the point of rivaling parental influence but rarely replacing it. Health professionals can use such data to reassure parents of normal adolescents and to indicate earlier evaluation and treatment for the troubled adolescent and his or her family.

Sexuality

Puberty is accompanied by the development of secondary sex characteristics and a change in the teen's self-concept. Young teens often feel frightened and overwhelmed by their lack of control over the rapid changes occurring in their bodies and self-conscious about differences between themselves and their peers. Body image is influenced not only by these rapid changes but also by perceived cultural norms. Adolescents who view their bodies as being less ideal than their peers' bodies may have less favorable feelings about themselves.[53]

Teenagers learn about body changes and develop sexual and social behavior through their peer relationships. In early adolescence a same-sex best friend is very important; intimate ideas and concerns are shared. Best friends experience a closeness that will develop into the capacity to form intimate heterosexual relationships.[53]

Adolescents become sexually active for a variety of reasons, which tend to change as they mature. Younger teens may use sexual experimentation as a way of being accepted into a specific peer group or as a means of bolstering their self-esteem. These youngsters are less likely to consider the long-term outcomes of their sexual activity. Conversely, older adolescents who have had opportunities to work through their sexual role are likely to be more comfortable with who they are and more capable of establishing intimacy in their relationships. Furthermore, these youngsters are more inclined to be thoughtful about the reasons for having intercourse, to plan for safe sex, and to use effective contraception.[37]

Impact of Diabetes on Psychologic Development

Since diabetes and its management are unavoidably intertwined with the complexities of growing up, an understanding of the normal process of adolescent development is essential for the health professional caring for teens with IDDM. In general, adolescents are highly concerned about their physical development, appearance, and emotions and are worried about being considered "normal." Teens with IDDM are faced with constant reminders that they are different each time that they inject insulin, monitor their blood sugar, or even eat a mouthful of food. The degree to which they and their families are able to meet the daily demands of self-management and still participate in life is a function of their coping.

Coping with diabetes

Diabetes management requires a degree of responsibility and behavioral control uncharacteristic of adolescents.[85] The daily demands of diabetes have an impact on the personal and public lives of adolescents, interacting with vital developmental tasks: independence, body image, identity, sexuality, responsibility, and self-esteem.[17] How well do young people and their families cope with the combination of diabetes and adolescence?

Psychosocial adjustment to diabetes has been the focus of considerable research. A number of earlier investigators reported that children and adolescents with diabetes, when compared with their healthy peers, were more often maladjusted and neurotic and had an inadequate self-image and weaker personality.[75,121] More recently, however, a growing body of research suggests that diabetes in children and adolescents does not typically lead to psychologic disruption and that these young people are in fact quite well adjusted.

The level of adjustment to diabetes is a reflection of the child and family's ability to cope with the additional tasks imposed by the disorder. According to Wexler,[130] families are required to master both cognitive/practical (e.g., develop a satisfactory understanding of diabetes, demonstrate an ability to apply the necessary skills) and certain psychosocial tasks. The latter include coping with the impact of the diagnosis, experiencing a sense of mastery over diabetes and thus maintaining good self-esteem, and finally striving for and attaining a balanced acceptance of diabetes with positive expectations for the immediate and long-term future.

Coping with the demands of diabetes is probably most difficult immediately after diagnosis but also continues to require considerable effort over time. Coping is influenced by past experience and life-style and is affected by strengths in the adolescent, the family, and the environment.

Initial coping. Kovacs and associates[77-79] investigated the course of adjustment of children and families to diabetes from the time of onset. Through interviews and psychometric testing, the coping responses and well-being of 74 children and their parents were assessed both in retrospect to and after diagnosis. They found that most children were no different from those in the nondiabetic population before diagnosis in terms of psychosocial functioning.

Furthermore, most children weathered the diagnosis and initial treatment quite well, although they typically exhibited some psychologic upset in the beginning. During the adaptation phase they typically experienced at least one of the following symptoms: periods of depression, feelings of friendlessness, irritability, anxiety, and some social withdrawal. These complaints declined within the first year of IDDM.

The study of Kovacs and others[79] showed that emotional and behavioral disturbances that met criteria for psychiatric disturbance were not the norm but were nonetheless quite prevalent (36%). Adjustment disorders with anxiety and depression were most common; a 50% recovery rate occurred within 3 months. Abnormal coping responses occurred more often in families from lower socioeconomic classes and in families who were experiencing severe marital difficulties. These children may have fewer coping resources available to them and are lacking in environmental and social assets or parental support.

Kovacs and associates[78] also studied the coping responses of parents of children with diabetes. When compared with a control group, mild to moderate depression was two to three times more common in mothers of children with diabetes. Mothers were also more preoccupied with diabetes than were fathers and "worried" all the time. Even when psychologic tests indicated that the parents were functioning well, they frequently became tearful, upset, and anxious and expressed feelings of hopelessness when asked about the child's diabetes. As with the children, the symptoms of depression and anxiety lessened over time.

The findings of this study demonstrate the emotional resilience of youngsters with diabetes and their families. Clinical experience and the reports of other investigators concur with Kovacs and colleagues' conclusions. For example, Jacobson and associates[62,63] assessed the psychosocial adjustment of children with recently diagnosed diabetes and found their levels of self-esteem, locus of control, and psychologic symptoms to be comparable to those of children with a recent, acute medical problem. In another study Hauenstein and co-workers[54] evaluated stress in parents of children with diabetes and demonstrated that most mothers of children with diabetes have coping skills that are adequate to deal with the added stress posed by diabetes.

Although healthy adaptation is the usual outcome for most children with diabetes, all these studies, particularly those of Kovacs and others, indicate that initially a negative emotional reaction should be expected. Health care professionals aware of these patterns of adjustment are better prepared to (1) help the child and family to anticipate the initial psychosocial effect of diabetes, (2) intervene with short-term supportive counseling knowing that most reactions are self-limited, and (3) identify those in need of more intensive psychosocial intervention.

Long-term coping. Current evidence also supports a picture of psychologic health for those adolescents with diabetes of longer duration. Sullivan[119] found no differences in the self-esteem of adolescent girls with and without diabetes. Kellerman and associates[70] reported a similar finding when they assessed the relationship between chronic illness and psychologic functioning in adolescents. The results of this study further suggest that, even though chronically ill adolescents report high levels of situational stress, they generally do not become chronically anxious or react with inordinate distress to the problems of daily living.

In examining a number of studies on the psychologic adjustment of adolescents to diabetes, Cerreto and Travis[17] found evidence to show that, on the whole, teens with diabetes view themselves as being similar to their peers in the areas of personal freedom and responsibility in their daily lives. The studies reviewed also indicate that most adolescents reported telling their friends about diabetes, developing occupational goals sooner than their nondiabetic peers, and planning to marry and have children.

Thus it would appear that for most adolescents, diabetes neither prevents nor seriously disrupts accomplishment of the developmental tasks viewed as essential for entry into psychologically healthy adulthood. Their sense of identity, self-esteem, autonomy, and future goal orientation seem to remain intact.

The documented evidence of healthy attitudes and lack of psychopathology in adolescents with diabetes is encouraging. Several authors postulate that this positive response is related to adolescents' denial of some of the harsh realities of their illness.[125] This denial, however, is not necessarily inappropriate; rather, it can be viewed as part of the adaptation process.

MANAGING DIABETES IN ADOLESCENTS: ROLE OF THE DIABETES HEALTH CARE TEAM

Not only should adolescents with IDDM have the opportunity for health care delivery by a multidisciplinary health care team experienced in their care, but they also should be integral members of the team. Other team members should include physicians, nurse educators, dietitians, behavioral specialists (e.g., social workers, psychologists, psychiatrists), public health nurses, and support groups (e.g., national diabetes associations, local teen support groups). Clearly, not all teens live in centers large enough to warrant such a comprehensive team. However, referral to such a center may be most beneficial at the onset of the disease and for those experiencing difficulty with one or more aspects of their diabetes care. Furthermore, as outlined earlier, the problems of these adolescents are sufficiently different from those of adults with the disorder that teens should not be lumped together with adults for education and care unless attention is paid to their specific needs. For example, information regarding foot care will be of much less relevance to a new-onset diabetic teen than will information about activities such as vigorous exercise, eating out, and partying.

The three components of health care that should be offered to teens with diabetes and their families by the health care team include education, support, and care. Each part of this package must be sensitive to the teen's increasing needs for self-responsibility, integrity of body image, and self-esteem.

Education

The overall goals of diabetes education for youth with IDDM are to ensure that they have the knowledge, skills, and support systems necessary to (1) maintain excellent health day to day, (2) make safe choices with regard to life-style issues, and (3) proceed in their development and their movement toward independence without undue interruption. Initial education requires that the teens and their families acquire an understanding of diabetes and the components of care essential to function adequately at home, such as insulin injection, self-monitoring of blood glucose (SMBG), urine ketone testing, hypoglycemia recognition and treatment, and nutritional planning. In the early weeks it is essential that they learn about and experience the various facets of diabetes management. Wexler[130] has referred to this period as the time for acquisition of "cognitive-practical tasks." Diabetes education for children and adolescents with IDDM starts at diagnosis and continues for the rest of their lives. For those who develop diabetes at a younger age, the onset of puberty signals an ideal time to update diabetes knowledge and to integrate developmental concepts into the discussion. Anticipatory guidance concerning psychosocial issues such as alcohol and drug use, smoking, sexuality, and normal parent-child conflict should be offered to all young teens and their families and reinforced regularly.

For adolescents the approach to diabetes education needs to be informal and interactional; both facts and feelings should be addressed. For example, it is natural for teens to have some difficulty with rules, but these are unavoidable with diabetes management. Diabetes educators should encourage teens to question these rules; this affords the opportunity to provide a solid rationale for each aspect of therapy and to discuss various options with them. Teens should also be encouraged to use a problem-solving approach to develop solutions to their diabetes-related dilemmas and to add flexibility to their routines.

Education and treatment goals must be practical and achievable and should take into account the teen's estimates of his or her own needs and abilities. Regardless of the adolescent's age, parents must be included in the learning process so that they can offer the appropriate level of support and guidance. Initially some teens may resist parental involvement in the diabetes education program. They want privacy and autonomy; it is important to respect these needs and spend at least some time in discussion with the teen alone. It is also essential that the youngster understand that inclusion of the parents in the education program is required to ensure consistency of understanding of diabetes in the teens and their parents and to promote self-efficacy. An often successful strategy is to encourage the teen to participate actively in teaching his or her parents about the diabetes. It is hoped such an approach will lessen family conflict about the diabetes and increase the parent's respect for and confidence in their teen's self-care abilities (Box 19-1).

BOX 19-1

CORNERSTONES OF DIABETES EDUCATION FOR ADOLESCENTS

Be informal and interactive.
Focus on facts *and* feelings.
Negotiate realistic goals.
Ensure matching expectations.
Involve parents.

Clearly, some teens welcome the chance to learn more about diabetes; it makes them feel one step closer to independence. Others, however, refuse all offers of diabetes education. For these teens, it is essential that parents remain responsible for daily diabetes management. At the same time, health professionals should maintain a nonjudgmental attitude when dealing with these youngsters and keep the door open for future opportunities to learn.

An excellent source of additional information for health professionals regarding specific educational strategies with a developmental focus is the *Diabetes Youth Curriculum: A Tool for Educators.*[91]

Support

Adolescents and their families must assume ultimate responsibility for daily diabetes management. The health care team, however, has an important role in enabling these families to cope with this onerous task. Some supportive and motivational strategies recommended or employed by health professionals include the use of the therapeutic relationship, contracting, social learning interventions, camps, counseling, and support groups.

The importance of a satisfying relationship between adolescents with diabetes and health care providers in promoting positive coping and enhancing compliance is well described.* Key to this *therapeutic alliance* is the health care providers' interest in and respect for the teen and his or her point of view. When social and psychologic issues are considered as carefully as physical concerns, caregivers are much more likely to arrive at an interpretation of facts that is congruent with that of the teen and family and thereby earn their trust. Once this has been established, teens and health care providers may be better able to negotiate realistic management goals and plan appropriate strategies to achieve them.

For many teens, *contracting* can be used to encourage good self-care behaviors. Contracting, which is addressed in detail in Chapter 15, involves an agreement that details specific rewards for specific behaviors. Contracts provide youths with an opportunity to become increasingly involved in planning their own care as they become more independent. They also provide a mechanism for clear communication and help all parties understand the division of responsibilities.[129]

Peer acceptance is extremely important during adolescence; thus peer group interventions may be effective in mediating health care goals. *Social learning strategies* are designed to provide groups of teens with opportunities to identify difficult situations, develop and practice creative solutions, and learn to counterargue. According to Kaplan and others,[68] such interventions have been used successfully to discourage smoking, truancy, and antisocial behavior in the adolescent population. Anderson and others[5] used an activity-based peer group intervention with teens with diabetes to prevent the expected deterioration in metabolic control during adolescence. Their strategy provided teens with the problem-solving skills and support needed for adjusting the insulin dose, exercising, and meal planning.

---

*References 13, 16, 50, 106, 120, 126.

Camps for youth with diabetes allow these youngsters to participate in a variety of new activities (e.g., marathon swimming, overnight canoe trips) and at the same time to consider their diabetes-related needs. The new learning that occurs during camp not only boosts their self-confidence but can also be applied to situations that youngsters encounter outside the camp environment.

It is critical that health professionals not limit their supportive efforts to the teens themselves. Families should be assessed for their adjustment and adaptive capabilities early in the course of the diabetes and periodically thereafter.[36,130] Most parents need help in finding the balance between the youngster's need to feel in charge and the need not to be abandoned. Once teens have assumed responsibility for their own routines, there is the risk that parents (and health providers) will pay only negative attention to the diabetes regimen, that is, nag when a task is not completed. Families should be encouraged to maintain a system of positive reinforcement throughout the youngsters' diabetes career. Youths and adults have a need to be recognized for their efforts. When adolescents and parents find themselves in a pattern of negative interaction to the extent that diabetes control suffers, *family counseling* may be indicated.[17]

Finally, parents and other family members may benefit from participation in *therapeutic and self-help groups.* Self-help groups for people with diabetes are frequently affiliated with organizations such as the American/Canadian Diabetes Associations or the Juvenile Diabetes Foundation. Such groups provide families with peer support, modeling, a sense of not being alone with diabetes, and an opportunity for sharing different attitudes and catharsis. Therapeutic groups refer to those organized and facilitated by experienced health professionals. Goals of the group are quite specific (e.g., to promote an understanding of emotional reactions to diabetes or to develop an awareness of the impact of diabetes on normal developmental tasks and learn ways of coping).

Care

Since diabetes is a lifelong disorder, continuity and consistency of care are important. This is particularly so during the adolescent years, when noncompliance, mistrust, and rebellion are most likely to be at a peak. In the ideal situation, some members of the health care team (physician, nurse educator, social worker/psychologist, dietitian) develop a relaxed, trusting, and caring relationship with the teen and parents. This is unlikely to occur at the first meeting and may take months or even years to develop. The clinic visits should be unhurried and focus on understanding the teen as an individual: what does he or she know about diabetes and its management, and what are his or her major fears and dislikes about the disorder?

It is necessary for the teen to begin to assume membership in his or her health care team. Decisions made by members of the team without consulting the teen will often be seen as arbitrary and intrusive and will likely be disregarded. When the teen's view is respected and incorporated into the treatment regimen, he or she is much more likely to comply. Noncompliance is virtually ensured when unrealistic goals and punitive action or judgmental attitudes are foisted on these youngsters.

BOX 19-2

GOALS OF THERAPY FOR ADOLESCENTS

1. To maintain normal growth and physical development.
2. To encourage normal psychosocial development, leading to acquisition of the cognitive and emotional skills necessary to carry out all aspects of self-care.
3. To control symptoms of hyperglycemia, such as polydipsia, polyuria, and nocturia.
4. To maintain normal blood lipid profiles.
5. To achieve acceptable metabolic control, as evidenced by most self-monitored blood glucose concentrations in the 70 to 180 mg/dl range preprandially and acceptable GHb levels.
6. To avoid severe hypoglycemia (mild, occasional hypoglycemia that can be easily recognized and treated is virtually ubiquitous) and ketoacidosis.

The tools of therapy (i.e., balance between insulin administration and food intake) are imprecise at best. Subcutaneous injection of insulin is nonphysiologic; for most teens, therefore, euglycemia is an unrealistic goal. The overzealous demand for tight control in the teen may lead to noncompliance with many or all aspects of diabetes care. Often it will lead to poor clinic attendance, fabricated test results, sneaking food, and so on. Box 19-2 lists the goals of therapy for adolescents.

No guidelines are available as to what constitutes acceptable glycemic control in adolescents with IDDM; *acceptable* implies blood glucose levels that may prevent the onset or progression of long-term complications, without serious risks. The results of the DCCT clearly show that the lower the GHb level, the lower the risk for both the onset and the progression of microvascular complications.[30-34] However, studies such as the DCCT underline the increased frequency of severe hypoglycemia associated with intensification of the treatment regimen in an attempt to achieve close to normoglycemia.[32-34] (For the results of the DCCT and the implications for care of adolescents with IDDM, see later discussion.)

At this time, complete normalization of blood glucose levels for adolescents with IDDM seems to be both an unrealistic and a potentially dangerous goal. Efforts (or demands) to keep preprandial glycemia in the 60 to 120 mg/dl range will ensure frequent levels less than 60 mg/dl, whether asymptomatic or symptomatic. Attention should focus not only on blood glucose targets, but also on the prevention of severe hypoglycemia (and diminution of episodes of asymptomatic or mild hypoglycemia as harbingers of more severe episodes); avoidance of repeat hospitalizations, whether for hypoglycemia, diabetic ketoacidosis (DKA), or generally poor overall control; and encouraging normal adjustment and optimal self-care practices as adolescence ends and young adulthood begins.

Insulin

Children and adolescents with new-onset IDDM typically begin on twice- (or three times–) daily injections of a short- and intermediate-acting insulin, with the first injection before breakfast and the second before the evening meal.

In nonadherent teens in poor metabolic control, caregivers are often tempted to intensify treatment to improve the situation, for example, by adding more insulin injections, demanding more frequent SMBG, or tightening up the nutritional plan. Such strategies are probably doomed to failure; increasing demands of the treatment regimen may lead to a vicious cycle of fabricated tests, insulin omission, worse control, more demands, and on and on.

Instead of a more complex treatment regimen, such situations often call for a back-to-basics approach in which a simpler regimen may actually lead to improvements. Increased parental support may be needed at this time as well. This approach requires two components: (1) what the teen is willing to do (as opposed to being told to do) and (2) support of the health care team to help the teen meet the mutually agreed-on (and often, at least initially, meager) goals.

Nutrition and exercise planning

Although the approaches to nutritional planning and exercise in individuals with diabetes are discussed in Chapters 4 and 5, this section highlights some issues relating to these that impact specifically on the adolescent with diabetes.

As described earlier, adolescence is a time of increasing independence from family, peer conformity, and experimentation. All these factors may significantly affect compliance with the treatment regimen and perhaps most importantly with the nutritional plan.[18,66] It becomes essential to keep adolescents with diabetes well informed about their diet and the reasons for consistency in timing of meals and snacks, amount, and types of food eaten. More important, however, is the need to provide a meal plan that provides sufficient calories to the rapidly growing adolescent and to provide these on an individual basis by tailoring each youngster's meal plan to his or her own needs. Similarly the plan must be flexible enough to accommodate "nonbasal" conditions, such as extra exercise, eating out, and partying. One thing that will ensure dietary noncompliance is provision of a meal plan that is inflexible and provides insufficient calories.

At the end of the growth spurt, adolescents in general and the females in particular may need a reduction in caloric intake to forestall excessive weight gain. The teen should be prepared for this in advance so that adjustment in his or her nutritional plan is not seen as punitive and can be carried out, wherever possible, before unwanted weight gain occurs.

Some adolescents, more often girls than boys, become concerned about their weight and want to lose a few pounds. At this time the health care professional must work along with the teen to establish realistic goals in terms of weight loss and to make rational adjustments in the meal plan to accommodate this change. Failure to support the adolescent's efforts in this way may result in fad diets or cycles of insulin omission, intentional glycosuria, bingeing, and so forth. Whenever the diet is decreased, insulin dosage must be adjusted appropriately to avoid hypoglycemia and excessive hunger that will jeopardize adherence. The role of SMBG to facilitate the changes in insulin dosage cannot be overemphasized.

Similarly, adolescents must learn to deal with the metabolic impact of extra exercise.[132] Whereas during earlier childhood most compensation is made by parents and other caregivers, during adolescence this task falls increasingly on the shoulders of the youngsters themselves.

They need to know not only about extra caloric intake before and during exercise, but also about the possibility of late postexercise hypoglycemia.[84,132] This latter condition most often occurs late at night or in the early-morning hours after a bout of strenuous exercise after the evening meal. What is needed in this situation is not necessarily extra calories during the exercise, but rather afterward to prevent the later decrease in blood glucose. An alternative approach is to decrease insulin dosage. Nevertheless, requirements may differ greatly from one individual to another, and only with the help of increased SMBG can the specific needs of each adolescent be addressed adequately.

Crisis Intervention

All teens with IDDM are susceptible to the acute complications of the disease, namely hypoglycemia and DKA, as well as to the impact of intercurrent illness on glucose homeostasis. Availability of medical personnel on an around-the-clock basis to help cope with such emergencies is therefore essential.

Hypoglycemia

Hypoglycemia is the most common acute complication of IDDM and therefore represents a significant and constant risk for all adolescents with the disease.[27] This subject is more fully dealt with elsewhere, but a few comments are pertinent here.

Virtually every individual with IDDM experiences some of the symptoms of hypoglycemia on a regular basis.[27,30,32] Many clinicians believe that the absence of any hypoglycemia may indicate metabolic control that is less than optimal[127]; mild occasional hypoglycemia that can be recognized and treated is therefore one of the prices to be paid in the achievement of acceptable levels of glycemic control. Teens, however, are often unwilling to pay this price. Their concern is not for the future; rather, they are more interested in avoiding any situation where they feel out of control, singled out, or inconvenienced. Thus overeating and insulin manipulation may represent their attempt to prevent even the mildest hypoglycemic reactions.

As much as teens want to avoid hypoglycemia, however, several important life-style factors put them at increased risk for reactions, including erratic physical activity, sleeping in, dieting, and experimenting with alcohol. Many teens refuse to wear their diabetes identification bracelet or necklace. When adolescents are secretive about their diabetes, the risk is compounded. In this situation there is more potential for missed snacks and delayed or inadequate meals. For example, one youngster became hypoglycemic during a sleepover at a friend's home because his friend's family was unaware of his diabetes. At dinner he failed to eat all his food choices because he did not want to "look like a pig." The embarrassing hypoglycemic episode might have been avoided had he discussed his diabetes and its requirements with his friend before the visit.

Severe hypoglycemia (defined by an episode of coma, convulsion, or confusion) is to be avoided at all costs, both because of its potential for morbidity and because of the anxiety that it creates in the teens and their families. For youngsters who have experienced severe insulin reactions, fear of hypoglycemia may be a source of more anxiety for them and their families than the fear of long-term diabetes-related complications. As a result, metabolic control may be compromised.

The frequency of episodes of severe hypoglycemia is unevenly distributed throughout the diabetic population.[45] Studies suggest that up to a third of those with IDDM will have an episode of severe hypoglycemia during their lifetime with the disease.[27,45] Many studies attest to tighter metabolic control as a risk factor for severe hypoglycemia.[27,30-34] For example, in the DCCT, those in the intensive treatment group were about three times more likely to experience an episode of severe hypoglycemia than were those receiving conventional treatment.[33] Data also suggest that between 4% and 20% of those with IDDM will suffer such an episode in any one year.[27] In our review of 311 children attending our clinic, we found that 31% had experienced a severe episode in the past and that in 16% at least one episode had occurred in a particular year. Younger age, longer duration of IDDM, and lower GHb levels were risk factors associated with the occurrence of severe hypoglycemia. Among adolescents in the DCCT, severe hypoglycemia occurred with a frequency of 19 episodes/100 patient years in the conventional group, but 62/100 patient years in the intensive treatment group.[34]

Most hypoglycemic episodes, whether mild or severe, are related to the known predisposing factors: decreased or missed meal or snack, extra exercise without additional caloric intake, or inadvertent (or occasionally intentional) insulin overdosage. However, there will always be a number of episodes that cannot be explained on the basis of these factors but likely relate to the variations in insulin dosage and absorption, food intake, and daily activity that are common in these children.

Although the potential exists for significant morbidity (and even mortality) from severe hypoglycemia, virtually all such episodes have an uneventful outcome in adolescents with IDDM. Furthermore, in the DCCT, there were no identifiable sequelae of severe hypoglycemia either in terms of neurocognitive development or in terms of interference with quality of life.[33] Nevertheless, these adolescents must be taught about the factors predisposing to hypoglycemia, how to recognize early warning symptoms, and what measures to take to prevent an episode from becoming more severe. Equally important, health professionals must explore the adolescent's concern about reactions and identify life-style factors that increase their risk of such events. Teens need to be engaged in active problem-solving around these issues. For example, they can be encouraged to take an extra late-night snack in anticipation of sleeping in on the weekend. They need to understand the effect of alcohol on blood glucose so that they will eat when they consume alcoholic beverages. Whenever possible, meals and snacks should be planned to fit in with the school schedule; if a snack must be eaten in class, the use of ''low-noise'' foods such as dried fruit can be suggested.

Teens need encouragement to carry some form of sugar with them at all times. Prepackaged dextrose either in tablet or gel form is convenient to carry and less likely to be consumed than candies, chocolate bars, and so on. Should a severe episode of hypoglycemia occur, parents need to know how to use glucagon. Unfortunately, research has shown that glucagon is used in only about one third of severe episodes.[27] Reasons for failure to use glucagon when required include inability to locate the glucagon at the time of the event, panic or fear during the event, absence of glucagon in the home and forgetfulness about its availability, or denial of the severity of the episode. Similar findings have been reported in adults with diabetes.[20] These findings underline the need to update the adolescent's and parents' understanding of hypoglycemia regularly and ensure that glucagon is available and accessible. We stress that glucagon can only help and not harm. When a glucagon vial expires, family members are encouraged to "practice preparing it" before discarding the outdated medication.

Somogyi phenomenon

Poor metabolic control in adolescents with diabetes is often ascribed to overinsulinization with the Somogyi phenomenon (i.e., posthypoglycemic hyperglycemia and ketonuria). A number of recent studies have shown this phenomenon to occur infrequently. A more likely explanation for fasting hyperglycemia (with or without ketonuria) is underinsulinization or waning of the effect of insulin in the early-morning hours.[55,82]

Diabetic ketoacidosis

DKA is a serious but preventable acute complication in the adolescent with IDDM who is well established on treatment and who is knowledgeable about diabetes management in general and illness management in particular. Most teens will not experience an episode of DKA. If this does occur, however, the incident should be used as an opportunity to explore the causes of DKA (e.g., intercurrent illness) and their prevention. Frequently parents need to be reminded that, although their teens manage their diabetes very responsibly when they are well, the same youngsters need extra help with their insulin and monitoring when sick or stressed. A second episode of DKA requires a more comprehensive approach (see later section on recurrent DKA).

The Case for Tight Metabolic Control

The DCCT has provided irrefutable evidence that individuals receiving intensive management achieve better metabolic control and show a delay in the onset and progression of microvascular disease.[30-34] This randomized control trial was initiated in the early 1980s to resolve the ongoing debate as to the validity of the "glucose hypothesis" for the pathogenesis of diabetes complications. The DCCT was the only trial of its kind to include an adolescent cohort. The trial was set up to answer two separate questions relating to the glucose hypothesis. The primary prevention question was, Would tight metabolic control prevent or delay the onset of complications? The secondary intervention question was, Would this therapy slow down or prevent the progression of the early manifestations of these complications? More than 1400 individuals, 13 to 39 years of age and with IDDM of 1 to 15 years' duration at the time the study started, participated in 27 centers across North America; 195 subjects were adolescents (13 to 18 years of age) at randomization. They were randomly assigned to receive either conventional management, designed to mimic the level of control achieved in typical diabetes clinics, or intensive therapy in an attempt to attain and maintain normoglycemia.

The study was a remarkable success: subject compliance and adherence to the treatment group was outstanding. Of importance, the two groups were separated by mean GHb concentrations of approximately 2%. In the total cohort the mean GHb was 8.9% in the conventional treatment group and 7.2% in the intensive group. These translate into mean blood glucose concentrations of 12.8 and 8.6 mmol/L, respectively. In the adolescent cohort, mean GHb was 9.8% in the conventional and 8.1% in the intensive group, with mean blood glucose levels of 14.4 and 9.8 mmol/L, respectively. Two points are worth noting: (1) the intensive treatment group did not, on average, achieve normoglycemia, and (2) the adolescents in both treatment groups were unable to achieve the same level of control as the total cohort.

Briefly, the DCCT demonstrated that intensive diabetes treatment reduced the risk of microvascular complication onset or progression by 25% to 75% for both primary prevention and secondary intervention groups. Risk reduction was similar in the adult and adolescent subgroups despite the different levels of metabolic control achieved. For example, among the adolescents, intensive treatment decreased the risk of having any retinopathy by 53% in the primary prevention group and decreased the risk of retinopathy progression by 70% and occurrence of microalbuminuria by 55% in the secondary intervention group.[34] The data relating to macrovascular disease were not significantly different, most likely because of the relatively young age and good general health of the study population at the start of the trial. Of note was the demonstration of an almost linear relationship between GHb and complication risk: any decrease in GHb was associated with a reduction in the risk of onset or progression of microvascular complications.

Two adverse effects of intensive diabetes treatment were documented in the DCCT: (1) an approximately threefold increase in the incidence of severe hypoglycemic events[32-34] and (2) a tendency for significant weight gain in the intensive treatment group.[31] Hypoglycemia was more likely in those with previous severe episodes and in those with lower GHb levels. Fortunately, no morbidity or mortality could be attributed to these hypoglycemic events. After 5 years, intensively treated adolescents had gained significantly more weight than their conventionally treated peers.

The study's findings provide cause for considerable optimism. First, the results show that any decrease in GHb is associated with a reduction in risk of complications. Thus a decrease in GHb from 10% to 8%, an imminently achievable goal, may reduce complication risk to a similar degree to that achieved by a decrease from 8% to 6%, a daunting prospect for even the most fastidious. Second, intensive treatment leading to improved metabolic control reduces risk of complications in both primary prevention and secondary intervention groups. Thus, at least in the adolescent population with IDDM, in whom microvascular disease would be expected to be in its early evolutionary stages, it is "never" too late to start intensive treatment.

Formulating an Intensive Diabetes Management Plan

Intensive diabetes management implies the employment of treatment strategies aimed at attaining and maintaining as close to normoglycemia as possible for the particular individual with diabetes. Box 19-3 outlines the different components of intensive management. Patient selection is of utmost importance; initiating intensive diabetes treatment in a recalcitrant

---

BOX 19-3

INTENSIVE DIABETES MANAGEMENT

Involves a multifaceted treatment plan that includes *all* of the following:
- Patient and family motivation and education
- Frequent contact between the patient and the multidisciplinary diabetes health care team
- Frequent daily SMBG
- Careful balance of food intake, activity, and insulin dosage
- A multiple daily insulin injection or subcutaneous insulin infusion regimen
- Self-adjustment of insulin dosage according to preset algorithms to meet blood glucose targets

---

adolescent from a dysfunctional family is doomed to failure. The intensive treatment regimen will only provide more opportunity for nonadherence and rebellion in such teens. In addition, it is probably unnecessary to introduce intensive therapy in an adolescent who is already achieving close to normoglycemia with conventional therapy. We do not support the argument that intensive treatment provides more flexibility in terms of diabetes care. In fact, to achieve the goals of intensive treatment, higher degrees of compliance and reliability are demanded, at least in the early stages of this management as the teen learns the new treatment approach. Thereafter, flexibility of routines with maintenance of excellent metabolic control will depend on a heightened understanding of the interrelationships among food types and amounts, exercise, and insulin.

Successful intensive diabetes management must start with careful assessment of the teen and family with respect to knowledge base and readiness to take on the added demands of this type of treatment. The key players in this process are the adolescent, family, and diabetes health care team. Encouraging teens to become involved in intensive treatment regimens depends on their understanding fully the risks and benefits of such a treatment approach, accepting the added burdens and responsibilities of the therapy, having their parents be supportive of the program, and having a diabetes health care team, including physician, diabetes nurse, and dietitian fully conversant with the intricacies of intensive therapy and who have a common treatment philosophy.

The cornerstones of intensive diabetes treatment include an enhanced understanding of the blood glucose targets, performance of more SMBG, establishment of an appropriate meal plan, and finally, setting up of an algorithm for insulin administration. These can often be introduced in a stepwise manner. An essential part of this program is frequent contact with the health care team.

1. *Blood glucose targets.* Individual goals need to be set for each individual, taking into account their life-style, exercise habits, and previous experience with and symptoms of severe hypoglycemia. In general, the following blood glucose targets are reasonable starting points for anyone initiating intensive therapy:

Preprandial	4-7 mmol/L (~70-140 mg/dl)
Postprandial	<10 mmol/L (<180 mg/dl)
3 AM (nadir)	>3.5 mmol/L (>~65 mg/dl)

2. *More SMBG.* To accomplish the goals of intensive treatment, it is essential that intensively treated teens be frequently aware of their blood glucose concentrations for three reasons: (1) it allows for appropriate adjustments in preprandial insulin dosage and food intake; (2) it helps to predict and prevent episodes of hypoglycemia; and (3) it encourages a much improved understanding of the impact of food intake and physical activity on glucose homeostasis. It brings a greater degree of immediacy to the entire decision-making process. A well-kept blood glucose logbook is an important component of care. Even though insulin adjustments are made on the basis of individual glucose levels, the overall insulin "algorithm" will change depending on patterns of control over a few days to a week or so.

Intensive treatment demands at least four daily blood glucose tests: before each meal and at bedtime. Regular (e.g., weekly) tests at 2 to 4 AM will help predict and prevent nocturnal hypoglycemia. Postprandial tests may be helpful to determine the glycemic response to specific foods or to problem-solve when GHb remains high despite preprandial blood glucose concentrations on target.

3. *Redefining the meal plan.* Teens starting multiple daily injection routines often have the impression that this will allow them "to eat when and what I want." This is a fallacy if the objective of this routine is the achievement of improved metabolic control. A thorough understanding of the meal plan, particularly the carbohydrate content of the foods to be ingested at each meal or snack ("carbohydrate counting"), is essential. The DCCT diet analysis clearly demonstrated that GHb levels were lowest in the most dietary compliant and knowledgeable subjects in the intensive treatment group.[29]

Patients with IDDM respond differently in terms of glycemic excursions to foods of different carbohydrate and other macronutrient content. One of the major purposes of the more frequent monitoring is to allow each individual to establish for himself or herself a profile of glycemic excursions to different meal types and sizes. This may be very difficult to conceptualize in the often noncompliant teens; nonetheless, it is a key to successful intensive treatment.

The dietary instruction includes information regarding the potential for significant weight gain with the introduction of improved glycemic control. Frequent reassessment of the meal plan and problem solving around such issues as eating out and fast foods is an important part of this component of intensive care. Intensive treatment is obviously contraindicated in the teenage or young adult female with IDDM who has an overt or even subclinical eating disorder. The introduction of further dietary restraint may trigger the cycle of binge eating, insulin omission, and induced glycosuria and further noncompliance in these individuals.[103] Specific dietary instruction around hypoglycemia treatment (i.e., avoiding the overtreatment of hypoglycemic reactions) is also an integral part of intensive treatment.

4. *The variable insulin dose schedule (VIDS).* An essential component of intensive diabetes management is the introduction of a more interactive insulin dosage schedule, almost invariably with more frequent insulin injections and dose adjustments based on ambient blood

glucose concentrations, intended caloric intake, and physical activity. The three frequently used approaches to intensive insulin treatment are as follows:

a. *Three dose-a-day routine:*

>NPH/Lente plus regular before breakfast
>
>Regular before supper
>
>NPH/Lente at bedtime

This regimen allows dose adjustment of the regular insulin before breakfast and supper according to blood glucose concentrations. The later intermediate-acting insulin may be helpful in reducing the risk of nocturnal hypoglycemia. This approach may be regarded as an intensification of conventional therapy and, for many teens, may be the first step in the introduction of a more aggressive insulin dose adjustment routine.

b. *Multiple daily injections (MDI)—"basal bolus" injection routine:*

>Regular before meals
>
>NPH/Lente at bedtime
>
>(Ultralente is sometimes given with the presupper regular.)

In the DCCT, this was the most frequently used intensive insulin delivery approach. Multiple daily injection routines allow patients to make greater use of handy insulin injection devices, specifically the insulin "pens."

c. *Continuous subcutaneous insulin infusions (CSII or "pump" therapy):*

>Basal infusion rate(s) are supplemented by premeal boluses.

This requires training in the use and care of the pump. Since the insulin used is short-acting regular insulin only, any breakdown in pump function will lead rapidly to insulinopenia and possible development of DKA.

To anyone with diabetes treated conventionally, the prospect of starting an intensive diabetes care program must seem overwhelming; this may be even more so in the teen juggling commitments to school, sports, family, friends, and so on. The diabetes team must be available to support the teen and family through the intense early learning phase and into the more chronic treatment period. Numerous adjustments will likely be needed to the VIDS, meal plan and testing schedule; problem solving around specific issues such as meter performance, recipe analysis, and hypoglycemia occurrence and prevention will be required. There will also be periods of frustration and disillusionment with the program, and these teens will need the encouragement and support of a qualified and nonjudgmental team.

Since the objective of intensive diabetes management is improved metabolic control, teens receiving this type of treatment must have regular GHb levels measured. It may be worthwhile to do these measurements monthly for the first few months. Both the patient and health care team will be encouraged by a falling level. GHb targets for intensive treatment patients should be within 20% to 25% of the upper normal range (e.g., if nondiabetic range is 4% to 6%, GHb in intensively treated patients should be less than 7.2% to 7.5%).

Failure to "induce" a decrease in GHb may be the first indication of difficulties in following the routines and in meeting the targets. In the adolescent whose GHb fails to fall or in whom the level rises after being near target, problems with compliance may be present, which may indicate the need to reassess the appropriateness of the intensive treatment program.

FACTORS ASSOCIATED WITH POOR HEALTH OUTCOME

Most adolescents with diabetes are healthy and well adjusted. A few teens, however, encounter serious problems characterized by persistently poor metabolic control and/or impaired psychologic functioning. This minority has been the focus of considerable attention both in the clinical setting and in the research literature, thus clouding the view of just how well most teens do. Box 19-4 lists factors associated with poor metabolic control.

What factors account for this difference in outcome? The roles of specific biologic and psychosocial variables in mediating health outcomes of teens with diabetes warrant further discussion.

Biologic Factors

As stated earlier, the adolescent with IDDM is less sensitive to the action of insulin than either children or adults with the disease.[4,12] In addition, epinephrine responses to moderate drops in blood glucose concentration occur earlier and to a greater extent than in adults.[122] These two factors may contribute not only to the higher insulin dose requirement, but also to some of the lability in metabolic control noted in some adolescents. Biologic factors are probably not central to the poorest level of metabolic control that characterizes a small group of adolescents with IDDM.

BOX 19-4

FACTORS ASSOCIATED WITH POOR METABOLIC CONTROL IN ADOLESCENTS WITH IDDM

A. Biologic
  1. Impaired insulin action ("insulin resistance") during adolescence
  2. Counterregulatory hormone responses
B. Medical
  1. Acute intercurrent disease (e.g., dental abscess, influenza)
  2. Chronic intercurrent disease
    a. Diabetes related (e.g., hypothyroidism, celiac disease)
    b. Unrelated to diabetes (e.g., chronic infection, malignancy)
C. Psychologic
  1. Lack of knowledge of diabetes and its management
  2. Poor social support, including unrealistic expectations for self-care
  3. Psychosocial issues
    a. Psychophysiologic response to stress
    b. Psychiatric disease
    c. Adolescent noncompliance
    d. Poor self-esteem and self-efficacy
    e. Family dysfunction
    f. Parental "collusion"
    g. Eating disorders: anorexia nervosa and bulimia and their subclinical variants

Medical Factors

Occasionally, intercurrent illnesses may interfere with the ability to achieve good blood glucose control (e.g., chronic pyelonephritis, malabsorption). These are relatively rare occurrences, but they do warrant a thorough evaluation before problems with blood glucose regulation are ascribed to the other causes listed.

Knowledge and Level of Cognitive Maturity

The daily demands of diabetes are complex, requiring technical competence with routines, comprehension of complicated concepts related to blood glucose balance, and an appreciation of future implications and complications. Knowledge about diabetes and the self-management routines is a prerequisite for self-care. Thus inadequate knowledge will potentially have an impact on metabolic control. Knowledge alone, however, is not sufficient to predict good diabetes control.

Many children develop diabetes at a time when their cognitive or emotional maturity is insufficiently developed to allow a thorough understanding of IDDM and its therapy.[75] It is essential to upgrade continuously the understanding and self-care skills of these youngsters to ensure that a simple "knowledge deficit" is not at the root of their inability to achieve adequate metabolic homeostasis. We believe that such a pure knowledge deficit is only occasionally the cause of metabolic deterioration. However, in these few individuals, correction of the deficit or misconception (e.g., timing of insulin injections, SMBG) can greatly improve their control. Educational efforts must be tailored to the specific cognitive capabilities of each teen and the family. Occasionally, specific learning disabilities hamper understanding of diabetes care. Such situations may warrant changes in the basic approach to self-care, for example, more frequent contact with the health care team to discuss insulin dose adjustment.

Supportive Factors

Two of the major causes leading to deterioration in adolescent diabetes control are (1) the setting of unrealistic expectations for treatment outcome (blood glucose and GHb levels) by parents and health care providers and (2) too early and too rapid transfer from parent- to adolescent-oriented diabetes care.

Many health care providers target unrealistic and unachievable goals such as euglycemia and normal GHb le ls in all children with IDDM. A number of studies have suggested just how unreasonable these goals are for most adolescents.[9,11,25,48] Rather, the diabetes regimen should be tailored to suit each individual adolescent and the family, taking into account their intellectual, economic, and social abilities. Health care providers should avoid being excessively judgmental in the way they deal with these youngsters and their families. Often the behavior of the health care provider leads directly to fabricated test results and implicit parental support for their noncompliant behaviors in an effort to satisfy the health care team.

The issue of when to encourage transfer of responsibility from parent- to self-oriented diabetes care has been dealt with in a number of studies.[1,75] For example, Ingersoll and colleagues[58] asked their adolescent patients to indicate who was making the adjustments in their insulin dosage: in children under 15 years of age, parents made some or all adjustments in 15 of 18 subjects; in those over 15 years, parents adjusted insulin in only 2 of 23 subjects. Nevertheless, increased self-management did not necessarily translate into "good" care. On the contrary, in some it led to deterioration in metabolic control.

It becomes clear that age is not the only criterion for transfer of responsibility; cognitive and emotional maturity are more important. The process is not and should not be sudden; that is, one day the parent gives the insulin injection and the next day the teen does it alone behind a closed door. Rather, a gradual evolution should take place, with direct parental involvement in the daily routines and decision making receding slowly as the adolescent demonstrates willingness *and* ability to take over. During times of stress (e.g., intercurrent illness), parental supervision once again becomes mandatory. By making responsibility contingent on performance, one hopes to reinforce appropriate self-care.

Psychosocial Issues

Since individuals with IDDM live their lives under the constant threat of both acute (hypoglycemia and DKA) and chronic (macrovascular and microvascular) complications, it is not surprising that attention would be focused on the psychosocial impact of this disease. The recent studies by Kovacs and Jacobson and their colleagues [62,63,77-79] are most reassuring in that they show that, after significant emotional trauma at the onset of their disease, most children with IDDM and their families learn to cope quite admirably. However, the presence of one or more psychosocial stresses may play havoc with metabolic stability.* Among the stresses that have been identified are those discussed next.

Psychophysiologic response to stress

Poor metabolic control has sometimes been blamed on a heightened physiologic response to stress. Laboratory studies have shown an increase in blood glucose levels and a release of free fatty acids in the blood during psychologic stress.[89] The clinical importance of this hormonal response as a direct cause of serious metabolic disturbances leading to DKA, however, has been overestimated. More recent studies link diabetes stability and control to the level of adherence with the treatment regimen.†

Psychiatric disease

Although overt psychopathology has not been shown to be more common in teenagers with IDDM or other chronic diseases, it is clear that the chance association of IDDM with a psychiatric disorder may lead to enormous difficulties with glycoregulation.[78]

Adolescent noncompliance

Haynes and colleagues[56] defined compliance as "the extent to which a person's behavior (in terms of taking medication, following a diet, or executing life-style changes) coincides with medical advice." For simplicity, we have chosen to abandon the semantic arguments for

---

*References 1, 14, 62, 70, 78, 119.
†References 44, 49, 67, 109, 131.

and against use of the terms *compliance* versus *adherence;* rather, we have used them interchangeably.

Poor adherence to health recommendations, particularly those that involve a life-style change, is widespread, perhaps more so in adolescents, including those with IDDM.[56,57,77] The factors that account for nonadherence are best understood within the context of normal adolescent development. Attitudes of experimentation, rebellion, and risk taking are often associated with the teen's struggle for control of his or her own destiny. It has been suggested that among adolescents with IDDM, management issues may become the battleground on which the struggle for independence is fought.[65]

Disregard for the diet, infrequent SMBG, and insulin dose manipulation are behaviors observed in many of these young people. SMBG is especially difficult for the nonadherent adolescent; tests are often missed and results fabricated. From the adolescents' perspective, this behavior is understandable, since test results may provide evidence of poor performance and reinforce lack of control. As one 15-year-old girl said, "I can't make myself test because if I do I'll see how bad I am and I'll have to do something about it and I'm not ready yet." This girl and other poorly adherent adolescents are at risk for deteriorating metabolic control that may jeopardize their future health. Few of them, however, will experience any immediate health consequences as a result of paying minimal attention to their diabetes regimen, and many of them will perceive an immediate reward, that is, acceptance into the peer group. Thus, for teenagers, the reasons *not* to follow good diabetes management practices may far outweigh those that promote compliance.

Parents and health care providers also play a role in adolescent noncompliance. As teens mature, there is often a mismatch between what is expected of them in terms of independent self-care and their own interest and capabilities in this regard.[51] Establishment of unrealistic goals for the adolescent frequently results in premature withdrawal of active parental involvement in daily diabetes management, contributing to poor adherence and poor metabolic control. Sometimes, noncompliance may represent a deliberate disruption to get other needs met, such as attention from parents and health care providers. It may also result from denial of the reality or implications of the disease, or it may be the result of genuine lack of knowledge or self-management mistakes.[64]

To a large extent, the health care providers rely on the information given to them by teens and their families to make suggestions regarding changes in the management regimen. Ability to offer safe, sensible advice depends on the teen's level of compliance and the reliability of his or her reporting to the team. Thus health care providers must be able to assess compliance accurately. Most adolescents respond to a direct, nonjudgemental approach. For example, to assess adherence to SMBG, one may ask, "How many times a week do you *manage* to check your blood sugar?" In assessing dietary adherence, we have most success when we begin by acknowledging how difficult it must be to follow a meal plan, by alluding to the problems that other teens have, especially when they are out with friends, and then by giving the teen an opportunity to discuss his or her own feelings, experiences, and concerns about food.

Extracting an admission from adolescents about noncompliant behavior rarely solves the problem. It is more important to find out what is interfering with their ability to care for their diabetes and to work with them and their families to develop strategies to deal with these issues.

Self-efficacy and self-esteem

Issues of personal control are important to adolescents with and without diabetes. Recent studies have shown that teens who are confident in their ability to control their diabetes are able to achieve better metabolic control than teens who feel overwhelmed and helpless in this regard.[52,83] The notion that self-perceived confidence in performing a task is a strong predictor of performance is termed *self-efficacy.* Adolescents with lower levels of self-efficacy also report less personal control and lower self-esteem. Poor self-efficacy and poor self-esteem may put youngsters at risk for depression.[52] Sullivan[118] has reported an association among depression, low self-esteem, and poor adjustment in adolescent girls with diabetes. All these factors may interfere with motivation to adhere to self-care routines and have a negative impact on metabolic control. Since self-reliance and instrumentality are critical issues during adolescent years, health care professionals should consider the teen's current estimation of his or her abilities and needs in planning treatment and education.

Family functioning

In her review of the psychologic aspects of diabetes in children and adolescents, Johnson[65] states that high levels of conflict, disorganization, and poor supervision within the family appear to be linked to poor health and adjustment to diabetes. Teens who do well generally report that their families are supportive, make them feel good about taking care of their diabetes, listen to their problems about having diabetes, and engage in efficient negotiation and problem solving. Conversely, adolescents who do poorly experience less effective communication within their families;[14,119] these adolescents frequently put on a facade of ignoring their parents, especially their mothers, or responding to them with arguments, heckling, or needling. In turn, mothers of poorly adherent adolescents often challenge their teens with examples of their misdemeanors, an approach that frequently leads to an escalation of conflict and increased alienation.[119] This pattern of interaction does not allow for discussion of deeper concerns, problem solving, or modification of behavior; thus adherence problems and resulting poor metabolic control persist.

Minuchin and colleagues[89] have done much to highlight pathologic family patterns in causing poor metabolic control. Some family characteristics of adolescents with unstable diabetes include (1) enmeshment to the extent that is no clear distinction exists between the role of the child and the role of the parents; (2) overprotectiveness; (3) rigidity for maintaining the status quo, leaving no room for decision making by the teen; and (4) lack of conflict resolution. In disturbed families the adolescent with diabetes sometimes assumes an important role in the family's attempt to avoid conflict; he or she becomes the scapegoat or the symptom bearer of the family. As long as the adolescent with diabetes remains unstable, the family can focus on the diabetes and avoid dealing with more threatening issues such as marital difficulties, alcoholism, or abuse.

Parental collusion

In certain families, parents can either implicitly or explicitly support the noncompliant behaviors of their children. The reasons for this are uncertain but most likely relate to their unwillingness to admit that either their children or they themselves may be less than "perfect." This is an exceptionally difficult situation to deal with, since attempts to increase parental supervision of routines are unlikely to be of any real benefit.

Eating disorders

Recent data suggest that eating disorders (anorexia nervosa, bulimia, and their subclinical variants) may be more common in teenage girls with IDDM than in the general population.[105,107] Based on the recognized risk factors for eating disorders, two aspects of IDDM have been identified that may contribute to the association between eating disorders and IDDM: (1) acute weight gain, which invariably follows the onset of insulin therapy or the institution of tight metabolic control, and (2) chronic dietary restraint and food preoccupation, which are integral parts of diabetes management.[103] Thus weight gain and dietary restraint may trigger or amplify the cycle of body dissatisfaction, dieting, binge eating, and purging (specifically, induced glycosuria from insulin omission or underdosing) in susceptible individuals, invariably girls in the adolescent or young adult age-groups.

Metabolic control in those girls with overt and subclinical eating disorders is likely to be poorer than in those without. Mechanisms for the deterioration in metabolic control include the direct metabolic effects of binge eating, self-induced vomiting or laxative abuse, and noncompliance with specific aspects of the diabetes treatment regimen. A high incidence of insulin omission with the specific intent of producing glycosuria and weight loss in these girls has been documented.[104] Thus, in young women with IDDM, poor metabolic control may be the result of eating pathology, with binge eating and insulin omission as common features. We have documented a higher incidence of long-term microvascular complications in these girls as they progress to young adulthood.

Recurrent Diabetic Ketoacidosis

During a 5-year period in the mid-1970s, a group of four teenage girls with IDDM provided our house staff with 130 opportunities to manage DKA. Careful attention to educational deficiencies and to the complex psychosocial situations of these four failed to break the pattern of recurrent DKA. This experience is certainly not unique.[40,44,49,131] More recently, however, health care professionals involved with IDDM in young people have become increasingly aware that intentional omission of insulin is overwhelmingly the most common immediate cause of recurrent DKA.[49,67] Schade and colleagues[109] developed a useful algorithm to determine the cause of life-threatening brittle diabetes: more than 90% of their subjects responded normally to insulin, administered subcutaneously or intravenously, effectively ruling out insulin resistance as a cause of this problem.

Golden and associates[49] pointed out that recurrent DKA is a problem of insulin omission; elaborate tests to diagnose its cause are unnecessary. When asked directly, most of these adolescents admit to either omitting or reducing their insulin dose. Weight loss by self-induced glycosuria, attempted suicide, and desire to get out of a dysfunctional family situation have been associated with this behavior. Episodes of DKA cease when responsibility for insulin administration is assumed by a reliable family member, while attempts are made to define and to deal with the underlying reasons. This approach to management of recurrent DKA is simple, logical, and effective. Nevertheless, it was overlooked until recently, with more emphasis placed on the physiologic response to stress as the cause of recurrent DKA rather than nonadherence to the insulin regimen. This way of thinking precluded any expectation that recurrent DKA would cease without long-term psychosocial intervention. Although individual or family therapy is a crucial part of management, this step alone rarely, if ever, eliminates the immediate risk of DKA. To reduce the risk requires guaranteed insulin administration.

Some health care providers still are unwilling to acknowledge or deal with the possibility of intentional insulin omission. They are often concerned about the risk of breaking the patient's or family's trust in the caregiver and interfering with normal adolescent development by asking parents to assume or resume responsibility for the diabetes routines. However, it is apparent from these youngsters' behavior that they need and want additional parental involvement. (See Case Presentation at end of the chapter.)

Surreptitious Insulin Administration

Most studies of youth with IDDM have focused on defining characteristics of those with poor compliance, including those who omit treatment (see recurrent DKA discussion). The opposite—repeated administration of extra insulin—secretly or surreptitiously, has received considerably less attention despite a number of reports in the literature.[6,96,109,128] The prevalence of this syndrome is unknown but most likely much higher than suspected.

The reasons for surreptitious insulin administration may be varied, but most would agree that this behavior invariably indicates a serious underlying psychologic disturbance.[96,109] This behavior may represent a suicidal attempt or gesture. It may also be a misguided attempt to manipulate family members and health care providers.

Suspicion of this syndrome should be triggered when hypoglycemia persists despite an unusually large decrease in perceived insulin dose requirement, particularly in adolescents with IDDM noted to have psychosocial difficulties. Direct confrontation of the adolescent and the family is essential to diagnose the problem. Psychiatric evaluation and therapy are mandatory.

CHRONIC COMPLICATIONS OF DIABETES

Based on the absence of either retinal microvascular changes or incipient nephropathy (defined by the presence of microalbuminuria) in the prepubertal child with IDDM, researchers have speculated that the years of diabetes before the onset of puberty contribute little, if at all, to the risk of the long-term complications related to diabetes.* Recent epidemiologic data support this notion, indicating that postpubertal diabetes duration is a more accurate determinant of the development of microvascular disease and diabetes-related mortality than total duration. For example, Kostraba and associates[76] examined the relationship between diabetic complications and duration, both before and after puberty, in three large cohorts of

---

*References 42, 71, 73, 76, 92.

subjects with IDDM: retinopathy, overt nephropathy, and mortality were all more prevalent in subjects diagnosed during or after puberty than in those diagnosed before puberty. Subtraction of the prepubertal years from the total duration led to disappearance of these differences. Similarly, Klein and associates[71] reported on the relationship between the time of menarche and diabetic retinopathy. The duration of diabetes after menarche conferred about 1.3 times the risk of retinopathy compared with duration before menarche. Murphy and others[92] found this risk to be even greater, about 4.8-fold.

The available data suggest that certain events occurring at puberty contribute or are related to the development of microvascular complications. Although glycemic control often deteriorates during adolescence, other factors would appear to be involved. Recent work suggests that IGF-1, similar to other growth factors, may contribute to angiogenesis and atheromatous lesions. Merimee[87] has postulated a direct association between IGF-1 and retinopathy. Whatever the reason, hyperglycemia and puberty are a potentially sinister combination. Correction of the hyperglycemia may require significant hyperinsulinemia, which is itself a further risk factor to hypertension and macrovascular disease.[103]

It is reassuring that the prepubertal years contribute so little to the development of complications. The fact that the clock starts ticking with puberty, however, highlights the need for health care professionals to be aware of the known and presumed/potential risk factors for the development of diabetes-related macrovascular and microvascular complications. These include (1) metabolic control, (2) hypertension, (3) lipid abnormalities, (4) smoking, and (5) obesity.[2,33,69]

The nature and risk of diabetes-related complications are very sensitive topics for adolescents, their families, and health care providers. However, it is essential that the realities of potential problems be discussed openly and honestly. Teens and their parents need to understand the importance of metabolic control and other factors that may contribute to the development of the complications so that they will have the opportunity to choose behaviors that may reduce their risk.

When adolescents do not adhere to the treatment regimen, parents and health care professionals are often tempted to threaten them with blindness, kidney failure, and loss of limbs. In our experience, threats have no impact on metabolic control and may lead to feelings of hopelessness and helplessness. Alternate and more successful strategies for enhancing compliance in these less mature teens include focusing on the immediate rewards for adherence (e.g., maintaining a high energy level, avoiding parents' nagging) and ensuring adequate parental support in daily diabetes management.

Advanced diabetes-related complications are rare during adolescence; thus it is essential that the focus be on anticipatory steps *(complication surveillance)*. These include routine blood pressure measurements and eye examinations, appropriate counseling that stresses avoidance of excess weight gain and cholesterol intake, avoidance of smoking, regular urine checks for protein, and measurement of GHb and serum lipid levels.[23]

Dietary counseling must include information regarding the relationship between hyperlipidemia and macrovascular disease. It is clear that improving metabolic control (by lowering GHb levels) will decrease serum cholesterol and triglyceride levels. However, in the

---

BOX 19-5

GUIDELINES FOR SCREENING FOR DIABETIC RETINOPATHY

1. Patients with type I diabetes should be screened annually for retinopathy beginning 5 years after the onset of diabetes. In general, screening is not indicated before the start of puberty.
2. Patients with type II diabetes should have an initial examination for retinopathy shortly after the diagnosis of diabetes is made.
   a. If dilated ophthalmoscopy is used, then examination should be repeated annually by an ophthalmologist or optometrist who is knowledgeable and experienced in the management of diabetic retinopathy.
   b. If skilled reading of seven-field stereo photographs is available and reveals no retinopathy at the initial screening, the next screening examination does not need to be done for 4 years.
   c. Patients with persistently elevated glucose levels or proteinuria should have yearly examinations. Care should be taken not to lose these patients to follow-up.
   d. After this 4-year examination, subsequent screening with stereo photographs or dilated ophthalmoscopy should be performed annually.
3. When planning pregnancy, women with preexisting diabetes should be counseled on the risk of development or progression of diabetic retinopathy. Women with diabetes who become pregnant should have a comprehensive eye examination in the first trimester and close follow-up throughout pregnancy. This does not apply to women who develop gestational diabetes, because such individuals are not at increased risk for diabetic retinopathy.
4. Patients with clinically significant macular edema, moderate to severe nonproliferative retinopathy, or any proliferative retinopathy require the prompt care of an ophthalmologist who is knowledgeable and experienced in the management of diabetic retinopathy.

Modified from American Diabetes Association position statement: *Diabetes Care* 18(suppl1): 21-23, 1995.

---

adequately "controlled" teen, lowering or maintaining lipid levels will depend on attention to a diet low in total cholesterol intake, specifically, decreasing saturated and increasing polyunsaturated fat intake. Snack foods are a major source of excess fat intake. Timely measurement of serum cholesterol and triglyceride concentrations will help facilitate dietary adjustments. Frequent dietary review in a nonthreatening manner may also help to forestall excess weight gain and the onset or worsening of obesity.

With respect to retinopathy, the American Diabetes Association has issued a position statement called *Eye Care Guidelines for Patients with Diabetes Mellitus.*[3] Box 19-5 lists guidelines of importance to the care of the adolescent with IDDM. These are consistent with the *Clinical Practice Guidelines for the Treatment of Diabetes Mellitus* issued by the Canadian Diabetes Advisory Board.[39]

Experience with teens with IDDM suggests that very few reach the stage of proliferative retinopathy requiring intervention with laser therapy. In teens who exhibit the poorest metabolic control, as evidenced by the presence of Mauriac syndrome, sudden improvement in glucose homeostasis may lead to a rapid deterioration in diabetic retinopathy.[26] This suggests that extra vigilance is required in such teenagers to diagnose and treat proliferative changes before sight is threatened. The reason for the deterioration has not been elucidated but may be related to changes in hormones, specifically GH and IGF-1, that occur during catch-up growth.

Just as the early detection and management of retinopathy may decrease visual loss by more than 80%, so may the detection and management of hypertension decrease the progression of diabetic nephropathy.[90] Whether reduction of blood pressure in normotensive adolescents with IDDM who have incipient nephropathy (microalbuminuria) will be equally effective remains under investigation.[22] The outcome of the latter investigations will dictate whether screening for microalbuminuria is indicated in the normotensive adolescent population with IDDM.[21] A number of studies have revealed that about 5% to 20% of all teens with IDDM have significant microalbuminuria (defined by albumin excretion rates greater than 20 μg/min), suggesting that they are at greatest risk for progression to overt nephropathy.

Reduction of the major risk factors for macrovascular disease (e.g., obesity, lipid abnormalities, hypertension, smoking) during adolescence may have a major positive effect in the long term. The importance of these risk factors in those adolescents with diabetes compared with that in the nondiabetic population is still being examined.

The role of health care providers of adolescents with IDDM is to be aware of the risk factors, provide anticipatory guidance, and detect complications as early as possible. Results of long-term trials will determine whether intensified insulin therapy or the use of specific agents such as those that decrease neuronal sorbitol levels (aldose reductase inhibitors) or intraglomerular pressure (angiotensin-converting enzyme inhibitors) will have a major impact on the development or progression of IDDM complications.

SPECIAL CONSIDERATIONS
Risk-Taking Behaviors

Risk taking is part of the natural expression of independence that all teenagers go through to some extent. Crucial to the psychologic maturation of adolescence is the pursuit of new activities and taking of initiative. Teens do much exploring at a time when their cognitive skills are insufficiently well honed to allow them to make decisions that will keep them out of trouble (e.g., sex without contraception, driving too fast or while drinking, illicit use of drugs and alcohol). They tend to have the idea that they are invulnerable; for example, if a teen drives a car while under the influence of alcohol and does not have an accident, he or she may begin to believe that this risk can safely be taken again. Conversely, for many teens, taking a drink, smoking cigarettes or marijuana, and having sex is, in fact, risk avoidant. It is sometimes easier for these teens to go along with their peers rather than running the risk of being shunned or ridiculed for not "indulging."

Teens with diabetes are no different from their nondiabetic peers in respect to the usual risk-taking behaviors of adolescence. However, the diabetes regimen itself may become a focus for risk taking (e.g., insulin omission, dietary and testing nonadherence). Furthermore, certain risks may be greater in those with diabetes (e.g., alcohol ingestion as a risk factor for acute hypoglycemia, marijuana use as a stimulus to increased food intake, smoking and unplanned pregnancies as risk factors for long-term complications).

Alcohol

Metabolic consequences of alcohol ingestion include inhibition of hepatic gluconeo-genesis, enhanced fatty acid and triglyceride synthesis, impaired hepatic fatty acid oxidation leading to fatty liver, diversion of fatty acids into ketone bodies producing ketosis, and enhanced conversion of pyruvate to lactic acid (producing lactic acidosis).[46] The impact of these metabolic changes on the individual with diabetes may include hypoglycemia (direct effect of alcohol on the liver), hyperglycemia and weight gain (if alcohol ingestion is accompanied by increased caloric intake), hyperlipidemia, gastrointestinal upset, and in the longer term, neurotoxocity and sexual dysfunction.

Adolescents with IDDM should be made aware of all these implications of alcohol use in a nonjudgmental manner. However, the dangers of alcohol use just listed do not imply that those with diabetes must abstain. As a general rule, it is better to educate appropriately about responsible alcohol use rather than to forbid it. Adolescents should be encouraged to wear identification that states that they have diabetes, to drink in moderation if they decide to drink, and not to drive when drinking. To avoid the alcohol-induced hypoglycemia, it is advisable never to drink on an empty stomach or after vigorous exercise. Also, although it may be important to "count" alcohol-derived calories when counseling teens, it is essential not to cut down on food intake during alcohol use.

Only Glasgow and associates[47] have commented on the frequency of alcohol use in teens with IDDM: of 101 adolescents surveyed, 49 denied any alcohol use, 26 admitted to having tried it, 19 to occasional use, and only 7 to alcohol use once or twice a week. Alcohol use was more common among older patients and among white compared with black youngsters.

Smoking and drug abuse

Most teens try smoking cigarettes or some form of tobacco use at some stage. Only some will become regular users. The same is likely also true for the use of street drugs. Educational programs are required that stress the risks of tobacco use and drugs in general and to the diabetic teen in particular (i.e., the relationship of smoking to the macrovascular and microvascular complications of the disease). Adolescents experiment with and continue to use these substances for a variety of reasons, including peer pressure, risk taking and experimentation, feeling "grown up," pleasurable relief from anxiety, and imitation of family members.

Primary prevention should start during the early school years and continue through adolescence. Education programs should focus on providing information to help young people make responsible decisions regarding the use of drugs and tobacco. If they are to be successful, such programs must take into account the teen's social context. Programs that use teen role models and peers are more likely to be successful than those that appear to the teen to be yet another example of the "establishment" preaching at them. Health care providers are obliged to ensure that their young patients are aware of the special hazards and risks in using these agents; tobacco use may accelerate the development of microvascular and macrovascular disease.

The impact of other "recreational drugs" in diabetes has been less extensively investigated. Nevertheless, certain drugs cause a change in appetite and alter level of awareness and concentration, effects that may interfere with safe diabetes management.[35] Because use of these agents is so common among adolescents, one should routinely ask about their use. Establishing open dialogue with these teens may allow them to seek sound answers to their questions and discuss their concerns. Indications of drug use, such as deterioration in school performance, personality change, mood swings, sleeplessness, or fatigue, should be assessed. When drug abuse is suspected, the issue needs to be addressed in a sensitive, nonjudgmental manner. The teen's motivation for drug use and extent of use must be explored. This information will help guide the health care provider in making appropriate decisions about the need for referral for further assessment or treatment.

Little information exists about the prevalence or incidence of concurrent diabetes and drug use or dependency.[113] In two studies of adult intravenous drug users, 1.4% of 2911 and 3.2% of 1780 individuals in Baltimore and New York, respectively, volunteered a history of diabetes.[15,94] In the report of Glasgow and colleagues,[47] only 1 of 97 consecutive urine specimens from adolescents with diabetes was positive for marijuana. This compares with a 24% positive rate among teens attending the adolescent clinic at the same hospital.[112] About 20% of teens in Glasgow's study reported having tried drugs, with none admitting to frequent use. The reported use of drugs in these studies is lower than might be expected from studies in the nondiabetic population.[15]

Contraception and avoidance of sexually transmitted diseases

Those involved in the continuing care of adolescents with diabetes have an excellent opportunity and an obligation to provide teens with accurate information and a forum for discussion of sexuality and sexual activity. No evidence indicates that youth with IDDM are more susceptible to sexually transmitted diseases (STDs). However, as with their peers, they need to be informed about the risks of STDs and how they can be prevented by safe-sex practices, including avoidance of sexual contact with an infected person and routine use of condoms.

Information and counseling regarding sexuality and contraception should not be limited to adolescent girls. Young men also need to understand methods of birth control and where to obtain advice and help. For example, one misguided adolescent male was responsible for his girlfriend's unplanned pregnancy because he believed himself to be sterile because of his diabetes. Furthermore, many teenage boys with diabetes fear the possibility of impotence. They should be reassured that this problem rarely affects the teenage population; however, the possibility that it may occur at a later stage in their lives should be addressed as questions arise.

In sexually active girls with IDDM, contraception is essential to avoid unwanted pregnancies. Again, anticipatory guidance is required. Although use of oral contraceptives may occasionally be associated with such complications as deterioration in metabolic control, hypertension, and hyperlipidemia, these agents constitute the preferred method of contraception for the adolescent with diabetes. In fact, recent data from Klein and associates[72] failed to reveal an association between either current or past use of oral contraceptives and severity of retinopathy, hypertension, or current metabolic control. Thus the risks of unwanted pregnancies and abortions most likely far outweigh those from use of oral contraceptives.

Driving

Most countries have laws that limit to some degree the rights of individuals with diabetes to operate motor vehicles in an unrestricted fashion. These restrictions have been based on the acute threat of hypoglycemia in insulin-requiring individuals and the chronic complications such as retinopathy, coronary disease, and hypertension in those with longer-standing disease. Unfortunately the laws are not based on appropriate data, and studies are under way to establish whether individuals with IDDM do in fact constitute an increased risk on the roads. A recent case control study by Songer and associates[114] attempted to examine accident rates for a cohort of individuals with IDDM and their relationship to hypoglycemia. In brief, the overall accident risk rate did not differ between persons with diabetes and control subjects; however, female drivers with diabetes did show a marked increased risk for accidents. Furthermore, in 9 of 11 individuals who admitted that a health-related problem was the cause of the accident, hypoglycemia was the recorded reason. In the other two, limited vision was the cause noted. Clearly, more data are required to assess the association between diabetes and accident risk.

Based on the available data, most countries require physician notification of the condition of the disease and the occurrence of any episodes of severe hypoglycemia, particularly while driving. In addition, many countries forbid insulin-requiring persons with diabetes from driving commercial vehicles.[100] Box 19-6 lists guidelines for safe driving.

Employment

Most health care providers are likely to be asked by their adolescents with IDDM about educational and employment opportunities. Even if not asked, these subjects should be broached as part of ongoing care. Two questions require attention: (1) Are there any jobs not available to individuals with IDDM? and (2) Do employers tend to be discriminatory in their hiring practice when it comes to employing these individuals? The answer to both questions is "yes."

A number of industries do not employ people with diabetes for specific jobs and will remove employees from such positions should they acquire diabetes. Since blanket rules prevent operation of commercial vehicles, trains, and aircraft by individuals with IDDM, employment in these positions is impossible in most places. Similarly, the military in many countries has traditionally denied employment to those with diabetes; recently in some countries, military employment in noncombat positions has been allowed. The same is true in many police forces. Before applying for a particular educational or employment opportunity, individuals with IDDM should inquire as to their employability in these areas. For example, it would be unwise for an adolescent to enter training in criminology at a college,

---

BOX 19-6

SAFE DRIVING GUIDELINES FOR ADOLESCENTS WITH DIABETES

1. Teens about to obtain their driver's permits should be fully informed once again about the hazards of hypoglycemia and its prevention.
2. They should be instructed to keep a source of concentrated carbohydrate readily available at all times (e.g., packet of glucose tablets in the glove compartment) as well as identification stating that they have diabetes.
3. They should avoid driving at a time when hypoglycemia is most likely, such as immediately after vigorous exercise. Rather, they should take some food to prevent possible hypoglycemia and monitor their blood glucose before driving again to ensure that it is in a "safe" range.
4. They should perform SMBG regularly as a method of preventing hypoglycemia.
5. They should have regular medical checkups and report immediately any episodes of severe hypoglycemia or visual problems.

---

only to find out years later that he or she is not eligible for employment by the local police force. The health care team can provide important counseling and support in these situations.

Employer discrimination has been documented in some recent reports both from the United States and United Kingdom.[102,115] Songer and others [115] report that individuals who told job interviewers about their diabetes were more likely to experience job refusal than were their nondiabetic siblings, whereas if they did not mention their diabetes, employment rates were similar.

Furthermore, Robinson[102] found that people with diabetes had to change their jobs more frequently because of their illness and (particularly shift workers) experienced more problems with their jobs than did control subjects. Absenteeism from work was similar in persons with diabetes and control subjects in both these studies.

In the report of Tebbi and associates,[126] young adults with IDDM appeared about as successful in obtaining and maintaining employment as a control group, despite an apparent deficit in their perceived general well-being. Those with diabetes seemed more likely to experience job-related problems; the results, however, did not suggest a pervasive deficit in overall job adjustment and performance.

The young person with IDDM seeking employment should be encouraged to stress personal qualifications, abilities, and ambitions to prospective employers. They should not withhold information about their diabetes from these employers and should not expect particular concessions, such as "better" shift rotations or more frequent sick leave. Satisfactory employment will depend on an enlightened attitude of both the employer and the employee. Diabetes should not be allowed to prevent productive employment. Young adults with diabetes, 18 years of age and older, who are experiencing difficulty acquiring and maintaining employment may be eligible for vocational rehabilitation services. These services vary from country to country and state to state but generally help with job training and placement. Individuals who believe they have suffered job discrimination should be encouraged to seek counsel from Human Rights Commissions or other employee advocate groups.

Transition From Pediatric to Adult Diabetes Care

Most children and adolescents with IDDM receive ongoing care from health professionals experienced in pediatric diabetes. This system, although ideal in many respects, ultimately leads to a disruption in the continuity of medical care. There comes a time when the teen must leave the nurturing environment of the pediatric center and establish himself or herself with an adult center. When the shift in care is abrupt and the adolescent and his or her family are poorly prepared to deal with transition, regular follow-up may cease. Recent data show that 25% of adolescents graduating from our diabetes clinic at age 18 years dropped out of medical care for months to years, resurfacing when they experienced a diabetes-related crisis that otherwise may have been averted.[41]

An extended transition period and anticipatory guidance may ease the teenager's transfer to adult diabetes care. Teens who are approaching "graduation" from the clinic should understand the reasons for ongoing regular medical care, specifically to maintain good metabolic control and screen for or treat the complications of IDDM. In addition, they should have the opportunity to discuss various options for ongoing care and be prepared for a health care approach that may differ from that used in the pediatric center. They may need coaching on how to be a "good" consumer of health services. Finally, the pediatric diabetes team can facilitate the teen's transition by making the first appointment at the adult center and contacting the teen after the visit to discuss the success of the transfer.

Perhaps the ideal method of providing comprehensive care to adolescents and young adults with IDDM is through a transition clinic where pediatric and adult specialists join forces to provide developmentally appropriate care. Baum and Kinmonth[7] have used this approach and described that it reduced the dropout rate from 20% to 3%.

RESEARCH DIRECTIONS

Several directions of research that should be encouraged to better understand and manage the adolescent with IDDM are as follows:

1. Studies of IDDM pathogenesis and immune modulation must necessarily include the late childhood and adolescent population because this is the group at greatest risk for developing the disease. Studies that employ only adults with new-onset IDDM may provide some confusing data because there may be contamination of the study group with non-insulin-dependent diabetic patients and also because IDDM has been noted to have a less severe course when it begins later in life.

2. Research must be directed at improving our understanding of the reasons for deteriorating metabolic control in the adolescent population. These studies must focus on the interaction between biologic and psychosocial factors.

3. Given the results of the DCCT, health care providers must focus efforts on finding and evaluating the most appropriate methods for ensuring a more intensive approach to the management and education of teens with diabetes.

4. The earliest lesions of diabetic microvascular disease must be sought in adolescents and methods developed for halting or slowing their progression.

SUMMARY

This chapter has reviewed both physical and psychologic factors having an impact on adolescents with diabetes. We have strived to paint a picture of hope: most teens with diabetes achieve adequate to good degrees of metabolic control and make a satisfactory transition to self-care and young adulthood. For those in whom adolescence is a stormy period, every effort must be made to define the cause(s) of their problems and construct therapeutic interventions that can best help them achieve mastery over their condition.

CASE PRESENTATION

A 15-year-old girl with IDDM of 3 years' duration was referred to our hospital after a 7-week admission to a community hospital following repeated episodes of moderate to severe DKA. Frequent attempts to discharge her from that hospital had been associated with hyperglycemia and ketosis, necessitating prolongation of the admission.

Of note is that her diabetes control had been very good from onset until about 15 months before referral. At that time her blood glucose concentrations became more erratic, and the episodes of DKA began to occur. At the same time her school attendance and performance deteriorated. Her local physician performed multiple tests, including thyroid, renal, and liver function tests; abdominal ultrasound; and insulin antibodies. When all these were found to be normal and her episodes of DKA increased in frequency, she was admitted to hospital. The continuation of poor control in hospital was the reason for her transfer to our center.

DISCUSSION

Our working diagnosis was that of insulin omission as the cause of recurrent DKA and poor metabolic control. Review of the practice at the community hospital revealed that this girl had been "giving" her own injections without supervision both at home for the past 18 months and during her hospital admissions. Attempts by the nursing staff to observe her injection technique were met with oppositional behavior, and each time the staff "backed off." We instituted a routine whereby *all* injections were given by the nursing staff, and the teen and her mother underwent psychosocial evaluation. The results in terms of metabolic control were immediate and impressive: frequent hypoglycemia demanded a decrease in her "prescribed" dose, and excellent metabolic control was established within a few days. Psychosocial evaluation was revealing in that her parents had separated 2 years before, and her mother had been seeing another man for the past year. The patient felt depressed, perhaps suicidal at times, and had become quite dissatisfied with "the way she looked." This had led to repeated cycles of binge eating and dieting, with insulin omission as an attempt to prevent weight gain and induce weight loss.

At discharge from the hospital, the mother was giving the insulin injections, metabolic control was stable, and ongoing family counseling had been instituted. Follow-up over the following 9 months revealed ongoing supervision of injections with stable diabetes control. However, problems were being encountered very frequently with regard to attendance at ongoing counseling, poor self-esteem, and occasional episodes of binge eating.

REFERENCES

1. Ahlfield JE, Soler NG, Marcus SD: The young adult with diabetes: impact of the disease on marriage and having children, *Diabetes Care* 8:52-56, 1985.
2. American Diabetes Association consensus statement: Role of cardiovascular risk factors in prevention and treatment of macrovascular disease in diabetes, *Diabetes Care* 12:573-579,1989.
3. American Diabetes Association position statement: Screening for diabetic retinopathy, *Diabetes Care* 18(suppl 1): 21-23, 1995.
4. Amiel S and others: Impaired insulin action in puberty: a contributing factor to poor glycemic control in adolescents with diabetes, *N Engl J Med* 315:215-219, 1986.
5. Anderson B and others: Effects of peer-group intervention on metabolic control of adolescents with IDDM: randomized outpatient study, *Diabetes Care* 12:179-183, 1985.
6. Arem R. Zogbhi W: Insulin overdose in eight patients: insulin pharmacokinetics and review of the literature, *Medicine* 64:323 332, 1985.
7. Baum JD, Kinmonth AL: *Care of the child with diabetes,* New York, 1985, Churchill Livingstone.
8. Beal C: Body size and growth rate of children with diabetes mellitus, *J Pediatr* 32:170-179, 1948.
9. Belmonte M and others: Impact of SMBG on control of diabetes as measured by HbA1:3-year survey of a juvenile IDDM clinic, *Diabetes Care* 11:484-488, 1988.
10. Bibace R, Walsh ME: Development of children's concept of illness, *Pediatrics* 66:912-917, 1980.
11. Blethen S and others: Effect of pubertal stage and recent blood glucose control on plasma somatomedin C in children with insulin-dependent diabetes mellitus, *Diabetes* 30:868-872, 1981.
12. Bloch C, Clemons P, Sperling M: Puberty decreases insulin sensitivity, *J Pediatr* 110:481-487, 1987.
13. Blum R: Compliance with therapeutic regimens among children and youth. In Blum RW, editor: *Chronic illness and disabilities in children and adolescence,* Orlando, Fla, 1984, Grune & Stratton.
14. Bobrow ES, AvRuskin TW, Siller J: Mother-daughter interaction and adherence to diabetes regimen, *Diabetes Care* 8:146-151, 1985.
15. Brown LS: Clinical aspects of drug abuse in diabetes, *Diabetes Spectrum* 4:45-47, 1991.
16. Bynam L, Vickery C: Compliance and health promotion, *Health Values* 12:5-12, 1988.
17. Cerreto MC, Travis LB: Implications of psychological and family factors in the treatment of diabetes, *Pediatr Clin North Am* 31:689-710, 1984.
18. Christensen N and others: Quantitative assessment of dietary adherence in patients with insulin-dependent diabetes mellitus, *Diabetes Care* 6:245-250, 1983.
19. Clarson C and others: The relationship of metabolic control to growth and pubertal development in children with insulin-dependent diabetes, *Diabetes Res* 2:237-341, 1985.
20. Collier A and others: Comparison of intravenous glucagon and dextrose in treatment of severe hypoglycemia in an accident and emergency department, *Diabetes Care* 10:712-715, 1987.
21. Cook J, Daneman D: Microalbuminuria in adolescents with insulin dependent diabetes mellitus, *Am J Dis Child* 144:234-237, 1990.
22. Cook J and others: Angiotensin converting enzyme inhibitor therapy to decrease microalbuminuria in normotensive children with insulin-dependent diabetes mellitus, *J Pediatr* 117:39-45, 1990.
23. Daneman D: Glycated hemoglobin in the assessment of diabetes control, *Endocrinologist* 4:33-43, 1994.
24. Daneman D, Ehrlich R: Children with insulin-dependent diabetes mellitus, *Med Clin North Am* 15:2926-2934, 1987.
25. Daneman D and others: Factors affecting glycosylated hemoglobin values in children with insulin-dependent diabetes, *J Pediatr* 99:847-853, 1981.
26. Daneman D and others: Progressive retinopathy with improved control in diabetic dwarfism (Mauriac syndrome), *Diabetes Care* 4:360-365, 1981.
27. Daneman D and others: Severe hypoglycemia in children with insulin-dependent diabetes mellitus: frequency and predisposing factors, *J Pediatr* 115:681-685, 1989.
28. Daniel WA: Impact of diabetes on adolescents, *Texas Med* 71:56-60, 1975.
29. Delahanty L, Halford BN: The role of diet behaviors in achieving improved glycemic control in intensively treated patients in the Diabetes Control and Complications Trial, *Diabetes Care* 16:1453-1458, 1993.
30. The Diabetes Control and Complications Trial (DCCT) Research Group: DCCT: results of feasibility study, *Diabetes Care* 10:1-19, 1987.
31. The Diabetes Control and Complications Trial (DCCT) Research Group: Weight gain associated with intensive therapy in the DCCT, *Diabetes Care* 11:567-573, 1988.
32. The Diabetes Control and Complications Trial (DCCT) Research Group: Epidemiology of hypoglycemia in the DCCT, *Am J Med* 90:450-459, 1991.
33. The Diabetes Control and Complications Trial (DCCT) Research Group: DCCT: the effect of

intensive treatment of diabetes on the development and progression of long-term complications in insulin-dependent diabetes mellitus, *N Engl J Med* 329:977-986, 1993.

34. The Diabetes Control and Complications Trial (DCCT) Research Group: Effect of intensive diabetes treatment on the development and progression of long-term complications in adolescents with insulin-dependent diabetes mellitus: DCCT, *J Pediatr* 125:177-188, 1994.

35. Dinwiddie S: Psychiatric aspects of drug abuse in diabetes, *Diabetes Spectrum* 3:353-356, 1990.

36. Drash A: *Clinical care of the diabetic child,* St Louis, 1987, Mosby.

37. Emans SJ: The sexually active teenager, *Dev Behav Pediatr* 4:37, 1983.

38. Erikson E: *Identity, youth and crisis,* New York, 1968, Norton.

39. Expert Committee of the Canadian Diabetes Advisory Board: Clinical practice guidelines for treatment of diabetes mellitus, *Can Med Assoc J* 147:697-712, 1992.

40. Flexner C and others: Repeated hospitalization for diabetic ketoacidosis, *Am J Med* 76:691-695, 1984.

41. Frank M, Perlman K, Ehrlich R: Factors contributing to non-compliance with medical follow-up after discharge from a pediatric diabetes clinic, *Diabetes* 39:55A, 1990.

42. Frank R and others: Retinopathy in juvenile-onset type 1 diabetes of short duration, *Diabetes* 31:874-882, 1982.

43. Freud A: Adolescence, *Psychoanal Stud Child* 13:255-278, 1958.

44. Fulop M: Recurrent diabetic ketoacidosis, *Am J Med* 78:54-60, 1985.

45. Gale E: The frequency of hypoglycemia in insulin-treated diabetic patients. In Serrano-Rios M, Lefebvre P, editors: *Diabetes,* Amsterdam, 1985, Elsevier.

46. Gaudiani L, Feingold K: Alcohol and diabetes: mix with caution, *Clin Diabetes* 2:121-132, 1984.

47. Glasgow AM and others: Alcohol and drug use in teenagers with diabetes, *Adolesc Health* 12:11-14, 1991.

48. Gokey D: Improving adherence: getting patients to stick to an intensive regimen, *Diabetes Spectrum* 6:140-145, 1992.

49. Golden M, Herold A, Orr D: An approach to prevention of recurrent diabetic ketoacidosis in the pediatric population, *J Pediatr* 107:195-200, 1985.

50. Goldstein D: Is glycosylated hemoglobin clinically useful? *N Engl J Med* 310:384-385, 1984.

51. Grossman HY: The adolescent with insulin-dependent diabetes mellitus: psychological considerations. In Brink SJ: *Pediatric and adolescent diabetes mellitus,* Chicago, 1987, Year Book.

52. Grossman HY, Brink S, Hauser ST: Self-efficacy in adolescent girls and boys with insulin-dependent diabetes mellitus, *Diabetes Care* 10:324-329, 1987.

53. Hancock LA, Fast GP: Adolescence. In Edelman C, Mandel C, editors: *Health promotion throughout the lifespan,* ed 2, St Louis, 1990, Mosby.

54. Hauenstein E and others: Stress in parents of children with diabetes mellitus, *Diabetes Care* 12:18-22, 1989.

55. Havlin C, Cryer P: Nocturnal hypoglycemia does not commonly result in major morning hyperglycemia in patients with diabetes mellitus, *Diabetes Care* 10:141-147, 1987.

56. Haynes RB, Taylor DW, Sackett DL: *Compliance in health care,* Baltimore, 1979, Johns Hopkins University Press.

57. Hays RD, DiMatteo MR: Patient compliance assessment, *J Compliance Health Care* 2:27-53, 1981.

58. Ingersoll G and others: Cognitive maturity and self-management among adolescents with insulin-dependent diabetes mellitus, *J Pediatr* 108:620-623, 1986.

59. Inhelder B, Piaget J: *The growth of logical thinking from childhood to adolescence,* New York, 1958, Basic.

60. Jackson R: Growth and development of children with diabetes mellitus, *Diabetes* 2:90-92, 1953.

61. Jackson R and others: Growth and maturation of children with insulin-dependent diabetes mellitus, *Diabetes Care* 1:96-107, 1978.

62. Jacobson A and others: Psychological adjustment of children with recently diagnosed diabetes mellitus, *Diabetes Care* 9:323-329, 1986.

63. Jacobson A and others: Psychologic prediction of compliance in children with recent onset of diabetes mellitus, *J Pediatr* 110:805-811, 1987.

64. Johnson S: Psychological aspects of childhood diabetes, *J Child Psychol Psychiatry* 29:729-738, 1988.

65. Johnson S, Rosenbloom A: Behavioral aspects of diabetes mellitus in childhood and adolescence, *Psychiatr Clin North Am* 5:357-369, 1982.

66. Johnson S and others: Assessing daily management in childhood diabetes, *Health Psychol* 5:545-564, 1986.

67. Kanimer Y, Robbins D: Insulin misuse: a review of an overlooked psychiatric problem, *Psychosomatics* 30:19-24, 1989.

68. Kaplan R, Chadwick M, Schimmel L: Social learning intervention to promote control in type 1 diabetes mellitus: pilot experiment results, *Diabetes Care* 8:152-155, 1985.

69. Keen H: Chronic complications of diabetes mellitus. In Galloway J, Potvin J, Shuman C, ed-

itors: *Diabetes mellitus,* ed 9, Indianapolis, 1988, Lilly.

70. Kellerman J and others: Psychological effects of illness in adolescence. 1. Anxiety, self-esteem, and perception of control, *J Pediatr* 97:126-131, 1990.

71. Klein B, Moss S, Klein R: Is menarche associated with diabetic retinopathy? *Diabetes Care* 13:1034-1038, 1990.

72. Klein B, Moss S, Klein R: Oral contraceptives in women with diabetes, *Diabetes Care* 13:895-898, 1990.

73. Klein R and others: Glycosylated hemoglobin predicts the incidence and progression of diabetic retinopathy, *JAMA* 260:2864-2871, 1988.

74. Knowles H and others: The course of juvenile diabetes treated with unmeasured diet, *Diabetes* 14:239-273, 1965.

75. Koski ML: The coping processes in childhood diabetes, *Acta Pediatr Scand* 188(suppl):7-56, 1969.

76. Kostraba J and others: Contribution of diabetes duration before puberty to development of microvascular complications in IDDM subjects, *Diabetes Care* 12:686-693, 1989.

77. Kovacs M and others: Initial coping responses and psychosocial characteristics of children with insulin-dependent diabetes mellitus, *J Pediatr* 106:827-834, 1985.

78. Kovacs M and others: Initial psychologic responses of parents to the diagnosis of insulin-dependent diabetes mellitus in their children, *Diabetes Care* 8:568-575, 1985.

79. Kovacs M and others: Children's self-reports of psychologic adjustment and coping strategies during first year of insulin-dependent diabetes mellitus, *Diabetes Care* 9:472-479, 1986.

80. Kurtz SM: Adherence to diabetes regimens: empirical status and clinical applications, *Diabetes Educ* 16:50-55, 1990.

81. Larsson Y, Sterky G: Long-term prognosis in juvenile diabetes mellitus, *Acta Pediatr Scand* 130(suppl S1):20-21, 1962.

82. Lerman I, Wolfsdorf J: Relationship of nocturnal hypoglycemia to daytime glycemia in IDDM, *Diabetes Care* 11:636-642, 1988.

83. Littlefield C and others: The relationship of self-efficacy and bingeing to adherence to diabetes regimen among adolescents, *Diabetes Care* 15:90-94, 1992.

84. MacDonald M: Postexercise late-onset hypoglycemia in insulin-dependent diabetic patients, *Diabetes Care* 10:584-588, 1987.

85. Marrero DG and others: Problem-focused versus emotion-focused coping styles in adolescent diabetes, *Pediatr Adolesc Endocrinol* 10:141-146, 1982.

86. Mauriac P: Hepatomegalies de l'enfants avecs troubles de la croissance et due metabolisme des glucide, *Paris Med* 2:525-528, 1934.

87. Merimee T: A follow-up of study of vascular disease in growth-hormone deficient dwarfs with diabetes, *N Engl J Med* 298:1217-1222, 1978.

88. Millstein SG, Adler NE, Irwin CE: Conceptions of illness in young adolescents, *Pediatrics* 68:834-839, 1981.

89. Minuchin S, Rosman B, Baker L: *Psychosomatic families,* Cambridge, Mass, 1978, Harvard University Press.

90. Mogenson C, Christensen C: Predicting diabetic nephropathy in insulin dependent patients, *N Engl J Med* 311:89-93, 1984.

91. Moynihan P and others: *Diabetes youth curriculum: a tool for educators,* Waysata, Minn, 1988, Diabetes Center.

92. Murphy R and others: The relationship of puberty to the onset of diabetic retinopathy, *Arch Ophthalmol* 108:215-218, 1990.

93. Natapoff JN: A developmental analysis of children's ideas of health, *Health Educ Q* 9:34-45, 1982.

94. Nelson KE and others: Diabetes is protective against HIV infections in IV drug users. In *Proceedings of the Sixth International Conference on AIDS,* San Francisco, 1990, Abstract FC 109.

95. Orr DP, Ingersoll GM: Adolescent development: a biopsychosocial review, *Curr Probl Pediatr* 18:441-499, 1988.

96. Orr D and others: Surreptitious insulin administration in adolescents with insulin-dependent diabetes mellitus, *JAMA* 256:3227-3230, 1986.

97. Perrin JM, MacLean WE: Children with chronic illness: the prevention of dysfunction, *Pediatr Clin North Am* 35:1325-1337, 1988.

98. Peyrot M, Rubin RR: Structure and correlates of diabetes-specific locus of control, *Diabetes Care* 17:994-1001, 1994.

99. Press M, Tamborlane W, Sherwin R: Importance of raised growth hormone levels in mediating the metabolic derangements of diabetes, *N Engl J Med* 310:810-815, 1984.

100. Ratner R, Whitehouse F: Motor vehicles, hypoglycemia, and diabetic drivers, *Diabetes Care* 12:217-222, 1989.

101. Reaven G: Role of insulin resistance in human disease, *Diabetes* 37:1595-1607, 1988.

102. Robinson N: Employment of people with diabetes in the United Kingdom, *Diabetes Care* 13:538-539, 1990.

103. Rodin G, Daneman D: Eating disorders and insulin-dependent diabetes mellitus: a problematic association, *Diabetes Care* 15:1402-1412, 1992.

104. Rodin G and others: Eating disorders in female adolescents with insulin-depdent diabetes mellitus, *Int J Psychiatr Med* 16:49-57, 1986.

105. Rodin G and others: Eating disorders and intentional insulin undertreatment in adolescent females with diabetes, *Psychosomatics* 32:171-176, 1991.

106. Rosenstock I: Understanding and enhancing patient compliance with diabetic regimens, *Diabetes Care* 8:610-616, 1985.

107. Rosmark B and others: Eating disorders in patients with insulin-dependent diabetes mellitus, *J Clin Psychol* 47:547-550, 1988.

108. Rutter M and others: Adolescent turmoil: fact or fiction? *J Child Psychol Psychiatry* 17:35-56, 1976.

109. Schade D and others: The etiology of incapacitating, brittle diabetes, *Diabetes Care* 8:12-20, 1985.

110. Schafer LC, Glasgow GE, McCaul KD: Adherence to IDDM regimens: relationship to psychosocial variables and metabolic control, *Diabetes Care* 6:493-498, 1983.

111. Schafer LC, McCaul K, Glasgow GE: Supportive and nonsupportive family behaviors: relationship to adherence and metabolic control in persons with Type 1 diabetes, *Diabetes Care* 9:179-185, 1986.

112. Silber TJ and others: Adolescent marijuana use: concordance between questionnaire and immunoassay for Cannabinoid metabolites, *J Pediatr* 111:299-303, 1987.

113. Sochett E and others: Factors affecting and patterns of residual insulin secretion during the first year of Type 1 diabetes mellitus in children, *Diabetologia* 30:453-459, 1987.

114. Songer T and others: Motor vehicle accidents and IDDM, *Diabetes Care* 11:701-707, 1988.

115. Songer T and others: Employment spectrum of IDDM, *Diabetes Care* 12:615-622, 1989.

116. Stanhope R, Brook C: An evaluation of hormonal changes at puberty in man, *J Endocrinol* 116:301-305, 1988.

117. Sterky G: Diabetic school children, *Acta Pediatr Scand* 144(suppl 1):1-36, 1963.

118. Sullivan B: Adjustment in diabetic adolescent girls. I. Development of the diabetic adjustment scale, *Psychosomat Med* 41:119-126, 1979.

119. Sullivan B: Adjustment in diabetic adolescent girls. II. Adjustment, self-esteem, and depression in diabetic adolescent girls, *Psychosomat Med* 41:127-138, 1979.

120. Surwit R, Scovern A, Feinglos M: The role of behavior in diabetes care, *Diabetes Care* 5:337-342, 1982.

121. Swift CR, Seidman F, Stein H: Adjustment problems in juvenile diabetes, *Psychosomat Med* 29:555-571, 1967.

122. Tamborlane W: Personal communication, 1991.

123. Tanner J: *Growth at adolescence,* ed 2, Oxford, 1962, Blackwell.

124. Tattersal R, Pyke D: Growth in diabetic children: studies in identical twins, *Lancet* 1:1105-1109, 1973.

125. Tattersall RB, Lowe J: Diabetes in adolescence, *Diabetologia* 20:517-523, 1981.

126. Tebbi C and others: Vocational adjustment and general well-being in young adults with IDDM, *Diabetes Care* 13:98-103, 1990.

127. Travis L: Hypoglycemia in insulin-dependent diabetes mellitus, *J Pediatr* 115:740-741, 1989.

128. Weintrob N and others: Severe hypoglycemia and hepatic dysfunction due to surreptitious insulin overdose, *J Pediatr Endocrinol* 3:277-280, 1989.

129. Wesolowski C: Self-contracts for chronically ill children, *Matern Child Nurs* 13:20-23, 1988.

130. Wexler P: The social worker and the child with juvenile diabetes mellitus. In Traisman HJS, editor: *Management of juvenile diabetes mellitus,* St Louis, 1980, Mosby.

131. White K and others: Unstable diabetes and unstable families: a psychosocial evaluation of diabetic children with recurrent ketoacidosis, *Pediatrics* 73:749-755, 1984.

132. Zinman B: Exercise in diabetes treatment, *Clin Diabetes* 1:18-22, 1983.

20 Diabetes Mellitus in Young and Middle Adulthood

James A. Fain and Gail D'Eramo-Melkus

Diabetes mellitus is a chronic illness that can occur at any age throughout the life span. The period of young adulthood (20s and 30s) is often thought to begin with separating from parents, seeking education and a career, and finding a partner with whom to share one's life. It is conceptualized as a time when individuals are willing to unite their identity with others. In general, by young adulthood, individuals reach the highest level of intellectual efficiency and cognitive development. Middle adulthood (40s and 50s) represents a stage of self-review—a time of questioning accomplishments, successes, and value to society. During both periods the impact of diabetes mellitus affects physical, cognitive, and psychosocial aspects of development.

This chapter discusses the physical, cognitive, and psychosocial tasks of young and

---

CHAPTER OBJECTIVES

- Identify physical changes associated with young and middle adulthood.
- Contrast the cognitive abilities of the young adult with those of the middle-age adult.
- Differentiate normal psychosocial tasks of development in young and middle adulthood.
- Discuss specific health needs of the young adult with diabetes.
- Describe the impact of drug and alcohol abuse in young adulthood.
- Discuss unique health problems associated with diabetes in middle adulthood.
- Outline sociocultural and economic factors that can affect young and middle-age adults with diabetes.
- Describe the role of the health care team in providing care to individuals in young and middle adulthood.

middle adulthood. It is important, however, that the health care team considers all changes as interrelated processes that affect and are affected by each other.

NORMAL PHYSICAL TASKS OF DEVELOPMENT IN YOUNG ADULTHOOD

Young adulthood is thought to be the healthiest time of life. During a 15-year span (20 to 35), the young adult's physical abilities are at a peak, with body systems compensating optimally during illness.[29] Physical growth is usually completed by age 20, and muscular strength is at peak efficiency by ages 25 to 30. The young adult can expect to have strong muscles and bones free from serious infections or degenerative disease. Physical stamina is usually sufficient to keep up with all the social, economic, and emotional tasks of this period.

Ninety percent of adult height and weight is attained during young adulthood.[29] Body shape and proportions finally reach their finished state, with the exception of weight and muscle mass. Fat accumulation and muscle mass are under more environmental influence (diet, exercise) and may fluctuate throughout a person's life. Skeletal development is completed as the long bones of the upper legs and arms finish their ossification process. Attainment of final adult height coincides with epiphyseal fusion. A few millimeters may be added to the width of some bones later by surface deposition. Head length and breadth, facial diameters, and the width of bones in the legs and hands may increase slightly by this process throughout life.

Muscles continue to gain strength throughout the 20s and reach peak strength at about age 30, depending on exercise and genetic endowment. Men have larger muscles that can produce more force than the muscle tissue of women. Men also have a greater capacity for carrying oxygen in the blood to the muscles and a greater capacity for neutralizing the chemical products of exercising muscle. Dental maturity is finally achieved in the 20s with the emergence of the last four molars, or wisdom teeth.

During young adulthood the senses are functioning appropriately. Ocular functioning is completely developed by age 20 and starts to decline during middle adulthood. Hearing is best at age 20, with higher-tone sounds tending to be gradually lost. The other senses of touch, smell, and taste remain intact until ages 45 to 50.[29]

The peak efficiency of cardiac output, which was achieved during adolescence, continues throughout the adult years to accommodate typical activity.[29] Changes in heart size and cardiac function occur with age and have a direct relationship to major risk factors, such as hypertension, diabetes, elevated serum cholesterol and lipids, lack of exercise, cigarette smoking, obesity, and stress.

AGE-RELATED VARIATIONS IN HEALTH PRACTICES
Health Practices in Young Adulthood

Young adulthood is a time when one searches for a place in society. Finding a mate, establishing a family, and initiating a career are major tasks to be accomplished.[38] In all instances the ability to integrate cognitive and socioemotional skills becomes critical. For some, their self-esteem and struggle for self-fulfillment will decrease when certain expectations are not met. Although physical health tends to be at a heightened stage, certain risk behaviors may develop, further affecting long-term health into middle adulthood. Within this period of development, health care providers must be aware of the individual's tendency and awareness for altering attitudes and behaviors that present major problems. Drug and alcohol abuse, automobile accidents, and stress-related illnesses present a major threat to the health of young adults.[29]

Drug Abuse

It is estimated that 58% of young adults have some experience in the use of marijuana, whereas 20% have tried stronger drugs, such as cocaine or hallucinogens. Medically prescribed drugs are another source of experimentation. Used alone or together, barbiturates, amphetamines, and sedative-hypnotics reportedly bring about feelings of physical and psychologic well-being. In contrast to adolescents, the young adult tends to restrict drug use, selecting only a few. Adolescents are more likely to experiment with a variety of drugs. Drug abuse continues to be associated with homicides, suicides, and inability to cope with adult responsibilities. Physical health problems account for more than 50% of the major acute and chronic problems of young adults who abuse drugs. Heroin users, for example, have a higher mortality rate because of overdosage or chronic disability associated with hepatitis, infections, contaminated supplies, and malnutrition.[49]

Alcohol Abuse

Many still consider alcohol to be a nondrug. It is readily available, inexpensive, and considered socially acceptable. Although young adults may drink less regularly than older adults, they tend to consume larger amounts of alcohol at one time. Alcohol-related accidents among young adults continue to be their leading cause of death. Alcohol is a factor in more than 10% of all deaths in the United States and in 60% of all highway fatalities involving young adults.[49]

Motor Vehicle Accidents

Despite the general good health in this period of life, motor vehicle accidents are a leading cause of death among young adults. In particular, they are responsible for more fatalities than all other causes of death combined. Most accidents occur in the late teenage years or early 20s, and males are involved in more accidents than females.[49]

Stress-Related Illnesses

Young adults encounter another type of risk to health: the pressure of achievement-oriented stress. This differs from stress in situational crises. The stress in an overachiever is brought about by internal pressures to succeed in relation to goals. Achievement stress often causes "workaholic" habits, including lack of sleep and omission of meals. If this behavior becomes extreme, physical exhaustion, nutritional problems, and burnout may occur. The individual may not perceive such behaviors, which often go undetected until changes in bodily functions occur.[29]

Many young adults enjoy some sort of physical activity and are usually health conscious and willing to alter life-styles and patterns of behavior according to their concept of health. It becomes important for young adults to recognize stress as a risk factor and behaviors such as increased anxiety, nervousness, depression, or somatic complaints as indicators of a problem.[29,49]

IMPACT OF DIABETES MELLITUS ON NORMAL PHYSICAL CHANGES IN YOUNG ADULTHOOD

It has become increasingly clear that vascular disease is associated with diabetes mellitus. Vascular disease is estimated to be 30 times more common in persons with diabetes, as evidenced by the risk of gangrene, which increases greatly among these persons.[3,5] The occurrence and progression of vascular disease may be directly related to prolonged elevation of blood glucose levels. Adults who have elevated blood glucose levels over years appear to be affected most by vascular changes. However, some adults with diabetes never develop complications despite prolonged elevations.[19]

Organ damage occurs in those tissues in which glucose transport across the cell membrane is not insulin mediated or dependent. Thus the vascular endothelium, the nerve sheath, the red blood cell, the lens of the eye, and other tissues are concentrated with amounts of glucose that are dependent on the degree of hyperglycemia. Such a situation can potentially lead to metabolic and functioning alterations within the cell structure.[2]

Although chronic or long-term complications of diabetes mellitus (degenerative cardiovascular changes, neuropathy, nephropathy, retinopathy) occur in less than 20% of those between ages 20 and 35, the impact of prevention, early diagnosis, and treatment is very important to young adults with insulin-dependent (type I) diabetes mellitus (IDDM).[2,19]

Diagnosis

Adults with IDDM usually have an abrupt onset of signs and symptoms of insulinopenia before age 30. Individuals with IDDM produce little or no insulin, depend on exogenous insulin, and account for approximately 10% of all individuals with diabetes. IDDM may occur at any age but usually is diagnosed before age 20. Adults typically experience an unexplained weight loss and test positive for urine ketones in conjunction with hyperglycemia.[5,17,23]

Individuals with non-insulin-dependent (type II) diabetes (NIDDM) at some point may require insulin for persistent hyperglycemia. NIDDM can occur at any age but usually is diagnosed after age 35 and is associated with obesity. Ketosis develops infrequently, unless precipitated by such factors as infection, surgery, stress, or trauma.[5,36] Box 20-1 lists goals related to the management of IDDM versus NIDDM in the adult.

NIDDM sometimes is present among children, adolescents, and young adults. This form of diabetes is referred to as *maturity-onset diabetes of the young* (MODY). MODY is a subtype of NIDDM that is inherited in an autosomal dominant manner. It is found in early adolescence

---

BOX 20-1

MANAGEMENT GOALS FOR ADULTS WITH IDDM VERSUS NIDDM

IDDM

Eliminate or avoid ketoacidosis.
Achieve metabolic control: minimize hyperglycemia while avoiding serious hypoglycemia.
Maintain normal growth and development.
Restore desired body weight.
Encourage physical and social activity appropriate to specific age-group.
Educate about pathophysiologic aspects of diabetes mellitus.

NIDDM

Achieve metabolic control.
Institute a plan of diet modification.
Increase physical activity appropriate to specific age-group.
Institute pharmacologic intervention with oral hypoglycemic agents or insulin if diet and
   exercise do not provide metabolic control.
Educate about pathophysiologic aspects of diabetes mellitus.

(9 to 14 years), particularly if sought on routine blood glucose testing, in the younger generations of families with more than one generation affected by NIDDM. Intake of excessive calories leading to weight gain and obesity is probably an important factor in its pathogenesis. In general, principles of management are the same as for adults with NIDDM. Diet therapy alone may be sufficient for some, whereas others may require sulfonylurea drugs.[18]

Hyperglycemia and ketonemia are more common in young adults with IDDM. Specific aspects of treatment are presented elsewhere in this text. In general, to minimize wide fluctuations in blood glucose, individuals should balance medication, diet, and exercise. Many acute episodes can thus be anticipated and prevented. Diabetes education helps to maintain a sense of well-being and prevent adverse stress and illness. This education should include both the individual with diabetes and his or her significant others.

Physical Effects

The young adult with diabetes may be susceptible to developing complications associated with microvascular or macrovascular disease, depending on these predisposing factors. As previously noted, diabetic complications tend to be associated with degree and duration of hyperglycemia. In addition, the role of genetics in diabetes and macrovascular disease cannot be ignored. Both conditions may be influenced by a common genetic aberration (see Chapters 7 and 8). Therefore much of the focus of diabetes management in young adulthood is on modification of factors that promote the development of long-term complications. With the advent of self-monitoring of blood glucose (SMBG), assessment of glycemic control allows individuals to note and evaluate the warning signs of hypoglycemia and hyperglycemia.

SMBG provides the individual and health care provider with immediate and accurate clinical data. After instruction, individuals are able to monitor and record their own blood glucose and make appropriate adjustments in diet, exercise, and medication. Such technology enables adults to manage their diabetes in consultation with the health care team. In addition, newer technology has allowed individuals to transmit blood glucose values via modem to a clinic's computer.[1] Assessment of glycemic control requires a system that both the health care provider and the individual can interpret. Compliance with SMBG is associated with understanding the results and responding appropriately. As such, adults with diabetes are prime candidates for learning SMBG as a tool for managing diabetes. However, careful education on how to monitor accurately and how to interpret and act on results is critical if the benefits of SMBG are to be realized.

Vascular Changes

As noted, young adults with diabetes are more susceptible to developing microvascular or macrovascular disease than their nondiabetic counterparts. The impact of *peripheral vascular disease* (PVD) in young adults with diabetes is enormous. Risk factors associated with PVD include hypertension, elevated serum cholesterol and lipids, smoking, and obesity.[19,36,39] The most significant factor is prevention of PVD by educating and encouraging specific interventions for health maintenance.

Hypertension in young adults with diabetes has prognostic significance. By monitoring blood pressure values, early identification and treatment may decrease long-term complications. In addition to immediate impacts associated with PVD, hypertension contributes substantially to the early cardiovascular morbidity and mortality of young adults with diabetes mellitus.[21] Cardiovascular and renal mortality accounts for 50% to 60% of diabetic deaths, and with advancing age and duration of the diabetes, the rate is greater than 70%. Young adults with diabetes who have hypertension need aggressive management and education to limit the likelihood of disease progression.[43]

Life-style Changes

Genetic factors are a major component in the development of disease, but life-style is also a major contributor. Young adults with modifiable risk factors should be targeted for extensive education and behavioral interventions to diminish the risk. Obesity is probably the major factor associated with hypertension and cardiovascular risk.[36,43] Young adults should be instructed to decrease their intake of salt and consider the high sodium content of commercially prepared foods, particularly the fast-food, convenient types they eat so frequently.

Elevated serum cholesterol and lipids are major components associated with *atherosclerosis*.[8] Since atherosclerosis is often associated with diabetes, periodic evaluation of fasting lipids should be done. Studies have shown that elevated plasma low-density lipoprotein (LDL) levels and suppressed high-density lipoprotein (HDL) concentrations are frequently seen in adults with diabetes.[4,11] In young adults with IDDM, this appears in the presence of hyperglycemia. The diet recommended by the American Heart Association is integrated into the diabetes meal plan to lower the intake of saturated fat and thereby lower cholesterol levels.

Limiting the use of dietary fat and adding fiber to meals may have a positive influence on the management of diabetes. The typical diet contains approximately 10 to 15 g of dietary fiber. An increase to 25 to 35 g of fiber per 1000 calories has been recommended by the American Diabetes Association (ADA) (see Chapter 4). There are two types of dietary fiber: water soluble and water insoluble. Water-soluble fibers include pectins and gums that are found in citrus fruits, oats, barley, and legumes. Water-insoluble fibers include cellulose and are found in leafy vegetables, wheat, cereal products, and most grains. Water-soluble fibers tend to form a gel within the gastrointestinal (GI) tract, slowing absorption of glucose across the intestinal mucosa and lowering cholesterol. Water-insoluble fibers increase bulk within the GI tract and help to relieve constipation.[8]

Elimination of cigarette smoking is another means of preventing peripheral vascular disease. Smoking is one of the strongest risk factors for intermittent claudication. Because the risk of cardiovascular complications is enormously greater in persons with diabetes, this should be an added deterrent to smoking. However, recent data suggest smoking remains a significant risk factor for adults with diabetes. Nicotine increases constriction of small blood vessels, further impeding an already diminishing circulation.[29]

Smoking tends to be initiated during adolescence. By young adulthood the habit is well entrenched by several years. It is crucial that persons with diabetes who smoke be strongly encouraged to quit. Smoking cessation strategies by the diabetes health care team or referral to appropriate resources, such as those found through the American Lung Association or American Cancer Society, should be implemented. Careful and systematic follow-up should also be done.[3,29]

Finally, exercise is an essential component of diabetes management for young adults. Exercise provides an excellent means of maintaining ideal body weight and avoiding the obesity typically associated with PVD. Although exercise alone is not an effective means of losing weight, since the caloric expenditure required to burn fat is enormous, it is an excellent method of "healthful stress" to the cardiovascular system. Exercise also promotes a sense of well-being, which is frequently needed when "getting into shape" (see Chapter 5).

NORMAL PHYSICAL TASKS OF DEVELOPMENT IN MIDDLE ADULTHOOD

Although 40 years of age has significance in chronologically demarcating the majority of persons with NIDDM from those with IDDM, it also signifies the beginning of middle adulthood, or "middlescence." This period of the life cycle connotes certain responsibilities and assumptions based on a normative system of age expectations. An age-graded system is socially defined and represents a means of rationalizing the life cycle and relevant events.

In contrast to the steady growth in adolescence, which peaks in young adulthood, physical changes among middle adults occur gradually and affect most body systems.[29,38] In general, the functional capacity of all systems begins to decrease. For example, in the GI tract, decreased metabolism leads to less enzyme production, resulting in lower hydrochloric acid levels and decreased tone in the large intestines. As a result, middle adults seem to complain more of acid indigestion with increased belching.[10] Also, more middle-age adults eat foods that are low in bulk, which may contribute to constipation. This, coupled with a sedentary life-style, diminishes motility through the GI tract.

Muscle size, strength, and reflex speed also begin a progressive decline. Size and strength that is lost from disuse, however, can be regained through rigorous exercise. Muscle strength of most men continues to be greater than that of most women throughout the life span.[29,38]

The bones lose further mass and density. As the cartilage between the vertebrae starts to degenerate from normal wear, the vertebrae become compressed, and the spinal column gradually begins to shorten. As adults age, they actually lose some of their height because of this compression of the spinal column. With increasing age, the cartilage in all joints has a more limited ability to regenerate.[10,38]

In addition to muscular and skeletal changes, age-related changes occur in the endocrine glands. Both the basal metabolic rate and the secretions of thyroid hormones decrease with age. Epinephrine and norepinephrine, the hormones of the sympathetic nervous system, are released more slowly in aging persons in response to stress. Evidence also indicates that the tissue response to these substances diminishes with age. Finally, glucose tolerance gradually declines and the prevalence of diabetes mellitus increases with age because of the tissue resistance to insulin that occurs with progressive weight gain.[38] Skin also begins to lose its resilience and elasticity.

Between ages 25 and 70 there is a 35% loss of nephron units. The remaining nephrons increase in size and undergo degenerative changes. The entire weight of the kidney decreases. With blood supply also diminished, the glomerular filtration rate is decreased by nearly one half.[10]

During middle adulthood the cardiovascular system undergoes several changes. The lungs and bronchi become increasingly less elastic, causing a progressive decrease in maximum breathing capacity. The heart muscle's ability to contract decreases, leading to a lower cardiac index (the cardiac output per minute per square meter of body surface).[38]

Blood vessels lose elasticity and become thicker, further contributing to elevated blood pressure. Middle-age adults are more prone to myocardial infarction, cerebrovascular accident (stroke), and hypertension, with heart disease being the leading cause of death for this age-group.[10,49]

IMPACT OF DIABETES MELLITUS ON NORMAL PHYSICAL CHANGES IN MIDDLE ADULTHOOD

Sensoriperceptual decline related to aging, which begins in the fourth decade of life, involves changes in vision, hearing, and cutaneous sensitivity. As an individual approaches the sixth decade of life, sensoriperceptual changes begin to take place relative to taste, smell, balance, and motor processes. These functions are responsible for the reception, interpretation, processing, and translation of new information and skills.[40] Similarly, diabetes-related changes as a result of microvascular and neuropathic complications may be found in vision, cutaneous sensitivity, balance, proprioception, and motor function. It is important to note that the degree of decline and resultant alteration in function vary among individuals depending on age, type (IDDM versus NIDDM), and duration of diabetes.

Vision

Presbyopia, the farsightedness of aging, begins in the fourth decade of life, causing most middle-aged adults to need corrective lenses. The lenses of the eyes gradually become less elastic with age, causing the eyes to lose their ability to bring near-point visual images into focus. At the same time, alterations in light perception begin to occur, which in turn affects night vision. These normal age-related changes in vision can be problematic for the individual with diabetes who is aware of and concerned with the potential for retinopathy. In addition, transient changes in lens refraction caused by fluctuations in blood glucose occur, which in turn affect visual acuity. Such refractive changes at high blood glucose levels result in myopia and at low blood glucose levels result in hyperopia.[19] These changes, whether age or diabetes related, represent a major source of stress in terms of the potential for visual impairment and loss of sight.

Diabetic retinopathy is the leading cause of new cases of blindness in the United States. The major source of stress related to potential loss of vision is apparent, since compared with individuals who do not have diabetes, those with diabetes are 29 times more likely to become blind.[19,48] When age is accounted for, the absolute risk of blindness from diabetic retinopathy increases with age, with the relative risk greater for persons ages 30 to 50. In terms of risk related to duration of disease, 80% of all persons with diabetes have some form of retinopathy 15 years after diagnosis.

The goal of diabetes self-care is the attainment of optimal metabolic control in an effort to prevent or minimize both acute and chronic complications of diabetes. When age and duration of disease are factored into the equation for potential visual impairment, good metabolic control alone is not the sole predictor of outcome.

Cutaneous System

The cutaneous system is responsible for tactile, temperature, and pain reception or sensitivity. Age-related changes occur in thermal and vibratory sensitivity; however, evidence suggesting a similar decline in pain sensitivity remains controversial. As an individual grows older and has increased duration of diabetes, the normal age-related changes are further compounded by the diabetes-related changes of peripheral neuropathy.

Diabetes-associated changes in vibratory, thermal, and pain sensitivity are related to peripheral neuropathy. Sensory and motor nerve conduction has been shown to be impaired early in the course of diabetes without any clinical symptomatology.[19] With disease progression, this asymptomatic state turns into one of minimal symptomatology characterized by paresthesias. This in turn predisposes individuals to painless injuries that increase the potential for ulceration, infection, and amputation.

Peripheral neuropathy affecting the lower extremities may interfere with one's ability to maintain a regular program of exercise and may also affect one's work role and involvement in social activities. Such impingements on activities of daily living can cause feelings of anxiety and depression, especially as one is confronted with the "middlescent" emotions of bodily decline and growing older.

The implication of such physiologic changes related to visual acuity and cutaneous sensitivity is that individuals may encounter difficulty when performing self-care tasks such as insulin injection, SMBG, and foot care. Problems with manual dexterity may be further complicated by the presence of osteoarthritis, which is a common chronic illness in middle-aged adults.

Kidney Function

Age-related changes that occur in the urinary tract are associated with arteriosclerosis and a decrease in muscle tone, nephrons, and renal tissue growth. The glomerular filtration rate begins to decline in midlife as renal blood flow decreases. In addition to the age-related changes, the kidneys of individuals with diabetes undergo many functional and morphologic changes. These changes occur before the clinical appearance of proteinuria. However, the occurrence of proteinuria is usually first noted 10 to 15 years after the diagnosis of IDDM. After a 15-year duration of diabetes, approximately one third of people with IDDM and one fifth of those with NIDDM will develop diabetic nephropathy.[5,19,48]

Because the incidence of diabetic nephropathy is associated with duration of disease, middle-age adults with diabetes feel vulnerable to nephropathy and perceive it as life-threatening. Hypertension may either precipitate or potentiate diabetic nephropathy. Many adults with diabetes develop hypertension that necessitates careful control.

Alterations in renal function related to aging and diabetes have implications for diabetes self-care. A decrease in renal excretion of drugs increases the half-life of drugs normally excreted by the kidneys. As a result, episodes of hypoglycemia may occur more frequently because of the increased half-life of oral sulfonylureas or insulin.

Table 20-1 summarizes various age-related changes that affect diabetes self-care activities.

Sexual Function

Sexual function is an important and integral part of middle adulthood as well as young adulthood. It is an essential component of a satisfying, intimate relationship with a significant other. Most young adults are concerned with the developmental task of childbearing, whereas middle-age adults typically are not.

It is theorized that the sexual element is decreasingly significant in middle adulthood as individuals redefine men and women as companions and partners.[10,38] However, this notion of socializing versus sexualizing in relationships does not negate the importance of an individual's sexuality relative to sexual performance.

Normal age-related changes that occur in women are associated with the menopausal period (late 40s to 50s). Changes occur in vaginal elasticity, with a reduction in vaginal

Table 20-1 Age and Diabetes Changes that Affect Self-Care

Age-associated changes	Complications of diabetes	Responses
Vision	Retinopathy	Decreased visual ac... Altered light perception Altered lens refraction
Cutaneous	Peripheral neuropathy	Altered tactile sensitivity Altered thermal sensitivity Altered vibratory sensitivity Decreased motor function
Renal	Nephropathy	Increased renal threshold Decreased renal clearance Increased drug half-life

SMBG, insulin injections, and foot care may be impaired by hypoglycemia/hyperglycemia.

lubrication. Males undergo changes in the time required for physical stimulation and for achieving an erection and in the time and force of ejaculations. In both men and women, no age-related decline is associated with libido.

Sexual dysfunction related to diabetes, however, is of great concern to the diabetic individual. Psychogenic impotence and organic impotence are common findings among men with diabetes. The prevalence rate for impotency has been reported to be as high as 60%. Organic impotence results from diabetic neuropathy and therefore could occur at any time after adolescence, depending on duration of disease. Proximal vascular insufficiency can be detected by examining the femoral pulses. However, localized obstruction of the penile artery must be examined by measurements of the brachial/penile blood pressure ratio using Doppler flow studies. Normal erections on awakening or impotence only with a certain partner suggests a psychogenic cause.[37]

Although sexual dysfunction has been widely studied in men, information is lacking on sexual function in women with diabetes. What has been described is that women are still functional and experience no decrease in libido or ability to achieve orgasm when compared with women without diabetes.

For many cultural groups the male holds the dominant sex role. Therefore sexual dysfunction often causes disruption in male self-image and self-esteem, which results in stress and conflict within significant intimate relationships. Individuals with a sexual dysfunction and their partners should be referred for sexual counseling. At that time, options for management can be discussed (e.g., alternative forms of mutual sexual gratification, penile prostheses).

Coronary Artery Disease

At least one third of all deaths occurring in individuals with diabetes after age 40 are caused by atherosclerotic heart disease.[5,19,36] Ischemic heart disease appears to be more prevalent

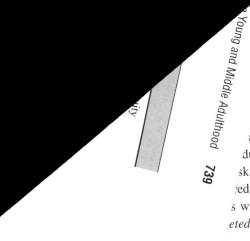

o have accelerated coronary atherosclerosis. Likewise, ,gressive premature macrovascular or microvascular chemic heart disease.[19] The risk of heart disease is two etes and is not necessarily associated with duration of

as previously described, increase the risk of premature duals with diabetes and coronary artery disease. Modification sk factors, such as smoking, obesity, elevated cholesterol and educe the risk of heart attack and stroke.

s with NIDDM are obese, the *importance of educational and eted at risk factor modification cannot be overemphasized.*

ES IN YOUNG AND MIDDLE ADULTHOOD

Intellectual ... itinues throughout adulthood. Young adults begin to acquire knowledge and develop skills that improve performance abilities gained as adolescents.[29] Piaget's stage of *formal operational thought* evolves from concrete operational thought in adolescence and extends into young adulthood.[41] During this developmental stage, young adults begin to analyze combinations of relations and construct hypotheses capable of being tested. It is a time when issues are approached realistically with important decisions being made. Young adults experiment with trial-and-error methodology and demonstrate use of problem-solving reasoning.

Piaget's stage of formal operational thought continues throughout middle adulthood with refinement in areas of spatial perception and problem-solving reasoning. Middle-age adults have the ability to deal more efficiently with complex problems of reasoning caused by life experiences and completion of adult developmental tasks.

IMPACT OF DIABETES MELLITUS ON COGNITIVE PROCESSES IN YOUNG AND MIDDLE ADULTHOOD

Fear of hypoglycemia is prevalent among individuals with diabetes and may be a motivating factor in the maintenance of elevated blood glucose levels to avoid risk of hypoglycemic episodes.[26] The transient or permanent impairments of brain function that can occur with repeated episodes of hypoglycemia are serious considerations. Central or peripheral nervous system dysfunction is the usual consequence of severe hypoglycemia. Individuals may exhibit symptoms of drowsiness or passivity; slow, confused thinking; impaired ability to judge the passage of time; impaired memory; impaired judgment; and slightly impaired auditory learning of declarative information.[12,26] In addition to memory and attention deficits, symptoms of hypoglycemia are unpleasant and often embarrassing. Such episodes can undermine an individual's credibility and reliability within the context of work and family roles. Frequent episodes may cause family, friends, and work associates to cast an individual into a traditional sick role, thus relieving this person of certain respon-sibilities.[25]

IMPACT OF DIABETES MELLITUS ON NORMAL PSYCHOSOCIAL DEVELOPMENT IN YOUNG ADULTHOOD

Erikson identified the development of self-esteem and self-satisfaction as major tasks during young adulthood. A sense of being open and capable of trusting others develops through the formation of intimate relationships. Erikson terms this period of psychosocial development as *intimacy versus isolation and loneliness*.[16] The concept of intimacy goes beyond sexual intimacy to a broader view of mutual psychosocial intimacy with peers, parents, and spouse. Intimacy requires mutual trust and involves reciprocal expression of affection. Young adults search for continuity and individuals in their lives who provide meaning. Those who are unsure of their identity may shy away from intimate contact with others, which can result in loneliness. Those with diabetes may be concerned about the quality of life and the impact of diabetes on establishing meaningful interpersonal relationships.

The strain faced by young adults dealing with newly diagnosed diabetes, or the focus on self-management issues associated with diabetes, may diminish or delay the accomplishment of developmental tasks as identified by Erikson. Table 20-2 outlines other aspects of Erikson's psychosocial development of young and middle adulthood.

Table 20-2   Erikson's Psychosocial Development of Young and Middle Adulthood

Young adulthood		
Intimacy	versus	Isolation
Intimacy is expressed in psychosocial terms such as *affiliation* and *partnership*. Affiliation indicates the meaning of intimacy as inclusive of friendships based on choice rather than family. Emotional intimacy refers to the capacity to perceive nondefensively the meaning of the emotion that the other person is expressing. Intellectual intimacy is the sharing of ideas without polarization of the relationship.		A lack of identity leads to a defensiveness that could polarize relationships. Unresolved identity questions lead to major problems with selecting a mate and finding a congenial social group. Expressive isolation is the self-protection of one's image. Individual may function within societal roles but may have difficulties in close relationships. Receptive isolation is defensiveness expressed in the distortion of social and environmental stimuli.

Middle adulthood		
Generativity	versus	Stagnation
Characterized by a concern with the establishment and setting forth guidelines for future generations. The virtue of *care* develops, as expressed by one's concern for others by wanting to take care of others and share knowledge and expertise.		Characterized by an absorption with the self to the extent that it excludes the welfare of others. When generativity is weak, the personality regresses and takes on a sense of impoverishment.

Modified from Erikson EH: *Adulthood,* New York, 1978, Norton.

Another psychosocial task of development during young adulthood is separation from parents. This task is usually accomplished by seeking education or pursuing a career away from home. Concerns about having diabetes may inhibit this developmental transition. It becomes critical to discuss with the young adult his or her perception of prognosis or quality of life in the context of long-term outcomes of diabetes. The health care team should also educate the young adult and the significant others as a means of encouraging optimal diabetes self-management.

Members of the health care team can assist young adults in being honest and realistic about the consequences of diabetes and the various options available. Employment can be a sensitive and critical issue for young adults with diabetes. Persons with diabetes may be restricted from pursuing certain jobs and should carefully consider career decisions in the light of their diagnosis. Federal and state legislation has been enacted in the last decade that limits discriminatory practices. Although most jobs are now open to those with diabetes, they should consider avoiding certain positions that may negatively affect long-term health. For example, the health care team should recommend the avoidance of jobs that require operating heavy machinery or working erratic schedules.[29] Some adults with diabetes had been working when their diabetes was diagnosed, which suggests the need for job counseling or retraining.

The decision to marry and have a family represents another developmental task of young adulthood. Young adults may question entering into marriage when their life span may be shorter with additional economic burdens. Their sense of self-worth and self-confidence may be decreased. Also, some may be ashamed of their condition and not willing to share various problems and complications with another individual within the context of a marriage and family. When entering into marriage, both the individual with diabetes and the spouse must learn what diabetes is, how to manage common crises, and what is involved with the treatment regimen. Discussion of long-term complications is also appropriate. Both should understand the risks of pregnancy for the woman with diabetes and the need for optimal glycemia at the time of conception to minimize the risk of congenital malformations.

For many women with diabetes, anxiety may surround the decision to have children or not. Specific management of diabetes during pregnancy includes preconception metabolic control, rigid glycemic control throughout gestation, and close monitoring of mother and fetus (see Chapter 11). Sensitive prepregnancy counseling for the woman with diabetes, along with her spouse, provides an essential foundation for a healthy and successful pregnancy.[33]

Gestational diabetes has been defined by the Second International Conference on Gestational Diabetes Mellitus as "carbohydrate intolerance of variable severity with onset of first recognition during the present pregnancy." Estimates of the incidence of gestational diabetes have ranged from 3% to 20%. A more accurate estimate is difficult because of the lack of population-based studies.[46] However, for most adult women (97%) this condition will rescind at the end of their pregnancy. With increased technology (e.g., SMBG, multiple-injection regimens, insulin pump therapy), many women with gestational diabetes are able to deliver healthy babies.

IMPACT OF DIABETES MELLITUS ON NORMAL PSYCHOSOCIAL DEVELOPMENT IN MIDDLE ADULTHOOD

In Erikson's theory of life span personality development, the middle adulthood period is characterized as a time of *generativity versus stagnation.*[16] Generativity is defined by an expansion of ego interests, productivity, and creativity. It can likewise be conceptualized as a sense of having contributed to the future versus a sense of ego stagnation. This developmental period is a time of valuing wisdom versus valuing physical powers and socializing versus sexualizing in human relationships (see Table 20-2).

Other expectations of middle adulthood include those of work, marriage, child-rearing, caring for aging parents, and legal and social responsibilities.[10] This period is characterized by a sense of accomplishment as the individual views his or her life within the context of family and career. At the same time, however, the person may sense bodily decline and growing old and recognize his or her mortality. Such feelings support the notion that individuals are aware of age norms and expectations in relation to their own patterns of tim-ing, and that timing plays an important role with respect to self-concept and self-esteem.

During young and middle adulthood, various developmental tasks must be achieved and accomplished for the individual to continue successfully on to the next stage of development. Box 20-2 lists specific tasks for both young and middle-age adults.[10,29,38]

BOX 20-2

DEVELOPMENTAL TASKS OF YOUNG AND MIDDLE-AGE ADULTS

Young adults

Accepting and stabilizing self-concept and body image
Establishing independence from parental home
Becoming established in a vocation or profession that provides personal satisfaction, economic independence, and a feeling of making a contribution to society
Expressing love responsibly through more than sexual contacts
Establishing an intimate bond with another individual
Finding a congenial social group
Formulating a meaningful philosophy of life

Middle-age adults

Accepting personal strengths and limits with a firm sense of identity
Striving for self-actualization; living up to highest potential
Ensuring security for later years, financially and emotionally
Drawing emotionally closer as a couple
Maintaining contact with grown children and their families
Participating in community life beyond the family
Reaffirming the values of life that have real meaning

Because self-concept and self-esteem are developed through interactions between an individual's ego and society, chronic illness inherently can alter such interactions. This is caused by the ambiguous and often stigmatized nature of chronic illness, in which society considers an individual either sick or well.

Strauss and Glaser[47] call such a phenomenon "identity spread" when the symptoms of a chronic illness are intrusive. Society may then assume that the ill individual cannot work, act, or be like an ordinary, "normal" individual. In essence, chronic illness lacks normative definition with corresponding rights and responsibilities. As a result, an individual may become isolated and nonproductive, contrary to a dominant cultural emphasis of active involvement and productivity. The potential for this is greatly increased among adults with diabetes-related complications. The central work role may be modified or lost because of disability or decreased capability for work role resumption. Similarly, the role within the family may be modified and altered.[15]

The coping responses of chronically ill persons are affected by the characteristics of the illness and by reactions of members of the family and society. Lazarus and Cohen[31] define *coping* as the process of managing demands that are appraised as taxing or exceeding the resources of the person. This definition emphasizes management rather than mastery, which is important in understanding the nature of living with a chronic illness such as diabetes. Diabetes self-management facilitates coping and adaptation. It is the reorganization of physical, psychologic, and social characteristics of an individual in such a way that one can resume well-adjusted living after the diagnosis of chronic illness or an incapacitating complication of illness.

When considering the long-term complications of diabetes, such as peripheral and autonomic neuropathy, retinopathy, nephropathy, and cardiovascular complications, a redefining of role obligations may be necessary to facilitate an individual's adaptation. Haber and Smith[20] identify this process as *normative adaptation,* which consists of three stages: (1) recognition of inadequacy, (2) attribution of responsibility, and (3) legitimacy of performance behavior. This process considers an individual's limitation, normalizing exceptional behavior within the framework of role obligations as a means of facilitating role maintenance. An individual's social and personal role obligations can be redefined so they are more in keeping with actual capabilities. An individual's performance can then be evaluated against redefined norms. Such an approach allows for a smoother transition into new roles while relinquishing previous roles relative to both work and family. Normative adaptation to the complications of diabetes may mean the difference between productive adaptation or surviving in a state of discouragement and invalidism.

Whether the diagnosis of diabetes mellitus occurs during middle adulthood or earlier, an individual is confronted with the issues of coping and adaptation within the context of negotiating middlescence. The diagnosis of diabetes-related complications during this time adds further to the conflict. The concerns of middle adulthood relative to bodily decline and a decreased sense of omnipotence are similar to the concerns and psychologic changes that can accompany illness. It is important, therefore, that members of the health care team understand the personal, familial, and social implications of living with a chronic illness such as diabetes mellitus.[27,28]

EDUCATIONAL AND BEHAVIORAL STRATEGIES

Diabetes education is a complex, multifaceted process that requires the adult learner's active participation. Because learning capacity continues throughout the life span, both young and middle-age adults are capable of learning new knowledge and skills. In designing various behavioral strategies for an educational intervention, members of the health care team must individualize care and educational goals according to young and middle adulthood. *An emphasis on preventive aspects of care and the importance of regular follow-up to monitor development or progression of complications is recommended.* The emphasis on changing behavior to eliminate modifiable risk factors (e.g., smoking, obesity) is important if the adult is to maintain an optimal level of health care.

Diabetes Care for Young and Middle-age Adults

Effective education requires that all adults be well informed about aspects of diabetes. For young or middle-age adults who are newly diagnosed, reassurance is vital, with the initial discussion of diabetes focused on "survival knowledge." Such knowledge allows the individual to possess information and skills that have immediate applicability and to participate in self-management. Adjusting to the diagnosis of diabetes may take weeks to months. Initially the individual may be preoccupied with fears of death, use of needles, and implications of the diagnosis. Thus it is unrealistic to expect adults to learn everything they need to know about their care in a few short days. Highest educational priorities for newly diagnosed young and middle-age adults should include encouraging them to talk about their fears and offer reassurances that they are understandable and possibly under their control. Regular contact with and availability of the health care provider for questions are important. Box 20-3 outlines basic diabetes concepts and survival skills.

Young adults who will most likely be diagnosed with IDDM, as well as those who have been diagnosed for at least 3 to 4 weeks, should receive more in-depth education, such as preventive aspects of care, exercise, prepregnancy counseling, complications, foot care, hygiene guidelines, career and job placement, travel guidelines, and driving a motor vehicle. Such information should be carefully documented and reviewed annually with the individual.[2] Information should be presented in small increments at a level the individual is capable of accepting. Too much information too soon may be overwhelming. A typical example is the individual who is told his tests indicate diabetes, followed by approximately 20 minutes of instruction on injecting insulin and a standard preprinted diet sheet. Once the individual arrives home, he is confused, depressed, and overwhelmed. Adequate time is needed to allow young adults to ventilate their perceptions of the condition and discuss various coping and educational strategies.

Middle-age adults with IDDM should be reevaluated every few years in terms of diabetes knowledge and self-care skills. Although they have typically had diabetes for several years, these individuals should be carefully evaluated as to their current knowledge and receive regular physical examinations to screen for complications. Additional health or financial problems or other concerns related to tasks associated with growth and development also

---

BOX 20-3

DIABETES CONCEPTS AND SURVIVAL SKILLS FOR ADULTS

Brief definition of and general information about diabetes

Basic principles of nutrition, essentials of nutrition management, and basic meal planning

Maintaining balance: food and stress increase blood sugar; insulin and activity lower blood sugar

"Honeymoon" (remission) phase for IDDM

Definition of hypoglycemia, including basic treatment and prevention

Information regarding function of insulin and/or hypoglycemic agents; how to draw up, mix, and administer insulin

Self-monitoring of blood glucose, with an introduction to meters

Guidelines for sick-day management, including suggested foods and liquids

Urine ketone testing

Supplies and identification

Emergency telephone numbers (when to call health care provider: blood glucose levels, symptoms)

---

require further evaluation by the health care team. (See Appendix D for a sample protocol for evaluation of diabetes status.)

Middle-age adults newly diagnosed with NIDDM experience many of the same reactions as any individual newly diagnosed with a chronic disease.[36] As with the young adult, information must be presented in frequent, small increments until the individual is able to comprehend the tasks involved with self-care.

Adults with NIDDM are also prone to other health problems and financial concerns. Likewise, if diagnosed with diabetes during middle adulthood, the person appears to be more vulnerable to sickness, loss of function, and possible disability than younger adults with diabetes. For these reasons, middle-age adults need to seek continuing support and periodic reeducation. Members of the health care team must take the time to understand each individual's situation and problems and be sensitive to these when designing a self-care plan. Care and education must be tailored to the individual's life-style if they are to be successful in promoting behavior change.

The success of care may depend on an individualized education approach. However, many adults may be suffering from emotional aspects of the diabetes that create barriers to the therapeutic regimen, contributing to poor metabolic control.[42] Improvement will ultimately depend on the health care team being able to identify and resolve underlying problems that interfere with self-management. Likewise, the individual's willingness to change is related to his or her perception of vulnerability to the complications of diabetes, sense of control over the condition, or the perceived benefits of adherence in delaying or preventing the long-term complications of diabetes. In particular, behavior-oriented education that focuses on problem solving and decision making and uses small-group strategies is effective.[34]

BOX 20-4
—

EDUCATIONAL STRATEGIES TO PROMOTE COMPREHENSION, RECALL, AND COMPLIANCE

Primacy and organization of material: most important information should be presented first.

Brevity: the time frame in which information is given should be short.

Specificity: information presented in specific terms rather than general terms is best understood and recalled.

Repetition.

Readability.

BOX 20-5
—

PATIENT EDUCATION PRINCIPLES FOR YOUNG AND MIDDLE-AGE ADULTS

- Build rapport.
- Provide a positive patient–health care provider relationship.
- Set educational goals that are specific, measurable, realistic, and attainable. Allow feedback from patients in negotiating goals.
- Concentrate on the most pressing needs or patients' questions first.
- Use appropriate educational tools, and educate based on relevant issues.
- Offer realistic outcomes of IDDM and NIDDM.
- Provide patients with a unified message from the health care team.
- Involve family members and significant others in the teaching process.

Adult Education

Effective diabetes education interventions use methods directed at the level of the learner (see Chapter 15). However, certain conditions must be met for adult learning to occur: (1) collaboration between teacher and learner, (2) learner-identified needs and objectives, (3) methods for learning, and (4) learner self-evaluation of the teaching-learning process.[27] Box 20-4 lists educational strategies that promote comprehension, recall, and compliance. Members of the health care team should use the educational principles presented in Box 20-5 when working with young and middle-age adults.

ADHERENCE ISSUES

One of the most significant issues in diabetes management is the inability or unwillingness of individuals with diabetes to adhere as closely to the recommended therapeutic program as is necessary to achieve control. Adequate knowledge does not guarantee that adults will adhere to the schedule that living with diabetes demands.[34,35,45]

BOX 20-6

STRATEGIES TO PROMOTE ADHERENCE

Reminders	Contingency contracting
Tailoring regimen	Self-monitoring
Gradual regimen implementation	Realistic, mutually agreeable goals
Active support of significant others	

In addition to readiness, willingness, and overall motivation, family support and cultural factors are critical determinants of patient motivation and adherence.[44] Patient satisfaction with the health care team and setting has been shown to affect adherence behavior. Barriers to adherence and compliance, both perceived and actual, must be assessed as part of the educational process. For example, if individuals believe and state that someone in their family has diabetes and is doing just fine, various consequences of diabetes need to be discussed. After correcting misconceptions, the health care provider should ensure that adequate information and skills necessary to follow a prescribed plan are presented and tailored to the individual's life-style.[30] Box 20-6 lists frequently used strategies to promote adherence.

All health care providers involved in the care of individuals with diabetes should be sensitive to specific areas that can affect patient adherence. For example, financial resources have an impact on compliance. Individuals who are unable to buy medications, certain types of food, and SMBG equipment may not comply with recommended therapeutic interventions. Health care providers must be prepared for the realities of society and possibly pursue avenues of financial assistance before educating individuals in basic survival knowledge.

Despite the many reasons why individuals have difficulty adhering to their regimen, the key to management is assessing factors that might be barriers or obstacles to adherence. Specifically, identifying barriers allows individuals to feel more in control. Daily decisions related to behavior modification become easier when barriers are identified. The grid illustrated in Fig. 20-1 allows an individual to check off appropriate obstacles. These obstacles are then prioritized to allow for step-by-step modification.

IMPLICATIONS OF THE DCCT FOR YOUNG AND MIDDLE-AGE ADULTS

The Diabetes Control and Complications Trial (DCCT)[13] established that intensive blood glucose control in patients with IDDM results in decreased rates of development and progression of retinopathy, neuropathy, and nephropathy. Although the DCCT is not the only study to support the link between lowering blood glucose levels and preventing or delaying complications associated with diabetes, it is the longest and largest. A total of 1441 individuals with diabetes enrolled in this multicenter, randomized, prospective clinical trial. The entire

Identified Adherence Problems

Obstacles to Adherence	Problem #1	Problem #2	Problem #3	Problem #4
Lack of knowledge or skill				
Competing priorities/ treatment costs				
Habit patterns				
Social support				
Stress				
Inappropriate cognitions				

Fig. 20-1   Identifying obstacles to adherence.

cohort was followed for a mean of 6½ years (range, 3 to 9 years), with 99% of the participants completing the study.

Based on DCCT results, the primary treatment goal for young adults with IDDM should be lowering blood glucose to or below the level seen in the trial's intensive treatment cohort (glycohemoglobin, 1% to 1.2% above nondiabetic range). If this goal is not achievable, the DCCT reports beneficial effects with any lowering of the glycohemoglobin level. Thus any degree of improved blood glucose control is beneficial to young adults.

Young adults with IDDM should strongly be advised to enter a program of intensive diabetes care and management. The DCCT showed that intensive management is not just "more insulin." Intensive management consists of intensive insulin therapy, intensive monitoring, intensive education, intensive medical intervention with the diabetes health care team, and intensive commitment from the individual with diabetes to focus daily on issues that affect blood glucose control.[13,24] Young adults with IDDM often are under the care of physicians who do not have extensive education and training in the field of diabetes. All health care providers are compelled to address the level of expertise and support available to individuals with IDDM and encourage collaboration with other specialists. Another consideration is that intensive management also means higher initial health costs for the patient. Particularly in young adulthood, that increased health care expense may not balance with the person's present resources.

> **BOX 20-7**
>
> ## COMMON ISSUES TO BE SHARED WITH THE HEALTH CARE TEAM
>
> Share and compare assessments and impressions about an individual's needs.
> Describe educational strategies that were useful to an individual.
> Advise team members how they can reinforce a constructive message by discussing what worked.
> Explain how a particular session with an individual may affect other team members' treatment plans.
> Note changes in individual outcomes.

Microvascular and neuropathic complications associated with IDDM presumably occur by the same pathophysiologic processes as in NIDDM.[14,22] Results of the DCCT provided evidence for tight blood glucose control in the prevention of diabetes-related complications. It was likewise suggested that middle-age adults with NIDDM would benefit from treatment directed at tight blood glucose control. This evidence is important information that should be used when educating adults about the benefits of self-care. Middle-age adults need to take reasoned actions, and the DCCT findings provide the necessary data for making informed decisions that result in positive self-care behaviors.[6]

ROLE OF THE DIABETES HEALTH CARE TEAM

Over the past 10 years, care of individuals with diabetes has shifted from acute, episodic care to more prevention and health maintenance and promotion. Along with a shift in the delivery of care, greater emphasis has been placed on multidisciplinary health care teams. The purpose of these teams is to promote self-management for individuals with diabetes through collaborative efforts.[32] One strategy is to have a weekly team conference during which team members discuss individuals and provide input and feedback to each other. In this way a consistent message is being given to individuals with diabetes, along with increased credibility from being associated with a team. The effectiveness of any multidisciplinary health care team is a function of its individual members. In a collaborative situation, individual patient goals become the team's goal. Box 20-7 outlines issues that need to be communicated to other members of the health care team.

ROLE OF THE FAMILY AND SOCIAL SUPPORT

Social factors and family functioning play an important role in facilitating an individual's adaptive responses to diabetes and self-care management. Families and significant social networks can foster independence and self-reliance through active support. If possible, families should be included in teaching; however, if families are dysfunctional, careful assessment and subsequent decision making as to the level of involvement are needed. In an effort to maximize support, it is important to discuss with the individual the advantages of involving significant others in diabetes education and nutrition counseling.

Social and family support have been studied in relationship to adherence and diabetes control. Studies suggest that the diabetic individual's perception of supportive behavior of family or significant others is predictive of compliance with the self-care regimen.[9] Similarly, studies of the influence of family function on diabetes control have demonstrated that individuals with diabetes in good metabolic control perceive the family environment to be more achievement oriented than do those in poor control.[7] Good family function is predictive of good diabetic control.[3]

The size of and satisfaction from the social support network are gender specific, serving different functions for men and women. As such, the concept of social support may vary among individuals. In general, social support is believed to effect positive outcomes for the individual with diabetes.[34]

SUMMARY

Diabetes during young and middle adulthood presents a variety of challenges to the individual with diabetes, his or her family, and the health care team. An understanding of not only the physical changes that occur but also the psychosocial implications associated with diabetes management in these age-groups need to be carefully assessed and individualized.

CASE PRESENTATIONS

The following vignettes highlight some clinical concerns of diabetes management and relate them to issues of growth and development.

Case Study 1

Ms. J. is a 31-year-old white female who has had IDDM since her early 20s and is presently a graduate student. She came to the office with erratic dietary patterns, often "forgetting to take her insulin." She volunteered detailed information about her background. Two years earlier she married a man somewhat older, which met with disapproval from her family. This caused some conflict, to the point where Ms. J. does not talk with her mother. She also talked about having difficulties at work and wanting to quit and start a family. On her first two visits, Ms. J. spoke very little about her diabetes and a recent episode of ketoacidosis that required hospitalization.

After several visits, Ms. J. became more communicative about her diabetes and what frightened her the most. She began to verbalize how difficult it would be to go through a pregnancy without the support of her mother, mentioning her real concerns about having diabetes and wanting children. Ms. J. received prepregnancy counseling and education. Months later, she became pregnant and started to become even more realistic about complications associated with pregnancy.

DISCUSSION

Individuals with diabetes often use denial as a way to cope with their condition. In Ms. J.'s situation, her use of denial was notable when she elected not to talk initially about her diabetes. Likewise, family and friends can use denial and create a conflict-laden situation, as with Ms. J. and her mother.

However, one aspect of Ms. J.'s condition possibly brought on her use of denial. As a young adult, Ms. J. was faced with great cultural pressure to marry and have children. Americans so value a "family" that unmarried adults are sometimes treated as incomplete. Besides the developmental task of establishing an intimate bond with another individual,[29,38] Ms. J. was seriously troubled about having diabetes and wanting children.

In helping young adults who are in denial, health care providers need to begin by conducting a thorough assessment, gathering facts and information regarding behaviors and feelings. While gathering such information, it is critical to be a good listener and assess when is the best time to impart knowledge or information. With Ms. J. the need for careful prepregnancy planning was identified. However, during periods of denial, individuals will not be receptive to the best teaching plan unless specific concerns and questions are addressed.

Case Study 2

Mrs. S. is a 43-year-old recent widow with an 8-year history of NIDDM. She lives alone and works as an executive secretary for a busy law firm. Her two daughters live in the same city with their families. Mrs. S. is 5 ft, 3 in and weighs 151 pounds. She has a history of osteoarthritis and peripheral neuropathy. She has been on a regimen of Diabenese, 500 mg daily, for the past 4 years. Over the past 4 months she has had a 20-pound weight loss. Her glycosylated hemoglobin is 12.6%, and a random blood glucose value is 297 mg/dl.

Two years ago Mrs. S. was taught SMBG but found it difficult to interpret the visual strips and therefore lost her motivation for monitoring. Her poor control warrants initiation of insulin therapy. She states that she will have difficulty self-administering insulin and probably will not perform SMBG.

DISCUSSION

As a first step, it would be appropriate to consider Mrs. S.'s perception of her diabetes. How does she view her diabetes? Does she have an adequate and accurate understanding of NIDDM and the treatment regimen prescribed for her thus far? Some adults perceive that NIDDM is the "milder" form compared with IDDM and not as serious unless one takes insulin. Assessing her beliefs and attitudes may also provide insight into how to structure further teaching.

In developing a teaching plan, it is essential to highlight the benefits of SMBG for adults with NIDDM. By using this information, Mrs. S. would be able to modify meal plans and exercise programs and achieve normal blood glucose and glycosylated hemoglobin levels. One might approach Mrs. S. by demonstrating a blood glucose monitoring meter that requires minimal manipulation. At the same time, show Mrs. S. various finger-lancing devices that she could manipulate in order to find one that is easiest to use. Once Mrs. S. finds the meter and finger-lancing device that best suit her needs, proceed with patient teaching, which includes a return demonstration.

If the meter and lancing devices are too difficult to manipulate, explore to what extent her daughters would be able to provide active support and assistance. This would also be an opportunity to explore Mrs. S.'s feelings of ambivalence and dependency relative to her diabetes and need for insulin. It would also provide an opportunity to address issues related to her recent widowhood and other avenues of social support.

Problems of manual dexterity caused by peripheral neuropathy and osteoarthritis that interfere with SMBG may also impede self-administration of insulin. Since Mrs. S.'s vision is good, she should have no problem in accurately drawing up the insulin if she is able to manipulate the insulin vial and syringe. If such manipulation is difficult, identify various aids for drawing up and injecting insulin.

Case Study 3

Mr. B. is a 52-year-old African American with a 10-year history of NIDDM. He is a first-level manager for a large manufacturing firm and works long hours that often extend into the weekend. He lives with his wife and three teenage children, ages 13, 15, and 17. A visit to his diabetes nurse practitioner reveals that he has gained 8 pounds since his last visit 4 months ago, his blood pressure is 148/94, and a random blood glucose value is 256 mg/dl. He states that his glycohemoglobin drawn 1 week before the visit was

9.6% and that he monitors his blood sugar three or four times a week, usually in the morning before breakfast. He has had less time to monitor blood glucose control and has stopped his usual exercise of walking 3 miles every other day because of work-related demands. It is important that he give 100% to work to maintain his job security. He says that he hopes to continue getting pay raises, especially with his children going to college in the near future.

DISCUSSION

Mr. B. is in middle adulthood, striving to live up to his highest potential in an effort to provide for his family. Erikson[16] defines this stage as generativity, in which an individual is concerned with caring for others and for a future generation. This is a time when men appraise their lives, decisions, failures, and accomplishments. It is a time for refining developmental tasks embarked on in the 40s.

Chronic illness and its demands take on a new meaning within this context. Mr. B. has put himself and his diabetes second. The challenge imposed by such a case confronts the diabetes care provider often when caring for the adult with NIDDM. Individuals with NIDDM are at increased risk for coronary heart disease. In addition, African Americans with NIDDM experience higher rates of cardiovascular morbidity and mortality. The health care provider needs to acknowledge Mr. B.'s goals and priorities while at the same time informing him of the health risks associated with taking less care of himself and his diabetes. Discussing ways in which he might begin to exercise again might be a first step, one that would help decrease weight, blood pressure, blood glucose, and stress. Mr. B.'s concern for his family's welfare is vitally important. Perhaps involving his wife as a means of support might also be helpful.

REFERENCES

1. Ahring KK and others: Telephone modem access improves diabetes control in those with insulin-requiring diabetes, *Diabetes Care* 15:971-975, 1992.
2. American Diabetes Association: *Physician's guide to insulin dependent (type I) diabetes: diagnosis and treatment,* Alexandria, Va, 1988, American Diabetes Association.
3. American Diabetes Association consensus statement: Role of cardiovascular risk factors in prevention and treatment of macrovascular disease in diabetes, *Diabetes Care* 13:53-59, 1989.
4. American Diabetes Association consensus statement: Detection and management of lipid disorders in diabetes, *Diabetes Care* 16:824-834, 1993.
5. American Diabetes Association: *Diabetes 1993: vital statistics,* Alexandria, Va, 1993, American Diabetes Association.
6. American Diabetes Association: Implications of the Diabetes Control and Complications Trial, *Diabetes Care* 16:1517-1520, 1993.
7. Anderson BJ and others: Assessing family sharing of diabetes responsibilities, *J Pediatr Psychol* 15:477-492, 1990.
8. Anderson J: Fiber and health: an overview, *Am J Gastroenterol* 81:892, 1986.
9. Auslander WF: Brief family interventions to improve family communications and cooperation regarding diabetes management, *Diabetes Spectrum* 6:330-333, 1993.
10. Behler D, Tippett T, Mandle CL: Middle adult. In Edelman CL, Mandle CL, editors: *Health promotion throughout the lifespan,* ed 3, St Louis, 1994, Mosby.
11. Bloomgarden ZT: A practical approach to lipid disorders in diabetes, *Pract Diabetol* 13:10-11, 1994.
12. Cryer PE: Hypoglycemia unawareness in IDDM, *Diabetes Care* 16:40-47, 1993.
13. DCCT Research Group: The effect of intensive treatment of diabetes on the development and progression of long-term complications in insulin-dependent diabetes mellitus, *N Engl J Med* 329:977-986, 1993.
14. DeFronzo RA, Bonadonna RC, Ferrannini E: Pathogenesis of NIDDM: a balanced overview, *Diabetes Care* 15:318-368, 1992.
15. Entmacher PS: Employment and insurance for those with diabetes. In Davidson JK, editor: *Clinical diabetes mellitus: a problem oriented approach,* New York, 1986, Thieme.
16. Erikson EH: *Adulthood,* New York, 1978, Norton.
17. Fain JA: National trends in diabetes: an epidemiologic perspective, *Nurs Clin North Am* 28:1-7, 1993.
18. Fajans SS: Recognizing maturity-onset diabetes of the young (MODY), *Pract Diabetol* 9:1, 1990.
19. Haas L: Chronic complications of diabetes mellitus, *Nurs Clin North Am* 28:71-85, 1993.
20. Haber L, Smith CT: Disability and deviance: normative adaptation of role behavior, *J Am Psychiatr Assoc* 15:344, 1971.

21. Haffner S and others: Cardiovascular risk factors in confirmed pre-diabetic individuals: does the clock for coronary heart disease start ticking before the onset of clinical diabetes? *JAMA* 263:2893-2898, 1990.

22. Harris MI: Undiagnosed NIDDM: Clinical and public health issues, *Diabetes Care* 16:642-652, 1993.

23. Hirsch IB, Farkas-Hirsch R: Type I diabetes and insulin therapy, *Nurs Clin North Am* 28:9-23, 1993.

24. Hodge C: The team approach to intensive insulin therapy, *Pract Diabetol* 12:13-16, 1993.

25. Holmes DM: The person and diabetes in psychosocial context, *Diabetes Care* 9:194-206, 1986.

26. Irvine AA, Cox DJ, Gorden-Frederick LA: Fear of hypoglycemia: relationship to glycemic control and psychological factors in IDDM patients, *Health Psychol* 11:135-138, 1992.

27. Knowles M: *The adult learner: a neglected species,* Houston, 1973, Gulf.

28. Krall LP, Entmacher PS, Drury TF: Life cycles in diabetes: socioeconomic aspects. In Marble A and others, editors: *Joslin's diabetes mellitus,* ed 12, Philadelphia, 1985, Lea & Febiger.

29. Kudzma EC, Quinn J: Young adult. In Edelman CL, Mandle CL, editors: *Health promotion throughout the lifespan,* ed 3, St Louis, 1994, Mosby.

30. Kurtz SM: Adherence to diabetes regimens: empirical status and clinical applications, *Diabetes Educ* 16:50-59, 1990.

31. Lazarus RS, Cohen JB: Environmental stress. In Altman L, Wohlwill JF, editors: *Human behavior and the environment: current theory and research,* ed 2, New York, 1979, McGraw-Hill.

32. Lorber DL, Lagana DJ: The health-care team in diabetes, *Pract Diabetol* 10:15-21, 1991.

33. Mann JI, Houston AC: Genetic factors in diabetes mellitus. In Davidson JK, editor: *Clinical diabetes mellitus: a problem oriented approach,* New York, 1986, Thieme.

34. Maxwell AE, Hunt IF, Bush MA: Effects of a social support as an adjunct to diabetes training on metabolic control and psychosocial outcomes, *Diabetes Care* 18:303-309, 1992.

35. McCaul KD, Glasgow RE, Schafer LC: Diabetes regimen behaviors: predicting adherence, *Med Care* 25(9):868-881, 1987.

36. Melkus G: Type II non-insulin dependent diabetes mellitus, *Nurs Clin North Am* 28:25-33, 1993.

37. Montague DK and others: Diagnostic evaluation, classification, and treatment of men with sexual dysfunction, *Urology* 14:545, 1979.

38. Papalia DE, Olds SW: *Human development,* ed 4, New York, 1989, McGraw-Hill.

39. Pecoraro RE, Reiber GE, Burgess EM: Pathways to diabetic limb amputations: bases for prevention, *Diabetes Care* 13:513, 1990.

40. Peirce AG, Fulmer TT, Edelman CL: Older adult. In Edelman CL, Mandle CL, editors: *Health promotion throughout the lifespan,* ed 3, St Louis, 1994, Mosby.

41. Piaget J: *The theory of stages in cognitive development,* New York, 1969, McGraw-Hill.

42. Rubin RR, Peyrol M, Savdek C: The effort of a diabetes education program incorporating coping skills training on emotional well-being and diabetes self-efficacy, *Diabetes Educ* 19:210-214, 1993.

43. Runyon JW: Co-existing hypertension and diabetes, *Pract Diabetol* 7:1-7, 1988.

44. Sackett DL, Haynes RB: *Compliance with therapeutic regimens,* Baltimore, 1976, John Hopkins University Press.

45. Seevers RJ: Diabetes support group: structure, function and professional roles, *Diabetes Educ* 17:401-406, 1991.

46. Sepe SJ and others: Gestational diabetes: incidence, maternal characteristics and prenatal care, *Diabetes* 34:13, 1985.

47. Strauss A, Glaser B: *Chronic illness and the quality of life,* St Louis, 1975, Mosby.

48. US Department of Health, Education and Welfare, Public Health Service: *Diabetes in America,* Pub No 85-1468, Washington, DC, 1985, US Government Printing Office.

49. US Department of Health and Human Services, Public Health Service: *Healthy People 2000: national health promotion and disease prevention objectives,* DHHS Pub No (PHS)91-5012, Washington, DC, 1990, US Government Printing Office.

21 Diabetes Mellitus and the Older Adult

Martha Mitchell Funnell and Jennifer Hayden Merritt

INTRODUCTION

Diabetes is surprisingly common among older adults, and thus health professionals who specialize in diabetes care and education need to understand the specific physiologic and sociocultural challenges that older persons encounter. In addition, health professionals who specialize in geriatric care and education need to keep abreast of advances in the treatment of diabetes. Diabetes is a serious disease, and its seriousness is often underestimated by the person with diabetes and occasionally by health care professionals, since its initial symptoms may make it appear harmless. However, persons with all types of diabetes risk developing all

---

CHAPTER OBJECTIVES

- Define the relationships among the impaired homeostasis of aging, impaired glucose tolerance, and diabetes.
- Describe the mechanism by which hyperosmolar nonketotic syndrome occurs.
- State two reasons why older persons are prone to concurrent disease interactions and polypharmacy.
- List the four areas of functional ability that need to be assessed with older adults.
- Define two developmental tasks related to this stage of the life span and the impact diabetes can have on each.
- Describe the psychosocial impact of diabetes on older adults.
- Describe the financial impact of diabetes on older adults.
- State three areas that need to be assessed before an educational program is initiated with newly diagnosed older adults.
- Describe two strategies that can be used to compensate for deficits related to the aging process when teaching older adults.
- State the value of an individualized diabetes care and education program for older persons.

its complications.[128] Also, the detection, treatment, and ongoing care of diabetes in the older population present a unique set of challenges.

Who are the older adults with diabetes? How does diabetes differ from glucose intolerance of aging? How does diabetes present atypically in older adults? How do other concurrent diseases, polypharmacy, functional decline, and sensory loss and the unique developmental and psychosocial issues of aging impact on the care of diabetes in older persons? What are the special considerations for the care of this age-group? What are the special considerations for the education of these persons? This chapter addresses these questions and describes the educational process for older adults with diabetes.

RELATIONSHIP BETWEEN DIABETES MELLITUS AND THE AGING PROCESS
Demographics

Currently, 12% of the population is over age 65, and studies show that the number of people over 65 is increasing at a rate three times greater than that of the general population. It is expected that by the year 2020, more than 20% of the population will be over age 65. Furthermore, persons over age 85 represent the fastest-growing segment of the population.[92] These demographic changes will have a profound impact on the U.S. health care system.

Data from the Framingham Heart Study reveal that the development of diabetes in later life is associated with hypertension, vascular disease, elevated very-low-density lipoprotein (VLDL) cholesterol, use of diuretics, and obesity. Subjects who were more than 40% overweight had a greater prevalence of diabetes compared with those of normal weight.[158]

Diabetes is increasingly common with age. It is almost 10 times as common among those over age 65 as those ages 20 to 44.[10] Based on the National Health Interview Survey (NHIS) data, it was estimated that from 1986 to 1988, 9.5% of all persons in the United States over age 65 were diagnosed with diabetes (Table 21-1). Alternatively, approximately 43% of all

Table 21-1 Number of Persons With Diagnosed Diabetes and Percentage of Persons Aged 45 Years and Older in the U.S. Population, 1986-1988

	Age (years)		
	45-64	65-74	75+
Number with diabetes (millions)			
Males	1.33	0.75	0.41
Females	1.30	0.90	0.65
Both sexes	2.63	1.65	1.06
Percentage of U.S. population			
Males	6.2	9.8	10.3
Females	5.5	9.3	9.5
Both sexes	5.8	9.5	9.8

From the National Health Interview Survey, 1986-1988, National Center for Health Statistics.

persons in the United States who were diagnosed with diabetes between 1986 and 1988 were over age 65.[61]

Prevalence of diabetes varies considerably by race. The NHIS data from 1980 to 1990 showed that the prevalence of non-insulin-dependent diabetes mellitus (NIDDM) is 50% higher among African Americans than Caucasians. African-American females show the highest prevalence, with a rate of 21%.[150] The higher prevalence is thought to result from a higher frequency of risk factors, a higher inherent susceptibility, or a greater effect of risk factors in this group.[22] Among Hispanic Americans the rate is even higher (Fig. 21-1).[61] African-American women over age 75 have the highest rate, with almost one in four having diabetes (Fig. 21-2).[150]

Many studies have attempted to determine the degree to which diabetes exists but is undiagnosed. The broadest study of this kind was the National Health and Nutrition Examination Survey II (NHANES II) of 1976 to 1980, in which more than 15,000 persons

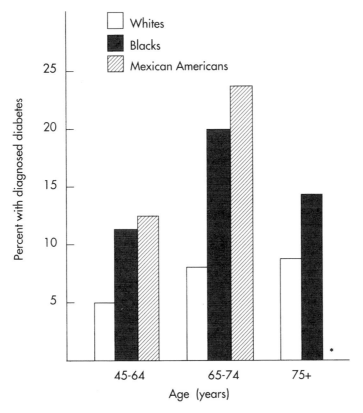

* Data not available

Fig. 21-1   Age-specific prevalence of physician-diagnosed diabetes among whites, blacks, and Mexican Americans in the U.S. population aged 45 years and older, 1982-1984. (From the National Health and Hispanic Health Nutrition Examination Survey, National Center for Health Statistics. In Harris MI: *Clin Geriatr Med* 6:703-729, 1990.)

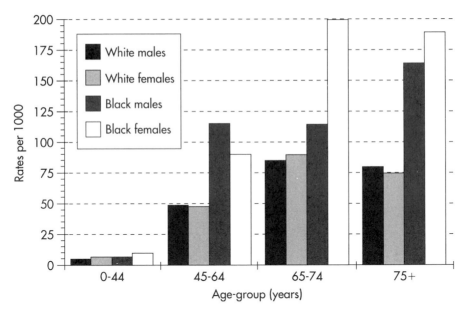

Fig. 21-2 Age-specific prevalence of diabetes by race, gender, and age, United States, 1988-1990. (From US Department of Health and Human Services: *Diabetes Surveillance, 1993,* Atlanta, 1993. Centers for Disease Control and Prevention.)

ages 20 to 74 participated in interviews and almost 12,000 had a physical examination and an oral glucose tolerance test. The data revealed that by World Health Organization (WHO) criteria, undiagnosed diabetes existed at essentially the same rate as a medical history of diabetes. In other words, half of all diabetes cases went undiagnosed. Table 21-2 shows the NHANES II data extrapolated to the U.S. population, 1986 to 1988.[61] Undiagnosed diabetes may be present in 10% to 20% of the U.S. population over age 50, with higher rates among Hispanic Americans and African Americans. An interim study in Finland revealed the prevalence of newly diagnosed NIDDM to be 7%, compared with about 10% of previously diagnosed NIDDM.[114] The onset of NIDDM may be at least 12 years before it is diagnosed, and retinopathy begins developing at least 7 years before NIDDM is detected. This represents a significant health risk for older adults, since the presence of macrovascular disease increases mortality rates for both diagnosed and undiagnosed diabetes.[62]

Because the NHIS has been conducted annually since 1958, one can see how the prevalence of physician-diagnosed diabetes has changed over several decades and can make projections about future prevalence. In the three decades from 1960 to 1990 the rate of diagnosed diabetes increased 2.5-fold among persons over 65 (Fig. 21-3). Harris[61] notes that this increase in prevalence is in addition to what can be expected as a result of the general aging of the population and projects that it will continue into the future.

IDDM Versus NIDDM

Largely because of improved survival rates, an increasing percentage of older adults have insulin-dependent diabetes mellitus (IDDM). To a lesser degree, IDDM may have its onset

Table 21-2   Estimated Prevalence of Undiagnosed Diabetes and Impaired Glucose Tolerance Among Persons Aged 45-75 Years in the U.S. Population, 1986-1988

	Age (years)	
	45-64	65-74
Undiagnosed diabetes*		
Number of persons (millions)		
Males	0.8	0.8
Females	1.6	0.8
Both sexes	2.4	1.6
Percentage of the U.S. population		
Males	3.9	10.4
Females	6.8	8.5
Both sexes	5.4	9.3
Impaired glucose tolerance†		
Number of persons (millions)		
Males	3.2	1.7
Females	3.5	2.2
Both sexes	6.7	3.9
Percentage of the U.S. population		
Males	14.8	22.5
Females	14.7	22.9
Both sexes	14.8	22.7

From the National Health and Nutrition Examination Survey II, 1976-1980, National Center for Health Statistics.
*Fasting plasma glucose ≥ 140 mg/dl and/or 2-hour plasma glucose after 75 g oral glucose ≥ 200 mg/dl.
†Fasting plasma glucose <140 mg/dl and 2-hour plasma glucose after 75 g oral glucose of 140-199 mg/dl.
Number of persons is computed by applying these rates to population estimates of the U.S. Bureau of the Census for 1986-1988.

in late life, or older persons with NIDDM may convert to IDDM during the course of the illness. The key diagnostic test is a C peptide test performed both at fasting and at 90 minutes after a glucose load. A very low serum C peptide level at both times indicates minimal beta-cell function and the presence of IDDM.[95] Since such tests are rarely done in routine outpatient care, limited data exist on the prevalence of IDDM among older adults. However, the vast majority of older persons show characteristics of NIDDM, such as a strong association with obesity, positive family history, and improved glycemia with diet, weight correction, and oral hypoglycemic agents. One study showed the prevalence of IDDM in older adults to be only 0.3%.[160]

Complications of Diabetes

Diabetes not only is common but also is serious, with long-term complications that are debilitating and demoralizing, especially as the person becomes more frail with advancing age.

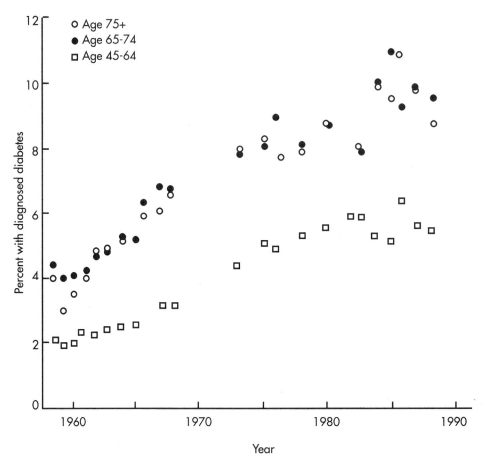

Fig. 21-3   Time trends in the percentage of the U.S. population aged 45 and older with physician-diagnosed diabetes, 1958-1988. (From the National Health Interview Survey, National Center for Health Statistics. In Harris MI: *Clin Geriatr Med* 6:703-729, 1990.)

When compared with persons of the same age without diabetes, those with diabetes are 25 times more likely to become blind, 17 times more likely to develop kidney disease, 20 times more likely to develop gangrene, 15 times more likely to require an amputation, and twice as likely to have a cerebrovascular accident (CVA, stroke) or myocardial infarction (MI).[25] The risk for developing these long-term complications of diabetes increases with longer duration of diabetes. Hospitalization rates and the rates for nursing home admissions are noted to be significantly higher for persons with diabetes compared with those without diabetes. Older adults with diabetes show a hospitalization rate 70% higher than that of the general population (Fig. 21-4).[61] Diabetes is also a significant risk factor for rehospitalization among older adults.[12] The rate of nursing home admissions is 1.2 times greater among persons with diabetes.[122] Mortality is increased as well; diabetes is the fifth ranking cause of death for Americans over age 65[149] and reduces the life expectancy of men by 9 years and women by 7 years.[124]

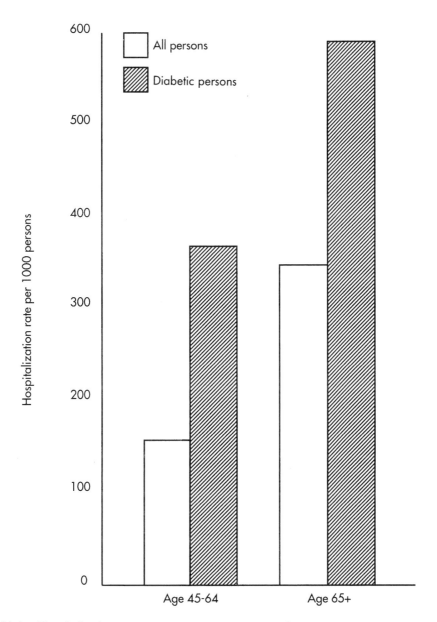

Fig. 21-4   Hospitalization rates among persons in the U.S. population aged 45 years and older, 1987. (From the National Hospital Discharge Survey, National Center for Health Statistics. In Harris MI: *Clin Geriatr Med* 6:703-729, 1990.)

BOX 21-1

CHALLENGES OF GERIATRICS

Impaired homeostasis	Iatrogenic disease
Atypical presentations	Physical and cognitive decline
Multiple concurrent disease interactions	Psychosocial and sociocultural issues
Geriatric pharmacology	Educational and behavioral issues

THE CHALLENGES OF GERIATRICS

Older adults experience common physical, cognitive, and psychosocial challenges as a result of the aging process and face similar developmental tasks as they near the end of their lives. Because of these inherent challenges, the needs of older persons tend to be different from those of younger adults, including health care needs. This has led to recognition of the field of geriatrics as a distinct specialty, similar to the way that pediatrics is recognized as a specialty. Box 21-1 outlines some of the common challenges of geriatrics. This chapter reviews the ways that these challenges apply to diabetes care for older adults.

Normal Physical Changes of Aging

Perhaps the first challenge of geriatrics is to understand what changes are "normal" aging and what changes represent a disease process. Physical changes related to aging that are considered normal are best described as universal, progressive, and irreversible.[44] Table 21-3 outlines systems affected by aging and the potential consequences of these changes.[43] It should be noted, however, that any changes or declines in ability should be evaluated for underlying pathology and not simply dismissed as normal.

Impaired Homeostasis of Aging

In individuals without diabetes, glucose homeostasis, or normoglycemia, is maintained by a complex of biochemical and hormonal mechanisms that balance glucose production with utilization. In the fasting state the amount of glucose produced in the liver by gluconeogenesis and glycogenolysis is equal to the amount utilized by the body's cells. In the postprandial state, when blood glucose levels are rising from digested food, the rise is limited by the release of insulin from the pancreas, which acts quickly to suppress gluconeogenesis and glycogenolysis and transport glucose into cells. As blood glucose then falls, so does the plasma concentration of insulin to maintain euglycemia. The counterregulatory hormones, including glucagon, epinephrine, growth hormone, and cortisol, work in concert to prevent hypoglycemia in this exquisite balancing act. With aging an impairment in this homeostatic mechanism often occurs, leading to higher causal glucose levels. The glucose levels may be sufficiently elevated for the diagnosis of *impaired glucose tolerance* (IGT).

Table 21-3 Physiologic Changes of Aging

System	Effect of aging	Consequences
Central nervous system	Decline in number of neurons and weight of brain Reduced short-term memory Takes longer to learn new information Slowing of reaction time	Do not impair function
Spinal cord/peripheral nerves	Decline in nerve conduction velocity Diminished sensation Decline in number of fibers in nerve trunks	Slowness of "righting" reflexes Diminished sensory awareness Reduced vibratory sensation
Cardiovascular system	Reduced cardiac output (normal?) Valvular sclerosis of aortic valves common Reduced ability to increase heart rate in response to exercise	Reduced exercise tolerance
Respiratory system	Decline in vital capacity Increased lung compliance Reduced ciliary action Increased residual volume Increased anteroposterior chest diameter	Diminished oxygen uptake during exercise Reduced pulmonary ventilation on exercise Increased risk of pulmonary infection Reduced exercise tolerance
Gastrointestinal tract	Decrease in number of taste buds Loss of dentition (normal?) Reduced gastric acid secretion Reduced motility of large intestine	Reduced taste sensation Possible difficulty in mastication Potential cause of iron deficiency anemia Constipation if coupled with low-fiber and low-fluid intake
Kidneys	Loss of nephrons Reduced glomerular filtration rate and tubular reabsorption Change in renal threshold Decreased concentrating ability	Decreased creatinine clearance Reduced renal reserve may lead to reduced glycosuria in presence of diabetes mellitus

Modified from Gambert SR, editor: *Handbook of geriatrics*, New York, 1987, Plenum.   *Continued.*

Table 21-3 Physiologic Changes of Aging—cont'd

System	Effect of aging	Consequences
Musculoskeletal system	Decreased number of muscle fibers	Poor mobility; pain
	Shortening of tendons	Decreased vertical height
	Slower turnover of bone	May predispose to fractures
	Loss of bone density (normal?)	Change in posture
	Diminished lean muscle mass	Reduced strength
Endocrine system/ metabolism	Reduced basal metabolic rate (related to reduced muscle mass)	Reduced caloric requirements
	Impaired glucose tolerance	Must distinguish from true diabetes mellitus
Reproductive system	Men: delayed penile erection, infrequent orgasm, increased refractory period, decreased sperm motility and altered morphology	Diminished sexual response
		Decreased reproductive capacity
	Women: decreased vasocongestion, delayed vaginal lubrication, diminished orgasm, ovarian atrophy	
Skin	Loss of elastic tissue	Increased wrinkling: senile purpura
	Atrophy of sweat glands	Difficulty in assessing dehydration
		Reduced sweating
	Hair loss	

With IGT, blood glucose ranges are greater than normal but less than values diagnostic of diabetes. IGT is so common that controversy exists as to whether it is a "normal" aging change or a typical abnormality (Fig. 21-5). However, because it is not seen in a significant subset of older persons, it is prudent to consider it an abnormality common among older adults, especially since increases in macrovascular disease are associated with IGT.[60] When detected, IGT warrants interventions such as weight reduction and exercise to decrease the risk of progression to NIDDM. In prospective studies, about 20% of those with age-related IGT developed overt diabetes, at a rate of up to 5% per year.[24] In the past, persons with glucose levels in the IGT ranges were told that they had "borderline diabetes." This term has now been replaced by IGT, since most do not develop diabetes. Blood glucose values of persons with normal glucose tolerance and diabetes are compared with values of persons with IGT, as now defined by the National Diabetes Data Group (NDDG) of the National Institutes of Health (NIH) (Table 21-4).[115]

Because serum insulin levels are higher among older persons with IGT (Fig. 21-6) and because insulin receptors are unchanged with aging alone, the belief has been that the primary defect that causes IGT is at the postreceptor site. However, this impairment is complex and

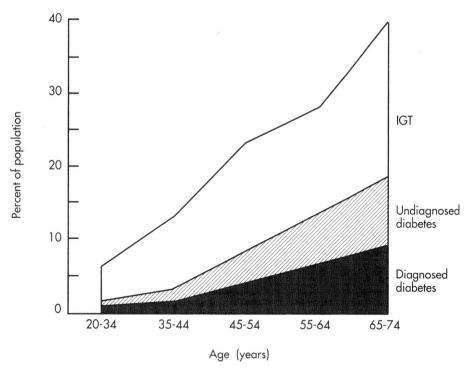

Fig. 21-5   Age-specific prevalence of diabetes and impaired glucose tolerance *(IGT)* in the U.S. population, 1976-1980. (From the National Health and Nutrition Examination Survey, National Center for Health Statistics. In Harris MI: *Clin Geriatr Med* 6:703-729, 1990.)

Table 21-4   Blood Glucose Values* Used to Differentiate Categories of Glucose Tolerance

	Normal	Diabetes mellitus	Impaired glucose tolerance
Fasting	<115	>140	<140
1 hour†	<200	>200	>200
2 hour	<140	>200	140-200

From National Diabetes Data Group: *Diabetes* 28:1039-1057, 1979.
*All figures refer to mg/dl venous plasma glucose levels in nonpregnant adults after a 75 g glucose load.
†Single reading at 30, 60, or 90 minutes.

not yet fully understood.[73] Research is currently under way to elucidate changes in insulin transport inside the cell that may be responsible for the defect. Regardless, the defects responsible for age-related IGT appear to be distinct from those associated with obesity and NIDDM (Table 21-5).[73]

Defects in the glucose homeostasis of NIDDM are even more intriguing, since it appears that the elevations in glucose further worsen insulin resistance, resulting in positive feedback or self-perpetuation of the abnormality.[30] Figure 21-7 illustrates this phenomenon.

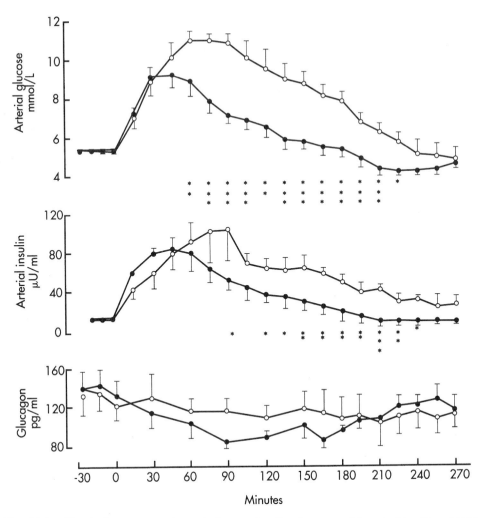

Fig. 21-6 Metabolic response to oral glucose loading in young (●) and older (○) subjects. *p <0.05; **p <0.01; ***p <0.001. (Reproduced with permission of the American Diabetes Association, Inc. From Jackson RA: *Diabetes Care* 13(suppl 2):9-19, 1990).

The diagnosis of IGT and diabetes are based on the NDDG criteria.[115] It is believed that age-specific screening criteria are not warranted.[11] The best screening test for older adults is determination of fasting glucose levels.[113] Two fasting blood glucose readings greater than 140 mg/dl are required to diagnose diabetes, unless there are unequivocal symptoms with a random glucose value greater than 200 mg/dl. A glycohemoglobin level 1% above the normal range is another indicator of an abnormality.[104] Generally, oral glucose tolerance tests are not recommended for older adults, since treatment will not be instituted if fasting glucose levels are lower than 140 mg/dl.[113]

Autonomic neuropathy, occurring as a complication of diabetes, can affect many other delicate homeostatic mechanisms. These include wider ranges in cardiac output, orthostatic

Table 21-5 Comparison of Metabolic Abnormalities in Aging, Obesity, and NIDDM

	Aging	Obesity	NIDDM
Glucose			
Basal	NC	NC	NC or ↑
Glucose tolerance	↓	NC	↓↓↓
Insulin			
Basal	NC	↑	↓ NC ↑
Glucose loading			
Initial response	D	↑	D
Later response	↑	↑↑↑	V
Feedback inhibition of secretion	↓	↓	↓
Triglyceride	NC	↑	↑
Site of defect			
Insulin receptor number	NC	↓	↓
Postreceptor defect	+	NC → +	+

Modified from Jackson RA: *Diabetes Care* 13(suppl 2):9-19, 1990.
NC, No change; ↑, increased; ↓, decreased; ↑↑↑, very increased; ↓↓↓, very decreased; *D,* delayed;
V, variable.

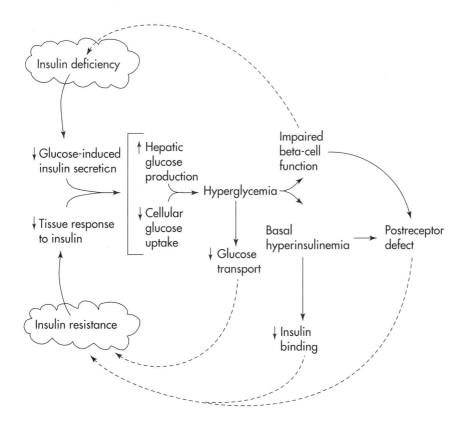

Fig. 21-7 Pathogenic sequence of events leading to development of insulin resistance in NIDDM. (Reproduced with permission of the American Diabetes Association, Inc. Modified from Defronzo RA: *Diabetes* 37:667-687, 1988.)

hypotension, abnormalities in thermoregulation, and a tendency for dehydration.[141] Impairments in the body's ability to maintain homeostasis with changing stresses significantly increases older persons' overall "frailty" and therefore their quality of life. With orthostatic hypotension, for example, many persons find it frustrating to have to arise slowly from a bed or chair to avoid dizziness, especially when they feel the urgency to urinate or answer the phone. This is an example of what may lead an elderly person to say, "It's awful to get old!"

Atypical Presentations of Diabetes and its Complications

Diabetes can present atypically in older adults, as can its acute and chronic complications. Whereas the classic symptoms of hyperglycemia in younger adults are polyuria, polydipsia, and polyphagia, these symptoms may be masked by other illnesses or entirely absent in older adults. Box 21-2 outlines symptoms of diabetes for younger and older adults. Detection of polyuria may be confounded by urinary incontinence. Thirst is typically blunted in older persons, increasing their chances of dehydration and electrolyte imbalance. Hunger may be blunted by the side effects of medication, depression, or gastrointestinal disease. Fatigue, also a common symptom of uncontrolled diabetes, may be discounted by the older person as "just part of getting old." Weight loss is sometimes profound but may be so gradual that it goes unnoticed for several years.

Acute complications of diabetes include *hypoglycemia, hyperosmolar hyperglycemic nonketotic syndrome* (HHNS), and *diabetic ketoacidosis* (DKA). These acute complications may present atypically in the older person, who may have a more difficult time physiologically coping with these challenges than a younger person. HHNS and DKA are relatively rare, especially DKA, since it occurs almost exclusively among persons with IDDM.[112] Efficient diagnosis and treatment are essential to reduce mortality but are often confounded by atypical presentations and the existence of other medical problems.

Hypoglycemia occurs almost exclusively in people taking insulin or sulfonylureas; thus those who are diet controlled are not usually at risk. The adrenergic symptoms of

---

BOX 21-2

TYPICAL PRESENTING SYMPTOMS OF DIABETES

Younger adults	**Older adults**
Polyuria	None; if present may include:
Polyphagia	Blurred vision
Polydipsia	Worsening urinary incontinence
Rapid weight loss	Increased nocturia
Diabetic ketoacidosis (DKA)	Gradual weight loss
	Presence of long-term complications

hypoglycemia that result from the release of epinephrine (shaking, sweating, nervousness), may be blunted or absent in older persons. As a result, medications that block beta-adrenergic receptors, such as propranolol, are not recommended. When hypoglycemia occurs without symptoms to prompt treatment, the reaction can progress to the point where the person with diabetes requires the assistance of another person. This is called *hypoglycemia unawareness.* It not only is frightening, but also may threaten the person's level of independence in the eyes of others. It is precisely this issue that causes many health professionals to be concerned about avoiding hypoglycemia, often to the point where they are hesitant to treat asymptomatic *hyper*glycemia. This is the basis of the debate about what glucose range is best, since many older adults have few symptoms of hyperglycemia, even with average blood glucose levels of 350 to 400 mg/dl.

Generally, older adults have symptoms of chronic complications that are similar to those experienced by younger persons. However, there are some caveats to note when working with older persons. First, a chronic complication of diabetes such as peripheral sensory neuropathy or impotence may be the initial symptom of NIDDM that has actually been present for years. Second, the presentation of chronic complications may be atypical, may be misinterpreted, or may be overshadowed by other conditions. For example, a person may think the discomfort of peripheral neuropathy is "rheumatism" and attempt numerous over-the-counter arthritis preparations before consulting a health care professional. Small cerebral or myocardial infarcts may present "silently" and be diagnosed only when the older man's son or daughter brings him in "because Dad has really slowed down." Symptoms of peripheral vascular occlusive disease such as claudication may not occur in a person who does not exercise enough to induce the related ischemia. Men may perceive impotence as a sign of aging and not mention it to their provider. Third, retinopathy may go undiagnosed and untreated in an older adult who has dense cataracts.

Multiple Concurrent Disease Interactions

Although some older adults have no chronic diseases or only one, most elderly persons have more than one chronic illness. The prevalence of vascular, musculoskeletal, neurologic, ocular, urinary, foot, and gastrointestinal diseases is almost twice as great in persons age 65 and over as those ages 45 to 64.[107] Progression of diabetes and other chronic diseases can lead to their long-term complications. Thus older adults are prone to multiple chronic conditions that may occur as primary disease entities or as secondary complications, and these may interact with each other as previously described.

Hypertension increases in incidence with age, particularly in the African-American population.[98] High blood pressure alone increases the incidence of renal, cardiovascular, and cerebrovascular disease; diabetes compounds the risk. Treatment of hypertension can be problematic in older adults with diabetes, since diuretics may further impair glucose tolerance and lead to electrolyte disturbances. Beta blockers can also have a negative effect on lipid and glucose levels and can mask symptoms of hypoglycemia. Therefore, calcium channel antagonists and angiotensin-converting enzyme (ACE) inhibitors are preferred for mono-therapy of hypertension. Of these, the ACE inhibitors appear to provide the greatest advantage because they show some nephroprotective effect in many studies and have few side effects. Generally, the earlier an ACE inhibitor is used, the better the protective effect on kidney function.[157] Current research is examining the question of whether ACE inhibition is indicated in the absence of hypertension when microalbuminuria is present.[97]

Coronary artery disease (CAD) is the most common condition present among older adults and, despite improvements in related mortality with the advent of cardiac intensive care units, it remains the number-one cause of death in people over age 65. CAD is more common among older persons with diabetes and has important implications for diabetes care. First, the avoidance of hypoglycemia is of particular importance for these persons. During a hypoglycemic reaction, the counterregulatory hormones that raise blood glucose also raise the blood pressure and pulse. This increases myocardial oxygen demands and can cause angina. Second, some research studies suggest that silent MIs are more common when diabetes is present, possibly as a component of autonomic neuropathy.[152] When an MI occurs without the usual manifestations of angina (chest tightness or pain, often radiating to the left arm or jaw), diagnosis and treatment are often delayed, increasing mortality. The prognosis is often poor for persons with diabetes who survive MI.[78] Survival rates at 1 and 5 years after MI are 82% and 58%, respectively, compared with 94% and 82% for people without diabetes.[98] Women with diabetes appear to have poorer survival rates than men.[55]

Diabetes is not a risk factor for osteoarthritis, but arthritic conditions are common in late life, and older persons may consider the related pain more serious than their diabetes. As an example, when an older woman with painful, debilitating osteoarthritis of the knees comes in for a routine appointment, advice about diet and blood glucose control may not seem relevant at that time. She may only want pain medication and instruction in using a cane. Also, arthritis pain may lead to depression, overeating, and decreased activity, which can worsen glycemic control in persons with NIDDM.

Parkinson disease, with its related tremors, muscular rigidity, and bradykinesia, can lead to difficulties with diabetes self-care practices. In its advanced stages the fine motor skills needed for self-monitoring of blood glucose (SMBG), insulin administration, and foot care may become impossible, causing frustration and an increased dependency on others. Dementia related to Parkinson disease, Alzheimer disease, or CVAs has a significant impact on diabetes self-care.

HHNS is an important example of an interaction in which acute and chronic diseases overlap. In this syndrome an older person with diabetes with compromised physiologic function usually has an acute insult such as pneumonia, MI, or CVA (Box 21-3).[112] The most common predisposing factor is infection.[153] The stress response to the insult leads to the secretion of stress hormones, including cortisol and epinephrine, which worsen hyperglycemia. As glucose is lost in the urine, dehydration and hyperosmolarity develop. The problem then becomes a self-perpetuating positive feedback loop instead of a self-correcting negative feedback loop; the more the person secretes stress hormones in an effort to cope with the stress, the more dehydration and hyperglycemia progress because of relative insulin insufficiency. In addition, older persons have a lower total body water content (60% or less) compared with young adults (70%) and may therefore have as much as 8 fewer liters of fluid with which to buffer changes in osmolarity.[99] Ketogenesis does not develop, partly because of the

> ## BOX 21-3
>
> ## RISK FACTORS FOR HYPERGLYCEMIC HYPEROSMOLAR NONKETOTIC SYNDROME (HHNS)
>
> | **Events** | **Drugs** |
> |---|---|
> | Infection | Diuretics |
> | Burn | Beta blockers |
> | Surgery | Glucocorticoids |
> | Cerebrovascular accident (CVA) | Anesthetic |
> | Renal failure | Diphenylhydantoin |
> | Pancreatitis | |
> | Myocardial infarction (MI) | |
>
> Modified from Morrow L, Halter J: *Geriatrics* 43(suppl):57-65, 1988.

availability of some circulating insulin; however, the mechanism is not fully understood. HHNS usually develops over the course of 1 to 2 weeks and has a significant mortality rate, reportedly as high as 40% to 70%, which is higher than in DKA.[83] The mortality rate is particularly high among older persons and those with higher serum osmolarities and more severe concomitant illnesses. One third of all cases of HHNS are diagnosed in persons with no prior history of diabetes.[153]

The person with HHNS may have a lower level of consciousness, such as acute confusion, lethargy, or even coma. Because the primary problem is profound dehydration from hyperglycemic osmotic diuresis, signs of dehydration, such as orthostatic hypotension, tachycardia, and dry skin with poor turgor, are generally present. Serum osmolarity is greater than 320 mOsm/L, indicating hypertonic dehydration. The plasma glucose value is typically more than 600 mg/dl and may be more than 1000 mg/dl.

The treatment of HHNS involves rehydration (which needs to be at a cautiously rapid rate in older adults), insulin, gradual reduction of hyperglycemia and osmolality, correction of electrolytes and pH, and diagnosis and treatment of the underlying cause. Table 21-6 summarizes the signs, symptoms, and treatment of HHNS. Health professionals need to be aware of the risk of HHNS in older persons with NIDDM and encourage them to monitor blood glucose levels, report any trends in high readings, and drink plenty of sugar-free fluids. HHNS is more common in nursing home residents and persons with dementia, so caregivers also need to be aware of signs and symptoms.[83] When a person with NIDDM is admitted to the hospital with infection or for surgery, glucose monitoring should be done frequently.

Geriatric Pharmacology

Persons over age 65 have an average of three prescriptions to manage and take 5.6 medications daily.[106] Although the 25 million Americans over age 65 constitute about 12% of the

Table 21-6 Hyperglycemic Hyperosmolar Nonketotic Syndrome (HHNS)

History/symptoms	Signs	Treatment
Complains of fatigue, weakness Caregivers note confusion, lethargy, or unresponsiveness Recent infection or other illness/injury 33% deny history of diabetes mellitus	Orthostatic hypotension Tachycardia Dry skin, tenting Poor skin turgor Cold extremities Glucose >600 mg/dl Serum osmolarity >320 mOsm/L	Rehydration Insulin Correct electrolytes and pH Treat underlying problem

population, they purchase 25% of drugs sold in the United States. Drug expenses may account for almost 20% of their personal budgets.[107] As a result, older persons with chronic conditions are at risk for problems related to *polypharmacy*. Not only does the possibility exist that a drug used to treat one illness may interact with another illness, but also that the drugs can interact with each other. To compound this problem, older adults are often taking a broad variety of over-the-counter (OTC) medications, such as antacids, pain relievers, cold preparations, and laxatives.

Performance errors with medications occur in all age-groups with alarming frequency, but there is no reason to believe that they occur more often among older adults than among younger persons.[4] However, because older persons take more medications and because of their greater frailty, the risks for negative effects as a result of these errors are of greater concern. Older adults typically experience other problems with medications, including receiving and sharing medications with peers and family members and receiving medications from several care providers.[92] Health professionals may fail to provide clear instructions about the correct use, dosage, and timing of medications they prescribe. Since older persons are often taking several medications, this increases the potential for errors. Many pills look alike, and one may be inadvertently substituted for the other. Discontinuing one drug to begin another is not always clearly explained, and individuals may take both. Therefore the use of both prescribed and OTC medications needs to be carefully assessed, including how, when, and why the person decides to take them.

Use of alcohol should not be overlooked in the challenge of geriatric pharmacology. Older adults often continue to enjoy alcohol in later life but may have a decreased tolerance. They are often unaware of the interactions between alcohol and other drugs, such as its synergistic effect with sedating medications, or that drinking alcohol may cause a mild Antabuse-like reaction when taking chlorpropamide. Depending on a broad array of factors, alcohol can promote hyperglycemia or hypoglycemia in the person with diabetes.[101]

The ingestion of alcohol, particularly for those with liver dysfunction, prolongs the hypoglycemic effect of many sulfonylurea agents (chlorpropamide, tolbutamide, acetohexamide, tolazamide, glipizide, glyburide).[141] Depression, which may affect older adults, may increase alcohol use. It is important that health professionals elicit information about alcohol use in a nonjudgmental way from all individuals, especially those with diabetes.

BOX 21-4

IMPORTANT SULFONYLUREA INTERACTIONS

May diminish hypoglycemic efficacy

Diuretics
Diphenylhydantoin
Glucocorticoids
Lithium
Rifampin
Isoniazid
Nicotinic acid

May enhance or prolong hypoglycemic effect

Sulfonamides
Salicylates
Clofibrate
Dicumarol
Monoamine oxidase inhibitors
Nonsteroidal antiinflammatory drugs
Beta-adrenergic blocking agents
Alcohol

Data from Halter JB, Morrow LA: *Diabetes Care* 13(suppl 2):86-92, 1990.

Sulfonylureas can have interactions with other drugs, and these interactions can affect glycemic control and are important considerations when working with older adults (Box 21-4).[58] The choice of oral agent is especially important for the older adult who may have altered hepatic and renal function. Table 21-7 shows the daily dose, duration of action, and route of elimination for various oral sulfonylurea agents. Generally, drugs with a short duration of action and inactive metabolites are considered safer. Thus chlorpropamide is not a drug of choice for older adults because of its long duration of action.

Iatrogenic Disease

Iatrogenic disease is any adverse condition that results from the efforts of health care professionals to treat an illness or other type of condition. These include the complications of immobility when a person is confined to bed in a hospital and nursing home, acute confusional states resulting from drugs and anesthesia, and nosocomial infections after surgeries and other procedures. The person with diabetes may be at increased risk for iatrogenic diseases because of compromised physiologic function and the worsening of blood glucose levels with stress hormones. For example, HHNS can be triggered iatrogenically by the use of certain medications, surgery, or infection secondary to procedures such as placement of an indwelling urinary catheter.

Table 21-7   Comparison of Oral Sulfonylurea Drugs

Drug	Daily dosage range (mg)	Approximate duration of action (hours)	Route of elimination
Tolbutamide	500-3000	6-12	Hepatic metabolism; renal excretion of less active metabolites
Glipizide	2.5-40	8-12	Hepatic metabolism; renal excretion of inactive metabolites
Tolazamide	100-1000	12-16	Hepatic metabolism; renal excretion of less active metabolites
Acetohexamide	250-1500	12-24	Hepatic metabolism; active metabolism (Hydroxyhexamide has half-life of 5 hours and is excreted renally.)
Glyburide	2.5-20	24	Hepatic metabolism; renal excretion of less active metabolites
Chlorpropamide	100-750	40-72	80% hepatic metabolism; renal excretion of parent drug and less active metabolites

From Morrow LA, Halter JB: Carbohydrate metabolism in the elderly. In: Sowers Jr, Felicetta JV, editors: *The endocrinology of aging,* New York, 1988, Raven.

FUNCTIONAL ABILITY AND THE AGING PROCESS

This chapter has discussed normal aging changes, the prevalence of diabetes, and how chronic conditions can interact. But what about function? Two older persons, both age 70 with diabetes, cataracts, cardiovascular disease, and arthritis, may be taking the same medications, but one may be independent while the other is totally dependent on a spouse for help. Why is one person able to function independently while the other is not? Obviously one's functional capacity is not solely determined by age or by health problems and medications.

Functional ability is the degree of independence with which a person is able to perform common activities of daily living (ADLs). Each person's total functioning is divided into four major areas: physical, cognitive, emotional, and psychosocial.[147] The body's organs and integrated physiologic function are essential for life. The mind's ability to learn, think, remember, communicate, and judge is essential for independence. Positive experiences and expression of emotion are essential for satisfaction. Contact with others and the fulfillment of vocational, leisure, social, financial, and cultural needs are essential for quality of life. Thus the ability to function in all areas has an impact on total health and the ability to care for oneself. Physical health impairments have been linked to depression in older adults.[6] In addition, the significant happenings in a person's life, the demands of family and friends, the environment of daily living, and personal values related to daily living all serve to make up a person's total functional ability.[42]

ADLs are divided into two areas: basic or personal ADLs and instrumental ADLs (IADLs). Personal ADLs relate to basic self-care; IADLs relate to what is necessary for independent living. Box 21-5 lists examples of each; both lists could be considerably longer.

BOX 21-5
_____

EXAMPLES OF ACTIVITIES OF DAILY LIVING (ADLS)

Basic ADLs	**Instrumental ADLs**
Eating	Writing
Bathing	Reading
Toileting	Cooking
Dressing	Menu planning
Grooming	Cleaning
Transferring (to/from bed/chair/bath)	Shopping
Ambulating (or other locomotion)	Doing laundry
Providing foot care	Climbing stairs
Monitoring blood glucose	Using the telephone
Communicating	Managing medications
	Managing insulin/hypoglycemia
	Managing money
	Traveling out of the home
	Maintaining upkeep of home

For example, basic ADLs could include shampooing hair and brushing teeth. IADLs could include cutting food, lifting pots, and turning faucets.

The essence of geriatrics is to assist each person to attain and maintain his or her optimal level of function, since cure of disease is often not possible.[118] In order for older persons to live as independently as possible for as long as possible, they require not only health care but often the care of many others, both professional and nonprofessional.

Physical Changes With Aging

Older adults vary as to the age and the extent that the normal physical effects of aging occur. Although there are generally declines in physical functioning, normal aging changes alone do not interfere with a person's ability to achieve and maintain a high level of independence and fulfillment.

Sensory declines, which are common among older adults, have important implications for functioning. Among people over age 65, 18% to 20% have visual impairments, and the incidence of color blindness increases.[84] Cataracts and macular edema or degeneration are the most common visual problems among people over 65, but their symptoms are rarely reported. Early cataract development leads to a yellowing or browning of the lens and color distortions. Later cataracts lead to bothersome glare and blurred vision. Macular edema may cause double vision, whereas macular degeneration results in a loss of central vision, causing difficult reading.[105] Presbycusis, leading to hearing deficits, is present in one fourth to one half of all older persons.[74,84] The number and size of taste buds may decrease and the sense of smell diminish, leading to a loss of interest in food.[43] Tactile sensation may also decrease.[84]

Cognitive Changes With Aging

Healthy older adults vary greatly in the extent to which their cognitive abilities change with age, but research has shown that a significant decline is not inevitable.[147] Cognitive impairment affects about 5% to 10% of persons over age 65 and is severe in only half of those.[92,155] Cognitive changes caused by normal aging include slowing but not elimination of the ability to create and retrieve memory, but no normal aging change by itself has to be a threat to an older person's ability to function independently.[147]

INTERACTION OF DIABETES AND FUNCTIONAL ABILITY
Physical Considerations

Older persons with diabetes are at an increased risk for functional limitations. Peripheral vascular disease, peripheral neuropathy, diminished proprioception, postural hypotension, obesity, and cardiac disease may interfere with the ability to walk, climb stairs, and perform other physical activities and may increase the likelihood of falls and their debilitating results. Peripheral neuropathy and decreased circulation increase the risks for foot ulcers, infections, and resulting amputations. Carpal tunnel syndrome and diabetic amyotrophy may limit the ability to use one's hands for cooking, dressing, and other fine motor tasks.[147]

The prevalence of diabetic retinopathy increases with aging, from 10% at age 55 to more than 30% by age 80.[111] The prevalence of glaucoma and cataracts also increases in older persons with diabetes. Visual impairment is a threat to independence because it impacts ADLs, work or hobby activities, the ability to drive, and social relationships.

Diabetes-related problems increase both the likelihood that older adults will need surgery and their risk for complications during and after a procedure. Frequent blood glucose monitoring is needed during all phases of the surgical process, and insulin may be needed until after the person has fully recovered.

Elevated glucose levels are associated with other conditions that are likely to impact the lives of older adults. Hyperglycemia leads to decreased red blood cell deformability, which may worsen peripheral vascular disease. Evidence indicates that elevated glucose levels increase platelet adherence, which increases the chances that a person may have an MI or CVA, and may also impair recovery from strokes.[111]

Persons with diabetes report pain more frequently than other chronically ill persons. It has been suggested that hyperglycemia heightens pain perception.[111] Pain from other chronic conditions and neuropathies may therefore be more difficult to manage for the older person with diabetes.

Loss of bladder control is generally devastating to the person's social and physical functioning. Hyperglycemia and the propensity for bladder infections among older adults with diabetes exacerbate difficulties with incontinence.[147]

Cognitive Considerations

It is fairly well established that persons with NIDDM perform more poorly on various cognitive tasks than those without diabetes.[147,148] One study of older persons with NIDDM and age-matched persons without NIDDM showed greater cognitive deficits among those with NIDDM even when they perceived themselves to be in good health.[129] All subjects were ambulatory, lived in the community, and were capable of undergoing several hours of cognitive testing. Poorer performance of relatively healthy older adults with NIDDM compared with the control subjects suggests that cognitive changes are related to the presence of NIDDM. Most of these differences parallel changes encountered with normal aging in that relatively minor differences are found for tests of immediate memory, whereas larger differences are found for more demanding tasks that require working memory. No significant diabetes-related differences have consistently been revealed in the realms of attention, short-term memory, or semantic memory. Although elevated glucose levels appear to contribute to cognitive deficits, the precise relationship is not clear. In addition, elevated triglycerides also appear to affect cognition negatively.[147] Older adults with more severe diabetes, as evidenced by higher glycosylated hemoglobin levels and peripheral neuropathy, show a relatively greater impairment in cognitive function.[120] However, verbal learning and memory may improve with better glycemic control,[53] although further research into the mechanism of this improvement is needed.[119] The presence of emotional problems such as anxiety and depression adversely affect cognitive measures in subjects with and without diabetes.

Cognitive abilities are essential to an older person's ability to maintain independence. When older adults who have diabetes and cognitive deficits are challenged to coordinate a complicated treatment program, their independence is likely to be threatened.

In its early stages, cognitive impairment can cause problems such as inconsistently taking medication to manage diabetes and other health problems, but it may not be recognized. Erratic eating patterns may lead to erratic blood glucose levels, weight loss, malnutrition, and dehydration, which in turn may further worsen cognitive function. Early detection of and intervention for cognitive deficits often lead to better health outcomes in older persons and can potentially help them stay in their own homes, if appropriate community resources are used.

In more advanced dementia, such as later stages of Alzheimer type of dementia or severe multiinfarct dementia, the diabetes treatment program often needs to be redefined. For example, if an older person with diabetes develops Alzheimer's disease with resultant weight loss, simply helping the person obtain adequate nutrition may be more important than avoiding moderate hyperglycemia. In this situation, most of the goal negotiation, education, and feedback needs to be between the health care team and the person's caregiver.

NORMAL PSYCHOSOCIAL DEVELOPMENT

The changes that occur during the aging process are not only biologic but social and psychologic as well. As the developmental tasks of middle adulthood are completed, the tasks related to the end of the life span are begun.

Several theorists have proposed tasks that are specific to this stage of life. Erikson[35] described this phase, beginning at age 50, as *integrity versus despair.* During this stage an individual reviews his or her life for relevance and meaningfulness and develops a sense of integrity or acceptance versus a sense of despair or rejection of one's life.[5] Havighurst[66] theorized that individuals must learn to adapt to new roles, situations, and relationships throughout the life span. He defined the adaptations of later maturity, beginning at age 60, as adjusting to a decline in strength and health, retirement, death of one's spouse, difficulty affiliating with one's age-group, and accepting death. More recently, Levinson and others[90] proposed a view of the life cycle as a series of eras, each lasting 20 to 25 years. The primary task of late adulthood, beginning at age 60, is to balance involvement with society with involvement with self.

The developmental tasks for this stage represent major life adjustments and many losses. Therefore this is one of the most stressful periods in the life span.[162] Depression is believed to be an extremely common response to these losses, although it is largely undetected and untreated. It is so common that it has been suggested that older adults go through a developmental depressive crisis, similar to the developmental crisis of adolescence.[42] The ability to make the many adjustments needed during this phase may be a function of what has occurred during the previous stages and whether earlier tasks were completed. This is not to say that growth and insight do not occur, because many older adults are able to review their lives, place events in perspective, and thus resolve lifelong conflicts.[79]

Older adults who are members of ethnic minorities appear to be at greatest risk for the negative impacts of the aging process on income, health, and some measures of life satisfaction. Interestingly, however, on some measures of quality of life, differences in scores between Caucasians and minority groups diminish with age.[79] Thus aging appears to both enhance and level off the problems associated with being part of a minority group. It is also important to note that members of every ethnic group are heterogeneous and culturally reflect both personal and shared experiences.

Family Relationships

The family is one of the most basic institutions within American society. Most people are born into a family, live much of their lives within a family, and consider it to be a high priority in their values system.[5] However, the family structure, roles and relationships within the family, and its purpose and function change over time.[79]

The family has a dynamic life cycle that begins with marriage and ends with the death of one spouse. Several models for the life cycle of a family exist, but the stages that generally occur among older adults begin when children start to leave home. In a model adapted by Atchley,[5] the last four phases are as follows:
1. Launching children (oldest child to youngest child leaving home)
2. Middle years (children gone to spouse's retirement)
3. Retirement (one spouse retired until start of disability)
4. Old age (one spouse disabled until death of one spouse)

The "empty-nest syndrome" is a relatively new phenomenon within the life of a family as people live longer and healthier lives. It generally refers to the years a couple spend together between the launching of their last child and the death of one spouse. Although the departure of the children is a disruption to the family and the parents, most research indicates that this is a time many parents look forward to, prepare for, and do not find exclusively stressful.[8]

Family units often include more than one generation. Research into family forms and functions has not borne out the expectation that the isolated nuclear family would emerge as the norm. With the increased longevity of the current population, four-generational families are becoming more and more common, and the generations frequently share many links. The common thread that binds the generations is a system of shared beliefs, norms, values, and cultural traditions in the family.[23]

Ethnicity appears to play a strong role in family relationships. It is often assumed that minority persons have more extended family ties, including aunts, uncles, siblings, nieces, nephews, and cousins, than do Caucasians. This appears to be true for African-American adults, with older African-American women playing an important role in this network.[143] However, this does not appear to be true for older Hispanic-American adults. Extended family life is the tradition of this culture, but it is rapidly becoming irrelevant with the increasing urbanization and assimilation of Hispanic-American families. Although this has led to some tensions between generations, it seems that older adults are still respected and revered.[79] Many older Asian-American and Native-American persons may be suffering from isolation for similar reasons. Members of the Asian-American minorities have generally been economically assimilated, but the simultaneous accommodation to American values has left some older members isolated and alienated from their families. Older Native-American adults are traditionally held in high esteem by younger tribe members. Although they still play an important role within the extended family, increased urbanization is also causing erosion in this family structure.[23]

The most important family relationship for many older adults is with their adult children.[143] About 80% of older Americans have living children, and most of them are not isolated from their offspring.[5] Most studies show that older adults and their children see each other quite often. Distance appears to be the strongest determinant for frequency of contact, and visitation is more frequent along the female line of the family.[79] Among older Caucasians, socioeconomic status is the most significant predictor of the informal support network, with persons at a high socioeconomic level more likely to have a supportive relationship with children.[143]

When asked, most parents and adult children report positive feelings for each other. Generally, older adults hold their children in high regard, and parents remain important to children throughout the life span. Most adult children are able to view their parents as individuals with strengths, limitations, and life histories.[5]

Despite these mutually strong feelings, almost all studies show that older adults prefer to live near, but not with, their children. Most appear to want "intimacy at a distance," citing the desire to preserve privacy and independence and to avoid conflict or interference with their children.[79] Most older parents are able to recognize that their children have the right to pursue their own lives.[5] Caucasian older adults are more likely to move in with their adult children, whereas older African-American and Hispanic-American persons are more likely to have adult children move in with them.[23]

Mutual aid is also considered to be a crucial intergenerational dimension. Research indicates that a two-directional flow of assistance occurs between parents and children. Financial and social support is provided by each generation to the other at different times over the years.[23] Parents generally attempt to provide emotional and financial support to their adult children as long as they are able and healthy.[5] The assistance provided consists of both informal, nonessential services (e.g., babysitting, transportation) and highly organized, essential services (e.g., financial aid, housing). The type of assistance offered and received depends on the gender of the parents and children, ethnicity, and social class.[80] For example, compared with other ethnic groups, African Americans are most likely to give or receive help and support across generations.[23] Older African Americans receive goods and services more often than younger ones, with reported frequency of help decreasing as age increases.[65]

The two-way flow of support may persist until the death of one spouse or extreme frailty in the older parent.[79] More attention is being given to the extent to which middle-age people experience being in the middle between their children and their parents. Feelings of a sense of duty underlie many intergenerational relationships during this time.[5] The expression "sandwich generation" identifies this dilemma. Many people believe that a role inversion or reversal occurs during this time. However, this should not be expected and may even be maladaptive. "Parentification" of the children and "infantilization" of the older parents not only leads to guilt, but also is demeaning to everyone involved. Such behavior is often a reflection on the past relationship between parents and children and conflicts that have never been resolved.[139]

About 80% of older persons have living brothers or sisters. With the advent of old age, the death of a spouse, and an "empty nest," many older adults seek to renew sibling relationships. Men are generally closest to sisters, and sister-sister relationships are often extremely close. Siblings are especially important in the lives of older adults who never married or had children, since spouses and children are generally viewed as the first lines of support.[5] Friends also serve a primary role in support networks for many older adults. Among African Americans, members of their churches are also a particularly important source of support and assistance.[144]

Marriage and Divorce

The number of older married couples is increasing because of the greater longevity of the population, particularly among men. The average couple can expect 15 years together after the departure of the last child.[79] Most older couples have grown old together, and their relationship is often the focal point in their lives.

Most studies have shown that the pattern of marital satisfaction is high in early adulthood, declines through middle age, and rises steadily again after childrearing. Happy couples provide great comfort and support to each other, show a high degree of interdependence, share many activities, remain sexually intimate, and exhibit greater equity between partners than unhappy couples.[5]

Marital satisfaction is a primary factor for overall satisfaction with life. One of the functions of couplehood involves intimacy, including a sense of belonging, mutual affection, regard, trust, and sex. Sexuality is an important but often neglected component of intimacy among older adults. Sexual activity reflects physical capacity, emotional needs, and social norms and means much the same to older persons as it does to others. For couples who remain physically healthy, the later years generally reflect feelings of greater appreciation and affection for each other and an increase in the time and opportunity for companionship. Diminished sexual function related to aging, poor health, or specific diseases, such as diabetes, can have a negative impact on marital happiness.[5]

Not all marriages become more satisfying over the years; a small proportion do not. The quality of the relationship and adjustments made in later life are probably a reflection of adjustments made earlier in life. Marriages among older couples reported as happy had generally been satisfying over the life span, whereas unhappy older couples reported difficulties from the beginning.[23] Higher proportions of unhappy couples reported children living at home, less than good communication, fewer mutual interests, differing values, poor communication, and low enjoyment of sex.[5]

The divorce rate is not high among older couples, but it has more than doubled since 1960. Older African Americans are almost twice as likely as older Caucasians to be divorced or separated.[34] The difficulty of adjusting to divorce increases as age increases, making it more stressful. Compared with younger divorced persons, older adults report greater unhappiness, fewer positive emotional experiences, greater pessimism, and long-term dissatisfaction.[79] Older women may experience a significant loss of income if they have no retirement funds of their own.[5]

Widowhood

The majority of older women are widows. The longevity gap between men and women has not been bridged completely, so the disproportion between the sexes increases with age.[139] The proportion of African-American and Hispanic-American widows is higher than Caucasians because of decreased longevity among African-American and Hispanic-American men.[23]

Considerable variation exists in the experience of widowhood. Almost everyone is emotionally impacted by the loss of a spouse, but some people are impacted more severely and for a longer time. Lopata[94] has proposed four stages in the adjustment to widowhood: (1) the official recognition of the event, which is a time of crisis and mourning; (2) the temporary disengagement stage; (3) limbo, when one confronts life without one's spouse; and (4) the reengagement stage with the establishment of a new life-style, when one reorganizes one's life as a single person.

Although controversial, the adaptation process and difficulties encountered appear to be similar for men and women. The concurrent loss of a widower's occupational role may compound the loss of his wife, while widows often experience a loss in income.[23] Widowhood affects all family interactions, and widowed parents must adjust to different relationships with their adult children.[5] For example, a widow may grow closer to an adult daughter. Loneliness is a primary problem, and having an effective social support network appears to soften the impact of a life event as stressful as widowhood.[23]

Grief is defined as a reaction to loss, and *bereavement* refers to the state of having sustained a loss.[80] Grief can include physiologic, psychologic, and sociologic responses.

People who experience a loss tend to go through predictable stages in the adjustment process, including protest, despair, detachment, and reorganization.[23]

Older adults in American society are not always provided with an opportunity to express their grief. Many people believe that since older persons should expect loss as inevitable, they should be able to "grin and bear it." The inability to express grief may lead to physical manifestations or symptoms that can be misinterpreted as dementia. Unresolved grief can also lead to increased risks for new illnesses, worsening of chronic illnesses, or even death.[121]

The person who becomes a widow(er) is confronted with a variety of personal and familial problems. Widowed persons consistently show higher rates of mortality, mental disorders, and suicides. The death of a spouse is particularly difficult for persons who depend heavily on their marital partner.[23] For persons with diabetes, this may be a time of worsening in blood glucose control because of stress, loss of support, or the gap left if the spouse was responsible for care activities or food preparation.

Remarriage

Remarriage may be desirable for many divorced or widowed older adults. The probability of remarriage decreases as age increases, however, partly because of the smaller numbers of eligible men among the older population. The opportunity for remarriage is even less for African Americans and Hispanic Americans.

The primary reason for marriage among older adults tends to be companionship. Some older persons remarry to allay their anxiety about poor health, to obtain financial security, and to avoid dependency on their adult children.[5]

Marriages between older adults generally appear to be successful, particularly when based on affection and mutual financial security. The approval of children also appears to contribute to success.[79] Having similar backgrounds and being well acquainted before marriage also increase the likelihood for success.[23] Impotence, which occurs frequently in men with diabetes, may hinder both the interest in and the success of a late-life marriage.

Grandparenting

Increased life expectancy, earlier marriages, shorter childrearing periods, and fewer children have exposed more middle-age and older adults to grandparenthood than ever before.[23] Many adults will spend 40 years as grandparents.[5] About 75% of older adults are grandparents, but only a few adults over age 65 have young grandchildren.

Neugarten and Weinstein[116] identified five major styles of grandparenting as the following:
1. Formal: maintain clearly defined lines between parenting and grandparenting and leave parenting exclusively to the mother and father
2. Fun seeking: informal and playful with an emphasis on mutual gratification
3. Distant figure: contact fleeting but benevolent
4. Surrogate parent: cares for children while mother works; usually grandmother
5. Reservoir of family wisdom: distinctly authoritative; usually grandfather

Older grandparents are more likely to have a more formal style of grandparenting, and women are more likely to look forward to the role of being a grandparent than men.[23]

More attention is now being paid to the growing number of great-grandparents in the United States. There appear to be two styles of great-grandparenting: remote and close. Many similarities exist between grandparenthood and great-grandparenthood, but increasing age, frailty, and distance have an impact on the relationship.[79]

Generally, grandchildren seem to have strong affection toward their grandparents.[79] Studies have shown that even as young adults, grandchildren rate relationships with their grandparents as very significant and keep in close contact.[5] Although not meaningful to all older adults, most come to enjoy the role because it involves a minimum of responsibility and much personal fulfillment.[23] The age at grandparenthood, concurrent life events, and ethnicity all influence grandparenting styles.[5]

Hispanic Americans have the largest number and report the most frequent contact with their grandchildren, while African Americans have more contact than Caucasians, except among the oldest groups.[79] More older African Americans appear to offer child-raising assistance with their grandchildren than Caucasians. Among older-adult households headed by African-American women, 41% include children under age 18, compared with 9% headed by older Caucasian women. Native Americans also appear to be influential in raising grandchildren, particularly those who live on reservations.[23] In cultures such as these, where NIDDM is prevalent and the influence of grandparents is strong, one approach that may be helpful is to teach the importance of childhood nutrition to the grandparents in an effort to prevent obesity and the subsequent development of diabetes.

Retirement

Work and retirement are highly significant aspects in the lives of many older adults. Work shapes an individual's daily activities and contributes to his or her self-concept and life satisfaction. Retirement is therefore a major event. It marks a change in daily activity and economic status and is a symbolic transition to old age.[162]

Retirement is a process that involves withdrawing from work and taking on the roles of a retired person. Being able to settle into a satisfying routine is important for retirement satisfaction. Atchley[5] describes phases that persons may go through when adjusting to retirement as follows:

1. Pre-retirement: concerns about the financial aspects and activities during retirement begin; includes remote and near phases
2. Honeymoon: immediately following retirement, when freedom is enjoyed
3. Rest and relaxation: temporary low level of activity
4. Disenchantment: a letdown during adjustment to a slower pace
5. Reorientation: refocus of activities and routines as persons pull themselves together
6. Termination: return to work or loss of retirement role through illness or disability

Retirement is somewhat different for women and minorities than for Caucasian men. Most older women have had discontinuous work histories or no employment history. Gains that occurred during the Civil Rights movement of the 1960s occurred too late to have much impact on the educational level or economic conditions of today's older minorities. As a result, older African Americans fare worse than Caucasians on a variety of economic indicators. The varied work histories of many African Americans, which include high levels of unemployment and overrepresentation in low-paying jobs, are reflected in their retirement incomes. Older African-American women generally have higher educational levels than African-American men but have generally had lower-paying jobs. African-American women are more likely to have worked steadily for all their adult lives than Caucasian women, but they are less likely to have retired.[79] Many older African Americans continue to work indefinitely and only yield to retirement because of health problems.[17] Older African Americans with a discontinuous work life and the economic need to work intermittently may be more likely to assume a disabled-worker role, which is viewed as more advantageous than a retired role. The "unretired-retired" are those 55 and older who are no longer working, generally because of disability, but who do not consider themselves to be retired.[47] This group appears to be the most deprived of the older African-American adults and may often need to work for economic reasons despite poor health or advancing age.[46]

Few Hispanic Americans have had lengthy work careers to prepare for retirement. The combined problems of low-paying, unskilled jobs and questionable citizenship or residential status has led to older Hispanic-American adults staying in the work force longer than older Caucasian adults.[79] In general, however, lower educational levels among minorities and past discrimination in the work place has led to lower incomes, lower Social Security benefits available, and the postponement of retirement for as long as possible.

Despite the grim picture that is often painted of retirement, studies show that most people look forward to retirement and see it as a positive time. The adjustment to retirement is thought to be determined in part by the person's attitude. Factors that impede the adjustment process include poor health, inadequate income, the inability to give up one's job gracefully, and any other situational changes that occur at the same time.[5] Research has shown that the health of retirees often improves rather than worsens, as is generally believed. Because older African Americans were more likely to have been shut out of meaningful occupational positions, they may be less likely to find retirement disruptive.[23]

Retirement before age 62 is considered to be early retirement. Very early retirees tend to be either in good health with high incomes or in poor health with very low incomes.[162] Unfortunately, early retirees among older adults with diabetes generally fall into the latter category, since the pathology and morbidity related to diabetes are risk factors for early retirement.[154]

Death and Dying

Death and the dying process are being viewed more and more as the terminal phase of the life cycle.[80] As people age and are confronted with the deaths of friends and family members, they are less able to avoid thinking about this stage in their own life and the inevitability of their own death.

The dying process is not conceptualized as an unbroken decline in health toward death. In the first or social stage, older persons are fighting the tendency of society to impose a premature social death. They may bargain to hold onto symbols that represent the future, such as a cane when they are no longer able to walk. In the second or terminal stage, death is more imminent, and the person may bargain directly with God.[80]

The meanings that people give to death vary as a function of age. Studies indicate that two meanings of death are of particular significance for older adults. One is death as an organizer of time. Anticipating the end of one's life may bring about a reorganization of time and priorities. The second is the meaning of death as loss. Facing death can make all possessions and other experiences appear to be transient and meaningless. The perception among older persons of the finitude of life is reinforced by both people and institutions. American society appears to perceive older persons as not deserving of a major investment of resources.[80] At the same time, health care professionals sometimes appear to value preservation of life whenever possible, whereas older persons who perceive their quality of life to be poor may want to avoid life-sustaining measures. The debate about how much societal values can supercede personal choice is increasingly an issue of concern among legislators and citizens.

Scientific studies about the effect of religious beliefs on attitudes toward death are inconclusive. The most common attitude toward death is fear, and the acceptance of death is viewed as true maturity. In general, studies have shown that older persons frequently are more accepting of death and have fewer anxieties about it. Among the aged population, those who report good health are most likely to be evasive about death, whereas those in poor health view death in a more positive manner.[23]

IMPACT OF DIABETES ON NORMAL PSYCHOSOCIAL DEVELOPMENT
Sociocultural Considerations

A complex interplay exists between the physical and sociocultural aspects of an illness among older persons.[23] Many of the negative events that occur to older adults are both physical and social and impact total functional ability. For example, because of the dietary demands of diabetes, older persons may isolate themselves from eating in restaurants or gatherings of family and friends, leading to loneliness and decreased support to cope with their illness. Diabetes-related impotence may lead to isolation from one's spouse and marital difficulties.

Very little work has been done on the sociocultural impact of diabetes on older adults. However, it is believed that the impact is generally less severe than among young persons. A study by Linn and colleagues[91] indicates that older adults are more likely to accept a chronic illness such as diabetes as a natural part of the aging process. Jenny[74] compared adaptation to diabetes among four age-groups: younger (mean age of 19.7), middle (mean age of 35.9), older (mean age of 57.3), and aged (mean age of 71.7) adults. The older and aged adults identified the fewest barriers to adherence and the least number of special concerns about diabetes. However, they also identified the greatest number of health problems that interfered with diabetes management and the least amount of social support. Among the four age-groups, diabetes was perceived as least severe by the aged subjects.

The issue of the sociocultural impact of diabetes is further complicated by differences in types of diabetes and treatment programs. One comparison of subjects with IDDM (mean age of 34.8), NIDDM using insulin (mean age of 58.7), and NIDDM not using insulin (mean age of 62.3) showed that subjects with NIDDM using insulin reported significantly more control problems, social problems, and barriers to adherence than persons with NIDDM not using insulin. IDDM and NIDDM participants using insulin reported similar perceptions of their risk for complications of diabetes, while NIDDM subjects not using insulin reported a significantly lower perceived risk.[27] Severity may also be related to glycemic control, with those in poorer control rating diabetes as more severe. In this sample, persons taking oral agents or insulin had higher glycated hemoglobin levels.[123] The perception of severity of diabetes compared with other chronic illnesses in late life has been largely unexplored.

Older adults' emotional response to diabetes is probably similar to that of younger persons. Depression appears more common among persons with either type of diabetes than among those without diabetes.[45] The older adult's self-esteem, bodily integrity, self-worth, autonomy, independence, and control all may be challenged by a diagnosis of diabetes. The ability to deal with these feelings is probably affected by previous coping style, social support, and economic factors.[147]

Family and social support appears to impact glycemic control and self-management behaviors among older adults. Persons with NIDDM generally report receiving more social support than those with IDDM,[86] and most samples of older adults report receiving adequate support to care for their diabetes,[19] although some report an increased sense of isolation. Little research has been done on how chronic illness impacts family relationships among older adults. Between husbands and wives, communication has been found to decrease and stress and loneliness increase. Many spouses (particularly wives) must accept care responsibilities and may find the demands overwhelming. The quality of the relationship between parents and adult children is also affected by a chronic illness. Negative feelings toward parents appear to increase as health declines and dependency increases.[89]

Very little is known about the impact of diabetes on the spouses and families of older adults. The response to NIDDM may be complicated because it tends to run in families.[147] Two potential negative effects are (1) increased dependency on family members due to increased care needs related to diabetes and (2) increased social isolation due to dietary and other demands of daily diabetes care.

The incidence of chronic conditions and levels of physical limitations may give the impression that older persons view themselves as being in poor health and unable to function. This is false perception. In a large study of older adults, most viewed themselves as being in good to excellent health compared with others their age.[79]

Socioeconomic Considerations

The importance of economic status among older adults cannot be overstated. Financial resources have a great impact on the ability to maintain control over one's life, participate in desired leisure activities, and adequately care for one's health.[79]

Although older adults have fewer expenses than during their child-raising years, they still have to pay for the same basic needs as other people. In addition, declining health, increasing medical care costs, and the financial costs of a chronic illness such as diabetes raise the economic needs of older adults.[23]

Older Americans consistently have lower incomes, about two-thirds that of younger adults. Newly retired persons (the young-old) are more likely to have adequate incomes than those over 75 (the old-old) years of age.[23] However, as a result of substantial improvements over the past 20 years, when noncash benefits are taken into account, a smaller percentage of older adults are now below the poverty line than the general population. Most older persons state that they are satisfied with their financial situation.[7]

Despite these gains, economic status clearly is a concern for many older adults. Hispanic Americans, African Americans, those living alone, those with less than 8 years of education, those living in central cities, and African-American women living alone are poorer than other older Americans. In the United States, older African Americans are the most economically disadvantaged of any group. Sixty-eight percent of rural, older African-American women live in poverty, compared with 21% of Caucasian females.[23] Because older adults spend proportionally more on health care, housing, and food than younger adults, these difficulties often manifest themselves in inadequate nutrition, housing, and medical care.[7] Older Asian Americans are most similar to Caucasians in income.[5]

Social Security is the major source of income for persons over age 65. Ninety percent of older adults receive income from this source, which constitutes 40% of their income. Assets, pensions, and other earnings make up the rest of the income. More older Americans who have low incomes rely on Social Security than do those with high incomes.[7]

Health Care Costs

U.S. health care costs have increased at a rapid pace, particularly among older persons. In 1981 the medical bill for the older population was three times that of other adults. One of the reasons medical costs are higher among older persons is the prevalence of chronic illnesses such as diabetes. It was estimated that the total health care costs for those with confirmed diabetes in 1992 was $85.7 billion, excluding nursing home costs.[137]

The largest health care expenditures among older adults are for hospitalizations, nursing home care, and medical care. Expenditures for medical care per person are 50% higher for those over 65 with diabetes than those without diabetes.[156] Persons with diabetes are twice as likely to be hospitalized as those without this illness and are prone to longer hospital stays.[79] The total amount spent on nursing home care for persons with diabetes in 1987 was $941.5 million.[122]

Diabetes is also expensive on a daily basis. An estimate of the annual per capita costs of diabetes in 1992 was about $9493 for all persons with diabetes and $11,157 for those with confirmed diabetes. For all cases of diabetes, per capita costs for persons ages 65 to 74 were $10,669 and $10,346 for those 75 and older.[137] For older adults, about 20% of total costs are out-of-pocket expenditures and can represent a substantial burden to persons with limited incomes.[156]

Insurance

Only about 8% of the total health care bill for older adults is covered by private insurance. The principal funding mechanisms for health care among older persons are Medicare and Medicaid.[79] Medicare was funded by Congress in 1966 to help alleviate medical costs incurred by older Americans. There are two parts to Medicare. Part A is compulsory hospital insurance and is provided at no cost to persons who receive Social Security, while Part B is optional and is available for a monthly fee. Part B partially covers physician visits, medical supplies, and other outpatient services. Per capita expenditures have tripled since the beginning of the program.[5]

Twenty-seven percent of the costs for diabetes in the United States is covered by Medicare.[137] Among a nationally representative sample of 2405 adults with diabetes, 98.8% of those 65 and over had health care coverage. Almost all those surveyed (96%) had Medicare coverage, and 71.7% had two sources of health insurance, generally Medicare and private fee-for-service plans.[63]

Medicare does not cover all medical costs; for example, prescription drugs, therapeutic shoes, eyeglasses, and hearing aids are excluded.[5] Medicare participants are still responsible for portions of their medical care costs through co-payments (usually 20%), deductibles, and uncovered expenses.[79] On average, 22% of the total expenses are paid out of pocket, and these costs can quickly become prohibitive. Some older adults augment their coverage with a "Medigap" or supplemental policy.[156] These policies generally cover the deductible and co-payment portions of hospital care and physician services and may provide coverage for medications and nursing home care. Such plans are expensive, are not extensively used, and have had limited impact. Alternatives to Medigap policies include major medical insurance, health maintenance organizations, and hospital indemnity policies.[5]

Sixteen percent of the costs for diabetes in the United States is covered by Medicaid.[137] Among adults with diabetes 65 years and older, 15.4% receive insurance coverage through Medicaid or other public assistance programs. Medicaid is available to low-income older adults and pays for some services not provided through Medicare, such as eyeglasses and prescription drugs.[23]

In the past, critics of Medicare and Medicaid maintained that it covered only acute problems and did not provide for many preventive services or the daily needs of caring for a chronic illness. In 1989 Congress attempted to offer a more equitable system by providing reimbursement for evaluation and management services. This system took effect in January 1992 and is expected to have a positive impact on services for chronic illnesses such as diabetes.[87] Coverage for diabetes-related supplies and equipment has also improved greatly in recent years, particularly for persons who take insulin, and home care services may be covered. Generally, annual eye examinations, treatment of retinopathy, routine foot care, outpatient education, and blood glucose meters and strips may be covered for those with diabetes.[1,15] Despite these difficulties, Medicare and Medicaid do represent legal entitlement to medical care for older adults.[79]

TEACHING AND LEARNING IMPLICATIONS

The daily care of diabetes is complex. Recommendations for diabetes treatment often initiate the need to incorporate meal planning, medications, exercise, and blood glucose monitoring into ADLs. Although some older adults find these self-care practices difficult because of decreased physical abilities, memory loss, or other cognitive deficits, others not only are capable of performing these tasks but are very interested in doing so. All older adults with diabetes should be offered an individualized treatment plan that includes education, nutrition counseling, an exercise program, and oral sulfonylureas or insulin as needed.[68]

It is important that health care professionals not be guilty of "agism" by assuming that older persons are unable to learn or unwilling to care for themselves. Most of the limits imposed by the effects of the aging process can be compensated for in some way through careful assessment, planning, and implementation of the teaching process.

Individualized Treatment of Goals for the Aged Population

As with other age-groups, it is important for all older persons with diabetes or the persons primarily responsible for their daily care to establish individual goals and priorities in collaboration with the health care team. The person's goals should then be used to initiate consciously a program of either basic diabetes care or more intensive diabetes care as the treatment strategy. The primary purpose of basic diabetes care is to prevent the acute complications of hyperglycemia by maintaining fasting blood glucose levels of less than 200 mg/dl. This treatment program includes meal planning, exercise, and an oral sulfonylurea when needed. In contrast, the primary purpose of intensive diabetes care is to prevent the long-term complications of diabetes through maintaining fasting blood glucose levels of less than 140 mg/dl. Insulin is often recommended, along with diet, exercise, and home blood glucose monitoring. Some persons can achieve this type of control with one or two shots per day of an intermediate-acting insulin, but others will benefit from the addition of a short-acting insulin. More than two shots per day are rarely required in this population.[113]

Although the Diabetes Control and Complications Trial (DCCT) established the value of tight blood glucose control to prevent complications in IDDM,[28] most older adults have NIDDM. However, the effect of blood glucose on the developing complications is believed to be similar, and it is recommended that otherwise healthy persons with NIDDM strive to achieve tight control.[2] Metabolic control has been shown to be predictive of the progression of retinopathy among older adults.[110] Although a short life expectancy is an argument used against more intensive insulin programs, a person age 65 has a life expectancy of 17 years, at age 75, 10 years, and at age 85, 6 years.[113] Therefore, although the link between hyperglycemia and the long-term complications of diabetes other than retinopathy has not been firmly established for older persons, their prevalence and resulting morbidity among this population means that this issue cannot be ignored.[57] It has been recommended that fasting blood glucose levels of less than 140 mg/dl, postprandial levels of less than 180 mg/dl, and hemoglobin (Hb) A_{1c} concentrations about 1% above the normal range be the targets for adults with NIDDM.[85]

The implementation of more intensive treatment programs is often challenging but can be facilitated by using a team approach and providing education and support.[41] Intensive insulin regimens have been shown to be feasible and efficacious in reducing glycohemoglobin levels among older adults without adversely impacting weight, blood pressure, lipid levels, and quality of life.[59] It is important to recognize that quality of life is a highly personal and individual perception, and health care professionals should not allow their own beliefs about the impact of these programs to influence the type of treatment offered. In addition, improvements in cognition with better glycemic control may actually enhance quality of life. As with all persons, older adults should be informed of treatment options, the costs and benefits of each option, and any other facts that they need to make a decision about their treatment programs.

The tools for the treatment of diabetes are the same for older adults as for other persons with IDDM and NIDDM. These include meal planning, weight control, exercise, and oral sulfonylureas or insulin. However, specific issues are related to older adults that need to be taken into account with each of these tools.

Diet is generally considered to be the cornerstone of metabolic control in diabetes. No differences exist in current dietary recommendations for older adults than for younger adults with diabetes, although age-related changes in functional and cognitive abilities do need to be taken into account.[38] Box 21-6 outlines dietary considerations for older persons with diabetes.

The basis for individual dietary recommendations may include achievement of an ideal or reasonable body weight, blood glucose control, a decrease in the intake of saturated fats and cholesterol, and a nutritionally adequate and balanced diet. The dietary intervention can involve a specific meal pattern to be more behaviorally focused. It is important to note, however, that radical dietary modifications are difficult at any age and may have a negative impact on quality of life.[125] The person needs to understand first and then weigh the potential advantages of any changes with costs and potential disadvantages.

Weight tends to decline gradually with age. In contrast to younger persons with diabetes, adult men over age 65 with NIDDM were found to be no more obese than age-matched controls but had more upper body fat mass.[108] Many persons with diabetes, particularly the very old, tend to have normal body weight or may actually be underweight. Among these persons, caloric restrictions may result in malnutrition. Eating similar amounts of food at regular times throughout the day may offer advantages in terms of blood glucose control. This can serve to smooth out blood glucose levels and prevent overtaxing a poorly functioning

---

BOX 21-6

SPECIAL DIETARY CONSIDERATIONS FOR OLDER ADULTS WITH DIABETES

Diabetes	Aging
Treatment methods and goals	Cost
Weight	Food preparation ability and skill
Merits of weight loss/control methods	Decreased taste and thirst sensations
Composition of recommended and current diet	Appetite
	Dental status
Cognitive ability	Constipation

pancreas.[136] Among persons with diabetes over age 60, 40% are overweight and an additional 15% are obese.[131] Caloric restrictions are recommended for older adults who are more than 20% above desired body weight.[138] These persons often achieve significant reductions in plasma glucose levels during periods of reduced calorie intake or with a modest weight loss.[131]

Older adults with diabetes have the same problems related to nutrition as other older persons. Loss of appetite caused by lack of activity, other chronic illnesses, poor dentition, medication interactions, depression, and diminished senses of taste and smell are factors that can negatively impact nutritional status.[131] Skipping meals has been shown to correlate with poorer metabolic control of diabetes, perhaps because it leads to snacking or overeating later in the day.[136] This can also impede weight loss. Many older persons, particularly those who live alone, are socially isolated, or have functional impairments that make food shopping and cooking difficult, may eat very little and tend to be malnourished. Approximately 16% of older Caucasian and 18% of older African-American adults consume fewer than 1000 calories per day. Among poor older persons, about twice as many consume less than 1000 calories per day.[131] Because eating patterns can be so variable among this population, it is particularly important that when insulin is required, the dose is planned to fit the person's usual eating habits, not vice versa.[126]

Increased physical activity may be effective in preventing NIDDM[67] and is generally believed to be a component of the treatment for diabetes. Few data address the effects of exercise training on older persons with diabetes. However, data on the positive effects of exercise among other groups of persons with NIDDM suggest that older adults could also receive the benefit of improved insulin action resulting from endurance training. Along with improved glucose utilization, the benefits of exercise for older adults include improved cardiovascular status, preservation and maintenance of joint mobility and range of motion, toning, improved appetite and bowel function, and an improved sense of well-being (Box 21-7). Because the potential risks of exercise related to diabetes are greater for older adults, a thorough history and physical assessment of diabetes control and complications are essential, and general exercise recommendations are usually more conservative. A complete physical examination and an exercise stress test should be done before an exercise program is initiated.[54] Aerobic exercises that do not cause excessive joint trauma, such as walking, swimming, or bicycling, are generally recommended.

Modifications may be needed to accommodate the reduced work capacity and special needs of older adults. An inactive person should begin at a low intensity for a short time, such as 50% of maximal capacity for 10 to 15 minutes, and gradually increase intensity and duration. Persons with peripheral vascular disease may benefit from a walk-rest-walk program.[54] Education about symptoms of cardiovascular distress, injury, prevention and treatment of hypoglycemia, and impact on long-term complications is particularly important for this population. Morning exercise programs may have the greatest benefit because this is the time of greatest insulin resistance; however, the timing of exercise needs to be individually planned, taking into account the person's treatment program and life-style.

Long-term adherence to exercise programs tends to be problematic for all ages, so every effort should be made for the exercise program to be a positive and enjoyable experience.[140] Walking with friends, a walking club, or exercise classes designed for senior citizens are

---

BOX 21-7

POTENTIAL BENEFITS AND RISKS OF EXERCISE FOR OLDER ADULTS WITH DIABETES

Benefits

Improved exercise tolerance
Improved glucose tolerance
Improved maximal oxygen consumption
Increased muscle strength
Decreased blood pressure
Decreased body fat and increased muscle mass
Improved lipid profile
Improved sense of well-being

Risks

Sudden cardiac death
Foot and joint injuries
Hypoglycemia

From Morrow LA, Halter JB: In Kahn CR, Weir GS, editors: *Joslin's diabetes mellitus,* ed 13, Philadelphia, 1994, Lea & Febiger.

---

strategies to increase the likelihood that persons with diabetes will choose to exercise. Activity is often a neglected topic for older adults because of assumptions that they are not able to exercise. It is important to ask about past exercise levels and what physical actvities the person is currently able and willing to do.

Oral sulfonylureas are widely used in the management of older persons with NIDDM. In fact, 50% of the oral hypoglycemics prescribed are for persons over age 65.[96] Of the second-generation agents, both glyburide and glipizide are effective in reducing blood glucose levels and are well tolerated by older adults.[135] However, sulfonylureas may not be adequate to achieve euglycemia in many persons. Also, the interaction of these pills with other medications that potentiate their hypoglycemic effects needs to be considered, particularly among older adults, who are frequently taking several medications for other chronic diseases.[58] Metformin has been tested in other countries and found to be effective in lowering blood glucose levels and has recently been approved for use in the United States.[18]

Hypoglycemia can occur with these medications, and older adults who tend to skip meals are particularly susceptible. These reactions are generally more severe and, because of their longer action time, are less amenable to treatment with a simple carbohydrate than those caused by insulin. Older adults taking either of the second-generation sulfonylureas are at risk for asymptomatic hypoglycemia.[16] Hyponatremia is another potential side effect of oral hypoglycemic medications in older adults. Use of thiazide diuretics and changes in water metabolism with aging appear to increase the risks in older persons.[113] Oral medications do offer the advantage of a medication in pill form rather than injections, making them easier to

---

BOX 21-8

SPECIAL CONSIDERATIONS FOR INSULIN THERAPY

Vision
Manual dexterity
Sensation in hands
Access to injection sites
Cost
Ability to perform self-monitoring of blood glucose (SMBG)
Cognitive function
Family support

From Morrow LA, Halter JB: In Kahn CR, Weir GS, editors: *Joslin's diabetes mellitus,* ed 13, Philadelphia, 1994, Lea & Febiger.

---

take. Although persons with diabetes prefer oral medications over injections, studies have shown that compliance with pills is no better than with insulin.[31] In addition, some oral agents are more costly than insulin.

Insulin treatment offers some advantages in that it is usually possible to lower plasma glucose values, and dosages can be more precisely adjusted to avoid symptoms and achieve the person's glucose goals. To avoid hypoglycemia, however, insulin needs to be implemented in small increments, with an appropriate meal plan; may require frequent physician visits for dose adjustment; and generally increases the importance and frequency of SMBG. Among older adults, opinions of health professionals, self-efficacy, SMBG, and knowledge about diabetes positively influence initiation and continuation of insulin therapy.[161] Because older adults may have diminished hypoglycemia symptom awareness,[103] the ability to detect and appropriately treat reactions are important considerations before implementing insulin treatment. Box 21-8 lists other special considerations for insulin therapy in older adults.

The person's functional ability to draw up and administer insulin successfully, perform SMBG, follow a meal pattern, and manage hypoglycemic reactions must be taken into account before insulin therapy is initiated.[125] Although no differences in outcomes were noted, older adults (mean age of 66.8) were found to make more dosage errors when mixing insulins themselves compared with using premixed insulins.[21] Functional factors are particularly important considerations when initiating insulin therapy on an outpatient basis, and the use of home care services may be a helpful and necessary resource during the initial phase. Visiting nurse assessment of the home environment for lighting, cleanliness, and insulin storage and use can be invaluable for care planning.

The use of insulin along with oral agents has been proposed for the treatment of some persons, particularly those with insulin resistance who do have some response to sulfonylureas. Although combination therapy has shown modest improvements in glycemic control,[127] benefits of its usefulness for older adults must be evaluated on an individual basis.

Older adults who are unable to achieve their desired glycemic control without excessive hypoglycemia or who are unable to recognize or treat hypoglycemia may be particularly good candidates. On the other hand, two different forms of therapy increase the complexity of the regimen and may increase the costs. Oral agents are often more costly than insulin and syringes. The benefits of using combination therapy for older adults remain controversial at this time.

Blood glucose testing is the recommended method for monitoring glycemic control. It can be used to achieve and maintain a specific level of glucose control, to assist in day-to-day decision making, to prevent and detect hypoglycemia and hyperglycemia, and to educate persons with diabetes about the impact of food, activity, medication, and stress on blood glucose. Older adults have shown acceptance of SMBG and report better medication compliance and no negative impact on quality of life.[49]

The frequency of monitoring schedules will vary based on the intensity of the regimen and glycemic stability. However, in order for SMBG to be effective, the person with diabetes must be capable of learning the proper technique, willing to expend the effort, and be educated about and committed to modifying the treatment plan based on the results.[3]

The number of adults not using insulin who monitor has increased from 2% to 31% over the past 10 years. Although the number of persons with NIDDM using insulin who practice SMBG with some regularity has increased from 6% to 82% in the past 10 years, only 21% use the information to make adjustments in insulin dosages. The number of older adults using insulin who monitor is similar to the number of younger adults, although those over 64 were told to monitor less often than those 45 to 64 years of age (70% versus 85%).[70] Diabetes education and more frequent physician visits positively impact the likelihood of blood glucose testing. Frequency of blood testing has been shown to be highly related to age, with the probability of SMBG decreasing with each decade.[64]

Although results of studies are mixed, evidence supports the value of home blood glucose monitoring for persons with NIDDM. In one study of persons with NIDDM (mean age of 56.3), less frequent blood glucose monitoring was significantly correlated with higher glycosylated hemoglobin values.[136] In another study of insulin-requiring NIDDM persons (mean age of 55.6), those who used daily fasting blood glucose measurements to make insulin dose adjustments based on an algorithm were able to bring their glycosylated hemoglobin values into the normal range.[36] Therefore older adults or their caregivers need to be taught not only how to perform home blood glucose monitoring, but also how to use the information to make adjustments in meal planning, activity, and insulin doses. SMBG can also be a useful tool for those taking oral medications and for those on diet therapy to provide information about asymptomatic hypoglycemia and concrete evidence to reinforce behavior. It may not be feasible because of the lack of reimbursement, but SMBG needs to be presented as an option, along with information about interpretation of the results. Meters that are more "user friendly" and less dependent on technique are generally most appropriate for older adults.

Educational Considerations

Older adults with diabetes appear to be a neglected population when it comes to diabetes self-management education. Jenny[74] found that aged adults (mean age of 71.7) received the least amount of diabetes instruction of any age-group. Older adults (mean age of 57.3) had the highest level of motivation and the second lowest level of instruction. Hiss[70] found that in a study of 393 persons with NIDDM, 62% of those age 64 or under had attended a diabetes educational program within the past 2 years, compared with 52% of persons over age 64. When specific areas of educational information were examined in this same study, it was found that persons 64 and older reported that they had been told to exercise more often (62% versus 58%) but told to follow a diet less often (83% versus 92%) and to take special care of their feet less often (54% versus 58%) than persons 45 to 64 years of age.

In a large study of 2405 adults with diabetes, of the 2268 subjects with NIDDM, 58.5% of insulin-treated adults ages 18 to 39 and 53.7% of those ages 40 to 64 had ever attended a class or program about diabetes, compared with only 41.2% of those age 65 or older. Among subjects with NIDDM not treated with insulin, 34.6% of those ages 18 to 39 and 25.1% of those ages 40 to 64 had attended diabetes education, compared with 21.3% of those 65 or older. Among this sample of persons with NIDDM, younger age, African-American race, Midwest residence, more education, and presence of complications were associated with having had diabetes education.[20]

Perhaps one of the reasons diabetes self-management education has been neglected among this population is because of the inherent difficulties of teaching older persons. Difficulty in comprehension does increase with age, and other cognitive and sensory deficits may be present.[74] However, this group deserves special attention and consideration because of the high incidence of diabetes in persons 65 and older and because they are at risk for developing its major complications. Interest in diabetes self-management education may actually increase as older adults face the inevitability of aging and become increasingly concerned about maintaining health and independence.

Older persons can be taught and can learn if educators adjust the teaching plan to meet their needs. Special considerations for teaching older adults include taking into account functional ability, particularly aspects that may be affected by the aging process; the treatment programs of any concomitant illnesses or diabetes-related complications; ethnic and cultural background; and the individual's personal strengths and goals related to health and treatment of diabetes. Older adults may be hesitant to ask questions and need to be encouraged to do so. Sitting down to talk during an appointment and listening carefully to what they have to say will help to build rapport.

Diabetes self-management does not occur in a vacuum and is carried out within the context of all aspects of a person's life. The educational program and choice of content needs to be selected based on jointly identified goals, interests, abilities, and needs.

Functional limitations among older adults have implications for both educational approaches and care practices. Visual or other sensory deficits may require the health care professional to make modifications to accommodate the needs of these persons. For example, if the teaching session involves using a chalkboard, white on black generally works best for persons with visual deficits. Glossy boards may create a glare, and colored markers may be difficult to see, especially red, yellow, blue, and orange.[81] Older adults with early cataracts and decreased ability to distinguish colors are not good candidates for visual methods of blood glucose monitoring. Insulin administration techniques may need to be modified to compensate for a decline in visual acuity or double vision. Magnifying glasses may be useful, particularly the types that attach to a syringe or can be worn around the neck, thus leaving the person's hands free. In some cases, insulin may need to be prepared by a family member or home care nurse ahead of time to be administered by the person with diabetes.

Booklets, pamphlets, videotapes, and other visual aids are frequently used as adjuncts to an educational program. Materials that use a lot of white space on each page, are written in a conversational style, use large type, and are black type on nonglossy white or yellow paper work best for older persons with visual deficits or impairments.[32] The educator should highlight key points or write them down if no appropriate materials are available. Glossy boards should not be used to project video images because of the potential for glare, and the sound needs to be carefully modulated. Video materials that can be played more than once or at home may be especially helpful for older persons who need a longer time to process new information.[81] Choosing written and videotape materials that feature both older adults and appropriate ethnic groups will increase the perception that the content is relevant to them.

Group classes may be less effective for persons with hearing deficits than one-to-one interactions, during which the educator can assess whether the individual is hearing what is said by asking him or her to repeat it back. In these interactions the educator should face the person and enunciate words clearly. Eliminating background noises and providing education in a quiet room is also helpful. Because the ability to hear high-pitched tones is often lost, speaking loudly does not necessarily help the person to hear better.[81]

Because of sensory and cognitive deficits, some older adults with diabetes respond more slowly to stimuli and may have a decreased ability to organize information. Adjustments in the teaching process need to reflect these changes to be effective. Content should be presented in a concrete, factual way so that it can be readily applied. Scheduling teaching sessions that are short, are focused on a limited number of concepts, are paced to allow time to synthesize, and provide adequate time to request responses so that understanding can be checked will increase the likelihood of success. Memory can be increased by helping the person "set the stage" for what is coming next by offering cues about the information that will be given.[32] External cues to serve as a reminder are useful for persons with specific memory deficits. The cues should be specific and active, for example, taping a syringe to the bathroom mirror.[42] Follow-up to education to evaluate knowledge deficits and difficulties with self-care practices is particularly important for this age-group to decrease self-care behavioral deficits.[147] Follow-up can be accomplished either in person or by telephone.

To care for diabetes, adults require knowledge, skills, appropriate tools, and practice. Many areas of care require both knowledge and skills. For example, participants need not only to hear about the importance of foot care, but also to have the opportunity to practice the associated skills before they can perform them at home.[39] When teaching skills to older adults, time must be given to process the instruction before the skill is performed. It is generally most effective to give the instructions and demonstrations one step at a time, allowing practice time between steps.[81] The practice time not only allows the person to enhance skills but also provides the educator with the opportunity to observe the person's ability to perform the skill. If physical limitations exist, the educator needs to suggest and teach alternative methods to carry out the skill. For example, persons with arthritis or tremors may find it easier to trigger a penlet device used to obtain the blood sample for monitoring by pressing the trigger down on a table top rather than trying to hold it steady to trigger the device.

The educational plan must take into account any concomitant acute or chronic illnesses and diabetes complications present. For example, with a person who has a prosthetic leg, getting up, putting on the leg, getting to the bathroom, doing a blood glucose test, taking medications, and finally getting to the kitchen, preplanning a simple breakfast or one that can be prepared the night before is an important consideration. The older person may also need assistance to manage several regimens, all of which may be complex and necessitate behavior change.

Ethnicity is an important consideration in the educational process. Individuals' ethnicity influences not only who they are, how they perceive themselves, and their moral beliefs, but also their beliefs and perceptions about health and health care. Food, language, and health care practices are all symbols of ethnicity and cultural beliefs. When health professionals and the person with diabetes are from different ethnic and cultural backgrounds, they may have different beliefs and expectations about health behaviors, which can lead to conflict. For example, many cultures have active folk medicine systems that may be tried first or along with conventional methods.[132] Health professionals may not recognize some self-care activities because they do not fit with the traditional medical model. Ethnic food preferences need to be incorporated into the meal pattern and folk medicine practices recognized as part of the diabetes care plan.

Incorrect health beliefs that stem from cultural influences need to be addressed. Many older adults' experiences with diabetes lead to the belief that its complications are inevitable. When combined with the fatalistic attitude toward illness and the strong "sense of present" common to many ethnic groups, education about preventive or self-care practices may seem irrelevant and may not be implemented.[71]

The educational program and materials need to be culturally sensitive and relevant to the persons for whom they are provided. The language and words used must match the person's language. Even among adults with English as the first language, words may be used differently or have a different meaning among members of some ethnic groups. Literal translations of English materials into other languages may not convey the actual message as appropriately as translating the material into words that express its meaning. Literacy both in the person's native language and in English must be taken into account. Some adults who speak more fluently in their native language may actually read better in English.

Group classes for diabetes education have become increasingly popular, partly because of reimbursement structures. Persons with limited social support may profit from the experiences of others, interactions with persons who face similar problems, and peer support. Older adults may be intimidated by an educational program that is too formal or too much like school.[81] However, older adults have been found to participate in and benefit from group educational programs.[41,48,51] Group classes are probably most appropriate for older adults who have basic knowledge about diabetes and no sensory or cognitive deficits. In addition, peer support groups may be useful to improve psychosocial outcomes and glycemic control for some older adults.[50,159]

One of the myths about aging is that older persons cannot learn. Health professionals and older persons alike may believe that the "elderly" are not educable. This is a false perception. Learning continues throughout the life cycle, although some older adults may learn more slowly and may be more discriminating about what is learned.[81] Education is an important part of the care of persons with diabetes, and older adults deserve the same opportunity to learn as their younger counterparts.

Behavioral Strategies

The purpose of education is to provide new knowledge and understanding, and the purpose of health education is positive behavioral change.[33] Most behavioral intervention studies have not included age as a factor, but it is reasonable to conclude that older adults living in the community are as amenable to behavioral strategies (e.g., contracting, goal setting) as their younger counterparts.[4] Teaching sessions that include a discussion of treatment benefits, techniques for making changes, specific information about ways to incorporate changes, and potential barriers may positively influence outcomes.[134] As examples, the *Sixty. . . Something* program developed targeted sessions for older adults with diabetes that emphasized social learning variables, particularly self-efficacy and problem-solving skills. Participants in the intervention were able to decrease weight, calorie intake, and percentage of calories from fat significantly and increase the frequency of blood glucose monitoring.[52] In PATHWAYS, African-American women (mean age of 57) were able to lose weight using goal-setting and problem-solving skills taught in the program.[102] In the DIABEDS study, a sample of older African-American females (mean age of 58) who were taught skill exercises and behavior modification techniques experienced significantly better self-care skills and adherence behaviors and improved metabolic control.[100] In addition, decreasing the complexity of the regimen and tailoring the intervention to the individual as much as possible are particularly relevant strategies for this age-group.[4]

Because older adults are prone to foot problems and resulting amputations, behavioral interventions to increase self–foot care behavior and influence provider behavior (e.g., remove footwear at all visits) can be effective in reducing abnormalities.[93] Although some older adults are hesitant to ask questions or speak up, it is likely that most are just as capable of becoming active participants in their diabetes care as younger adults, and strategies that help to activate and empower persons with diabetes are equally appropriate for both groups. Affirming the older adult as a person and recognizing self-care efforts are less likely to result in reporting behaviors to please the health professional (e.g., falsified monitoring records) than providing positive reinforcement for self-care outcomes.[40]

It is important to recognize any underlying social, functional, and psychologic changes related to the aging process when working with older adults. All aspects of functional states as well as all other acute and chronic illnesses must be taken into account when implementing any behavioral or life-style change programs.[4] If significant cognitive impairment exists, a complex regimen requiring extensive education, behavior change, and personal involvement is likely to fail.[88]

Assessment and Planning

As outlined in Table 21-8, assessment is the first step in the educational process. Appendix 21a at the end of this chapter provides an example of an educational assessment for older adults. The assessment may appear to be lengthy and time consuming, but it is an essential beginning to education. Ultimately the assessment can save time by assisting the health professional to focus the teaching process and plan for a more formal and extensive education program. Using information gleaned from the assessment prevents stereotyping of older persons into predetermined categories and allows the educational intervention to be tailored for individual needs. The assessment of newly diagnosed persons is extensive and provides a baseline diabetes and functional profile of each individual. However, the health status and functional abilities of older adults are not static and need frequent reevaluation. Thus the assessment process must be ongoing and incorporated into each interaction.[39] Noting the person's functional, sensory, cognitive, psychosocial, and educational status on a diabetes flow chart or education record is an effective strategy that not only helps the health care professional to follow the person's progress but also serves as a reminder for reassessment.[117]

Newly Diagnosed Older Adults

The initial assessment needs to include a review of the individual's existing functional abilities, including knowledge and beliefs about diabetes and its care, physical function, sensory ability, cognitive ability, literacy, emotional status, social support system, cultural factors, financial status, and readiness to learn. During the assessment, participants should be given the opportunity to express their own interests, beliefs, treatment goals, values, emotions, and attitudes about diabetes.[133]

Diabetes knowledge and beliefs

Even when newly diagnosed, older adults have frequently had experience with diabetes through spouses, family members, or friends. Some have seen the harmful effects of the complications of diabetes and believe that diabetes automatically means blindness or an amputation. Other adults may view diabetes as a natural part of the aging process and not take it very seriously. Still others have learned inaccurate information or seen people with diabetes receive poor care or not take care of themselves. These experiences and beliefs can impact both the educational process and the person's willingness to care for his or her diabetes. Asking if the person has ever known anyone with diabetes and what effect it had on the individual is one way to obtain this information. Misconceptions about diabetes may need to be clarified and advancements in treatment options presented as the first step in the educational process. Beliefs about the impact of diabetes on longevity also need to be assessed.[29] Written knowledge tests might also provide some of this information, but their usefulness has not been fully evaluated among older persons.[39]

Physical function

Age-related changes in physical function can affect diabetes self-care activities. These include anorexia, leading to hypoglycemia and inadequate nutrition; arthritis or tremors,

Table 21-8   Educational Process for Older Adults With Diabetes

Area	Assessment strategy	Educational strategy	Follow-up/reassessment strategies
Diabetes knowledge	"Have you ever attended a formal diabetes education program?" "What areas of diabetes would you like to learn more about?"	Develop plan. Provide specific content. Use teachable moments.	Evaluate educational progress and self-care skills and behaviors.
Current health practices	"What are you doing now to take care of your diabetes?" "Describe your typical daily activities and eating patterns."	Demonstrate skills and provide feedback. Provide specific content.	
Current health beliefs	"What are you doing to take care of your feet?" "Do you know anyone with diabetes?" "How does it affect them?" Ask the costs and benefits of treatment.	Concentrate on most pressing needs or questions first. Establish long-term and short-term goals.	Evaluate progress toward goals.
Physical function/ sensory ability	Ask what, when, and how the person performs skills. Observe participant performing a skill, (e.g., drawing up insulin, foot care routines).	Help identify ways to incorporate skills into daily activities.	
Cognitive ability	Summarize what was taught and ask participant to explain in own words.	Select appropriate teaching methods and materials.	
Literacy	Ask participant to read some diabetes-related information and then explain it to you.		

Category	Assessment questions	Intervention
Emotional status	"What are your thoughts and feelings about having diabetes?" "What do you fear most about having diabetes?"	Listen and encourage expression of feelings and fears through reflective statements. Monitor emotional status and any changes.
Social environment and support	Observe if family members are present at appointments and educational sessions. "Who helps and supports you with your diabetes care?" "What community and diabetes resources do you currently use?"	Encourage expression of thoughts and feelings related to diabetes and aging. Coordinate diabetes home care and community resources.
Cultural factors	"What do you think caused your illness?" "How serious do you believe diabetes is?" "How should a person with diabetes act?"	Plan education program interventions that are culturally relevant.
Financial status	"What impact has diabetes had on your financial status?" "Does your insurance pay for the diabetes care supplies you need?"	
Readiness to learn	"Are you interested in learning more about diabetes?" "What are your feelings and thoughts about having diabetes?"	

Modified from Funnell MM: *Diabetic Care* 13(suppl 2):60-65, 1990; Funnell MM, Anderson RM: *Pract Diabetol* 12(2):22-25, 1993.

interfering with insulin administration, SMBG, foot care, and food shopping and preparation; and concurrent illnesses with complex regimens that can interfere with the person's ability to implement them.[111] Many of these physical impairments can be compensated for, and strategies can be recommended to overcome deficits, if they are noted.

The person's ability to perform ADLs needs to be assessed. This assessment can range from informal questions to observing task performance to formal questionnaires. Because health professionals tend to overestimate functioning, a more systematic assessment is probably useful.[117] Many functional assessment tools that measure items related to physical function in various ways are available, but no single tool is appropriate for all persons.[42,76,117] Different tools uncover different problems to different degrees. The assessment instrument included in Appendix 21a includes questions related to overall physical functioning. Instruments specifically designed to test the functional capacity of older adults to perform self-management tasks, such as the Assessment of Diabetes Ability Performance Tool (ADAPT), may be useful.[26] This initial assessment needs to be followed up with repeat administrations of the tool or direct observations of the person's ability to carry out diabetes care tasks at each visit.

Pain from arthritis, peripheral neuropathy, or other problems may be present and more severe in older adults. The experience of pain has important implications for older adults and their ability to care for themselves, but it is difficult to measure. Because pain is completely subjective, asking about the presence of pain and how it limits ability to perform ADLs should be part of the assessment process. Pain may lead not only to decreased activity but also to sporadic intake of food and overeating, which can affect glycemic control. Treatment for any painful conditions is based on etiology.

Impotence occurs in 95% of the men with diabetes who are over age 70.[111] Because sexual functioning can play such an important role in marital happiness and total quality of life at any age, it needs to be assessed and addressed for both older men and older women.

Sensory ability

Altered vision can interfere with insulin administration and SMBG. Standardized visual acuity and color vision tests can be administered. In addition, asking participants to read

Table 21-9 An Informal Hearing Test for Older Adults With Diabetes

Test words	Response in hearing-impaired person
fill	fine
catch	cat
thumb	fun
heap	heat
wise	wives
wedge	red
fish	fifth
snows	phones
bed	bugs

Data from Miller LV: *Clin Diabetes* 4:74-76, 90, 1985.

standard newsprint or numbers on a syringe or to repeat back what was said to them can provide information to assist the health professional to adjust the teaching or care program. Annual ophthalmologic examinations are recommended for older adults, just as they are for all adults with diabetes.

Diminished hearing can negatively impact the ability to hear and understand the information needed for self-care. Informal tests of hearing can be conducted by standing behind the person, saying a list of key words, and asking the person to repeat what was said.[106] Table 21-9 lists an informal test of key words and common responses that would indicate mild to moderate hearing impairments. Some types of hearing loss can be helped through the use of hearing aids, and it is recommended that all persons with hearing deficits be referred to an audiologist for testing.

Cognitive ability

Cognitive abilities have an impact on the older person's ability both to learn about diabetes care and to carry out the treatment program. For example, choosing and measuring foods and deciding when to call a health care professional about a skin infection or blood glucose readings require both knowledge and judgment. Memory deficits are of particular concern for persons taking insulin. The ability to remember to take the insulin and whether a dose has been given or not has obvious safety implications for these persons. Principal areas of cognitive function that need to be assessed among older persons include orientation, attention, language, recall, calculation, and visuospatial ability.[107] All these can be screened with standard mini-mental status examinations such as the Folstein Mini-Mental State (see Appendix 21b at the end of this chapter) or other tests.[37,42] Subtle changes in cognitive function usually require formal neuropsychologic testing, which can also help to identify the degree to which depression is affecting cognitive impairment. Frequent reassessment of cognitive ability is important for older adults to detect any changes.

Literacy

Older adults may have more difficulty comprehending diabetes print materials than younger persons.[82] A survey of 105 persons with diabetes over age 64 found that 21% read at less than an eighth-grade level, 30% at an eighth- to twelfth-grade level, and 49% at above the twelfth-grade level.[69] Tests of frequently used diabetes education booklets revealed that the booklets were written at a mean grade level of 10.2, because the nature of health-related information and terminology skews reading level toward the higher grades.[9,142] These studies demonstrate the importance of determining literacy and matching educational materials to each participant's reading and cognitive abilities. Simple tools of reading ability are available and can be incorporated as part of the assessment.

Emotional status

Depression is common in older adults but is not always recognized. Affective changes seen in younger persons may not be present in older adults. Signs and symptoms of depression, such as an unkempt appearance, decreased attention, reduced memory, and lack of initiative, are often mistaken for dementia. Standardized tests, such as the Geriatric Depression Scale, are available to assess levels of depression.[42,163] In addition, asking participants about their moods and feelings not only provides the health care professional with information but also lets participants know that these are important areas for discussion.

Older persons do experience strong feelings about having an illness such as diabetes, and these feelings need to be acknowledged and discussed. Because many older adults were brought up to be stoic and not to discuss their emotions, asking that they tell you their thoughts about diabetes may elicit more of a response than asking how they "feel" about it. The educator should use active listening techniques and reflective statements and should avoid attempting to make participants feel better by minimizing negative feelings.

Social support system

The lack of social support identified by older persons has already been discussed. Asking participants who helps them with their diabetes care and who they turn to in times of trouble can provide information about the amount of support participants perceive is available to them. In addition, asking who shops for and cooks most of the food is important when planning an educational intervention related to nutrition. Among many ethnic groups, extended families, friends, and church groups are likely sources of social support that need to be considered.

Cultural factors

The major values, beliefs, and behaviors related to diabetes that are culturally influenced must be assessed. General areas include ethnic affiliation, religious beliefs and practices, family patterns, food preferences, and health care practices.[145]

Financial status

As already noted, diabetes is an expensive disease. Because income and expenditures are often less clearly defined among older persons, it is generally more useful to ask if their income is adequate or inadequate for their needs rather than to ask the amount of the annual income. Information about insurance coverage for diabetes care and supplies is also important before recommendations are made for a particular care program. In addition, persons with diabetes may not be aware of benefits to which they are entitled under changing Medicare and Medicaid guidelines and may benefit from this information.

Readiness to learn

Readiness to learn involves emotional and experiential readiness and reflects the individual's background of experiences, skills, attitudes, and ability to learn. Readiness can be affected by both physical health and current emotional status and can reflect health beliefs.[130] For example, individuals who are experiencing strong emotions (e.g., shock, denial) are rarely ready to learn. The educator needs to be sensitive to the fact that these factors are subtle and may not be readily apparent in the assessment process.[133]

Ongoing Care

The continuing assessment during ongoing care provides the opportunity to answer questions, reinforce previous learning, and give positive feedback on self-care strengths. Asking participants to tell what they are doing to care for their diabetes and observing their self-care skills, such as insulin administration and blood testing, are useful indicators of both changes from the initial assessment and current care practices. This information can be used to offer individualized recommendations and suggestions in areas of self-management declines or deficits. It is important, however, that the educator be nonjudgmental, be noncritical of the person's self-care efforts, and reflect a positive and caring attitude.[133]

The ongoing assessment also includes continued follow-up with the individual to determine progress in meeting goals and to determine if other referrals or resources are needed.

Implementation and Evaluation

Specific diabetes content areas for the educational program are no different for older adults than other persons with diabetes. The content needs to be relevant to the type of diabetes they have, their stated interests, and treatment regimen and goals. Whenever possible, diabetes content should be presented sequentially over time and at a pace that meets the individual's needs. Because of the amount of content needed for diabetes self-management, one approach that may be useful is to divide the content into manageable sections to make it less overwhelming and to provide time for assimilation of new information.

One recommendation is to divide the content into three levels: initial management, home management, and home improvement in life-style. The *initial management* level includes only the survival skills needed for diabetes care. The person who is newly diagnosed, the person who has had diabetes for a time but has received limited formal education, or the person who is experiencing a major change in treatment (e.g., starting insulin) is generally at this level. The second, or *home management,* level contains information that can be used to perform the daily care of diabetes and to enhance persons' ability to manage their illness in a more flexible, realistic, and appropriate way. This level includes most of the content areas. The third level, *improvement in life-style,* contains information for individuals who have learned to manage their diabetes successfully on a daily basis and who need information on specific topics.[56] Table 21-10 provides an example of appropriate topics for each of these levels. The definition of each of these levels can vary according to individual needs, and some topics may need to be presented at more than one level in varying degrees of complexity.

Adherence Issues

No clear-cut evidence indicates that age is positively or negatively correlated with adherence. Issues that impact adherence among younger persons, such as regimen complexity, provider relationship, health beliefs, and social support, appear to have similar effects on older adults' adherence behaviors.[4] In addition, the need to manage more than one complex regimen is more likely to impact adherence negatively among older persons, as are the physical limitations imposed by other chronic illnesses.

Older adults appear to identify the least number of barriers to adherence,[74] although cost may be a significant factor in ability to adhere for some older adults.[123] The perception of NIDDM as less threatening than IDDM or as just part of the aging process may also lead to

Table 21-10 Sample Educational Program for Older Adults With Diabetes

Initial management	Home management	Improvement in life-style
What is Diabetes?	More facts about diabetes	Tips for changing your health habits
Feelings about diabetes	Balance of food, exercise, and medicines	Coping with stress
What foods should you eat?	Living with diabetes	Your exercise program
Weight loss	How families can help	Travel
Diabetes pills	Why a "diet"?	What's in food?
Giving insulin	Healthy food choices	The exchange diet
Monitoring your diabetes	Practical tips for planning meals	What does the label say?
Foot care	Physical activity	Special diet foods and sweeteners
	Facts about insulin	Eating away from home
	How to use monitoring information	Fiber
	Low blood sugar (hypoglycemia)	Alcohol and diabetes
	High blood sugar (hyperglycemia)	Taking charge of your diet
	Sick-day care	Sexual health
	Personal care	Taking care of diabetes with other illnesses
	Long-term problems and risk factors	Older person with diabetes
	Complications of diabetes	Community resources
		Being a smart shopper
		Working with your health care team

decreased adherence with the treatment plan, particularly among those who do not use insulin.[27] Reinforcing that diabetes is a serious disease, without using "scare tactics," may be appropriate when working with some persons. Assisting older adults to cope with the demands and limitations of other illnesses and to organize self-care behaviors for all aspects of their health is also helpful to enhance adherence.

Role of the Diabetes Health Care Team

The diabetes health care team for older adults should include the same members as any other care team for adults with diabetes, with the addition of an expert in gerontology. Because most older adults strive to maintain their independence, social workers have a particularly important role to play. Appropriate referral to community resources can help older persons to remain in their preferred environment for as long as possible.

Nurse members of the team may include an advanced-practice nurse with expertise in diabetes and/or geriatrics, a nurse case manager, a diabetes educator, and a home health nurse. The advanced-practice nurse can provide primary care for routine and chronic illnesses, along with comprehensive health assessment, planning, and intervention and health education and counseling. Nurses in advanced roles are prepared to provide holistic care that integrates the psychosocial and physical components of the person and his or her health status.[72] The prevalence of chronic illnesses among older adults supports the value of advanced-practice nurses as the preferred primary care providers among this population. The nurse case manager can integrate and coordinate care for the older person with diabetes; provide comprehensive patient assessment; develop, implement, and modify the care plan; provide direct patient care; and facilitate communication with other members of the health care team.[13] Both the advanced-practice nurse and the nurse case manager offer client-centered, cost-effective care that maximizes the team approach and minimizes fragmentation of care.

The role of the health care team is first to assess functional ability and put functioning, the severity of diabetes, and other health problems in perspective with the older adult's total health status. Treatment goals should be established by the person with diabetes and those involved with his or her daily care. The role of the team is then to assist older persons to carry out the diabetes care program, to meet their care goals, to maximize their self-care abilities, and to remain safe and independent for as long as possible. The team's activities include diabetes care and education, coordination of community resources and referrals, and communication with other health care providers who are involved in the person's total health care. This may include contact with pharmacists, podiatrists, neighbors, and extended family members, as well as community agencies.

For older adults who require foster, nursing home, or other institutional care, the health care team needs to provide information and serve as a resource to the facility staff. If desired, in-service educational programs that are either targeted for the specific needs of that individual or more general in nature can be provided.

Role of the Person With Diabetes and the Family

Diabetes is a chronic illness that requires long-term active participation to maintain metabolic control. The need for the older adults with diabetes to carry out daily self-management behaviors is no less important simply because they are older. However, many older adults do have unique difficulties and needs because of the physical limitations that may be imposed by the aging process and the presence of other chronic illnesses and complications. Although these events do cause some difficulties, many can be either treated or compensated for in some way.

Educational programs designed to meet the specific needs of older adults and their families need to be developed and provided. Including family members in the teaching process is of particular importance for older adults because of the likelihood that impairments related to the aging process will increase their need for assistance. It may be beneficial to assist individuals with diabetes and their family members to develop strategies to minimize the problems of social isolation related to diabetes, such as leaving insulin or monitoring supplies at a family member's house where they often eat dinner. In addition, it has been demonstrated that including spouses in diabetes education class for older male adults (ages 65 to 82) significantly improved metabolic outcomes, diabetes knowledge, and family involvement and reduced stress.[48]

Although families can provide much assistance with and support for the diabetes care regimen, it is important to recognize that spouses may be frail or have chronic illnesses of their own and therefore may be unable to support or care for a spouse with diabetes adequately. The daily nature of diabetes management may make it difficult for adult children with other family and work responsibilities to be involved in the routine aspects of care. In these situations the person with diabetes may need referral to outside resources for assistance. Home care agencies, visiting nurse associations, Meals-on-Wheels, or other community resources may be available to provide daily support. It may be helpful to suggest to family members that they can recognize the person's positive efforts toward self-care and still provide support and reinforcement even when daily assistance is not possible.

Outcome Evaluation

A number of measures have been suggested as outcome evaluation criteria for diabetes care and education. These include metabolic control, adherence, knowledge, skills, behavior, attitudes, use of health services, days missed from work, hospitalizations, complications, and costs. None of these has been found to be entirely satisfactory criteria.[75,77] This is especially true for older adults, who frequently have concomitant medical problems and other disabilities. Evaluation measurements for older persons may be based best on maintenance or improvement in health status, quality of life, personal progress, goal attainment, and the ability of the individual or caregiver to manage diabetes effectively on a daily basis.[39]

EXTENDED CARE

In 1977 it was estimated that 14.5% of U.S. nursing home residents had a diagnosis of diabetes. Rates of nursing home admissions are two times greater among people with diabetes, and residents with NIDDM tend to be in poorer health than demographically similar residents who do not have diabetes.[151] In 1992 nursing home costs for people with diabetes were estimated to be $1.83 billion, and this amount is expected to increase dramatically over the next 20 years.[1]

Although two thirds of nursing home residents are treated with either insulin or oral hypoglycemic agents, intensity of treatment and appropriate blood glucose goals remain controversial.[151] However, because of the increased risks for acute complications and decreased visual acuity and cognition that may occur as a result of hyperglycemia, blood glucose control aimed at control of hyperglycemia and prevention of symptoms and acute complications is appropriate.[113] Control of hyperglycemia is achieved through diet and medications for most extended care facility residents, with exercise playing only a limited role. Because extended care facilities generally provide consistent meal patterns at regular times, no special dietary restrictions are recommended.[38] The decision to use sulfonylureas or insulin is based on achievement of glucose goals and symptom control.[113] Blood glucose monitoring is needed for patients taking insulin, particularly those who are unable to recognize or report hypoglycemia. The monitoring schedule should be individualized and based on the resident's stability.[109] Frequent foot inspection and care are important components of treatment for these persons, who are vulnerable to injury, gangrene, and amputation. Because nursing home residents with diabetes are also vulnerable to bedsores and other infections, skin care and hygiene are also important considerations. Monitoring for complications should be done with the same regularity as for other persons with diabetes.[113]

Foster care may be an option for some older adults with diabetes. Although some foster care facilities may be unable or unwilling to accept persons taking insulin, others will accept insulin-taking residents if appropriate support is provided by the health care team. Persons with diabetes requiring hospice care should be kept symptom free and comfortable.[14]

RESEARCH IMPLICATIONS

Research in diabetes among older adults and its impact is a newer area of interest, and much work still needs to be done. General areas include the physiologic impact of hyperglycemia in older persons; intensive treatment and other appropriate treatment modalities for older adults; the concomitant physical and psychosocial effects of diabetes, its complications, and other illnesses among this age-group; and educational and behavioral strategies that are most effective with this population.

Specifically, the effects of metabolic control on the long-term health of older adults need to be explored further. Persons with NIDDM and health professionals often do not appear to consider diabetes to be a serious disease in older adults. Documentation of the effects of diabetes are needed to verify or alter this perception. Also, studies of the treatment methods to achieve the needed levels of glycemic control for this population are needed. Insulin use and particularly intensive insulin programs remain controversial for treating older persons, and the efficacy, costs, and benefits of such programs require additional study and clarification. Because older adults frequently experience diabetic complications or have other chronic illnesses along with diabetes, both the physical and the psychosocial impacts of multiple health problems in this population need to be explored.

The psychosocial impact of diabetes and the personal meaning that older persons and their families attach to it require further study. Strategies that can be used to increase the effectiveness of teaching efforts when working with older adults need to be tested and implemented. Educational materials specifically for older adults and methods that would enhance learning among this population need to be developed and tested. Behavioral strategies that could be used to assist older adults to achieve their diabetes and other health care goals need to be designed and evaluated. In short, almost all components of diabetes care and treatment need further exploration for this special population.

COMMUNITY RESOURCES

In addition to diabetes-specific resources that may be available in a community, additional resources may be available especially for older adults. Most are located in the Yellow Pages under "senior citizens" or "social service agencies." Some examples include the following:

Senior Citizens Centers

Senior citizens centers provide activities, classes, and programs for those ages 55 and older. Some offer meals on a regular basis, and some have public health nursing services available.

Meals on Wheels

Meals on Wheels provides one meal a day for homebound or invalid people who qualify. They may offer special diets in some places.

Easter Seals, Elks, Lions, Kiwanis, Rotary Clubs

These community service groups are often helpful in finding money for equipment, clinic visits, or other needs.

Goodwill Industries, United Way, Salvation Army, Volunteers of America

These organizations offer a variety of social services as well as opportunities for volunteerism outside the home.

Churches

Local churches may be able to help with transportation, care for brief periods of an older person who cannot be left alone, and emergency needs such as food, clothing, and shelter. Churches sometimes sponsor diabetes or other support groups.

Several national organizations for older adults also provide information and other services including the following:

The National Institute on Aging (NIA)

The NIA publishes a *Resource Directory for Older People.* It includes addresses and telephone numbers of national organizations that offer health information, legal aid, self-help programs, educational opportunities, social services, consumer advice, or other assistance.

Resource Directory for Older People
National Institute on Aging
9000 Rockville Pike
Bethesda, MD 20898
(301) 496-1752

The American Association of Retired Persons (AARP)

AARP is a nonprofit organization for older persons. Its goal is to help people cope better with growing older. Persons age 50 and older, retired or not, are eligible to belong for a small fee. AARP offers information, publications, discount coupons, help with tax forms, a prescriptive and nonprescriptive drug service, and insurance plans.

American Association of Retired Persons
National Headquarters
601 E St. NW
Washington, DC 20049
(202) 434-2277

National Council of Senior Citizens
The National Council of Senior Citizens offers low-cost insurance, support groups, and other types of help.

National Council of Senior Citizens
1331 F St. NW
Washington, DC 20005
(202) 347-8800

National Association of Area Agencies on Aging (NAAAA)
NAAAA represents agencies that offer services to older adults. For information about agencies in your area, contact:

National Association of Area Agencies on Aging
Suite 100
1112 16th St. NW
Washington, DC 20036
(202) 296-8130

Gray Panthers
Gray Panthers is an organization to help older adults learn about and become politically active in health care and social issues.

Gray Panthers
Suite 602
1424 16th St. NW
Washington, DC 20036
(202) 387-3111

Children of Aging Parents
Children of Aging Parents is a national group for information and referral services. They also offer support groups for caregivers of their parents.

Children of Aging Parents
1609 Woodburn, Suite 302
Levittown, PA 19056
(215) 945-6900

American Society on Aging
The American Society on Aging is a nonprofit, membership organization that informs the public and health professionals about issues that affect the quality of life for older persons and promotes innovative approaches to meeting their needs.

American Society on Aging
Suite 512
833 Market St.
San Francisco, CA 94103
(415) 882-2910

National Association of Meal Programs

The National Association of Meal Programs is a group of professionals and volunteers who provide congregate and home-delivered meals to people who are frail, disabled, or homebound.

National Association of Meal Programs
206 E St. NE
Washington, DC 20002
(202) 547-6157

Self-Help for Hard of Hearing People, Inc. (SHHH)

SHHH is a nonprofit, educational organization devoted to the welfare and interests of those who have hearing impairments.

Self-Help for Hard of Hearing People, Inc.
7800 Wisconsin Ave.
Bethesda, MD 20814
(301) 657-2248 (Voice)
(301) 657-2249 (TDD)

The National Shut-In Society, Inc.

The National Shut-In Society is a private, nonprofit organization whose members work to bring cheer and comfort to members with chronic illnesses.

The National Shut-In Society, Inc.
1925 North Lynn St.
Rosslyn, VA 22209
(703) 516-6770

Concerned Relatives of Nursing Home Patients

Concerned Relatives of Nursing Home Patients is a consumer group whose goals are to maintain quality care and improve services for all nursing home residents.

Concerned Relatives of Nursing Home Patients
3130 Mayfield Rd.
Cleveland Heights, OH 44118
(216) 321-0403

National Association for Home Care (NAHC)
NAHC is a professional organization that represents a variety of agencies that provide home care services, including home health agencies, hospice programs, and homemaker/home health aid agencies.

National Association for Home Care
519 C St. NE
Washington, DC 20002
(202) 547-7424

National Association for Hispanic Elderly (Asociación Nacional por Personas Mayores)
The National Association for Hispanic Elderly works to ensure that older Hispanic citizens are included in all social service programs for older Americans.

National Association for Hispanic Elderly
Asociación Nacional por Personas Mayores
Suite 800
3325 Wilshire Blvd.
Los Angeles, CA 90010-1724
(213) 487-1922

National Indian Council on Aging
The National Indian Council on Aging, a nonprofit organization funded by the U.S. Administration on Aging, works to ensure that older Indian and Alaskan Native Americans have equal access to quality, comprehensive health care, legal assistance, and social services.

National Indian Council on Aging
City Centre, Suite 510W
6400 Uptown Blvd. NE
Albuquerque, NM 87110
(505) 888-3302

National Caucus and Center on Black Aged, Inc.
The National Caucus and Center on Black Aged is a nonprofit organization that works to improve the quality of life for older black Americans.

National Caucus and Center on Black Aged, Inc.
Suite 500
1424 K St. NW
Washington, DC 20005
(202) 637-8400

National Pacific/Asian Resource Center on Aging

The National Pacific/Asian Resource Center on Aging is a private organization that works to improve the delivery of health care and social services to older members of the Pacific/Asian community across the United States.

National Pacific/Asian Resource Center on Aging
Melbourne Tower, Suite 914
1511 Third Ave.
Seattle, WA 98101
(206) 624-1221

Organization of Chinese Americans (OCA)

OCA works to ensure equal opportunities for Americans of Chinese ancestry.

Organization of Chinese Americans
Room 707
1001 Connecticut Ave. NW
Washington, DC 20036
(202) 223-5500

Japanese American Citizens League (JACL)

JACL is a nonprofit, educational organization that works to ensure equal opportunities for Americans of Japanese ancestry.

Japanese American Citizens League
1765 Sutter St.
San Francisco, CA 94115
(415) 921-5225

Older Women's League (OWL)

OWL seeks to educate the public about the problems and issues of concern to middle-age and older women.

Older Women's League
Suite 700
666 11th St. NW
Washington, DC 20001
(202) 783-6686

Catholic Golden Age

Catholic Golden Age sponsors charitable work and offers religious worship opportunities for older people.

Catholic Golden Age
430 Penn Ave.
Scranton, PA 18503
(717) 342-3294

B'nai B'rith International

B'nai B'rith International is a voluntary service organization that helps people of all faiths.

B'nai B'rith International
1640 Rhode Island Ave. NW
Washington, DC 20036
(202) 857-6600

CASE PRESENTATION

Mrs. J., 78 years old, has NIDDM and is treated with glipizide, 10 mg twice daily. She came to the clinic to participate in a new Diabetes Care Program for older adults. Her past medical history is positive for hypertension for 25 years, congestive heart failure (CHF) for 4 years, degenerative joint disease (DJD), cataracts, constipation, mild stress, and urinary incontinence. In addition to glipizide, she also takes captopril, 25 mg three times daily; furosemide, 40 mg every day; potassium chloride, 20 mEq every day; ibuprofen once or twice a day; Metamucil, 1 tsp every day. Her glycated hemoglobin is 15% (normal, 6% to 8%); total cholesterol, 210 mg; high-density lipoproteins (HDLs), 44 mg; triglycerides, 326 mg; and creatinine, 1.4 mg/dl, without proteinuria. She is 5 ft, 1 in tall and weighs 160 pounds. Her mother had diabetes and developed blindness as a result.

Mrs. J. was born to French-Canadian parents and speaks French and English fluently. She earned a high-school diploma. She is married, worked for 26 years in a factory, and has two sons. One son is now in his late 40s and lives nearby; the other in his early 50s and lives more than 1000 miles away. Mrs. J. has four grandchildren and one great-grandchild.

Her husband is in reasonably good health, and they own their home. Mrs. J. enjoys retirement immensely. She sleeps each day until 10 AM and stays up until the early hours of the morning. She stays active going to church, traveling, playing cards, visiting with friends and family, and eating out. She has Medicare, which helps pay for health care visits and glucose monitoring equipment, but it does not cover medications, eyeglasses, and certain other costs.

Mrs. J. has a 30 pack-year smoking history but quit 15 years ago. She has no particular exercise or diet plan and avoids strenuous exercise because of her CHF. She eats little or no breakfast but eats lunch, dinner, and a bedtime snack. She loves to cook French food and chooses foods high in fats and sugars. She does not want any of the food substitutes, saying, "I'll either have the real thing or skip it altogether." She drinks one or two cups of coffee a day and rarely has social alcohol intake.

Mrs. J. perceives that she is susceptible to the complications of diabetes and realizes their severity, partly out of her experience with her mother's diabetic retinopathy. She comes an hour each way to the clinic to receive care for her diabetes to avoid blindness, amputation, or illness. She sees the benefits of more intensive therapy as outweighing the barriers.

Mrs. J. began with 20 U human NPH insulin every morning. She did not like to perform SBGM but did it twice a day and kept a record. She met with the dietitian and agreed to spread out food intake and eat at more consistent time intervals. Her insulin dose was gradually increased. After 6 months she was taking 42 U NPH in the morning only, and her glycated hemoglobin level had decreased to 10.1%.

To achieve better control, an evening injection of NPH was added. After 12 months, she was taking 60 U NPH in the morning and 12 U NPH in the evening and had a glycated hemoglobin level of 6.8%. She rarely had symptoms of low glucose and was able to manage it without problems.

Mrs. J. and her husband are active participants in the diabetes education program, asking many questions and appearing to benefit from the information and interaction with other group members.

DISCUSSION

In many ways, Mrs. J. is very typical of older adults with diabetes. Despite a glycated hemoglobin level of 15%, insulin had not been recommended because she was asymptomatic. She did not monitor glucose levels, knew very little about diabetes, and had not been referred to a dietitian. Mrs. J. is also representative of many older adults with diabetes in other ways, as follows:

Asymptomatic insidious onset and course. At the time of diagnosis, Mrs. J. had no symptoms. Her diabetes was discovered during an unrelated hospitalization, so it is likely that she had undiagnosed diabetes for years and was largely asymptomatic.

Overweight. She fits the criteria for obesity, and her excess adipose tissue may have contributed to insulin resistance. She gained 12 pounds in a year with intensive insulin therapy.

After 12 months, her lipid profile showed improvement with better glucose control: total cholesterol, 186 mg; HDLs, 40 mg; and triglycerides, 205 mg.

Hypertension. More than 2.5 million Americans have both diabetes and hypertension. The coexistence of diabetes and hypertension increases the risk for developing cardiovascular, cerebrovascular, peripheral vascular, and renal disease.

Multiple other concurrent chronic diseases. This poses certain challenges in optimizing glucose control. For example, Mrs. J.'s DJD and CHF kept her from exercising. She showed a mild elevated creatinine without proteinuria, probably because of hypertensive effects, indicating a need for even more rigorous blood pressure control. Many older adults have developed other diseases or complications of diabetes that can impact their ability to care optimally for their diabetes.

Polypharmacy. Mrs. J. is taking several drugs, and without careful attention by all prescribers, she is at risk for drug interactions. For example, furosemide promotes hyperglycemia, but the need for it outweighed this effect and could be compensated for with insulin. Diuretics may also contribute to volume depletion with hyperglycemia in the early stages of HHNS. Thus her glucose levels and hydration status required careful monitoring. Nonsteroidal antiinflammatory agents can promote renal insufficiency and gastrointestinal bleeding, so minimal use is encouraged in older adults. Sulindac, which is somewhat less nephrotoxic, was prescribed for Mrs. J.

Functional status. Mrs. J. was referred for and benefited from cataract surgery. She had hearing loss of upper frequencies (presbycusis) but managed without a hearing aid. She needed no help other than her spouse in personal or instrumental ADLs, although she preferred not to drive. If she or her husband becomes disabled, the health care team will need to make further assessment to help her maintain independence.

Full cognitive capacity. Mrs. J. showed no memory impairments and had good learning abilities. Dementing illnesses are common among older persons, but most retain good cognitive function. High and low glucose levels can affect cognitive function negatively and should be avoided as much as possible.

Mrs. J. did well on her more intensive regimen and greatly improved her diabetes control. She was able to manage the insulin injections, hypoglycemia, and monitoring. She was not able to exercise regularly and gained 12 pounds in 1 year on insulin therapy. Although she disliked food substitutes and gained weight, she also made many positive changes in her diet, such as greater consistency and reducing portion sizes. She also had great difficulty decreasing her salt intake. Despite the weight gain, her glucose and lipid levels and blood pressure all decreased. Mrs. J. is fortunate to have a healthy husband and many close friends. She showed great pride in achieving good glucose control and continues to attend the diabetes support group with her husband.

REFERENCES

1. American Diabetes Association: *Direct and indirect costs of diabetes in the United States in 1992,* Alexandria, Va, 1993, American Diabetes Association.

2. American Diabetes Association: Position statement: implications of the Diabetes Control and Complications Trial, *Diabetes Care* 16:1517-1520, 1993.

3. American Diabetes Association: Consensus statement: self-monitoring of blood glucose, *Diabetes Care* 17:81-86, 1994.

4. Anderson LA: Health-care communication and selected psychosocial correlates of adherence in diabetes management, *Diabetes Care* 13(suppl 2):66-76, 1990.

5. Atchley RC: *Social forces and aging,* ed 6, Belmont, Calif, 1991, Wadsworth.

6. Badger TA: Physical health impairment and depression among older adults, *Image* 25:325-330, 1993.

7. Bahr SJ: The economic well-being in aging families. In Bahr SJ, Peterson ET, editors: *Aging and the family,* Lexington, Mass, 1989, Heath.

8. Barber CE: Transition to the empty nest. In Bahr SJ, Peterson ET, editors: *Aging and the family,* Lexington, Mass, 1989, Heath.

9. Barr P, Hess G, Frey ML: Relationships between reading levels and effective patient education, *Diabetes* 35(suppl 1):48A, 1986.

10. Barrett-Connor E: Commentary, *Diabetes Spectrum* 2:164-166, 1989.

11. Blunt BA, Barrett-Connor E, Wingard DL: Evaluation of fasting plasma glucose as a screening test for NIDDM in older adults, *Diabetes Care* 14:989-993, 1991.

12. Boult C and others: Screening elders for risk of hospital admission, *J Am Geriatr Soc* 41:811-817, 1993.

13. Bower KA: *Case management by nurses,* Kansas City, Mo, 1992, American Nurses Publishing.

14. Boyd K: Diabetes mellitus in hospice patients: some guidelines, *Palliative Med* 7:163-164, 1993.

15. Bransome ED Jr.: Financing the care of diabetes mellitus in the US: background, problems, and challenges, *Diabetes Care* 15(suppl 1):1-5, 1992.

16. Brodows RG: Benefits and risks with glyburide and glipizide in elderly NIDDM patients, *Diabetes Care* 15:75-80, 1992.

17. Coleman LM: The black Americans who keep working. In Jackson JS, Chatters LM, Taylor RJ, editors: *Aging in black America,* Newbury Park, Calif, 1993, Sage.

18. Colwell JA: Is it time to introduce metformin in the US? *Diabetes Care* 16:653-655, 1993.

19. Connell CM: Psychosocial contexts of diabetes and older adulthood: reciprocal effects, *Diabetes Educ* 17:364-371, 1991.

20. Coonrod BA, Betschart J, Harris MI: Frequency and determinants of diabetes patient education among adults in the US population, *Diabetes Care* 17:852-858, 1994.

21. Coscelli C and others: Use of premixed insulin among the elderly, *Diabetes Care* 15:1628-1630, 1992.

22. Cowie CC and others: Effect of multiple risk factors on differences between blacks and whites in the prevalence of non-insulin-dependent diabetes mellitus in the United States, *Am J Epidemiol* 137:719-732, 1993.

23. Cox HG: *Later life: the realities of aging,* ed 2, Englewood Cliffs, NJ, 1988, Prentice-Hall.

24. Davidson MB: Diabetes in the elderly: diagnosis and treatment, *Hosp Pract* 17:113-120, 125, 128-129, 1982.

25. Davidson MB: The impact of diabetes in the elderly, *Diabetes Educ* 8:10, 65, 1983.

26. Davis WK, Dedrick RF, Anderson L: Assessing patients' functional capacity to perform diabetes self-management tasks, *Diabetes* 39(suppl 1):305A, 1990.

27. Davis WK and others: Psychosocial adjustment to and control of diabetes mellitus: differences by disease type and treatment, *Health Psychol* 6(1):1-14, 1987.

28. The DCCT Research Group: The effect of intensive treatment of diabetes on the development and progression of long-term complications in insulin-dependent diabetes mellitus, *N Engl J Med* 329:977-986, 1993.

29. Deakins DA: Teaching elderly patients about diabetes, *Am J Nurs* 94(4):38-42, 1994.

30. DeFronzo RA: The triumvirate: β-cell, muscle, liver: a collusion responsible for NIDDM, *Diabetes* 37:667-687, 1988.

31. Diehl AK, Sugarek NJ, Bareer RL: Medication compliance in non-insulin dependent diabetes: a randomized comparison of chlorpropamide and insulin, *Diabetes Care* 8:219-223, 1985.

32. Doak CC: Communicating with the elderly, *Diabetes Educ* 8:45-47, 64, 1983.

33. Dudley J: Health education and perceived patient needs, *Diabetes Educ* 15:154-155, 1989.

34. Engram E, Lockery SA: Intimate partnerships. In Jackson JS, Chatters LM, Taylor RJ, editors: *Aging in black America,* Newbury Park, Calif, 1993, Sage.

35. Erikson E: *Childhood and society,* New York, 1963, Norton.

36. Floyd JC Jr and others: Feasibility of adjustment of insulin dose by insulin-requiring type II

diabetic patients, *Diabetes Care* 13:386-392, 1990.

37. Folstein MF, Folstein SE, McHugh PR: Mini-Mental State: a practical method for grading the cognitive state of patients for the clinician, *J Psychiatr Res* 12:189-198, 1975.

38. Franz MJ and others: Nutritional principles for the management of diabetes and related complications: a technical review, *Diabetes Care* 17:490-518, 1994.

39. Funnell MM: Role of the diabetes educator for older adults, *Diabetes Care* 13(suppl 2):60-65, 1990.

40. Funnell MM, Anderson RM: Patient education in a physician's office, *Pract Diabetol* 12(2):22-25, 1993.

41. Funnell M and others: Participation in a diabetes education and care program: experiences from the Diabetes Care for Older Adults Project (DCOAP), *Diabetes* 43(suppl 1):20A, 1994.

42. Gallo JJ, Reichel W, Anderson L: *Handbook of geriatric assessment,* Rockville, Md, 1988, Aspen.

43. Gambert SR, editor: *Handbook of geriatrics,* New York, 1987, Plenum.

44. Gambert SR: Atypical presentation of diabetes mellitus in the elderly, *Geriatr Clin North Am* 6:721-730, 1990.

45. Gavard JA, Lustman PJ, Clouse RE: Prevalence of depression in adults with diabetes: an epidemiological evaluation, *Diabetes Care* 16:1167-1178, 1993.

46. Gibson RC: Retirement. In Taylor RJ, editor: *Life in black America,* Newbury Park, Calif, 1991, Sage.

47. Gibson RC: The black American retirement experience. In Jackson JS, Chatters LM, Taylor RJ, editors: *Aging in black America,* Newbury Park, Calif, 1993, Sage.

48. Gilden JL and others: The effectiveness of diabetes education programs for older patients and their spouses, *J Am Geriatr Soc* 37:1023-1030, 1989.

49. Gilden JL and others: Effects of self-monitoring of blood glucose on elderly diabetic patients, *J Am Geriatr Soc* 38:511-515, 1990.

50. Gilden JL and others: Diabetes support groups improve health care of older diabetic patients, *J Am Geriatr Soc* 40:147-150, 1992.

51. Glasgow RE, Toobert DJ, Hampson SE: Participation in outpatient diabetes education programs: how many patients take part and how representative are they? *Diabetes Educ* 17:376-380, 1991.

52. Glasgow RE and others: Improving self-care among older patients with type II diabetes: the Sixty. . . Something Study, *Patient Educ Counsel* 19:61-64, 1992.

53. Gradman TJ and others: Verbal learning and/or memory improves with glycemic control in older subjects with non-insulin-dependent diabetes mellitus, *J Am Geriatr Soc* 41:1305-1312, 1993.

54. Graham C: Exercise and aging: implications for persons with diabetes, *Diabetes Educ* 17:189-195, 1991.

55. Greenland P and others: In-hospital and 1-year mortality in 1,524 women after myocardial infarction: comparison with 4,315 men, *Circulation* 83:484-491, 1991.

56. *Guidelines for diabetes care,* New York, 1981, American Diabetes Association/American Association of Diabetes Educators.

57. Halter JB, Christensen NJ: Introduction: diabetes mellitus in elderly people, *Diabetes Care* 13(suppl 2):1-2, 1990.

58. Halter JB, Morrow LA: Use of sulfonylurea drugs in elderly patients, *Diabetes Care* 13(suppl 2):86-92, 1990.

59. Halter J and others: Intensive treatment safely improves glycemic control of elderly patients with diabetes mellitus, *Diabetes* 42(suppl 1):146A, 1993.

60. Harris MI: Impaired glucose tolerance in the US population, *Diabetes Care* 12:464-474, 1989.

61. Harris MI: Epidemiology of diabetes mellitus among the elderly in the United States, *Clin Geriatr Med* 6:703-729, 1990.

62. Harris MI: Undiagnosed NIDDM: clinical and public health issues, *Diabetes Care* 16:642-652, 1993.

63. Harris MI, Cowie CC, Eastman R: Health insurance coverage for adults with diabetes in the US population, *Diabetes Care* 17:583-591, 1994.

64. Harris MI, Cowie CC, Howie LJ: Self-monitoring of blood glucose by adults with diabetes in the United States population, *Diabetes Care* 16:1116-1123, 1993.

65. Hatchett SJ, Cochran DL, Jackson JS: Family life. In Taylor RJ, editor: *Life in black America,* Newbury Park, Calif, 1991, Sage.

66. Havighurst RJ: *Developmental tasks and education,* ed 2, New York, 1972, McKay.

67. Helmrich SP and others: Physical activity and reduced occurrence of non-insulin-dependent diabetes mellitus, *N Engl J Med* 325:147-1452, 1991.

68. Henry RR, Edelman SV: Advances in treatment of type II diabetes mellitus in the elderly, *Geriatrics* 47(4):24-30, 1992.

69. Hiss RG, editor: *Diabetes in communities,* Ann Arbor, 1986, University of Michigan, Diabetes Research and Training Center.

70. Hiss RG, editor: *Diabetes in communities II,* Ann Arbor, 1992, University of Michigan, Diabetes Research and Training Center.

71. Hussey LC, Gilliland K: Compliance, low literacy and locus of control, *Nurs Clin North Am* 24:605-611, 1989.

72. Inglis AD, Kjervik DK: Empowerment of advanced practice nurses: regulation reform needed to increase access to care, *J Law Med Ethics* 21:193-205, 1993.

73. Jackson RA: Mechanisms of age-related glucose intolerance, *Diabetes Care* 13(suppl 2):9-19, 1990.

74. Jenny JL: A comparison of four age groups' adaptation to diabetes, *Can J Public Health* 75:237-244, 1984.

75. Johnson SB: Methodological issues in diabetes research, *Diabetes Care* 15:1658-1667, 1992.

76. Kane RA, Kane RL: *Assessing the elderly: a practical guide to measurement,* Lexington, Mass, 1981, Heath.

77. Kaplan RM, Davis WK: Evaluating the costs and benefits of outpatient diabetes education and nutrition counseling, *Diabetes Care* 9:81-88, 1986.

78. Karlson BW, Herlitz J, Hjalmarson A: Prognosis of acute myocardial infarction in diabetic and non-diabetic patients, *Diabetic Med* 10:449-454, 1993.

79. Kart CS, editor: *The realities of aging: an introduction to gerontology,* ed 3, Boston, 1990, Allyn & Bacon.

80. Kart CS, Metress ES: Death and dying. In Kart CS, editor: *The realities of aging: an introduction to gerontology,* ed 3, Boston, 1990, Allyn & Bacon.

81. Kick E: Patient teaching for elders, *Nurs Clin North Am* 24:681-686, 1989.

82. Kicklighter JR, Stein MA: Factors influencing diabetic clients' ability to read and comprehend printed diabetic diet materials, *Diabetes Educ* 19:40-46, 1993.

83. Kitabchi AE and others: Diabetic ketoacidosis and the hyperglycemic, hyperosmolar nonketotic state. In Kahn CR, Weir GS, editors: *Joslin's diabetes mellitus,* ed 13, Philadelphia, 1994, Lea & Febiger.

84. Knight PV, Kesson CM: Educating the elderly diabetic, *Diabetic Med* 3:170-172, 1986.

85. Kovisto VA: Insulin therapy in type II diabetes, *Diabetes Care* 16(suppl 3):29-39, 1993.

86. Kvam SH, Lyons JS: Assessment of coping strategies, social support, and general health status in individuals with diabetes mellitus, *Psychol Rep* 68:623-632, 1991.

87. Lasker RD: Payment for diabetes care under the Medicare fee schedule, *Diabetes Care* 15(suppl 1):62-65, 1992.

88. Laufer IJ: Diabetes in the elderly, *Pract Diabetol* 4(3):7-9, 1985.

89. Leifson J: Physical health of the elderly: impact on families. In Bahr SJ, Peterson ET, editors: *Aging and the family,* Lexington, Mass, 1989, Heath.

90. Levinson DJ and others: *The seasons of a man's choice,* New York, 1978, Knopf.

91. Linn M, Linn BS, Stein AR: Satisfaction with ambulatory care and compliance in older patients, *Med Care* 20:606-614, 1982.

92. Lipson LG: Diabetes in the elderly: diagnosis, pathogenesis and therapy, *Am J Med* 80(5A):10-21, 1986.

93. Litzelman DK and others: Reduction of lower extremity clinical abnormalities with noninsulin-dependent diabetes mellitus: a randomized controlled trial, *Ann Intern Med* 119:36-41, 1993.

94. Lopata H: *Widowhood in an American city,* Cambridge, Mass, 1973, Schenkman.

95. Madsbad S: Classification of diabetes in older adults, *Diabetes Care* 13(suppl 2):93-95, 1990.

96. Martin DB, Quint AR: Therapy for diabetes. In *Diabetes in America: diabetes data compiled 1984,* NIH Pub No 85-1468, 1985, National Diabetes Data Group, US Department of Health and Human Services.

97. Mathiesen ER and others: Efficacy of captopril in postponing nephropathy in normotensive insulin-dependent diabetic patients with microalbuminuria, *Br Med J* 303:81-87, 1991.

98. Matz R: Diabetes mellitus in the elderly, *Hosp Pract* 21(3):195-218, 1986.

99. Matz R: Summaries and comments, *Diabetes Spectrum* 2:173-174, 1989.

100. Mazzuca SA and others: The diabetes education study: a controlled trial of the effects of diabetes patient education, *Diabetes Care* 9:1-10, 1986.

101. McDonald J: Alcohol and diabetes, *Diabetes Care* 3:629-637, 1980.

102. McNabb WL, Quinn MT, Rosing L: Weight loss program for inner-city black women with non-insulin-dependent diabetes mellitus: PATHWAYS, *J Am Diet Assoc* 93:75-77, 1993.

103. Meneilly SG, Cheung E, Toukko H: Counterregulatory hormone responses to hypoglycemia in the elderly patient with diabetes, *Diabetes* 43:403-410, 1994.

104. Messena MD, Beizer JL: Diabetes in the elderly, *Pract Diabetol* 10(1):1-4, 1991.

105. Miller LV: Educating the elderly diabetic, *Diabetes Educ* 10:67-69, 1984 (special issue).

106. Miller LV: Managing the elderly patient with diabetes, *Clin Diabetes* 4:74-76, 90, 1985.

107. Minaker KL: What diabetologists should know about elderly patients, *Diabetes Care* 13(suppl 2):34-46, 1990.

108. Mooradian AD: The nutritional status of ambulatory elderly type II diabetic patients, *Age* 13:87-89, 1990.

109. Mooradian AD: Caring for the elderly nursing home patient with diabetes, *Diabetes Spectrum* 5:318-322, 1992.

110. Morisaki N and others: Diabetic control and progression of retinopathy in elderly patients: five year follow-up study, *J Am Geriatr Soc* 42:142-145, 1994.

111. Morley JE: Diabetes in elderly patients, *Pract Diabetol* 7(5):6-10, 1988.

112. Morrow L, Halter J: Diabetes mellitus in the older adult, *Geriatrics* 43(suppl):57-65, 1988.

113. Morrow LA, Halter JB: Treatment of the elderly with diabetes. In Kahn CR, Weir GS, editors: *Joslin's diabetes mellitus,* ed 13, Philadelphia, 1994, Lea & Febiger.

114. Mykkanen L and others: Prevalence of diabetes and impaired glucose tolerance in elderly subjects and their association with obesity and family history of diabetes, *Diabetes Care* 13:1099-1105, 1990.

115. National Diabetes Data Group: Classification and diagnosis of diabetes mellitus and other categories of glucose intolerance, *Diabetes* 28:1039-1057, 1979.

116. Neugarten BL, Weinstein KK: The changing American grandparents, *J Marr Fam* 26:199-204, 1964.

117. O'Connor PJ, Jacobson AM: Functional status measurement in elderly diabetic patients, *Clin Geriatr Med* 6:865-882, 1990.

118. Pace WD: Geriatric assessment in the office setting, *Geriatrics* 44:29-35, 1989.

119. Perlmuter LC: Choice enhanced performance in non-insulin dependent diabetics and controls, *J Gerontol Psychol Sci* 46:218-223, 1991.

120. Perlmuter LC and others: Decreased cognitive function in aging non-insulin-dependent diabetic patients, *Am J Med* 77:1043-1048, 1984.

121. Pitcha BW, Larson DC: Elderly widowhood. In Bahr SJ, Peterson ET, editors: *Aging and the family,* Lexington, Mass, 1989, Heath.

122. Polin SS: Paying for health care: the high cost of diabetes, *Clin Diabetes* 3:108-116, 1985.

123. Polly RK: Diabetes, health beliefs, self-care behaviors, and glycemic control among older adults with non-insulin dependent diabetes mellitus, *Diabetes Educ* 18:321-327, 1992.

124. Poplin LE: Diabetes that first occurs in older people, *Nutr Today* 17(5):4-13, 1982.

125. Porte D Jr, Kahn SE: What geriatricians should know about diabetes mellitus, *Diabetes Care* 13(suppl 2):47-54, 1990.

126. Powers MA, Kohrs MB, Raimondi MP: Diabetes nutrition and management for the elderly, *Diabetes Educ* 8:26-33, 1983.

127. Pugh JA and others: Is combination sulfonylurea and insulin therapy useful in NIDDM patients?: a meta-analysis, *Diabetes Care* 15:953-959, 1992.

128. Reaven GM: *Clinician's guide to non-insulin dependent diabetes mellitus,* ed 2, New York, 1989, Dekker.

129. Reaven G and others: Relationship between hyperglycemia and cognitive function in older NIDDM patients, *Diabetes Care* 13:16-21, 1990.

130. Redman BK: *The process of patient teaching in nursing,* ed 4, St Louis, 1980, Mosby.

131. Reed RL, Mooradian AD: Nutritional status and dietary management of elderly diabetic patients, *Clin Geriatr Med* 6:883-901, 1990.

132. Rempusheski VF: The role of ethnicity in elder care, *Nurs Clin North Am* 24:717-725, 1989.

133. Resler MM: Teaching strategies that promote adherence, *Nurs Clin North Am* 18:799-811, 1983.

134. Rosenstock IM: Understanding and enhancing patient compliance with diabetic regimens, *Diabetes Care* 8:610-615, 1985.

135. Rosenstock J and others: Diabetes control in the elderly: a randomized, comparative study of glyburide versus glipizide in non-insulin dependent diabetes mellitus, *Clin Ther* 15:1031-1040, 1993.

136. Rost FM and others: Self-care predictors of metabolic control in NIDDM patients, *Diabetes Care* 13:1111-1113, 1990.

137. Rubin RJ, Altman WM, Mendelson DN: Health care expenditures for people with diabetes mellitus, 1992, *J Clin Endocrinol Metab* 78:809A-809F, 1994.

138. Ruoff G: The management of noninsulin-dependent diabetes mellitus in the elderly, *Fam Practitioner* 36:329-335, 1993.

139. Schwartz AN, Snyder CL, Peterson JA: *Aging and life: an introduction to gerontology,* ed 2, New York, 1984, Holt, Rinehart & Winston.

140. Schwartz RS: Exercise training in the treatment of diabetes mellitus in elderly patients, *Diabetes Care* 13(suppl 2):77-84, 1990.

141. Sherman RA: Diabetes and its complications, *Diagnosis,* May 1985, pp 127-136.

142. Streif LD: Can clients understand our instructions? *Image* 18:48-52, 1986.

143. Taylor RJ: The extended family as a source of support to elderly blacks, *Gerontologist* 25:488-494, 1985.

144. Taylor RJ, Keith VM, Tucker MB: Gender, marital, familial, and friendship roles. In Jackson JS, Chatters LM, Taylor RJ, editors: *Aging in black America,* Newbury Park, Calif, 1993, Sage.

145. Tripp-Reimer T, Brink PJ, Saunders JM: Cultural assessment: content and process, *Nurs Outlook* 32(2):78-82, 1984.

146. Tu K-S, McDaniel G, Templeton J: Diabetes self-care knowledge, behaviors, and metabolic control of older adults: the effect of a post-educational follow-up program, *Diabetes Educ* 19:25-30, 1993.

147. Tun PA, Nathan DM, Perlmuter LC: Cognitive and affective disorders in elderly diabetics, *Clin Geriatr Med* 6:731-746, 1990.

148. U'ren RC and others: The mental efficiency of the elderly person with type II diabetes, *J Am Geriatr Soc* 38:505-510, 1990.

149. US Department of Health and Human Services: *Diabetes in the United States: a strategy for prevention,* Atlanta, 1993, Centers for Disease Control and Prevention.

150. US Department of Health and Human Services: *Diabetes surveillance 1993,* Atlanta, 1993, Centers for Disease Control and Prevention.

151. VanNostrand JF: Nursing home care for diabetics. In *Diabetes in America: diabetes data compiled 1984,* NIH Pub No 85-1468, 1985, National Diabetes Data Group, US Department of Health and Human Services.

152. Vinik AI and others: Diabetic neuropathies, *Diabetes Care* 15:1926-1975, 1992.

153. Wachtel TJ: The diabetic hyperosmolar state, *Clin Geriatr Med* 6:797-806, 1990.

154. Waclawski ER: Ill-health retirement and diabetes mellitus, *J Soc Occup Med* 41:80-82, 1991.

155. Weick HH and others: Senile dementia in geriatrics. In Platt D, editor: Geriatrics, New York, 1982, Springer.

156. Weinberger M and others: Economic impact of diabetes mellitus in the elderly, *Clin Geriatr Med* 6:959-970, 1990.

157. White JR Jr: Angiotensin converting enzyme inhibitors, their potential role in diabetes care. Research to practice: introduction and conclusion, *Diabetes Spectrum* 6:169-200, 1993.

158. Wilson PW, Anderson KW, Kannel WB: Epidemiology of diabetes in the elderly: The Framingham Study, *Am J Med* 80(5A):3-9, 1986.

159. Wilson W, Pratt C: The impact of diabetes education and peer support upon weight and glycemic control of elderly persons with noninsulin dependent diabetes mellitus (NIDDM), *Am J Public Health* 77:634, 1987.

160. Wingard D and others: Community based study of prevalence of NIDDM in older adults, *Diabetes Care* 13(suppl 2):3-8, 1990.

161. Wolffenbuttel BH, Drossaert CH, Visser AP: Determinants of injecting insulin in elderly patients with type II diabetes mellitus, *Patient Educ Counsel* 22:117-125, 1993.

162. Woodruff-Pak DS: *Psychology and aging,* Englewood Cliffs, NJ, 1988, Prentice-Hall.

163. Yesavage JA: Geriatric depression scale, *Psychopharmacol Bull* 24:709-711, 1988.

PATIENT FORM

To help us work with you, we would like you to fill out this form about yourself, the way you live, and the things you do at home to take care of yourself. Your answers to these questions are very important and help us to get to know you better. If you do not understand a question or are unsure of your answer, please leave it blank and we will review it with you.

1. Have you ever attended a formal diabetes education program?
   ☐ No
   ☐ Yes   Date _____

2. How would you rate how much you know about diabetes?
   ☐ Good
   ☐ Fair
   ☐ Poor

3. Are you interested in learning more about diabetes and its care?
   ☐ No
   ☐ Yes

4. If you have been given information on the following topics, please check all that apply.

		Yes	If so, when:	Would like more information
a.	Feelings about diabetes			
b.	Meal planning			
c.	Exercise			
d.	Insulin			
e.	Blood sugar testing			
f.	Low blood sugar			
g.	High blood sugar			
h.	Personal health habits			
i.	Sick-day care			
j.	Complications of diabetes			
k.	Risk factors (smoking, etc.)			
l.	Other			
m.				

5. Do you ever seek out information about diabetes (e.g., TV programs, magazine articles, books)?
   ☐ No
   ☐ Yes

6. What other people have you known with diabetes? _____

_____

_____

7. How did diabetes affect them? _____

_____

_____

8. How has having diabetes affected your life? _____

_____

_____

9. How is your diabetes treated?
   ☐ Diet only
   ☐ Diabetes pills: Name of pill _____ Time taken _____
   ☐ Insulin: How many times a day _____
                       Types of insulin _____
                       Who gives your shot? _____

10. On the average, how many *days* out of a week do you:

a. Eat breakfast?	None	1	2	3	4	5	6	7
b. Eat lunch?	None	1	2	3	4	5	6	7
c. Eat dinner?	None	1	2	3	4	5	6	7

11. Mark the times at which you *usually* eat by placing a B (breakfast), L (lunch), D (dinner),
    or S (snack) in the box below the times.
    Record times that you usually take diabetes medication by circling the hour.
    Record times that you usually exercise by placing an E in the box below times.

	AM						Noon									PM			
5	6	7	8	9	10	11	12	1	2	3	4	5	6	7	8	9	10	11	12

12. Do you eat your meals at the same time every day?
    ☐ Never
    ☐ 1-3 times/week
    ☐ 4-7 times/week
    ☐ More than 7 times/week

13. If you eat less than three meals a day, are you willing to eat more meals per day?
    ☐ No
    ☐ Yes

14. Do you follow any kind of special diet?
   - ☐ No
   - ☐ Yes   If yes, what? _____

15. Do you take any vitamin, mineral, or other nutritional supplements?
   - ☐ No
   - ☐ Yes   If yes, what? _____

16. How long have you been at your current
    weight? _____

17. On the average, how often in a week do you eat sugar foods like candy, cookies, pie, and so forth
   - ☐ Never
   - ☐ 1-3 times/week
   - ☐ 4-7 times/week
   - ☐ More than 7 times/week

18. Do you have a regular exercise plan?
   - ☐ No   Why not? _____
   - ☐ Yes   What is it? _____
            How many days of the week do you do it? _____
            How many minutes do you do it each time? _____

19. Would you like to have an exercise plan?
   - ☐ No
   - ☐ Yes   If yes, what would you be able to do? _____
   _____

20. Do you test your blood sugar at home?
   - ☐ No
   - ☐ Yes   What do you use to do the tests? _____
            How many days of the week do you test? _____
            On days you do tests, how often do you test? _____
            What times of the day? _____
            Who does the tests? _____

21. Do you test your urine for ketones at home?
   - ☐ No
   - ☐ Yes   What do you use to do the tests? _____
            Who does the tests? _____

22. Do you change your diet, exercise, or medicine dose as a result of the tests?
    ☐ No   Would you like to learn to make changes? _____
    ☐ Yes   What do you change? _____
            How do you change it? _____

23. Do you take special care of your feet?
    ☐ No
    ☐ Yes   What do you do? _____
            Who does your foot care? _____

24. a. Do you ever have **low** blood sugar?
       ☐ No
       ☐ Yes   If yes, about how often? _____
    b. How do you feel when your blood sugar is **low**? _____
       _____

    c. What do you do if your blood sugar is **low**?
       ☐ Nothing
       ☐ Something, which is _____
       _____

25. a. Do you ever have **high** blood sugar?
       ☐ No
       ☐ Yes   If yes, about how often? _____
    b. How do you feel when your blood sugar is **high?** _____
       _____

    c. What do you do if your blood sugar is **high?**
       ☐ Nothing
       ☐ Something, which is _____

26. Most of the time, how well do you follow your treatment plan? (Circle one.)

	No plan	**Not well**	**Fairly well**	**Very well**
a. Diabetes medication	0	1	2	3
b. Meal plan	0	1	2	3
c. Testing for sugar	0	1	2	3
d. Exercise plan	0	1	2	3

27. Do you wear or carry diabetes identification?
    ☐ No
    ☐ Yes

28. Place an X in the box to show whether or not you need help and whether or not you get help for each of the following:

	Do not need help	Need and get help	Need help but don't get it
a. Diabetes care (shots, tests, foot care)			
b. Care for other health problems			
c. Dressing			
d. Bathing			
e. Cooking			
f. Housework			
g. Yardwork			
h. Shopping			
i. Handling finances			
j. Transportation			
k. Seeing			
l. Hearing			
m. Walking			
n. Sleeping			
o. Eating			
p. Remembering			
q. Reading			
r. Writing			

29. If you get help, from whom?
(Check all that apply.)   Specify from whom:

    a. ☐ Family   _____

    b. ☐ Friends   _____

    c. ☐ Visiting nurse   _____

    d. ☐ Hired help   _____

e. ☐ Volunteer help   _____

f. ☐ Community services   _____

g. ☐ Other   _____

INTERVIEW FORM

30. Do you have someone you can talk to about your diabetes?
    ☐ No
    ☐ Yes. If yes, who? _____

31. How often do you see or talk to family or friends?
    ☐ Daily
    ☐ 1-3 times a week
    ☐ 4-6 times a week
    ☐ Less than once a week
    ☐ Less than once a month

32. Whom do you feel close to?

33. Do you see them as often as you would like?

34. What makes it hard to live with your diabetes?

35. What helps you live with diabetes?

36. What would make it easier to live with your diabetes?

37. a. How would you rate the stress you are under using the following scale?
    - ☐ Little or no stress
    - ☐ Fair amount of stress
    - ☐ Lot of stress

    b. What do you think is causing your stress?

    c. What do you do about your stress?

38. a. Do you ever have feelings of fear or anxiety?
    - ☐ No
    - ☐ Yes

    b. Describe how you feel.

    c. What do you feel fear or anxiety about?

    d. What do you do about it?

39. a. Do you ever feel down or depressed?
    - ☐ No
    - ☐ Yes

    b. Describe how you feel.

c. What do you feel down or depressed about?

d. What do you do about it?

40. Have there been any major changes in your life in the last few years?
    ☐ No
    ☐ Yes

41. How do you deal with things that worry you?

42. What do you do in your leisure time (groups, friends, regular activities)?

43. Are you active in any groups?

44. What good things are going on in your life?

45. Do you have any other comments or concerns at this time?
    ☐ No
    ☐ Yes   If yes, what? _____
    _____

EDUCATIONAL PLAN

Areas of strength:

Areas of weakness:

Educational problem list:

Problem	Plan	Date Resolved Signature	Date Identified Signature

Other pertinent data (e.g., functional status, knowledge, test scores, psychosocial information, reading level):

_____

_____

_____

_____

_____

Instructions for Administration of Mini-Mental State Examination (test follows on p. 833)

ORIENTATION

1. Ask the person for the date. Then ask specifically for parts omitted, such as, "Can you also tell me what season it is?" One point for each correct answer.
2. Ask in turn, "Can you tell me the name of this hospital (town, county, etc.)?" One point for each correct answer.

REGISTRATION

Ask the person if you may test his or her memory. Then say the names of three unrelated objects, clearly and slowly, about 1 second for each. After you have said all three, ask the person to repeat them. This first repetition determines the score (0 to 3), but keep saying them until he or she can repeat all three, up to six trials. If the person does not eventually learn all three, recall cannot be meaningfully tested.

ATTENTION AND CALCULATION

Ask the person to begin with 100 and count backward by 7. Stop after five subtractions (93, 86, 79, 72, 65). Score the total number of correct answers.

   If the person cannot or will not perform this task, ask him or her to spell the word "world" backward. The score is the number of letters in correct order (e.g., dlrow = 5, dlorw = 3).

RECALL

Ask the person if he or she can recall the three words you previously asked him or her to remember. Score 0 to 3.

LANGUAGE

Naming: Show the person a wristwatch and ask what it is. Repeat for pencil. Score 0 to 2.
Repetition: Ask the person to repeat the sentence after you. Allow only one trial. Score 0 or 1.
Three-stage command: Give the person a piece of plain blank paper and repeat the command. Score 1 point for each part correctly executed.
Reading: On a blank piece of paper, print the sentence, "Close your eyes," in letters large enough for the person to see clearly. Ask him or her to read it and do what it says. Score 1 point only if the person actually closes the eyes.

Modified from Folstein MF, Folstein SE, McHugh PR: *J Psychiatr Res* 12: 189-198, 1975.

Writing: Give the person a blank piece of paper and ask him or her to write a sentence for you. Do not dictate a sentence; it is to be written spontaneously. It must contain a subject and verb and be sensible. Correct grammar and punctuation are not necessary.

Copying: On a clean piece of paper, draw intersecting pentagons, each side about 1 inch, and ask the person to copy it exactly as it is. All 10 angles must be present, and two must intersect to score 1 point. Tremor and rotation are ignored.

Estimate the person's level of sensorium along a continuum, from alert on the left to coma on the right.

Patient _____ Examiner _____ Date _____

Maximum	Actual Score	Orientation	Maximum	Actual Score	Recall

Orientation

5 ( ) 1. What is the (year) (season)(date) (day)(month)?

5 ( ) 2. Where are we (state)(county) (town)(clinic)(floor)? Give 1 point for each correct answer.

Registration

3 ( ) Name three objects: 1 second to say each. Then ask the patient all three after you have said them. Give 1 point for each correct answer. This first repetition determines his score (0 to 3), but keep saying them until he can repeat all three, up to six trials. Count trials and record.

Trials: _____

Attention and Calculation: Serials 7's

5 ( ) Go back from 100 by 7's. 1 point for each correct. Stop after 5 answers. If the patient cannot or will not perform this task, ask him to spell the word "world" backwards. The score is the number of letters in correct order e.g. dlrow = 5, dlorw = 3

Recall

3 ( ) Ask for the three objects repeated above. Give 1 point for each correct answer.

Language

2 ( ) Name a pencil and a watch

1 ( ) Repeat the following: "No ifs, ands or buts"

3 ( ) Follow a 3-stage command: "Take a paper in your right hand, fold it in half, and put it on the floor"

1 ( ) Read and obey "CLOSE YOUR EYES" below

1 ( ) Write a sentence on the line below

1 ( ) Copy design below

30 Total score _____

Indicate level of consciousness:

Alert   Drowsy   Stupor   Coma

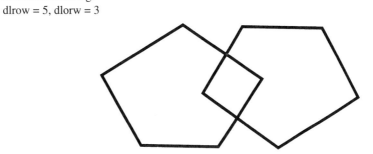

X _____

CLOSE YOUR EYES

A Diabetes Resources

PUBLICATIONS

A complete listing of diabetes-related materials can be obtained from:
National Diabetes Information Clearinghouse
  Box NDIC
  Bethesda, MD 20892
  1-301-468-2162

ORGANIZATIONS

American Dietetic Association
  216 W. Jackson Blvd., Suite 800
  Chicago, IL 60606-6995
  1-312-899-0400

The International Diabetes Center
  Diabetes Center, Inc.
  P.O. Box 739
  Wayzata, MN 55391

American Diabetes Association (ADA) is a nonprofit, voluntary health agency supported by donations. The ADA offers funding for research, free screening programs, physician referrals, written materials, support groups, education, and recognition of education programs that meet certain standards. The national office address is:
American Diabetes Association, Inc.
1660 Duke St.
Alexandria, VA 22314
1-800-ADA-DISC (1-800-232-3472)

Juvenile Diabetes Foundation (JDF) is a nonprofit, voluntary health agency supported by donations. Money is used for educational programs, camping programs, and support groups. The national office address is:
Juvenile Diabetes Foundation International
432 Park Ave. South
New York, NY 10016
1-212-889-7575
1-800-223-1138

American Association of Diabetes Educators
American Association of Diabetes Educators
500 North Michigan Ave.
Suite 1400
Chicago, IL 60611
1-312-661-1700

The Diabetes Care and Education Practice Group of the American Dietetic Association
216 West Jackson Blvd., Suite 800
Chicago, IL 60606-6995
1-312-899-0040

Diabetes Research and Training Centers
National Diabetes Information Clearinghouse
Box NDIC
Bethesda, MD 20892
1-301-468-2162

International Diabetic Athletes Association. The purpose of the IDA is to promote healthful participation in sports and vigorous exercise by diabetic persons. Membership includes a subscription to *The Challenge: Newsletter of the International Diabetic Athletes Association.*
International Diabetic Athletes Association
P.O. Box 10010
Phoenix, AZ 85064

SPECIAL GROUPS
Visually Impaired

American Council for the Blind
1211 Connecticut Ave. NW
Washington, DC 20036
1-800-424-8666

American Foundation for the Blind
  15 West 16th St.
  New York, NY 10011
  1-212-620-2000

National Association for the Visually Handicapped
  221 West 21st St.
  New York, NY 10010

National Society to Prevent Blindness, Inc.
  79 Madison Ave.
  New York, NY 10016

The National Library Service for the Blind and Physically Handicapped of the Library of Congress provides a lending service from a collection of Braille and talking books and magazines. For more information contact:
National Library Service for the Blind and Physically Handicapped
  Library of Congress
  1291 Taylor St. NW
  Washington, DC 20542
  1-202-287-5100

The LIONS Clubs also offer services for blind persons. Contact your local group or:
LIONS Club International
  300 Twenty-Second St.
  Oakbrook, IL 60570
  1-312-571-5466

Kidney Disease

National Kidney Foundation
  2 Park Ave.
  New York, NY 10016
  1-212-889-2210

Heart Disease

American Heart Association
  7320 Greenville Ave.
  Dallas, TX 75231
  1-214-750-5300

Smoking

American Cancer Society (ACS)

Call the local ACS unit listed in your telephone book for more information about publications and services. Programs include the following:

- *Fresh Start.* A group smoking cessation program consisting of multiple sessions.
- *Smart Move!* A single-session smoking cessation program.

  Both programs are offered to the public free of charge by trained volunteers in ACS units nationwide. ACS also provides materials for youth of all age-groups, from preschool through high school.
- *50 Questions . . . Smoking and Health . . . and Answers.* Brochure that compiles questions most frequently asked about smoking.

National Cancer Institute (NCI)

Office of Cancer Communications
Building 31, Room 1OA24
Bethesda, MD 20893
Cancer Information Service: 1-800-4-CANCER

American Lung Association (ALA)

Call the local lung association for more information about publications and services. Some selected information includes the following:

- *Freedom from Smoking.* A 7-week behavior modification program for people who want to quit, offered to the public by trained members of the local lung associations nationwide.
- *A Healthy Beginning: The Smoke Free Family Guide for New Parents.* A handbook for health care professionals on counseling new parents to quit.
- *A Lifetime of Freedom from Smoking.* A self-help booklet that includes many coping strategies for relapse prevention.
- *Freedom from Smoking for You and Your Family.* A self-help manual.

National Heart, Lung, and Blood Institute (NHLBI)

Information Center
4733 Bethesda Ave., Suite 530
Bethesda, MD 20814
1-301-951-3260

Office on Smoking and Health (OSH)

Parklawn Building, Room 1-16
5600 Fishers Lane
Rockville, MD 29857
Patient Education: 1-301-443-5287
OSH continually develops new patient, public, and professional education materials that are available while supplies last. Some materials are produced in both English and Spanish.

SOCIAL SECURITY

The **Social Security Administration** is a government agency that may provide income when family earnings are stopped or reduced because of retirement, disability, or death.

MEDICARE

Medicare provides hospital and medical insurance for those age 65 and over or for persons of any age who are blind or disabled and who have received Social Security disability checks for 24 months in a row.

Disability benefits—These benefits provide monthly checks to workers who are disabled.

Survivor's benefits—Monthly checks or a one-time payment may be made to some family members when a person becomes disabled or dies.

Supplemental security income (SSI)—Monthly checks may be provided to people in need who are over age 65 or to blind or disabled persons of any age.

DEPARTMENT OF SOCIAL SERVICES

The **Department of Social Services** is the agency that makes financial and medical help, food stamps, and social services available to people who qualify. Those most useful for people with diabetes are the following:

Medicaid—This is a medical assistance program for persons who have a low income.

Aid to Families with Dependent Children (ADC)—This is a program of financial aid for families with children under 18 years when either one or both parents are missing or one or both parents are disabled for 90 days or more.

Food stamps—The food stamp program enables low-income families to buy more food for the same amount of money.

Social services—This agency provides a broad range of social and other services.

Veterans' Administration—Veterans of the Armed Forces can call their local Veterans' Administration (VA) for information about benefits.

COMMUNITY HEALTH CARE RESOURCES

Planned Parenthood—Planned Parenthood provides birth control advice and services for men and women, pregnancy tests, and problem pregnancy counseling. It is listed in the white pages of the phone book under "Planned Parenthood" and in the yellow pages under "Clinics" and "Birth Control Information Centers."

County public health departments—Health departments generally offer a wide range of services for people who live in that county. They offer education about diet, health problems, sex, birth control, and alcohol abuse. Public health departments are usually listed in the white pages of the phone book under "County government."

Visiting nurse associations—Visiting nurses provide nursing care and education in your home. Third-party payment (Medicare, Medicaid, Blue Cross, other insurance) will often pay for these services. Look in the white pages under "Visiting Nurse Association" or in the yellow pages under "Nurses."

Home health care—Many home health agencies are available. The types of services, expertise, and requirements vary from agency to agency. Some services may be covered by insurance.

Meals on Wheels—Meals on Wheels provides one meal a day for homebound or invalid people who qualify. Look under "Meals on Wheels" in the white pages of the phone book, or contact the Department of Social Services for information.

Lawyer Referral Service—This service provides a list of lawyers available in your area. The service can be reached at 1-800-292-7850.

SPECIAL CONCERNS

Weight loss programs—The American Dietetic Association can provide information about meal-planning and weight loss programs. They can be reached by calling or writing:
American Dietetic Association
430 North Michigan Ave.
Chicago, IL 60611
1-312-280-5000

SUBSTANCE ABUSE PROGRAMS

Alcoholics Anonymous (AA)—AA is a self-help group for people who want to stop drinking or using drugs. Look in the white pages of the phone book for local groups, or contact:
Alcoholics Anonymous
P.O. Box 459
Grand Central Station
New York, NY 10163
1-212-686-1100

DIABETES IDENTIFICATION

Medic Alert Foundation is a charitable, nonprofit organization that provides identification through the Medic Alert emblem. This tag is worn as a bracelet or necklace.
Medic Alert Foundation
Turlock, CA 95381
1-209-632-2371
1-800-344-3226

EMPLOYMENT

Vocational Rehabilitation is a federally funded program for vocationally handicapped persons. Individuals with diabetes are eligible for their services, which include the following:

- Medical and psychologic services
- Vocational testing
- Job counseling
- Job training and placement
- Help with employer problems

B Types of Diabetes Mellitus and Other Categories of Abnormal Glucose Metabolism

Clinical Classes	Distinguishing Characteristics
Diabetes mellitus Insulin-dependent diabetes mellitus (IDDM or type I)	Patients may be of any age, are not usually obese, and often have abrupt onset of signs and symptoms with insulinopenia before age 30. These patients often have strongly positive urine ketone tests in conjunction with hyperglycemia and depend on insulin therapy to prevent ketoacidosis and to sustain life.
Non-insulin-dependent diabetes mellitus (NIDDM or type II) (obese or nonobese)	Patients usually are over age 30 years at diagnosis, are obese, and have relatively few classic symptoms. They are not prone to ketoacidosis except during periods of stress. Although not dependent on exogenous insulin for survival, they may require it for adequate control of hyperglycemia.
Secondary and other types of diabetes	Patients with secondary and other types of diabetes mellitus have certain associated conditions or syndromes.
Malnutrition-related diabetes mellitus*	Patients are young (ages 10 to 40 years), usually symptomatic, and not prone to ketoacidosis, but most require insulin therapy.
Impaired glucose tolerance (IGT) (obese or nonobese)	Patients with impaired glucose tolerance have plasma glucose levels that are higher than normal but not diagnostic for diabetes mellitus.
Gestational diabetes mellitus (GDM)	Patients with gestational diabetes mellitus have onset or discovery of glucose intolerance during pregnancy.

*Recommended as a separate clinical class of diabetes mellitus by the World Health Organization (WHO).

Modified from *Medical management of insulin dependent (type I) diabetes,* ed 2, Alexandria, Va, 1994, American Diabetes Association.

C Indications and Criteria for Screening Tests

Indications

Screening tests for diabetes mellitus may be indicated when the individual has (is) the following:

- Strong family history of diabetes mellitus
- Obese
- Morbid obstetric history or a history of babies over 9 lb at birth
- Pregnant (between 24 and 28 weeks)
- History of recurrent skin, genital, or urinary tract infections

- Over 65 years old
- Hypertension or hyperlipidemia
- Of certain races (American Indian, Hispanic, African American)
- Previously identified impaired glucose tolerance (IGT)

Diagnosis of Diabetes Mellitus in Nonpregnant Adults

Diagnosis of diabetes mellitus in nonpregnant adults should be restricted to those who have *one* of the following:
- Random plasma glucose level of 200 mg/dl (11.1 mM) or higher *plus* classic signs and symptoms of diabetes mellitus, including polydipsia, polyuria, polyphagia, weight loss, and blurred vision
- Fasting plasma glucose level of 140 mg/dl (7.7 mM) or higher on at least two occasions
- Fasting plasma glucose level less than 140 mg/dl (7.7 mM) *plus* sustained elevated plasma glucose levels during at least two oral glucose tolerance tests. The 2-hour sample and at least one other between 0 and 2 hours after 75 g glucose dose should be 200 mg/dl (11.1 mM) or higher. Oral glucose tolerance testing (OGTT) is not necessary if patient has fasting plasma glucose level of 140 mg/dl (7.7 mM) or higher.*

Diagnosis of Diabetes Mellitus in Pregnant Women

An oral glucose challenge (does not have to be fasting) with a 50 g glucose load is recommended for screening. A plasma glucose level of 140 mg/dl (7.8 mM) or higher 1 hour later is considered an indication for diagnostic testing.

---

*An OGTT is rarely needed to diagnose type I diabetes.

Modified from *Medical management of insulin dependent (type I) diabetes,* ed 2, Alexandria, Va, 1994, American Diabetes Association.

APPENDIX

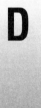

D Sample Diabetes Care Protocol

Guide to Initial Evaluation

Initial visit and evaluation
Medical history

- Symptoms
- Results of laboratory tests and special examination results related to the diagnosis of diabetes
- Prior glycated hemoglobin records
- Eating patterns, nutritional status, and weight history; growth and development in children and adolescents
- Details of previous treatment programs, including nutrition and diabetes self-management training
- Current treatment of diabetes, including medications, meal plan, and results of glucose monitoring and patients' use of data
- Exercise history
- Frequency, severity, and cause of acute complications such as ketoacidosis and hypoglycemia
- Prior or current infections, particularly skin, foot, dental, and genitourinary
- Symptoms and treatment of chronic complications associated with diabetes
- Other medications that may affect blood glucose levels
- Risk factors for atherosclerosis

- History and treatment of other conditions, including endocrine and eating disorders
- Family history of diabetes and other endocrine disorders
- Gestational history
- Life-style, cultural, psychosocial, educational, and economic factors that may influence the management of diabetes

Physical examination

- Height and weight (and comparison with norms in children and adolescents)
- Sexual maturation (during peripubertal period)
- Blood pressure determination, including orthostatic measurements when indicated, and comparison with age-related norms
- Ophthalmoscopic examination, preferably with dilation
- Oral examination
- Thyroid palpation
- Cardiac examination
- Abdominal examination
- Evaluation of pulses by palpation and with auscultation
- Hand/finger examination
- Foot examination
- Skin examination
- Neurologic examination

Modified from *Medical management of insulin dependent (type I) diabetes,* ed 2, Alexandria, Va, 1994, American Diabetes Association. *Continued.*

Guide to Initial Evaluation—cont'd

Initial visit and evaluation—cont'd
Laboratory evaluation

- Fasting plasma glucose (A random plasma glucose level may be obtained in an undiagnosed symptomatic patient for diagnostic purposes.)
- Glycated hemoglobin
- Fasting lipid profile, including total cholesterol, high-density lipoprotein cholesterol, triglycerides, and low-density lipoprotein cholesterol
- Serum creatinine
- Urinalysis for glucose, ketones, protein, and evidence of infection
- Determination for microalbuminuria
- Urine culture if evidence of infection is present
- Thyroid function test(s) when indicated

Self-management plan

The self-management plan should include information/strategies regarding the following:

- Statement of philosophy and goals
- General facts about IDDM and NIDDM
- Stress and psychosocial adjustment
- Family involvement/social support
- Nutrition
- Exercise/activity
- Medications
- Monitoring
- Relationships among nutrition, exercise, medication, and blood glucose levels
- Prevention, detection, and treatment of acute complications (hypoglycemia, hyperglycemia, illness)
- Prevention, detection, treatment, and rehabilitation of chronic complications
- Foot, skin, and dental care
- Behavior change strategies
- Benefits, risks, and treatment options for improving blood glucose
- Preconception care and pregnancy
- Use of health care system/community resources

APPENDIX

E Principles of Diabetes Patient Education

Microvascular Health

Retinopathy

- Inform patients that sight-threatening eye disease is a common complication of diabetes and may be present even with good vision. Remind them to report all ocular symptoms, since essentially any symptoms may be diabetic in origin. Blurred vision while reading may indicate macular edema. The presence of floaters may indicate hemorrhage, and flashing lights may indicate retinal detachment. Inform patients that early detection and appropriate treatment of diabetic eye disease greatly reduce the risk of visual loss.
- Explain the relationship between glycemic control and the subsequent development of ocular complications.
- Discuss the importance of not smoking. Counsel patients who smoke on strategies for achieving cessation.
- Inform patients about the association between hypertension and diabetic retinopathy. Stress the importance of the diagnosis and continuing treatment of hypertension.
- Explain the natural course and treatment of diabetic retinopathy and the importance of yearly eye examinations.
- Inform patients with diabetic retinopathy about the availability and benefits of early and timely laser photocoagulation therapy in reducing the risk of visual loss.
- Inform patients about their higher risks of cataract formation, open-angle glaucoma, and neovascular glaucoma.
- Discuss with patients who have any visual impairment (including blindness) the availability of visual, vocational, and psychosocial rehabilitation programs.

Nephropathy

- Inform patients about the potential renal complications of diabetes.
- Explain the relationship between poor glycemic control and the development of diabetic renal disease.
- Discuss the importance of not smoking. Counsel patients who smoke about strategies for achieving cessation.

Modified from *The prevention and treatment of complications of diabetes: a guide for primary care practitioners,* Atlanta, 1991, Department of Health and Human Services, Centers for Disease Control.

Microvascular Health—cont'd

Nephropathy—cont'd

- Inform patients about the association between hypertension and accelerated renal disease. Discuss the need for regular blood pressure measurements and the importance of treating hypertension.
- Explain the potential role that excessive protein in the diet may play in the pathogenesis and progression of diabetic nephropathy.
- Emphasize the importance of achieving and maintaining ideal body weight.
- Encourage regular physical exercise as a strategy for preventing hypertension and improving glycemic control.
- Review with patients the symptoms of urinary tract infection. Instruct patients to contact their health care provider if such symptoms occur.
- Review with patients which drugs are potentially nephrotoxic. Explain the danger of radiographic dye studies.
- Review the natural history of clinical diabetic nephropathy with patients who have this condition. Discuss the therapeutic options—dialysis versus transplantation—for end-stage renal disease (ESRD).

Neuropathy

- Explain the relationship between poor glycemic control and the subsequent development of diabetic neuropathy.
- Explain possible risk factors (e.g., consumption of alcohol) that may hasten the development or progression of diabetic neuropathy.
- Discuss the importance of not smoking. Counsel patients who smoke about strategies for achieving cessation.
- Discuss the importance of routine evaluation as necessary even for patients who have no symptoms of neuropathy.
- Explain that diabetic neuropathy can contribute to the development of other complications, including loss of limb.
- Discuss the signs and symptoms of autonomic neuropathy.
- Explain the benefits of treatment to patients with autonomic neuropathy.

Macrovascular Health

Cardiovascular disease

- Explain the relationship between glycemic control and the subsequent development of macrovascular complications.
- Inform patients with diabetes that their risk of developing cardiovascular disease is higher than that of persons without diabetes.
- Discuss the importance of not smoking. Counsel patients who smoke about strategies for achieving cessation.
- Emphasize to patients the importance of following dietary principles appropriate for their conditions (e.g., hypertension or hyperlipidemia).

Continued.

Macrovascular Health—cont'd

Cardiovascular disease—cont'd

- Discuss with patients the importance of treating hypertension and hyperlipidemia vigorously.
- Tell patients to immediately report symptoms of cardiovascular disease (e.g., chest or leg pain) so that investigation and treatment can begin promptly.

Foot care

- Instruct patients on the importance of regular foot care.
- Explain the importance of maintaining glycemic control to avoid complications. Discuss the relationships among glycemic control and neuropathy, peripheral vascular disease, and foot ulcers.
- Urge patients to avoid risk factors associated with worsening of neuropathy.
- Discuss the importance of not smoking. Counsel patients who smoke on strategies for achieving cessation.
- Inform patients who have lost sensation in their feet about the importance of caring for their feet, wearing proper shoes, and performing appropriate exercise.
- Inform patients about special shoes for preventing or treating foot problems.
- Refer patients to a certified pedorthist if they have foot deformities or otherwise need special shoes.
- Inform patients about the availability of podiatric services; encourage patients to use these services.

Special Issues in Diabetes Management

For patients with diabetic ketoacidosis (DKA)

- Be sure your patients with diabetes know if they are at risk for DKA.
- Be sure your patients with diabetes know when they are most susceptible to DKA.
- Be sure your patients with diabetes know what they can do to prevent DKA.
- Be sure your patients with diabetes know when they should contact you.

For patients with hyperglycemic hyperosmolar nonketotic coma

- Remind persons responsible for the older adults or chronically ill persons to look for the signs and symptoms of diabetes when their patients do not thrive.
- Recommend routine blood glucose screening.

For patients with hypoglycemia

- Discuss with patients who use oral hypoglycemic agents or insulin the signs, symptoms, causes, and treatment of hypoglycemia.
- Instruct patients who use oral hypoglycemic agents or insulin to wear a bracelet or necklace that identifies them as having diabetes.
- Instruct patients to carry sugar or some other source of simple carbohydrate that can be used to treat hypoglycemia promptly.
- Advise patients to tell close friends and co-workers about their diabetes, how to recognize hypoglycemia, and what to do if an emergency occurs.

Special Issues in Diabetes Management—cont'd

For patients with hypoglycemia—cont'd

- Advise patients to have glucagon available. Teach family members and friends how to administer it.
- Instruct patients with diminished awareness of the signs and symptoms of hypoglycemia to monitor their blood glucose levels at frequent intervals.
- Consider changing the level of diabetes control in the following patients:
    Those who do not or cannot recognize the early warning signs of hypoglycemia
    Those who do not understand the educational details of avoiding or treating hypoglycemia
    Those whose life-style makes them vulnerable to life-threatening episodes of hypoglycemia

Pregnancy and Diabetes

For patients with pregestational diabetes

- Emphasize the importance of prepregnancy care.
- Work with the patient, her partner, her family, and other health care providers to improve the patient's nutrition, exercise program, and glucose control.
- Recommend that conception be delayed until the patient's blood glucose control is excellent and the glycosylated hemoglobin level is normal or near normal.
- Explain the risks of birth defects and adverse perinatal outcomes and the need for fetal surveillance.
- Recommend that the patient's vascular condition be thoroughly evaluated before she becomes pregnant.
- Explain that pregnancy may exacerbate advanced diabetic retinopathy but generally does not permanently worsen diabetic nephropathy.
- Explain that, overall, pregnancy does not shorten the life expectancy of a woman with diabetes but does increase her risk for hypoglycemia and ketoacidosis and for associated mortality.
- Inform patients with coronary atherosclerosis that their risks for morbidity or mortality may be greater during pregnancy.
- Discuss the emotional and financial demands of pregnancy with the patient, her partner, and her family.
- Emphasize that patients should not consume alcoholic beverages or smoke before or after becoming pregnant.

For patients with gestational diabetes

- Work with the patient, her partner, her family, and other health care providers to improve the patient's nutrition, exercise program, and glucose control.
- Explain the risks of adverse perinatal outcomes and the need for fetal surveillance.
- Inform patients that they are at increased risk both for developing gestational diabetes during future pregnancies and for developing overt diabetes later in life.
- Encourage physical activity and postpartum weight loss to decrease the likelihood of developing diabetes later in life.

Continued.

Pregnancy and Diabetes—cont'd

For patients with gestational diabetes—cont'd

• Recommend an evaluation at 6 to 8 weeks postpartum, and annually thereafter, for detecting the development of diabetes.

For patients with a history of gestational diabetes

• Recommend screening for overt diabetes before subsequent pregnancies.
• Recommend early screening for the onset of carbohydrate intolerance during subsequent pregnancies.

Other Issues of Health and Diabetes Management

Periodontal disease

• Explain the importance of maintaining glycemic control.
• Instruct patients to:
  Brush their teeth with a soft toothbrush and a fluoridated toothpaste at least twice a day, especially before going to sleep.
  Rinse their toothbrush thoroughly after each brushing, and replace it at least every 3 months. (Toothbrushes can harbor bacteria.)
  Use dental floss, bridge cleaners, water sprayers, or other cleaning aids recommended by their dentist.
• Emphasize the importance of seeking regular preventive dental care at least every 6 months (or according to the dentist's recommended schedule).
• Instruct patients to see a dentist if they have bad breath, an unpleasant taste in the mouth, bleeding gums, sore gums or teeth, red or swollen gums, difficulty chewing, or loose teeth.
• Instruct patients to inform their dentist that they have diabetes and to remind their dentist of this when they make appointments.
• Instruct patients to give their dentist their health care provider's name and telephone number.
• Stress the importance of scheduling dental appointments that do not interfere with the patient's insulin and meal schedule. Tell patients not to skip a meal or insulin before an appointment.

F Education Modules for Children With Diabetes Mellitus

EDUCATION MODULES FOR CHILDREN WITH DIABETES MELLITUS

Session I: Initial family assessment

Date	Initial	
_____	_____	Introduce self, unit staff, dietitian, and social worker.
_____	_____	Give basic explanation of treatment and length of hospitalization.
_____	_____	Interview family in regard to support systems: other family members, main caregivers, babysitters, working parents, religious beliefs, other diabetic relatives, educational background, daily family routines of parents and child, and when parents can be present for education.
_____	_____	Assess financial status and medical insurance benefits.
_____	_____	Assess signs and symptoms of hyperglycemia experienced in the last 2 months.
_____	_____	Assess diabetic ketoacidosis experienced in last 2 months.
_____	_____	Assess for signs and symptoms of hypoglycemia experienced; if so, when and which ones occurred.

If diagnosed with diabetes before this hospitalization, assess:

Date	Initial	
_____	_____	Meals and snacks (exchanges)
_____	_____	Use of waiting times
_____	_____	Relationship of exercise to blood glucose levels
_____	_____	Blood glucose testing times
_____	_____	Knowledge of insulin times
_____	_____	Knowledge of insulin dosage adjustments

Basic physiology and ketoacidosis

Date reviewed	Initial	Date reinforced	Initial	
_____	_____	_____	_____	IDDM versus NIDDM
_____	_____	_____	_____	Genetics and triggers that stimulate diabetes in children
_____	_____	_____	_____	Basic physiology of pancreas, insulin, and cells

---

Modified from St. Louis Children's Hospital, 1991.   *Continued.*

EDUCATION MODULES FOR CHILDREN WITH DIABETES MELLITUS—cont'd

Basic physiology and ketoacidosis—cont'd

Date reviewed	Initial	Date reinforced	Initial	
_____	_____	_____	_____	Why insulin cannot be given as a pill
_____	_____	_____	_____	Importance of insulin
_____	_____	_____	_____	"Honeymoon" period: explanation of and presence of unexplained hypoglycemia
_____	_____	_____	_____	Signs of hyperglycemia (thirst, increased urination, exhaustion, headache) and reasons for their appearance
_____	_____	_____	_____	Signs of ketoacidosis (nausea, vomiting, stomachache, Kussmaul respirations, acidotic breath) and reasons for their appearance

Session II: Hypoglycemia/insulin reactions

_____	_____	_____	_____	Signs and symptoms of insulin reactions (shaky, sweaty, sleepy, *very* hungry, pale, dizzy, combative) during the day and reasons why
_____	_____	_____	_____	Signs, symptoms, and causes of hypoglycemia (restless, sleepwalking, sleep talking) at night and reasons why
_____	_____	_____	_____	Causes of insulin reaction (miss meal or snack, increased exercise, too much insulin).
_____	_____	_____	_____	Treatment of low blood sugar
_____	_____	_____	_____	Role of epinephrine (adrenalin) and glucagon in increasing blood sugar level
_____	_____	_____	_____	Glucagon use and storage in cool place required; not to exceed 85° F and not to freeze
_____	_____	_____	_____	If child passes out or has seizure, intramuscular glucagon administered

Insulin actions

Date reviewed	Initial	Date reinforced	Initial	
_____	_____	_____	_____	Types of insulin (beef, pork, human)
_____	_____	_____	_____	Actions of regular insulin begin in ½ hour and peak in 2 to 3 hours.
_____	_____	_____	_____	Actions of NPH insulin begin in 1 hour and peak in 6 to 8 hours.
_____	_____	_____	_____	Time actions of Ultralente insulin
_____	_____	_____	_____	Importance of peak insulin times in relation to hypoglycemia
_____	_____	_____	_____	Effect of circardian rhythms on nighttime blood glucose levels, especially decreased hormones and decreased blood sugar, particularly with NPH peak at 2 to 4 AM and increased hormones, increased blood sugar, and decreased insulin at 5 to 8 AM

EDUCATION MODULES FOR CHILDREN WITH DIABETES MELLITUS—cont'd

Insulin actions—cont'd

Date reviewed	Initial	Date reinforced	Initial	
_____	____	_____	____	Relationship of blood glucose and ketone testing to time and actions of insulin (i.e., need to test for blood sugar level less than 60 mg/dl and when insulins are peaking)
_____	____	_____	____	Relationship of food, exercise, and insulin injections to blood glucose levels (food increases blood sugar; exercise decreases blood sugar; insulin decreases blood sugar)
_____	____	_____	____	Times and reasons for blood glucose testing and urine ketone testing at home
_____	____	_____	____	Determination of individualized diabetic regimen schedule for both usual school and weekend home schedule
_____	____	_____	____	Determination of individualized diabetic regimen for summer (i.e., changes in exercise schedule and increased need to check for decreased glucose sugars, possibility of need to increase snacks)

Session III: Diabetic skills—mixing and injecting insulin and demonstration of blood glucose monitoring machines

Date reviewed	Initial	Date reinforced	Initial	
_____	____	_____	____	Explanation of insulin syringe parts: plunger, barrel, unit markings, 3/10 ml syringe, 5/10 ml syringe, 1 ml syringe, needle, bevel
_____	____	_____	____	Differences in types of insulin syringes: BD, Terumo, Monoject
_____	____	_____	____	Demonstration of mixing regular and NPH insulin by nurse
_____	____	_____	____	Demonstration of insulin injection technique by nurse, including pinching up skin and fat, inserting at a 90-degree angle, aspirating to check for blood, and rotating syringe before removing needle
_____	____	_____	____	Injection sites and importance of rotating sites (from arms to abdomen one week to legs and abdomen the next week)
_____	____	_____	____	Return demonstration of mixing and injecting insulin by parents
_____	____	_____	____	Return demonstration of mixing and injecting insulin by child

Continued.

EDUCATION MODULES FOR CHILDREN WITH DIABETES MELLITUS—cont'd

Session III: Diabetic skills—mixing and injecting insulin and demonstration of blood glucose monitoring machines—cont'd

Date reviewed	Initial	Date reinforced	Initial	
_____	_____	_____	_____	Return demonstration of mixing and injecting insulin by significant other(s)
_____	_____	_____	_____	Demonstration of urine ketone testing using Ketostix
_____	_____	_____	_____	Return demonstration of urine ketone testing
_____	_____	_____	_____	Storage of insulin (environmental temperature not to exceed 85° F)
_____	_____	_____	_____	Demonstration of the use of two or three blood glucose monitoring meters
_____	_____	_____	_____	Demonstration of two to three different types of blood glucose strips
				Return demonstration on meter and blood glucose strips of choice:
_____	_____	_____	_____	By child
_____	_____	_____	_____	By parents
_____	_____	_____	_____	By significant other(s)

Session IV: Insulin dose adjustments

Date reviewed	Initial	Date reinforced	Initial	
_____	_____	_____	_____	Explanation of times that dose will need to be increased or decreased: illness, puberty, growth spurts, increased or decreased activity, menses, times of stress
_____	_____	_____	_____	Need to keep accurate daily records of blood sugar tests
_____	_____	_____	_____	Explanation of what and how necessary information needs to be recorded in relation to insulin dosages and blood glucose values, exercise, dose adjustments, and other notes
_____	_____	_____	_____	Discussion of principles of dose adjustments
				Explanation of how much the dose will need to be increased or decreased:
_____	_____	_____	_____	Change by ½ U with preschoolers
_____	_____	_____	_____	Change by 1 U with school-age children
_____	_____	_____	_____	Change by 1 to 2 U with adolescents
				Practice in making dose adjustments by role playing with blood glucose diary:
_____	_____	_____	_____	Mother
_____	_____	_____	_____	Father
_____	_____	_____	_____	Child
_____	_____	_____	_____	Significant other(s)

EDUCATION MODULES FOR CHILDREN WITH DIABETES MELLITUS—cont'd

Session IV: Insulin dose adjustments—cont'd

Date reviewed	Initial	Date reinforced	Initial	
_____	_____	_____	_____	Identification of patterns of blood glucose levels and when to call for insulin dose changes
_____	_____	_____	_____	Meaning of glycated hemoglobin and hemoglobin A_{1c}
				Problem solving with concrete age-appropriate situations:
_____	_____	_____	_____	Hypoglycemia:
_____	_____	_____	_____	Shopping mall
_____	_____	_____	_____	Park
_____	_____	_____	_____	Float trip
_____	_____	_____	_____	Camping
_____	_____	_____	_____	Skiing
_____	_____	_____	_____	Sport events
_____	_____	_____	_____	Movie theater
				Nighttime
_____	_____	_____	_____	Hyperglycemia:
_____	_____	_____	_____	Before sport events/activities
_____	_____	_____	_____	After sport events/activities
				During infections and growth
_____	_____	_____	_____	Ketoacidosis (before and after):
_____	_____	_____	_____	Sports events
_____	_____	_____	_____	Infections
_____	_____	_____	_____	Exercise
_____	_____	_____	_____	With normal blood glucose values
_____	_____	_____	_____	With low blood glucose values
				With high blood glucose values
_____	_____	_____	_____	Snacks
				In relation to low bedtime blood glucose values
_____	_____	_____	_____	In relation to bedtime glucose of 150 to 250 mg/dl
_____	_____	_____	_____	In relation to high bedtime blood glucose
				Whether or not to include AM and PM snack
_____	_____	_____	_____	When you need to increase/decrease a snack:
_____	_____	_____	_____	Morning
_____	_____	_____	_____	Afternoon
_____	_____	_____	_____	Bedtime
_____	_____	_____	_____	With exercise
				Use of waiting times to keep blood glucose levels even

Continued.

EDUCATION MODULES FOR CHILDREN WITH DIABETES MELLITUS—cont'd

Session V: Sick-day management

Date reviewed	Initial	Date reinforced	Initial	
_____	_____	_____	_____	**What to do:**
				If blood glucose value is greater than 250 mg/dl, check for ketones in urine.
_____	_____	_____	_____	If have stomach/abdominal pain, telephone endocrine physician on call.
_____	_____	_____	_____	If ketones present, drink 8 to 12 oz fluid every 2 hours and retest, and if ketones still present, telephone endocrine physician on call.
_____	_____	_____	_____	If child vomits twice or more, telephone endocrine physician on call.
_____	_____	_____	_____	If blood glucose value in range and has ketones, call for insulin dose.
_____	_____	_____	_____	If nighttime hypoglycemia occurs, give ½ glass orange juice.
_____	_____	_____	_____	**How to handle emergencies:**
				When to call _____
				Who to call _____
				If no one answers, telephone _____ and ask for diabetes physician on call immediately.
_____	_____	_____	_____	If child cannot eat, use full-liquid and/or clear-liquid diet.

Discharge planning

Date reviewed	Initial	Date reinforced	Initial	
_____	_____	_____	_____	Diabetes Quiz taken and passed with 80% accuracy
_____	_____	_____	_____	Discharge prescriptions given: insulin, glucagon, and blood-testing supplies
_____	_____	_____	_____	Follow-up appointment made to outpatient endocrine offices (call _____ to make this)
_____	_____	_____	_____	Family instructed to call the endocrine physician or nurse daily for dose adjustment

EDUCATION MODULES FOR CHILDREN WITH DIABETES MELLITUS—cont'd

Nutrition Checklist
Day 1

___   Take nutritional history and compare with hospital-ordered meal pattern.

___   Make change in hospital diet to reflect child's usual eating pattern.

___   Provide family and patient, if age appropriate, with rationale of meal pattern, focusing on need for balance, timing of meals, and consistency required.

___   Give exchange booklet and begin explanation of content.

Day 2

___   Explain American Diabetes Association (ADA) exchanges and guidelines.

___   Explain importance of carbohydrate (CHO) distribution throughout day.

___   Emphasize need for balance of 20% protein, 30% fat, and 50% CHO (approximate balance).

___   Provide instruction on exchanges with booklet.

___   Explain how various foods affect the blood glucose level differently.

___   Provide rationale for keeping fat less than 30% of kilocalories.

___   Discuss "diet," "light," and "dietetic" foods.

___   Have patient fill out hospital menu according to exchanges allowed and write appropriate amounts of each item. Child should do this with parent, if appropriate cognitive development present.

___   Have patient write out a typical menu for use at home.

Day 3

___   Review explanation of diet

___   Review menu and discuss corrections if needed.

___   Give *Eats and Treats* booklet and discuss.

___   Provide sick-day management and basic explanation of replacement CHO.

___   Prepare sick-day menu to replace CHO at each meal.

___   Explain exercise guidelines.

___   Discuss holiday or special day's menus.

___   Discuss importance of label reading.

___   Discuss how to convert a product with an appropriate label to exchanges.

Day 4

___   Discuss use of "fast foods."

___   Prepare one meal of "fast foods" into allotted exchanges.

___   Provide phone number for questions, and encourage family to contact if any questions should arise.

_____

Dietitian

_____

Date

Continued.

EDUCATION MODULES FOR CHILDREN WITH DIABETES MELLITUS—cont'd

Psychosocial/family/child assessment

Initial

_____ Assess parents' emotional response to diagnosis, family structure and supportiveness, ability to communicate with each other, life-style including daily routine, ability to learn, problem-solving ability, financial status, and cultural or religious considerations.

_____ Assess parent/child relationship.

_____ Assess child's reaction to diagnosis and medical procedures, behavior at home and school, grades, possible learning problems, and attendance record.

_____ Identify family factors or stresses that might interfere with adjustment and adherence to the regimen (i.e., single-parent family, other health problems in the family, financial problems). Did family respond appropriately to child's symptoms before diagnosis?

Education/support

Initial

_____ Discuss emotional reactions to diagnosis. Explain grief process.

_____ Discuss previous knowledge of diabetes and parents' fears. Correct misconceptions.

_____ Reassure patient and family of competence and support of medical staff. Familiarize them with diabetes program and functions of diabetes team.

_____ Discuss reactions of parents and child to medical procedures (e.g., testing, injection). Suggest ways to ease trauma and reinforce child's efforts. Teach parents behavioral reinforcement techniques.

_____ Discuss possible effects of diabetes on child's behavior, home life, social life, and school performance. Discuss importance of maintaining appropriate discipline.

_____ Discuss possible effects of diabetes on parents and siblings.

_____ Discuss patient's return to school. Provide teacher literature. Discuss ways to keep diabetes from interfering with school experience.

_____ Help child anticipate return to school, including telling friends, sticking to the diet, parties, and outings. Discuss child's feelings, fears, and concerns.

_____ Help family plan diabetes care task assignments (i.e., who will do what at home). Be sure father is included and child is assigned age-appropriate tasks.

_____ Discuss problem-solving approach to diabetes care and realistic expectations of diabetes control.

_____ Familiarize patient and family with community supports and support groups.

_____ Give family opportunity to discuss their concerns. What problems do they anticipate? Help with beginning problem-solving efforts or refer to appropriate staff for assistance.

_____ Help shape effective parenting behaviors by reinforcing parents' efforts to use knowledge from diabetes classes and counseling.

G National Standards for Diabetes Self-Management Education Programs and American Diabetes Association Review Criteria

In 1993, the National Diabetes Advisory Board charged the American Diabetes Association (ADA) to coordinate a task force of representatives of diabetes and other organizations to review, and revise if indicated, the National Standards for Diabetes Patient Education Programs. The task force consisted of representatives from the following organizations: The American Association of Diabetes Educators, ADA, American Dietetic Association, the Centers for Disease Control and Prevention (CDC), the Department of Defense, the Department of Veterans Affairs, the Diabetes Research and Training Centers, the Indian Health Service, and the Juvenile Diabetes Foundation, Inc. The task force decided to revise the standards to reflect recent research and current health care trends. Thus the standards were revised and are now termed the National Standards for Diabetes Self-Management Education Programs. These revised standards have been endorsed by the organizations involved in their development.

American Diabetes Association. Reprinted from *Diabetes Care* 18:737-741, 1995.

Diabetes mellitus is a chronic metabolic disorder. Individuals affected by diabetes must learn self-management skills and make life-style changes to manage diabetes effectively and avoid or delay the complications associated with this disorder. For these reasons, self-management education is the cornerstone of treatment for all people with diabetes. These National Standards, which were developed in collaboration with diabetes organizations, provide guidance for the establishment and maintenance of quality diabetes self-management education programs.

The process whereby people with chronic diseases, such as diabetes, learn to take care of these disorders has traditionally been termed "patient education." Over time, however, this designation has changed and is currently termed *self-management training* and *self-management education* as well as patient education. This document uses the term *self-management education* to refer to the process whereby individuals learn to manage their diabetes.

These standards provide:

1. Diabetes educators with the means to do the following:

- Develop quality self-management education programs.
- Assess the quality of their education programs.
- Identify areas in their programs where changes and improvements are needed.

2. People with diabetes with the means to do the following:
   - Assess the quality of the diabetes-related services they receive.
   - Gain an understanding of the skills needed for self-management.

3. Referral sources, insurers, employers, government agencies, and the general public with the following:
   - A description of quality self-management education services for people with diabetes
   - An awareness of the importance of comprehensive self-management education to enable people with diabetes to manage this disorder effectively

Quality diabetes self-management education programs can be measured in terms of structure, process, and outcomes. Each of these program components includes one or more elements with specific standards. The broad outline of the National Standards for Diabetes Self-Management Education Programs is as follows:

Structure

- Organization
- Needs assessment
- Program management
- Program staff
- Curriculum
- Participant access

Process

- Assessment
- Plan and implementation
- Follow-up

Outcomes

- Program outcome evaluation
- Participant outcome evaluation

STRUCTURE

The structure necessary to provide quality diabetes self-management education consists of the human and material resources and the management systems needed to achieve program and participant goals. Such structure includes the support and commitment of the organization that is sponsoring the program, the program administration and management systems, the qualifications and diversity of the personnel involved in the program, the curriculum and instructional methods and materials, and the accessibility of the program.

Organization

The sponsoring organization must provide the support and structure within which the program functions. Organizational commitment to self-management education, including operational support, adequate space, personnel, budget, and materials, must be clearly evident. Since multiple health care professionals from a variety of disciplines are involved in diabetes care, clear line of authority and efficient communication systems should be established.

Standard 1.

The sponsoring organization shall have a written policy that affirms education as an integral component of diabetes care.

Review criterion

1-1. A written statement from the sponsoring organization reflects that self-management education is an integral component of diabetes care.

Standard 2.

The sponsoring organization shall identify and provide the educational resources required to achieve its educational objectives in terms of its target population. These resources include adequate space, personnel, budget, and instructional materials.

Review criterion

2-1. For both individual and group instruction, resources, including space, staff, budget, and educational materials are adequate to support the programs offered and the participants served.

Standard 3.

The organizational relationships, lines of authority, staffing, job descriptions, and operational policies shall be clearly defined and documented.

Review criteria

3-1. The sponsoring institution's organizational chart delineates the placement of the diabetes program, staff, and advisory committee.

3-2. There is a description of the following for the coordinator and each instructional staff member:
   • Role in the program
   • Teaching responsibilities
   • Other program responsibilities
   • Amount of time spent in the program

3-3. There are written policies approved by the advisory committee concerning the operation of the program.

Needs Assessment

A successful program is based on the needs of the population that the program is intended to serve. Because diabetes popula-

tions vary, each organization should assess its service area and match resources to the needs of the defined target population. Needs assessments should guide program planning and management. Periodic reassessment should be done to allow the program to adapt to changing needs.

Standard 4.

The service area shall be assessed to define the target population and determine appropriate allocation of personnel and resources to serve the educational needs of the target population.

Review criterion

4-1. The target population is defined (specifically the potential number to be served, types of diabetes, age range, language, ethnicity, unique characteristics, and special educational needs) based on an assessment of the service area.

Program Management

Effective management is essential to implement and maintain a successful program and to ensure that resources are adequate for the defined tasks. To ensure that management policies and program design reflect broad perspectives relevant to diabetes, the organization should designate a standing advisory committee that includes health care professionals and people with diabetes to assist staff with program planning and review. Involvement and support from the medical community are also necessary. At times, resources outside the sponsoring institution may be required to enable individuals affected by diabetes to maximize their health outcomes.

Standard 5.

A standing advisory committee consisting of a physician, nurse educator, dietitian, an individual with behavioral science expertise, a consumer, and a community representative, at a minimum, shall be established to oversee the program.

Review criteria

5-1. The advisory committee members just specified attend at least two meetings a year.

5-2. The health professional members include at least one physician, one nurse educator, and one dietitian, each with expertise in diabetes.

5-3. The individual with behavioral science expertise is any professional with academic preparation in the behavioral sciences (e.g., counseling, health behavior, psychology, social work, sociology).

5-4. The consumer is any individual with diabetes or the person's caregiver.

5-5. The community representative is any individual not employed by the institution.

5-6. A written policy lists the membership and responsibilities of the advisory committee.

5-7. The advisory committee minutes document that the committee is fulfilling its responsibilities to approve the program plan, recommend and approve policy, and review the program annually.

Standard 6.

The advisory committee shall participate in the annual planning process, including determination of target audience, program objectives, participant access mechanisms, instructional methods, resource requirements (including space, personnel, budget, and materials), participant follow-up mechanisms, and program evaluation.

Review criterion

6-1. The advisory committee minutes document the approval each year of a written program plan that includes the items just specified.

Standard 7.

Professional program staff shall have sufficient time and resources for lesson planning, instruction, documentation, evaluation, and follow-up.

Review criterion

7-1. The instructors' available hours and resources are adequate to meet the needs of the program and the participants.

Standard 8.

Community resources shall be assessed periodically.

Review criterion

8-1. There is a list (including name, address, and telephone number) of community resources within the service area that serve the target population and their families. This list is updated yearly.

Program Staff

Qualified personnel are essential to the success of a diabetes self-management education program. The sponsoring organization should identify the program personnel, which must include a program coordinator who has overall responsibility for the program. Because diabetes is a chronic disorder requiring life-style changes, instructors need to be skilled and experienced health care professionals with recent education in diabetes, educational principles, and behavior change strategies.

Standard 9.

A coordinator shall be designated who is responsible for program planning, implementation, and evaluation.

Review criteria

9-1. The job description for the program coordinator includes his or her responsibility for the following:

- Acting as a liaison between the program staff, the advisory committee, and the administration of the institution
- Providing and/or coordinating the orientation and continuing education for the professional program staff
- Participating in the planning and review of the program each year
- Participating in the preparation of the program budget
- Evaluating program effectiveness
- Serving as the chair or a member of the advisory committee

9-2. The program coordinator is a certified diabetes educator (CDE) or has completed at least 24 hours of approved continuing education that includes a combination of diabetes, educational principles, and behavioral strategies.

Standard 10.

Health care professionals with recent didactic and experiential preparation in diabetes clinical and educational issues shall serve as the program instructors. The staff shall include at least a nurse educator and a dietitian who collaborate routinely. Certification as a diabetes educator by the National Certification Board for Diabetes Educators (NCBDE) is recommended.

Review criteria

10-1. Program instructors are professional staff who routinely teach in the diabetes self-management education program and include at least one nurse educator and one dietitian.

10-2. Program instructors are health care professionals with a valid license, registration, or certification and who are CDEs or have completed at least 16 hours of approved continuing education that includes a combination of diabetes, educational principles, and behavioral strategies.

Standard 11.

Professional program staff shall obtain education about diabetes, educational principles, and behavioral change strategies on a continuing basis.

Review criterion

11-1. The program coordinator and all instructors complete at least 6 hours per year of approved continuing education that includes a combination of diabetes, educational principles, and behavioral strategies.

Curriculum

A quality diabetes self-management education program should provide comprehensive instruction in the content areas relevant to the target population and to the participants being served. The curriculum, instructional methods, and materials should be appropriate for the specified target population, considering type and duration of diabetes, age, cultural influences, and individual learning abilities.

Standard 12.

Based on the needs of the target population, the program shall be capable of offering instruction in the following content areas:

a. Diabetes overview

b. Stress and psychosocial adjustment

c. Family involvement and social support

d. Nutrition

e. Exercise and activity

f. Medications

g. Monitoring and use of results

h. Relationships among nutrition, exercise, medication, and blood glucose levels

i. Prevention, detection, and treatment of acute complications

j. Prevention, detection, and treatment of chronic complications

k. Foot, skin, and dental care

l. Behavior change strategies, goal setting, risk factor reduction, and problem solving

m. Benefits, risks, and management options for improving glucose control

n. Preconception care, pregnancy, and gestational diabetes

o. Use of health care systems and community resources

Review criteria

12-1. A written curriculum includes educational objectives, content outline, instructional methods and materials, and the means for evaluating achievement of the objectives for each content area or session of the program.

12-2. The curriculum is current and includes all 15 content areas as appropriate for the identified target population.

Standard 13.

The program shall use instructional methods and materials that are appropriate for the target population and the participants being served.

Review criterion

13-1. Instructional methods and materials are appropriate for the target population and participants in terms of cultural relevance, age, language, reading level, and special educational needs.

Participant Access

Quality programs must be readily accessible to those in need of education. The sponsoring organization should facilitate access to self-management education for the target population identified in the needs assessment. Access is promoted by a commitment to inform referral sources and the target population routinely of the availability and benefits of the program.

Standard 14.

A system shall be in place to inform the target population and potential referral sources of the availability and benefits of the program.

Review criterion

14-1. The program informs its identified target population and potential referral sources about the program at least once a year.

Standard 15.

The program shall be conveniently and regularly available.

Review criterion

15-1. Program utilization, attrition rates, and waiting periods are assessed yearly.

Standard 16.

The program shall be responsive to requests for information and referrals from consumers, health care professionals, and health care agencies.

Review criterion

16-1. A written policy and procedure stipulate that all requests for information and referrals receive a timely response.

PROCESS

Process refers to the methods or means by which resources are used to attain stated goals. The process of providing diabetes self-management education involves the integration of an individual assessment, goal setting, education plan development, implementation, evaluation, and follow-up. Each component requires documentation that can be evaluated.

Assessment

Because individuals are unique, their educational needs will vary with age, disease processes, culture, and life-styles. Effective instruction can only be accomplished by a collaborative effort between educators and participants to identify individualized educational needs.

Standard 17.

An individualized assessment shall be developed and updated in collaboration with each participant. The assessment shall include relevant medical history, present health status, health service or resource utilization, risk factors, diabetes knowledge and skills, cultural influences, health beliefs and attitudes, health behaviors and goals, support systems, barriers to learning, and socioeconomic factors.

Review criteria

17-1. An initial assessment of the items just specified is documented in the education record and updated as needed.

17-2. The participant's preprogram knowledge of and skill level in each of the appropriate content areas of the National Standards are documented in the education record and updated as needed.

Plan and Implementation

For the educational experience to meet the participant's needs, an individual assessment should be used to develop the education plan. All information about the educational experience should be documented in the participant's permanent medical or education record. Since different health care professionals may be involved in the provision of the educational experience, effective communication and coordination are essential.

Standard 18.

An individualized education plan, based on the assessment, shall be developed in collaboration with each participant.

Review criterion

18-1. An education plan, developed in collaboration with the participant and based on the educational needs identified in the initial assessment, is documented in the education record.

Standard 19.

The participant's educational experience, including assessment, intervention, evaluation, and follow-up, shall be documented in a permanent medical or education record. There shall be documentation of collaboration and coordination among program staff and other providers.

Review criteria

19-1. The participant's progress through the program is documented in the education record and includes the following:

- The initial assessment and education plan as just specified
- An indication of the content taught, dates of instruction, and the instructors
- A postprogram assessment of the participant's knowledge and skill level of each of the appropriate content areas of the National Standards
- Behavior change goals
- A plan for follow-up
- Communication of participant's progress and any follow-up recommendations to the primary care provider
- Follow-up assessment and any resulting nterventions

19-2. Each program instructor documents his or her own interventions with the participants.

19-3. Communication and collaboration among program staff are facilitated by and documented in the education record.

19-4. There is a written policy that the education record is made available to external health care providers with permission from the participant.

19-5. There is a written policy that participants are given a copy or summary of their education record, if requested.

Follow-Up

Because diabetes is a chronic disorder requiring a lifetime of self-management, follow-up services are needed. Participants' life-styles, knowledge, skills, attitudes, and disease characteristics change over time, so that ongoing education is necessary and appropriate. Programs should be able to offer periodic reassessment and education as part of comprehensive services.

Standard 20.

The program shall offer appropriate and timely educational interventions based on periodic reassessments of health status, knowledge, skills, attitudes, goals, and self-care behaviors.

Review criteria

20-1. There is a written policy for the provision of follow-up assessment of the items just specified and any resulting interventions.

20-2. At least one follow-up assessment of the items previously specified and any interventions are documented in the education record.

20-3. Participant achievement of behavior change goals is assessed and documented 1 to 3 months after goal setting.

OUTCOMES

Outcomes are the desired results for the program and participants. For programs, the desired results include achievement of stated objectives, reaching the defined target population, and helping participants improve their health outcomes. For participants, outcomes include the knowledge and skills necessary for self-management, desired self-management behaviors, and improved health outcomes. Assessing outcomes and using the assessments in regular program evaluation and subsequent planning are essential to maintain quality programs.

Program Outcome Evaluation

The advisory committee should periodically review the program to ascertain that the program continued to meet the National Standards for Diabetes Self-Management Education Programs. The results of this review should be documented and used in subsequent program planning and modification.

Standard 21.

The advisory committee shall review program performance annually, including all components of the annual program plan and curriculum, and use the information in subsequent planning and program modification.

Review criteria

21-1. The advisory committee minutes document the results of an annual review of the program, including the following:

- Program objectives
- The curriculum, instructional methods, and materials
- Actual audience compared with the target population
- Participant access, as well as follow-up mechanisms
- Program resources (space, personnel, and budget)
- Program effectiveness and participant outcomes.

21-2. The results of the annual review are reflected in the next annual program plan.

Participant Outcome Evaluation

Participant outcomes, such as success in incorporating self-management into their life-styles, should be periodically reviewed. The specific outcomes evaluated will vary with the program, but the program's effectiveness in helping participants improve their health outcomes should be documented and used for future program planning and modification.

Standard 22.

The advisory committee shall annually review and evaluate predetermined outcomes for program participants.

Review criteria

22-1. Participants' outcomes are measured and evaluated, specifically the degree to which the participants achieve their behavior change goals and *one* other outcome measure (e.g., monitoring for complications, lost work or school days, metabolic control, others).

22-2. The program's effectiveness at improving outcomes among participants is evaluated by the advisory committee, and the results of this evaluation are reflected in the next annual program plan.

Index